617.55059 C

Laparoscopic Surgery

LAPAROSCOPIC SURGERY

Jorge Cueto-García, MD
Professor of Surgery (Minimally Invasive)
University of Anahuac School of Medicine
Coordinator of Laparoscopic Surgery
Angeles Lomas Hospital
American British Cowdray Hospital
Mexico City, Mexico
Adjunct Associate Professor of Surgery
Louisiana State University
New Orleans, Louisiana

Moisés Jacobs, MD
Laparoscopic Center of South Florida
Coral Gables, Florida

Michel Gagner, MD
Franz W. Sichel Professor of Surgery
Director, Minimally Invasive Surgery Center
Chief, Division of Laparoscopic Surgery
Mount Sinai School of Medicine
New York, New York

McGraw-Hill
Medical Publishing Division

New York   Chicago   San Francisco   Lisbon   London   Madrid   Mexico City
Milan   New Delhi   San Juan   Seoul   Singapore   Sydney   Toronto

Laparoscopic Surgery

1 2 3 4 5 6 7 8 9 0 KGP KGP 0 9 8 7 6 5 4 3

ISBN 0-07-136481-1

This book was set Palatino by Matrix Publishing Services.
The editors were Marc Strauss, Kathleen McCullough, and Karen Davis.
The production supervisor was Phil Galea.
The cover designer was Aimée Nordin.
The index was prepared by Robert Swanson.
Quebecor Kingsport was printer and binder.

This book is printed on acid-free paper.

Cataloging-in-Publication data is on file for this title at the Library of Congress.

Contents

Contributors

Kranthi K. Achanta, MD
Department of Surgery
University of Southern California
School of Medicine
Los Angeles, California
Chapter 20

J. Arturo Almeida, MD
Advanced Laparoscopy Fellow
Texas Endosurgery Institute
San Antonio, Texas
Chapters 42, 56, 63

Ahmet Alponat, MD
Associate of Endoscopic and Laparoscopic Surgery
Minimally Invasive Surgical Center
National University Hospital
Singapore
Chapter 23

Valeriu Eugen Andrei, MD
Robert Wood Johnson University Hospital
St. Peter's University Hospital
New Brunswick, New Jersey
Chapter 76

Ronald J. Aronoff, MD
General Laparoscopic Surgery and Vascular Surgery
Medical City Dallas Hospital
Dallas, Texas
Chapter 96

S. Azagra, MD
Saint Pierre University Hospital
Charleroi, Belgium
Chapter 22

C. Balaguè, MD
Hospital Clinic
University of Barcelona
Barcelona, Spain
Chapter 43

J.G. Balique, MD
University of Valencia
Valencia, Spain
Chapter 22

Carlos Ballesta-Lopez, MD
Director, Laparoscopic Center of Barcelona
Barcelona, Spain
Chapter 24

Jorge E. Balli, MD
Laparoscopic General Surgeon
Department of Surgery of Hospital San Jose
Technological Institute of Monterrey
Monterrey, Mexico
Chapters 42, 56, 63, 93

Carlos A. Baptista, MD
Laparoscopic Clinic of South Florida
Coral Gables, Florida
Chapter 45

Tomas Barrientos-Fortes, MD
Director, School of Medicine
University of Anahuac
San Miguel Chapultepec
Mexico City, Mexico
Chapter 90

X. Bastida-Vila, MD
Head Surgeon
General and Digestive Surgery Department
Bellvitage Hospital
Barcelona, Spain
Chapter 24

C. Bettonica-Larrañaga, MD
General and Digestive Surgery Department
Bellvitage Hospital
Barcelona, Spain
Chapter 24

I.N. Bicha-Castelo, MD
University of Valencia
Valencia, Spain
Chapter 22

Laurent Biertho, MD
Minimally Invasive Surgery Center
Department of Surgery
Mount Sinai School of Medicine
New York, New York
Chapters 9, 34

Thomas Birdas, MD
West Penn Allegheny Health System
Pittsburgh, Pennsylvania
Chapter 44

Francisco Blanes-Masson, MD
Chief, Hepatic Surgery Section
Hospital "Dr. Peset"
Valencia, Spain
Chapter 31

Alexis Bolio, MD
Chief Resident in Surgery
Hospital Central Sur de Alta Especialidad
Mexico City, Mexico
Chapter 87

Henirich J. Bonjer, MD
Professor of Surgery
Vice-Chair, Department of Surgery
Erasmus Medical Center
Rotterdam, The Netherlands
Chapter 39(2)

Luigi Brusciano, MD
Resident of General Surgery
1st Division of General and Gastrointestinal Surgery,
    School of Medicine
Second University of Naples
Naples, Italy
Chapter 14

Robert N. Cacchione, MD
Department of Laparoscopic Surgery
Staten Island University Hospital
Staten Island, New York
Chapter 73

Luis G. Castañeda, MD
Department of Orthopedic Surgery
American British Cowdray Hospital
Mexico City, Mexico
Chapter 97

Pablo Castañeda, MD
Resident in Orthopedic Surgery
American British Cowdray Hospital
Mexico City, Mexico
Chapter 97

W. Ricardo Castañeda, MD
Fellow
Department of Imagenology
Louisiana State University
Charity Hospital
New Orleans, Louisiana
Chapters 30(2), 37, 38, 80

Wilfrido R. Castañeda, MD
Professor and Chairman
Department of Radiology
Louisiana State University
New Orleans, Louisiana
Chapters 37, 38

Antoni Castells, MD, PhD
Department of Gastroenterology
Institute of Digestive Disorders
Hospital Clinic
Barcelona, Spain
Chapter 43

Octavio Castillo, MD
Clinica las Nieves
Santa Maria de Manquehue
Santiago, Chile
Chapter 79

F. Casto-Sousa, MD
Department of Surgery
Medical and Dental School
University of Valencia
Valencia, Spain
Chapter 22

Philip Caushaj, MD, FACS, FCRS
Professor of Surgery
Yale University School of Medicine
New Haven, Connecticut
Chapter 44

Albert K. Chin, MD
Vice-President of Research
Guidant Corporation
Menlo Park, California
Chapter 6

Ralph Clayman, MD
Department of Surgery
Division of Urology
Department of Radiology
Mallinckrodt Institute of Radiology
St. Louis, Missouri
Chapter 78

Atila Csendes, MD
Chief of Surgery Department
Clinical Hospital
University of Chile
Santiago, Chile
Chapters 10, 15

Miguel A. Cuesta, MD
Department of Surgery
Academic Hospital
Free University
Department of Surgery
Afdeling Heelkunde
Amsterdam, The Netherlands
Chapters 48, 60, 61

Jorge Cueto-García, MD
Professor of Surgery (Minimally Invasive)
University of Anahuac School of Medicine
Coordinator of Laparoscopic Surgery
Angeles Lomas Hospital
American British Cowdray Hospital
Mexico City, Mexico
Adjunct Associate Professor of Surgery
Louisiana State University
New Orleans, Louisiana
Chapters 7, 9, 12(1), 18, 21, 25, 27, 28, 29, 30(1),
    39(1), 55, 94, 98

Maximo Cunillera, MD
Department of Surgery
National Institute of Perinatology
Mexico City, Mexico
Chapter 67

Myriam J. Curet, MD
Associate Professor of Surgery
Stanford University Medical Center
Stanford, California
Chapter 71

Danilo Cuttitta, MD
Resident of Gastrointestinal Surgery
1st Division of General and Gastrointestinal Surgery,
    School of Medicine
Second University of Naples
Naples, Italy
Chapter 14

Gregory F. Dakin, MD
Mount Sinai Medical Center
New York, New York
Chapter 3

Bernard Dallemagne, MD
Chirurgie de l'Appareil Digestif
Les Cliniques Saint Joseph ASBL
Liege, Belgium
Chapters 13, 40

S. Delgado, MD
Hospital Clinic
University of Barcelona
Barcelona, Spain
Chapter 43

Fernando Delgado-Gomez, MD
Department of Surgery
Medical and Dental School
University of Valencia
Valencia, Spain
Chapter 31

Alberto del Genio, MD
Professor of General Surgery, FACS
1st Division of General and Gastrointestinal Surgery,
    School of Medicine
Second University of Naples
Naples, Italy
Chapter 14

Ricardo Di Segni, MD
Fellow
Department of Imagenology
Louisiana State University
Charity Hospital
New Orleans, Louisiana
Chapters 37, 38, 80

Ives-Marie Dion, MD
California Surgical Associates
General and Vascular Surgeon, Minimally Invasive Surgery
Pleasanton, California
Chapter 82

Carlos Eduardo Domene, MD
Department of Digestive and Laparoscopic Surgery and
    Coloproctology
School of Medicine
Sao Paulo, Brazil
Chapter 19

Mikhail Dvorochin, MD
Department of Anesthesia
Saint Luke's-Roosevelt Hospital
New York, New York
Chapter 4

Michael Edye, MD
Associate Professor
New York University School of Medicine
New York, New York
Chapter 76

P. Espalieu, MD
Department of Surgery
Medical and Dental School
University of Valencia
Valencia, Spain
Chapter 22

Rahila Essani, MD
Department of Surgery
University of Southern California School of Medicine
Los Angeles, California
Chapter 20

E. Estour, MD
Department of Surgery
Medical and Dental School
University of Valencia
Valencia, Spain
Chapter 22

Richelle J.F. Feet-Bersma, MD
Academic Hospital
Free University
Amsterdam, The Netherlands
Chapter 48

Edward Félix, MD
Assistant Clinical Professor of Surgery
University of California at San Francisco
San Francisco, California
Surgical Laparoscopy and Endoscopy
Director, The Center for Hernia Repair
Fresno, California
Chapters 62, 94

Carlos Fernández del Castillo, MD
Professor
Department of Surgery
Harvard Medical School
Massachusetts General Hospital
Boston, Massachusetts
Chapter 49

George S. Ferzli, MD
Professor of Surgery
State University of New York at Brooklyn
Brooklyn, New York
Director, Laparoscopic Surgery
Staten Island, New York
Chapter 73

Morris E. Franklin, Jr., MD
Director, Texas Endoscopic Institute
Professor of Surgery
University of Texas Health Sciences Center, San Antonio
San Antonio, Texas
Chapters 42, 56, 63, 93

Melanie H. Freilander, MD
Fellow
Department of Surgery
USC, School of Medicine
Los Angeles, California
Chapter 20

Angeles Fuentes del Toro, MD
Department of Surgery
Hospital #60
IMSS
Mexico City, Mexico
Chapter 98

Daniel Gagné, MD
West Penn Allegheny Health System
Pittsburgh, Pennsylvania
Chapter 44

Michel Gagner, MD
Franz W. Sichel Professor of Surgery
Director, Minimally Invasive Surgery Center
Chief, Division of Laparoscopic Surgery
Mount Sinai Medical Center
New York, New York
Chapters 3, 8, 9, 26, 27, 34, 35, 36, 50, 51, 52, 54, 81

Sashidhar Ganta, MD
Harvard Regional Bariatric Center
Harvard Memorial Hospital
Harvard, Illinois
Chapter 47

J.C. García-Valdecasas, MD
Hospital Clinic
University of Barcelona
Barcelona, Spain
Chapter 43

Denzil Garteiz-Martínez, MD
Department of Surgery
Hospital Angeles de las Lomas
Mexico City, Mexico
Chapters 5, 89

Mounir Gazayerli, MD
Laparoscopic Laser Surgeon Institute
Detroit, Michigan
Chapter 18

Paolo Gentileschi, MD
Division of Laparoscopic Surgery
Mount Sinai School of Medicine
New York, New York
Chapters 26, 36, 54

Carlos Roberto Gimenez, MD
Department of Imagenology
Louisiana State University
Charity Hospital
New Orleans, Louisiana
Chapter 30(2)

Peter M.Y. Goh, MD
Chairman Associate Professor, Consultant Surgeon,
   Chief of Surgical Endoscopy
Department of Surgery
Minimally Invasive Surgical Centre
National University Hospital
Singapore
Chapter 23

Jeffrey A. Goldstein, MD
Seaport Orthopaedic Associates Spine Center
New York, New York
Chapter 85

Eddie Gómez, MD
Laparoscopic Center of South Florida
Coral Gables, Florida
Chapters 47, 87

Fernando Gómez-Ferrer Bayo, MD
Department of Surgery
Medical and Dental School
University of Valencia
Valencia, Spain
Chapter 22

Carlos R. Gracia, MD
Chief of Miniinvasive Surgery
University of California at Los Angeles
Los Angeles, California
Chapter 82

Steven W. Grant, MD
Fellow
Department of Surgery
University of Southern California School of Medicine
Los Angeles, California
Chapter 20

Frederick Greene, MD
Chairman, Departments of General Surgery
Surgical Oncology, Endoscopy Surgery
Carolinas Medical Center (Health Care System)
Charlotte, North Carolina
Chapter 59

Valerie J. Halpin, MD
Fellow, Department of Surgery
Washington University, School of Medicine
St. Louis, Missouri
Chapter 53

Rene F. Hartmann, MD
Laparoscopic Clinic of South Florida
Coral Gables, Florida
Chapter 45

Juan David Hernandez Restrepo, MD
Hospital de Medellin
Medellin, Columbia
Chapter 57

Marcos Herrera, MD
Fellow, Department of Imagenology
Louisiana State University
Charity Hospital
New Orleans, Louisiana
Chapters 37, 38, 80

Daniel M. Herron, MD
Assistant Professor of Surgery
Division of Endoscopic Surgery
Mount Sinai School of Medicine
New York, New York
Chapter 11

David M. Hoenig, MD
Chief of Weiler Division
Director, Laparoscopy and Endourology
Assistant Professor
Department of Urology
Montefiore Medical Center
Albert Einstein School of Medicine
New York, New York
Chapter 78

Santiago Horgan, MD
Director, Minimally Invasive Surgery
Director, Swallowing Center
Department of Surgery
University of Illinois at Chicago
Chicago, Illinois
Chapter 17

Carlos Hurtado, MD
Chief Department of Anesthesia
American British Cowdray Hospital Mexico
Mexico City, Mexico
Chapter 88

Valentin Ibarra, MD
Department of Gynecology and Obstetrics
National Institute of Perinatology
Mexico City, Mexico
Chapter 67

William B. Inabnet, III, MD
Division of Laparoscopic Surgery
Mount Sinai School of Medicine
New York, New York
Chapter 81

Giuseppe Izzo, MD
Associate Professor of Surgery
1st Division of General and Gastrointestinal Surgery,
    School of Medicine
Second University of Naples
Naples, Italy
Chapter 14

J.J. Jackimowicz, PhD, FRCS(Ed)
President, European Association of Endoscopic Surgery
Veldhoven, The Netherlands
Chapter 86

Moisés Jacobs, MD
Laparoscopic Center of South Florida
Coral Gables, Florida
Chapters 1, 27, 28, 29, 30(1), 41, 46, 47, 87, 92, 93

Gregg H. Jossart, MD
Director, Minimally Invasive Surgery
Advanced Laparoscopic and Endocrine Surgery
California Pacific Medical Center
San Francisco, California
Chapter 35

Alberto Kably, MD
Chief Department of Gynecological Surgery
Assisted Reproduction
Hospital Angeles Lomas
Mexico City, Mexico
Chapter 69

Namir Katkhouda, MD
Professor of Surgery, Chief
Division of Emergency Non-trauma Surgery
Healthcare Consultation Center
Los Angeles, California
Chapter 20

Geert Kazemier, MD
Department of Laparoscopic Surgery
University Hospital Rotterdam/Dijkzigt
Rotterdam, The Netherlands
Chapter 39(2)

Won Woo Kim, MD
Minimally Invasive Surgery Center
Mount Sinai Medical Center
New York, New York
Chapter 8

Subhash Kini, MD, FRCS (Eng), FRCS(Ed), FRCS(Glas)
Division of Endoscopic Surgery
Mount Sinai School of Medicine
New York, New York
Chapter 27

Owen Korn, MD, FACS
Assistant Professor of Surgery
Clinical Hospital
University Hospital
Santiago, Chile
Chapter 10, 15

Jorge Kunhardt, MD
Medical Director, National Institute of Perinatology
Lomas Virreyes, Mexico
Chapter 67

Antonio Ma de Lacy, MD
Associate Professor of Surgery
Gastrointestinal Surgery
Institute of Digestive Diseases
Hospital Clinic
University of Barcelona
Barcelona, Spain
Chapter 43

Luis Landa-Verdugo, MD
Gastroenterologist
Former Chief of the Department of Internal Medicine
National Medical Center
IMSS
Mexico City, Mexico
Chapter 12(3)

David Lasky-Marcovich, MD
Department of Surgery
American British Cowdray Hospital
Mexico City, Mexico
Chapter 97

Giuseppe Mario Lentini, MD
Florence Center of Ambulatory Surgery
Florence, Italy
Chapter 70

Raimundo Llanio-Navarro, MD
General Hospital
Gastroenterologic Institute
Havana, Cuba
Chapter 58

Mary Beth Lobrano, MD
Fellow
Department of Imagenology
Louisiana State University
Charity Hospital
New Orleans, Louisiana
Chapter 38

Armando Lopez-Ortiz, MD
Department of Imagenology
American British Cowdray Hospital
Mexico, DF
Chapter 30(3)

Cristina Lopez-Peñalver, MD
Laparoscopic Center of South Florida
Coral Gables, Florida
Chapter 92

Beatriz Loscertales, MD
Fellow
Department of Imagenology
Louisiana State University
Charity Hospital
New Orleans, Louisiana
Chapters 37, 38, 80

Henry J. Lujan, MD, FACS
Laparoscopic Clinic of South Florida
Coral Gables, Florida
Chapter 46

Vincenzo Maffettone, MD
Surgical Researcher
1st Division of General and Gastrointestinal Surgery,
  School of Medicine
Second University of Naples
Naples, Italy
Chapter 14

Javier Martin-Delgado, MD
Department of Surgery
Medical and Dental School
University of Valencia
Valencia, Spain
Chapter 31

Juan Manuel Marina, MD
Department of Urology
Spanish Hospital
Mexico City, Mexico
Chapter 75

Raúl Martinez, MD
Fellow
Department of Imagenology
Louisiana State University
Charity Hospital
New Orleans, Louisiana
Chapter 30(2)

Sergio Martinez, MD
Department of Surgery
Jackson Memorial Hospital
University of Miami
Miami, Florida
Chapter 45

Wagner C. Marujo, MD
Liver Transplantation Unit
Albert Einstein Hospital
Faculty of Medicine
University of Sao Paulo
Sao Paulo, Brazil
Chapter 64

Paul C. McAfee, MD
The Scoliosis and Spine Center
St. Joseph Medical Center
Baltimore, Maryland
Chapter 85

Donald J Mehan, MD
Saint Louis University Health Sciences Center
Department of Surgery
Division of Urology
St Louis, Missouri
Chapter 74, 77

Sybren Meijer, MD
Fellow
Department of Surgery
Academic Hospital
Free University
Amsterdam, The Netherlands
Chapters 48, 60

Luca Mencaglia, MD
Director, Florence Center of Ambulatory Surgery
Florence, Italy
Chapter 70

Jesús Merello-Godino, MD
United Surgical Partners
San Camilo Clinic
Madrid, Spain
Chapters 83, 84

Roberto Millán-Sandoval, MD
Department of Surgery
General Hospital
Gastronterologic Institute
Havana, Cuba
Chapter 58

Robert G. Moore, MD
Saint Louis Health Sciences Center
Department of Surgery
Division of Urology
Saint Louis, Missouri
Chapters 74, 77

Jean Mouiel, MD
Former President of EAES
Hospital Archet
Nice, France
Chapter 20

Vincenzo Napolitano, MD
Surgical Researcher
1st Division of General and Gastrointestinal Surgery,
    School of Medicine
Second University of Naples
Naples, Italy
Chapter 14

Roberto Nevarez-Bernal, MD
Resident
Department of Gynecology and Obstetrics
National Institute of Perinatology
Mexico City, Mexico
Chapters 12(3), 18, 67

Camran Nezhat, MD
Institute for Special Pelvic Surgery
Atlanta, Georgia
Stanford University School of Medicine
Department of Obstetrics and Gynecology
Stanford, California
Chapter 95

Ceana H. Nezhat, MD
Institute for Special Pelvic Surgery
Atlanta, Georgia
Stanford University School of Medicine
Department of Obstetrics and Gynecology
Stanford, California
Chapter 95

Farr Nezhat, MD
Institute for Special Pelvic Surgery
Atlanta, Georgia
Stanford University School of Medicine
Department of Obstetrics and Gynecology
Stanford, California
Chapter 95

Joseph Ostroski, MD, FACS, FRCSC
Laparoscopic Center of South Florida
Coral Gables, Florida
Chapter 1

Enrique Palacios, MD
Fellow
Department of Imagenology
Charity Hospital
Louisiana State University
New Orleans, Louisiana
Chapter 30(2)

Pavlos Papasavos, MD
West Penn Allegheny Health System
Pittsburgh, Pennsylvania
Chapter 44

Raul O. Parra, MD
Adjunct Professor of Surgery
Oregon Health Sciences University
Department of Surgery
Division of Urology
Portland, Oregon
Chapters 74, 77

Carlos A. Pellegrini, MD
Professor of Surgery and Chairman, Department of Surgery
University of Washington Medical School
Seattle, Washington
Chapter 17

Jacques Perissat, MD, FACS
Professor
Membre d l'Académie Française de Chirugie
Honorary Fellow of the American Surgical Association
President of the International Federation Societies
   Endoscopic Surgeons
Bordeaux, France
Chapter 91

Jeffrey H. Peters, MD
Assistant Professor of Surgery Chief
Section of General Surgery
School of Medicine
University of Southern California
Los Angeles, California
Chapter 16

Ricardo Pettinari, MD
Department of Surgery
Hospital Privado Comunitario
Mar del Palata
Chubut, Argentina
Chapter 33

J.M. Piqué, MD
Head of Gastroenterology Department
Institute of Digestive Diseases
Hospital Clinic, University of Barcelona
Barcelona, Spain
Chapter 43

Gustavo Plasencia, MD
Professor of Surgery
University of Miami, School of Medicine
Medical Director
Colorectal Physiology Laboratory
Miami Baptist Hospital
Miami, Florida
Chapters 41, 46

Luis Poggi, MD
Laparoscopic General Surgeon
Angloamerican Clinic
Guillermo Almenara, Hospital
Lima, Peru
Chapter 32

Alfons Pomp, MD
Associate Professor of Surgery
Division of Endoscopic Surgery
Mount Sinai School of Medicine
New York, New York
Chapter 50

Carlos Quesnel, MD
Associate Professor
Department of Gynecological Surgery
National Institute of Perinatology
Mexico City, Mexico
Chapter 67

Theresa M. Quinn, MD
Instructor in Surgery
Mount Sinai School of Medicine
Mount Sinai Medical Center
New York, New York
Chapter 51

Jorge Ramirez, MD
Fellow
Department of Imagenology
Louisiana State University
Charity Hospital
New Orleans, Louisiana
Chapter 37

Alexander Raschke-Febres, MD
Fellow
Department of Surgery
Angeles de las Lomas Hospital
Huixquilucan, Edo, Mexico
Chapters 6, 18, 98

Harry Reich, MD
Assistant Clinical Professor
Columbia-Presbyterian Medical Center
Kingston, Pennsylvania
Assistant Clinical Professor
Tufts University
Boston, Massachusetts
Chapter 68

D. Rodero, MD
Department of Surgery
Medical and Dental School
University of Valencia
Valencia, Spain
Chapter 22

Sergio Roll, MD, PhD
Director of Laparoscopic Surgery
Department of General Surgery
Heliopolis Hospital
University of Santos School of Medicine
São Paulo, Brazil
Former Visiting Professor of Surgery
National University of Nordeste
Corrientes, Argentina
Former Visiting Professor of Surgery
National University of Plata
La Plata, Argentina
Chapter 64

James Ross, PhD, MD
Clinical Professor
UCLA School of Medicine
Director, Center for Reproductive and Laparoscopic Surgery
Salinas, California
Chapter 72

Gianluca Rossetti, MD
Resident of Gastrointestinal Surgery
1st Division of General and Gastrointestinal Surgery,
    School of Medicine
Second University of Naples
Naples, Italy
Chapter 14

Gianluca Russo, MD
Resident of Gastrointestinal Surgery
1st Division of General and Gastrointestinal Surgery,
    School of Medicine
Second University of Naples
Naples, Italy
Chapter 14

Raul José Salgueiro, MD
Department of Urology
Spanish Hospital of Mexico
Mexico City, Mexico
Chapter 75

Rodolfo Sánchez, MD
Chief, Centre for Land Use and Environmental Sciences
Department of Surgery
San Jose and Santa Engracia Hospital
Monterrey, Mexico
Chapter 25

Julián Sánchez-Cortázar, MD
Medical Director, American British Cowdray Medical
    Center of Mexico
Mexico City, Mexico
Chapter 30(3)

Richard M. Satava, MD
Professor of Surgery
Yale University School of Medicine
New Haven, Connecticut
Chapter 2

Daniel Seidman, MD
Chaim Sheba Medical Center
Sackler School of Medicine
Tel-Hashomer, Israel
Chapter 95

Michael R. Seitzinger, MD
CHN Women's Medical Services
Berlin, Wisconsin
Chapter 66

Ariek Shalhan, MD
Fellow in Endourology and Extracorporeal Shockwave Lithotripsy
Washington University School of Medicine
Saint Louis, Missouri
Chapter 78

Colin Sietses, MD
Department of Surgery
Academic Hospital
Free University
Amsterdam, The Netherlands
Chapter 61

Nathaniel J. Soper, MD
Professor of Surgery
Washington University School of Medicine
St. Louis, Missouri
Chapter 53

Miguel A. Statti, MD
Head, General Surgery
Private Community Hospital
Mar del Plata, Argentina
Chapter 33

Ewout W. Steyerberg, PhD
Erasmus University
Rotterdam, The Netherlands
Chapter 39(2)

Lee Swanstrom, MD
President Elect of SAGES
Santa Monica, California
Program Director, Minimally Invasive Surgery
Oregon Clinic General Surgery Division
Portland, Oregon
Chapter 12(1), 12(2)

Pablo Tarazona-Velutini, MD
Department of Orthopedic Surgery
American British Cowdray Hospital
Mexico City, Mexico
Chapter 97

Ennio Tiso, MD
Florence Center of Ambulatory Surgery
Florence, Italy
Chapter 70

Martín Salvador Valencia-Reyes, MD
Department of Surgery
Angeles Lomas Hospital and
American British Cowdray Hospital
Mexico City, Mexico
Chapters 5, 9, 25, 89

Daniel Valle, MD
Fellow
Department of Imagenology
Louisiana State University
Charity Hospital
New Orleans, Louisiana
Chapter 80

Rafael F. Valle, MD
Department of Obstetrics and Gynecology, Reproductive
   Endocrinology
Northwestern Medical Faculty Foundation, Inc.
Chicago, Illinois
Chapter 65

Daniel G. Vanuno, MD
Laparoscopic Surgery
Minimally Invasive Surgery Center
Department of Surgery
University of Illinois at Chicago
Chicago, Illinois
Chapter 17

José Antonio Vázquez-Frías, MD
Department of Surgery
Angeles de las Lomas Hospital and
American British Cowdray Hospital
Mexico, DF
Chapters 6, 7, 9, 18, 21, 25, 30(1), 39(1), 55, 56, 94, 98

Manuel Viamonte, III
Laparoscopic Center of South Florida
Coral Gables, Florida
Chapter 41

Anne Waage, MD
Mount Sinai Medical Center
Department of Surgery
Division of Laparoscopic Surgery/Minimally Invasive
   Surgery
New York, New York
Chapter 52

Alejandro Weber-Sánchez, MD
Department of Surgery
Angeles de las Lomas Hospital
Mexico, DF
Chapters 5, 89

Natan Zundel Majerowick, MD
Consultant Surgeon in Minimally Invasive Surgery
Fundación Santa Fe de Bogatá
Assistant Professor of Surgery
Escuela Colombiana de Medicina
Assistant Professor of Surgery
Universidad del Rosario
Assistant Professor of Surgery
Universidad Javeriana
Bogatá, Columbia
Chapter 57

*F*oreword

2002 was the tenth anniversary of the real start on a worldwide scale of minimally invasive or laparoscopic surgery.

In 1992, during the Third World Congress of Endoscopic Surgery, 3000 surgeons from every part of the world gathered in Bordeaux to meet about 50 pioneers who had opened the door to new territories of surgery during the past six years. The key to this progress was not a new surgical trick but a technological innovation, a small and light video camera, adapted to the laparoscope, used until then as an instrument of exploration. This camera transmitted in real time on a TV screen the images of what happens inside the human body, without damaging its envelope.

This camera, held by an assistant, freed the two hands of the surgeon, making it as easy as open surgery to perform the necessary maneuvers for real surgical operations. Everybody knows the incredible popularity that surrounded this method. These successes came more from the satisfaction of the surgery patients than from the opinion of the academic medical community, which was very critical towards a new surgery that upset established concepts and ideas.

Thus, we saw, as usual when a leap forward occurs in the evolution of surgery, the confrontation between conservatism and innovation, the surgical community becoming divided in two clans: the "laparo-skeptics" and the "laparo-enthusiastics." Such a controversy, which is still running, has been greatly beneficial. It obliged the most enthusiastic ones to have more moderation and a real scientific control on their innovative process. It obliged the most reluctant ones to revise gradually their points of view, the major argument often being for them the very constant drop in the number of patients seated in the waiting room of their offices.

Since 1992, many well-structured educational programs for laparoscopic surgery were set up; irrefutable scientific evaluations of laparoscopic treatments were delivered. Those efforts must continue. As to education, so many people have no access to the benefit of laparoscopic surgery around the world because of a lack of well-trained surgeons that we must extend our education programs.

As to research, we must be partners in the development of high technologies and integrate them into our operating rooms. The tasks are immense.

After ten years of constant improvements, the time has come for a remarkable milestone on the road of evolution of this surgery. This book fills this task perfectly. It offers a vision at once panoramic and at the same time detailed on what is today the state of the art in Laparoscopic Surgery. It even includes recent specialties to laparoscopic approach such as surgery of the spine, plastic surgery, neurosurgery and, in futuristic domains, robotics, remote controlled surgery, and others interventional techniques.

Among the authors of the various chapters the readers will find the names of pioneers and those who followed them who conquer new fascinating territories everyday. This book is an excellent springboard for surgeons, still not totally convinced, to jump onto the train. It must be one of the major reference books for residents in training. They will read, thanks to the talent of the editors, well-balanced chapters placed both in historical and futuristic perspectives and presented in an excellent didactic way. This work does great credit to the editors and contributors. They are mostly from North and Latin America with a special mention to Mexico. This book testifies to the excellence and vitality of the laparoscopic surgical teams in that part of the world.

Evolution of laparoscopic surgery is where it is because of one simple reason: it considers one of the greatest concerns of human beings—to be better healed with less adverse side effects.

The time has come to teach new generation of surgeons a new state of mind: "the minimally invasive spirit," which places the comfort of the patient in the foreground. The surgeons who master laparoscopic techniques have proven their work is as or even more effective than work by open surgery. Teachers will find in this book all the necessary materials to understand this innovative new minimally invasive surgery.

Professor Jacques Perissat, MD, FACS

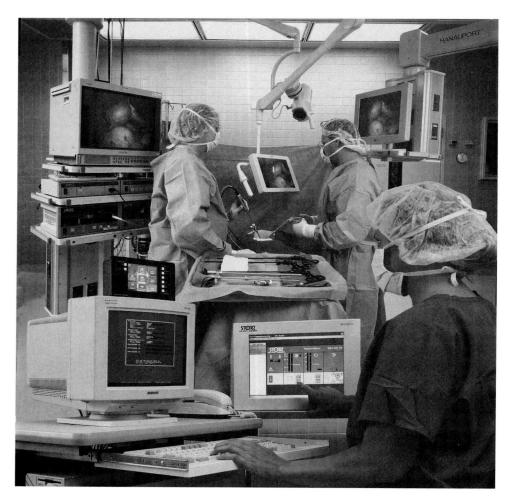

Courtesy of K. Storz, Germany. See Color Section.

Preface

The impressive advances of endoscopic surgery continue and it is our intention to present a comprehensive and authoritative book that synthesizes such progress into today's modern practice of surgery. As more clinical experience is accumulated, it is evident that many endoscopic surgical procedures have become the new "gold standard" of our practice. This is true in the areas of adrenal surgery, various bariatric procedures, and the diagnosis and treatment of acute abdomen, etc. In the sections on endocrine, thoracic, vascular, gynecologic, and urologic surgery, an assessment of the efficacy of these operations is also made, as well as others that are presently considered controversial. Likewise, certain diseases that are considered unusual or rare are covered here by groups that deal with them frequently. Discussions of these are supported by modern surgical references.

As anticipated, laparoscopic surgery is now commonplace in every hospital worldwide. New surgical residents are now familiar with its ever-growing list of applications, as they receive training daily in the basics and frequently assist in advanced endoscopic surgical operations. Several clinical and experimental projects have confirmed the enormous training potential of virtual reality models, although due to economic constraints, this modality is currently available in only a few teaching institutions. It is very likely that it will gain widespread acceptance in the future. To provide support for this aspect, some chapters describe the current methods of credentialing, including the use of the experimental laboratory for training and basic research. This applies not only to general surgery, but also to the subspecialty areas of gynecologic, thoracic, pediatric, and urologic surgery, as well as many others as described in the book.

The book does not intend to replace the existing atlases of operative technique or standard textbooks of surgery. Rather, an effort has been made by the authors, representatives of many internationally known surgical groups, to describe in an objective manner a rationale for the use of endoscopic surgery over conventional open procedures. Emphasis is made throughout of the potential benefits to patients and the cost savings relationship that is omnipresent in our daily practice.

The largest and most important section is devoted to the prevention, early diagnosis and treatment of complications of endoscopic surgery. Those that have plagued the field since its inception are ascribable mainly to the increased morbidity related to laparoscopic cholecystectomy. In retrospect, problems associated with this operation were due primarily to the lack of proper training and supervision and the use of deficient equipment and instrumentation. Efforts are now being made to avoid these same mistakes and problems extensively throughout the world, although the prevalence of these complications still remains unacceptably high in some parts.

As mentioned, the invited authors were selected for their expertise in their respective fields. Most of them are distinguished members of SAGES, EAES, ALACE, AMCE, and others. Updated consensual conclusions of these associations have been included in various chapters, even though some have only been presented in recent congresses. This is the case of the 2000 Consensus of Experts of the EAES, in which the laparoscopic treatment of large bowel cancer is introduced. The authors and editors appreciate the efforts made by the staff of McGraw-Hill to coordinate the work of many experts from different parts of the world.

If an objective analysis is made of the world literature from 1990 on, it is clear that minimally invasive surgery has made a dramatic and beneficial change in modern surgical practice. We are convinced that the technologic advances that we continually witness, and the ingenuity and talent of many devoted surgeons and their staffs, will ensure that this new modality will continue to make progress and find broader application and appeal. This will in turn help to achieve our main goal, which is to provide more and substantial benefits to our patients. This is, then, the chief purpose of publishing *Laparoscopic Surgery*.

Jorge Cueto-García
Moisés Jacobs
Michel Gagner

Dedicated to

My Children Maru, Gracy and Jorge Luis

My Wife Gabriela

For Their Patience and Never Ending Support

Jorge Cueto-Garcia

My Mother and Father,

Who Have Taught Me
That Through
Dedication, Hard Work, and Love,
Everything is Possible

Moisés Jacobs

My Lovely Family

My Wife Lapointe

My Sons Xavier, Guillaume, and Maxime

My Mother Louise Duchaine

My Father Raymond Gagner, MD,
Pioneer of Laparoscopic Gynecology in Quebec

Michel Gagner

General Considerations

Chapter One · · · · · ·

*H*istory of Laparoscopy

JOSEPH OSTROSKI and MOISÉS JACOBS

Laparoscopic surgery has created a revolution in the field of surgery in the past 10 years, even though in the last century we have witnessed the discovery and widespread use of sterile surgery, microsurgery, cardiac surgery, organ replacement, and reconstructive surgery. Where did this all begin and what are the historical milestones?

Laparoscopy owes much of its development to physicians as far back as the 11th century (Albukasimi) and later in the 1800s (Bozzini), who used endoscopic instruments to examine body orifices. Later in that century, tube endoscopes were being used to examine the urinary bladder and urethra (Desonneaux, 1853) and not long after, the lung by Kussmaul and Nitze. In 1901, in order to observe the effect of pneumoperitoneum on the abdominal organs, German-born Georg Kelling introduced a cystoscope into a dog's abdominal cavity and performed the first laparoscopy. In 1910, Hans Christian Jacobaeus in Stockholm, Sweden, carried out the first clinical laparoscopy and thoracoscopy. In 1913, Jacobaeus, an internist, lysed adhesions under thoracoscopic vision. Then in the 1930s, Heinz Kalk, an internist of Berlin, occasionally used the laparoscope to lyse adhesions within the abdomen. The first known textbook, *Laparothoroscopy*, was published in Munich by Korsbach in 1927. Despite the fact that laparoscopic sterilization was first performed in 1941 in the United States and the discovery of major advances in gynecologic instrumentation such as the CO_2 insufflator, "cold light" endoscopy, and egg harvesting for fertilization, laparoscopy remained largely a gynecologist's tool. Interest in laparoscopy languished with academic centers being the only source for residency training in endoscopic techniques.

The era of modern laparoscopic surgery was catalyzed in the University Women's Clinic in Kiel headed by Kurt Semm. He developed an automatic insufflation device (1963), a heat-transfer system, thermocoagulation (1973), and invented an irrigation device and an electronic insufflator. He also developed the endosuture and instruments for more advanced procedures. Semm performed the first laparoscopic appendectomy (1980), but numerous prominent surgeons were harsh critics of the new procedure.

Fascinated by Semm's technique, Erich Mühe, a general surgeon in Böblingen, Germany, used Semm's instruments to perform the world's first laparoscopic cholecystectomy on September 12, 1985. In April 1987, Mühe presented 97 laparoscopic cholecystectomies to the Congress of German Surgeons. This was made possible by the introduction in 1986 of a computer chip that allowed magnification and projection of endoscopic images onto television screens. Videoendoscopy allowed surgeons to stand upright and use both hands to perform surgery. It was easier to follow the magnified image, and the entire operating team could view their work.

This news reached French surgeons Phillipe Mouret (Lyon), Francois Dubois (Paris), and Jacques Perissat (Bourdeaux), who introduced laparoscopic cholecystectomy in their clinics, and it was Perissat who presented this work at a SAGES (Society of American Gastrointestinal Endoscopic Surgeons) meeting in Louisville in April of 1989, thus establishing what many called the "French technique."

In 1988, when Semm presented the videotape of his laparoscopic appendectomy at a gynecologic meeting in Baltimore, he gave impetus to McKernan and Saye of Marietta, Georgia, to carry out the first laparoscopic cholecystectomy in the United States. They were followed shortly by Reddick and Olsen of Nashville, Tennessee. These pioneers brought acceptance of this use of laparoscopic surgery not only by surgeons, but by the general population as well. Within less than 2 years gallbladder removal would be changed dramatically. Thousands of surgeons retrained in cholecystectomy. The era of "big surgeon—big incision" ended.

The early 1990s also saw the introduction of numerous laparoscopic procedures into general surgery, and during this period laparoscopic surgery became incorporated into general surgical thinking. The introduction and spread of laparoscopy is one of the greatest success stories in the history of modem medicine, and is significant for many reasons. The use of laparoscopy marked the beginning of the end of the era of traditional open surgery. It also revitalized general surgery, reshaped approaches in other branches of surgery, and accelerated the development of surgical instrumentation. The success of laparoscopic cholecystectomy encouraged surgeons to consider new perspectives on their practice. It also encouraged surgeons to collaborate with physicians in other specialties. Around the world, surgeons have begun an active search for new ways to apply endoscopic techniques. The number of endoscopic procedures increased rapidly in all branches of surgery in the early 1990s.

The role of the medical industry in the development and increased use of endoscopy cannot be overstated. Companies such as Storz, U.S. Surgical, and Johnson & Johnson have been pivotal in advancing laparoscopy through their contributions in education and in the design of more complex instrumentation for all specialties in the field of minimally-invasive surgery. Without an adequate technological base, the rise of laparoscopic surgery would have been impossible.

Because of their greater financial resources, much of the explosive growth of laparoscopy was carried out in private hospitals, and academic institutions lagged behind. These institutions were startled to discover that the majority of laparoscopic techniques and procedures performed in this country were not being taught in the controlled setting of a residency or fellowship training program. Over the past 10 years, this divergence between private and academic institutions is slowly disappearing as they work together with industry to train the future surgeons of the world, thus assuring the consistent teaching and proper use of laparoscopic procedures. Still, as of 1999 only 7% of residency programs taught advanced laparoscopic surgery in a consistent fashion.

The quantum leap in the use of laparoscopy in the late 1980s led to the innovations of the 1990s and the discoveries of more successful laparoscopic techniques such as:

- The astounding contributions to laparoscopic biliary tract surgery made by Karl Zucker;
- The advancements in reflux surgery made by Dallegmane of St. Joseph's Clinic in Liege, Belgium;
- The exciting improvements in gastric surgery made by Katkhouda;
- The contributions made by Flowers of Baltimore and Phillips of Los Angeles to improving techniques for handling splenic disorders;
- The discoveries made by Gagnier in laparoscopic adrenal surgery; and
- The improvements made by Jacobs and Plasencia of Miami and Franklin of San Antonio in pioneering techniques for colon surgery for both benign disease and malignancies.

It is impossible not to be fascinated by the diverse indications for laparoscopic surgery, including its use in tumor diagnosis and staging, to remove adrenal tumors, and even for pediatric patients and those requiring vascular surgery. The revolution may be slowing somewhat, but refinements are still taking place; just think what will be achieved in this new millennium—surgery performed by remote-controlled robots. Will the direct touch of the surgeon's hands no longer be necessary? We doubt that these advancements, however great, will ever make the human touch unnecessary. Just think of the excitement that future surgeons will have as they operate on a molecular level. Will they feel the same thrill as Kelling did in 1901? We think so.

Chapter Two ● ● ● ● ● ●

*T*he New Technology

RICHARD M. SATAVA

INTRODUCTION

Laparoscopic surgery has provided a revolutionary niche in the annals of surgery. It initially appeared that minimally invasive surgery was going to be the standard of surgery toward which all procedures would migrate. Within a decade, the majority of surgical procedures that were performed using traditional open surgery had been accomplished through minimally invasive techniques, at least in a few isolated reported cases. However, the limitations for the vast majority of surgeons in performing the more advanced procedures became apparent, and today laparoscopic surgery is either limited to a few simple procedures performed by most general surgeons, or more advanced procedures being performed by a very few surgeons who specialize in laparoscopic surgery.

However, progress is being made to overcome the factors that prevent all minimally invasive surgery from becoming available to all surgeons. This is being accomplished through the use of innovative technological solutions to overcome the barriers. These barriers have been reported on extensively, and they include the inability to visualize in three-dimensions, a lack of the sense of touch, decreased dexterity, and very poor human–machine interfaces. The surgeon has traded direct visualization and sensitive manual manipulation for an extremely awkward means of indirectly viewing and handling tissues. One of the main reasons is the reliance upon modified traditional instruments that use technologies from the Industrial Age rather than seeking out solutions from the high technology available in the Information Age.[1] The only Information Age technology currently incorporated into laparoscopic surgery is the use of video monitoring systems. In addition, minimally invasive procedures require special educational and training systems, and to date this has been accomplished using conventional training methods. New computer and network technologies such as virtual reality and the World Wide Web will provide enhanced training methods.

There are two approaches to the solutions for the barriers noted above; those that are requirements-driven (recognized problems for which there are solutions) and those that are opportunity-driven (emerging technologies which will provide new opportunities). The requirements-driven solutions provide unique solutions through the use of computers, imaging, robotics, and telecommunications. These changes are being made today, and will continue into the future. The opportunities-driven solutions are revolutionary new technologies that may provide some answers to today's problems, but more likely will extend a surgeon's capabilities into new areas through the use of advancements in genetics, microelectromechanical systems (MEMS), tissue engineering, or nanotechnology. Many of these will replace current surgical procedures and must be evaluated as to whether they are to be incorporated into the realm of general surgery, or if they will be taken over by nonsurgical specialties. This dilemma here is obvious in light of the rapid rise of interventional radiologic procedures such as percutaneous drainage of abscesses, catheter angioplasties, endoscopic stent placement, and endovascular grafts that have become the realm of nonsurgical specialists.

THE NEXT GENERATION

Information Age technologies have enabled the transition of laparoscopic surgery to the next generation of minimally invasive surgery. This requires incorporating 3-D visualization and newer data-fusion techniques to improve vision; the addition of force feedback to improve the sense of touch, perception of scale, reduce tremors, and allow additional degrees of freedom (DOF) for instruments; and more intuitive interfaces that more closely resemble open surgery. Preoperative planning and surgical training are enhanced through the use of virtual reality. Surgical education and training are benefiting from telementoring and distant education over the Internet and World Wide Web. All of these technologies can be incorporated into systems which are computer-assisted and/or robotically controlled and represent the next major revolution in surgery.

Vision and Visualization

The next generation of tools have incorporated new 3-D stereoscopic displays into their systems. The purpose of these displays, such as

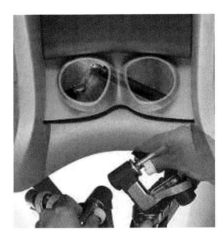

Figure 2–1. Stereoscopic view in the surgeon's console. *(Courtesy of Fred Moll, M.D., Intuitive Surgical, Inc., Menlo Park, CA.)*

the surgeon's console on the Intuitive Surgical system (Fig. 2–1), is to provide the depth perception which is lost with the standard 2-D monitors currently used with laparoscopic systems. This allows for more precise positioning of the instruments. Other systems integrate 3-D data fusion, such as the image-guided system of GE Medical Research Corporation (Fig. 2–2). For neurosurgeons, this is accomplished by overlaying the preoperative magnetic resonance imaging (MRI) image over the brain, permitting the visualization of the exact tumor margins with 0.5-mm accuracy in the open MRI-guided neurosurgical procedures by Dr. Ferenc Jolesz of Brigham Women's Hospital.[2] This demonstrates the return of normal 3-D visualization as well as extending the ability to "see through tissue" with the use of data fusion. These are investigational systems which have nearly completed their final clinical trials and approval process and should soon be widely available. The RoboDoc system for hip replacement uses the image-guided principle to create a more accurate re-creation of the femoral shaft cavity to allow precise positioning of the correct prosthesis.[3] Other systems for prostate surgery and knee surgery that are in the experimental phase use various data-fusion modalities for precision location.

Sense of Touch

Current laparoscopic systems do not have feedback for the sense of touch. The telepresence systems (below) incorporate a simple force feedback from the instrument as a whole back to the handles on the surgeon's console. The force feedback is rather basic, and measures the amount of pressure against the instrument tip and sends this force to the computer, which then applies this amount of force against the handles in the console. This provides a sense of resistance as the tissues are poked or pulled, but does not give the sensation of how firmly the tissue is being grasped nor the consistency and elasticity of the tissue. To address this problem, a prototype system by Dr. Blake Hannaford of University of Washington (Fig. 2–3) incorporates tiny sensors in the tips of the grasper which record the amount of pressure exerted by the grasper tips, and provides this resistance to the fingers of the surgeon.[4] Because such as system is computer-controlled, it can even scale up the amount of pressure imparted to the fingers, providing a sensitivity greater than that of simple direct palpation. The sense of touch is much more complicated than simply the amount of pressure. Clinical testing will be required to determine if increasing the sensitivity actually does improve the sense of touch, and ultimately the performance, of the surgeon. Other possibilities for microsensors embedded on various instruments include vibration and tangential stress (shearing forces) to detect the slipping of tissue, temperature for coagulation to prevent overcoagulation of tissues, and accelerometers to detect blood vessel pulsation in tissues. The result will be a new generation of instruments that can compensate for the sensory input that was lost with laparoscopic surgery, and long-range research might provide sensory information not available even in open surgery (see below).

Dexterity and Precision

The growth of laparoscopic surgery quickly demonstrated to every surgeon the incredible dexterity and precision of the human hand. The loss of this control with minimally invasive procedures resulted in long, arduous training sessions, as well as increased operative time. Precision was lost because of the instrument's long shaft which is manipulated over a fulcrum, as well as the amplifi-

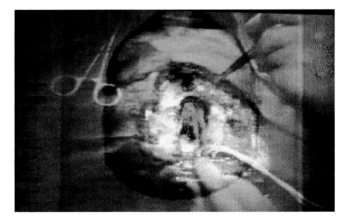

Figure 2–2. Data fusion of a MRI image over the video image of a patient with a brain tumor. *(Courtesy Dr. Ferenc Jolesz, Brigham Women's Hospital, Boston, MA.)*

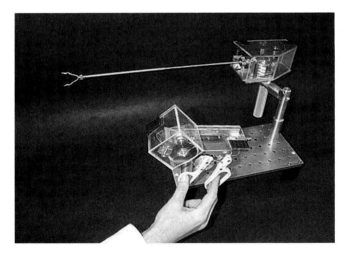

Figure 2–3. Prototype grasper with microsensors in the tips that transmit the pressure to the fingertips via the handle. *(Courtesy of Dr. Blake Hannaford, University of Washington, Seattle, WA.)*

cation of tremor by such long instruments. Dexterity was lost because of the severe restriction of the amount of degrees of freedom (DOF) of the instruments. The DOF can be simplistically thought of as the number of different directions in which an instrument (or the hand) can be moved. As joints are added to an instrument, they permit more directions in which the instrument can be moved (the hand has 23 DOF). A laparoscopic instrument typically can be moved through a trocar with 4 DOF (in/out, left/right, up/down, and rotate). Adding grasper or scissor tips (open/close) results in 5 DOF. The difficulty is that with only 4 to 5 DOF, the instruments cannot be manipulated into all the positions needed to perform a procedure, and many of the points of anatomy are reached only with very awkward maneuvers. The addition of a "wrist" for the sixth DOF to the instrument greatly increases the points that can be reached, as well as improving the ease with which the instrument can be used. Construction of an instrument that can be manipulated through more than 5 DOF is extremely difficult; however, controlling such an instrument with more DOF by a computer is quite feasible. Thus the newer computer-assisted robotic systems are incorporating an additional DOF via an internal "wrist" to provide this dramatic increase in dexterity (Fig. 2–4). Obviously, the increasing number of DOF creates an increasing level of complexity to control. Whether adding a seventh DOF via an "elbow" inside the patient's abdomen would provide additional dexterity has not been evaluated. Higher levels of DOF could be added by creating additional "fingers" on the tips of the manipulators, resulting in an instrument such as a 3-fingered grasper. The success of such 6-DOF systems depends also upon the hand controller, which must permit the manipulation of the instrument in a fashion that is intuitive and mimics natural hand motions. As most surgeons are aware, a significant part of the difficulty with laparoscopic instruments is that they are manipulated as much with the elbow and shoulder (which are designed for powerful motion) as with the hands (which are designed for fine manipulation). Ramon Berguer has devoted a significant amount of his ergonomics research to studying the effects of this awkward positioning in laparoscopic surgery.[5]

Precision

The ability to precisely position the tip of an instrument depends on a combination of many factors, including the visual perception of the position of the target, the number of DOF of the instrument, the stability of the instrument, the control of the surgeon's hand and fatigue with prolonged use, to name only a few. Many of these factors can result in tremor, the small movements of the tip of the instrument. In microsurgical procedures, tremor can be reduced by stabilizing the hand against a support to reduce fatigue and improve coordination. Also, during prolonged procedures that create fatigue, intention tremor becomes manifest. Computer-assisted robotic systems are able to compensate for the flailing of the surgeon's arms as well as the tremor that comes with fatigue. By sitting comfortably at a console with support for the hands, the surgeon's movements can be stabilized. (See a new instrument, Figure 2–5.) In addition, the normal intention tremor that occurs at 8 to 14 Hz can be filtered out of the motion of the instruments, providing a steady and precise trajectory for the tip of the instrument.

Human Interface Issues

As indicated above, at first laparoscopic surgery adapted existing instruments for use in laparoscopic procedures without regard to the needs of the surgeon. Initially, laparoscopic cholecystectomy was performed by looking at a monitor which was placed wherever it could fit into the operation room, and surgeons frequently had to strain their necks in order to see the image. The importance of the direct hand–eye axis was demonstrated, and it was a significant improvement. However, the surgeon was still unable to directly view the site where the hands were performing the surgery. Computer-assisted robotic systems have provided the ideal solution by having the surgeon look directly past the hands at the image, thereby returning the natural hand–eye axis. With the addition of the mechanical "wrist" to the instruments inside the abdomen, the surgeon can now use the fine motions of the hands rather than the awkward motions of the elbows and shoulders to control the instruments. Finally, the surgeon sits comfortably at the console, rather than the fatigue-inducing standing position at the operative table. All of these modifications using the improved human interface technology of the telepresence surgical systems have dramatically improved the ability to perform the procedures while reducing the fatigue of the surgeon.

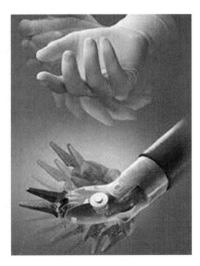

Figure 2–4. The EndoWrist provides an additional DOF for a surgical instrument. *(Courtesy of Fred Moll, Intuitive Surgical Inc., Menlo Park, CA.)*

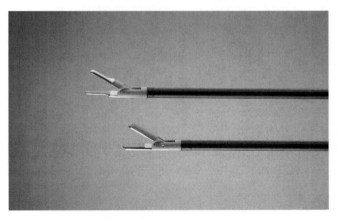

Figure 2–5. A new instrument. *(Courtesy of K. Storz, Germany.)*

Preoperative and Intraoperative Assistance

Computed tomography (CT) and MRI scans have given us the ability to represent the patient's anatomy via three-dimensional images of their actual organs and tissues. This provides the opportunity to perform preoperative planning of difficult procedures. For example, Altobelli[6] uses the preoperative scans of patients with craniofacial dysostosis to measure the degree of asymmetry of the two sides of the face by overlaying a mirror image of the normal side of the face over the deformed side. By visualizing the difference between the two sides he can create a prosthesis which will exactly match the defect. Using similar principles, Stephanides, Montgomery, and Schendel have devised a preoperative planning system for microsurgical reconstruction of the mandible.[7] Marescaux[8] is using 3-D segmented and reconstructed images from CT scans of liver tumors (Fig. 2–6) to provide both preoperative planning and rehearsal of the procedures, some of which can be performed laparoscopically.

Virtual Reality Simulations for Training

The technology of virtual reality as applied to medicine consists of 3-D representations of anatomic structures by a computer system that permits an individual to interact with the image as if it were real. Some of the anatomic models are graphic representations, while others are derived from CT or MRI scans of an individual, such as the Visible Human Project of the National Library of Medicine.[9] In creating the visual representations, there is a trade-off that limits the realism of the simulation. Simple graphic images require a small amount of computing power, but provide the opportunity to interact with the image in real time in a realistic fashion—the images behave as if they were real, but they do not look real. On the other hand, ultrarealistic images with very high visual fidelity cannot be manipulated in real time—the images look real, but they do not behave realistically. This is due to the limitations on computing power. Powerful though the computers of today may be, there is still not enough power to do all the calculations required; thus there is a trade-off of either improved visual realism or improved real-time interactivity. This will likely continue for a decade or more, even though computer power is doubling about every 18 months (Moore's law). The reason is that the human body is so complex, that increases in orders of magnitude in computing power will be required to represent the visual, physiologic, kinematic, haptic, and other properties which we take for granted in our daily world. Nevertheless, there are a number of simulators which have been developed in pursuit of the ultimate real-time realistic imaging sys-tem. One of the earliest was the abdominal simulator for cholecystectomy by Satava[10] (Fig. 2–7). Other simulators have been developed for laparoscopic cholecystectomy,[11] hysteroscopy,[12] ENT sinusoscopy,[13] and anastomosis,[14] among others. The latest generation of simulators, such as the anastomosis simulator or the Minimally Invasive Surgery Trainer–VR (MIST-VR),[15] have begun incorporating automatic objective grading of performance. What has been learned from these early generations of simulators is that both visual realism and real-time interactivity are critical to training surgeons to perform complex surgical procedures. None of the existing simulators can meet these expectations. Therefore it is essential to take the level of realism that is available and use it to develop a curriculum that is within the limitations of these simulators. Rather than developing skills by training on ultrarealistic simulations of entire procedures, simpler tasks must be used for training (such as the anastomosis simulator), thus enhancing the training of young surgeons in standard procedures. As simulators improve, the complexity of these tasks can be improved. We must not abandon the use of virtual reality simulators because they are in their early phases of development. The lesson learned from history is that the first flight simulators were no more than modified carnival rides to which a structured training program was applied; even though the simulators bore no resemblance to the real aircraft, the training programs were able to reduce crash landings in the dark or in bad weather by 90%. From today's meager beginnings and as computer power increases, so too will surgical simulators become ultrarealistic.

Telementoring and Distant Learning

Because laparoscopic surgery is performed via images on a video monitor, the opportunity to remotely train novice surgeons gave rise to telementoring. Early demonstrations of remote telementoring by Kavoussi et al[16] and Go et al[17] proved that the concept was valid. Subsequently, Rosser et al[18] incorporated telementoring into their

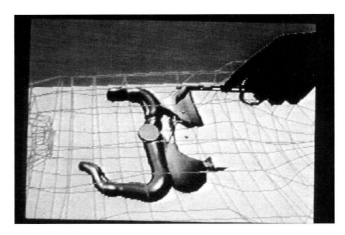

Figure 2–7. Early surgical simulator of a cholecystectomy. *(Photo courtesy of the author.)*

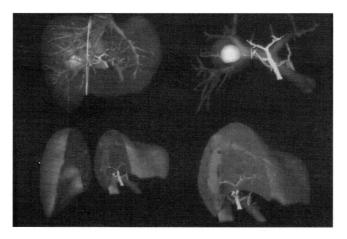

Figure 2–6. Three-dimensional reconstruction of a patient's liver tumor, with the hepatic vascular anatomy separated to allow preoperative planning or surgical simulation. *(Courtesy Jacques Marescaux, European Telesurgical Institute (ETIS), Strasbourg, France.)*

laparoscopic training courses originating from Yale University, both within their local region in the northeast U.S. and in distant countries such as Ecuador and the Dominican Republic. Marescaux conducts similar telementoring training for many western European countries from the European Telesurgical Institute in Strassbourg, France. The purpose and advantage of telementoring is that it provides an opportunity for the distant student to receive real-time feedback during the procedures. Another option for distant learning that is growing dramatically is Internet-based education on the World Wide Web. In addition to structured interactive lectures that reside on web pages, live video clips have been added. Thus text, graphics, and stored video can be combined to provide an information-rich learning experience. Investigations are ongoing into providing continuing medical education credit for courses taken on the web. Issues such as security, user validation (verification that the person taking the test is actually the person who signed up for the course), and even administrative issues such as payment are still being addressed. The expectation is that in the future there will be many different levels of education and training, and the web-based courses will have the advantage of being asynchronous—they can be taken at a time convenient to the student, and not limited to scheduled periods as in telementoring or real-time video conferencing.

Image-Guided, Computer-Assisted, Robotic, and Telesurgery Systems

The era of robotic and computer-assisted surgical systems began in the early 1990s, just as laparoscopic surgery was experiencing exponential growth. Early pioneers were Hap Paul, William Bargar, and Russell Taylor,[3] who designed the first system called "RoboDoc" (Fig. 2–8). This is a sophisticated robotic arm with a drill attached, used to core out the femur for a femoral prosthesis in hip replacement. This system has an accuracy of 97%, compared to the traditional broach method, which has an accuracy of 75%.

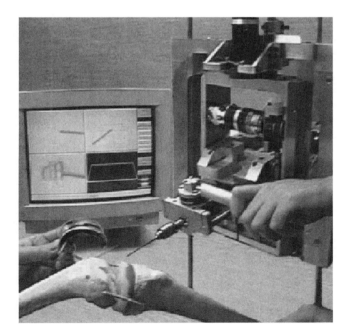

Figure 2–8. RoboDoc, the first robotic surgical system. *(Courtesy Hap Paul, University of California at Davis, Davis, CA.)*

Image-guided systems are most commonly used in neurosurgical procedures. Bucholz[19] has been using image-guided systems in stereotactic neuronavigation with an accuracy of 2 mm during resection of deep-seated brain tumors. In these computer-assisted systems (either image-guided or robotically controlled), the surgeon preoperatively plans the procedures from patient-specific x-rays or CT scans, and feeds the coordinates into the system. After the operative site has been exposed and the registration process (matching the location on the patient to the coordinates in the robot's computer) has been completed, the robot can precisely perform that portion of the procedure (in image-guided neurosurgery, the surgeon uses the system to achieve precise placement of the tip of the scalpel or probe according to predetermined coordinates) while the surgeon serves a supervisory role. The surgeon then completes the operation. The advantage of such systems is that they allow for a level of accuracy well beyond that of the unaided human hand. The telesurgical systems are significantly different; the surgeon holds the master control handles and directly manipulates the tips of the instruments. These systems include motion tracking, motion and vision scaling, dexterity enhancement, and tremor reduction as the computer augments the surgeon's own hand motions. There is no preprogramming, nor is there any relinquishing of control to the robotic system as with the devices mentioned above. There is real-time instant response by the robot to the surgeon's most delicate hand motions. The earliest system was the Green Telepresence system by SRI International,[20] a firm that explores telesurgical systems for open and laparoscopic surgery. Subsequent commercial systems have been derived from these early prototypes, and the first report of a telesurgical procedure was published by Himpens and Cardiere[21] in Brussels, Belgium in 1997. Within a year, Carpentier[22] had performed over 150 cardiac coronary artery bypass procedures using the improved Intuitive Surgical system (Fig. 2–9). The second commercially available telesurgical system, developed by Computer Motion, employed similar concepts and likewise focused on minimally invasive surgical procedures, allowing markedly enhanced dexterity in performing minimally invasive tubal reanastomoses, with an accuracy of 2 mm (Fig. 2–10). As indicated above, the addition of a "wrist" joint to the surgical instruments permits the extra DOF that results in increased dexterity. Since these are the pioneering systems for telesurgery, it can be expected that additional capabilities will be added, such as additional DOF, microsensors on the tips of the instruments to simulate the sense of touch, and visualizing and analytic instruments that will exceed human sensory perception, such as ultrasound, infrared, and noninvasive spectroscopy. The surgical systems of the future will not only extend our human capabilities, but provide visual, tactile, and other sensory information beyond normal human capacity.

All of the aforementioned surgical systems are computer-mediated; signals are transmitted from the surgeon to a computer, and then to a robotic manipulator. Thus the surgeon does not have to be in the same room, or even the same city, to perform the surgical procedure. This is the "tele" part of telesurgery. The expectation is that it will be possible to remotely perform surgery in distant places such as Third World countries or even in outer space. With our current understanding of the laws of physics, this is not currently possible. This is due to the delay time (or latency or lag) between the movement of the surgeon's control handles and the transmission of the signal to the tip of the instrument. With the surgeon's console directly wired to the manipulators in the operating

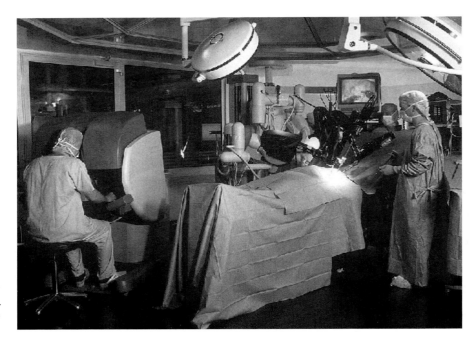

Figure 2–9. Telesurgical system set-up in operating room. *(Courtesy Fred Moll, MD, Intuitive Surgical Inc., Menlo Park, CA.)*

room, the transmission time is less than 25 milliseconds (msec). In order to transmit the same signal to a system located in a underdeveloped country, the signal must go to a satellite (which is 22,000 miles above the earth) and then back down to the ground, for a minimal total trip time of more than a second. Experiments have demonstrated that the maximum delay that is tolerable by a system is approximately 200 msec, beyond which the system becomes unstable. In addition, with transmission times over 200 msec, the surgeon cannot compensate for the delay. At 25 msec the surgeon is not aware of the delay, at 50 msec the surgeon knows something isn't quite right but automatically compensates, and at 100 msec the surgeon is aware of the delay and employs strategies (such as slowing down hand motions) to compensate for the delay. However at 200 msec, even these strategies are inadequate, and critical structures such as blood vessels could move between the time the motion was initiated and when the scalpel actually cuts. Thus for the near term, any remotely-conducted surgery will have to be conducted with de-

lay of 200 msec or less, which is geographically estimated to be within about 200 kilometers with a dedicated wired connection or approximately 35 km by wireless connections. But even more important than the technical considerations are the practical issues. Is there a medical center that is willing to place many of these systems in remote areas, where the number of surgical procedures requiring the expertise of a specialist surgeon may be small? Experience in telemedicine has shown that many of the anticipated uses of remote consultation did not succeed when faced with the practical matters of a small number of patients utilizing the system, cost effectiveness, reimbursement, and other nontechnical issues. However, if these systems became inexpensive enough that many could be distributed in remote areas, widespread remote telesurgery could certainly become a reality.

EMERGING TECHNOLOGIES FOR THE TWENTY-FIRST CENTURY

The above discussion focused on those technologies, principally Information Age technologies, that are available today and can provide specific solutions to currently identified problems and barriers. There are a number of emerging technologies in the earlier stages of development that may or may not impact upon the way surgery will be performed in the future. These technologies reflect a new approach to scientific research, and may be the heralds of a new era. There is no name for this new revolution, so we shall use the term BioIntelligence Age until a more accurate description of these new technologies can be clarified. The basic premise is that the Information Age is not the future; the Information Age is the present. The future belongs to interdisciplinary research. Figure 2–11 is a Venn diagram illustrating this new trend in science. Until recently, scientific advancements have been made by individuals or teams within one of the three main branches of science (biological, physical, or information). Today, universities are forming new departments, and corporations are forming new divisions, that

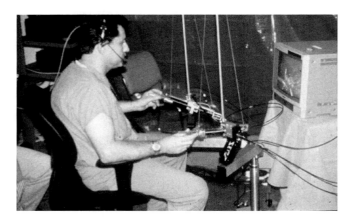

Figure 2–10. Surgeon at work on telesurgical system. *(Courtesy Yulun Wang, Computer Motion, Inc., Goleta, CA.)*

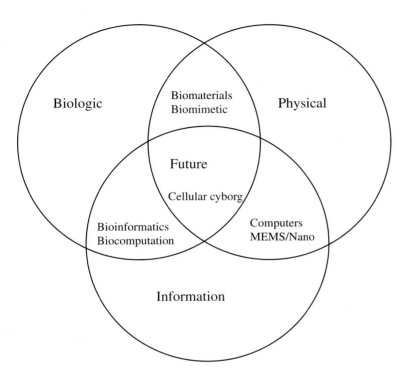

Figure 2–11. The BioIntelligence Age Venn diagram.

are combinations of at least two of the sciences. For example, the intersection of biologic and physical sciences gives birth to biosensors, biomaterials, and biomimetic systems. Combining physical and information sciences brings forth interdisciplinary teams for microelectromechanical systems (MEMS), nanotechnology, and autonomous robotics. Blending information and biologic sciences yields bioinformatics, biocomputation, genomics, and proteinomics. These interdisciplinary efforts are required to solve the diverse problems that are facing all of the scientific disciplines. By blending the biologic (adaptability, flexibility, self-assembling, and self-regulating), the physical (robust, precise, reproducible, and work-generating) and the information (intelligent, distributed, and networked) worlds, goals can be achieved which no single discipline can accomplish. This combining is possible as we become more able to fit devices into smaller packages, or as we enter the micro and nano worlds. For example, cell membranes can generate a membrane potential from 20 to 100 millivolts. The newest MEMS machines can be powered by as little as 50 millivolts. Thus, theoretically (and in certain laboratory experiments) it could be expected that cells (by changing their membrane potential) could "communicate" directly with a machine, and with an information system to provide artificial intelligence, could actually control the MEMS device. Stem cells can be programmed to sense levels of glucose, and MEMS devices with microwells (Fig. 2–12) could release drugs or biochemicals (such as insulin). It is hypothesized that growing stem cells that sense glucose on the surface of these microchips, with an information system to interpret the signal from the cell and release the insulin, could result in an artificial pancreatic beta cell. Although this has not yet been accomplished, all the technologies exist to create such a device. Such a device would be so small that it could be implanted. Another research area is implanting microsensors into

insects (Fig. 2–13), such as this honeybee from the University of Montana. This insect is carrying a device which contains a sensor for bacterial agents and a tiny transmitter. When the honeybee encounters a biologic agent, it is sensed by the sensor and the information is transmitted back to the receiving station. Combining biologic and physical systems provides capabilities beyond any single system. Tissue engineering offers the opportunity to grow synthetic organs from precursor lines. Cells and tissues need a blood supply since diffusion occurs only in cells near the surface of a tissue. Va-

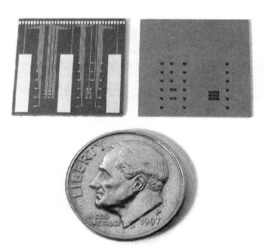

Figure 2–12. A microelectromechanical system (MEMS) microwell device which can be programmed to release minute doses of drugs or biochemicals. *(Courtesy John Santini, MicroChips, Inc., Boston, MA.)*

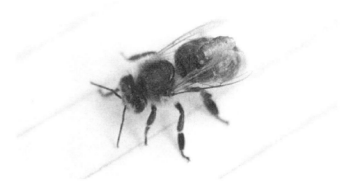

Figure 2–13. Honeybee with implanted sensor and radio transmitter. *(Courtesy of University of Montana.)*

canti has devised a method of taking biocomputed maps of branching blood vessels and creating a 3-D scaffold using biopolymers impregnated with vascular endothelial growth factors (Fig. 2–14). This scaffold will be seeded by vascular endothelial cells to form a matrix of supporting blood vessels. The next step is to add cells of the required organ type (e.g., hepatocytes, nephrocytes, etc.) to make a functioning organ. The implication for surgeons is that we might be able to transplant synthetically-grown organs in the near future. The new field of nanotechnology is defined as building structures molecule by molecule. The first success in this area was fabrication of carbon nanotubules, which resemble the structures built by living organisms such as diatoms or coral. These carbon nanotubules have 10 times the strength and one-seventh the weight of stainless steel. They can be arranged into a number of different configurations, depending on the requirements of the desired structure. We may see new surgical instruments that are microscopic in size or new devices to implant into patients. All the above technologies are so new that their potential is highly speculative. Yet it is critical to be aware of these new directions because technology is developing so fast that opportunities could be missed if we are not prepared for the next revolution. It will be up to the individual

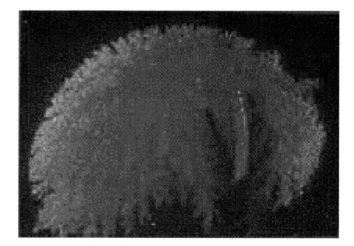

Figure 2–14. Scaffold prototype of vessels to support an artificial liver. *(Courtesy Dr. Joseph Vacanti, Massachussetts General Hospital, Boston, MA.)*

surgeon—academic, research, or clinical—to seek out these opportunities and help guide these new technologies.

CONCLUSIONS

The future of laparoscopic surgery will involve a combination of enhancing current systems, adapting laparoscopic procedures so that they may be performed by computer-assisted robotic devices, and replacement of certain techniques using emerging technologies. There will always be a niche for laparoscopic procedures; the question is one of how many of the procedures we perform laparoscopically today will evolve into other procedures, and which will remain the standard of surgical practice.

The overall direction of research is moving toward making devices that are more intelligent, using biosensors and networking; toward making things more visible, with new imaging modalities and data fusion; toward making things more dexterous, by using computers and robotics; toward making things easier to use, by creating a better human interface with surgical consoles or 3-D displays; toward making procedures more accurate, by preoperative planning and simulation using virtual reality and 3-D visualization tools; and toward better surgical training, with virtual reality simulators. As the systems become more complex, the issues of ergonomics and the human interface will become even more critical; it will be necessary to make using the new systems absolutely intuitive and transparent to the surgeon, creating the illusion of performing a surgical procedure in the traditional fashion while allowing the computer to translate the surgeon's actions into minimally invasive or noninvasive motions. Just as critical will be the building of more sophisticated surgical simulation systems, to provide a structured learning environment that delivers a uniform training experience to all students, and which can be expanded to include all the surgical procedures required for thorough training, rather than the haphazard training available today. Finally, it is essential to be aware of the new science that is being created in the laboratories today—basic science discoveries not within the medical arena, but which will nonetheless revolutionize the future of surgical health care. It is not inconceivable that the surgeon of the future will no longer use a scalpel, but rather various noninvasive tools and energy-directed instruments. The surgeon may no longer go to an operating suite, but instead to a "control room" from which telesurgical procedures are transmitted. Some of these speculative events will not come to pass; however, the history of laparoscopic surgery tells us that there may well be a revolutionary discovery that may be considered unacceptable today (even as laparoscopic surgery was decried as recently as two decades ago), but which will once again fundamentally change the direction of surgery. Surgeons must be willing to look at the technologies with an open mind, stringently subject them to rigid scientific evaluation, and then be willing to embrace those that provide our patients a higher quality of health care.

REFERENCES

1. Satava RM. Cybersurgery: A new vision for general surgery. In: Satava RM ed. *Cybersurgery.* John Wiley & Sons:1998;3.
2. Jolesz FA. Image guided procedures and the operating room of the future. *Radiology* 1997;204:601.
3. Paul HA, Bargar WL, Mittlestadt B, et al. Development of a surgical robot for cementless total hip arthroplasty. *Clin Orthop.* 1992;285:57.

4. MacFarlane M, Rosen J, Hannaford B, et al. Force feedback grasper helps restore the sense of touch in minimally invasive surgery. *J Gastrointest Surg.* 1999;3:278.
5. Berguer R. Surgery and ergonomics. *Arch Surg.* 1999;134:1011.
6. Altobelli DE, Kikinis R, Mulliken JB, et al. Computer assisted three dimensional planning in craniofacial surgery. *Plast Reconstruct Surg.* 1993;92:576.
7. Stephanides M, Montgomery K, Schendel S. Microsurgical reconstruction of the mandible using a new 3D surgical planning system. Computer Assisted Radiology and Surgery (CARS) 1999, Paris, France.
8. Marescaux J, Clement JM, Tassetti V, et al. Virtual reality applied to hepatic surgery simulation: The next revolution. *Ann Surg.* 1998;228:627.
9. Spitzer VM, Whitlock DG. Electronic imaging of the human body. Data storage and interchange format standards. In: Vannier MW, Yates RE, Whitestone JJ, eds. *Proceedings of the Electronic Imaging of the Human Body Working Group,* March 9–11, 1992:66.
10. Satava RM. Virtual reality surgical simulator: The first steps. *Surg Endosc.* 1993;7:203.
11. McGovern K. The virtual clinic: A virtual reality surgical simulator. *Proceedings of the Medicine Meets Virtual Reality II.* San Diego, January 27–30, 1994.
12. Levy JS. Virtual reality hysteroscopy. *J Am Assoc Gynecol Laparosc.* 1996;3(Suppl):S25.
13. Edmond CV, Wiet GJ, Bolger B. Surgical simulation in otology. *Otolaryngol Clin North Am.* 1998;31:369.
14. Raibert M, Playter R, Krummel TM. The use of a virtual reality haptic device in surgical training. *Acad Med.* 1998;73:596.
15. Gallagher AG, McClure N, McGuigan J, et al. Virtual reality training in laparoscopic surgery: a preliminary assessment of Minimally Invasive Surgical Trainer—Virtual Reality (MIST VR). *Endoscopy* 1999; 31:310.
16. Kavoussi LR, Moore RG, Partin AW, et al. Telerobotic assisted laparoscopic surgery: Initial laboratory and clinical experience. *Urology* 1994;44:15.
17. Go PMN, Payne JH, Satava RM, et al. Teleconferencing bridges two oceans and shrinks the surgical world. In: Zoltan S, Lewis JE, Fantini GA, eds. *Surgical Technology International IV.* Universal Medical Press:1995;29.
18. Rosser JC, Wood M, Payne JH, et al. Telementoring. A practical option in surgical training. *Surg Endosc.* 1997;11:852.
19. Bucholz RD, Greco DJ. Image-guided surgical techniques for infections and trauma of the central nervous system. *Neurosurg Clin North Am.* 1996;7:187.
20. Green PS, Satava RM, Hill JR, et al. Telepresence: Advanced teleoperator technology for minimally invasive surgery (Abstr). *Surg Endosc.* 1992;6:90.
21. Himpens J, Leman G, Cardiere GB. Telesurgical laparoscopic cholecystectomy. *Surg Endosc.* 1998;12:1091.
22. Carpentier A, Loulmet D, Aupecle B, et al. Computer-assisted cardiac surgery [letter]. *Lancet* 1999;353:379.

Chapter Three · · · · · ·

Mini-Endoscopic Surgery

GREGORY F. DAKIN and MICHEL GAGNER

INTRODUCTION

For the past 15 years, patients have increasingly enjoyed the many benefits of minimally invasive surgery, including quicker recovery, decreased length of hospital stay, decreased pain, and improved cosmesis. In an effort to further enhance these benefits, surgeons have recently turned towards smaller mini-instruments that are 2 to 3 mm in diameter. These "needlescopic" instruments and endoscopes were first used in the early 1970s by gynecologic surgeons for performing diagnostic procedures.[1] At the time, the relatively poor optical quality of these endoscopes limited their usefulness. Today, however, commercial interest in minimally invasive surgery has led to the development of mini-instruments sophisticated enough to perform not only diagnostic procedures, but many complex therapeutic procedures as well. The further refinement of these mini-endoscopic instruments may allow surgeons and patients to further expand the benefits of minimally invasive surgery.

While mini-endoscopic surgery has many potential benefits, strong supporting evidence has been lacking to date. Recent work, however, has begun to provide some comparative data to support its use. This chapter will review the potential benefits of mini-endoscopic surgery and describe the currently available technology. In addition, we will review the technical details and outcomes of common mini-endoscopic procedures in general surgery, paying particular attention to recently available comparative data.

TERMINOLOGY

The rapid emergence of these mini-endoscopic instruments and techniques has led to considerable confusion regarding terminology. Synonyms often used include mini-laparoscopy, micro-laparoscopy, micro-endoscopic surgery, needlescopic surgery, and micro-invasive surgery. We prefer to use the general term **mini-endoscopic surgery** when not referring to a specific body site, and more specific terms such as mini-laparoscopy or mini-thoracoscopy as needed. The broadest definition of mini-endoscopic surgery is any procedure that predominantly uses endoscopic instruments less than 5 mm in diameter.

BENEFITS AND LIMITATIONS OF MINI-ENDOSCOPIC SURGERY

There are many potential or presumed benefits of mini-endoscopic surgery. Improved cosmesis is one eagerly anticipated effect. A recent prospective, randomized study of 50 patients comparing mini-laparoscopic cholecystectomy to standard laparoscopic cholecystectomy demonstrated a modest improvement in cosmetic score using an analog scale.[2] Other groups have reported no scarring at all after mini-endoscopic procedures.[3] The small size of the trocar sites eliminates the need for suturing wounds and may therefore lead to a decreased incidence of wound infection. The small trocar sizes should also reduce the incidence of trocar-site hernias, though no data currently exist to support this. Mini-endoscopic instruments may afford the surgeon additional operative flexibility as well. Because of the small size, the surgeon may elect to place an additional trocar at very little expense, possibly enhancing exposure and visualization.

Much interest has focused on the potential of mini-endoscopic surgery to reduce operative and postoperative pain. A recent randomized double blind trial in 26 patients comparing mini-laparoscopic cholecystectomy with standard laparoscopic cholecystectomy showed a significant improvement in postoperative pain in the mini-laparoscopic group.[4] While this study is limited by the small number of patients and a high rate of conversion to standard laparoscopy, it does show the potential of the mini-laparoscopic approach. Another retrospective study showed that postoperative analgesic requirements were 70% lower in patients operated on with mini-laparoscopic instruments.[3]

The small size of mini-endoscopic instruments and subsequent reduction in pain may also reduce the requirement for general anesthesia, further expanding the role of mini-endoscopic surgery. Many diagnostic and therapeutic mini-endoscopic procedures have been performed under local anesthesia with or without intravenous sedation.[5] Though no direct comparison exists, eliminating general anesthesia from certain diagnostic procedures should certainly lower costs. While decreased cost is another potential benefit of mini-endoscopic surgery, this has yet to be definitively shown.

There are several potential limitations as well. Though image quality has vastly improved, there is decreased field of vision and depth perception when compared with traditional rod-lens endoscopes. The need to repeatedly change cameras from the standard 10-mm endoscopes to the mini-endoscope during a procedure may also contribute to increased operative times. One retrospective study showed a 20% increase in OR time for mini-laparoscopic cholecystectomy,[3] while other studies have shown comparable times in performing mini-laparoscopic procedures.[6]

The increased costs of instruments may be a limitation of mini-endoscopic surgery. Many varieties of disposable and reusable mini-instruments exist, with a wide range of prices. Though unit costs are comparable to standard instruments, the fragility of mini-endoscopic instruments may lead to more frequent repair or replacement charges. Also, these instruments are understandably more delicate and require a finer touch. Though improved from earlier models, they may still be inadequate to grasp thick, inflamed tissues. Finally, mini-endoscopic staplers, clip-appliers, and ultrasonic cutting devices do not currently exist.

INSTRUMENTATION

Mini-endoscopic surgical equipment is readily available from many manufacturers: Karl-Storz Endoscopy, Stryker Endoscopy, Olympus, Ethicon, Microfrance, Wolf Medical Instruments, Aesculap, US Surgical Corporation, and others. Endoscopes range in size from 1.9 mm to 3.3 mm and have a range of viewing angles (Fig. 3–1). Most mini-endoscopes today use fiber-optic technology. While this has improved light transmission and flexibility, these endoscopes have a lower resolution and depth-of-field when compared to standard rod-lens scopes.[1] Resolution of the newer mini-endoscopes is steadily improving, however, with many having as many as 50,000 pixels. Operative instrumentation is increasingly available as well. Most manufacturers provide a variety of reusable and disposable trocars, mini-endoscopic graspers, dissectors, scissors, blunt retractors, suction devices, and pre-tied endoloops. More recently, mini-endoscopic needle-drivers became available (Fig. 3–2). Though the unit costs of these instruments are comparable to those of standard endoscopic instruments, their life expectancy may be shorter. Despite these advances, still lacking are mini-versions of endoscopic staplers, clip-appliers, and ultrasonic scissors.

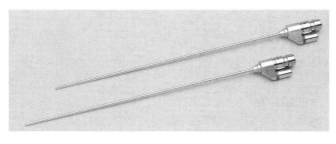

Figure 3–1. Examples of mini-laparoscopes. *(Courtesy of Karl-Storz Endoscopy.)*

DIAGNOSTIC MINI-ENDOSCOPIC SURGERY

The potential of mini-endoscopic surgery to reduce pain and anesthetic requirements has led to its application in several areas of general surgery. Though in its infancy, application of these techniques may increase diagnostic accuracy and prevent unnecessary procedures.

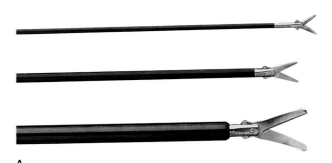

A

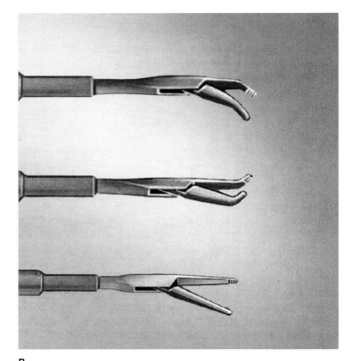

B

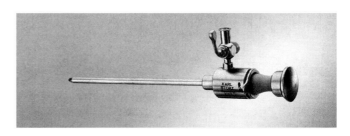

C

Figure 3–2. A. Photo of a 3.5-mm endoscopic scissors (*top*) with 5-mm and 10-mm scissors (*middle and bottom*) for comparison. **B.** Photo of three different mini-endoscopic dissectors. **C.** Photo of a 3-mm trocar. *(Courtesy of Karl-Storz Endoscopy.)*

Mini-Laparoscopy Under Local Anesthesia

Though this chapter focuses on general surgical applications, it is worth mentioning the contributions of gynecologic surgeons in the area of office mini-laparoscopy. The miniaturization of these instruments has nearly allowed the mini-laparoscope to become a standard tool of the physical examination, not unlike the otoscope or opthalmoscope. Office mini-laparoscopy under local anesthesia has been used since the early 1990s with encouraging results. Specifically, mini-laparoscopy for chronic pelvic pain, diagnosis of infertility, and sterilization has shown excellent patient tolerance and efficacy. These data are thoroughly summarized elsewhere.[5]

Diagnostic mini-laparoscopy holds promise for the general surgeon as well. One area of particular interest is in the diagnosis of liver disease. Because blind or ultrasound-guided liver biopsies may fail to make a diagnosis of cirrhosis in as many as 25% of cases,[7] many investigators are turning towards laparoscopic liver biopsy to improve success rate. One recent randomized study showed that mini-laparoscopy was comparable to standard laparoscopy for diagnosing cirrhosis in terms of success and complication rates. The procedures were performed under conscious sedation and may lead to improved patient outcome.[7]

Trauma

There has been much interest in the role of mini-laparoscopy in the evaluation of blunt abdominal trauma. It is no more invasive than diagnostic peritoneal lavage (DPL) and may offer the advantage of a rapid, specific diagnosis, thereby eliminating unnecessary procedures or surgery. A prospective, randomized multi-center trial has shown that the diagnostic specificity of mini-laparoscopy under local anesthesia in blunt abdominal trauma was 94% compared to 88% for DPL (sensitivity was 100% in both groups).[8] Another study showed similar effectiveness of mini-laparoscopy in blunt abdominal trauma.[9] Additional studies will be needed, however, to compare the efficacy of mini-laparoscopy to CT scan, which is now more widely used than at the time of these studies.

Acute Abdominal Pain

While there is considerable support for the use of mini-laparoscopy for chronic pelvic pain and infertility, there are fewer data on its use in acute abdominal conditions. Evidence is conflicting; some groups claim that the diagnostic accuracy in the evaluation of right lower quadrant pain is too low to recommend routine use, while others have had more favorable results.[10,11] Clearly, further study is needed to evaluate the utility of mini-laparoscopy in the acute abdomen. Another area of significant interest will be in the intensive care unit where conventional diagnostic laparoscopy is gaining popularity.

THERAPEUTIC MINI-ENDOSCOPIC SURGERY

As instruments continue to be refined, mini-endoscopic surgery will be applied to a wider variety of procedures. This discussion is limited to common general surgical procedures for which there are some supportive data in the literature. It should be noted that the majority of these procedures, while certainly performed safely, have not undergone rigorous, prospective comparison to standard endoscopic techniques.

Mini-Laparoscopic Cholecystectomy

For this procedure we use a 10-mm umbilical port and three subcostal miniports (a fourth may be added if cholangi-ography is necessary) (Fig. 3–3). A standard 10-mm 30° laparoscope is used in conjunction with mini-instruments to dissect the cystic duct and artery. Once these structures are isolated, the camera is switched to the mini-laparoscope and the cystic duct and artery are clipped and divided via the umbilical port using standard 5-mm instruments. Once this is accomplished the camera is then shifted back to the standard 10-mm laparoscope and the gallbladder is taken off its bed with the mini-instruments. Finally, the camera is again exchanged for the mini-laparoscope so that the gallbladder can be removed through the umbilical port.

Mini-laparoscopic cholecystectomy is the most commonly performed mini-laparoscopic procedure and has shown promising results in prospective studies.[12] One group has shown slight improvements in postoperative pain and cosmetic outcome with no change in operative time when prospectively comparing a mini-laparoscopic cholecystectomy group to standard laparoscopy.[2] A retrospective report of 60 patients showed similar improvements in postoperative analgesia requirements and scar score when compared to historic controls, though they experienced a 20% increase in operative time.[3] A separate report of 50 patients undergoing mini-laparoscopic cholecystectomy showed promising improvements in postoperative pain and subjective assessment of cosmetic outcome.[1]

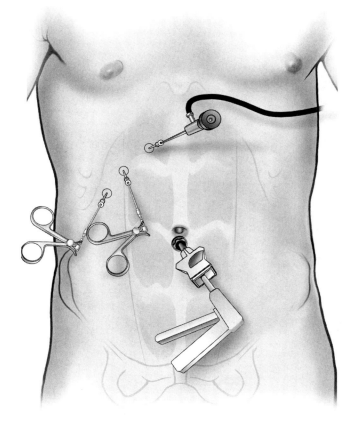

Figure 3–3. Trocar placement during mini-laparoscopic cholecystectomy, illustrating the use of the mini-laparoscope while a 5-mm clip-applier is introduced through the umbilical port for clipping the cystic duct and artery.

Mini-Laparoscopic Fundoplication

We place the patient in supine, split-leg position with the surgeon between the legs. A 10-mm trocar is placed through the umbilicus and 4 to 5 miniports are placed in the upper abdomen (Fig. 3–4). Dissection of the gastroesophageal junction is performed with a 10-mm 45° laparoscope and mini-instruments. To fully mobilize the gastric fundus, the camera is shifted to a mini-port and the short gastric vessels are divided via the umbilical port with an ultrasonic coagulator. We introduce a Penrose drain under mini-laparoscopic vision through the umbilical port, and the wrap is around the distal esophagus to isolate the gastroesophageal junction and aid in exposing the crura. If a hiatal hernia is present, mini-endoscopic needle-drivers are used to close the defect intracorporeally with 0 silk sutures. A 180° gastric wrap is fashioned and anchored anteriorly with 2-0 silk sutures sewn intracorporeally. Several groups have reported excellent outcomes in small numbers of patients, though long-term follow-up and comparative studies are lacking.[1,3]

Mini-Endoscopic Inguinal Herniorraphy

We perform a preperitoneal repair using a 10-mm umbilical port and 2 paramedian miniports (Fig. 3–5). Dissection of the preperitoneal space is aided by the use of a balloon dissector deployed via the umbilical port. The hernia sac is identified and reduced endoscopically with mini-dissectors. A polypropylene mesh is introduced via the 10-mm port and then unrolled to cover the hernia defect under mini-endoscopic vision. The mesh is secured in place with a standard 5-mm tacking stapler via the umbilical port, again under vision of the mini-endoscope. Transabdominal approaches have also been performed with mini-endoscopic instruments. The only series reported thus far, of 30 patients undergoing preperitoneal mini-endoscopic inguinal hernia repair, has shown excellent results with no complications, though follow-up is short and no comparison to standard laparoscopic repair is made.[13]

Mini-Laparoscopic Appendectomy

We use a 12-mm umbilical trocar and 2 miniports in the lower abdomen (Fig. 3–6). The procedure begins with a 10-mm laparoscope via the umbilical trocar. The appendix is identified and a window through the mesoappendix is created with mini-dissectors. The camera is changed to a mini-laparoscope and a linear stapler is introduced through the umbilical port to divide the mesentery and appendix. The appendix is placed in an endobag and removed via the umbilical site while still under mini-laparoscopic vision. While several groups have reported success with this technique in limited numbers of patients, no large comparative studies exist.[3,14]

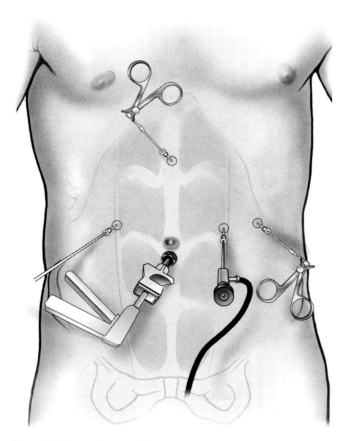

Figure 3–4. Trocar placement for mini-laparoscopic fundoplication. The camera is shown here through a miniport so the short gastric vessels can be clipped with a standard 10-mm clip-applier or divided with a harmonic scalpel via the umbilical port.

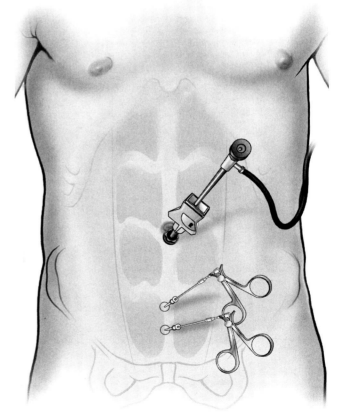

Figure 3–5. Trocar placement in mini-endoscopic inguinal herniorraphy. The camera is changed during the procedure to one of the mini-ports so a polypropylene mesh can be introduced through the umbilical port.

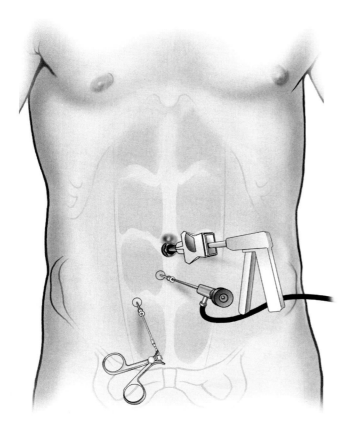

Figure 3–6. Trocar placement in mini-laparoscopic appendectomy, illustrating the use of a mini-laparoscope while the appendix is divided with a linear cutting stapler introduced through the umbilical port.

Mini-Laparoscopic Splenectomy

We place the patient in the right lateral decubitus position. A 10-mm 45° laparoscope is introduced through the umbilicus and three miniports are placed in the left upper quadrant (Fig. 3–7). Mini-endoscopic instruments are used to mobilize the attachments to the spleen. We leave a portion of the splenorenal ligament attached to the spleen to facilitate its manipulation. We have found that grasping these attachments minimizes trauma to the fragile spleen, especially when working with the delicate mini-instruments. Once the hilum is isolated, the camera is shifted to one of the miniports and a linear stapler is used to divide the hilum. The

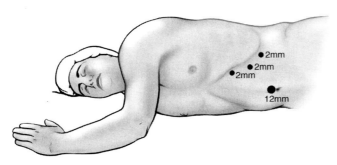

Figure 3–7. Trocar placement during mini-laparoscopic splenectomy. The trocar arrangement is similar for mini-laparoscopic left adrenalectomy.

spleen is placed in an endobag and morcellated for extraction. We have safely performed this procedure in several patients for a variety of hematologic indications. There are no large series reporting results of mini-laparoscopic splenectomy.

Mini-Laparoscopic Adrenalectomy

We place the patient in the decubitus position with a 10-mm 45° laparoscope via the umbilicus and 3 to 4 miniports in the upper abdomen (Fig. 3–7). We use a transperitoneal approach. Gravity will displace the liver or spleen towards the midline. The retroperitoneum and lateral border of the adrenal gland are dissected with mini-instruments. The gland is gently retracted cephalad and the dissection proceeds along the inferior border medially. Whenever necessary, the laparoscope is switched to one of the mini-ports so the arterial branches may be clipped via the umbilical port. The adrenal vein is similarly clipped. The gland is removed via an endobag. We have performed this procedure on several patients with good results; however, no large comparative series exist.

Mini-Endoscopic Neck Surgery

We currently use mini-instruments to perform endoscopic thyroidectomy and parathyroidectomy in select patients. The surgical approach is similar for either procedure, and is carried out under general anesthesia with the patient in the supine position and the neck extended. A 5-mm incision is made in the midline just above the sternal notch and carried sharply through the platysma. A 5-mm trocar is inserted and secured with a purse-string suture. The subplatysmal space is developed by gentle blunt dissection using the tip of a standard 5-mm 30° endoscope. Dissection of this plane is concentrated on the side of the neck that has been targeted with preoperative imaging studies. Once enough space has been created, 2 to 3 additional 3-mm ports are placed in the lateral neck, approximately 1 cm medial to the sternocleidomastoid (Fig. 3–8). The strap muscles are divided vertically and retracted laterally with an endoscopic hook and cautery. When necessary, the camera is switched to the mini-endoscope to improve visualization and to allow the surgeon to approach the dissection from whichever angle is most appropriate. Dissection proceeds lateral to the thyroid, carefully identifying the recurrent laryngeal nerve. If a thyroid lobectomy is planned, the camera is again switched for a mini-endoscope and the thyroid tissue is divided with a 5-mm harmonic scalpel. If a parathyroidectomy is planned, the involved gland is mobilized and its pedicle is doubly clipped with a 5-mm clip-applier. Still under vision of the mini-endoscope, the specimen is placed into a small bag (fashioned from the cut finger of a sterile glove) and removed via the 5-mm port.

Endoscopic endocrine surgery in the neck is becoming more commonplace. There are several different techniques, ranging from video-assisted gasless techniques to totally endoscopic procedures as described above.[15,16] We have performed the totally endoscopic procedure on more than 20 patients with primary hyperparathyroidism with excellent surgical outcome and patient satisfaction. To date, no large prospective series exists comparing the mini-endoscopic approach with more traditional thyroid and parathyroid procedures.

SUMMARY

There are many other areas of surgery that have made use of mini-endoscopic surgical techniques. Increasing numbers of pediatric surgeons are using mini-laparoscopes for a variety of procedures, from

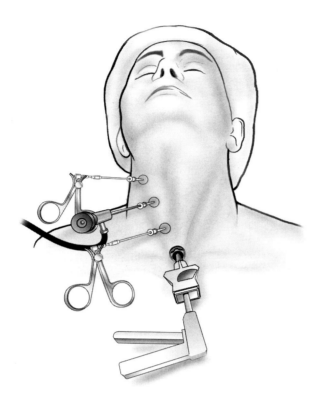

Figure 3–8. Trocar placement for mini-endoscopic neck surgery. In this illustration, the mini-endoscope is used while a vascular pedicle is clipped with a standard 5-mm clip-applier.

inguinal hernia repair to pyloromyotomy. Several reports exist on the use of mini-endoscopes in thoracic and neurosurgical cases as well. There are many potential benefits of mini-endoscopic surgery, including improved cosmesis, decreased pain, decreased anesthetic requirements, and decreased costs. Successful application of these techniques to a variety of diagnostic and therapeutic procedures is beginning to provide supportive evidence for these potential benefits. A clear benefit to the technology remains to be proven with further prospective comparative studies on large numbers of patients. The eventual acceptance of mini-endoscopic surgery will depend on the elaboration of this data, and on the effectiveness of these techniques in comparison to standard endoscopic surgery.

REFERENCES

1. Schauer PR, Ikramuddin S, Luketich JD. Minilaparoscopy. *Semin Laparosc Surg.* 1999;6:21.
2. Schwenk W, Neudecker J, Mall J, et al. Prospective randomized blinded trial of pulmonary function, pain, and cosmetic results after laparoscopic vs microlaparoscopic cholecystectomy. *Surg Endosc.* 2000;14:345.
3. Gagner M, Garcia-Ruiz A. Technical aspects of minimally invasive abdominal surgery performed with needlescopic instruments. *Surg Laparosc Endosc.* 1998;8:171.
4. Bisgaard T, Klarskov B, Trap R, et al. Pain after microlaparoscopic cholecystectomy: a randomized double-blind controlled study. *Surg Endosc.* 2000;14:340.
5. Palter SF. Office microlaparoscopy under local anesthesia. *Obstet Gynecol Clin North Am.* 1999;26:109.
6. Garcia FAR, Steinmetz I, Barker B, et al. Economic and clinical outcomes of microlaparoscopic and standard laparoscopic sterilization: a comparison. *J Reprod Med.* 2000;45:372.
7. Schneider AR, Benz C, Adamek HE, et al. Minilaparoscopy versus conventional laparoscopy in the diagnosis of hepatic diseases. *Gastrointest Endosc.* 2001;53:771.
8. Cuschieri A, Hennessy TPJ, et al. Diagnosis of significant abdominal trauma after road traffic accidents: preliminary results of a multicentre clinical trial comparing minilaparoscopy with peritoneal lavage. *Ann Roy Coll Surg Engl.* 1988;70:153.
9. Berci G, Dunkelman D, Michel SL, et al. Emergency minilaparoscopy in abdominal trauma: an update. *Am J Surg.* 1983;146:261.
10. Mutter D, Navez B, Gury JF, et al. Value of microlaparoscopy in the diagnosis of right iliac fossa pain. *Am J Surg.* 1998;176:370.
11. Rosser JC, Palter SF, Rodas EB, et al. Minilaparoscopy without general anesthesia for the diagnosis of acute appendicitis. *JSLS.* 1998;2:79.
12. Sarli L, Costi R, Sansebastiano G. Mini-laparoscopic cholecystectomy vs laparoscopic cholecystectomy: a matched case-control study. *Surg Endosc.* 2001;15:614.
13. Vara-Thorbeck C, Toscano R, Felices M. Preperitoneal hernioplasty performed with needlescopic instruments (microlap-aroscopy). *Surg Laparosc Endosc Percutan Tech.* 1999;9:190.
14. Croce E, Olmi S, Russo AR. Laparoscopic appendectomy and mini-laparoscopic approach: a retrospective review after 8-years' experience. *JSLS.* 1999;3:285.
15. Miccoli P, Benedinelli C, Vignali E, et al. Endoscopic parathyroidectomy: report of an initial experience. *Surgery.* 1998;124:1077.
16. Naitoh T, Gagner M, Garcia-Ruiz A, et al. Endoscopic endocrine surgery in the neck: an initial report of endoscopic subtotal parathyroidectomy. *Surg Endosc.* 1998;12:202.

ADDITIONAL READING

Almeida OD Jr. Current state of office laparoscopic surgery. *J Am Assoc Gynecol Laparosc.* 2000;7:545.

Cheah WK, Goh P, Gagner M, et al. Needlescopic retrograde cholecystectomy. *Surg Laparosc Endosc.* 1998;8:237.

Faber B, Coddington CC. Microlaparoscopy: a comparative study of diagnostic accuracy. *Fertil Steril.* 1997;67:952.

Faggioni A, Moretti G, Mandrini A, et al. Mini-laparoscopic cholecystectomy. *Hepatogastroenterology* 1998;45:1014.

Kovacs GT, Baker G, Dillon M, et al. The microlaparoscope should be used routinely for diagnostic laparoscopy. *Fertil Steril.* 1998;70:698.

Paulson JD, Oliver KA. A new technique for performing a laparoscopic hysterectomy using microlaparoscopy: microlaparoscopic assisted vaginal hysterectomy (mLAVH). *JSLS.* 2000;4:91.

Pellicano M, Zullo F, DiCarlo C, et al. Postoperative pain control after microlaparoscopy in patients with infertility: a prospective randomized trial. *Fertil Steril.* 1998;70:289.

Roth JS, Park AE, Gewirtz R. Minilaparoscopically assisted placement of ventriculoperitoneal shunts. *Surg Endosc.* 2000;14:461.

Unger SW, Paramo JC, Perez M. Microlaparoscopic gallbladder surgery. Surg Endosc. 2000;14:336.

Yamamoto H, Kanehira A, Kawamura M, et al. Needlescopic surgery for palmar hyperhidrosis. *J Thorac Cardiovasc Surg.* 2000;120:276.

Zadrozny D, Draczkowski T, Lichodziejewska-Niemierko M. Two-millimeter minisite mini-laparoscopy for rescue of dysfunctional continuous ambulatory peritoneal dialysis catheters. *Surg Laparosc Endosc Percut Tech.* 1999;9:369.

Zullo F, Pellicano M, Zupi E, et al. Minilaparoscopic ovarian drilling under local anesthesia in patients with polycystic ovary syndrome. *Fertil Steril.* 2000;74:376.

Zupi E, Marconi D, Sbracia M, et al. Is local anesthesia an affordable alternative to general anesthesia for minilaparoscopy? *J Am Assoc Gynecol Laparosc.* 2000;7:111.

Chapter Four • • • • • •

A nesthesia for Laparoscopic Surgery

MIKHAIL DVOROCHKIN

INTRODUCTION

Instituted in the early 1970s as a procedure for diagnosis and treatment of various gynecologic conditions, laparoscopic surgery has greatly expanded in scope and volume over the last two decades. Laparoscopic cholecystectomy, appendectomy, and hernia repair are today some of the most commonly performed procedures. It is apparent that laparoscopy has many benefits compared with open procedures. Its use has been extended to more complex procedures such as colectomy, splenectomy, nephrectomy, and adrenalectomy.

Although considered a minor surgical procedure that is frequently used to treat several disorders, laparoscopy may present a significant challenge for an anesthesia team. The pneumoperitoneum and the position of the patient required for laparoscopy produce multiple pathophysiologic changes, which though well tolerated by young and healthy patients, could be devastating in elderly and infirm patients.

RESPIRATORY CHANGES

Ventilatory Changes

The pneumoperitoneum causes significant respiratory changes involving lung and chest wall mechanics, pulmonary volumes, and gas exchange. With abdominal insufflation, intra-abdominal pressure (IAP) increases, commonly up to 15 mm Hg, and results in cephalad displacement of the diaphragm, limitation of diaphragmatic and anterior abdominal wall movement, decreased lung volumes, atelectasis, and increase in peak inspiratory pressure (PIP), shunt fraction, and dead space ventilation.

The functional residual capacity (FRC), already reduced by induction of general anesthesia, decreases even further, by 20 to 25%, 5 min after abdominal insufflation. Respiratory compliance decreases by 30 to 50% in healthy patients. The reduction in respiratory compliance is due to decreases in lung (up to 38%) and chest wall compliance (up to 45%).[1,2] The respiratory resistance increases as much as 79% 5 min after abdominal insufflation due

to a marked increase in lung and chest wall resistance. In contrast, the airway resistance is not significantly affected by abdominal insufflation. The duration of pneumoperitoneum has no significant effect on pulmonary mechanics unless complications such as bronchospasm or subcutaneous emphysema occur. Both respiratory compliance and resistance return to preinsufflation levels approximately 15 min after abdominal deflation.[1–7]

Abdominal wall lift (AWL), a technique utilizing a fan retractor, was proposed for use during laparoscopic procedures to reduce the hemodynamic and respiratory effects of abdominal insufflation. This technique allows a decrease in the IAP of more than 50%. Application of AWL during laparoscopic cholecystectomy significantly improves peak airway pressure and total resistance of the respiratory system. However, the elastance of the respiratory system remains elevated, probably due to an AWL-induced impairment of anterior abdominal wall and diaphragmatic mechanics.[8]

Healthy patients tolerate pneumoperitoneum well, despite the respiratory changes described above. The data suggest that there are no clinically significant changes in shunt fraction or dead space ventilation even in a 10 to 20° head-up or head-down position. Oxygen saturation remains stable, and PaO_2/PAO_2 as well as $ETCO_2/PaCO_2$ gradients are not significantly affected.[1–3,9,10]

When there is a baseline decrease in lung volumes and low respiratory compliance, as is often seen in obese American Society of Anesthesiologists (ASA) III to IV patients and patients with pulmonary disease, superimposed pneumoperitoneum could produce dramatic changes in pulmonary mechanics by shifting the lungs to a flat, noncompliant portion of the pressure-volume curve. Ventilation-perfusion (V-Q) mismatch, high PIP, and increased physiologic dead space make adequate ventilation and elimination of CO_2 difficult.[11–13] Hypoventilation, combined with increased intrathoracic pressure and decreased cardiac output, might result in inadequate oxygenation.

Increase in $PaCO_2$

Carbon dioxide is the gas most commonly used when creating a pneumoperitoneum. In patients under general anesthesia and controlled mechanical ventilation, $Paco_2$ progressively increases and reaches a plateau 15 to 30 min after the beginning of CO_2 insufflation.[1,2,14-17]

The rate of absorption of a gas depends on its solubility in tissue, pressure gradients across membranes containing the gas, the absorption area, and the diffusion constant of the gas. CO_2 is much more soluble in body fluids than oxygen (ratio 23:1) or nitrogen (ratio 35:1). During laparoscopy $Paco_2$ values may increase despite continued hyperventilation due to absorption of a large amount of carbon dioxide.[17-19] Hypercarbia was not observed when helium or N_2O was used for insufflation.[20-22] The level of $Paco_2$ reflects the balance between production, endogenous (metabolism) and exogenous (absorption), and elimination. This balance is controlled primarily via the lungs (Table 4–1).

The rate of CO_2 absorption is higher at the beginning of insufflation. Elevated IAP may impair the local perfusion of the abdominal wall, limiting the rate of CO_2 absorption. Abdominal decompression at the end of the procedure allows CO_2 that has accumulated in collapsed vessels to reach the circulation, and this may produce a transient increase in $Paco_2$, followed by a rapid fall in $Paco_2$ levels.[19]

Although permissive hypercarbia has become an accepted approach to treatment of certain medical conditions, one should make a reasonable attempt to maintain relatively normal levels of $Paco_2$ during laparoscopic procedures.

General anesthesia with mechanical ventilation allows relatively easy control of the elimination of CO_2 in healthy patients under normal circumstances. A 20 to 30% increase in minute ventilation is usually sufficient to compensate for CO_2 absorption.[17-19] Hyperventilation should be achieved by increasing the respiratory rate rather then the tidal volume. An increase in tidal volume might produce a significant increase in PIP due to high IAP and changes in pulmonary mechanics. The desire to maintain relatively normal CO_2 values should be weighed against the potential risks of significantly increasing airway pressure. Dramatic changes in pulmonary mechanics in patients with obesity and some pulmonary diseases could make hyperventilation almost impossible. Moderate hypercarbia is acceptable. Intermittent decompression of the abdomen will allow reasonable control of $Paco_2$. Positive end-expiratory pressure (PEEP) of 5 to 10 cm H_2O is advocated by many to prevent atelectasis, increase FRC, and improve oxygenation.

If laparoscopy is performed under local anesthesia, $Paco_2$ remains unchanged because of significantly increased spontaneous minute ventilation. The awake patient undergoing discomfort pro-

duced by the pneumoperitoneum may require a high level of sedation, which can result in respiratory depression, an unpredictable rise of $Paco_2$, and a fall in oxygen saturation.[23]

Capnography provides valuable information about changes in $Paco_2$. Although the $Paco_2/ETCO_2$ gradient increases during laparoscopy, it does not change significantly in healthy patients.[1,2,9,14,15,24] However, in morbidly obese ASA III and IV patients with hemodynamic instability, and patients under general anesthesia breathing spontaneously, end-tidal CO_2 might not be a reliable indicator of $Paco_2$.[13,25-27] Increased dead space ventilation, as is often seen in pulmonary disease such as emphysema or conditions associated with decreased cardiac output, results in an increased $Paco_2/ETCO_2$ gradient. Low or normal $ETCO_2$ could be an indicator of difficulty in elimination of CO_2 rather than a reflection of actual $Paco_2$ levels. A sudden drop in $ETCO_2$ might reflect a dramatic fall in cardiac output, as seen in pulmonary embolism. In these situations, frequent arterial blood gas sampling is required to accurately assess $Paco_2$.

Physiologic Effects of Carbon Dioxide

Hypercarbia produces considerable physiological alterations. In awake, healthy individuals, breathing a gas mixture containing 3% CO_2 produces a feeling of discomfort. Breathing 5 to 7% CO_2 causes acute distress with disorientation, dyspnea, and anxiety.[28] Narcosis occurs with a $Paco_2$ greater than 90 mm Hg.

Hypercarbia causes a predictable increase in cerebral blood flow (CBF). For each 1-mm Hg increase in $Paco_2$, CBF increases 1.8 mL/100 g/min and cerebral blood volume increases 0.04 mL/100 g. As $Paco_2$ increases from 40 to 80 mm Hg, CBF doubles. In patients with intracranial lesions and increased intracranial pressure, these changes in CBF and cerebral blood volume could be disastrous.

The enzyme systems of the body require tight control of the acid–base balance for proper function. Under normal circumstances, a narrow range of pH, 7.36 to 7.44, is maintained despite a wide variation in acid production. The Henderson-Hasselbalch equation defines the relationship between pH, Pco_2, and HCO_3^-:

$$pH = 6.1 + \log[HCO_3^-]/0.0301 \times Pco_2$$

In the acute situation, as seen with CO_2 pneumoperitoneum,[29,30] for every 10-mm Hg change in $Paco_2$ the pH will change 0.08 units in the opposite direction. Acidemia and elevated $Paco_2$ shifts potassium from the intracellular to the extracellular compartment. Although clinically insignificant in healthy individuals, a rise in plasma K^+ concentration might reach dangerously high levels in patients with impaired potassium regulation, such as in renal failure or hypoaldosteronism.

The $Paco_2$ level has the major regulatory effect on ventilation via central mechanisms, and to a much lesser degree via stimulation of peripheral chemoreceptors in the carotid and aortic bodies. The chemosensitive area, located in the ventral surface of the medulla, is extremely sensitive to hydrogen ions. However, the blood–brain barrier is relatively impermeable to hydrogen ions. Thus CO_2, which easily crosses the blood–brain barrier, indirectly controls this region by formation of carbonic acid, which dissociates to produce HCO_3^- and H^+. The activation of receptors in the chemosensitive area results in stimulation of the inspiratory center, and increases the rate of respiration. The maximal stimulation is attained at a $Paco_2$ level of about 100 mm Hg. Any further

TABLE 4–1. FACTORS AFFECTING $Paco_2$ LEVEL

Increase in Production of CO_2	Decrease in Elimination of CO_2
Absorption of exogenous CO_2 <ul><li>Level of intra-abdominal pressure</li><li>Extent of dissection</li><li>CO_2 subcutaneous emphysema</li><li>CO_2 pneumothorax</li></ul> Endogenous CO_2 production <ul><li>Metabolic state</li><li>Light anesthesia</li></ul>	Changes in pulmonary mechanics V-Q mismatch Increased dead space ventilation Inadequate mechanical ventilation Inadequate muscle relaxation Reduced cardiac output Respiratory depression during spontaneous ventilation

increase results in respiratory depression.[31] Many anesthetic drugs cause respiratory depression by altering the ventilatory response to CO_2. Volatile agents and sedative/hypnotic drugs decrease the slope of the CO_2 response curve, while all opioids produce a dose-dependent respiratory depression by shifting the CO_2 response curve to the right, and resetting the respiratory centers to respond to a higher level of Pa_{CO_2}.

In addition to its ventilatory effects, hypercarbia influences the pulmonary circulation. It increases pulmonary vascular resistance and locally augments hypoxic pulmonary vasoconstriction, probably by causing acidosis. In a case of preexisting pulmonary hypertension, superimposed pulmonary vasoconstriction from a high level of CO_2, causes an additional stress on the right ventricle, and potentially could lead to a right ventricular failure in a poorly compensated heart.

CO_2 produces excitation of the sympathetic nervous system and provokes multiple responses. Many of the sympathetic effects of CO_2 are directly related to stimulation of the medullary vasomotor centers. In addition, stimulation of chemoreceptor areas of the carotid and aortic bodies triggers sympathetic responses. High levels of CO_2 influence the release of catecholamines from the adrenal medulla. The plasma concentrations of norepinephrine and epinephrine may rise two- to threefold. The mechanism is unclear, but both decreased pH and increased Pa_{CO_2} have been implicated.[32,33]

The cardiovascular effects of hypercarbia are the result of a balance between the direct cardiodepressant effect of CO_2 and the increased activity of the sympathetic nervous system. The depressant effect of CO_2 is possibly secondary to the pH changes.[34]

Activation of the sympathetic nervous system by CO_2 in healthy individuals overcompensates for the direct cardiodepression. When CO_2 is added to a breathing gas mixture under controlled conditions to produce a Pa_{CO_2} range of 39 to 50 mm Hg, there is a significant increase in cardiac output, cardiac index, heart rate, stroke volume, and myocardial contractility. Left ventricular work and myocardial oxygen consumption are increased up to 20%.[35] Coronary blood flow is autoregulated to match metabolic requirements. Accordingly, high Pa_{CO_2} and low pH produce coronary vasodilatation. If perfusion pressure remains constant, coronary blood flow increases, compensating for the increased metabolic requirement.[36] When there is significant coronary disease, additional vasodilatation becomes impossible. Failure to maintain myocardial balance between supply and demand leads to myocardial ischemia.

Although the threshold level of Pa_{CO_2} that produces cardiac arrhythmias is high, there is an increased risk of arrhythmias when hypercarbia is accompanied by electrolyte disturbances, or superimposed on preexisting cardiac conduction abnormalities. Some anesthetic agents, such as halothane, may increase the risk of CO_2-induced arrhythmias. Vasodilatation produced by CO_2 results in a 14% fall of the peripheral vascular resistance with a 10-mm Hg increase in Pa_{CO_2}.[35] The effect on systemic blood pressure is the result of a balance between increased cardiac output and decreased peripheral resistance. The usual effect is a mild to moderate increase in mean blood pressure, but the responses may vary from slight hypotension to marked hypertension.

PATIENT POSITION

It is a common practice to alter the patient's position to facilitate surgical exposure during laparoscopy. The Trendelen-burg position is usually used for pelvic laparoscopy, while the head-up position is routine for upper abdominal surgery. In addition, the lithotomy position and right or left tilt can be utilized. Some procedures require multiple position changes. These simple maneuvers may be responsible for, or contribute to, the pathophysiologic changes observed during laparoscopy. The steepness of the tilt, associated cardiac disease, anesthetic drugs, and the patient's intravascular volume status have a major effect on the magnitude of these changes. The effects of position are more marked in obese, elderly, and ill patients.

Cardiovascular Changes

As the patient is tilted head-up or head-down, the effect of gravity on blood flow and redistribution becomes quite significant. The Trendelenburg position results in an increase in venous return, central venous pressure, and cardiac output. In response to increased hydrostatic pressure, the baroreceptor reflex triggers systemic vasodilatation and bradycardia.[37] As a result, in healthy normovolemic subjects who were placed in a 15° head-down position, central displacement of the blood volume of only 1.8% occurred and no significant hemodynamic changes were observed.[38–40] However, central blood volume and pressure changes may be greater in patients with cardiovascular diseases. This might lead to an increase in myocardial stress and oxygen demand, and potentially to myocardial ischemia in patients with coronary disease.

The reverse Trendelenburg position produces the opposite effect. In anesthetized patients, a steep head-up position causes decreased venous return, decreased central venous pressure, and a fall in cardiac output. Increases in both systemic vascular resistance (SVR) and pulmonary vascular resistance (PVR) are probably a compensatory response, triggered by the sympathetic nervous system and renin-angiotensin-aldosterone system activation.[39,41–43] The venous capacitance system is not affected, which promotes pooling of blood in the peripheral circulation.[44] Hypotension, tachycardia, decreased organ perfusion, and fluid and electrolyte retention may result. The changes are more dramatic if significant hypovolemia is present. Epidural or spinal anesthesia, pneumoperitoneum, and an abrupt change from the Trendelenburg to head-up position aggravate the hemodynamic changes.

Impaired venous drainage from the head, neck, and upper body is an additional concern of the steep Trendelenburg position, especially in patients with high IAP and obesity. Patients at special risk are those with intracranial pathology accompanied by decreased intracranial compliance.[45,46] Elevation of the intraocular pressure, which may occur with pneumoperitoneum in the Trendelenburg position,[47] has to be considered in patients with acute glaucoma. A prolonged steep head-down tilt may result in edema of the face and upper airway. The possibility of upper airway obstruction upon extubation should be anticipated in these patients.

Venous stasis and deep venous thrombosis (DVT) in the lower extremities may result from blood pooling due to a head-up position and high IAP. Elastic stockings or venous compression devices are routinely used to decrease this effect.

Respiratory Changes

In the head-down position, gravity-shifted abdominal viscera and cephalad displacement of the diaphragm lead to a decrease in FRC, development of atelectasis, and an increase in airway pressure. Decreased effective ventilation and an increased shunt fraction may result. In the head-up position, the abdominal viscera shift away from the diaphragm, which improves lung mechanics. However, a head-up position of up to 25° does not seem to have significant benefit in morbidly obese patients undergoing surgical laparoscopy.[26]

Other Concerns

Endotracheal tube displacement, air embolism, and ventilator circuit and IV line disconnections are all potential complications of changing patient position. Position-related peripheral nerve injuries are a significant source of peri-operative morbidity and a common reason for medical malpractice claims. The combined efforts of all operating room personnel are required to prevent these serious complications.

HEMODYNAMIC EFFECTS OF PNEUMOPERITONEUM

The effects of pneumoperitoneum on the cardiovascular system have been studied extensively in experimental and clinical investigations. While some investigators have shown minimal changes, others have reported significant alterations in hemodynamics with increased SVR and a dramatic fall in cardiac output. These broad variations in effects are probably a result of a complex interaction of several factors that affect the hemodynamic response during laparoscopy (Fig. 4–1).

Early studies suggested that a mild to moderate increase in IAP during CO_2 insufflation in the head-down position facilitates venous return, increases effective cardiac filling pressure, and might increase cardiac output. When the IAP was raised further, a fall in cardiac output was observed.[48] More recent studies utilizing pulmonary artery catheterization, thoracic electrical bioimpedance, and transesophageal echocardiography have demonstrated significant hemodynamic alterations with an IAP of 10 mm Hg or higher. Although the degree of these disturbances varies, most have shown a fall in cardiac output, increased SVR and PVR, and elevated mean arterial blood pressure in the head-up or head-down position.[40,49–51]

D'Ugo et al[52] reported minimal hemodynamic changes in ASA I and II patients during laparoscopic cholecystectomy in the reverse Trendelenburg position. An interesting finding was their observation of mitral valve backflow with the onset of abdominal insufflation. Others have demonstrated 16 to 35% increases in mean arterial pressure (MAP), up to 30% increases in central venous pressure (CVP) and pulmonary capillary wedge pressure (PCWP), 10 to 30% drops in cardiac index and stroke volume index, and increases of up to 50% in systemic vascular resistance (SVR).[41,42,49–51,56] Joris et al[53] found that in otherwise healthy, nonobese adults, a combination of general anesthesia, pneumo-peritoneum at an IAP of 14 mm Hg, and a head-up position may result in a frightening 50% fall in cardiac output, as much as a 65% increase in SVR, and up to a 90% increase in pulmonary vascular resistance.

Myre et al[54] tried to eliminate the effects of position and hypovolemia on the hemodynamic response to increased IAP. They

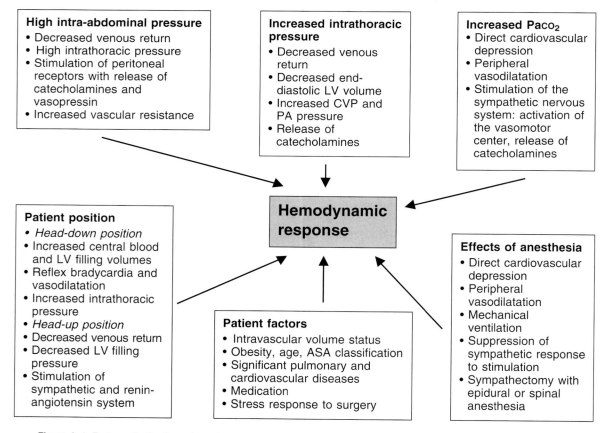

Figure 4–1. Factors affecting hemodynamic response during laparoscopy. ASA, American Society of Anesthesiologists; CVP, central venous pressure; LV, left ventricular; PA, pulmonary artery.

produced a pneumoperitoneum of 15 mm Hg after Ringer's lactated solution was administered to reach a PCWP of 10 mm Hg, with all measurements being obtained in the supine position. While the cardiac index, left ventricular end-diastolic index (LVEDI), and SVR did not change significantly, increases in MAP (median 24%), CVP (median 75%), PCWP (median 70%), and pulmonary arterial pressure (PAP) (median 44%) were observed. Dorsay et al[43] reported a 10% decrease in LVEDI and stroke volume index (SVI), and unchanged cardiac index (CI) and left ventricular ejection fraction (LVEF) upon abdominal insufflation. With the addition of a 20° tilt and the reverse Trendelenburg position, the CI, SVI, and LVEF fell by an additional 11%, 78% (from baseline), and 12%, respectively. The heart rate was unchanged or mildly increased in most studies, and all hemodynamic indices returned to baseline levels after abdominal desufflation.

Although the precise mechanisms of the hemodynamic responses seen during laparoscopy have yet to be determined, preload and afterload alterations seem to play a major role. At an IAP of 10 mm Hg or higher, caval compression, pooling of blood in the legs, and an increase in venous resistance all produce a significant decrease in venous return, which is accentuated by a head-up position and increased intrathoracic pressure. The decline in venous return results in a reduction left ventricular end-diastolic volume (LVEDV) and cardiac output. A markedly increased CVP and PCWP do not reflect filling volume, and are therefore not reliable indicators of LVEDV during pneumoperitoneum.

Activation of the sympathetic system, a result of increased CO_2, a reflex response to decreased venous return and stimulation of peritoneal receptors, as well as mechanical factors are probably responsible for increased PVR. Mean arterial pressure increases, while cardiac output falls. Activation of the renin-angiotensin system and release of arginine vasopressin (AVP) may contribute to an increase in afterload. Up to a fivefold increase in AVP concentration is probably due to mechanical stimulation of peritoneal receptors and is correlated with changes in intrathoracic pressure and right atrial pressure.[51,55]

Despite this significant stress, patients with healthy hearts tolerate the preload-afterload alterations well. Appropriate anesthetic management allows a stable intraoperative course with minimal fluctuation of hemodynamic parameters. ASA III and IV patients may experience similar or even more significant changes in hemodynamics with dramatic increases in CVP, PCWP, and SVR, and a fall in cardiac output.[56,57] Mixed venous saturation was decreased in 50% of patients despite the preoperative hemodynamic optimization.[58] Unlike ASA I patients, patients with poor preoperative cardiac performance sustaining a further decrease in cardiac output may demonstrate inadequate oxygen delivery, inadequate tissue perfusion, and cardiovascular collapse. Patients with significant coronary disease are at risk for ischemia due to increased myocardial stress and changes in the balance of oxygen supply and demand. However, with preoperative optimization, careful intraoperative hemodynamic control, and continued monitoring during the immediate postoperative period, laparoscopic procedures can be safely performed in high-risk cardiac patients.[57,59–61]

COMPLICATIONS OF PNEUMOPERITONEUM

Subcutaneous Emphysema

Subcutaneous emphysema is a frequent complication of laparoscopy. It is result of accidental or intentional (e.g., during inguinal hernia repair) extraperitoneal insufflation. The incidence of clinically significant subcutaneous emphysema varies, and can be as high as 60% during laparoscopic fundoplication.[62] Because of the large area of absorption, subcutaneous emphysema causes a rapid and dramatic increase in $ETCO_2$ and $PaCO_2$, reportedly as high as 100 mm Hg.[63] Sufficient hyperventilation might become virtually impossible. When significant emphysema develops in the upper body (face, neck, and chest), it can cause compression and obstruction of the upper airway.[64] Peak airway pressure, unchanged initially, might increase with a decrease in chest wall compliance. However, even extensive subcutaneous CO_2 emphysema will readily resolve after abdominal de-sufflation. Patients can be safely extubated at the end of the surgery, assuming that the $ETCO_2$ has returned to acceptable levels.[64,65]

CO$_2$ Pneumothorax

Pneumothorax can occur at any time during laparoscopy. Possible sources of pneumothorax include embryonic abdominal wall channels, defects and weak points in the diaphragm, and pleural tears created during surgical manipulations.[65] Right-sided pneumothorax is more likely with cholecystectomy, and left-sided pneumothorax occurs more often during fundoplication. The clinical presentation includes marked hypercarbia, increased peak airway pressure, and hypoxemia. Subcutaneous emphysema is usually present as well.[65,66] Chest x-ray and auscultation will confirm the diagnosis. Tension pneumothorax must be ruled out in patients with hemodynamic instability. CO_2 pneumothorax, without associated pulmonary trauma, will resolve spontaneously 30 to 60 minutes after abdominal desufflation. Treatment of CO_2 pneumothorax includes ventilation with 100% oxygen, a reduction in IAP, or discontinuation of the pneumoperitoneum and application of PEEP.[66] Thoracocentesis might become necessary in the event of significant hypoxemia and hemodynamic instability.

Gas Embolism

Gas embolism is a dangerous and potentially lethal complication of surgery. The consequences of gas embolism depend on the type of gas used, and the amount and rate of intravascular entry. Certain procedures such as craniotomy in the sitting-up position are associated with a high incidence of air embolism. Although rare, massive air embolism can occur during laparoscopic procedures as well.[67] The clinical presentation of massive air embolism is cardiovascular collapse and hypoxemia. While precordial Doppler and transesophageal echocardiography are the most sensitive indicators, an abrupt decrease in $ETCO_2$, appearance of nitrogen on the gas analyzer, a high PAP, a "mill-wheel" murmur, and electrocardiogram (ECG) changes are characteristic of air embolism.

CO_2 embolism during laparoscopy can be the result of a needle or trocar puncture of a vessel or insufflation into an abdominal organ. This complication usually develops during initiation of pneumoperitoneum.[68,69,72] CO_2 is more soluble in blood than air, N_2O, or helium. This increases the margin of safety in the event of an inadvertent intravascular injection.[71] The rate of insufflation has a major effect on the amount of gas entering the vascular bed. Abdominal insufflation must therefore be started slowly to reduce the possible consequences of embolism. Unlike air embolism, CO_2 embolism produces an initial rise in $ETCO_2$ followed by a fall in $ETCO_2$ and an increase in the $ETCO_2/PaCO_2$ gradient secondary to cardiovascular collapse.[65]

Treatment of CO_2 embolism consists of immediate cessation of insufflation, release of pneumoperitoneum, discontinuation of N_2O, ventilation with 100% O_2, and cardiovascular support. Patients should be placed in a head-down position with left tilt, which may help decrease the amount of gas entering the pulmonary circulation. Aspiration of CO_2 via a central line might be attempted.[65,68,70] Although CO_2 embolism can be fatal,[67,71] the high solubility and rapid elimination of CO_2 account for the rapid recovery of clinical signs seen with prompt treatment.[68–70]

ALTERNATIVES TO CO2 PNEUMOPERITONEUM

N_2O and Inert Gases

Laparoscopy using N_2O or an inert gas such as helium produces similar changes in pulmonary mechanics as those seen with CO_2 pneumoperitoneum. However, it does not result in hypercarbia or acidosis.[21,29] Therefore, hyperventilation is not required, which might be beneficial when managing obese patients and patients with significant pulmonary diseases. It might also permit laparoscopy under local or regional anesthesia,[73] as it allows a higher level of IV sedation.

Helium or nitrous oxide insufflation does not offer any significant hemodynamic advantages over CO_2 pneumo-peritoneum. It causes a similar fall in cardiac output with a smaller increase in SVR, which makes hypotension more likely.[20,22]

Although the data are insufficient, the lower solubility of helium and N_2O raises the issue of safety in the event of pneumothorax or gas embolism with these gases.[71,74]

Gasless Laparoscopy

Abdominal wall lift is a relatively new technique that utilizes a fan retractor during laparoscopy. This technique avoids many of the respiratory and hemodynamic effects of abdominal insufflation and preserves renal and splanchnic perfusion.[8,75–78] AWL may be useful in patients with significant cardiac, pulmonary, or renal disease. A recent report indicates that gasless laparoscopy might be advantageous in patients with increased intracranial pressure.[79] The ability to perform laparoscopy under epidural or spinal anesthesia is an additional benefit of AWL.[80,81]

Although gasless laparoscopy offers many advantages as compared to the standard procedure, it compromises surgical exposure and increases technical difficulties. A low-pressure pneumoperitoneum could be combined with AWL to improve surgical exposure.

LAPAROSCOPY DURING PREGNANCY

Although pregnancy was initially considered a contraindication to laparoscopy, recent experience suggests that laparoscopy may be a safe and efficient approach to treatment of surgical conditions during pregnancy. Pregnancy is associated with a variety of physiologic changes, including significant alternations in the respiratory and cardiovascular systems. Creation of a pneumoperitoneum and changes in patient position may produce significant effects during pregnancy.[82] Uterine flow is not autoregulated, and is proportional to the mean perfusion pressure, which might be affected by increased IAP. CO_2 pneumoperitoneum induced significant fetal acidosis in an animal model.[83] Clinically, however, laparoscopy

appears to be well tolerated by pregnant patients, and does not seem to alter the fetal outcome when compared to open procedures.[80,84–87] Further studies are necessary to ensure the safety of laparoscopic surgery during pregnancy.

The anesthetic management of the parturient during laparoscopy can be quite challenging, especially in late pregnancy. Difficulty with positioning, risk of aortocaval compression, tight hemodynamic and respiratory control, an altered response to anesthetic drugs, an increased risk of aspiration, and the possibility of a difficult airway are among the many concerns of laparoscopic surgery performed during pregnancy.[82] Fetal monitoring during laparoscopic surgery may be performed using transvaginal ultrasonography, and should be considered to ensure fetal viability.

Gasless laparoscopy may be a valuable alternative to CO_2 pneumoperitoneum in the pregnant patient. It avoids the potential side effects of abdominal insufflation, and can be managed with regional anesthesia.[80]

LAPAROSCOPY IN CHILDREN

Laparoscopy is being successfully performed in infants and children. A growing number of reports have shown the efficacy, safety, and cost effectiveness of diagnostic and surgical laparoscopy in children.[88–90]

Although the data are limited, recent investigations suggest that pneumoperitoneum may produce significant respiratory and hemodynamic effects in infants and children. In a study of the hemodynamic consequences of a 10-mm Hg CO_2 pneumoperitoneum in healthy infants, using continuous esophageal aortic blood flow echo-Doppler, Gueugniaud et al[91] showed more than a 60% decrease in aortic blood flow and stroke volume, and up to a 162% increase in SVR. Many investigators have reported significant increases in peak airway pressure and $ETCO_2$ with abdominal insufflation.[91–95] However, most investigators have demonstrated no significant changes in blood pressure, heart rate, or oxygen saturation, with the return of all hemodynamic parameters to preinsufflation levels after release of the pneumoperitoneum.[91–95]

Although general anesthesia with endotracheal intubation remains a standard approach in managing pediatric patients, several reports have demonstrated that general/laryngeal mask airway (LMA) or general/mask anesthesia combined with caudal block could be an alternative anesthetic technique for laparoscopic procedures of short duration.[92,95]

ANESTHESIA

Preparation for Anesthesia

Preoperative Evaluation. In the era of outpatient surgery and surgery performed on the same day as admission, the anesthesiologist usually sees a patient for the first time no more than 10 to 15 minutes prior to the actual procedure. It is up to the surgeon to provide an appropriate medical evaluation. The goals in the preoperative evaluation should be to identify, evaluate, and optimize coexisting medical conditions that the patient may have. The age of the patient, his or her past medical history, and the complexity of the planned operation should be considered in determining which preoperative ambulatory tests must be undertaken.

Routine preoperative testing, as traditionally required by many institutions, has a very low yield despite considerable cost. Positive findings in otherwise asymptomatic patients are rare, and anesthetic or surgical implications are usually minimal.[96–98] The incidence of abnormal testing and subsequent alternation of anesthetic management increases with patient age and ASA status.[97,99] Generally, for young, healthy adults who are undergoing routine elective procedures, a detailed history and physical examination are usually sufficient, with the addition of a hematocrit and pregnancy test for menstruating women of childbearing age. Many advocate obtaining a 12-lead ECG for men over 45 and women over 50, and CBC and blood chemistry test (e.g., SMA-7) for healthy patients older than 50 years old.

With the development and rapid expansion of laparoscopy, it has become a common part of the care of older patients who are likely to have chronic medical conditions, undiagnosed diseases, and diminished cardiopulmonary reserve. The laparoscopic approach tends to be advocated for these patients because of its multiple benefits in comparison with open procedures. Despite the less complicated postoperative period and faster recovery, the intraoperative course for these patients might be difficult, and the hemodynamic and respiratory effects of pneumoperitoneum can be devastating. Preoperative evaluation of patients for laparoscopic procedures must be at least as thorough, and possibly even more thorough, than for open surgery.

The American Society of Anesthesiologists classifies patients by their physiologic status (Table 4–2). Although the ASA classification was not originally designed as a risk predictor, it has been shown to be a reliable indicator of perioperative morbidity.[101–103] The preoperative evaluation should target specific aspects of the patient's medical history. The functional status and level of control of extant conditions are more important than the actual diseases in question.

Laboratory Tests. A complete blood count (CBC) and blood chemistry (e.g., SMA-7) should be obtained for most patients of ASA II and higher. Many comorbid conditions and their therapies may cause fluid and electrolyte imbalances. Significant abnormalities may require preoperative compensation or modification of anesthetic technique. More extensive laboratory studies are usually unnecessary, and should be directed by the patient's medical condition. Coagulation studies are necessary if the patient has been on an anticoagulant or has a history of a coagulation disorder or unusual bleeding. They are also indicated if significant hepatic, renal, or other organ dysfunction is present. Some anesthesiologists, in addition to evaluating the platelet count via CBC, will routinely request a PT and PTT if epidural or spinal anesthesia is planned.

Medication. Current drug therapy must be carefully reviewed during the preoperative evaluation. Discontinuation of most drugs is not necessary, and may even be dangerous. The safety of maintaining current drug therapy should be based on the anesthesiologist's knowledge of potential adverse drug interactions rather than on modification of the drug regimen. Optimal control of comorbid conditions with antihypertensive and antianginal medications, digitalis, anticonvulsants, and hormone replacement should be continued throughout the perioperative period. Drugs without implications if withdrawn for a short time, such as drugs used to treat HIV or cholesterol-lowering medications, can be withheld on the day of surgery. Diuretics and oral antihyperglycemics are also usually discontinued on the day of surgery. NPH insulin is given at one-third to one-half of the usual dose on the morning of surgery, and is coupled with blood glucose monitoring in the perioperative period. In most situations, aspirin should be discontinued 7 days, and coumadin 5 days prior to surgery. When anticoagulation medications cannot be stopped, the patient needs to be admitted for heparin administration. Discontinuation of heparin for 4 to 6 hours is usually sufficient to achieve reversal of anticoagulation.

Medical Consultations. Although medical clearance or a consultation with a specialist is unnecessary in many cases, they should be obtained if significant cardiac or pulmonary disease is present. Detailed assessment of the patient's functional status and preoperative optimization are the primary goals of specialist consultations.

Preoperative evaluation by the anesthesiologist is essential in cases of significant comorbidity. This will allow for the development of an appropriate anesthetic plan and preparations for possible complications.

Cardiac Evaluation. In 1996 the American College of Cardiology and the American Heart Association jointly published guidelines for perioperative cardiovascular evaluation for noncardiac surgery. These guidelines are an excellent tool for planning the preoperative evaluation of a patient suspected to have clinically significant cardiac disease.[104] Cardiac function should be evaluated in light of the hemodynamic changes induced by pneumoperitoneum. The potential benefits of laparoscopy versus laparotomy should be balanced against the risk of further deterioration of cardiac function due to abdominal insufflation and position changes. Gasless or low-pressure laparoscopy might be an alternative for these patients.

Pulmonary Diseases. Patients with significantly decreased pulmonary function might benefit from a laparoscopic procedure

TABLE 4–2. THE AMERICAN SOCIETY OF ANESTHESIOLOGISTS PHYSICAL STATUS CLASSIFICATION

ASA I	A healthy patient.
ASA II	A patient with mild systemic disease, without functional limitation. *Examples:* Well-controlled hypertension, diabetes mellitus, bronchial asthma; moderate obesity, smoking, advanced age
ASA III	A patient with severe systemic disease that limits activity, but is not incapacitating. *Examples:* Poorly controlled hypertension, diabetes mellitus with vascular or renal complications, stable angina pectoris, prior myocardial infarction, morbid obesity, severe pulmonary disease
ASA IV	A patient with incapacitating systemic disease that is a constant threat to life. *Examples:* Unstable angina pectoris, uncompensated congestive heart failure, advanced pulmonary, renal, or liver dysfunction
ASA V	A moribund patient who is not expected to survive with or without the operation. *Examples:* A patient with multiple organ failure on ventilator and vasopressor support who needs exploratory laparotomy for ischemic bowel
E	Any patient who requires emergency surgery. *Examples:* 45-year-old male with history of well-controlled hypertension who requires surgery for acute appendicitis, ASA IIE

From ASA.[100]

instead of open surgery, especially for upper abdominal procedures. Relative preservation of pulmonary function in the postoperative period counterbalances difficulty with ventilation and gas exchange during pneumoperitoneum. Laparotomy under epidural or spinal anesthesia should be considered when it is preferable to avoid airway manipulation, as in a patient with severe bronchial asthma.

Preoperative pulmonary evaluation consists of a detailed history and assessment of functional status. Chest x-ray, baseline arterial blood gases (ABG), and pulmonary consultation directed at optimization of the patient's condition can be very helpful.

Premedication

The once-common practice of routinely premedicating and sedating patients in the preanesthesia period has become less popular today; this is a reflection of a shift to outpatient and same-day surgery. Primary goals for premedication include anxiolysis, sedation, analgesia, and amnesia, and to decrease salivation, increase gastric pH, decrease gastric fluid volume, and attenuate sympathetic nervous system response. Although it is unnecessary in most circumstances, pharmacologic premedication may facilitate induction of anesthesia and improve outcomes in certain situations. H_2-antagonists, nonparticulate antacids, and stimulants of gastric motility are indicated for patients at risk of pulmonary aspiration of gastric contents. Because laparoscopy may increase the chance of regurgitation, aspiration precautions should be taken seriously in these patients. β_2-agonists are administered prior to induction of anesthesia in an attempt to decrease the risk of bronchospasm during manipulation of the airway in asthmatic patients. Short-acting benzodiazepines such as midazolam provide sedation, anxiolysis, and amnesia, and may be given shortly before induction of anesthesia.

Monitoring

Standard intraoperative monitors should include a noninvasive blood pressure monitor, 5-lead ECG, pulse oximeter, end-tidal capnograph, temperature probe, and precordial or esophageal stethoscope. Modern anesthesia ventilators incorporate airway pressure, tidal volume, and FIO_2 monitors, as well as a number of safety alarms. Use of an inspiratory/expiratory gas analyzer and neuromuscular stimulator completes the list of routine monitors.

Arterial line placement should be considered when tight hemodynamic control is desirable, as in patients with significant cardiac disease. Invasive blood pressure monitoring substantially decreases the response time to changes in blood pressure, and is especially beneficial during critical periods of anesthesia, such as induction, abdominal insufflation, changes of patient position, or with significant blood loss. Arterial access simplifies blood sampling for laboratory tests. Frequent ABG analysis may be necessary in some situations, such as with severe pulmonary disease, morbid obesity, or poor cardiac function. ABG monitoring may be needed in situations when ETCO$_2$ values are less reliable, and adequate oxygenation and ventilation more difficult.

Although invasive cardiac monitoring may be necessary in patients with decreased cardiac function, the effects of pneumoperitoneum on CVP and PCWP complicate the interpretation of the data. In these cases pulmonary artery catheterization with cardiac output measurement, rather than CVP line placement, is usually indicated. Transesophageal echocardiography may be more reliable in monitoring the volume status and cardiac function during

laparoscopy and should be considered in patients with severe cardiac disease.[60]

Anesthetic Techniques

The choice of anesthesia for laparoscopic procedures depends on the type of procedure, the patient's medical condition, and surgeon and patient preference. The surgeon's technical skill and style are very important, as is his or her understanding of the benefits and limitations of different anesthetic techniques. General, regional, and local anesthesia have been used successfully for laparoscopic procedures (Table 4–3).

General Anesthesia

General anesthesia, with muscle relaxation, endotracheal intubation, and controlled mechanical ventilation, is the most commonly used technique for laparoscopic surgery. It provides optimal operating conditions and allows respiratory and hemodynamic control.

The choice of a specific anesthetic agent probably does not affect the outcome after laparoscopic surgery.[105–113] The decision is usually based on the patient's medical condition, the side effects of anesthetic agents, inpatient versus outpatient status, and the personal experience of the anesthesiologist.

Anesthetic agents that are direct cardiovascular depressants should be avoided in patients with compromised cardiac function. A narcotic-based anesthetic technique might be preferable in these cases. The concomitant administration of vasodilating agents will reduce the hemodynamic effects of pneumoperitoneum and might facilitate management of cardiac patients.[54,114] Delayed recovery from general anesthesia can be avoided by using ultra-short-acting narcotics such as remifentanil.[111,115]

Nitrous oxide is routinely used in maintenance of anesthesia for laparoscopic surgery. Omitting this agent does not offer any clinically significant advantage,[107,108,113] with the possible exception of intestinal surgery, when bowel distention due to diffusion of N_2O might interfere with surgical exposure. The use of N_2O during laparoscopic cholecystectomy does not seem to affect operating conditions.[113,116] Although the contribution of nitrous oxide to postoperative nausea and vomiting is controversial,[107,108,117] it is reasonable to avoid N_2O in patients with a previous history of postoperative nausea and vomiting (PONV).

Narcotics, an important part of a balanced anesthesia technique, can interfere with certain aspects of laparoscopic cholecystectomy. All narcotics except pentazocine increase intrabiliary pressure, and have been reported to cause spasm of the choledochoduodenal sphincter (sphincter of Oddi). Although the incidence is relatively small (3% in one study[118]), spasm of the sphincter

TABLE 4–3. ANESTHETIC TECHNIQUES USED FOR LAPAROSCOPIC PROCEDURES

- General anesthesia with endotracheal intubation
- General/LMA with mechanical ventilation
- General anesthesia with spontaneous ventilation, with or without airway devices
- Regional anesthesia, spinal or epidural
- Local anesthesia with or without IV sedation
- Combined general/regional anesthesia

LMA, laryngeal mask airway.

may produce findings characteristic of a common bile duct stone during intraoperative cholangiography. However, the narcotic-induced spasm of the sphincter of Oddi is readily reversible. Several drugs including naloxone, glucagon, and nalbuphine can be used to reverse this narcotic effect.

After institution of pneumoperitoneum, ventilation should be adjusted to maintain the $ETCO_2$ at approximately 35 mm Hg. Adequate muscle relaxation and deep anesthesia facilitate hyperventilation. In some cases, high peak airway pressure may be required. Mild to moderate hypercarbia may be permitted to avoid barotrauma to the lungs or a decrease in cardiac output.

Hemodynamic control is usually achieved by adjustment of the level of anesthesia and/or use of vasoactive medications. The combined β- and α-blocking properties of labetalol make this drug especially useful for control of hypertensive responses to abdominal insufflation. When β blockers are contraindicated, calcium channel blockers or peripheral vasodilators may be used. Significant hypotension during laparoscopy might indicate a severe drop in cardiac output. Administration of a combination of inotropic agents and vasodilators may become necessary.[57,114] Occasionally, desufflation of the abdomen will be required to stabilize a patient and allow time for adjustment of the depth of anesthesia and administration of fluids or appropriate drugs.

An oro- or nasogastric tube is routinely placed after induction of general anesthesia and endotracheal intubation. Its use is more important for upper abdominal surgery, especially for procedures involving the small intestine. Decompression of the stomach improves surgical conditions for laparoscopy and may decrease the incidence of PONV[117] and regurgitation. Positive-pressure ventilation via a mask prior to intubation of the trachea can inflate the stomach, which poses some risk for passive regurgitation or gastric perforation during trocar placement.

Urinary bladder catheterization is not necessary for upper abdominal procedures of short duration. However, it is recommended for pelvic laparoscopy, procedures of long duration, and when significant blood losses or fluid shifts are expected.

Positioning an anesthetized patient requires a team effort by all OR personnel. It must be done with great care to prevent nerve injuries and falls. Tilting must be slow and progressive to avoid sudden hemodynamic and respiratory changes. Correct placement of the endotracheal tube, infusion lines, and respiratory circuit must be verified after any change in patient position.

The laryngeal mask airway (LMA) has proven to be a safe and efficient airway control device for general anesthesia.[119] It offers several advantages in comparison to endotracheal intubation, especially for patients with reactive upper airway disease, or those for whom endotracheal intubation would be difficult. However, its suitability for laparoscopic surgery is controversial and somewhat limited. Some patients who undergo laparoscopy are at increased risk of gastroesophageal regurgitation. Laparoscopy often requires stomach decompression with an oro- or nasogastric tube, and even when positioned properly the LMA does not give the same degree of airway protection from aspiration as a cuffed endotracheal tube, nor does it allow easy placement of the nasogastric tube. The changes in pulmonary mechanics that occur during abdominal insufflation may result in an airway pressure that far exceeds the LMA sealing pressure (approximately 20 cm H_2O). Inadequate ventilation and stomach inflation can be a real hazard in this situation. LMA dislodgment during repositioning of the patient adds yet another potential problem to the use of an LMA for laparoscopy. However, the LMA can be an acceptable alternative to endotracheal intubation for certain procedures, such as pelvic laparoscopy or laparoscopic hernia repair.[120–123] Recent investigations have shown no difference in the incidence of gastroesophageal reflux during gynecologic laparoscopy with an LMA versus endotracheal intubation.[121,123] The LMA-ProSeal™, the newest modification of the LMA, has an additional lumen for passage of a gastric tube. The LMA-ProSeal's higher airway sealing pressure (up to 50% higher than that of a standard LMA)[124–125] offers more effective positive-pressure ventilation, and the presence of the gastric tube may prevent regurgitation and aspiration.[126] Although more clinical studies are necessary to prove its safety and efficacy, the LMA-ProSeal may become a valuable option in the management of anesthesia for abdominal surgery, including laparoscopic procedures.

Although it is not a common practice, for some laparoscopic procedures of short duration, general anesthesia can be performed with spontaneous ventilation via the patient's natural airway.[26,92,127] Avoidance of manipulations of the airway, positive-pressure ventilation, and administration of muscle relaxants may offer some benefits. However, an unprotected airway, insufficient CO_2 elimination due to respiratory depression and changes in pulmonary mechanics, the lack of correlation between end-tidal and arterial CO_2 tension, the danger of upper airway obstruction, and the inability to control the airway make this approach less attractive.[25,128]

Local and Regional Anesthesia

Local anesthesia has been successfully used for outpatient laparoscopic gynecological procedures[129,130] as well as laparoscopic extraperitoneal herniorrhaphy.[131,132] It offers several advantages, including quicker recovery, avoidance of the side effects and complications of general anesthesia, and considerable financial advantages and scheduling flexibility. However, even with the best technique, patients experience significant discomfort with abdominal insufflation, positioning, and manipulation of the internal organs. Occasionally vagal reflexes with bradycardia, hypotension, and nausea may complicate the procedure. In addition, local anesthesia provides less than optimal surgical conditions. Intravenous administration of sedatives and narcotics are commonly needed to facilitate the procedure. Excellent results and high patient satisfaction have been reported when local anesthesia was combined with intravenous sedation.[129,130] However, the level of sedation is greatly limited by the risk of hypoventilation. Combining pneumoperitoneum and IV sedation may result in significant hypercarbia and hypoxemia.[23] A motivated patient, a skillful surgeon, a low IAP, short duration of the procedure, minimal organ manipulation, and careful sedation are the necessary components of a successful laparoscopic procedure performed under local anesthesia.

Epidural or spinal anesthesia might be a suitable alternative to general anesthesia for some gynecologic procedures, laparoscopic herniorrhaphy, and gasless laparoscopy.[73,80,81,133–135] Pursnani et al[136] reported six uneventful cases of laparoscopic cholecystectomy under epidural anesthesia in patients with severe pulmonary disease. A desire to avoid general anesthesia (e.g., to avoid manipulation of the airway) rather than convenience should be the primary motivation for choosing this type of anesthesia. Shoulder tip pain secondary to diaphragmatic irritation and discomfort with changes in position might mandate IV sedation. The high level of sensory block (T4–T5) necessary for laparoscopy results in paralysis of the intercostal muscles. This, together with a pneumoperitoneum and tilted position, can cause dyspnea. Excessive IV sedation in this situation might lead to hypoventilation. However, in cases of gasless lower abdominal laparoscopy, an epidural or spinal block should provide sufficient anesthesia and abdominal muscle relaxation.[80,81] Patient cooperation, as well as the surgeon's understanding of the limitations of regional anesthesia, is very important for successful anesthesia.

Postoperative Concerns

Postoperative Pain. Although significantly less than after laparotomy, patients may experience a considerable amount of pain after laparoscopic procedures.[137] Right upper quadrant and port wounds appear to be the most painful areas in the first 24 hours after laparoscopic cholecystectomy. Shoulder tip pain is the leading site on the second postoperative day.[137,138] The incidence of shoulder tip pain has been reported at about 30 to 40%, but may be as high as 100%.[139,140]

The mechanism of pain after laparoscopy is not well understood, and is probably multifactorial. Mechanical, chemical, and inflammatory effects of pneumoperitoneum might be responsible for shoulder and visceral pain. Several factors may influence the degree of pain. The type, total volume, and temperature of gas used, level of IAP, volume of residual gas retained after desufflation, and rate of insufflation have been implicated.[141–145] The type of procedure may affect the level of pain as well. Different interventions have been proposed to reduce postoperative pain (Table 4–4). Despite extensive investigations, the effectiveness and clinical significance of these interventions remain controversial.

It appears that low pressure insufflation, multimodal analgesia, and mesosalpinx/tubal block may offer clinically relevant benefits, while other modalities have only modest short-term effects.[146,147]

Postoperative Nausea and Vomiting

Postoperative nausea and vomiting is a common anesthetic problem. It may delay discharge and result in unanticipated hospital admission.[151–153] PONV is frequently listed by patients as one of their most important perioperative concerns. The overall incidence of PONV is 25 to 40% during the first 24 hours after surgery, but is reportedly as high as 60 to 70% in some investigations.[154–160] The etiology of PONV is complex and multifactorial, and several independent risk factors are associated with its development. These include a previous history of PONV or motion sickness, younger age, female sex, general anesthesia, nonsmoking status, duration of anesthesia, plastic surgery, and administration of opioids postoperatively.[117,161] Although the data are somewhat conflicting, patients who undergo laparoscopic procedures may also be at increased risk for PONV.[117,156,158,161,162]

A wide variety of antiemetics have been used for prophylaxis and treatment of PONV, including anticholinergics (scopolamine), phenothiazines (promethazine), butyrophenones (droperidol), benzamides (metoclopramide), and steroids (dexamethasone). The newest additions to antiemetics are the 5-HT$_3$ receptor antagonists (ondansetron, dolasetron, granisetron, tropisetron). It is evident that 5-HT$_3$ receptor antagonists have efficacy and side effect profiles superior to other drugs.[157,162–166] Dexamethasone may be as effective as droperidol, at least after gynecologic laparoscopy.[155,167] Combinations of 5-HT$_3$ antagonists with droperidol or dexamethasone may give better results than these medications alone.[156,168]

A less traditional approach to the management of PONV includes infusion of propofol and use of acupressure. Propofol is an anesthetic agent with a relatively low incidence of PONV.[109,169,170] Whether propofol has antiemetic properties per se remains controversial. While some have failed to show any significant benefits of subhypnotic doses of propofol,[171,172] others have demonstrated that propofol is highly effective in the treatment of PONV.[173,174]

Although not uniform in results, several investigations targeting a nonpharmacologic approach have shown that stimulation of acupuncture points might significantly reduce PONV.[159,160,175]

The choice of specific anesthetic agents does not seem to have a clinically significant effect on outcomes after laparoscopic surgery.[105–113] However, modification of the anesthetic

TABLE 4–4. PAIN MANAGEMENT IN LAPAROSCOPIC SURGERY

Pain Management Modalities	Clinical Implication
Perioperative NSAIDs	Minimal effect to statistically significant early (6 to 24 h) decrease in narcotic requirement; pain and nausea reduction. Multiple contraindications to NSAIDs use.
Intraperitoneal local anesthetics	No effect to modest pain reduction for 2 to 24 h. Seems to be more effective for pelvic laparoscopy than for laparoscopic cholecystectomy.
Wound infiltration with local anesthetic	No benefit to some pain reduction for 4 to 18 h. Peritoneal combined with subcutaneous infiltration is better than subcutaneous alone.
Removal of insufflation gas	No benefit to some reduction in shoulder tip pain for up to 3 days.
Intraperitoneal normal saline irrigation	Large volume (25–30 mL/kg) with or without bupivacaine more effective than local anesthetic alone.
Insufflation modification	
Gasless laparoscopy	Reduction in shoulder tip pain. Some investigations have shown no benefit.
Low IAP	Significant reduction in pain and analgesic requirement for 1 to 6 days.
Low-flow insufflation	Less shoulder pain for up to 3 days.
N$_2$O pneumoperitoneum	Pain reduction up to 24 h.
Heated and humidified CO$_2$	From increase in shoulder tip pain to prolonged pain reduction (up to 10 days), and earlier return to activities.
Phrenic nerve block	Significantly decreased incidence of shoulder tip pain, but not analgesic requirement.
Mesosalpinx/tubal block	Significant pain reduction (up to 24 h) after laparoscopic sterilization.

From Joris et al,[138] Salman et al,[140] Aitola et al,[142] Wallace et al,[143] Berberoglu et al,[144] Mouton et al,[145] Wills et al,[146] Moiniche et al,[147] Slim et al,[148] Korell et al,[149] and Elhakim et al.[150]

technique, including propofol-based anesthesia, ultra-short-acting narcotics, and stomach decompression with a gastric tube, as well as avoiding N_2O, muscle relaxant antagonists, and postoperative narcotics, might be justified in patients who are at high risk for PONV.[117,155,156,159–161]

SUMMARY

Laparoscopy has become one of the most common surgical interventions. Along with multiple postoperative benefits, it presents a significant challenge in high-risk patients. Pneumoperitoneum and altered patient position result in complex pathophysiologic changes that may cause cardiovascular and/or respiratory decompensation. Thorough preoperative evaluation, optimization of the patient's medical condition, careful monitoring, and understanding and appropriate management of cardiopulmonary disturbances are essential for successful management of patients who undergo laparoscopic surgery. General anesthesia with muscle relaxation and endotracheal intubation remains the most commonly used technique for laparoscopic procedures. Several other techniques have been successfully used, mostly for gynecologic procedures. Local or regional anesthesia, or general anesthesia with an LMA, may be an acceptable alternative in selected cases.

REFERENCES

1. Pelosi P, Foti G, Cereda M, et al. Effects of carbon dioxide insufflation for laparoscopic cholecystectomy on the respiratory system. *Anesthesia* 1996;51:744.
2. Koivusalo AM, Lindgren L. Respiratory mechanics during laparoscopic cholecystectomy. *Anesth Analg.* 1999;89:800.
3. Hirvonen EA, Nuutinen LS, Kauko M. Ventilatory effects, blood gas changes, and oxygen consumption during laparoscopic hysterectomy. *Anesth Analg.* 1995;80:961.
4. Kendall AP, Bhatt S, Oh TE. Pulmonary consequences of carbon dioxide insufflation for laparoscopic cholecystomies. *Anesthesia* 1995;50:286.
5. Obeid F, Saba A, Fath J, et al. Increases in intra-abdominal pressure affects pulmonary compliance. *Arch Surg.* 1995;130:544.
6. Fahy BG, Barnas GM, Flowers JL, et al. The effects of increased abdominal pressure on lung and chest wall mechanics during laparoscopic surgery. *Anesth Analg.* 1995;81:744.
7. Oikkonen M, Tallgren M. Changes in respiratory compliance at laparoscopy: Measurements using side stream spirometry. *Can J Anesth.* 1995;42:495.
8. Carry PY, Gallet D, Francois Y, et al. Respiratory mechanics during laparoscopic cholecystectomy: The effects of the abdominal wall lift. *Anesth Analg.* 1998;87:1393.
9. Bures E, Fusciardi J, Lanquetot H, et al. Ventilatory effects of laparoscopic cholecystectomy. *Acta Anesthesiol Scand.* 1996;40:566.
10. Tan PL, Lee TL, Tweed WA. Carbon dioxide absorption and gas exchange during pelvic laparoscopy. *Can J Anesth.* 1992;39:677.
11. Fox LG, Hein HAT, Gawey BJ, et al. Physiologic alternation during laparoscopic cholecystectomy in ASA III-IV patients. *Anesthesiology* 1993;79(Suppl. 3A):A55.
12. Yasinski P, Joris J, Desaive C, et al. Respiratory changes during CO_2 pneumoperitoneum in morbidly obese patients. *Acta Anaesthesiol Belg.* 1995;46:P189.
13. Domsky M, Wilson RF, Heins J. Intraoperative end-tidal carbon dioxide values and derived calculations correlated with outcome: prognosis and capnography. *Crit Care Med.* 1995;23:1497.
14. Baraka A, Jabbour S, Hammoud R, et al. End-tidal carbon dioxide tension during laparoscopic cholecystectomy. *Anaesthesia* 1994;49:304.
15. Nyarwaya JB, Mazoit JX, Samii K. Are pulse oximetry and end-tidal carbon dioxide tension monitoring reliable during laparoscopic surgery? *Anaesthesia* 1994;49:775.
16. Mullet CE, Viale JP, Sagnard PE, et al. Pulmonary CO_2 elimination during surgical procedures using intra- or extraperitoneal CO_2 insufflation. *Anesth Analg.* 1993;76:622.
17. Wahba RW, Mamazza J. Ventilatory requirements during laparoscopic cholecystectomy. *Can J Anaesth.* 1993;40:206.
18. McMahon AJ, Baxter JN, Kenny G, et al. Ventilatory and blood gas changes during laparoscopic cholecystectomy. *Br J Surg.* 1993;80:1252.
19. Hirvonen EA, Nuutinen LS, Kauko M. Ventilatory effects, blood gas changes, and oxygen consumption during laparoscopic hysterectomy. *Anesth Analg.* 1995;80:961.
20. Fleming RY, Dougherty TB, Feig BW. The safety of helium for abdominal insufflation. *Surg Endosc* 1997;11:230.
21. Neuberger TJ, Andrus CH, Wittgen CM, et al. Prospective comparison of helium versus carbon dioxide pneumoperitoneum. *Gastrointest Endosc.* 1996;43:38.
22. Rademaker BM, Odoom JA, de Wit LT, et al. Haemodynamic effects of pneumoperitoneum for laparoscopic surgery: a comparison of CO_2 with N_2O insufflation. *Eur J Anaesthesiol.* 1994;11:301.
23. Brady CE, Harkleroad LE, Pierson WP. Alteration in oxygen saturation and ventilation after intravenous sedation for peritoneoscopy. *Arch Intern Med.* 1989;149:1029.
24. Bhavani-Shankar K, Steinbrook RA, Brooks DC. Arterial to end-tidal carbon dioxide pressure difference during laparoscopic surgery in pregnancy. *Anesthesiology* 2000;93:370.
25. Cheng KI, Tang CS, Tsai EM, et al. Correlation of arterial and end-tidal carbon dioxide in spontaneously breathing patients during ambulatory gynecologic laparoscopy. *J Formos Med Assoc.* 1999;98:814.
26. Casati A, Comotti L, Tommasino C, et al. Effects of pneumoperitoneum and reverse Trendelenburg position on cardiopulmonary function in morbidly obese patients receiving laparoscopic gastric banding. *Eur J Anaesthesiol.* 2000;17:300.
27. Frei FJ, Konrad R. [The arterial-end tidal CO_2 partial pressure difference during anesthesia]. *Anaesthesist* 1990;39:101.
28. Welkowitz LA, Rapp L, Martinez J, et al. Instructional set and physiologic response to CO_2 inhalation. *Am J Psychiatry.* 1999;156:745.
29. Kuntz C, Wunsch A, Bodeker C, et al. Effect of pressure and gas type on intraabdominal, subcutaneous, and blood pH in laparoscopy. *Surg Endosc.* 2000;14:367.
30. Iwasaka H, Miyakawa H, Yamamoto H, et al. Respiratory mechanics and arterial blood gases during and after laparoscopic cholecystectomy. *Can J Anaesth.* 1996;43:129.
31. Guyton AC: *Textbook of Medical Physiology*, 8th ed. WB Saunders:1991.
32. Staszewska-Barczak J, Dusting GJ. Importance of circulating angiotensin II for elevation of arterial pressure during acute hypercarbia in anesthetized dogs. *Clin Exp Pharmacol Physiol.* 1981;8:189.
33. Rasmussen JP, Daucot PJ, de Aplma RG, et al. Cardiac function and hypercarbia. *Arch Surg.* 1981;113:1196.
34. Wexels JC, Mjos OD. Effects of carbon dioxide and pH on myocardial function in dogs with acute left ventricular failure. *Crit Care Med.* 1987;15:1116.
35. Cullen DJ, Eger EI. Cardiovascular effects of carbon dioxide in man. *Anesthesiology* 1974;41:345.
36. Eliades D, Weiss HR. Effect of hypercapnia on coronary circulation. *Cardiovasc Res.* 1986;20:127.
37. Sibbald WJ, Paterson NAM, Holliday RL, et al. The Trendelenburg position: Hemodynamic effects in hypotensive and normotensive patients. *Crit Care Med.* 1979;7:218.

38. Bivins HG, Knopp R, dos Santos PA. Blood volume distribution in the Trendelenburg position. *Ann Emerg Med*. 1985;14:641.

39. Hirvonen EA, Nuutinen LS, Vuolteenaho O. Hormonal responses and cardiac filling pressure in head-up or head-down position in patients undergoing operative laparoscopy. *Br J Anaesth*. 1997;78:128.

40. Hirvonen EA, Nuutinen LS, Kauko M. Hemodynamic changes due to Trendelenburg position and pneumoperitoneum during laparoscopic hysterectomy. *Acta Anaesthesiol Scand*. 1995;39:949.

41. Hirvonen EA, Poikolainen EO, Paakkonen ME, et al. The adverse hemodynamic effects of anesthesia, head-up tilt, and carbon dioxide pneumoperitoneum during laparoscopic cholecystectomy. *Surg Endosc*. 2000;14:272.

42. McLaughlin JG, Scheeres DE, Dean RJ, et al. The adverse hemodynamic effects of laparoscopic cholecystectomy. *Surg Endosc*. 1995; 9:121.

43. Dorsay DA, Greene FL, Baysinger CL. Hemodynamic changes during laparoscopic cholecystectomy monitored with transesophageal echocardiography. *Surg Endosc*. 1995;9:128.

44. Matzen S, Perko G, Groth S, et al. Blood volume distribution during head-up tilt induced central hypovolemia. *Clin Physiol*. 1991;11:411.

45. Halverson A, Buchanan R, Jacobs L, et al. Evaluation of mechanism of increased intracranial pressure with insufflation. *Surg Endosc*. 1998;12:266.

46. Rosenthal RJ, Hiatt JR, Phillips EH, et al. Intracranial pressure. Effects of pneumoperitoneum in a large-animal model. *Surg Endosc*. 1997;11:376.

47. Lentschener C, Benhamou D, Niessen F, et al. Intra-ocular pressure changes during gynaecological laparoscopy. *Anaesthesia* 1996;51:1106.

48. Kelman GR, Swapp GH, Smith I, et al. Cardiac output and arterial blood-gas tension during laparoscopy. *Br J Anaesth*. 1972;44:1155.

49. Sharma KC, Brandstetter RD, Brensilver JM, et al. Cardiopulmonary physiology and pathophysiology as a consequence of laparoscopic surgery. *Chest* 1996;110:810.

50. Wahba RWM, Beique F, Kleiman SJ. Cardiopulmonary function and laparoscopic cholecystectomy. *Can J Anaesth*. 1995;42:51.

51. Walder AD, Aitkenhead AR. Role of vasopressin in the hemodynamic response to laparoscopic cholecystectomy. *Br J Anaesth*. 1997;78: 264.

52. D'Ugo D, Persiani R, Pennestri E, et al. Transesophageal echocardiographic assessment of hemodynamic function during laparoscopic cholecystectomy in healthy patients. *Surg Endosc*. 2000;6:120.

53. Joris JL, Noirot DP, Legrand MJ, et al. Hemodynamic changes during laparoscopic cholecystectomy. *Anesth Analg*. 1993;76:1067.

54. Myre K, Buanes T, Smith G, et al. Simultaneous hemodynamic and echocardiographic changes during abdominal gas insufflation. *Surg Laparosc Endosc*. 1997;7:415.

55. Herruzo SJA, Castellano G, Larrodera L, et al. Plasma arginine vasopressin concentration during laparoscopy. *Hepatogastroenterology* 1989;36:499.

56. Fox LG, Hein HAT, Gawey BJ, et al. Physiologic alterations during laparoscopic cholecystectomy in ASA III & IV patients. *Anesthesiology* 1993;79(3a):Suppl.

57. Hein HA, Joshi GP, Ramsay MA, et al. Hemodynamic changes during laparoscopic cholecystectomy in patients with severe cardiac disease. *J Clin Anesth*. 1997;9:261.

58. Safran D, Sgambati S, Orlando R: Laparoscopy in high-risk cardiac patients. *Surg Gynecol Obstet*. 1993;176:548.

59. Stuttmann R, Paul A, Kirschnic M, et al. Preoperative morbidity and anaesthesia-related negative events in patients undergoing conventional or laparoscopic cholecystectomy. *Endosc Surg Allied Technol*. 1995;3:156.

60. Portera CA, Compton RP, Walters DN, et al. Benefits of pulmonary artery catheter and transesophageal echocardiographic monitoring in laparoscopic cholecystectomy patients with cardiac disease. *Am J Surg*. 1995;169:202.

61. Dhoste K, Lacoste L, Karayan J, et al. Haemodynamic and ventilatory changes in elderly ASA III patients. *Can J Anaesth*. 1996;43:783.

62. Chiche JD, Joris J, Lamy M. Respiratory changes induced by subcutaneous emphysema during laparoscopic fundoplication. *Br J Anaesth*. 1994;72:A37.

63. Pearce DJ. Respiratory acidosis and subcutaneous emphysema during laparoscopic cholecystectomy. *Can J Anaesth*. 1994;42:314.

64. Chien GL, Soifer BE. Pharyngeal emphysema with airway obstruction as a consequence of laparoscopic inguinal herniorrhaphy. *Anesth Analg*. 1995;80:201.

65. Wahba RWM, Tessler MJ, Kleiman SJ. Acute ventilatory complication during laparoscopic upper abdominal surgery. *Can J Anaesth*. 1996;43:77.

66. Joris J, Chiche JD, Lamy M. Pneumothorax during laparoscopic fundoplication: Diagnosis and treatment with positive end-expiratory pressure. *Anesth Analg*. 1995;81:993.

67. Greville AC, Clements EAF, Erwin DC. Pulmonary air embolism during laparoscopic laser cholecystectomy. *Anesthesia* 1991;46:113.

68. Cottin V, Delafosse B, Viale JP. Gas embolism during laparoscopy: a report of seven cases in patients with previous abdominal surgical history. *Surg Endosc*. 1996;10:166.

69. Moskop RJ Jr, Lubarsky DA. Carbon dioxide embolism during laparoscopic cholecystectomy. *South Med J*. 1994;87:414.

70. Herron DM, Vernon JK, Gryska PV. Venous gas embolism during endoscopy. *Surg Endosc*. 1999;13:276.

71. Yau P, Watson DI, Lafullarde T, et al. Experimental study of effect of embolism of different laparoscopy insufflation gases. *J Laparoendosc Adv Surg Tech*. 2000;10:211.

72. Lantz PE, Smith JD. Fatal carbon dioxide embolism complicating attempted laparoscopic cholecystectomy—case report and literature review. *J Forensic Sci*. 1994;39:1468.

73. Spivak H, Nudelman I, Fuco V, et al. Laparoscopic extraperitoneal inguinal hernia repair with spinal anesthesia and nitrous oxide insufflation. *Surg Endosc*. 1999;13:1026.

74. Roberts MW, Mathiesen KA, Ho HS, et al. Cardiopulmonary responses to intravenous infusion of soluble and relatively insoluble gases. *Surg Endosc*. 1997;11:341.

75. Golberg JM, Maurer WG. A randomized comparison of gasless laparoscopy and CO_2 pneumoperitoneum. *Obstet Gynecol*. 1997;90:416.

76. Koivusalo AM, Kellokumpu I, Ristkari S, et al. Splanchnic and renal deterioration during and after laparoscopic cholecystectomy: a comparison of the carbon dioxide pneumoperitoneum and the abdominal wall lift method. *Anesth Analg*. 1997;85:886.

77. Ninomiya K, Kitano S, Yoshida T, et al. Comparison of pneumoperitoneum and abdominal wall lifting as to hemodynamics and surgical stress response during laparoscopic cholecystectomy. *Surg Endosc*. 1998;12:124.

78. Schulze S, Lyng KM, Bugge K, et al. Cardiovascular and respiratory changes in laparoscopic colonic surgery: comparison between carbon dioxide pneumoperitoneum and gasless laparoscopy. *Arch Surg*. 1999;134:1112.

79. Moncure M, Salem R, Moncure K, et al. Central nervous system metabolic and physiologic effects of laparoscopy. *Am Surg*. 1999;65:168.

80. Tanaka H, Futamura N, Takubo S, et al. Gasless laparoscopy under epidural anesthesia for adnexal cyst during pregnancy. *J Reprod Med*. 1999;44:929.

81. Ohta J, Kodama I, Yamauchi Y. Abdominal wall lifting with spinal anesthesia vs pneumoperitoneum with general anesthesia for laparoscopic herniorrhaphy. *Int Surg*. 1997;82:146.

82. Steinbrook RA, Brooks DC, Datta S. Laparoscopic cholecystectomy during pregnancy. Review of anesthetic management, surgical considerations. *Surg Endosc*. 1996;10:511.

83. Hunter JG, Swanstrom L, Thornburg K. Carbon dioxide pneumoperitoneum induces fetal acidosis in a pregnant ewe model. *Surg Endosc*. 1995;9:272.

84. Curet MJ. Special problems in laparoscopic surgery. Previous abdominal surgery, obesity and pregnancy. *Surg Clin North Am.* 2000;80:1093.

85. Conron RW, Abbruzzi K, Cochrane SO, et al. Laparoscopic procedures in pregnancy. *Am Surg.* 1999;65:256.

86. Lachman E, Schienfild A, Boldes R, et al. Pregnancy and laparoscopic surgery. *J Am Assoc Gynecol Laparosc.* 1999;6:347.

87. Nezhat FR, Tazuke S, Nezhat CH, et al. Laparoscopy during pregnancy: a literature review. *J Soc Laparoendosc Surg.* 1997;1:17.

88. Luks FI, Logan J, Breuer CK, et al. Cost-effectivness of laparoscopy in children. *Arch Pediatr Adolesc Med.* 1999;153:965.

89. Montupet P, Esposito C. Laparoscopic treatment of congenital inguinal hernia in children. *J Pediatr Surg.* 1999;34:420.

90. Stringel G, Berezin SH, Bostwick HE, et al. Laparoscopy in the management of children with chronic recurrent abdominal pain. *J Soc Laparoendosc Surgeons.* 1999;3:215.

91. Gueugniaud PY, Abisseror M, Moussa M, et al. The hemodynamic effects of pneumoperitoneum during laparoscopy in healthy infants: assessment by continuous esophageal aortic blood flow echo-Doppler. *Anesth Analg.* 1998;86:290.

92. Tobias JD, Holcomb GW 3rd, Brock JW 3rd, et al. General anesthesia by mask with spontaneous ventilation during brief laparoscopic inspection of the peritoneum in children. *J Laparoendosc Surg.* 1994;4:379.

93. Laffon M, Gouchet A, Sitbon P, et al. Difference between arterial and end-tidal carbon dioxide pressure during laparoscopy in paediatric patients. *Can J Anaesth.* 1998;45:561.

94. Hsing CH, Hseu SS, Tsai SK, et al. The physiological effect of CO_2 pneumoperitoneum in pediatric laparoscopy. *Acta Physiol Sinica.* 1995;33:1.

95. Tobias JD, Holcomb GW 3rd, Rasmussen GE, et al. General anesthesia using the laryngeal mask airway during brief, laparoscopic inspection of the peritoneum in children. *J Laparoendosc Surg.* 1996;6:175.

96. Perez A, Planell J, Bacardaz C, et al. Value of routine preoperative tests: a multicenter study in four general hospitals. *Br J Anaesth.* 1995;74:250.

97. Vogt AW, Henson LC. Unindicated preoperative testing: ASA physical status and financial implications. *J Clin Anesth.* 1997;9:437.

98. Meneghini L, Zadra N, Zanette G. The usefulness of routine preoperative laboratory tests for one-day surgery in healthy children. *Paediatr Anaesth.* 1998;8:11.

99. Munro J, Booth A, Nicholl J. Routine preoperative testing: a systematic review of the evidence. *Health Technol Assess.* 1997;1:i, 1.

100. American Society of Anesthesiologists. New classification of physical status. *Anesthesiology* 1963;24:111.

101. Sidi A, Lobato EB, Cohen JA. The American Society of Anesthesiologists Physical Status: category V revisited. *J Clin Anesth.* 2000;12:328.

102. Prause G, Offner A, Ratzenhofer-Komenda B, et al. Comparison of two preoperative indices to predict perioperative mortality in noncardiac thoracic surgery. *Eur J Cardiothorac Surg.* 1997;11:670.

103. Wolters U, Wolf T, Stutzer H, et al. ASA classification and perioperative variables as predictors of postoperative outcome. *Br J Anaesth.* 1996;77:217.

104. American College of Cardiology/American Heart Association. Guidelines for perioperative cardiovascular evaluation for non-cardiac surgery. *JACC.* 1996;27:910.

105. Kirsch MA, Carrithers JA, Ragan RH, et al. Effects of a low-cost protocol on outcome and cost in a group practice setting. *J Clin Anesth.* 1998;10:416.

106. Nelskyla K, Eriksson H, Soikkeli A, et al. Recovery and outcome after propofol and isoflurane anesthesia in patients undergoing laparoscopic hysterectomy. *Acta Anaesthesiol Scand.* 1997;41:360.

107. Arellano RJ, Pole ML, Rafuse SE. Omission of nitrous oxide from a propofol-based anesthetic does not affect the recovery of women undergoing outpatient gynecologic surgery. *Anesthesiology* 2000;93:332.

108. Tang J, Chen L, White PF, et al. Use of propofol for office-based anesthesia: effect of nitrous oxide on recovery profile. *J Clin Anesth.* 1999;11:226.

109. Raeder J, Gupta A, Pedersen FM. Recovery characteristics of sevoflurane- or propofol-based anesthesia for day-care surgery. *Acta Anaesthesiol Scand.* 1997;41:988.

110. Delogu G, Famularo G, Luzzi S, et al. General anesthesia mode does not influence endocrine or immunologic profile after open or laparoscopic cholecystectomy. *Surg Laparosc Endosc Percutan Tech.* 1999;9:326.

111. Juckenhofel S, Feisel C, Schmitt HJ. TIVA with propofol-remifentanil or balanced anesthesia with sevoflurane-fentanyl in laparoscopic operations. Hemodynamics, awakening and adverse effects. *Anaesthesist* 1999;48:807.

112. Jakobsson J, Rane K, Ryberg, G. Anaesthesia during laparoscopic gynaecologic surgery: A comparison between desflurane and isoflurane. *Eur J Anaesthesiol.* 1997;14:148.

113. Jensen AG, Prevedoros H, Kullman E, et al. Perioperative nitrous oxide does not influence recovery after laparoscopic cholecystectomy. *Acta Anaesthesiol Scand.* 1993;37:683.

114. Duale C, Bazin JE, Ferrier C, et al. Hemodynamic effects of laparoscopic cholecystectomy in patients with coronary disease. *Br J Anaesth.* 1994;72(Suppl S1):A31.

115. Song D, Whitten CW, White PF. Remifentanil infusion facilitates early recovery for obese outpatients undergoing laparoscopic cholecystectomy. *Anesth Analg.* 2000;90:1111.

116. Taylor E, Feinstein R, White PF, et al. Anesthesia for laparoscopic cholecystectomy. Is nitrous oxide contraindicated? *Anesthesiology* 1992;76:541.

117. Apfel CC, Roewer N. [Risk factors for nausea and vomiting after general anesthesia: fictions and facts]. *Anaesthesist* 2000;49:629.

118. Jones RM, Detmer M, Hill AB, et al. Incidence of choledochoduodenal sphincter spasm during fentanyl-supplemented anesthesia. *Anesth Analg.* 1981;60:638.

119. Verghese C, Brimacombe JR. Survey of laryngeal mask airway usage in 11,910 patients: safety and efficacy for conventional and nonconventional usage. *Anesth Analg.* 1996;82:129.

120. Ho BY, Skinner HJ, Mahajan RP. Gastro-oesophageal reflux during day case gynaecological laparoscopy under positive pressure ventilation: laryngeal mask vs. tracheal intubation. *Anaesthesia* 1998;53:921.

121. Bapat PP, Verghese C. Laryngeal mask airway and the incidence of regurgitation during gynecological laparoscopies. *Anesth Analg.* 1997;85:139.

122. Brimacombe J. Laparoscopy and the laryngeal mask airway. *Br J Anaesth.* 1994;73:121.

123. Swann DG, Spens H, Edwards SA, et al. Anaesthesia for gynaecological laparoscopy—a comparison between the laryngeal mask airway and tracheal intubation. *Anaesthesia* 1993;48:431.

124. Brimacombe J, Keller C. The ProSeal laryngeal mask airway: a randomized, crossover study with the standard laryngeal mask airway in paralyzed, anesthetized patients. *Anesthesiology* 2000;93:104.

125. Brain AI, Verghese C, Strube PJ. The LMA "ProSeal"—a laryngeal mask with an oesophageal vent. *Br J Anaesth.* 2000;84:650.

126. Keller C, Brimacombe J, Kleinsasser A, et al. Does the ProSeal laryngeal mask airway prevent aspiration of regurgitated fluid? *Anesth Analg.* 2000;91:1017.

127. Kurer FL, Welch DB. Gynaecological laparoscopy: Clinical experience of two anaesthetic techniques. *Br J Anaesth.* 1984;54:1207.

128. Peterson HB, DeStefano F, Rubin GL, et al. Death attributable to tubal sterilization in the United States, 1997–1981. *Am J Obstet Gynecol* 1983;146:131.

129. Milki AA, Tazuke SI. Office laparoscopy under local anesthesia for gamete intrafallopian transfer: technique and tolerance. *Fertil Steril.* 1997;68:128.

130. Miller GH. Office single puncture laparoscopy sterilization with local anesthesia. *J Soc Laparoendosc Surg.* 1997;1:55.

131. Ferzli G, Sayad P, Vasisht B. The feasibility of laparoscopic extraperitoneal hernia repair under local anesthesia. *Surg Endosc.* 1999;13:588.

132. Pendurthi TK, DeMaria EJ, Kellum JM. Laparoscopic bilateral inguinal hernia repair under local anesthesia. *Surg Endosc.* 1995;9:197.

133. Topel HC. Gasless laparoscopic assisted hysterectomy with epidural anesthesia. *J Am Assoc Gynecol Laparosc.* 1994;1:S36.

134. Vaghadia H, McLeod DH, Mitchell GW, et al. Small-dose hypobaric lidocaine-fentanyl spinal anesthesia for short duration outpatient laparoscopy. I. A randomized comparison with con-ventional dose hyperbaric lidocaine. *Anesth Analg.* 1997;84:59.

135. Chilvers CR, Vaghadia H, Mitchell GW, et al. Small-dose hypobaric lidocaine-fentanyl spinal anesthesia for short duration outpatient laparoscopy. II. Optimal fentanyl dose. *Anesth Analg.* 1997;84:65.

136. Pursnani KG, Bazza Y, Calleja M, et al. Laparoscopic cholecystectomy under epidural anesthesia in patients with chronic respiratory disease. *Surg Endosc.* 1998;12:1082.

137. Ure BM, Troidl H, Spangenberger W, et al. Intensity and localization of pain and analysis of predictors in preoperative symptoms and intraoperative events. *Surg Endosc.* 1994;8:90.

138. Joris J, Thiry E, Paris P, et al. Pain after laparoscopic cholecystectomy: characteristics and effect of intraperitoneal bupivacaine. *Anesth Analg.* 1995;81:379.

139. Cason CL, Seidel SL, Bushmiaer M. Recovery from laparoscopic cholecystectomy procedures. *AORN J.* 1996;63:1099.

140. Salman MA, Ercan Yucebas M, Coskun F, et al. Day-case laparoscopy: a comparison of prophylactic opioid, NSAID or local anesthesia for postoperative analgesia. *Acta Anaesthesiol Scand.* 2000;44:536.

141. Jackson SA, Laurence AS, Hill JC. Does post-laparoscopy pain relate to residual carbon dioxide? *Anaesthesia* 1996;51:485.

142. Aitola P, Airo I, Kaukinen S, et al. Comparison of N_2O and CO_2 pneumoperitoneum during laparoscopic cholecystectomy with special reference to postoperative pain. *Surg Laparosc Endosc.* 1998;8:140.

143. Wallace DH, Serpell MG, Baxter JN, et al. Randomized trial of different insufflation pressure for laparoscopic cholecystectomy. *Br J Surg.* 1997;84:455.

144. Berberoglu M, Dilek ON, Ercan F, et al. The effect of CO_2 insufflation rate on the postlaparoscopic shoulder pain. *J Laparoendosc Adv Surg Tech Part A* 1998;8:273.

145. Mouton WG, Bessell JR, Millard SH, et al. A randomized controlled trial assessing the benefit of humidified insufflation gas during laparoscopic surgery. *Surg Endosc* 1998;13:106.

146. Wills VL, Hunt DR. Pain after laparoscopic cholecystectomy. *Br J Surg.* 2000;87:273.

147. Moiniche S, Jorgensen H, Wetterslev J, et al. Local anesthetic infiltration for postoperative pain relief after laparoscopy: A qualitative and quantitative systematic review of intraperitoneal, port-site infiltration and mesosalpinx block. *Anesth Analg.* 2000;90:899.

148. Slim K, Bousquet J, Kwiatkowski F, et al. Effect of CO_2 gas warming on pain after laparoscopic surgery: a randomized double-blind controlled trial. *Surg Endosc.* 1999;13:1110.

149. Korell M, Schmaus F, Strowitzki T, et al. Pain intensity following laparoscopy. *Surg Laparosc Endosc.* 1995;6:375.

150. Elhakim M, Elkott M, Ali NM, et al. Intraperitoneal lidocaine for postoperative pain after laparoscopy. *Acta Anaesthesiol Scand.* 2000;44:280.

151. Gold BS, Kitz DS, Lecky JH, et al. Unanticipated admission to the hospital following ambulatory surgery. *JAMA.* 1989;262:3008.

152. Isenberg SJ, Apt L, Yamada S. Overnight admission of outpatient strabismus patients. *Ophthalm Surg.* 1990;21:540.

153. Watcha MF, White PF. Postoperative nausea and vomiting: its etiology, treatment, and prevention. *Anesthesiology* 1992;77:162.

154. Iitomi T, Toriumi S, Kondo A, et al. Incidence of nausea and vomiting after cholecystectomy performed via laparotomy or laparoscopy. *Masui* 1995;44:1627.

155. Wang JJ, Ho ST, Liu HS. Prophylactic antiemetic effect of dexamethasone in women undergoing ambulatory laparoscopic surgery. *Br J Anaesth.* 2000;84:459.

156. Wu O, Belo SE, Koutsoukos G. Additive anti-emetic efficacy of prophylactic ondansetron with droperidol in out-patient gy-necological laparoscopy. *Can J Anaesth.* 2000;47:529.

157. Kovac AL. Prevention and treatment of postoperative nausea and vomiting. *Drugs* 2000;59:213.

158. Henzi I, Sonderegger J, Tramer MR. Efficacy, dose-response, and adverse effects of droperidol for prevention of postoperative nausea and vomiting. *Can J Anaesth* 2000;47:537.

159. Harmon D, Gardiner J, Harrison R, et al. Acupressure and the prevention of nausea and vomiting after laparoscopy. *Br J Anaesth.* 1999;82:387.

160. Schlager A, Boehler M, Puhringer F. Korean hand acupressure reduces postoperative vomiting after strabismus surgery. *Br J Anaesth.* 2000;85:267.

161. Sinclair DR, Chung F, Mezei G. Can postoperative nausea and vomiting be predicted? *Anesthesiology* 1999;91:109.

162. Fujii Y, Tanaka H, Kawasaki T. Randomized clinical trial of granisetron, droperidol and metoclopramide for the treatment of nausea and vomiting after laparoscopic cholecystectomy. *Br J Surg.* 2000;87:285.

163. Tang J, Wang B, White PF, et al. The cost effect of timing of ondansetron on its efficacy, cost-effectiveness, and cost-benefit as a prophylactic antiemetic in the ambulatory setting. *Anesth Analg.* 1998;86:274.

164. Swiatkowski J, Goral A, Dzieciuch JA, et al. Assessment of ondansetron and droperidol for the prevention of post-operative nausea and vomiting after cholecystectomy and minor gynaecological surgery performed by laparoscopy. *Eur J Anaesth.* 1999;16:766.

165. Loewen PS, Marra CA, Zed PJ. 5-HT3 receptor antagonists vs traditional agents for the prophylaxis of postoperative nausea and vomiting. *Can J Anaesth.* 2000;47:1008.

166. Polati E, Verlato G, Finco G, et al. Ondansetron versus metoclopramide in the treatment of postoperative nausea and vomiting. *Anesth Analg.* 1997;85:395.

167. Rothenberg DM, McCarthy RJ, Peng CC, et al. Nausea and vomiting after dexamethasone versus droperidol following outpatient laparoscopy with a propofol-based general anesthetic. *Acta Anaesth Scand.* 1998;42:637.

168. Eberhart LH, Morin AM, Georgieff M. [Dexamethasone for prophylaxis of postoperative nausea and vomiting. A meta-analysis of randomized controlled studies.] *Anaesthesist* 2000;49:713.

169. Soppitt AJ, Glass PS, Howell S, et al. The use of propofol for its antiemetic effect: a survey of clinical practice in the United States. *J Clin Anesth.* 2000;12:265.

170. Randel GI, Levy L, Kothary SP, et al. Propofol versus thiaminalenflurane anesthesia for outpatient laparoscopy. *J Clin Anesth.* 1992;4:185.

171. Harper I, Della-Marta E, Owen H, et al. Lack of efficacy of propofol in the treatment of early postoperative nausea and vomiting. *Anaesth Intensive Care.* 1998;26:366.

172. Scuderi PE, D'Angelo R, Harrish L, et al. Small-dose propofol by continuous infusion does not prevent postoperative vomiting in females undergoing outpatient laparoscopy. *Anesth Analg.* 1997;84:71.

173. Borgeat A, Stirnemann HR. Antiemetic effect of propofol. *Anaesthesist* 1998;47:918.

174. Gan TJ, Glass PS, Howell ST, et al. Determination of plasma concentration of propofol associated with 50% reduction in postoperative nausea. *Anesthesiology* 1997;84:779.

175. Agarwal A, Pathak A, Gaur A. Acupressure wristbands do not prevent postoperative nausea and vomiting after urological endoscopic surgery. *Can J Anaesth.* 2000;47:319.

Chapter Five • • • • • •

Establishing the Pneumoperitoneum

**ALEJANDRO WEBER-SÁNCHEZ, DENZIL GARTEIZ-MARTÍNEZ,
and SALVADOR VALENCIA-REYES**

The peritoneal cavity is only a potential operating space, and it must be transformed into a actual space in order to allow laparoscopic surgical maneuvers, exposure, and safe manipulation of the instruments, with minimum risk to the patient. Thus the first step in any laparoscopic procedure is the induction of pneumoperitoneum. The introduction of the Veress needle into the abdomen, the insufflation of gas, and the placement of trocars, all involve risks that the surgeon must always bear in mind. An appropriate pneumoperitoneum facilitates the procedure and avoids dangerous and even fatal complications. Therefore, it is important to pay special attention and remember certain useful details during this initial part of the procedure.[1,2]

TYPES OF GAS USED FOR PNEUMOPERITONEUM

The surgeon must be familiar with the characteristics of the different gases used for pneumoperitoneum. Ambient air was used for many years, but proved to be inconvenient in several aspects: It is highly irritating to the peritoneum, air and oxygen carry a greater risk of air embolism, and their presence increases the probability of thermal lesions, especially with the use of electrocautery. Nitrous oxide was also used some years ago. Recent studies have reported fewer arrhythmias with nitrous oxide than with CO_2,[3–5] and its anesthetic properties help to reduce the discomfort of abdominal wall distention, but its rapid and uncontrollable absorption into the bloodstream can cause worsening of ileus and cerebral edema. Although initially believed to support combustion, studies have refuted this. The concentration of flammable gases produced during pneumoperitoneum with nitrous oxide is less than 5% of the amount necessary to cause combustion.[3,4] An exception to this would be the presence of a colonic perforation with a subsequent increase in methane concentrations. Theoretically, methane in combination with an oxidizing agent like nitrous oxide and a spark could cause an explosion; thus it is of critical importance to avoid this risk. In rare cases, inert gases such as helium have also been used to create pneumoperitoneum, but their use is not widespread.

Carbon dioxide has become the gas of choice for pneumoperitoneum during laparoscopic procedures because it is readily available, inexpensive, and easily absorbed into the bloodstream with minimal risk of air embolism. Its effects on blood pH can be measured by capnography and manipulated by the anesthesiologist by changing the ventilatory rate. Finally, the fact that it is not an inflammable gas allows the use of electrocautery or laser during the procedure.

PHYSIOLOGIC EFFECTS OF CARBON DIOXIDE

Carbon dioxide is highly diffusable and very soluble in blood. It is metabolized quickly through respiration. Up to 100 mL could be injected directly into the bloodstream per minute without significant metabolic effects, thus allowing the anesthesiologist to cleanse it from the blood by increasing ventilation. CO_2 causes vasodilatation, which could be misinterpreted as indirect evidence of peritoneal inflammation in some patients. Its uncontrollable absorption through the peritoneum or subcutaneous tissue causes acidosis and hypercapnia. Capnographic monitoring is essential during all laparoscopic procedures and in order to avoid changes in pH, and the anesthesiologist must increase minute ventilation when P_{CO_2} is higher than 40 mm Hg. This margin may change depending on the patient's status.[6,7]

The cardiopulmonary effects of hypercapnia are caused by sympathetic reflexes which increase heart rate and contractility as well as cause vasoconstriction of some blood vessels. This causes increased cardiac output and blood pressure. Also, abdominal overdistention due to pneumoperitoneum interferes with venous return and lung compliance. Therefore it is important to maintain close surveilance of all these parameters during the entire procedure.[8]

At the beginning of the twentieth century, surgeons performed laparoscopic diagnostic procedures by simply introducing air with a syringe into the abdominal cavity.[9] Today, high-flow automatic insufflators can pump gas at rates of up to 15 to 20 liters per minute and allow constant abdominal distention during the procedure. The optimal intra-abdominal pressure has not been established, but the general consensus is to work with pressures below 15 mm Hg. This reduces problems with mechanical ventilation or other cardiopulmonary adverse effects. The authors prefer to use pressures below 10 to 12 mm Hg, especially in patients with restrictive lung problems or those undergoing hiatal surgery, in order to avoid respiratory complications and subcutaneous emphysema.

Working with low pressure is also useful when laparoscopic procedures are carried out with regional anesthesia and during pregnancy. With regional anesthesia and sedation, patients develop breathing complications and therefore many surgeons have resisted the idea of performing laparoscopic procedures in this manner. Nonetheless, the enthusiasm for diagnostic laparoscopic procedures in an outpatient facility has increased, particularly in gynecological practice, with the use of insufflation pressures between 6 and 10 mm Hg. Recently, Curet et al[9] published the results of laparoscopic procedures on pregnant women, such as cholecystectomy and appendectomy, and recommends the use of low insufflation pressures to preserve the fetoplacental blood flow and to avoid the fetal acidosis related to hypercapnia. Studies with a pregnant ewe model show that apparently, in spite of maternal changes, the placental perfusion pressure, blood flow, pH, and blood gases are not affected by insufflation or deflation, suggesting that laparoscopic procedures in pregnancy are safe.[10]

CONSIDERATIONS OF PNEUMOPERITONEUM INDUCTION

Before pneumoperitoneum is induced, the surgeon must examine the patient for evidence of previous surgery, possible adhesions, or ileus. All these situations increase the risk of intra-abdominal lesions with the conventional needle induction method. Other techniques should be considered in these cases.

Patients with No Previous Abdominal Surgery

If there is no history of previous surgery, a small incision is made with the tip of the scalpel (blade no. 15) at the base of the navel. The tip of the Veress needle is introduced through this incision while the abdominal wall is lifted on both sides of the umbilicus. In obese or muscular patients, towel clamps may be used to aid in lifting the abdominal wall.[11,12] The needle is introduced slowly in order to feel, hear, and see the penetration into the umbilical fascia and parietal peritoneum. Most needles have a protective mechanism that helps to signal when penetration is complete. Before gas is introduced, it is important to verify that no damage has been produced with this blind puncture. While maintaining the abdominal wall with upward traction (Fig. 5–1), the following maneuvers should be performed with the needle in the intraperitoneal space:

1. Feel the free tip of the needle upon gentle motion.
2. Infuse a small amount of physiologic solution through the needle and observe its passage without difficulty.
3. Aspirate the same amount of solution back into the syringe and observe for blood, urine, or intestinal contents.
4. Remove the syringe from the needle and observe the free passage of solution toward the abdominal cavity.
5. Connect the needle to the tube that carries the CO_2 and begin insufflation. The insufflator should indicate an initial intra-abdominal pressure of less than 5 mm Hg. Higher pressures indicate obstruction of gas flow that may be due to needle tip

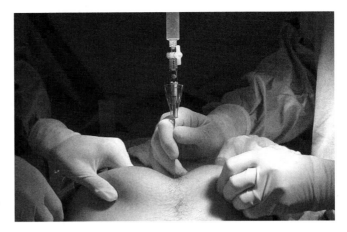

Figure 5–1. Suggested method of Veress needle introduction. While lifting the abdominal wall, the needle is carefully introduced at a slight angle to avoid intra-abdominal visceral injury.

occlusion or extraperitoneal placement. In this case it is advisable to withdraw the needle and repeat all steps.

Note that high intra-abdominal pressure may be recorded in spite of proper needle insertion. This may happen when extrinsic compression on the abdominal wall is applied, when liquid is present in the insufflator's tubing, when the tube is bent or obstructed, or when the patient has not been appropriately anesthetized by the anesthesiologist. If there is any doubt about the needle's position, it is advisable to repeat the procedure or use another technique.[13]

Patients with Previous Abdominal Surgery

When a patient has had previous abdominal or pelvic surgery, the risk of adhered intra-abdominal organs is higher, and therefore other options should be used to induce pneumoperitoneum. If the surgical scar is far from the navel, pneumoperitoneum induction could be attempted in the manner described above. If, on the other hand, the scar is around the navel, the needle may be introduced in the left upper quadrant as taught by Jacques Perissat, being careful to avoid forceful penetration. Midline needle insertions above the umbilicus should be avoided because of possible placement of the needle tip in the falciform ligament.

Another option is the open technique described by Hasson, which involves making a larger incision in the navel skin, fascia, and peritoneum, and entering the abdomen under direct vision. A finger is introduced to remove adhesions and a purse-string suture is placed on the fascia to close the orifice around a special trocar that allows preservation of the pneumoperitoneum. Additional sutures may be placed to secure the trocar in place.

Semm describes a technique in which an incision is made through the skin and fascia of the navel, without entering the peritoneum. A 10-mm trocar is introduced along with the laparoscope to examine for possible omental or visceral adhesions. When a free area is located, the laparoscope and trocar are inserted together under direct vision while maintaining traction on the abdominal wall, avoiding intra-abdominal lesions. If necessary, the skin is sutured around the trocar to avoid gas leaks.

The authors describe a technique that is used mainly in cases in which needle pneumoperitoneum induction cannot be established, such as in very thin patients or in patients with ileus. The

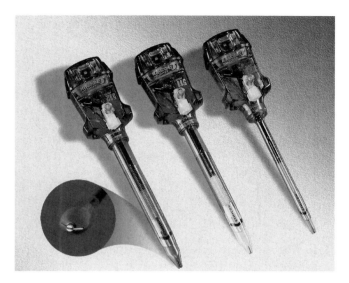

Figure 5–2. Different sizes of disposable retractable-tipped trocars. See Color Plates. *(Photo courtesy of Johnson & Johnson Ethicon.)*

incision is made at the base of the umbilicus, where skin and fascia join together, and depending on the size of the trocar to be used (Fig. 5–2), is extended for 10 to 11 mm in the midline of the umbilical scar. Using Kelly forceps, the tissues are dissected until abdominal cavity is entered. With the aid of the forceps, it is ascertained that no adhesions are present. To avoid injuries from the trocar, the safety mechanism is activated outside of the abdomen and the trocar introduced while maintaining traction on the abdominal wall with towel clamps. If there is any doubt about the penetration of the abdominal cavity, the trocar along with the laparoscope is introduced as in Semm's technique. Gas leaks with this technique are minimal, since the incision adjusts to the size of the trocar. However, if there is a gas leak, a screw-type adapter (Fig. 5–3) or a balloon-tipped trocar may be used.[14–15] This technique has a low bleeding and infection rate, is very secure, and has better cosmetic results than other techniques.

Insufflation of the Abdominal Cavity

Insufflator parameters should be preset with a maximum intra-abdominal pressure of 15 mm Hg and gas flow of 1 to 2 L/min. Pneumoperitoneum is induced slowly, making sure that there are no changes in the patient's status. Once this is ascertained, gas flow may be increased up to the capacity of the insufflator. The authors prefer to insert the trocars with an intra-abdominal pressure of 15 mm Hg to avoid organ or vascular injury. Once the trocars are placed, the rest of the procedure is carried out with pressures between 8 and 12 mm Hg. Use of higher pressures may be dangerous due to adverse cardiopulmonary and metabolic effects. Continuous surveillance of intra-abdominal pressure is of great importance.

Trocar Placement

The use of disposable trocars is advisable, especially for surgeons who are new to laparoscopic procedures, because their sharp tips and security mechanisms facilitate introduction. Most are equipped with a plastic shield that covers the sharp tip as soon as it penetrates the abdominal cavity. Reusable trocars may lose their sharpness with

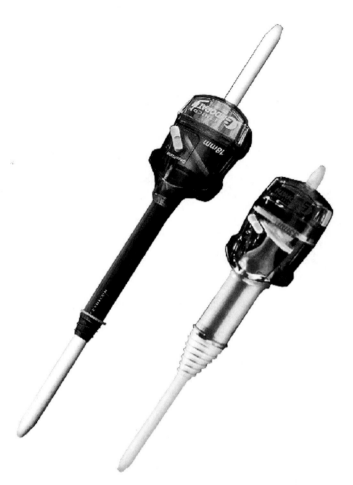

Figure 5–3. Different sizes of blunt-tipped trocars with screw-type adapters. *(Photo courtesy of Johnson & Johnson Ethicon.)*

time and have blunter tips. They may require a more forceful abdominal entry with a higher risk of injuring the viscera or major blood vessels. Once pneumoperitoneum is established, the trocar is held on the palm of the hand, with the index finger on the shaft of the trocar. The finger helps to direct the trocar, control the force of entry, and limit the depth of its introduction. Introduction should be smooth, with a gentle rotating motion and never with excessive force. Care must always be taken during this procedure because even disposable trocars are not completely fail-safe.

With the first trocar in place, the laparoscope is introduced. The abdominal cavity is inspected for possible inadvertent injuries, with special attention paid to the sites of needle and trocar insertion. The introduction of the accessory trocars should always be made under laparoscopic vision and placed wherever they are required. According to the size of the trocar, a small skin incision is made, avoiding the epigastric blood vessels by transillumination of the abdominal wall.[16]

Pneumoperitoneum Leaks

The most frequent cause of sudden loss of vision during the procedure is a pneumoperitoneum leak. This can be ascertained by examining the abdominal wall of the patient and the intra-abdominal pressure reading of the insufflator. In this case, it is necessary to find the site of the leak, correct it, and wait for the pressure to recover before continuing the procedure. If the leak is found at the site between the trocar and the skin incision, the skin may be sutured to close the leak. Other options include screw adapters for the trocar shaft or use of balloon-tipped trocars. If the leak cannot be easily controlled, a higher gas flow may be required to maintain the intra-abdominal pressure. This may be achieved with an insufflator of higher flow capacity or the use of two insufflators at the same time.

Evacuation of Pneumoperitoneum

At the end of the procedure, pneumoperitoneum is evacuated by opening one of the valves of a trocar. A complete evacuation of the gas should be assured in order to diminish the postoperative abdominal distention and shoulder pain that is seen in some cases. Trocars should be withdrawn carefully and under laparoscopic vision in order to avoid herniation of the omentum or an intestinal loop into the incision site as well as unnoticed bleeding at the trocar site.

SURGERY WITHOUT PNEUMOPERITONEUM

To avoid the potential problems associated with CO_2 pneumoperitoneum, in 1991 Japanese surgeons introduced the gasless laparoscopy technique.[17] They described a device for mechanical elevation that is introduced through the peritoneum and placed under the anterior abdominal wall. To date, several devices for this purpose have been used: wires inserted in the subcutaneous tissue of the abdominal wall, hooks, and T- or fan-shaped retractors, among others. These instruments are introduced using open technique and they are placed under direct vision, permitting ambient air to enter the abdominal cavity. This system also allows use of conventional instruments through mini-incisions or laparoscopic instruments through trocars. Unfortunately, these devices produce an uneven elevation of the abdominal wall, causing anatomical distortion, and thus surgical exposure is often not optimal. It is advisable to make the accessory trocar incisions after the abdominal wall has been elevated. Recently, several clinical reports have been published showing the physiologic advantages of these devices for abdominal wall elevation and compared them to pneumoperitoneum. The results showed fewer hemodynamic and metabolic alterations, less hypercapnia and acidosis, and less interference with cardiac output and central venous pressure. In spite of these advantages, gasless laparoscopy has not had wide acceptance. The disadvantages of devices for gas-less laparoscopy include high cost, the requirement for additional incisions, an increase of postoperative pain, and abdominal wall distortion. Pneumoperitoneum produces better operative field vision by creating an upward displacement of the abdominal wall and a downward displacement of the viscera. Nevertheless, patients with special conditions such as impaired lung function or intracranial lesions may benefit from the gasless techniques.

SUGGESTIONS FOR A SAFER APPROACH TO MINI-INVASIVE TECHNIQUES

Experience has led the authors to refine certain details that have been helpful in the performance of endoscopic surgical procedures and the avoidance of complications. Although some of these resources are applied intuitively by other surgeons with experience in this field, we offer the following suggestions.[18,19]

Preoperative Preparations

- *Antibiotic prophylaxis*: In general, a single dose of a third-generation cephalosporin is used an hour before the procedure, to lower the incidence of infectious complications, mainly of the abdominal wall.
- *Verification of operating table function*: During mini-invasive procedures, the operating table is frequently moved into different positions in order to accommodate to the surgeon's position and to displace viscera away from the operating field. It is important to verify the adequate function of the operating table before the procedure begins.
- *Fastening of the patient to the operating table.* Some procedures require forced side, Fowler, or Trendelenburg positions, and if the patient is not adequately fastened, he or she may fall off the table. This is particularly common in colon, hiatal, and thoracic surgery. If cholangiography is planned during the procedure, the patient must be adequately attached to the table to allow placement of the fluoroscopic arch.
- *Prevention of venous thrombosis*: Due to the increased intra-abdominal pressure caused by the pneumoperitoneum and the forced position of the patient, venous thrombosis prophylaxis should always be considered. Many reports favor routine administration of antithrombotic agents. The use of elastic stockings or intermittent compression devices are useful in high-risk patients.
- *Nasogastric and urinary catheters*: Although nasogastric and urinary catheter placement was initially recommended for all patients, the decision now depends on the procedure and surgeon's judgment, as in open surgery.

Position of the Patient and the Surgical Team

- *Patient position*: The patient can be placed in the European position (legs spread apart) so that one of the members of the surgical team can stand between the legs, or the American position (legs together), with the members of the surgical team working at both sides of the patient. The position of the arms should be also considered, mainly in pelvic and hernia surgery, because they can interfere with the procedure.
- *Monitor position*: When there are two monitors, they should be placed before the operation begins. Vision should not be obstructed by members of the surgical team or other obstacles. They should be placed on wheeled carts so they can be moved as needed during the procedure.
- *Position of surgical team*: The surgical team should work with comfort. The authors prefer the European position for all procedures except for gynecologic procedures, hernia surgery, and appendectomy, for which they use the American position.

During the Operation

- *Trocars*: Choice of trocar placement is similar to planning the incision in open surgery; it should be adjusted to the morphology of the patient and the type of procedure. A single pattern suitable for all cases does not exist. In patients suspected to have adhesions, it is useful to insert the first trocar far from the previous scar and then, under laparoscopic vision, introduce the rest of the trocars as adhesions are detached. The number and sites of trocars vary depending upon the procedure. The surgeon must keep in mind that an additional trocar could make the difference between conversion or continuing with the laparoscopic procedure. This extra port could be useful for retraction, aspiration-irrigation, or the use of bipolar forceps in case of bleeding.

- *Laparoscopic vision*: The assistant that holds the camera must be considered the eyes of the entire surgical team. It is important that this technician be acquainted with the steps of the procedure, so that the operation can proceed with maximum efficiency. The tips of the surgeon's instruments must always be in the center of the screen, and their movements should be followed carefully. Using the laparoscope zoom is of particular utility, mainly in situations which require greater precision, such as dissection or section of fine structures and suturing, among others. However, it is also important to show panoramic views periodically, in order to guide the surgeon in the operative field.
- *Clarity of vision*: A frequent problem seen in laparoscopic procedures is blurring of the image, especially in cases with acute inflammation, bleeding, or hyperthermia. The high temperature inside the abdominal cavity causes the laparoscope to fog in spite of repeated cleaning of the lens. Although special cleansing solutions exist, the authors prefer to dip the laparoscope in sterile hot water to heat the lens.[15]
- *Instrument manipulation in the trocars*: Sometimes movements and manipulation of the instruments through the trocars is difficult. In these cases it is useful to lubricate them with sterile mineral oil, which facilitates their motion through the trocar.
- *Use of bipolar energy*: It has been proven that use of bipolar energy is safer and more effective than monopolar energy, especially when used near important anatomical structures. Bipolar energy limits the passage of the electric current between the two electrodes, requires less voltage, and produces less smoke.
- *Harmonic scalpel*: The recent introduction of this instrument has provided major advantages for laparoscopic procedures. It allows section and dissection of structures with minimal bleeding, even with larger blood vessels.

Finishing the Procedure

1. *Final cavity inspection*: Before the procedure is finished and the trocars withdrawn, inspection of the operative field and the entire abdominal cavity is necessary. Any previously undetected problem should be corrected at this time.
2. *Retrieval of specimens*: In certain circumstances it is important to remove tissues or organs in extraction bags to prevent wound contamination. This is particularly necessary in cancer surgery and septic processes like appendicitis or acute cholecystitis. In other situations, such as splenectomy for hematological problems, it avoids splenosis. Although commercial devices exist for this propose, their cost and lack of appropriate sizes have forced surgeons to use sterile condoms, glove fingers, or plastic bags. The authors have used the common zipper-type plastic bags, which have a rigid opening that facilitates the introduction of the specimens, are inexpensive, and present no problems for sterilization. They are easy to obtain and are available in many sizes.[15]
3. *Bupivacaine instillation*: At the end of the procedure, the authors instill a bupivacaine solution (2 mg/kg of body weight) in both subdiaphragmatic spaces. This has been useful in reducing postoperative shoulder and abdominal wall pain.[19,20,21]
4. *Trocar withdrawal*: Trocar withdrawal should always be done under laparoscopic vision, before evacuating the pneumoperitoneum. If the abdomen is desufflated and trocars are removed blindly, the omentum or an intestinal loop may be suctioned by the trocar and pulled through the orifice, producing a hernia or even an intestinal obstruction.
5. *Closing of the mini-incisions*: All incisions greater than 10 mm should be sutured to prevent complications. Skin may be sutured in the usual manner, but in general the authors use a subdermal absorbable fine suture and approximate the skin borders with sterile tape strips.

REFERENCES

1. Cueto GJ, Serrano BF, Ramírez AG, et al. Colecistectomía por laparoscopia. *Cirujano General*. 1991;13:52.
2. Serrano BF, Cueto GJ, Weber SA. 160 casos de colecistectomía laparoscøpica. *Anales M, dicos del Hospital ABC*. 1993;38:147.
3. Hunter JG, Staheli J, Oddsdottir M, et al. Nitrous oxide pneumoperitoneum revisited. *Surg Endosc*. 1995;9:501.
4. Staheli J, Bordelon B, Hunter JG. Nitrous oxide pneumo-peritoneum: No need to fear. *Surg Endosc*. 1991;1:26(abstract).
5. Scott DB, Julian DG. Observation on cardiac arrhythmias during laparoscopy. *Br Med J*. 1972;1:411.
6. Liu S, Leighton T, Davis I, et al. Prospective analysis of cardiopulmonary responses to laparoscopic cholecystectomy. *Laparoendosc Surg*. 1991;1:241.
7. Safran D, Sgambati S, Orlando R. Laparoscopy in high risk cardiac patients. *Surg Gynecol Obstet*. 1993;176:548.
8. Shantha TR, Harden J. Laparoscopic cholecystectomy: Anesthesia-related complications and guidelines. *Surg Laparosc Endosc* 1991;1:173.
9. Curet CJ, Allen D, Josloff RK, et al. Laparoscopy during pregnancy. *Arch Surg*. 1996;131:546.
10. Barnard JM, Chaffin D, Droste S, et al. Fetal response to carbon dioxide pneumoperitoneum in the pregnant ewe. *Obstet Gynecol* 1995;85:669.
11. Cohen R, Schiavaon CA, Schaffa TD. Avoiding complications in closed pneumoperitoneum (umbilicus lifting) insufflation, retaining good cosmetic results. *Surg Endosc* 1995;9:543(letter).
12. Biojo RG, Manzi GB. Safe laparoscopic surgery: Tubal ligation without prior pneumoperitoneum. *Surg Laparosc Endosc*. 1995;5:105.
13. Weber SA, Cueto GJ. *Manual para la Enseñanza de la Colecistectomía Laparoscópica*, 1a. ed. Weber A, ed. Johnson & Johnson (EUA): 1993;17.
14. Ballesta C, Bastida X, Bettonica C. El posoperatorio en el paciente con laparotomías previas. In: Ballesta LC ed. *Posoperatorio en Laparoscopia Quirúrgica*, 1a. ed. Video Médica S.L.:1996;281.
15. Weber A, Rojas O, Garteiz D, et al. Cuidados posoperatorios en cirugía laparoscópica de las urgencias abdominales. In: Ballesta LC, ed. *Posoperatorio en Laparoscopia Quirúrgica*, 1a. ed. Video Médica S.L.:1996;263.
16. Weber SA, Serrano BF, Cueto GJ. Técnicas de neumoperitoneo. In: Sepúlveda AC, ed. *Cirugía Laparoscópica Avanzada*, Tomo 2. Ediciones Video Cirugía:1997;273.
17. Nagai H, Inabo T, Kamiya S. A new method of laparoscopic cholecystectomy: An abdominal wall lifting technique without pneumoperitoneum. *Surg Laparosc Endosc*. 1991;1:26(abstract).
18. Weber SA, Serrano BF, Cueto GJ. Puntos claves para facilitar la técnica en cirugía endoscópica. *Cirujano General*. 1994;16:25.
19. Weber SA, Serrano BF, Cueto GJ. Puntos claves para facilitar la técnica en cirugía endoscópica. *Cirujano General*. 1994;17:88.
20. Pasqualucci A, Contardo R, Broid GDB, et al. The effects of intraperitoneal local anesthetic on analgesic requirements and endocrine response after laparoscopic cholecystectomy: A randomized double-blind controlled study. *J Laparoendosc Surg*. 1994;4:405.
21. Jones DB, Clery MP, Soper NJ. Strangulated incisional hernia at trocar site. *Surg Laparosc Endosc*. 1996;6:152.

Chapter Six • • • • • • •

Gasless Laparoscopic Surgery

**ALBERT K. CHIN, ALEXANDER RASCHKE-FEBRES,
and JOSÉ ANTONIO VÁZQUEZ-FRÍAS**

INTRODUCTION

Mechanical techniques of lifting the abdominal wall for endoscopic surgery offer benefits associated with conventional open surgery which previously were unavailable with traditional laparoscopy using a pneumoperitoneum. With relatively simple procedures such as laparoscopic cholecystectomy, these benefits may be unnecessary. However, more technically demanding endoscopic procedures demonstrate the utility of approaches that do not use insufflation. Increased instrument control, improved surgical manipulation, and simplified technical requirements make gasless laparoscopy an attractive alternative to traditional laparoscopy.

HISTORICAL BACKGROUND

Various groups of laparoscopic surgeons have approached the development of mechanically assisted laparoscopy. The first efforts employed mechanical lifting as an adjunct to pneumoperitoneum in patients with factors complicating conventional laparoscopy, such as morbid obesity. In 1991 Gazayerli[1] described the use of a T-shaped retractor which provided localized point lifting to augment gas insufflation. Semm and Lehmann-Willenbrock[2] developed a similar hinged retractor (ACE System, WISAP) which is placed through a trocar sleeve in a straight configuration, pivoting to form an inner cross member for abdominal lifting.

The next stage of development in mechanical abdominal wall retraction involved devices whose placement was preceded by establishment of a pneumoperitoneum. Once these devices were correctly positioned, the pneumoperitoneum was either decreased or completely desufflated. In 1992, Francois and Mouret[3] wrote about the use of a rigid wire form (Tri-X System) which is inserted into the abdomen via a single incision and suspended from an overhanging arm. The wire form lifts a broad length of abdominal wall to create a flat ceiling-like plane of elevated tissues. In that same year, Kitano et al[4] devised a U-shaped retractor which is placed through the abdominal wall by means of a curved 5-mm-diameter needle which enters the abdomen at the subxiphoid region, pierces through the falciform ligament, and exits inferior to the tip of the 12th rib. This tubular retractor, which is placed under endoscopic guidance, is lifted by a winch attached to a rigid frame assembled over the chest wall. The retractor contains openings in its central portion to allow evacuation of smoke. A wire suspension system was developed[5] that resembles a coat hanger, which is introduced via a small incision lateral to the epigastric vessels, to provide a linear area of lift extending transversely across the abdomen.

Mechanical abdominal retraction without prior gas insufflation has been applied using two different types of techniques. The first technique, employed by several different investigators in Japan, involves inserting lifting cables or wires through multiple puncture sites in the abdominal wall. In 1991, Nagai et al[6] reported on the use of Kirschner wires placed through the skin and subcutaneous tissue just below the right costal margin and at the supraumbilical area. Hoisting chains attached to the Kirschner wires are lifted by winches on a framework connected to the side rail of the operating table.

Hashimoto et al[7] described a similar technique in 1993. Starting at a small incision in the right anterior axillary line midway between the costal margin and the iliac crest, two Kirschner wires are tunneled through the subcutaneous space; one passes along the costal margin, and the second courses medially to the midline before it curves superiorly to intersect the first wire. Four suture strands are then placed through the skin to hold the wires and to suspend them from the arched crossbeam of a Kent retractor, which attaches to the operating table via two vertical posts.

The second technique, developed by Chin and Moll[8] in 1993, involves inserting a two-bladed fan (Laparofan™, Origin Medsystems, Inc., Menlo Park, CA) into the abdominal cavity via a 15-mm periumbilical incision. The fan blades spread apart to form a triangular outline for abdominal lifting (Fig. 6–1). The fan is elevated by an electrically powered arm (Laparolift,™ Origin Medsystems, Inc., Menlo Park, CA) which clamps to the operating table. The arm is designed with a force limiter which halts vertical travel when the lifting force is equivalent to that achieved with

41

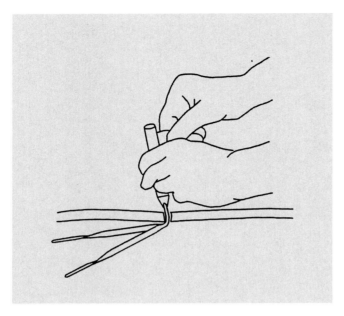

Figure 6–1. Fan retractor.

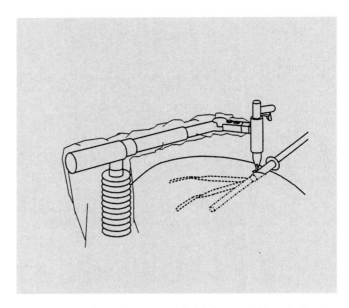

Figure 6–2. The Ligasure™ system (Valleylab, TYCO Healthcare) with a laparoscopic instrument. The system can be used with a different grasper in open procedures.

conventional gas insufflation of 15 mm Hg. An inflatable ring may also be used instead of the fan, to increase the lifting surface area and improve surgical exposure.

The advantages of the permanent vessel occlusion achieved with the Ligasure System (Fig. 6–2) include:

- It can be used to ligate vessels up to 7 mm in diameter
- It causes minimal thermal spread (its effect is confined to the target tissue)
- It seals tissue bundles without dissection and isolation
- It reduces sticking and charring
- It minimizes the need for multiple applications
- There are no dislodged clips or foreign material left behind

To date, several systems for gasless laparoscopic surgery have been used.[9,10]

RATIONALE FOR GASLESS LAPAROSCOPY

Simplification of laparoscopic technique was the primary motivation for development of gasless laparoscopy. The use of pneumoperitoneum in laparoscopy presents two issues that do not exist with open surgery. First, each instrument introduced into the surgical site must pass though a trocar port which has a valve to maintain gas pressure within the peritoneal cavity. Second, separation of the abdominal wall from abdominal contents during gas insufflation leads to a need for elongated surgical instruments that make manipulation more difficult. The need for the gas seal means that tasks such as suturing and knot tying become difficult when a laparoscopic approach is used, and learning curves are long for new procedures. Organ and bowel retraction require insertion of multiple instruments, as broad retractors can-not be placed through small trocar ports. Digital palpation and finger dissection are also impossible in an insufflated abdomen.

Surgical exposure and visualization in laparoscopy are directly related to the degree of pneumoperitoneum present during the procedure. The use of suction aspiration to clear electrocautery smoke, irrigation fluid, and blood is limited by the need to preserve an adequate pneumoperitoneum for laparoscopic visualization.

Use of carbon dioxide gas insufflation is associated with a certain degree of danger to the patient. There are reports of reactive bradycardia during CO_2 infusion in the literature,[11–13] as well as cases of gas embolism.[14,15] Although rare, these complications generally result in death. Other cardiovascular effects attributed to gas insufflation include venous stasis[16] as a result of increased intra-abdominal pressure. Pulmonary compromise may also be a by-product of pneumoperitoneum.[17] Pneumothorax has been reported in routine laparoscopy,[18] and the potential for pneumothorax should always be considered when laparoscopic evaluation of a blunt trauma patient is undertaken. Postoperative changes in respiratory function have been seen; however, these changes do not appear to occur as much as in postceliotomy patients.[19]

Insufflation of pressurized gas into the abdominal cavity creates a need for positive-pressure ventilation and general anesthesia during the procedure. This requirement makes the use of laparoscopy controversial for procedures which may be performed open under local or regional anesthesia. Thus, transabdominal laparoscopic inguinal hernia repair has less of an advantage over outpatient open herniorrhaphy. Other anesthetic considerations which are the direct result of a pneumoperitoneum include acid-base disturbances due to carbon dioxide absorption.[20,21] The magnitude of the disturbance and its consequences depend on pre-existing comorbidities, such as obstructive pulmonary disease and coronary artery disease. Occurrence of subcutaneous emphysema during the procedure also affects the acid-base balance.[22,23]

Gasless laparoscopy addresses these potential problems with gas insufflation. In terms of the operative technique, mechanical abdominal lifting allows shorter instruments to be used.[24] The systems that lift the abdominal wall in a planar fashion (e.g., Laparolift, Tri-X) allow the surgeon to be closer to the operative field than is possible with gas insufflation, which distends the abdomen equally in all directions. Since no gas pressure needs to be maintained, a valveless flexible sleeve or simple abdominal wall incision may be used for instrument access. Standard hinged, straight, or curved instruments may be easily inserted into the abdominal cavity. Endoscopic suturing is facilitated by the use of conventional needle-holders, and knot tying may be accomplished by a gloved finger rather than a knot pusher. Instruments with irregularly shaped cross-sections may be used, because they do not need to fit through the circular valves used in laparoscopic trocar seals. Tissue palpation is possible through an entry incision, permitting evaluation of vascular and lymphatic structures.

Abdominal wall lifting also avoids potential complications due to gas insufflation. CO_2-related cardiac rhythm disturbances, subcutaneous emphysema, gas embolism, pneumothorax, pneumomediastinum, venous stasis, and acidosis are no longer problems with mechanical abdominal lifting. Gasless laparoscopy also allows local and regional anesthesia to be considered in a wider range of endoscopic cases.

As does any surgical technique, gasless laparoscopy has its limitations. Previous abdominal surgery that resulted in widespread abdominal adhesions preclude the insertion of lifting devices and the formation of a laparoscopic cavity. Extreme obesity limits the ability to achieve an adequate intra-abdominal operating space, but this limitation also applies to use of a pneumoperitoneum. One disadvantage of mechanical lifting that is less prevalent in the presence of gas insufflation is the occurrence of bowel distention leading to a compromised laparoscopic cavity. The positive pressure of a pneumoperitoneum aids in controlling bowel distention; this pressure is absent in gasless laparoscopy. Other measures for bowel control must thus be used. These include favorable patient positioning, such as a Trendelenburg or reverse Trendelenburg for pelvic or upper abdominal procedures, respectively. Placement of multiple laparoscopic retractors or multiple moist laparotomy pads on the surface of the bowel may also be needed. Mechanical abdominal wall retraction results in a truncated pyramid-shaped cavity, as opposed to the spherical cavity obtained with a pneumoperitoneum. The pericolic gutters are obscured with mechanical lifting, and manipulation in the lateral reaches of the abdominal cavity require rotation of the patient towards the opposite side.

TECHNIQUE

Each type of mechanical retractor requires its own individualized method of insertion and elevation. The use of the Laparolift will be detailed, as it is a typical example of gasless laparoscopy.

Lift Placement

The patient is placed in a supine position on the operating table. The lifting arm (Laparolift) is clamped to the side rail of the operating table on the side opposite the primary surgeon, near the patient's shoulder level. A sterile drape is provided with the fan retractor (Laparofan); the drape is attached to the end of the wrist portion and pulled the length of the arm and the vertical post which elevates the arm.

A 12-mm incision is made at the umbilicus. Blunt dissection is carried down through the subcutaneous tissue to expose the linea alba,

which is incised to allow the peritoneum to be grasped with two hemostats. The peritoneum is incised, and an index finger inserted into the incision and swept circumferentially to detach any adhesions.

If a fan retractor is to be used, it is inserted into the incision in a closed position at a 45° angle. Once the distal portion of the fan has been inserted, the blades are angled to lie parallel with the abdominal wall. The closed blades are swept in both directions, and unimpeded movement rules out the presence of adhesions or entrapment of bowel or omentum. The blades are locked in an open position, oriented superiorly for upper abdominal procedures and inferiorly for pelvic surgery. The passive telescopic lifting arm is brought into position, connected to the fan retractor, and elevated using the control button on its wrist joint. Abdominal lifting is continued until adequate laparoscopic visualization is achieved or until maximal lifting force has been applied, at which point the motor shuts off. A sleeve is placed into the incision, behind the elbow of the fan retractor, to provide clear access for the endoscope. The operating table is tilted to allow bowel to fall away from the surgical site. If additional bowel retraction is needed, one or more inflatable retractors may be inserted into the abdomen through separate incisions. These inflatable retractors are covered by a 10-mm sleeve in a deflated state. Following insertion, they are inflated with air to form broad contact surfaces for bowel and organ manipulation and retraction.

An inflatable lifting ring (Airlift™) may be used to lift the abdominal cavity instead of the fan retractor. The lifting ring, whose packaging is cylindrical in shape, is advanced through the periumbilical incision until it lies entirely within the abdomen. Upon inflation with a hand pump, a perforated plastic sheath splits open and the ring deploys to form a planar lifting surface which extends concentrically about the incision. Tethering cords attached to the ring are connected to the Laparolift, and the abdominal wall elevated as above. The laparoscope is inserted through the hole in the center of the ring and additional instrument ports may be placed, taking care to avoid puncturing the ring.

The inflatable lifting ring provides a larger area of abdominal elevation compared to the fan retractor, as its area of lift encircles the umbilicus, rather than being limited to a supraumbilical or infraumbilical distribution. The wider plane of lift allows a greater mass of bowel to fall away from the surgical site upon rotation of the operating table, enhancing laparoscopic visualization. The smooth surface of the ring and its compressibility provide an atraumatic lifting surface. Bowel slides off the sides of the ring, making it less likely to be trapped by the lifting device upon elevation. Upon completion of the procedure, the ring is deflated and a strap attached to its outer edge is pulled out of the incision to remove the device.

CLINICAL APPLICATIONS

Laparoscopic Cholecystectomy

Laparoscopic cholecystectomy was one of the earliest applications of mechanical lifting, with several papers published by Japanese researchers in the 1990s. In 1991, Nagai[6] described the use of his Kirschner wire abdominal suspension system for laparoscopic cholecystectomy, and in 1993 followed it up with a report on 111 successful cholecystectomies.[25] Kitano et al[26] completed a prospective randomized trial in 1993, favorably comparing his use of a U-shaped retractor with pneumoperitoneum in 83 patients. Hashimoto[27] detailed his use of subcutaneous wires suspended from a Kent retractor, and its application in 415 laparoscopic chole-cystectomy patients between June 1991 and June 1994. Only two of the first fifteen cases required conversion to an open procedure, both due to common bile duct injuries; the remaining 400 cases were successfully completed using a gasless lifting technique.

The widespread use of gasless laparoscopy for laparoscopic cholecystectomy in Japan may be related to a body habitus favorable to mechanical lifting in the right upper quadrant. Paolucci[28] described a series of 78 laparoscopic cholecystectomies using the Laparolift in Frankfurt, Germany. In 70 cases, cholecystectomy was completed using mechanical lifting and conventional surgical instruments. Three cases were converted to the use of pneumoperitoneum in order to achieve sufficient exposure in the right upper abdomen. An additional 5 cases were converted to open surgery due to pre-existing causes such as empyema of the gallbladder. In patients with marked obesity and thick abdominal walls, mechanical lifting provides limited lifting of the lateral paracolic regions, making it more difficult to elevate the liver and expose the infundibulum of the gallbladder and the cystic duct. Increased retraction of bowel at the site of the gallbladder may compensate for limited liver elevation in gasless laparoscopic cholecystectomy. The inflatable retractor may be used to displace and compress bowel overlying the hepatic flexure to maximize gallbladder exposure. Use of a substantially reversed Trendelenburg position may also increase the exodus of bowel from the surgical area. A systematic approach to gaining operative experience with mechanical abdominal lifting is most helpful in achieving a positive result with gasless laparoscopic cholecystectomy. Initial cases should be performed on thin patients, to allow the surgeon to gain familiarity with the instrumentation without the added complexity of limited right upper quadrant visualization due to a thick abdominal wall. Subsequent cases with increased degrees of difficulty may then be approached with more confidence.

Laparoscopic Colectomy

Use of mechanical lifting has many advantages over laparoscopic colectomy. Several graspers and clamps may be inserted through a single incision to manipulate and dissect the bowel. Exteriorization of the bowel loop for resection allows application of open anastomotic stapling devices, with considerable cost savings compared with use of laparoscopic gastrointestinal staplers.

Laparoscopic colectomy was initially performed in a pneumoperitoneum. Redwine and Sharpe[29] first described segmental resection of the sigmoid colon for treatment of endometrial implants, and Cooperman et al[30] published a case report of laparoscopically-assisted removal of a villous adenoma of the ascending colon. In the former case, the resected segment was removed transanally, and in the latter case sigmoid colon extraction was performed via a transabdominal incision. In both procedures, the anastomoses were performed in an end-to-end fashion using staplers.

Quattlebaum et al[31] published a series of 20 patients undergoing laparoscopically-assisted colectomy in which sufficient colonic mobilization was attained under gas insufflation to allow exteriorization of the isolated bowel segment through an abdominal incision. Bowel resection and subsequent anastomosis were performed outside the abdominal cavity, allowing application of conventional linear stapling devices. Increased surgical control and decreased operative time during the anastomotic phase of the procedure was the result of bowel exteriorization, in contrast to colectomy performed entirely laparoscopically.

Laparoscopic colectomy remains controversial for two reasons. First, debate exists over the advisability of using laparoscopic colectomy in the treatment of malignant lesions. This controversy centers not only on the ability to obtain adequate margins during colonic resection in a confined space, but also on the completeness of lymph node dissection under laparoscopic guidance. Second, there are increasing reports of port site wound metastasis following laparoscopic resection. It has been postulated that CO_2 insufflation is associated with movement of tumor cells to trocar sleeves with subsequent seeding of port entry sites, though some reports have concluded otherwise.[32,33]

A gasless approach addresses both of these concerns regarding laparoscopic colectomy. Abdominal lifting simplifies bowel mobilization, making it easier to isolate a generous segment of colon for exteriorization, thus ensuring adequate margins of resection. A gloved index finger may be introduced via a small incision, and digital palpation of lymph nodes is possible, aiding in assessment of metastatic lymphatic involvement. With mechanical abdominal lifting, there is no movement of gas within the belly, and dislodgment and aerosol spread of tumor cells should not be any greater than in conventional open cancer surgery.

In gasless laparoscopic colectomy, the lifting fan retractor or lifting balloon is placed at the umbilicus.[34] For a right hemicolectomy, an instrument access port is placed in the midline, halfway between the umbilicus and the symphysis pubis. A 3-cm muscle-splitting incision is made in the right lower quadrant to be used for specimen removal.

The laparoscope is inserted behind the blades of the fan retractor in the umbilical incision and several instruments may be introduced via both of the two access incisions. These access incisions are also used for a sigmoid colectomy if a transanal anastomosis is planned. If an extracorporeal anastomosis is to be performed following sigmoid resection, the specimen removal port is made in the left lower quadrant.

For abdominoperineal resection, the fan retractor is introduced via the umbilical incision, and the ancillary access sites are placed in the lower midline and lower quadrants on either side. The specimen removal site doubles as the colostomy site. Transverse colectomy is performed with the umbilical fan retractor blades directed cephalad. Working ports are placed on both sides at the midabdominal region, and the specimen removal incision is made in the midline of the upper abdomen.

The operating table is rotated to allow the bowel to roll away from the area of dissection. For a right-sided lesion, the table is rotated to the left, and vice versa. The patient is placed in the Trendelenburg position for access to the cecum, and in reverse Trendelenburg for manipulation of the hepatic or splenic flexures.

Mobilization of the colon involves the release of the flexure on the appropriate side. Mesenteric vessels are ligated with a ligate/divide/staple (LDS) device, vascular clips, or suture ties. For standard suture ligatures, the index finger may be advanced through the abdominal wall incisions to tighten the knot directly. An endoscopic or standard gastrointestinal anastomosis (GIA) stapler is advanced through the specimen removal incision to section the bowel and allow exteriorization of the segment. Bowel excision and anastomosis are accomplished using conventional open stapling techniques or hand suturing. The lifting fan retractor may be lowered to maximize bowel evisceration during resection and anastomosis. The fan retractor is elevated following completion of the extracorporeal anastomosis, to allow final examination of the abdominal cavity for bleeding sites.

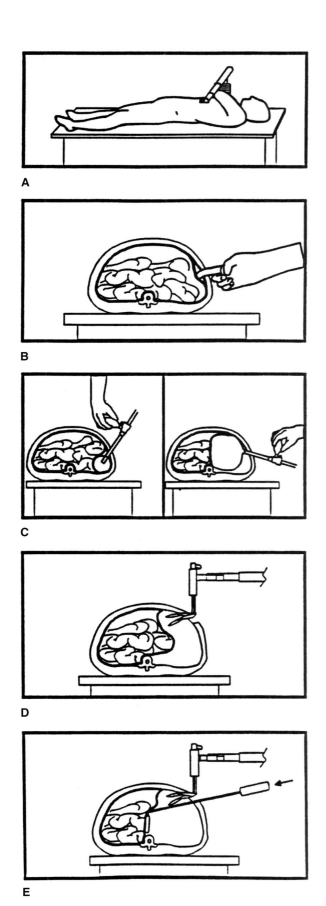

Laparoscopic Gynecologic Surgery

The earliest clinicians to apply laparoscopy on a widespread basis were gynecologists, who performed diagnostic pelvic examination and tubal sterilization under endoscopic guidance. At the same time that laparoscopic cholecystectomy underwent explosive growth, operative pelviscopy also saw additional advancements. Laparoscopically-assisted vaginal hysterectomy,[35] ovarian surgery,[36] and colposuspension for treatment of stress urinary incontinence[37] were procedures that were initially performed using a pneumoperitoneum.

In addition to the technical benefits it shares with standard surgical procedures, gasless laparoscopy confers several other advantages over gas insufflation in gynecologic surgery. In laparoscopically-assisted vaginal hysterectomy, incision through the vaginal cuff during uterine resection causes loss of gas pressure, deflation of the abdominal cavity, and subsequent loss of visualization in the middle of the procedure. With mechanical abdominal lifting, the endoscopic cavity remains unchanged throughout the procedure, and simultaneous internal and external visualization is possible. Paracervical incision may be performed from a vaginal approach, with the laparoscope providing an intra-abdominal view to guide the dissection and prevent bladder or bowel injury.

Gasless laparoscopy also allows extraction of large tissue masses during myomectomy or ovarian cystectomy. Long-handled scalpels and electrocautery units with extended blades may be inserted via small abdominal incisions to section tissue for direct removal, avoiding the lengthy morcellation process required during performance of the same procedures under gas insufflation.

Mechanical lifting is also beneficial when laparoscopic surgery is contemplated in the pregnant patient.[38] Concerns about the effects of CO_2 insufflation on the fetus are alleviated. Spinal or epidural anesthesia may be used, eliminating the risk of fetal exposure to general anesthetic agents. Reduced postoperative pain and decreased need for postoperative analgesics make gasless laparoscopy an attractive alternative to laparotomy during pregnancy.

Laparoscopic Retroperitoneal Surgery

Retroperitoneal endoscopic procedures may be performed by using a dissection balloon to create a retroperitoneal cavity, followed by support of the cavity using mechanical lifting.[39] Retroperitoneoscopy using a balloon dissection technique was first described by Gaur,[40] who performed nephrectomy under a pneumoretroperitoneum. The advantages of mechanical lifting in a retroperitoneal cavity was recognized by the author (Chin), who developed a balloon-assisted endoscopic, retroperitoneal, gasless (BERG) approach for more complex laparoscopic procedures, including aorto-bifemoral bypass grafting[41] and lumbar discectomy and spinal fusion. In these technically-demanding procedures, increased vascular control and the ability to apply conventional surgical instrumentation simplifies previously difficult surgeries.

The initial approach is the same for retroperitoneal gasless aortic reconstruction and lumbar spinal surgery (Fig. 6–3). The patient is placed in a supine position on the operating table, and a sandbag

Figure 6–3. Description of the balloon-assisted, endoscopic, retroperitoneal, gasless (BERG) approach to the aorta and anterior spine. **A.** Make an incision in the left flank at the anterior axillary line. **B.** Perform digital dissection in the pararenal space. **C.** Perform balloon dissection under direct vision. **D.** Use a mechanical lift to increase exposure. **E.** Use supplemental retraction for medial exposure.

is placed under the left hip. A 2-cm incision is made in the midaxillary line, midway between the costal margin and the iliac crest. The incision is carried down to the muscle, and the oblique and transversus muscles are bluntly dissected to expose the perirenal fat layer. The dissection balloon is advanced into the posterior pararenal space, and inflated under endoscopic vision to form a 1-liter cavity in the retroperitoneum. The dissection balloon is removed, the fan retractor is inserted into the incision, and the ceiling of the cavity is elevated with the mechanical lift. An inflatable bowel retractor and the laparoscope are inserted into the flank incision, behind the fan blades. The retractor is inflated and used to displace the peritoneum and abdominal contents medially, providing an operating cavity that exposes the left kidney and ureter, aorta, and lumbar spine.

Aortobifemoral Bypass

Placement of a standard bifurcated aortic graft may be accomplished through 4 or 5 small flank incisions. Following dissection of the retroperitoneal cavity, a 10-cm-long fan retractor is inserted via the initial incision and deployed medially. The laparoscope is inserted behind the blades of the fan retractor. An incision is made 2 cm distal to the fan insertion site, and a balloon retractor is placed against the lateral aspect of the balloon-dissected peritoneum and pushed medially to retract the side of the periaortic cavity. Two additional incisions are made; one lies several centimeters superior, and the other lies lateral to the first incision. These incisions are used to insert needle-holders and graspers. The last, most superior incision accommodates the aortic cross-clamp, which is applied to the infrarenal aorta. Exposure and isolation of the aorta may be performed using long right angled clamps or laparoscopic dissectors. Lumbar branches emanating from the aorta may be clipped and transected using a right angled laparoscopic clip-applier. A right angled clip-applier is used rather than a straight applier, because it can more easily be used to control branches located in deep cavities and tight spaces. The aorta is transected, and an end-to-end anastomosis is performed, starting at the far wall of the vessel and proceeding to the near side. Suturing can be done using either conventional long vascular needle-holders or laparoscopic needle-drivers.

The distal aortic stump may be ligated using a laparoscopic linear stapler (Endo GIA,™ United States Surgical Corp., Norwalk, CT), a laparoscopic suture loop (Endo-Loop,™ Ethicon, Inc., Somerville, NJ), or it may be oversewn.

Following completion of the proximal anastomosis, tunnels are formed from both groins back into the retroperitoneal cavity for passage of the femoral limbs of the graft. Long curved clamps are introduced at the femoral incision sites and advanced underneath the inguinal ligament, coursing along the common iliac artery to the aortic bifurcation. The retroperitoneal cavity remains supported by the mechanical lift, allowing the surgeon to direct the tunneling clamp into the endoscopic periaortic cavity. When the tips of the clamp enter the endoscopic cavity, they are used to grasp the distal end of the bifurcated graft and pull each limb out to the femoral anastomotic site. The distal anastomoses are completed in the customary open fashion.

Use of a gasless technique is imperative in endoscopic aortic reconstruction, as it allows the vascular control essential to this potentially hazardous procedure. Mechanical lifting allows conventional vascular clamps to be applied for secure aortic occlusion. Unanticipated bleeding may be controlled by application of direct pressure using surgical clamps or sponge sticks, maneuvers which

are difficult to perform through trocar ports in the presence of gas insufflation. High-flow suction aspiration may be used to clear the field of blood without loss of visualization or loss of the operating cavity, and saline irrigation may be used liber-ally. Once abdominal lifting and peritoneal retraction have established a stable operating field, the remainder of the procedure may proceed without concern for fluctuations in the working space due to gas leakage. The most difficult portion of the procedure, anastomotic suture of the proximal end of the graft, is aided by the ability to apply vascular needle-holders in an endoscopic environment.

Lumbar Discectomy and Spinal Fusion

This procedure is generally a cooperative effort between the vascular surgeon and the spinal surgeon. Formation of the retroperitoneal cavity is performed by the vascular surgeon, with identification of the aorta, vena cava, and iliac vessels. This is done through a single flank incision, which accommodates the lifting fan retractor, the balloon retractor, and the endoscope. A second incision is made medial to the first incision, to admit a vessel retractor and various spinal instruments. The aortic bifurcation and iliac vessels are isolated and retracted medially to allow the spinal surgeon to safely access the anterior spine. Fibers of the iliopsoas muscle overlying the spine are retracted using periosteal elevators, to expose the anterior longitudinal ligament, which is incised using a long-handled scalpel. A Steinmann pin is inserted into the disc space, and operative fluoroscopy is used to confirm the level of the repair. Lumbar segmental vessels that appear in the field of dissection are isolated using right angled clamps, ligated with the right angled laparoscopic clip-applier, and transected with scissors or endoscopic shears. In the lumbosacral region, the median sacral artery may be ligated and transected in a similar manner. Conventional open spinal instruments are used to perform the discectomy. Pituitary rongeurs and curets excise the disc in a fashion similar to that used in open discectomy, and osteotomes are used to prepare adjacent vertebral surfaces to receive the implant.

Anterior fusion may be performed using any of a number of implants, including cortical femoral allograft packed with cancellous autograft harvested from the iliac crest, titanium cages filled with harvested autograft, or implants impregnated with prosthetic bone substitutes. The placement of a few of these implants requires a true anterior approach, while the majority may be inserted via an anterolateral incision. Access via a true anterior approach requires dissection of the peritoneum as far medial as the linea alba. This may be performed from the retroperitoneal cavity, with the laparoscope angled upwards to identify the peritoneal reflection, followed by dissection of the peritoneal edge towards the midline using an endoscopic Kittner probe.

BERG discectomy and fusion allows the spinal surgeon to repair the spine from an anterior approach, using familiar spinal instruments to simplify an otherwise difficult laparoscopic endeavor. The retroperitoneal approach enables repairs at multiple levels, and concomitant repairs at the L4–5 and L5–S1 levels are routinely performed. The approach described above was used in over 100 patients between September 1995 and May 1997.[42] A gasless environment offers the same benefits in terms of vascular control as those cited above for endoscopic aortobifemoral bypass surgery. The proximity of the spine to the great vessels renders this control necessary, as inadvertent vascular injuries sometimes occur during the application of bulky spinal hard-ware. A gasless approach helps circumvent these potential complications.

DISCUSSION

Gasless laparoscopy, which was initially used in simple procedures such as laparoscopic cholecystectomy, today has broader applications to increasingly sophisticated techniques. With some of the more demanding procedures such as aortic or spinal reconstruction, mechanical lifting may be the technology that allows once-challenging endoscopic procedures to be more easily accomplished on a routine basis.

Gasless laparoscopy has both benefits and disadvantages. Disadvantages include truncated exposure on the sides of the abdominal cavity, and loss of the compressive effect of insufflation that helps counteract bowel distention. These disadvantages relate to the means used to establish the laparoscopic operating cavity. With gasless laparoscopy, increased preparation must occur at the beginning of the procedure, to ensure that adequate endoscopic visualization and operative exposure are present before proceeding with surgical dissection. If an effort is made to carefully prepare the operative cavity through proper placement of the abdominal lifting retractor, proper patient tilt and position, and ancillary bowel retraction, the remainder of the gasless procedure should go smoothly. The benefits of gasless laparoscopy include manipulation of standard open surgical instruments through valveless incisions, accommodation of multiple instruments in each abdominal entry site, the ability to liberally use irrigation and aspiration as well as digital palpation, the ability to tighten knots intra-abdominally, and an enhanced ability to remove large masses of tissue through small incisions.

Gasless retroperitoneal endoscopic surgery appears to be promising as a technique for operating on structures that are difficult to access via a transabdominal route. The use of the balloon-dissected peritoneum to contain bowel for simple retraction using one or two inflatable retractors significantly reduces the time spent controlling bowel and achieving exposure of retroperitoneal organs. Vascular, urologic, and orthopedic procedures become simpler through use of gasless retroperitoneal surgery, facilitated by a team of a laparoscopic surgeon and a surgical specialist. More sophisticated techniques for obtaining surgical exposure are required for these procedures, including a combination of balloon dissection and balloon retraction in addition to mechanical abdominal lifting.

To sum up, gasless laparoscopy has evolved from simple beginnings using single-point lifting and wire suspension techniques to multistep procedures involving peritoneal dissection and displacement, that make possible more complex surgical procedures that require more delicate surgical control. Expanded uses for gasless endoscopic surgery will be found as a result of continuing technical advancements and surgical innovations are discovered. These advancements will affect all areas of the many surgical subspecialties, leading to less invasive procedures and increased comfort and benefits to the patient.

REFERENCES

1. Gazayerli MM. The Gazayerli endoscopic retractor model 1. *Surg Laparosc Endosc.* 1991;1:98.
2. Semm K, Lehmann-Willenbrock E. Pelvioscopy and laparoscopy without overpressure—the aspiration pneumoperitoneum. In: Paolucci V, Schaeff B, eds. *Gasless Laparoscopy in General Surgery and Gynecology.* Thieme:1996.
3. Francois Y, Mouret P. Suspenseur de paroi et coeliochirurgie. *J Chir. (Paris)* 1992;129:492.
4. Kitano S, Tomikawa M, Iso Y, et al. A safe and simple method to maintain a clear field of vision during laparoscopic cholecystectomy. *Surg Endosc.* 1992;6:197.
5. Schaeff B. Abdominal wall lifting systems in laparoscopy. In: Paolucci V, Schaeff B, eds. *Gasless Laparoscopy in General Surgery and Gynecology.* Thieme:1996.
6. Nagai H, Inabo T, Kamiya S, et al. A new method of laparoscopic cholecystectomy: an abdominal wall lifting technique without pneumoperitoneum. *Surg Laparosc Endosc.* 1991;1:26.
7. Hashimoto D, Nayeem SA, Kajiwara S, et al. Laparoscopic cholecystectomy: A new approach without pneumoperitoneum. *Surg Endosc.* 1993;7:54.
8. Chin AK, Moll FH, McColl MB, et al. Mechanical peritoneal retraction as a replacement for carbon dioxide pneumoperitoneum. *J Am Assoc Gynecol Laparosc.* 1993;1:62.
9. Gutt CN, Daume J, Schaeff B, et al. Systems and instruments for laparoscopic surgery without pneumoperitoneum. *Surg Endosc.* 1997;11:868.
10. Leuzinger J, Nussbaumer P, Blessing H. The laparo-hook for use in gas-free laparoscopy. *Swiss Surg.* 1997;3:3.
11. Myles PS. Bradyarrhythmias and laparoscopy: A prospective study of heart rate changes with laparoscopy. *Aust NZ Obstet Gynaecol.* 1991;31:171.
12. Motew M, Ivankovich AD, Bieniarz J, et al. Cardiovascular effects and acid-base and blood gas changes during laparoscopy. *Am J Obstet Gynecol.* 1973;115:1002.
13. Doyle DJ, Mark PW. Laparoscopy and vagal arrest. *Anesthesiology* 1989;44:448.
14. Clark CC, Weeks DB, Gusdon JP. Venous carbon dioxide embolism during laparoscopy. *Anesth Analg.* 1977;56:650.
15. Yacoub OF, Cardona I, Coveler LA, et al. Carbon dioxide embolism during laparoscopy. *Anesthesiology* 1982;57:533.
16. Beebe DS, McNevin MP, Crain JM, et al. Evidence of venous stasis after abdominal insufflation for laparoscopic cholecystectomy. *Surg Gynecol Obstet.* 1993;176;443.
17. Barnett RB, Gordon S, Drizin GS, et al. Pulmonary changes after laparoscopic cholecystectomy. *Surg Laparosc Endosc.* 1992;2:125.
18. Pascual JB, Baranda MM, Tarrero MT, et al. Subcutaneous emphysema, pneumomediastinum, bilateral pneumothorax and pneumopericardium after laparoscopy. *Endoscopy* 1990;22:59.
19. Putensen-Himmer G, Putensen C, Lammer H, et al. Comparison of postoperative respiratory function after laparoscopy or open laparotomy for cholecystectomy. *Anesthesiology* 1992;77:675.
20. Brown DR, Fishburne JI, Roberson VO, et al. Ventilatory and blood gas changes during laparoscopy with local anesthesia. *Am J Obstet Gynecol.* 1976;124:741.
21. Holzman M, Sharp K, Richards W. Hypercarbia during carbon dioxide gas insufflation for therapeutic laparoscopy: a note of caution. *Surg Laparosc Endosc.* 1992;2:11.
22. Kent RB. Subcutaneous emphysema and hypercarbia following laparoscopic cholecystectomy. *Arch Surg.* 1991;126:1154.
23. Pearce DJ. Respiratory acidosis and subcutaneous emphysema during laparoscopic cholecystectomy. *Can J Anaesth.* 1994;41:314.
24. Tsoi EKM, Organ CH Jr. Abdominal wall lifting devices as alternatives to pneumoperitoneum. *Semin Laparosc Surg.* 1995;2:205.
25. Nagai H, Kondo Y, Yasuda T, et al. An abdominal wall-lift method of laparoscopic cholecystectomy without pneumoperitoneal insufflation. *Surg Laparosc Endosc.* 1993;3:175.
26. Kitano S, Iso Y, Tomikawa M, et al. A prospective randomized trial comparison of pneumoperitoneum and U-shaped retractor elevation for laparoscopic cholecystectomy. *Surg Endosc.* 1993;7:311.
27. Hashimoto D. Abdominal wall lifting in laparoscopic cholecystectomy: Subcutaneous wiring and adjustable plate lifting. In: Paolucci V, Schaeff B, eds. *Gasless Laparoscopy in General Surgery and Gynecology.* Thieme:1996.
28. Paolucci V. Cholecystectomy. In: Paolucci V, Schaeff B, eds. *Gasless Laparoscopy in General Surgery and Gynecology.* Thieme:1996.
29. Redwine DB, Sharpe DR. Laparoscopic segmental resection of the sigmoid colon for endometriosis. *J Laparoendosc Surg.* 1991;1:217.

30. Cooperman AM, Katz B, Zimmon D, et al. Laparoscopic colon resection: A case report. *J Laparoendosc Surg*. 1991;1:221.

31. Quattlebaum X Jr., Flanders HD, Usher CH III. Laparoscopically assisted colectomy. *Surg Laparosc Endosc*. 1993;3:81.

32. Wittich PH, Marquet RL, Kazemeier G, Bonjer HJ. Port-site metastases after CO_2 laparoscopy. Is aerosolization of tumor cells a pivotal factor? *Surg Endosc*. 2000;14:189.

33. Ishida H, Murata N, Yamada H, et al. Influence of trocar placement and CO_2 pneumoperitoneum on port site metastasis following laparoscopic tumor surgery. *Surg Endosc*. 2000;14:193.

34. Swanstrom LL. Gasless laparoscopic colectomy. In: Smith RS, Organ CH Jr., eds. *Gasless Laparoscopy With Conventional Instruments: The Next Phase in Minimally Invasive Surgery*. Norman Publishing:1993.

35. Reich H, DeCaprio J, McGlynn F. Laparoscopic hysterectomy. *J Gynecol Surg*. 1989;5:213.

36. Nezhat C, Winer WK, Nezhat F. Laparoscopic removal of dermoid cysts. *Obstet Gynecol*. 1989;73:278.

37. Liu CY, Paek W. Laparoscopic retropubic colposuspension (Burch procedure). *J Am Assoc Gynecol Laparosc*. 1993;1:31.

38. Pelosi MA III, Pelosi MA, Giblin S, et al. Gasless laparoscopy under epidural anesthesia for adnexal surgery in pregnancy. *Gynaecological Endosc*. 1997;6:17.

39. Chin AK, Moll FH. Balloon-assisted extraperitoneal surgery. In: Darzi A, ed. *Retroperitoneoscopy*. Isis Medical Media:1996.

40. Gaur DD. Laparoscopic operative retroperitoneoscopy: use of a new device. *J Urol*. 1992;148:1137.

41. Chin AK, Dion Y-M. Retroperitoneal laparoscopic aorto-bifemoral bypass. In: Darzi A, ed. *Retroperitoneoscopy*. Isis Medical Media:1996.

42. Thalgott JS. Personal communication. Columbia Sunrise Hospital and Medical Center, Las Vegas, NV, May 1997.

Chapter Seven ● ● ● ● ● ●

*C*losure of Mini-Incisions

JORGE CUETO-GARCÍA AND JOSÉ ANTONIO VÁZQUEZ-FRÍAS

Given the advances in laparoscopic surgery, thousands of mini-invasive procedures are carried out every year worldwide. Unfortunately, complications do occur, and port sites are a potential place for them. To date, complications related to the port closure after laparoscopic surgery have been reported in 0.23 to 6.3% of patients,[1] with hernias being the most feared. Incisional hernia is estimated to occur in 3% of major laparoscopic procedures.[2]

It is a well-known fact that suturing 10-mm and 12-mm mini-incisions can be a difficult task, particularly in obese patients, regardless of the instruments and suture materials used. Many times surgeons just close fatty tissue without incorporating the fascia, which can lead to the development of a hernia (Fig. 7–1). Other factors such as a chronic increase in pressure in the peritoneal cavity (due to weight gain, cellulitis, or bronchitis, among other factors), malnutrition, and prolonged procedures using trocars larger than 10 mm have been implicated in the etiology of laparoscopic incisional hernias.[3] Reports of several of these complications have been already published, including cases of intestinal obstruction with gangrene and peritonitis.[4–16] Recently, even herniation through 5-mm trocar incisions has been reported.[17]

The problem of herniation of bowel loops with obstruction can be complicated by the fact that many patients that had a good result of the laparoscopic procedure do not return for follow-up, and obese patients or those with a deep subcutaneous plane may not have the typical deformity (soft mass) seen in incisional hernia or the initial symptoms of a complication, such as bowel necrosis or obstruction.

A recent study[18] comparing the prevalence of incisional hernias in laparoscopic versus open surgery showed a lower (though not significant) incidence in the laparoscopic group; the literature reporting this sort of comparison is scarce. Most, but not all, port-site herniations occur in the midline.

Often, mini-incisions are closed by hand suture. In such cases the needle may break, and in an effort to recover the fragments, anesthesia time can be prolonged and costs increased if x-rays are necessary to retrieve the pieces.

In order to avoid hernia complications at the port sites, several instruments and techniques have been designed to close them.[2,19–31] Their advantages and disadvantages should be analyzed by each surgical team. Some of these devices require pneumoperitoneum and the video camera in order to verify that the invasive end of the instrument introduced into the abdomen (generally a modified needle-type of instrument) does not cause any lesion or injury. What the surgeon needs is a device with which he or she can place a suture that includes the fascial layer of the abdomen wall in a quick and safe way that will not prolong surgical time. The authors have designed a hook-type instrument (Cueto-needle; Karl Storz, Germany)[32] that satisfies the above-mentioned requirements (Fig. 7–2). Whichever instrument the surgeon decides to use, the general recommendation is to systematically suture all incisions 10 mm or larger, including the fascia, and attempt to do the same with 5-mm incisions.

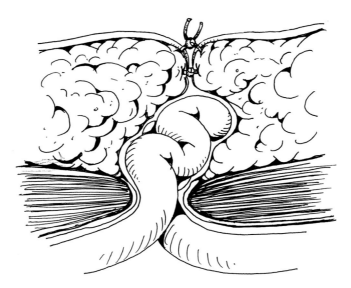

Figure 7–1. Poor wound closure. A loop of bowel that herniates through the fascial defect may not be apparent on inspection, especially in obese patients.

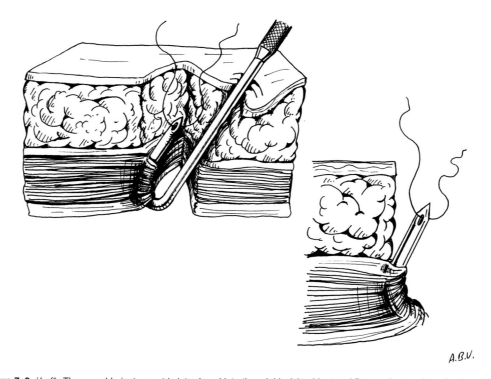

A.B.V.

Figure 7–2. (*Left*): The reusable instrument is introduced into the mini-incision blunt end first, and upward traction is applied in order to hook the fascia and thread the suture. The hook is removed and the maneuver is repeated on the other end of the incision. (*Right*): The distal part of the hook has a hole to facilitate the threading of suture. Neither pneumoperitoneum nor laparoscopy is needed

REFERENCES

1. Osama ME, Nakada SY, Wolf JF, et al. Comparative clinical study of port-closure techniques following laparoscopic surgery. *J Am Coll Surg*. 1996;183:335.
2. Chatzipapas IK, Hart RJ, Magos A. Simple technique for rectus sheath closure after laparoscopic surgery using straight needles, with review of the literature. *J Laparoendosc Adv Tech A*. 1999;9:205.
3. Coda A, Bossotti M, Ferri F, et al. Incisional hernia and fascial defect following laparoscopic surgery. *Surg Laparosc Endosc*. 2000; 10:34.
4. Bourke JB. Small intestinal obstruction from a Richter's hernia at the site of insertion of a laparoscope. *Br Med J*. 1977;2:1393.
5. Mealy K, Hylar J. Small bowel obstruction following laparoscopic cholecystectomy. *Eur J Surg*. 1991;157:675.
6. Larson GM, Vitale GC, Casry J, et al. Multipractice analysis of laparoscopic cholecystectomy in 1983 patients. *Am J Surg*. 1992;163:221.
7. The Southern Surgeons Club. A prospective analysis of 1518 laparoscopic cholecystectomies. *N Engl J Med*. 1991;324:1073.
8. Nord HJ. Complications of laparoscopy. *Endoscopy* 1992;24:693.
9. Plans WJ. Laparoscopic trocar site hernias. *J Laparoendosc Surg* 1993;3:567.
10. Hass BE, Schrager RE. Small bowel obstruction due to Richter's hernia after laparoscopic procedures. *J Laparoendosc Surg*. 1993;3:421.
11. Wegener ME, Chung D, Crans C, et al. Small bowel obstruction secondary to incarcerated Richter's hernia from laparoscopic hernia repair. *J Laparoendosc Surg*. 1993;3:173.
12. Jenkins DM, Paluzzi M, Scott TE. Postlaparoscopic small bowel obstruction. *Surg Laparosc Endosc*. 1993;3:139.
13. Patterson M, Walters D, Browder W. Postoperative bowel obstruction following laparoscopic surgery. *Am Surg* 1993;59:656.
14. Félix EL, Michas CA, McKnight RL. Laparoscopic herniorrhaphy. Transabdominal preperitoneal floor repair. *Surg Endosc*. 1994;8:100.
15. Huang ShM, Wu ChW, Lui WY. Intestinal obstruction after laparoscopic herniorrhaphy. *Surg Laparosc Endosc*. 1997;7:288.
16. Ohta J, Yamauchi Y, Yoshida Sh, et al. Laparoscopic intervention to relieve small bowel obstruction following laparoscopic herniorrhaphy. *Surg Laparosc Endosc*. 1997;7:464.
17. Eltabbakh GH. Small bowel obstruction secondary to herniation through a 5 mm laparoscopic trocar site following laparoscopic lymphadenectomy. *Eur J Gynaecol Oncol*. 1999;20:275.
18. Sanz-Lopez R, Martinez-Ramos C, Nunez-Pena JR, et al. Incisional hernias after laparoscopic vs. open cholecystectomy. *Surg Endosc*. 1999;13:922.
19. Hampel N, Selzman AA. A new technique for closing abdominal fascial openings after laparoscopic surgery. *Surg Laparosc Endosc*. 1994; 4:436.
20. Carter JE. A new technique of fascial closure for laparoscopic incisions. *J Laparoendosc Surg* 1994;4:143.
21. Jager RM. Safe repair of umbilical fascial wounds after laparoscopy. *J Laparoendosc Surg* 1994;4:199.
22. Monk BJ, Gordon NS, Johnsrud JM, et al. Closure of fascial incisions made at the time of laparoscopy: development of a device. *J Laparoendosc Surg*. 1994;4:257.
23. Grice OD, Garzotto MG, Newman RC, et al. Closure of laparoscopic trocar sites using spring loaded needles. *J Urol*. 1994;151:462A.
24. Berguer RA. A technique for full thickness closure of laparoscopic trocar sites. *J Am Coll Surg*. 1995;180:227.
25. Weiland DE, Cheung P, Heilbron MJ. An inexpensive, quick, and easily learned technique for closure of abdominal trocar wounds after laparoscopy. *J Am Coll Surg*. 1995;180:224.
26. Nadler RB, McDougall EM, Bullock AD, et al. Fascial closure of laparoscopic port sites: a new technique. *Urology* 1995;45:1046.
27. Rumstadt B, Sturm J, Jentschura D, et al. Trocar incision and closure: daily problems in laparoscopic procedures—A new technical aspect. *Surg Laparosc Endosc*. 1997;7:345.
28. Critchlow JT. Trocar site closure: a simple, inexpensive technique. *JSLS*. 1997;1:273.
29. Hasson HM. Laparoscopic cannula cone with means for cannula stabilization and wound closure. *J Am Assoc Gynecol Laparosc*. 1998;5:183.
30. Chapman WH III. Trocar site closure: a new and easy technique. *J Laparoendosc Adv Surg Tech A*. 1999;9:499.
31. Petrakis I, Sciacca V, Chalkiadakis G, et al. A simple technique for trocar site closure after laparoscopic surgery. *Surg Endosc* 1999;13:1249.
32. Cueto J, Weber A. A simple and safe technique for closure of trocar wounds using a new instrument. *Surg Laparosc Endosc* 1996;6:392.

Chapter Eight ∎ ∎ ∎ ∎ ∎ ∎

*T*raining and Credentialing in Laparoscopic Surgery

WON WOO KIM and MICHEL GAGNER

LAPAROSCOPIC SURGERY FOR SURGICAL RESIDENCY TRAINING

Laparoscopic operations are a primary component of general surgery. Opportunities to perform laparoscopic operations currently vary widely among surgical training programs. As utilization of minimal access procedures increases in the future, residents will more readily learn the skills necessary to safely accomplish these operations.

General concepts for training in laparoscopic surgery should consist of (1) laparoscopic operations comprise a core component of general surgery; (2) training of general surgeons in laparoscopic surgery should occur within the 5 years of general surgery residency; (3) general surgical training should include a number of basic laparoscopic operations (diagnostic laparoscopy, laparoscopic cholecystectomy, and laparoscopic appendectomy); (4) advanced laparoscopic operations are a scarce commodity in most general surgical residency programs. Advanced laparoscopic operations should not, at this time, be designated as a separate category (postresidency program); (5) program directors should be granted the flexibility to focus the residency experience in advanced laparoscopic surgery on those individuals who are committed to a career in general surgery.

CURRICULUM GUIDELINES IN ADVANCED LAPAROSCOPIC SURGERY

Basic laparoscopic operations include laparoscopic cholecystectomy, laparoscopic appendectomy, and diagnostic laparoscopy. All other laparoscopic operations are defined as advanced. Prior to learning or performing advanced laparoscopic operations, the resident must be familiar with and experienced in basic laparoscopy.

Laparoscopic operations, as with all operations, are appropriately learned in the broad context of surgical science and practice. Critical educational components include: pathophysiology of disease, diagnosis, operative indications and contraindications, familiarity with alternative treatments, comprehensive principles of pre- and postoperative care and understanding of the prevention, diagnosis, and treatment of complications. In addition, the relative advantages and disadvantages of both open and minimal access approaches must be known.

SKILLS ACQUISITION FOR ADVANCED LAPAROSCOPIC OPERATIONS

Training to learn advanced laparoscopic operations begins with acquisition of skills in basic laparoscopy. There is a core group of technical skills common to all advanced laparoscopic operations. Such skills are best acquired in the operating room or alternatively, through skills laboratories involving surgical trainers, animal models, or other simulated operating conditions. Examples of such skills include two-handed dissection, intracorporeal suturing, and intra- and extracorporeal knot tying. Mastery of these advanced laparoscopic skills by the resident is encouraged prior to initiating the performance of advanced laparoscopic operations. Experience in the performance of a specific operation via celiotomy will also facilitate mastery of the similar laparoscopic procedure using a minimal access approach.

Since many advanced laparoscopic skills are common to all advanced laparoscopic operations, experience in a specific operation enhances the acquisition of skills necessary to perform others. Therefore it is the combined experience in advanced procedures that should be emphasized during training, rather than the mastery of any one individual procedure.

METHODS TO INTEGRATE ADVANCED LAPAROSCOPY TRAINING INTO GENERAL SURGERY RESIDENCY

Residents should ultimately learn these procedures in the operating room under the direction of skilled faculty instructors. Until such time as complete integration is possible, we believe the following measures can help accomplish this goal:

- Train faculty;
- Train residents;
- Provide guidelines for postresidency training for prospective faculty.

Faculty Training

Courses. Hands-on courses are useful for conveying the techniques of laparoscopic operations to those who are proficient in similar open operations. Faculty members interested in obtaining advanced laparoscopic training may benefit from advanced laparoscopic courses.

Faculty Mentoring. Faculty who have already acquired the fundamental skills in advanced laparoscopic surgery and who desire to learn a new or modified laparoscopic operation will benefit from observing and interacting with a peer who is skilled and accomplished in that specific operation.

Fellowships. Postgraduate training in advanced laparoscopic surgery is another means by which faculty or faculty candidates may obtain experience. Such programs should not detract from the experience of surgical residency training where they co-exist.

Resident Training

Courses. Courses in advanced laparoscopic procedures are one method of introducing skills. Appropriate candidates for such courses are:

- Residents who plan a career in general surgery;
- Residents who have already achieved a mastery of basic laparoscopic surgery;
- Residents who are unlikely, based on their program's current practice patterns, to obtain significant experience in advanced laparoscopic surgical techniques;
- Faculty from programs that do not have faculty to teach the procedure in question may elect to send a faculty member to the course.

Skills Labs. The creation of inanimate and animal training facilities in individual programs is encouraged to provide supplemental teaching of advanced laparoscopic surgical skills.

Needs Assessment

Reexamination of Residency Training. Optimal training in a general surgery residency should include adequate experience in both advanced open and laparoscopic procedures. Data suggest that the case load is insufficient to provide such an experience. The appropriate leadership organizations should consider reexamining the flexibility of the general surgery residency training in order to optimize the availability of such advanced cases for residents planning a career in general surgery.

Educational Resources. These include postgraduate courses, annual meetings, a video library, and guidelines for credentialing, training, and standards of practice.

POSTRESIDENCY LAPAROSCOPIC SURGERY TRAINING

Objective

The primary purpose of postresidency laparoscopic surgical education is to ensure safe, high-quality patient care.

Definitions

Some of the terms used here were carefully selected to indicate the relative weight attached to each statement.

- **Must or shall:** Indicates a mandatory or indispensable recommendation.
- **Should:** Indicates a highly desirable recommendation.
- **May or could:** Indicates an optional recommendation; alternatives may be appropriate.
- **Competence:** Competence is defined as the minimum level of skill, knowledge, and/or expertise, derived through training and experience, required to safely and proficiently perform a task or procedure.
- **Credentials:** Documents provided following successful completion of a period of education or training.
- **Clinical privileges:** Authorization by a local institution (usually hospital) to perform a particular procedure.
- **Pretest:** A quantifiable examination of a trainee's level of clinical knowledge, manual skills, or technical proficiency prior to commencing a training course.
- **Posttest:** A quantifiable examination of a trainee's level of clinical knowledge, manual skills, or technical proficiency upon completion of a training course.

Policy Statements

Use of Inanimate Training Models. Inanimate, ex vivo models or simulators may be preferable to animate models. Animate models may be necessary to simulate clinical situations when teaching certain surgical skills or techniques.

Educational Grants. Educational grants provided by industry or other organizations or sources, to support any educational program, course, skills laboratory, or preceptorship must be clearly noted in promotional and educational materials.

Investigational Procedure. A procedure is considered investigational if it has not been accepted into clinical practice, has not been critically assessed in peer-reviewed medical literature, and has not been presented and discussed at suitable scientific meetings. By contrast, a procedure is not investigational if sufficient studies are available to prove its efficacy and safety.

Surgical progress would be impeded if every surgical innovation were required to be tested by randomized trials prior to clinical use. The surgeon should use his or her judgment to determine when such study is appropriate. Introduction of an investigational procedure may, however, require the approval of the appropriate institutional review board (IRB). Self-training in new procedures must take place on a background of basic surgical skills. The surgeon should recognize when and how much additional training in each new procedure is necessary.

Certification. Successful completion of any one or more training components or objectives does not necessarily signify an individual's clinical competence in a specific procedure or technique.

Components of Postresidency Surgical Education

Basic Training. Completion of an Accreditation Council for Graduate Medical Education (ACGME) accredited surgical residency training program in surgery is mandatory. International medical graduates must have satisfied additional requirements to secure licensure.

Courses

Definition. A course is a limited period of instruction with defined objectives designed to educate participants in clinical skills, techniques, or procedures. Course structure and duration may vary according to the course objectives.

Objectives. The course must have a stated set of objectives. The objectives must be defined as tasks, successful completion of which can be quantitatively and qualitatively assessed.

Qualifications of Faculty. The course director and the faculty members must have appropriate clinical and/or laboratory expertise to educate participants in the stated objectives. When clinical procedures are taught, instructors must have clinical experience in those procedures. The course must have a written policy on disclosure of faculty-industry relationships, according to ACCME/AMA guidelines, and an appropriate ratio of faculty to participants.

Qualifications of Participants. Participants should have appropriate fundamental knowledge, skills, and clinical experience relevant to course content in order to meet the stated objectives by the course's conclusion.

Site/Operations. A course site must be physically adequate to meet the stated objectives and to accommodate the course's enrollment. A course may be conducted at an industry facility, provided it is operated in affiliation with a hospital, medical institution, university, or medical association that is qualified to grant continuing medical education (CME) credits.

Curriculum. A course must contain didactic instruction in the following areas as they may apply to the stated objectives:

- Patient selection;
- Indications and contraindications;
- Instrumentation;
- Techniques;
- Documentation;
- Pre- and postoperative care;
- Follow-up;
- Outcome;
- Self-assessment exercises;
- Complications and their avoidance and treatment;
- Course evaluations according to ACCME essentials;
- Components that should be included are printed materials (syllabus, reprints, bibliography), and pre- and posttesting;

- Components that may be included are practice on inanimate models, practice on animate tissues and organs, animate laboratory instruction/practice, video instruction/practice, procedure observation, and simulator models.

In the future, skills may also be developed using simulation technology (e.g., virtual reality scenarios). The use of telemedicine technology may also play a role in skill development.

Endorsement. Course directors should provide continuing medical education (CME) credits and/or obtain endorsement by appropriate medical organizations.

Documentation. Documentation for certain courses consisting of only didactic instruction may consist of verification of attendance.

Skills Laboratories

Definition. A facility in which a practicing physician acquires, refines, or improves his or her ability to perform specific medical and surgical tasks or procedures. Skills are the foundation upon which procedures are constructed. A skills laboratory may teach one skill or the entire set of skills required to perform a procedure. A skills laboratory is usually a continuing resource that can be revisited.

Mission Statement. Every skills laboratory must have a mission statement defining objectives, curriculum, eligibility for training, and an evaluation process.

Objectives. The skills laboratory must have a set of objectives. The objectives must be defined as tasks which can be quantitatively and qualitatively assessed.

Qualifications of Faculty. Faculty must have comprehensive practical and teaching experience in the skills outlined in the curriculum.

The skills laboratory director has the overall responsibility for setting objectives, curriculum development, faculty and staff appointment, and development of evaluation criteria. There must be an appropriate ratio of faculty to trainees in order to assure that progress is made and to enable documentation of achievement of objectives.

Qualifications of Trainees. The skills laboratory must define eligibility for participation. The trainee must have appropriate background knowledge, basic skills, and clinical experience relevant to the tasks to be learned.

Site/Operations. The skills laboratory may be located at an industrial site that is operated in affiliation with an organization which is qualified to grant CME credits.

Curriculum. There must be a curriculum statement that should include a list of tasks, definitions of skill levels, and a defined method of progressing from one skill level to the next. The curriculum must also include the learning components and their requirements. The curriculum may also include use and maintenance of medical instruments and equipment.

Appropriate components of a skills laboratory may include, but are not limited to:

- Inanimate model practice;
- Ex vivo and simulator models;

- Videotapes;
- Audio tapes;
- CD-ROM;
- An interactive computer program;
- Self-assessment exercises.

Clinical case observation or clinical tapes may be used to reinforce the principles learned. In the future, skills may also be developed using simulation technology such as virtual reality scenarios and/or telesurgery or teleconferencing.

Duration of Training. The duration of training is not fixed but should be determined by the participants' mastery of the requisite skills. The trainee may demonstrate these by passing the posttest(s). The duration may also be determined by needs assessment and evaluations completed by past participants.

Assessment. The posttest should quantitatively and qualitatively evaluate the participant's acquisition of skills as defined by the program's objectives. The curriculum may be modified based on the performance during participation in the skills laboratory curriculum. Such modifications may include a series of exercises, tasks, or maneuvers which can be learned and later practiced outside the laboratory.

Documentation. The instructor or laboratory director must document mastery of the defined objectives and provide both qualitative and quantitative descriptions of the trainees' experiences.

Preceptorship

Definitions

Preceptorship. An individual educational program in which the physician acquires additional skills and/or judgment to improve his or her performance of specific medical or surgical techniques and/or procedures. The preceptorship should define eligibility for participation.

Preceptor. An expert surgeon who undertakes to impart his or her clinical knowledge and skills in a defined setting to a preceptee. The preceptor must be appropriately privileged, skilled, and experienced in the procedures and techniques in question. In order to serve as a preceptor in a specific procedure or technique, the surgeon (preceptor) must be a recognized authority (e.g., via publications, presentations, or extensive clinical experience) in the particular field of expertise.

Preceptee/Trainee. A surgeon with appropriate basic knowledge and experience seeking individual training in skills and/or procedures not learned in prior formal training. The trainee must have the appropriate background knowledge, basic skills, and clinical experience relevant to the proposed curriculum. The trainee should be board eligible or certified in the appropriate specialty or possess equivalent board certification from outside the United States.

Objectives. The preceptorship must have stated objectives. The objectives must include a program outline and a proposed list of tasks and skills to be addressed during the training period.

Role of Preceptor. The preceptor has the overall responsibility for setting objectives, developing curriculum, overseeing instruction and practice of skills, demonstrating technique and clinical procedures, and evaluating the trainee. The preceptor has primary patient care responsibility and is obliged to supervise not only procedures in which the trainee participates, but also the appropriate perioperative care. This relationship must be reflected in the informed consent documentation.

Role of Trainee/Preceptee. The trainee must be involved in: (1) learning the skills and knowledge required to perform a technique or procedure, and (2) both preoperative and postoperative patient care. Completion of a preceptorship denotes adequate training in the patient's complete preoperative, operative, and postoperative care.

Site/Operations. The preceptorship site must have sufficient clinical material and facilities to adequately educate the trainee. The preceptorship may be operated by or in affiliation with an accredited hospital, medical institution, university, or a medical association which is qualified to grant CME credits.

Curriculum. The preceptor-trainee relationship should be analogous to residency training and include factual, technical, and judgmental components. This training is based on clinical experience; however, the experience may be supplemented with teaching tools at the preceptor's discretion. Teaching aids utilized by the preceptor may include:

- Inanimate models and simulators;
- Ex vivo tissues;
- Videotapes;
- Audio and video tools;
- CD-ROM;
- An interactive computer program;
- Self-assessment exercises;
- Animate laboratories.

In the future, skills may also be developed using simulation technology (e.g., virtual reality scenarios). Telementoring may also be used as an adjunct for skill development.

Documentation. The preceptor must document in writing both qualitative and quantitative descriptions of the trainees' experiences. This should include skills acquired and the number of procedures in which the trainee assisted or served as primary operator. Documentation stating that the procedures were satisfactorily performed must be provided to the preceptee. A certificate of training should be provided by the preceptor.

Indemnity. It is the dual responsibility of the preceptor and the trainee to secure appropriate authorization and indemnity through their own institution(s) or through independent sources in order to protect the patient.

Program Assessment

Each program must regularly evaluate the degree to which its goals are being met through a formal assessment process. Such evaluation should be ongoing and systematically documented. The goal of each program should be to prepare qualified surgeons. The assessment process should include faculty evaluation by trainees.

Privileging

Credentialing/Privileging Committee. The trainee's local hospital or institutional body is charged with granting of privileges as defined by the Joint Commission on Accreditation of Healthcare

Organizations (JCAHO). In conjunction with standard JCAHO guidelines for granting hospital privileges, the structure and process remain the individual responsibility of each institution. Having completed formal residency and postresidency training, privileging guidelines may include:

- Consideration of clinical experience and postresidency training and education;
- Privileging in comparable alternative procedures;
- Appropriate ability and experience to manage common complications.

Appeals Mechanisms. As part of its responsibility, the privileging committee must establish appropriate mechanisms of appeal for individuals denied privileges.

Renewal of Privileges. Surgeons' experience and skills vary, therefore clinical privileges must be periodically re-evaluated. The hospital privileging committee must have a written policy concerning renewal of privileges. The written policy should indicate if renewal of privileges is a part of, or separate from, hospital reappointment. It is suggested that privileges be renewed every 2 years. Renewal should be contingent upon a stated level of clinical activity in specific procedures, in addition to satisfactory performance as assessed by quality assurance monitoring.

Documentation of Continuing Education. Continuing medical education related to the field should be required as part of the periodic renewal of privileges. Attendance or participation at appropriate local, national, or international meetings and courses should be encouraged and documented.

Proctoring

Definition. Traditionally, a proctor is a person who supervises or monitors students. As defined here, a proctor differs from a consultant or a preceptor in that he or she functions as an observer and evaluator, does not directly participate in patient care, and receives no fees from the patient. Proctoring may be an element of the privileging process.

Qualifications of the Proctor. A proctor must be a physician/ surgeon who has recognized proficiency or documented expertise in the specialty being proctored. The proctor should be free of perceived or actual conflicts of interest, which might create a bias in favor of or against the applicant. A proctor may work at the same or at another institution.

When a Proctor May Be Required. A proctor should be available to the privileging committee when a surgeon requests initial or extended privileges, during the review process, or for special quality assurance situations.

Proctoring Process. The proctor should always be appointed by, and serve as an agent of, the medical staff's privileging committee. The privileging committee should determine the extent of proctoring. It is the hospital's responsibility to indemnify the proctor and so advise in writing.

It may be necessary to have more than one proctor evaluate the candidate at different times. The proctor must certify the trainee's competence in the procedure's performance. The proctors' evaluations must be documented in writing and submitted directly to the privileging committee. The evaluation should include the type and number of procedures observed, and whether these were sufficient to enable the proctor to render an opinion concerning the applicant's performance. The committee should develop a formal written protocol and maintain detailed records. The proctoring document must be kept confidential.

Criteria of competency should be established in advance. These should include:

- Patient selection;
- Preoperative evaluation and preparation;
- Familiarity with instrumentation;
- Surgical skills and judgment;
- Safe, expeditious completion of the procedure;
- Postoperative plan;
- Complication avoidance.

The Proctor's Responsibility. The proctor's sole responsibility is to the medical staff's privileging committee. There must be no financial obligation to the proctor from the surgeon or the patient.

Intervention. The issue of whether and to what extent a proctor should intervene in a procedure is complex and unsettled. Certain clinical situations, or simple humanitarian concerns, may dictate that the proctor become a consultant to the applicant or actually intervene to assist in a procedure gone awry. The proctor must realize that if she or he goes beyond merely observing the procedure, she or he has undertaken a duty to the patient which can result in liability arising from sequelae of the procedure. The proctor's involvement should be disclosed on the patient's chart and in the proctor's confidential report to the privileging committee. In situations in which an applicant has an associate who holds privileges in the procedure being proctored, some hospitals have encouraged the associate to be present to assist (if necessary) in the procedure and to avoid the necessity for the proctor to become involved. The proctor may or may not be included in the patient's informed consent, recognizing that such inclusion may expose the proctor to risk beyond that of mere proctoring.

CURRICULUM GUIDELINES IN LAPAROSCOPIC SURGERY

The teaching of advanced laparoscopic surgical procedures, as with the teaching of all surgical procedures to treat pathologic conditions, is appropriately taught only in a setting of an understanding by the surgical trainee of the general principles and practice of surgical science as well as the specific pathophysiology of the disease process being treated. Without such a scientific approach to surgical therapy, its practice becomes a technical exercise only. As such, all conditions treated using laparoscopic surgical techniques should be fully understood in terms of the spectrum of disease, and the role of surgical therapy in its treatment. The indications and contraindications to performing any given procedure must be understood, as well any appropriate alternative treatment procedures and approaches. In particular, when an advanced laparoscopic procedure may be done alternatively using a traditional celiotomy approach, the surgeon-in-training must understand the relative merits of both approaches, and specific instances where one approach should be favored over another. In addition, the surgical trainee should, whenever possible, have adequate experience with and exposure to the alternative or traditional approach to the procedure that allows that approach to be a part of his or her treatment armamentarium, and allows for a safe intraoperative conversion from one approach to another should that be in the patient's best interest.

The principles of appropriate preoperative and postoperative care for a given surgical procedure, whether traditional or laparoscopic, must be mastered by the surgical resident prior to the initiation of any significant operative experience with performing that procedure. Similarly, the appreciation of potential complications is necessary, as well as their treatment.

Prior to initiating an experience with advanced laparoscopic procedures, the resident should be familiar with and experienced in basic laparoscopy and basic laparoscopic procedures. These are defined as diagnostic laparoscopy, laparoscopic cholecystectomy, and laparoscopic appendectomy. Since basic principles incorporated in the safe performance of these procedures are inherent in the similar performance of advanced procedures, a brief list and description of important aspects of these basic procedures which should be mastered during the surgical residency training are given below:

Basic Laparoscopy

Physiology of Laparoscopy

Mechanical Effects of Abdominal Distention
- Decreased lung volume;
- Higher airway pressure;
- Abdominal compartment distention.

Pharmacologic Effects of CO_2
Local effects:

- Decreased visceral blood flow;
- Decreased portal venous flow;
- Decreased venous return to heart.

Systemic effects:

- Decreased cardiac index;
- Respiratory and metabolic acidosis;
- Increased SVR, decreased PVR;
- Exacerbation of cardiac arrhythmias.

All effects are rapidly reversible and their clinical significance is unclear.

Immunologic Response to Laparoscopy
- May be different than open procedure;
- Evaluation continues.

Preoperative Patient Evaluation
- Overall physiologic performance;
- Cardiorespiratory parameters;
- Coagulation parameters;
- Abdominal factors (prior to surgery);
- Gasless laparoscopy as an alternative.

Equipment Requirements

Insufflation
- CO_2 preferred (NO_2, He, Ar, N, and others possible);
- High-flow (10 to 15 L/min) pressure valves, visible flow rates, and patient pressure monitors.

Camera
- Single/triple chip;
- Three-dimensional;
- Printers and video recorders.

Video Monitors

Light Sources
- Safety precautions to prevent thermal injury.

Laparoscopes
- Size: 10 mm to 1.4 mm (needlescopes); smaller size = less light;
- Angles (0, 24, 30, and 45 degree).

Instrumentation

Disposable vs. Reusable
- Cost, sterility, reliability, availability.

Trocars
- Hasson, shielded, versatility.

Graspers/Dissectors/Scissors
- Traumatic, atraumatic, specially-designed;
- Electrocautery-capable.

Retractors
- Size, application.

Tissue Approximation Devices
- Clip-appliers;
- Linear staplers (staple size, applications);
- Specialty devices.

Hemostatic Devices
- Monopolar cautery;
- Bipolar cautery;
- Harmonic scalpel;
- Lasers.

Suturing
- Devices;
- Pre-tied sutures;
- Needle types;
- Needle-holders.

Trocar Closure Devices

Other
- Dissecting balloons;
- Gasless abdominal wall retractors;
- Specimen containment devices.

Diagnostic Laparoscopy
The surgical resident should be knowledgeable regarding the following:

- Indications and contraindications;
- Role in diagnosing liver disease, fever of unknown origin, abdominal or pelvic pain of unknown etiology;
- Staging and assessing intra-abdominal tumors;
- Evaluating ascites;
- Selective role in penetrating and blunt trauma;
- Evaluating intestinal viability or ischemia;
- Complications specific to laparoscopy, including subcutaneous emphysema, air embolism, pneumothorax, cardiac arrhythmias, injury from Veress needle or trocar insertion to abdominal viscera, trocar-site bleeding or hematoma, and trocar-site incisional hernia;
- Methods of safe creation of a pneumoperitoneum using the Veress needle technique;

- Creating a pneumoperitoneum using an open technique with a Hasson trocar;
- Appropriate port placement principles with respect to telescope and working port relationships, including alignment of axis of telescope with monitor;
- Principles of safe organ handling using laparoscopic instruments;
- Safe techniques of enterolysis when previous surgical adhesions preclude visual assessment or access;
- Techniques of liver and other organ biopsy.

Laparoscopic Cholecystectomy

The resident must gain a firm understanding of the following:

- Indications for the procedure;
- Contraindications to the approach;
- Trocar placement;
- Appropriate exposure of infundibulum and triangle of Calot;
- Indications for intraoperative cholangiography and its safe conduct and appropriate interpretation;
- Indications for intraoperative ultrasound as an alternative or adjunctive procedure to cholangiography, and where possible its safe conduct and appropriate interpretation;
- Understanding of potential anatomic anomalies and their potential contribution to procedural complications;
- Recognition of the cystic duct/gallbladder junction;
- Technique of division of cystic artery and duct;
- Technique of dissection of gallbladder off liver bed;
- Removal of gallbladder from abdominal cavity;
- Role of the first assistant in gaining proper exposure;
- Special considerations in patients with pregnancy, severe obesity, previous upper abdominal surgery, and potential choledocholithiasis;
- Complications peculiar to laparoscopic cholecystectomy and their treatment;
- Indications for conversion to an open procedure.

Laparoscopic Appendectomy

The resident must master a firm understanding of the following:

- Indications for appendectomy and laparoscopic versus open approaches;
- Contraindications to appendectomy or the laparoscopic approach;
- Trocar placement;
- Exposure of the appendix for dissection;
- Evaluation of other potential sources of right lower quadrant abdominal pain;
- Technique of laparoscopic appendectomy using endo-loops;
- Technique of laparoscopic appendectomy using a stapler;
- Removal of appendix from the abdomen;
- Treatment of appendiceal abscess;
- Indications for conversion to an open procedure;
- Complications of the procedure and the approach and their treatment.

ADVANCED LAPAROSCOPIC PROCEDURES

Principles and Skills

The initiation of experience in advanced laparoscopic surgical procedures for the surgical trainee should only begin once the skills of basic laparoscopy have been mastered. While individual training programs will likely have a different mix of cases in which advanced laparoscopic approaches are used, there is a core group of

technical skills that should be mastered through the performance of a variety of such procedures. Such skills can be appropriately introduced and taught through preliminary, and if needed concurrent, additional skills laboratories involving surgical trainers, animal models, or other simulated operating conditions. These skills include, but are not limited to, the following:

- Two-handed surgical manipulations;
- Two-handed dissection;
- Intracorporeal suturing;
- Intra- and extracorporeal knot tying;
- Intracorporeal tissue approximation with sutures and staples;
- Achieving hemostasis after unexpected hemorrhage;
- Exposure of all intra-abdominal and retroperitoneal organs.

Mastery of these core advanced skills, coupled with adequate experience in the performance of a procedure using a traditional approach (e.g., open Nissen fundoplication) will likely allow the surgical trainee to master the particular advanced laparoscopic procedure (e.g., laparoscopic Nissen fundoplication) in a setting requiring fewer supervised or assisted cases than if those skills were not yet completely mastered before embarking on an experience with the advanced procedure.

The greater the experience of the resident in all types of advanced laparoscopic procedures, the greater the likelihood that the ability to learn and perform additional advanced procedures will occur with safety and facility. Thus it is the combined experience in advanced procedures that should be emphasized, rather than necessarily the mastery of any one individual procedure. However, it is also expected that the case mix and availability will on some occasions allow the resident a significant enough experience in one of the procedures below to serve as a basis for mastery of its performance.

Laparoscopic Inguinal Herniorrhaphy

The resident should become familiar with the following concepts and aspects of this procedure:

- Indications for performing a laparoscopic versus an open inguinal herniorrhaphy; relative advantages and disadvantages of each approach;
- Situations in which advantages are likely to outweigh disadvantages (i.e., recurrent and bilateral hernias for the laparoscopic approach);
- Methods currently used: transabdominal preperitoneal and total extraperitoneal; relative advantages and disadvantages of each approach;
- Trocar placement;
- Knowledge of inguinal anatomy from the laparoscopic view;
- Proper dissection techniques;
- Placement of prosthetic mesh and securing it appropriately in place;
- Coverage of mesh;
- Complications specific to laparoscopic herniorrhaphy and their prevention and treatment;
- Expected long-term results.

Laparoscopic Antireflux Procedures

The resident should be knowledgeable about the following aspects of these procedures:

- Indications for performing antireflux surgery;
- Interpretation of preoperative tests for GERD;

- Understanding modifications of operations based on preoperative testing;
- Expected benefits and efficacy of antireflux surgery;
- Knowledge of anatomy of the proximal gastric/distal esophageal area, including the ability to locate and easily identify major structures including both vagal trunks;
- Technical performance of the procedure, including trocar placement; division of short gastric vessels; crural and esophageal dissection; suturing diaphragmatic crura; positioning of wrap; and suturing of wrap;
- Potential intraoperative and postoperative complications, and their recognition and treatment.

Laparoscopic Gastric Surgery

The resident should be familiar with the following aspects of laparoscopic gastric surgery, with the recognition that based on current practice patterns, the experience in such procedures will likely be limited:

- Situations and diagnoses in which a laparoscopic approach to gastric resection or vagotomy is appropriate;
- Relative benefits of the laparoscopic approach in performing vagotomy or resection;
- Knowledge of the anatomy of the vagus nerves and stomach and recognition of these structures under laparoscopic conditions;
- Trocar placement and exposure;
- Mobilization and division of the gastric blood supply;
- Division of the branches of the vagus nerve;
- Division of the stomach;
- Anastomotic techniques: stapled, stapled and sewn, and sewn;
- Potential complications, operative and postoperative, especially those peculiar to a laparoscopic approach, and their diagnosis and treatment;
- Indications, preoperative selection, and appropriateness of a laparoscopic approach for selected patients undergoing bariatric surgical procedures, along with the expected operative results and potential complications;
- Techniques currently used to perform such procedures and differences from the celiotomy approach.

Laparoscopic Colon or Intestinal Resection

The resident should be familiar with the following and have a working knowledge of, and if possible a practical experience with, the following:

- Indications for performing a laparoscopic resection or procedure for pathologic conditions of the colon and small intestine;
- Appropriate indications for surgery based on the individual disease or condition;
- Role of resection, bypass, and diversion as treatment options;
- Appropriate trocar placement based on condition;
- Techniques of intestinal mobilization and exposure;
- Knowledge of the anatomy, including blood supply and retroperitoneal structures relevant to performing appropriate surgical intestinal resection;
- Dissection techniques for the bowel;
- Mesenteric vascular division techniques;
- Intestinal division techniques;
- Anastomotic techniques: intracoroporeal vs. extracorporeal;
- Anastomotic techniques: stapled vs. sewn;

- Relevant concerns of using laparoscopy for treatment of malignant conditions;
- Technique of laparoscopic creation of colostomy/ileostomy;
- Technique of laparoscopic enteroenterostomy/enterocolostomy using the above anastomotic techniques;
- Indications for surgical treatment of rectal prolapse and specific instances in which laparoscopic rectopexy is the preferred or appropriate treatment for rectal prolapse;
- Potential intraoperative and postoperative complications of laparoscopic intestinal surgery, and their recognition and treatment.

Laparoscopic Hepatobiliary Surgery (Other Than Cholecystectomy)

The resident should be exposed to laparoscopic exploration of the common bile duct, should have a working knowledge of the following, and in most cases have some hands-on experience with laparoscopic common duct exploration:

- Interpretation of cholangiography and ultrasonographic findings during laparoscopic cholecystectomy that indicate a likely presence of choledocholithiasis or bile duct pathology;
- Thorough knowledge of portal hilar anatomy and its variations;
- Technique of dilating cystic duct for transcystic exploration of the common bile duct;
- Technique of choledochoscopy and use of choledochoscopic instruments for stone clearance;
- Use of transcystic baskets and balloons for stone clearance;
- Technique of laparoscopic dissection of the portal area, including exposure of the common duct and choledochotomy;
- Laparoscopic placement of a T-tube and closure of a choledochotomy;
- Laparoscopic biliary-enteric anastomosis, including cholecysto-jejunostomy using stapled or sewn technique;
- Laparoscopic treatment of hepatic cysts, including localization using intraoperative laparoscopic ultrasound, drainage, resection, and destruction of the cyst wall or placement of omental pedicle in a cyst;
- Technique of laparoscopic use of special hepatic dissecting instruments including the ultrasonic surgical aspirator and the argon beam coagulator;
- Technique of hepatic wedge resection.

Laparoscopic Splenectomy and Adrenalectomy

The resident should become familiar with the following aspects of these solid organ removal procedures:

- Indications for performing adrenalectomy;
- Indications for using a laparoscopic approach for adrenalectomy;
- Indications for performing splenectomy;
- Indications for using a laparoscopic approach for splenectomy;
- Relevant anatomy of the spleen, especially as viewed laparoscopically from anterior and lateral positions;
- Anatomy and surrounding structures of left adrenal and right adrenal glands, including blood supply;
- Techniques for exposing left and right adrenal glands;
- Techniques for removing left and right adrenal glands, including vein ligation and division;
- Techniques for performing laparoscopic splenectomy, including division of short gastric vessels and splenic hilar vessels;
- Techniques of removal of adrenals from the abdominal cavity;

- Techniques of removal of the spleen from the abdominal cavity;
- Potential intraoperative and postoperative complications peculiar to this operation and operative approach, and their recognition and treatment.

Laparoscopic Gastrostomy and Jejunostomy

The resident should be expected to have experience with these procedures to some extent, and be fully knowledgeable regarding the following:

- Indications for performing gastrostomy or jejunostomy, and the relevant differences and preferences for each type of access;
- Contraindications to placing feeding access tubes;
- Indications for preference of using a laparoscopic approach to placing enteral access tubes;
- Trocar placement for laparoscopic gastrostomy;
- Technique of laparoscopic gastrostomy;
- Trocar placement for laparoscopic jejunostomy;
- Technique of laparoscopic jejunostomy;
- Potential intraoperative and postoperative complications arising from these procedures and their management;
- Postoperative management of enteral access tubes.

CREDENTIALING OF SURGEONS IN LAPAROSCOPIC SURGERY

Principles of Credentialing

There is a need for surgeons to be proficient in emerging and evolving technologies. In the course of patient care, surgeons need to accurately identify anatomy and pathologic processes. Evolving technologies in laparoscopic surgery, including endoscopic surgery, are a natural extension of the surgeon's capability to adequately evaluate these critical factors in patient care. In surgical training, all surgeons obtain extensive exposure to understanding of the spatial relationship of organs, vasculature, and lymphatics in the peritoneal and thoracic cavities. Over the course of a 5-year residency, the surgeon additionally obtains intensive experience in pathophysiology, natural history, and management (both medical and surgical) of the many disease processes affecting the gastrointestinal system. This background of extensive hands-on experience with the organs and pathology involved will greatly facilitate surgeons' incorporation of these new advanced techniques into their practice.

Purpose. The purpose of this is to assist hospital credentialing committees in their task of granting privileges to surgeons for the performance of laparoscopic surgical techniques, in conjunction with the standard JCAHO guidelines for granting hospital privileges.

Uniformity of Standards. Uniform standards that are applicable to all surgeons should be developed by the credentialing committee. Criteria must be established that are medically sound, and not unusually stringent, taking into account the skills a surgeon already possesses as part of his or her surgical training.

Responsibility for Credentialing. The credentialing structure and process are the responsibility of each hospital. It should be the responsibility of the department of surgery, through its chief, to recommend individual surgeons for privileges in laparoscopic surgery as for other procedures performed by members of his or her department.

Guidelines for Credentialing

In the United States, there are no nationally accepted standards for the credentialing of surgeons in laparoscopic surgery. However, the Society of Gastrointestinal Endoscopic Surgeons has helped to develop basic guidelines for granting privileges to surgeons in advanced laparoscopic techniques. This is a summary of their statement of guidelines: (1) The practicing surgeon may recognize, or a privileging committee may mandate, when additional formal education is required. Examples include a procedure new to the surgical community at large or new to part of the surgeon's current repertoire; (2) The components of training must result in a surgeon who is comfortable performing a new procedure; (3) Training must be uniformly structured to provide sufficient information to objectively document the results of training. Hospital accreditation committees are beginning to use such guidelines to grant privileges in the more advanced, less common laparoscopic procedures. Just as with other advanced surgical procedures, complex advanced laparoscopic procedures should be performed by surgeons with advanced laparoscopic training.

ADDITIONAL READING

1. Airan MC. Effectiveness of strict credentialing and proctoring guidelines on outcomes of laparoscopic cholecystectomy in a community hospital. *Surg Endosc.* 1994;8:196.
2. Arregui ME, Fitzgibbons RJ Jr., Katkhourda N, et al. *Principles of Laparoscopic Surgery—Basic and Advanced Techniques.* Springer-Verlag:1995.
3. American Society of Gastrointestinal Endoscopy. Proctoring and hospital endoscopy privileges. *Gastrointest Endosc.* 1991;37:666.
4. Azziz R. Operative endoscopy: The pressing need for a structured training and credentialing process [editorial]. *Fertil Steril.* 1992;58:1100.
5. Barnes RW, Lang NP, Whiteside MF. Halstedian technique revisited. Innovations in teaching surgical skills. *Ann Surg.* 1989;210:118.
6. Berci G, Cuschieri A. *Practical Laparoscopy.* Bailliere Tindall:1986.
7. Brooks DC. *Current Review of Laparoscopy*, 2nd ed. Current Medicine:1995.
8. Chekan EG, Pappas TN. *Textbook of Surgery: Minimally Invasive Surgery.* WB Saunders:2001.
9. Cuschieri A, Berci G. *Laparoscopic Biliary Surgery.* Blackwell (Mosby, Philadelphia):1990.
10. Dent TL, Strodel WE, Turcotte JG. *Surgical Endoscopy.* Year Book Medical Publishers:1985.
11. Dent TL. Training, credentialing, and granting of clinical privileges for laparoscopic general surgery. *Am J Surg.* 1991;161:399.
12. Dent TL. Training, credentialing, and evaluation in laparoscopic surgery. *Surg Clin North Am.* 1992;72:1003.
13. Greene FL, Ponsky JL. *Endoscopic Surgery.* WB Saunders:1994.
14. Hunter JG, Sackier JM. *Minimally Invasive Surgery.* McGraw-Hill:1993.
15. Joint Commission on Accreditation of Health Care Organizations. *The 1993 Joint Commission Accreditation Manual for Hospitals.* JCAHO:1992.
16. Lewis BS, Pace WD. Qualitative and quantitative methods for the assessment of clinical preceptors. *Fam Med.* 1990;22:356.
17. Pennsylvania Medical Society, Hospital Medical Staff Section. New procedure credentialing protocol, 1994.

18. Peters JH, DeMeester TR. *Minimally Invasive Surgery of the Foregut.* Quality Medical:1994.

19. Pickleman J, Schueneman AL, et al. Legal interfaces in tele-medicine technology. *Military Med.* 1996;161:280.

20. Ponsky JL. *Atlas of Surgical Endoscopy.* Mosby Year Book:1992.

21. Rosser JC, Wood M, Payne JH, et al. Telementoring: A practical option in surgical training. *Surg Endosc.* 1997;11:852.

22. Schueneman AL, Pickleman J, Freeark RJ. Age, gender, lateral dominance, and prediction of operative skill among general surgery residents. *Surgery* 1985;98:506.

23. Schulam PG, Docimo SG, Saleh W, et al. TeleSurgical mentoring. Initial clinical experience. *Surg Endosc.* 1997;11:1001.

24. Scott-Conner CE. Laparoscopic surgery. *Surg Clin North Am.* 1996; 76:437.

25. Society of American Gastrointestinal Endoscopic Surgeons (SAGES). *Granting of Privileges for Gastrointestinal Endoscopy by Surgeons.* SAGES:1992.

26. Society of American Gastrointestinal Endoscopic Surgeons (SAGES). Guidelines for submission of continuing medical education seeking SAGES endorsement for courses in laparoscopic surgery. *Surg Endosc.* 1993;7:372.

27. Society of American Gastrointestinal Endoscopic Surgeons (SAGES). Framework for post-residency surgical education and training—A SAGES guideline. *Surg Endosc.* 1994;8:1137.

28. Society of American Gastrointestinal Endoscopic Surgeons (SAGES). Guideline for the Granting of Endoscopic Ultrasonography Privileges for Surgery—A SAGES Guideline. SAGES:1996.

29. Society of American Gastrointestinal Endoscopic Surgeons (SAGES). Guidelines for the surgical practice of tele-medicine. *Surg Endosc.* 1997;11:789.

30. Statement on emerging surgical technologies and the evaluation of credentials. *Bull Am Coll Surg.* 1994;79:40.

31. Toouli J, Gossot D, Hunter JG. *Endosurgery.* Churchill Livingstone:1996.

32. Zucker KA, Bailey RW, Graham SM, et al. Training for laparoscopic surgery. *World J Surg.* 1993;17:3.

33. Zucker KA. *Surgical Laparscopy Update.* Quality Medical Publishing:1993.

Chapter Nine ■ ■ ■ ■ ■ ■

Experimental Animal Models in Laparoscopy

LAURENT BIERTHO, MICHEL GAGNER, JORGE CUETO-GARCÍA, JOSÉ ANTONIO VÁZQUEZ-FRÍAS, and MARTÍN SALVADOR VALENCIA-REYES

INTRODUCTION

Virtually all medical innovations of the last century have been based to a significant extent upon the results of animal experimentation. With the growth of laparoscopy nearly 15 years ago, a whole generation of surgeons had to rapidly adapt their surgical skills to a new laparoscopic approach for gallbladder resection. This was mainly accomplished by using animal models, which raised problems both for surgical training and for the animals. This was followed by the institution of new regulations for animal training, credentialing, experimentation, and finally by the development of nonanimal models.

Refinement, Reduction, and Replacement

The general guiding principles for animal experimentation, refinement, reduction, and replacement,[1] are partially motivated by concern to improve the welfare of experimental animals. **Refinement** is achieved by improving the skill of the researchers and the advancement of the techniques used. **Reduction** of the number of subjects is possible when measures are taken to increase the reproducibility and precision of the experiments. **Replacement** is only possible when the basic knowledge is available for the production and testing of biological substances to use as a model.[2]

We shall review the indications and characteristics of the animals most commonly used in laparoscopic research.

ANIMALS AS RESEARCH SUBJECTS

The Mouse and Rat Model

The mouse (*Mus musculus*) and rat (*Rattus norvegicus*) have made large contributions to scientific advances.[3] The areas of research in which they have been useful are diverse: bacteriology, virology, genetics, molecular biology, immunology, oncology, radiobiology,

pharmacology, behavioral genetics, and many more. In 1993, Gutt et al[4] used the rat as an experimental model in minimally invasive surgery, and many laparoscopic experiments followed using that model. The main advantages of using the rat are that their physiological parameters have been thoroughly studied, genetically similar strains are available, they are inexpensive, easy to handle, and available worldwide.

For laparoscopic surgery, once anesthetized, the animal is affixed to a piece of board using adhesive bands, exposing the previously-shaved abdomen. Pneumoperitoneum is then created with a pressure of 3 to 4 mm Hg. Pediatric laparoscopic instruments (2- to 5-mm trocars) are used to perform the operations.

These animals have been primarily used as a physiopathological model for laparoscopy, to refine technical aspects of laparoscopic surgery, to assess immunologic modifications and risks associated with laparoscopy (especially in oncology), and to develop new procedures such as laparoscopic hepatectomy and splenectomy.[5–7] They also offer opportunities to develop advanced laparoscopic skills and to do research at an affordable price.

Canine Model

The dog (*Canis familiaris*) has long been the traditional model used for transplantation (e.g., liver, kidney, or pancreas transplantation), hepatobiliary and pancreatic surgery, and gastrointestinal surgery. However, the pig, which is more biologically similar to man, is relatively cheap, and is much less popular as a pet, is replacing it.

A Medline review shows that during the last 12 months, 70 studies involving animals as a model in laparoscopic surgery have been performed. Of this total, 30 used swine, 25 small animals (mainly rats and mice), 7 sheep, and 5 dogs. Other less-frequently animals used were calves and nonhuman primates.

The canine models have been used recently in laparoscopic surgery for physiopathological studies, hepatobiliary surgery, upper GI surgery, colonic surgery, and vascular surgery.[8–10] Their advantages are the same as those of the pig, except perhaps ease of handling and better compliance.

Porcine Model

The pig (*Sus scrofa domestica*) has become increasingly popular as a research model in recent years because of its physiological, metabolic, anatomic, and nutritional similarities to humans. Moreover, its size and resistance to infection have made it the ideal subject on which to perform new laparoscopic procedures, as well as use for training and physiological studies. Because it is the most commonly used animal in laparoscopic research, we will examine the pig's characteristics as a model for use in laparoscopic surgery in more detail.

Most of the hematologic and biochemical values for the different species are widely available,[11] and porcine anatomy has also been extensively studied.[12,13] The choice of a breed depends on the biological characteristics necessary to conduct the experiment. The most common breeds found in the literature are Yorkshire, Landrace, Duroc, and crossbred animals. Miniature swine (Yucatan) and micro varieties (Hanford, Gottingen) offer different advantages (e.g., size, cost, weight gain for long survival studies) and are also commonly used. Most laparoscopic procedures can be performed in swine weighing 25 to 35 kg.

Preoperatively. The pig is fasted in order to facilitate approach to the organs and to prevent vomiting. The stomach and intestine may generally be considered empty after 8 to 12 hours, but larger animals may require 48 hours. The same laparoscopic instrumentation used in humans can be used in pigs.

The pig is usually placed in the supine position, but the position used depends on the procedure being attempted (Fig. 9–1). Pneumoperitoneum is created using an open approach or with a Verres needle. The usual insufflation pressure is 12 to 14 mm Hg.

Swine can be used for almost any laparoscopic procedure. We shall now point out the major anatomical differences between the pig and human, and discuss some of the operations reported.

Gastrointestinal Tract. The main differences in the pig are (1) the torus pyloricus (a muscular and glandular structure adjacent to the pylorus, involved in the closure of this orifice), (2) the mesenteric vessels, which form arcades in the subserosa of the intestine rather than the mesentery, creating a fan-like appearance, and (3) the spiral colon (the descending colon is arranged in a series of coils in the left upper quadrant of the abdomen). The gastric and colon wall is thicker than in humans, but procedures can be performed on the GI tract by using, for example, a larger stapler. Swine have been used to perform procedures involving the

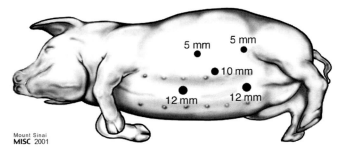

Figure 9–1. Position and trocar placement for laparoscopic aortorenal bypass in pig.

stomach, small or large bowel, and for bariatric studies (e.g., gastric bypass or biliopancreatic diversion).[14–16]

Liver and Biliary System. From a surgical point of view, the pig's liver and gallbladder have relatively few differences from the human organs. The main differences are that the bile duct enters the duodenum separately from the pancreatic duct, and that the liver is composed of six lobes. Laparoscopic cholecystectomy was one of the first procedures performed in pigs.[17,18] Cannulation of the common bile duct, liver biopsy, and partial hepatectomy have also been performed laparoscopically before these procedures were attempted in humans.[19]

Pancreas and Spleen. The porcine pancreas is similar to that in the human, except that the pancreatic duct is composed of two separate ducts that drain the tail and body (they join immediately prior to entering the pancreatic sphincter), and that the pancreas encircles the portal and superior mesenteric veins. The spleen is more elongated and usually bigger in pigs than in humans, but has the same anatomical relationships and vascular supply. Laparoscopic pancreatic surgery (distal pancreatectomy and robotically-assisted pancreaticojejunostomies) and spleen resections have been performed in pigs, and they interesting models for these procedures.[20,21]

Urinary System and Adrenal Glands. The pig's kidneys are similar to those of humans, except in that the blood supply is divided into cranial and caudal segments rather than into longitudinal halves. The adrenal glands are associated with the medial surface toward the cranial pole of each kidney. The right adrenal gland adheres tightly to the caudal vena cava. The arterial supply to the gland is either from the aorta or branches of the lumbar arteries, and the venous drainage is into either the vena cava or the renal veins. Despite those difficulties, a laparoscopic model for adrenal resection has been created and proved to be useful.[22] Numerous urologic procedures have also been described (hand-assisted or totally laparoscopic nephrectomy, cystic resection, and cystoprostatectomy with ileal conduit).[23,24]

Reproductive System. There are many similarities between the porcine and human oviduct. The reproductive tract of the female is typical of a bicornuate species. The ovaries are located caudal to the kidneys and are loosely attached by a thin ovarian ligament. Ovarian vessels are the last branches from the aorta and vena cava. The fallopian tubes are long and tortuous. This favors the use of swine, particularly for training surgeons in reconstructive surgical techniques of the oviduct.[25] The sheep model is usually preferred for ovulation and fertility studies (when superovulation is needed).[26]

Transplantation. The pig has become one of the most commonly used animals in transplantation studies. With the development of laparoscopy, swine have been used to develop a model for laparoscopic kidney harvesting, and even laparoscopic transplantation.[27]

Abdominal Wall. Ventral or inguinal hernia models have been developed in swine, to train young surgeons, and to develop new techniques and instruments.[28]

Vascular Surgery. The similarities in size and anatomy of the porcine vasculature to those of humans have allowed development of laparoscopic models for vascular procedures (e.g., splenorenal shunt, aortical aneurysm repair, and kidney transplantation).[29,30]

Swine have also been used to study many other aspects of laparoscopic surgery: to reduce the risk of laparoscopy in oncologic surgery,[31] to study gas embolism and physiological changes that occur due to pneumoperitoneum,[32,33] to develop new instruments,[34] for training purposes,[35] for telesurgery, and many more.

CONCLUSION

Progress in laparoscopic surgery has been, and remains, dependent on animal research. However, it should be the concern of all researchers involved in animal study to ask if the study is really worth animal experimentation, and if so, to ensure that the animals are maintained under the best possible conditions, and that they undergo only the minimum discomfort necessary to the accomplish the study.

REFERENCES

1. Russel WMS, Burch RL. *The Principles of Humane Experimental Technique*, 2nd ed. Methuen:1992.
2. Obrink KJ, Rehbinder C. Animal definition: a necessity for the validity of animal experiments? *Lab Anim* 2000;34:121.
3. Gay WI. *Health Benefits of Animal Research.* Foundation for Biomedical Research:1984.
4. Gutt CN, Berguer R, Stiegman GV. Laparoscopic surgery in the rat: description of a new technique. *Zentralbl Chir* 1993;118:631.
5. Gutt CN, Kim ZG, Schmandra T, et al. Carbon dioxide pneumoperitoneum is associated with increased liver metastases in a rat model. *Surgery* 2000;127:566.
6. Krahenbuhl L, Feodorovici M, Renzulli P, et al. Laparoscopic partial hepatectomy in the rat: a new resectional technique. *Dig Surg* 1998;15:140.
7. Targarona EM, Espert JJ, Bombuy E, et al. Laparoscopic splenectomy in a rat model: developing an easy technique. *J Laparoendosc Adv Surg Tech A.* 1999;9:503.
8. Tittel A, Schippers E, Anurov M, et al. Shorter postoperative atony after laparoscopic-assisted colonic resection? An animal study. *Surg Endosc.* 2001;15:508.
9. Byrne J, Hallett JW Jr., Ilstrup DM. Physiologic responses to laparoscopic aortofemoral bypass grafting in an animal model. *Ann Surg.* 2000;231:512.
10. Sakuramachi S, Kimura T, Choudhury NA. Laparoscopic highly selective vagotomy using CO_2 laser: experimental study in dogs. *Surg Laparosc Endosc.* 1996;6:355.
11. Radin JM, Weiser MG, Fettman MJ. Hematologic and serum biochemical values for Yucatan miniature swine. *Lab Anim Sciences* 1986;36:425.
12. Swindle M. *Surgery, Anesthesia, & Experimental Surgery in Swine.* Iowa State University Press:1998.
13. Swindle M, Adams R. *Experimental Surgery and Physiology: Induced Animal Models of Human Disease.* Williams & Wilkins:1998.
14. Watson DI, Mathew G, Pike GK, et al. Efficacy of anterior, posterior and total fundoplication in an experimental model. *Br J Surg.* 1998;85:1006.
15. Jorgensen LS, Langkilde NC, Moller PK, et al. Aseptic laparoscopic colon resection with intraabdominal anastomosis. An experimental study in pigs. *Surg Endosc.* 1998;12:1245.
16. Potvin M, Gagner M, Pomp A. Laparoscopic Roux-en-Y gastric bypass for morbid obesity: a feasibility study in pigs. *Surg Laparosc Endosc.* 1997;7:294.
17. Soper NJ, Barteau JA, Clayman RV, et al. Safety and efficacy of laparoscopic cholecystectomy using monopolar electrocautery in the porcine model. *Surg Laparosc Endosc.* 1991;1:17.
18. Rodriguez J, Kensing K, Cardenas C, et al. Laparoscopy guided subhepatic cholecystectomy: a feasibility study in swine. *Gastrointest Endosc.* 1993;39:176.
19. Wu JS, Strasberg SM, Luttmann DR, et al. Laparoscopic hepatic lobectomy in the porcine model. *Surg Endosc.* 1998;12:232.
20. Soper NJ, Brunt LM, Dunnegan DL, et al. Laparoscopic distal pancreatectomy in the porcine model. *Surg Endosc.* 1994;8:57, discussion 60.
21. Uranus S, Pfeifer J, Schauer C, et al. Laparoscopic partial splenic resection. *Surg Laparosc Endosc.* 1995;5:133.
22. Park A, Gagner M. A porcine model for laparoscopic adrenalectomy. *Surg Endosc.* 1995;9:807.
23. Fergany AF, Gill IS, Kaouk JH, et al. Laparoscopic intracorporeally constructed ileal conduit after porcine cystoprostatectomy. *J Urol.* 2001;166:285.
24. Barret E, Guillonneau B, Cathelineau X, et al. Laparoscopic partial nephrectomy in the pig: comparison of three hemostasis techniques. *J Endourol.* 2001;15:307.
25. Margossian H, Garcia-Ruiz A, Falcone T, et al. Robotically assisted laparoscopic microsurgical uterine horn anastomosis. *Fertil Steril.* 1998;70:530.
26. Calvano CJ, Moran ME, Mehlhaff BA, et al. Minimally traumatic techniques for in utero access and fetal surgery. *JSLS.* 1998;2:227.
27. Meraney AM, Gill IS, Kaouk JH, et al. Laparoscopic renal autotransplantation. *J Endourol.* 2001;15:143.
28. Garcia-Ruiz A, Naitoh T, Gagner M. A porcine model for laparoscopic ventral hernia repair. *Surg Laparosc Endosc.* 1998;8:35.
29. Gentileschi P, Gagner M, Kini S, et al. Laparoscopic aortorenal bypass using a PTFE graft: survival study in the porcine model. *J Laparoendosc Adv Surg Tech A.* 2001;11:223.
30. Dion YM, Cardon A, Gracia CR, et al. A model for laparoscopic aortic aneurysm resection. *Surg Endosc.* 1999;13:654.
31. Schneider C, Jung A, Reymond MA, et al. Efficacy of surgical measures in preventing port-site recurrences in a porcine model. *Surg Endosc.* 2001;15:121.
32. Nagelschmidt M, Holthausen U, Goost H, et al. Evaluation of the effects of a pneumoperitoneum with carbon dioxide or helium in a porcine model of endotoxemia. *Langenbecks Arch Surg.* 2000;385:199.
33. Ho HS, Saunders CJ, Gunther RA, et al. Effector of hemodynamics during laparoscopy: CO_2 absorption or intra-abdominal pressure? *J Surg Res.* 1995;59:497.
34. Platt RC, Heniford BT. Development and initial trial of the minilaparoscopic argon coagulator. *J Laparoendosc Adv Surg Tech A.* 2000; 10:93.
35. Watson DI, Treacy PJ, Williams JA. Developing a training model for laparoscopic common bile duct surgery. *Surg Endosc.* 1995;9:1116.

*E*sophageal Surgery

Chapter Ten ▪ ▪ ▪ ▪ ▪ ▪

*P*reoperative Evaluation of Patients with Gastroesophageal Reflux Disease

OWEN KORN and ATTILA CSENDES

The majority of patients with gastroesophageal reflux disease (GERD) who are candidates for surgical treatment have been undergoing medical treatment for many years. Few of them have had a complete laboratory evaluation. The persistence and progression of this disease are usually the main indications for surgery, and they usually imply an advanced illness with severe functional and anatomic damage to the lower esophageal sphincter and the body of the esophagus. Thus surgery can be the only alternative for a long-term cure. This treatment can alter the natural history of this disease, and it is essential to offer the patient an appropriate and complete anatomic and functional evaluation of the foregut before surgery.

Any surgeon who is going to perform antireflux surgery should order the following laboratory studies, which not only are useful to establish the correct preoperative diagnosis, but also are essential in choosing the most appropriate technique for each particular case:

- Complete medical history
- Endoscopy and biopsy
- Computerized manometry
- 24-hour pH monitoring
- 24-hour bilirubin monitoring
- Various radiologic studies

CLINICAL EVALUATION

The need for a complete and diligent medical history is not new, but it is necessary, even if the patient has already been diagnosed with GERD, and especially if the patient is seen by the surgeon for the first time. The cardinal symptoms such as heartburn, regurgitation, and dysphagia not only should be solicited, but also analyzed exhaustively. The presence, frequency, severity, and particular characteristics of each symptom can be of great help in determining the clinical profile of the patient.

Oligosymptomatic patients or patients with atypical symptoms can be a real challenge to the surgeon, and their condition should not be underestimated or undervalued. On the other hand, in very symptomatic patients, who usually have strong emotions about the condition, it is mandatory to objectively and carefully evaluate the diagnosis and the feasibility of surgical treatment, because the results in these patients are frequently inadequate.

Findings of retrosternal pain are unusual among patients with GERD, and frequently indicate the presence of motor disorders of the esophagus. It is necessary to exclude a cardiac origin for this pain before proposing an antireflux procedure in these cases, since such misdiagnosis could have disastrous results. A specialist must evaluate respiratory and/or laryngeal symptoms before considering them as manifestations of GERD.

The response to medical treatment must be critically evaluated, because currently-used drugs can frequently provide relief of symptoms. Special care should be taken to avoid automedication, which may occur due to the many advertisements for drugs to treat GERD. Contrary to what was supported even a few years ago, the best results are obtained in patients who are drug-dependent and who have recurrence of symptoms as soon as they stop taking their medication. On the other hand, the surgeon must be careful with patients who do not improve despite proper medication; usually in these cases there also are severe psychiatric symptoms, and they are bad candidates for surgery.

Other data obtained from the past medical history, such as chronic use of NSAIDs, bronchodilators, calcium channel blockers, or anxiolytics, the presence of alcoholism, diabetes, neurological disease, or scleroderma, and previous surgery of the foregut must be well known and carefully evaluated before surgery.

ENDOSCOPY AND BIOPSY

The first diagnostic approach is via endoscopy. It is very useful and is mandatory in every patient with suspected GERD. At one time, endoscopy was employed to make the diagnosis of GERD by demonstration of erosive esophagitis or by taking biopsy specimens of the esophageal mucosa above the Z line, especially in cases with no macroscopic evidence of esophageal injury. However, it is now well known that 40 to 50% of patients with GERD do not have erosive esophagitis; therefore endoscopy is still essential to ascertain the grade of esophagitis and is a useful tool to evaluate the effectiveness of any therapy that is used. The use of endoscopy must be even more widespread.

Although endoscopy is essential to confirm or refute other co-existing diagnoses and to survey the severity, progression, and consequences of the injury that the pathologic reflux has produced in the distal esophagus, it is not the ideal way to confirm the presence of pathologic gastroesophageal reflux. What is most important is the search for Barrett's esophagus, either uncomplicated or complicated by ulcer, stricture, or dysplasia. The concept of Barrett's esophagus has evolved and is now defined as the presence of metaplasia below the squamous columnar junction or Z line, independent of its extension, but clearly visible on endoscopic evaluation.[1] It is a particularly important finding, because the presence of metaplasia is associated with dysplasia and eventually with adenocarcinoma. Therefore, under this new definition, the endoscopist should not take biopsy specimens above the Z line, but rather below it, even if there is a stricture. It is essential to dilate the stricture and then take biopsies at and below the level of the stricture. As its length increases, Barrett's esophagus should be considered a premalignant condition and a very close surveillance should be maintained.

MANOMETRY

The conventional or computerized manometric study of the esophagus and the lower esophageal sphincter (LES) cannot confirm the diagnosis of GERD. Its utility is in demonstrating manometric alterations of the LES and motor abnormalities of the esophageal body that are seen in advanced stages of the disease or in Barrett's esophagus.

Several years ago, DeMeester et al[2] introduced the concept of a mechanically incompetent lower esophageal sphincter, defining it as a sphincter that has one or more of the following features:

- A resting pressure $\leq$6 mm Hg
- A total length $\leq$20 mm
- An abdominal length $\leq$10 mm

LES incompetence is not synonymous with GERD, but the likelihood of having pathologic reflux increases progressively with the presence of one or more of the above parameters. Until now, the concept of mechanical incompetence of the LES has been based on these standardized manometric characteristics.

Clinical experience has demonstrated that these parameters are difficult to find in many patients with a mechanically incompetent sphincter, so a new concept has been introduced, "sphincter pressure vector volume,"[3] a value obtained by computerized manometry. It has been established that in normal control subjects, the mean value of this parameter is 5700 mm $Hg^2 \times$ mm. Values below 1200 indicate the presence of an incompetent LES (Fig. 10–1). While this value

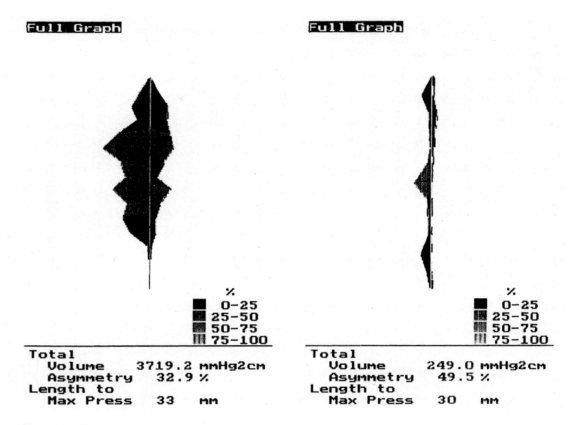

Figure 10–1. The three-dimensional manometric lower esophageal sphincter image in a normal subject (*right*), and in a patient with gastroesophageal reflux disease (*left*).

is a better indicator of the extent of disease, its use is still limited and the parameters of conventional manometry are still being employed.

In light of its limitations, the most important part of the manometric study is the search for a mechanically incompetent lower esophageal sphincter, which implies severe and profound anatomic and functional damage to the sphincter. This condition indicates that it is highly unlikely that medical treatment will be able to correct the defect, leaving surgery as the only logical therapeutic approach.

24-HOUR INTRAESOPHAGEAL pH MONITORING (24-HOUR pH STUDY)

This test is the gold standard in establishing the presence of GERD, defined as the excessive exposure of the esophageal lumen to gastric juices.[4]

This study is performed by placing a small pH sensor that is introduced nasally 5 cm proximal to the upper limit of the LES, which has been previously determined by manometry. This sensor is connected to an external device that can store all the pH readings taken over a 24-hour period, for a total of 22,000 pH measurements. This patient remains ambulatory so that he or she is able to carry out his or her normal activities, only with certain limitations on the foods eaten during the test. The patient must keep track of when meals are taken, as well as when they are prone or supine, so the effect of these actions on the pH can be noted. A special computer program allows the analysis of all stored data, and gives a profile of the reflux episodes in the patient, and calculates a score which combines 6 parameters:

- Total time with pH <4
- Total time with pH <4 in prone position
- Total time with pH <4 in supine position
- Number of reflux episodes
- Number of reflux episodes longer than 5 minutes
- Reflux episodes of longer duration

A combined score of 14 or lower is normal, which was the 95th percentile obtained in 50 healthy volunteers. The most useful value is the total time when the intraesophageal pH is less than 4, with a normal value being less than 4% (55 minutes).

It is important to observe the profile of reflux periods, because this allows us to evaluate the relationship between reflux periods and symptoms, and also helps to determine if there were methodological problems, such as a reading period less than 24 hours or intragastric positioning of the electrode. Currently, this is the most objective test to establish the presence of pathologic GERD, and every patient who is a candidate for surgery should undergo this evaluation. It is also the most useful method of determining the success rate of surgery and to detect eventual failures (Fig. 10–2).

RADIOLOGY

Initially, radiological studies were used to document GERD, using barium sulfate as a contrast medium. However, the demonstration of GERD with a contrast study only shows the reflux event, and only gives a quantitative determination, and not the magnitude or frequency of the phenomenon.[5] Until now, radiologic evaluation has been very useful in detecting anatomic and functional alterations not only in the esophagus, but also in the stomach and/or duodenum. It is essential that the radiologist has experience with these patients, because frequently there is confusion between Barrett's esophagus and a hiatal hernia (a problem that usually results in overdiagnosis of the latter) due to the dynamic nature of the contrast examination and to the motility of the gastroesophageal junction. To summarize, radiologic intervention is very useful in preoperative evaluation of the following:

- Esophageal motility disorders
- Evaluation of esophageal clearance
- Determination of a stricture (length and internal diameter)
- Anatomic dilatation of the gastroesophageal junction or cardia

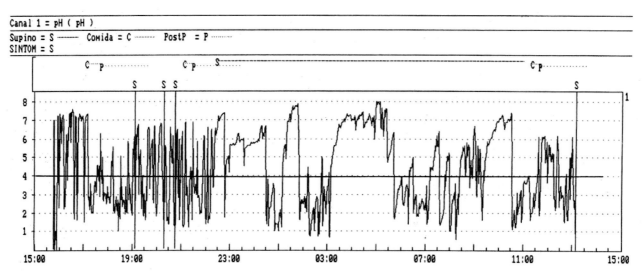

Figure 10–2. Record of 24-hour pH monitoring of the distal esophagus in a patient with esophagitis. The record shows a high number of reflux episodes (intraesophageal pH below 4), both in the upright and supine position, some of them with prolonged clearing time.

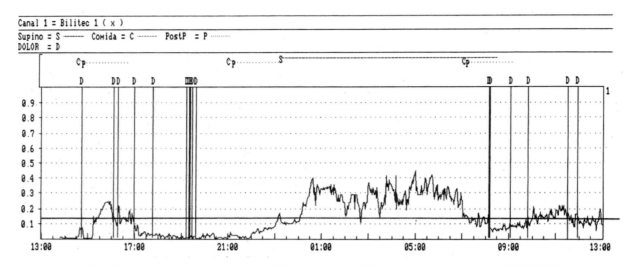

Figure 10–3. Tracing generated by intraesophageal 24-hour ambulatory bilirubin monitoring of duodenogastroesophageal reflux in a patient with Barrett's esophagus. The tracing shows a large percentage of time with bilirubin absorbance ≥0.14 absorption units in the distal esophagus.

- Presence of a true hiatal hernia
- Motility and gastric emptying
- Permeability of the pyloric and duodenal segment

24-HOUR BILIRUBIN MONITORING OF THE DISTAL ESOPHAGUS

The importance of duodenal reflux into the esophagus in the pathophysiology of GERD and its complications is well recognized. Initially, it was believed that an intraesophageal pH determination above 7 was a good indication of this event, and an alkaline reflux was considered diagnostic of reflux of duodenal contents. Later it was shown that in 95% of cases, a pH above 7 was not due to reflux of duodenal contents into the esophagus, but rather to retention of saliva, food, or dental sepsis, and the demonstration that duodenal reflux could occur at a pH between 2 to 4 made it necessary to search for another method to prove the reflux of duodenal contents. A new method was developed, based on 24-hour intraesophageal monitoring of bilirubin, which is present only in the duodenal juices,[6] and is a very reliable endogenous marker for the detection of duodenal reflux.

The design of an optical-electronic data tracking system, which processes all data from a fiberoptic sensor placed at the distal end of the esophagus, allows the detection of bilirubin due to its peculiar absorbance of light from a diode at the end of the sensor. It is thus possible to evaluate the circadian cycle of duodenal reflux and to measure its magnitude and relationship to other clinical and diagnostic parameters.

Although this test is not a routine procedure, it should be employed in every patient with the suspicion of duodenal reflux, especially in patients with Barrett's esophagus, and in patients with GERD symptoms but with a normal 24-hour pH study (Fig. 10–3).

REFERENCES

1. Sampliner RE. Practice guidelines on the diagnosis, surveillance, and therapy of Barrett's esophagus. The Practice Parameters Committee of the American College of Gastroenterology. *Am J Gastroenterol*. 1998; 93:1028.
2. Zaninotto G, DeMeester TR, Schwiser W, et al. The lower esophageal sphincter in health and disease. *Am J Surg*. 1988;155:104.
3. Stein HJ, DeMeester TR, Naspetti R, et al. The three-dimensional lower esophageal sphincter pressure profile in gastroesophageal reflux disease. *Ann Surg*. 1991;214:374.
4. Jamieson JR, Stein HJ, DeMeester TR, et al. Ambulatory 24-hour esophageal pH monitoring: Normal values, optimal thresholds, specificity, sensitivity, and reproducibilty. *Am J Gastroenterol*. 1992;87: 1102.
5. Stein HJ, DeMeester TR, Hinder RA. Outpatient physiologic testing and surgical management of foregut motility disorders. *Curr Prob Surg*. 1992;29:415.
6. Bechi P, Paucciani F, Baldini F. Long-term ambulatory enterogastric reflux monitoring. Validation of a new fiberoptic technique. *Dig Dis Sci*. 1993;38:1297.

Chapter Eleven ▪ ▪ ▪ ▪ ▪ ▪

*L*aparoscopic Antireflux Surgery: Indications and Patient Selection

DANIEL M. HERRON

Gastroesophageal reflux disease (GERD) is the most common disorder of the upper gastrointestinal tract, accounting for approximately 75% of esophageal pathology.[1] About 44% of Americans suffer heartburn at least once per month, and 18% treat themselves with nonprescription medication on a regular basis.[2] The majority of these patients do not need antireflux surgery; many will be adequately treated with behavioral changes, antacids, H_2 blockers, or proton pump inhibitors alone or in combination. Swanström found that of all patients referred to him for antireflux surgery, 17.5% were inappropriate candidates based on 24-hour pH monitoring, esophageal manometry, or upper endoscopy.[3] In order to obtain the best possible results from antireflux surgery, it is imperative to identify the indications for surgery carefully, perform a thorough preoperative work-up, and educate the patient regarding the expected outcome.

The ideal candidate for laparoscopic antireflux surgery is a young, healthy individual with substantial symptoms attributable to GERD. The patient's symptoms are well controlled with proton pump inhibitors but reappear shortly after stopping medical therapy. Manometry demonstrates normal motility in the esophageal body and a short, low-pressure lower esophageal sphincter (LES) that relaxes normally with swallowing. The 24-hour pH study reveals an elevated DeMeester score and excellent correlation between reflux episodes and GERD symptoms.

Unfortunately, the majority of patients referred for laparoscopic antireflux surgery differ substantially from this theoretical ideal. The selection of any given individual as a candidate for laparoscopic antireflux surgery must address not only their anatomy and physiology, but also other considerations such as lifestyle and economic issues. This chapter reviews the anatomic and physiologic indications for antireflux surgery as well as the nonmedical factors to be considered in patient selection.

SYMPTOMS

All patients referred for antireflux surgery will complain of some combination of typical and atypical GERD symptoms. The typical symptoms—heartburn, regurgitation, and dysphagia—are fairly straightforward to elicit. Atypical symptoms may be substantially more varied, including asthma, chronic cough, frequent pneumonia and pneumonitis, hoarseness, globus hystericus, and excessive salivation or water brash.

Most patients presenting to the surgeon's office have been previously treated with medical therapy for their GERD, including a regimen of H_2 blockers or proton pump inhibitors. Indeed, failure of medical therapy for reflux has traditionally been considered the primary indication for surgical intervention. However, the specific nature of the "failure" needs to be carefully elicited. Specifically, did the patient's symptoms improve substantially while on proton pump inhibitor therapy? Did the symptoms disappear entirely while on medical therapy but return on cessation of treatment? The patient who answers "yes" to either of these questions is more likely to have a satisfactory outcome from laparoscopic antireflux surgery than one who had no improvement with medical treatment.

The proper duration of initial medical therapy prior to consideration of laparoscopic antireflux surgery is debated. However, most GERD patients are only referred for surgical intervention after they have completed a 2- to 3-month course of maximal medical management with proton pump inhibitors. If symptoms are not fully relieved by that time, or if they recur upon completion of this course of therapy, then surgery is indicated.

ENDOSCOPIC FINDINGS

The most common indication for referral for laparoscopic antireflux surgery is continued typical or atypical GERD symptoms despite proton pump inhibitor therapy.[4] The majority of these patients will have a major abnormal finding on upper endoscopy, such as erosive esophagitis, stricture, or Barrett's esophagus. While severe esophagitis may respond to intensive medical therapy with proton pump inhibitors, such an approach requires careful monitoring of therapy and adjustment of dosages as needed.[5] Because this level of follow-up care may be difficult to achieve in practice, a laparoscopic antireflux procedure should be strongly considered in the setting of severe esophagitis.

Severe esophagitis may ultimately result in the formation of a stricture. A stricture should be biopsied to rule out a malignant etiology. If benign, the stricture should be progressively dilated up to 19 mm diameter (60F). Since a longstanding stricture may cause esophageal body dysmotility, manometry should always be performed to assess the amplitude and coordination of esophageal peristalsis. This will facilitate a "tailored approach" to the selection of an appropriate antireflux procedure.[4] Laparoscopic antireflux surgery has been demonstrated to diminish the need for further dilatation of esophageal strictures refractory to medical therapy, and result in good patient satisfaction.[6]

Barrett's esophagus is another common reason for patient referral for laparoscopic antireflux surgery. Barrett's changes are frequently associated with a severely dysfunctional LES. While there is no evidence to date that surgery reverses the disease, most surgeons feel that an antireflux procedure will at least slow its progression and help to heal the erosions or strictures that may accompany it. In the presence of moderate- to high-grade dysplasia, an esophageal resection or ablative procedure is more appropriate than an antireflux operation.

Some patients may present for laparoscopic antireflux surgery with a completely normal upper endoscopy. If their reflux is confirmed by 24-hour pH study, and their symptoms correlate well with the documented reflux episodes, then these patients should still be considered viable candidates for surgery.

ESOPHAGEAL MANOMETRY FINDINGS

The valve effect of the LES depends on the resting pressure of the sphincter, its overall length, and the length of the intra-abdominal portion of the sphincter. Since the surgical therapy of GERD is based on mechanical restoration of the LES, the optimal candidate for surgery will demonstrate a mechanically deficient sphincter. Preoperative evaluation of the LES may be performed using either a water-perfused or solid-state esophageal manometry system. Whichever system is used, it is important to compare the patient's manometric measurements against an age-matched group of normal subjects evaluated using a similar technique.

Richter's 1987[7] study of 95 normal adult volunteers demonstrated a mean LES pressure of 15 mm Hg at end expiration. DeMeester's group[8] compared the LES characteristics of 50 normal subjects with 622 GERD patients. They defined the *mechanically defective LES* as one demonstrating one or more of the following manometric features:

- Mean pressure <6 mm Hg
- Overall length <2 cm
- Intra-abdominal length less than 1 cm

These values represent the 2.5th percentile for LES pressure and overall length, and the fifth percentile for intra-abdominal length. The greater the number of these manometric findings, the higher the likelihood that significant gastroesophageal reflux will be present.

A 1987 study by Lieberman[9] examined a group of patients with longstanding reflux esophagitis treated with cimetidine and metoclopramide. Patients with a mechanically defective LES were

more likely to experience recurrent symptoms after medication was tapered or discontinued than those with intact sphincters.

In addition to measuring the defective LES, manometry is useful to identify esophageal body motility disorders. If peristalsis is absent or severely disorganized (greater than 50% simultaneous contractions) or if the amplitude of esophageal body contractions is less than 20 mm Hg, most surgeons would consider a partial fundoplication such as a Toupet or Dor.[4] Nonetheless, the laparoscopic surgeon must approach this type of procedure with caution; a partial wrap, while less likely to cause dysphagia, will also provide less protection against reflux.[10]

The patient with endoscopically-confirmed esophagitis who possesses a manometrically normal LES presents a difficult situation. It must be remembered that a manometric evaluation is a snapshot of the esophagus at a single point in time, and that normal LES pressures during the study do not necessarily imply normal LES pressures during the remainder of the day. However, this finding must raise the surgeon's suspicion that a different mechanism—inadequate esophageal clearance of refluxate or delayed gastric emptying—may be responsible for the esophagitis. Further diagnostic studies including repeat manometry or a gastric emptying scan may be warranted. If the surgeon elects to proceed with surgery, the patient must understand that an excellent outcome is less likely than in a patient whose reflux is due to a deficient LES.

24-HOUR pH STUDY FINDINGS

It is important to perform 24-hour pH monitoring on all patients being considered for antireflux surgery. This study is the gold standard for identifying whether acid reflux is present and whether such reflux correlates temporally with the patient's symptoms. In this examination, a thin catheter is inserted transnasally until a pH probe near the tip is located 5 cm above the upper boundary of the LES. The pH is then recorded electronically over a 24-hour period by a portable device worn on the patient's belt. Upon completion of the study the stored data is downloaded to a desktop computer.

The single most useful numerical result is the percentage of time during which the pH drops below 4. A value greater than 4%—approximately 1 hour out of the 24-hour period—suggests pathologic reflux. The "DeMeester score," a value calculated from 6 different pH study parameters, summarizes the amount of reflux in a single number. Computed automatically by most 24-hour pH systems, the score should be 14 or less in a normal individual.

It is important to remember that while manometry gives a snapshot of the esophageal physiology at one point in time, the pH study provides continuous monitoring over a 24-hour period. For this reason, many surgeons consider it to be the single most helpful study in the objective evaluation and quantification of GERD. Objective correlation of acid reflux episodes with subjective complaints of heartburn confirms that a patient's symptoms are indeed caused by GERD.

An abnormal 24-hour pH study should be an absolute prerequisite for surgical intervention in the treatment of acid reflux disease. In the less common situation in which endoscopically-confirmed esophagitis is identified in the patient with a normal pH study, the possibility of bile reflux may be entertained. This situation should prompt referral for a 24-hour esophageal bilirubin study.

LIFESTYLE AND ECONOMIC CONSIDERATIONS

Some GERD patients may experience resolution of symptoms with medical therapy, but wish to avoid the need for daily medication. Other patients may have unpleasant side effects from medical therapy. Economically disadvantaged patients may not have adequate insurance or the financial means to obtain optimal medical therapy on a long-term basis. These patients may be considered for laparoscopic antireflux surgery based on such nonmedical grounds.

REFLUX AND MORBID OBESITY

The morbidly obese patient with GERD presents a special situation. Because obesity is known to exacerbate reflux, obese GERD patients are commonly counseled to lose weight. In patients whose body mass index is greater than 35 kg/m^2, their chance of losing this weight permanently by dietary and behavioral management alone is extremely poor. If a morbidly obese patient with GERD qualifies for a bariatric procedure, a Roux-en-Y gastric bypass can treat their obesity and reflux simultaneously. Like antireflux surgery, this procedure can be performed laparoscopically with minimal morbidity and mortality. This type of patient should be referred to an obesity surgery center for definitive treatment.

CONCLUSION

Most patients with GERD have mild disease which responds relatively well to behavioral, dietary, and medical management. It is the patients who fail this approach, or whose symptoms recur upon tapering of medical therapy, who present to the surgeon's office for minimally invasive surgical management. In order to optimize the outcome of a laparoscopic antireflux procedure, it is imperative to fully evaluate both the severity and underlying physiologic basis of the disease with endoscopy, esophageal manometry, and a 24-hour pH study. Additionally, patients must be carefully educated regarding the expected side effects of any surgical procedure, and the potential for requiring continued medical therapy even after surgery.[11]

REFERENCES

1. DeMeester TR, Stein HJ. Gastroesophageal reflux disease. In: Moody FG, Carey LC, Jones RC, eds. *Surgical Treatment of Digestive Disease.* Year Book:1989;65.
2. Jamieson GC, Duranceau A. *Gastroesophageal Reflux.* WB Saunders:1988;65.
3. Swanstrom L, Wayne R. Spectrum of gastrointestinal symptoms after laparoscopic fundoplication. *Am J Surg.* 1994;167:538.
4. Hunter JG, Trus TL, Branum GD, et al. A physiologic approach to laparoscopic fundoplication for gastroesophageal reflux disease. *Ann Surg* 1996;223:673.
5. Klinkenberg-Knoll EC, Festen HPM, Jansen JB, et al. Long term treatment with omeprazole for refractory reflux esophagitis: efficacy and safety. *Ann Int Med.* 1994;121:161.
6. Klingler PJ, Hinder RA, Cina RA, et al. Laparoscopic antireflux surgery for the treatment of esophageal strictures refractory to medical therapy. *Am J Gastroenterol.* 1999;94:632.
7. Richter JE, Wu WC, Johns DN, et al. Esophageal manometry in 95 healthy adult volunteers. *Dig Dis Sci.* 1987;32:583.
8. Zaninotto G, DeMeester TR, Schwizer W, et al. The lower esophageal sphincter in health and disease. *Am J Surg.* 1988;155:104.
9. Lieberman DA. Medical therapy for chronic reflux esophagitis. Long-term follow-up. *Arch Int Med.* 1987;147:1717.
10. Horvath KD, Jobe BA, Herron DM, et al. Laparoscopic Toupet fundoplication is an inadequate procedure for patients with severe reflux disease. *J Gastrointest Surg.* 1999;3:583.
11. Spechler SJ, Lee E, Ahnen D, et al. Long-term outcome of medical and surgical therapies for gastroesophageal reflux disease. *JAMA.* 2001;285:2331.

Chapter Twelve (Part One) ● ● ● ● ● ●

Antireflux Procedures

JORGE CUETO-GARCÍA and LEE SWANSTROM

INTRODUCTION

Gastroesophageal reflux disease (GERD) is one of the most common foregut disorders, affecting more than 40% of the adult population of the United States and Europe on at least an occasional basis.[1-3] It is well known that the number of patients requiring prescription drugs to control it is increasing[4] and that since the introduction of laparoscopic surgery the number of antireflux operations has increased sharply in most parts of the world.[3,5] Associated complications, including Barrett's esophagus and Barrett's-related adenocarcinoma, are concurrently increasing. The treatment of GERD and its complications is becoming a critical healthcare issue worldwide.

NATURAL HISTORY OF GASTROESOPHAGEAL REFLUX DISEASE (GERD)

Experience has shown that some patients can have many years of GERD symptoms without developing complications whereas other patients with no history of reflux complaints will present first to the physician with symptoms from a complication of GERD. The reasons behind this disparity in presentation are poorly understood but are currently an area of intense genetic study.[6]

The elegant, well-planned, and frequently cited long-term longitudinal studies done by Monnier et al in Switzerland[7] have shown that 77% of patients with GERD have only isolated episodes or recurrent nonprogressive disease whereas 23% will have a recurrent progressive disease associated with the risk of development of complications such as ulcers, Barrett's esophagus, strictures, and a short esophagus. Furthermore, in related studies long-term follow-up has clearly demonstrated the progressive nature of the disease, diagnosed both by endoscopy and pathological examination, with irritation progressing to ulceration which subsequently heals by fibrosis or by replacement with metaplastic columnar epithelium occurring in 19% of cases during a median follow-up of 3 years.[7]

The work of several groups has identified the breakdown of the antireflux barrier due to a defective lower esophageal sphincter (LES) as the etiologic factor that leads to esophageal reflux of acid contaminated with duodenal contents that can subsequently lead to mucosal injury. In fact, very low LES pressures are associated with all of the complications mentioned above.[3,5,7,8]

The cause and effect relationship between reflux disease and Barrett's esophagus is well established and has recently been associated with the reflux of acid and alkaline duodenal contents, and this in turn is likewise related to stenosis, ulcers, shortening of the esophagus, and bleeding.[9-14] A recently published nationwide population-based study from Sweden has clearly demonstrated a strong and probably causal relationship between GERD and esophageal adenocarcinoma.[15] In fact, most countries have noticed a relative and absolute increase of adenocarcinoma of the lower esophagus associated with Barrett's disease.

In some patients, but particularly those at both extremes of age, the regurgitation of gastric juice into the respiratory tract—bronchial aspiration—can produce varied symptoms, and in some cases serious complications.[16] Rarer complications of GERD include chronic anemia, dental erosions, adult asthma and laryngeal cancer. The contribution of *Helicobacter pylori* to GERD, if any, is unknown at present.[17]

INDICATIONS FOR SURGERY

Gastroesophageal reflux symptoms in most patients can be controlled with dietary and lifestyle modifications or with drug therapy.[1-5,8] However, it is important to identify the minority of patients (8 to 10%) who have a more virulent type of disease that is characterized by more severe or uncontrollable symptoms, complications of GERD in spite of maximal medical control, or frequent relapses after discontinuing therapy.[3,5-8,15,18-22] These patients should have a thorough and complete evaluation, particularly if they are young. One must also consider that some patients will be unable to comply with the dietary adjustments and medical therapy, and that others will not want long-term medical treatment of their symptoms. Still others will be unable to tolerate the medication or will be unable to afford it. As stated by Heading, "the selection for therapeutic strategies for long-term management of reflux disease should involve considerations of patient preferences and opinions."[23]

Since the introduction of the proton pump inhibitors (PPIs), it has been shown that a large group of patients (90%) with GERD can have satisfactory symptom control often associated with healing of superficial esophagitis. However, approximately 80% of these patients will have a relapse after the drug is suspended, a few patients will have a partial or no response, and there is concern that chronic use, which is known to produce achlorhydria and hypergastrinemia, will create other complications. The economic and emotional burden of having to take medication on a chronic basis may also play an important limiting role, but the crucial aspect is that they cannot—as Spechler put it—cure the underlying most important factor that produces GERD: a mechanically deficient LES.[20]

The demonstration that a mechanically deficient LES is the main cause for GERD in a large group of patients—a physiologic deficit that obviously cannot be corrected with long-term drug therapy—has challenged the classic indications for antireflux surgery. The authors agree with DeMeester and others that at the present time, the main indication for surgery can no longer be considered "when medical therapy fails,"[3,5,8,21,22,24] since short- and intermediate-term follow-up has shown that surgical treatment is curative in 85 to 93% of patients.[3,5,24] If a patient fails to have a satisfactory response after a 12-week trial with drug therapy, has an early relapse, or if the dosages of the medications have to be increased, there is a clear indication for a complete work-up that includes endoscopy, a barium swallow, esophageal manometry, and in some cases pH monitoring. If a mechanically deficient LES is found, there is an indication for antireflux endoscopic surgery, which should now be considered the gold standard of therapy.[3,5,24–28]

Respiratory complications such as aspiration and asthma are indications for antireflux surgery as well. Patients with Barrett's esophagus, stenosis, ulcers, and short esophagus are also candidates for surgical treatment, although from the onset a different type of result is to be expected in many of these complicated patients. Paraesophageal hernias, which require repair in order to avoid gastric volvulus, also are an indication for a fundoplication, even though they are seldom associated with GERD. In this case the fundoplication is performed to prevent postoperative reflux and to minimize the chance of recurrence.

Previous prospective and well-controlled studies have shown that surgical treatment of GERD is superior to medical therapy, although there has been no comparison between PPI use and laparoscopic surgery, the current standards of therapy.[26,27–30]

PREOPERATIVE EVALUATION

It is well known that the more thorough the evaluation of the patient with GERD, the better the postoperative result. If the patient does not have an adequate preoperative evaluation, even a well-performed surgical procedure can have a poor outcome. Preoperative studies also serve as a baseline for postoperative follow-up studies, increasingly an important aspect of surgical care.

Although most patients have typical gastrointestinal symptoms of GERD such as heartburn, regurgitation, and dysphagia, others present with atypical symptoms, mainly respiratory complaints, such as chronic infections, adult-onset asthma, or chest pain that is frequently confused with cardiac disease. Several studies have shown that the patient population with typical gastrointestinal reflux symptoms and a good response to medical therapy will have a better postoperative result.[26,31]

Endoscopic examination with biopsy is necessary in every case to document the presence of esophageal mucosal injury, assess the anatomy, and rule out malignancy. Barrett's esophagus, an important indication for antireflux surgery, can only be detected with endoscopy and must be carefully biopsied to rule out high-grade dysplasia. Endoscopy allows the severity of the disease to be graded, the presence of complications such as strictures, dilatation, ulcers, shortening, or diverticuli to be detected, and the type and size of hiatal hernia to be documented. Gastric or duodenal pathology such as peptic ulcer disease, Cameron's ulcers, and pyloric stenosis are also detected during endoscopic examination. However, it must be kept in mind that a group of patients with GERD documented by other methods may not show macro- or microscopic evidence of mucosal injury, particularly if they have been on acid-suppressing medication. In cases of severe esophagitis or peptic strictures diagnosed by endoscopy, intensive medical treatment along with progressive dilatation should be attempted for at least 10 days before the operation.

A barium swallow is mainly useful to assess the anatomy, particularly the size and type of hiatal hernia or the presence and severity of strictures. Abdominal ultrasound to look for cholelithiasis may also be useful because as many as 8% of our patients have concomitant cholecystitis or cholelithiasis.

Manometric studies of the esophagus are of paramount importance as a diagnostic and prognostic tool. They provide information on the status of the LES: its resting pressure (normal, 15 to 25 mm Hg), length (3 to 4 cm), and location (intra-abdominal or intrathoracic), and provide measurements of esophageal peristalsis, the integrity of which can be used to determine the type of antireflux surgery reqired.[3,5]

The routine use of pH monitoring is more controversial, with some authors advocating its use only for patients with atypical symptoms, when endoscopy fails to show gross evidence of esophagitis, or for the evaluation of those with a failed previous antireflux procedure. Other authors advocate routine use, arguing that it provides a basis of comparison for follow-up testing and that it remains the most accurate way to document actual reflux.[8,24,26,31]

Other tests, such as gastric emptying studies, pulmonary function tests, gastric acid assays, and provocative challenge testing (Bernstein test) are only done in selected cases and for specific indications.

A complete cardiopulmonary evaluation should be considered for patients 40 years of age or older, particularly when chest pain is one of the presenting symptoms.

SURGICAL TREATMENT

The goal of any surgical treatment of GERD is to provide an efficient and adequate antireflux valve for the patient while minimizing untoward side effects or surgical morbidity. To this end, the ability to perform fundoplications laparoscopically, which dramatically reduced patient pain, hospital stay, and recovery period, represented an enormous improvement in patient care. Selection of the appropriate antireflux procedure is also directly related to the patient's outcome and should be carefully considered. There are several different laparoscopic antireflux procedures available to the surgeon treating GERD but, in general, the three most commonly described are: the 360° "floppy" Nissen fundoplication, the 270° posterior partial fundoplication (often called the Toupet), and the partial anterior or Dor hemifundoplication.[3,5,31–39]

The 360° "short, floppy Nissen" which incorporates changes introduced and popularized by DeMeester et al[3,5,8,24,31,32] is currently the benchmark for antireflux repair. There is currently much controversy regarding the place of the partial fundoplication as a routine repair. Some authors have advocated these repairs as a more physiologic and better-tolerated alternative to the Nissen.[33,34,36,37] There is little dispute that partial wraps are indicated in patients with named motility disorders such as scleroderma and achalasia. They may also be preferred in the elderly, and perhaps for patients with poorly-defined motility disorders.[3,5,22,27,33–38] There are, however, several practitioners who have long favored the primary use of partial fundoplications for open or laparoscopic antireflux surgeries. In particular, several Scandinavian and French groups such as Guarner and others have reported very satisfactory results in long-term follow-up (up to 30 years) with various forms of partial wraps.[39–46] Watson et al reported excellent postoperative results in the treatment of GERD with his variation of a partial fundoplication when compared with a 360° wrap.[44] Recently Laws et al, in a prospective randomized study showed that patients with adequate mobilization of the gastric fundus (i.e., with division of the short gastric vessels) randomly selected at the time of the operation to receive either a 360° or a 270° Nissen fundoplication had similar postoperative results.[47] On the other hand, several other investigators have shown that partial wraps have a greater incidence of late failure and recommend that the floppy Nissen fundoplication should be used in all cases with normal motility.[24,31–33,48–52] This raises questions about possible variations in technique, such as the length or degree of fundoplication, which might explain the unsatisfactory results.

Other laparoscopic procedures such as the posterior gastropexy or Hill operation, and the thoracoscopic Belsey operation, which have proven to be highly successful in conventional surgery, require further evaluation of endoscopic approaches.[53,54]

SURGICAL TECHNIQUE

All surgeons have their own variations on the technical details of laparoscopic fundoplications. Below is a description of our technique which encompasses the common tenets of the procedure and also presents some technical tips derived from a decade of experience with laparoscopic antireflux surgery.

The patient is usually admitted the morning of surgery and a first-generation cephalosporin given intravenously. Precautions against deep venous thrombosis should be taken. The operating table should allow for the surgeon to stand between the legs of the patient (European position) and the assistants and nurse to be positioned at the right and left side. Usually two monitors are placed to allow optimal viewing at both sides of the head of the table (Fig. 12–1).

An orogastric tube is introduced for gastric decompression and pneumoperitoneum is established with either a Veress needle or by an open Hasson technique. Pneumoperitoneum pressure should be maintained between 10 and 12 mm Hg throughout the procedure. If the patient has had previous upper abdominal surgery

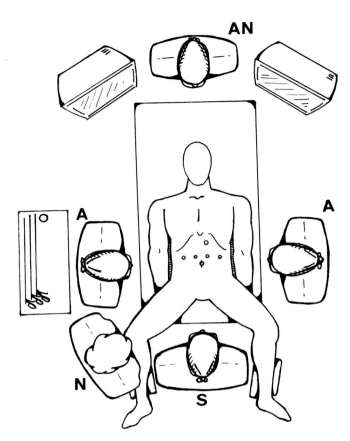

Figure 12–1. Positioning of the surgical team. AN, assistant nurse; A, assistant surgeon; S, surgeon.

(6% in our series) the left upper quadrant port site should be chosen for the initial puncture. The approximate placement of 4 to 6 trocars is shown in Fig. 12–2. Before insertion, all of the trocar sites are infiltrated with 2% lidocaine with epinephrine. Though in the past the majority of access ports for a fundoplication were 10 mm in diameter, there is a recent trend toward the use of 5-mm access ports to minimize scarring and postoperative pain from the incisions. Certainly for pediatric patients the trocars can be 5 or even 3 mm in diameter, but for these patients the pneumoperitoneum should be kept at no more than 5 to 6 mm Hg.

If the distance between the umbilicus and the xiphoid is extremely short, the initial trocar can be placed as low as the umbilical area; however, more often this trocar should be placed to the right and 3 to 5 cm above the umbilicus in order to reach the hiatus without undue effort. After the liver retractor is introduced in the right subcostal area, a 10-mm 0° laparoscope is introduced in the subxiphoid port site. The left subcostal port is used for a Babcock-type instrument to provide traction by the assistant surgeon, which leaves the two paraumbilical ports for both hands of the surgeon. If needed, in difficult cases where severe scarring, fibrosis, obesity, or other findings make exposure difficult, a sixth 5-mm trocar port can be placed in the left upper quadrant for additional traction, suction, or a bipolar electrocautery scalpel.

The procedure is begun with a thorough exploratory laparoscopy, and then the patient is placed in a steep reverse Trendelenburg position to provide exposure to the upper abdomen. The most appropriate description of the procedure is the careful dissection

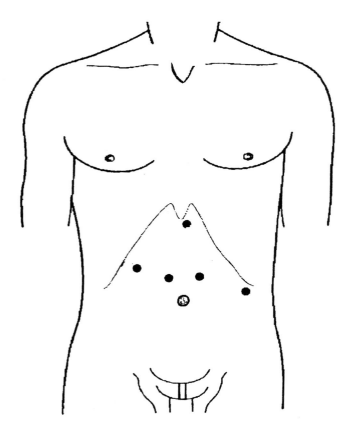

Figure 12–2. Approximate placement of the trocars.

and exposure of both crura, reduction of the esophagogastric junction into the abdominal cavity, construction of a antireflux valve without tension, and the closure of the diaphragmatic defect.

Although there are no definitive rules that determine the order of the dissection, which to a large extent will depend on the conditions found upon initial exploration, in most cases the dissection will be started anteriorly with the division of the phrenoesophageal ligament. This membrane is divided widely in order to identify the right crus. In cases without periesophagitis, the gastrohepatic ligament with vagal and left gastric artery branches is spared. In our experience, however, the gastrohepatic ligament has to be divided to gain access to the right crus in more than two-thirds of the cases, due to the fibrosis found in patients with severe, chronic reflux. This dissection is usually accomplished with the ultrasonic coagulating scissors but can also be done with bipolar electrocautery and clips. We do not use, or recommend the use of, monopolar electrocautery in operations carried out near the esophageal hiatus.

The surgeon next grasps the right crus with his left hand using a Babcock-type instrument (Fig. 12–3), and with blunt and sharp dissection enters the mediastinum and begins to clear the crura inferiorly to the origin of both the left and right crura (the "V"). This dissection should be carried cephalad into the mediastinum for 4 to 5 cm, staying away from the esophageal wall and identifying and preserving the right vagus nerve. The dissection is then extended lateral to the left wall of the esophagus until the left crus is identified. At this time the surgeon retracts the

gastroesophageal (GE) junction to the left and inferiorly in order to complete the dissection of the left crus. It is very important to divide all the adhesions between the GE junction and the uppermost aspect of the greater curvature of the stomach to the diaphragm (or even the spleen in cases of severe periesophagitis). The assistant can then retract the left crura outward, allowing the surgeon to dissect the left side of the mediastinal esophagus under direct vision. Along the base of the left crus there is occasionally a branch of the phrenic artery, which requires careful control. In the next step of the procedure, the assistant holds the GE junction and provides upward traction toward the patient's left, to allow the surgeon to clear the retroesophageal area using blunt and sharp dissection. This part of the procedure should be done with extreme care to avoid injury to the esophagus or stomach, which would result in mediastinitis with its high morbidity and mortality rates. Such injuries can be the result of a direct laceration or retraction injury or a delayed perforation from occult trauma. A 30° scope can be very useful during this (and other) parts of the procedure. The retroesophageal window created must be wide enough to easily allow the passage of the fundus of the stomach for the fundoplication. A soft Penrose drain can be used to retract the GE junction and allow completion of the retroesophageal window dissection. There is no difference between placing the wrap around or inside the right vagus nerve, although there are advocates of both methods. It is critical, however, that the vagus nerves not be injured during the procedure, and this mandates minimal manipu-

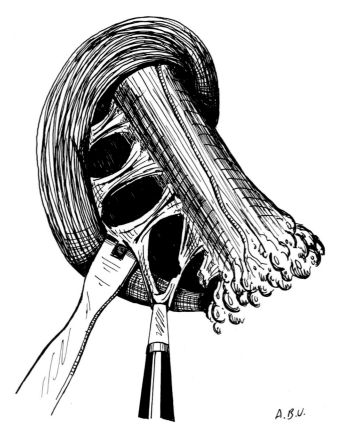

Figure 12–3. The surgeon provides outward traction with his left hand in the right crus. The dissection must be done very carefully, close to the pillars and away from the esophageal wall.

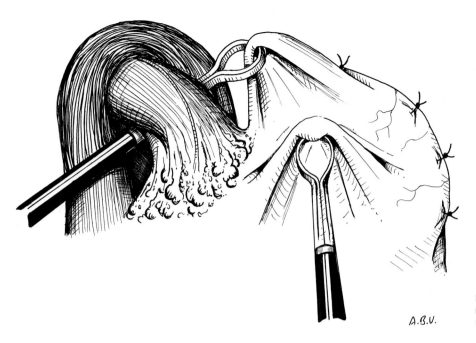

A.B.V.

Figure 12–4. The mobilization of the gastric fundus must be complete to provide a loose wrap. This may require division of the short gastric vessels.

lation. Once the periesophageal dissection is complete, the anesthesiologist irrigates the GE junction through a nasogastric tube in order to rule out a perforation.

The mobilization of the greater curvature is important regardless of the type of wrap employed (Fig. 12–4). Critical elements include division of all adhesions between the left diaphragm and adjacent structures including the distal esophagus, GE junction, and the proximal gastric fundus. All dissection should be done under direct vision, which is facilitated by using an angled laparoscope (30° or 45°). Care must be used when dividing the gastrosplenic ligament to avoid injury to the spleen, a complication that frequently results in splenectomy and was common in the era of conventional surgery but is fortunately rare in the era of laparoscopic fundoplication. The issue of division of the short gastric vessels to ensure adequate mobilization of the gastric fundus, a defining step for the floppy Nissen fundoplication, remains somewhat controversial.[5] On the whole, the literature seems to indicate that there are more postoperative side effects—namely dysphagia and the gas bloat syndrome—as well as a higher reflux recurrence rate, when the short gastric vessels are not divided.[32,49,50,52,55,56] Thus the general recommendation is to do it in all cases of a 360° wrap and in cases of partial wraps that require it to prevent tension on the repair. A very useful maneuver of assessing the need for further fundal mobilization was described by Dallemagne[50] in 1991: After the fundus of the stomach is gently passed around the esophagus (Fig. 12–5) it is released and observed to see if it stays in place or if it retracts rapidly to its original location. Rapid retraction implies excess tension and a wrap constructed under such conditions will produce more dysphagia (whether or not it was constructed around a large bougie), which may require dilatation or surgical revision, or lead to herniation or disruption of the repair. The fear of dissection and division of the short gastric vessels that was once present has been minimized by the introduction of the harmonic scissors, which has made this part of the procedure simpler, faster, and safer. The basic technique of gastric fundus mobilization requires careful dissection with traction maintained by the assistant on the gastrosplenic ligament superiorly and to the

left of the patient, while the surgeon provides gentle countertraction on the stomach with an atraumatic grasper. A curved dissector (5 or 10 mm) is used to make windows between the blood vessels, which can then be divided using the harmonic scissors or bipolar electrocautery and staples.

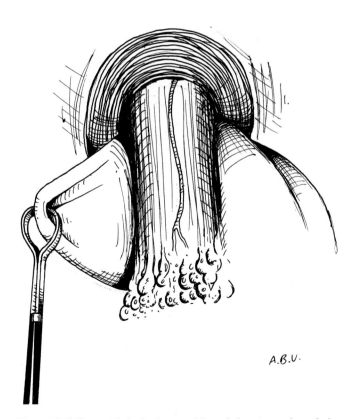

A.B.V.

Figure 12–5. The gastric fundus is passed through the retroesophageal window without undue tension.

The 2- to 2.5-cm long 360° wrap is constructed using 3 or 4 stitches of 00 nonabsorbable suture (Fig. 12–6). All but one suture will include both sides of the wrap as well as a bite of the anterior esophageal wall. Extracorporeally-tied knots are used for the most part. An intraesophageal bougie is routinely used by many groups to gauge the looseness of the fundoplication. Because of the risk of iatrogenic trauma from bougie insertion we prefer to assess the wrap's looseness by inserting an atraumatic instrument between the wrap and the esophagus. If a bougie is used, it must be passed with extreme care to avoid a perforation. Early in one's experience or in complicated procedures, an endoscopy should be done after the procedure is complete to ensure that there is no laceration, obstruction, angulation, or other problem. When a partial fundoplication is done—and many groups firmly believe that there are indications for it—the esophagus and fundus of the stomach are mobilized in the same way as for the 360° wrap. The short vessels are not divided routinely; this is only done if there is tension on the wrap. The suture line on each side should be at least 4 cm long, which requires 4 to 5 nonabsorbable sutures on each side. Care must be taken not to injure the vagus nerves during suturing (Fig. 12–7).

Nonabsorbable sutures are also used to close the diaphragmatic defect posteriorly (Fig. 12–8) to prevent postoperative paraesophageal herniations. This usually requires 2 or 3 stitches that should not be placed too tightly or the result may be postoperative obstructive symptoms that are notoriously resistant to dilatation, and could lead to a reoperation to remove a suture.

At the completion of the procedure, hemostasis should be ascertained and 30 to 40 mL of bupivacaine instilled in both subdiaphragmatic areas to decrease referred postoperative pain in the shoulder and/or neck.[57] All trocars are removed under direct vision and all 10-mm fascial incisions are closed with absorbable sutures.[58]

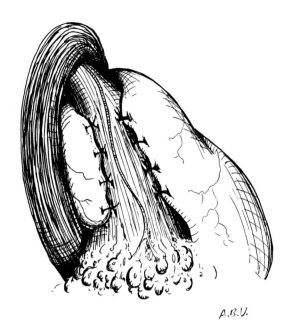

Figure 12–7. A partial fundoplication.

ADDITIONAL PROCEDURES

GERD often is a result of, or is exacerbated by, coexisting GI dysfunction. It is important for the surgeon to recognize the contributing role of gastric or biliary pathology and to treat it at the same time as the fundoplication if necessary. The most common associated problem is symptomatic cholelithiasis. Peptic ulcer

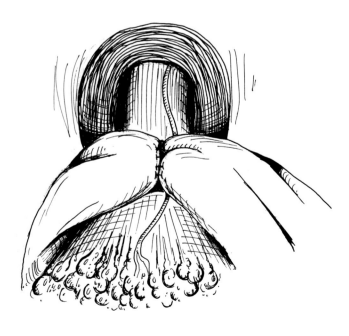

Figure 12–6. A 360° Nissen-DeMeester fundoplication.

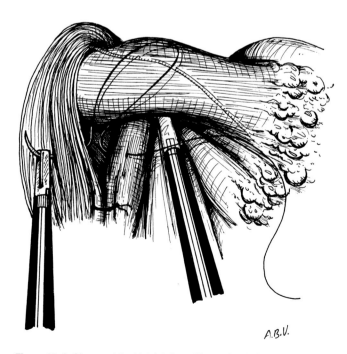

Figure 12–8. Closure of the hiatal defect with nonabsorbable sutures without producing stenosis of the esophagus.

disease and delayed gastric emptying, either from a mechanical outlet obstruction or from a gastric motility disorder, can also cause reflux and can result in poor outcomes (gas bloating) if not treated. Likewise, peptic ulcer disease, if it is not *Helicobacter pylori*–related, may result in the patient continuing to require medical therapy if it is not treated at the time of the antireflux procedure. Based on our experience of 503 antireflux procedures, the need for an additional procedure at the time of fundoplication occurs around 14% of the time. We have had 40 patients (8%), (28 females and 12 males) who required a cholecystectomy. In addition, 18 males and 2 females (4%) were found to have inguinal hernias, 10 of which were repaired during the same operation. Five patients (1%) had a parietal cell vagotomy for chronic (4) or acute (1) duodenal ulcerations; one of the former bled in spite of PPI administration on the seventh postoperative day, and required emergency endoscopy and overnight hospitalization.[59] Two female patients also had a bilateral laparoscopic tubal division. We have not found it necessary to perform esophageal lengthening (Collis gastroplasty) or gastric emptying procedures, although these additional procedures have been reported in other series.[60,61]

POSTOPERATIVE CARE

Patients are taken to the recovery room and, if the procedure was long or particularly complicated, a portable chest film is taken. The nasogastric tube is removed when the patient is transferred from recovery to their room. Postoperatively, pain control is achieved with IV parenteral nonsteroidal anti-inflammatories (ketorolac, thrometamine, etc.); it is rare that more than two doses are needed. Ice chips and sips of water are given the same night and most patients are encouraged to sit in a chair and to ambulate with assistance. The vast majority of patients—more than 90%, are discharged next day on 2 weeks of a full liquid diet. Peptic medications are given for a week if there is a history of peptic ulcer disease, and cisapride is also given on a short-term basis when patients have symptoms of delayed GI motility.

RESULTS

The short- and intermediate-term follow-up of laparoscopic fundoplication patients has shown results that compare favorably with the ones obtained with conventional open surgery.[3,5,22,31,33,49–51] In fact, the majority of reports document that the complications and recurrence rates—most of which happen in the first 2 years—are lower than with conventional surgery.[62]

Table 12–1 summarizes the complications we observed in our series of 503 patients. Our experience began in April 1991 after having performed more than 200 laparoscopic cholecystectomies and several dozen diagnostic or basic procedures.[22,33] Most of the major complications and conversions to laparotomy occurred during the first 2 years (during our first 120 procedures). Since then, 2 patients have had gastroesophageal lacerations; both were recognized at the time of surgery when the anesthesiologist injected the nasogastric tube with air and saline. Both injuries were repaired with 000 nonabsorbable sutures and no postoperative complications were seen.

DISCUSSION

The recent well-designed epidemiologic report from Sweden that clearly associated chronic symptomatic GERD with the development of esophageal carcinoma (objective confirmation of an old clinical observation) has created a public demand for more information about the disease and has focused the interest of clinicians and researchers on finding a definitive treatment for the problem.[15] Laparoscopic access has become established as the new gold standard for GERD treatment because it is both effective and well tolerated.[28] (See Table 12–2.)

In spite of the advantages laparoscopic fundoplication provides patients, there remain individuals who are challenging to treat with this "patient-friendly" approach, including those with paraesophageal hernias, motility disorders, shortened esophagus, or redo fundoplications. For these patients, one can elect to use an open approach, attempt the procedure laparoscopically, or use alternative options such as reverting to a hand-assisted operation that entails somewhat less postoperative pain and cosmetic damage, as discussed elsewhere.

As for the best type of operation to use, the 360° Nissen-DeMeester fundoplication is likely the procedure of choice, but as in most other types of surgery, it is almost certainly not a good idea to try to apply a single procedure to all patients. It is well known that GERD patients are a heterogeneous group having a wide range of presenting symptoms and idiosyncrasies, ranging from basic GERD without complicating factors, to a group of complicated disorders that include atypical symptoms, poorly-defined motility disorders, and congenital and acquired mechanical disorders of the esophagus, stomach, or LES. Tailoring the approach and technique to each patient's physiology and symptomatology is the best approach.[63]

As previously stated, the literature describes excellent results whether the procedure is done open, laparoscopically, or using

---

TABLE 12–1. MORBIDITY OF ANTIREFLUX SURGERY: EXPERIENCE WITH 503 PATIENTS, APRIL 1991–APRIL 2000

Mortality: 0	
Major complications: 9 (1.7%)	1 obstruction converted by laparoscopy to a partial fundoplication
	1 postoperative case of pneumonia requiring transfer to the ICU
	1 esophageal laceration requiring conversion
	1 laceration of a jejunal loop requiring laparotomy
	2 late reoperations for detachment of a partial fundoplication
	1 postoperative paraesophageal hernia requiring laparotomy elsewhere
	1 postoperative hemorrhage, treated medically
	1 perforation of the gastric fundus on the sixth postoperative day requiring laparotomy elsewhere
Minor complications: 57 (11.3%)	Temporary dysphagia (30), pneumothorax (4), massive subcutaneous emphysema, umbilical cellulitis, others

TABLE 12–2. RESULTS OF LAPAROSCOPIC NISSEN FUNDOPLICATION

		Number of Patients	Complications (%)	Reoperations (%)	Conversions (%)	Hospital stay (days)	Dysphagia[2] (%)	% Patient Satisfaction
Watson	1996	174	5.2	5.7	9.2	3	6.2	91
Laws	1997	23	4.4	0	4.4	2.7	8.7	91.3
Cattey	1996	100	8	0	2	2.3	4	92
Paluzzi	1997	103	11	3.9	3.9	2.3	1.9	96
Anvari	1995	168	8.9	1.5	2.3	2.7	2.4	92
Coster	1995	52	4	4	6	2.3	2	98
Hunter	1996	252	7.1	3.1	1	2	4	—
Peters	1996	34	0	—	—	4.7	8.8	—
Cadiere	1994	80	7.4	1.3	3.8	3	0	91
Hinder	1994	198	8	2.5	4	3	6	97
Hinder	1995	150	6	—	0	—	—	—
Jamieson	1994	155	2.6	6.5	12.3	2.6	17.6	97
Pitcher	1994	70	11.3	4.3	2.9	3	7	91
Perdikis	1997	2453	5.9	3.1	5.8	3	5.5	98
Cueto	2000	503	12	3	2.8	1.5	5	90
TOTAL		4515	6.78	3.00	4.31	2.72	5.65	93.27

Modified from Chae and Stiegmann.[21]

**Persistent more than 4 weeks

hand-assisted techniques. The role of partial vs. total fundoplication does continue to be controversial, with differing results reported from different centers. Our own experience with long partial fundoplications, when the fundus is well mobilized, seems to indicate that the repair offers durable long-term results. Recently, Watson et al[44] also presented evidence of favorable results with anterior hemifundoplication, even when the procedure was compared with the 360° wrap. By contrast, other groups have shown that there was up to a 50% failure rate for partial fundoplication based on objective follow-up and using reduced acid reflux as an endpoint for success. These centers advocate the use of the partial repairs only for cases of severe esophageal dysmotility.[26,31,32,48] The controversy has been further complicated by the demonstration that in many patients, the peristaltic function of the esophageal wall is improved following a successful antireflux operation.[64] This makes the preoperative selection of patients who absolutely require a partial fundoplication even more difficult.

Finally in this era of cost containment, the cost-benefit advantages of laparoscopic surgery vs. chronic palliative treatment need to be stressed, particularly for young patients.[65,66]

NEWER ENDOSCOPIC PROCEDURES

Recently , several groups have reported their initial experience with different methods altering the G-E junction in order to prevent GERD, such as the new purely endoscopic antireflux procedures, the application of radiofrequency, and the injection of collagen via endoscopy, with varying degrees of success and complications.[67,68,69] It is very early to make a solid judgment as to the long-term durability and efficacy of these endoscopic methods and the role that they eventually could have in the clinical management of patients with gastroesophageal reflux disease. From a surgical point of view and in reference to the endoscopic antireflux procedures, it is known that for the fundoplications to be successful, it is necessary to achieve an adequate dissection, mobilization, and

descent of the gastroesophageal junction to the abdomen—particularly in the presence of hiatal hernias—which certainly cannot be done using the endoscopic method alone. Additionally, it may appear that to suture superficially the wall of the esophagus and stomach using this approach may result in breakdown with recurrence of the disease even more often than with laparoscopic surgery.

CONCLUSIONS

The etiology of GERD remains unknown. What is known is that there has been a dramatic increase in the incidence of patients who suffer from GERD and its complications and that this ultimately has an impact on the number of patients who will die of esophageal cancer. Fortunately, the majority of these patients can be controlled satisfactorily with medical therapy and by lifestyle modifications. It is important, however, to identify a small group of patients that have a more aggressive type of disease that is resistant to drug treatment, with more relapses, and those that do not comply with the treatment prescribed or who refuse to live with a palliative therapy for the rest of their lives.

The experience of the past 10 years has shown that when a patient is properly diagnosed and evaluated, and when the appropriate surgical procedure is adequately performed, laparoscopic antireflux surgery is a safe, cost-effective therapy that provides significant advantages when compared with conventional surgery or chronic medical treatment.

The impact of all therapies, surgical or pharmacologic, on the development of complications of the disease, including Barrett's esophagus and esophageal cancer, remains unknown.

REFERENCES

1. Castell DO, Vault KR. Diagnosis and treatment of gastro-esophageal reflux disease. *Mayo Clin Proc.* 1994;69:867.

2. Richter JE. Management of gastroesophageal reflux disease, 1995. Dis Esophagus 1994;7:223.

3. SAGES Committee on Standards of Practice: SAGES Guidelines for surgical treatment of gastroesophageal reflux disease. Surgical Treatment of Gastroesophageal Reflux Disease (GERD). October 1996.

4. Castell DO. Management of gastroesophageal reflux disease 1995. Maintenance medical therapy of gastro-esophageal reflux—which drugs and how long? *Dis Esophagus*. 1994;7:230.

5. Eypasch E, Neugebauer E. Laparoscopic antireflux surgery for gastroesophageal reflux disease (GERD) Results of a Consensus Development Conference of the European Association of Endoscopic Surgery. *Surg Endosc*. 1997;11:413.

6. Katada N, Hinder RA, Smyrk TC, et al. Apoptosis is inhibited early in the dysplasia-carcinoma sequence of Barrett esophagus. *Arch Surg*. 1997;132:728.

7. Monnier P, Ollyo JB, Fontolliet C, et al. Epidemiology and natural history of reflux esophagitis. *Sem Laparosc Surg*. 1995;2:2.

8. DeMeester TR, Johnson LS, Koseph GJ, et al. Patterns of gastroesophageal reflux in health and disease. *Ann Surg*. 1976;184:459.

9. Haggitt RC. Adenocarcinoma in Barrett's esophagus: a new epidemic? *Hum Pathol*. 1992;23:475.

10. Stein HJ, Barlow AP, De Meester TR, et al. Complications of gastroesophageal reflux disease: Role of the lower esophageal sphincter, esophageal acid and acid/alkaline exposure, and duodenogastric reflux. *Ann Surg*. 1992;216:35.

11. Stein HS, Hoeft S, DeMeester TR. Functional foregut abnormalities in Barrett's esophagus. *J Thorac Cardiovasc Surg*. 1993;105:107.

12. Savary M, Monnier P. Diagnosis, pathophysiology and adenocarcinogenesis of Barrett's esophagus. In: *Esophageal Disorders,* DeMeester TR, Skinner DB, eds. Raven Press, New York:1985;121.

13. Katz D, Rothstein R, Schned A, et al. The development of dysplasia and adenocarcinoma during endoscopic surveillance of Barrett's esophagus. *Am J Gastroenterol*. 1998;95:536.

14. DeMeester TR. Barrett's esophagus. *Surgery* 1993;113:239.

15. Lagergren J, Bergstrom R, Lindgren A, et al. Symptomatic gastroesophageal reflux as a risk factor for esophageal adenocarcinoma. *N Engl J Med*. 1999;340:825.

16. Allen CJ, Anvari M. Gastro-oesophageal reflux related cough and its response to laparoscopic fundoplication. *Thorax* 1998;53:963.

17. Kuipers EJ, Lundell L, Klinkenberg-Knol EC, et al. Atrophic gastritis and *Helicobacter pylori* infection in patients with reflux esophagitis treated with omeprazole or fundoplication. *N Engl J Med*. 1996;334: 1018.

18. Ortiz-Hidalgo C, De la Vega G, Aguirre-Garcia J. The histopathology and biologic prognostic factors of Barrettss esophagus. *J Clin Gastroenterol*. 1998;26:324.

19. Csendes A, Braghetto I, Maluenda F, et al. Peptic ulcer of the esophagus secondary to reflux esophagitis: clinical, radiological, endoscopic, histological, manometric and isotopic studies in 127 patients. *Gullet* 1991;1:177.

20. Spechler SJ. Drug therapy of reflux esophagitis. Society for Surgery of Alimentary Tract Postgraduate Course. May 14, 1995. San Diego, California.

21. Currie RA, Cueto GJ. The surgical treatment of hiatal hernia. *W V Med J*. 1967;64:101.

22. Cueto GJ. Hernia hiatal y esofagitis por reflujo. *Rev Gastroent Mex*. 1972;37:299.

23. Heading RC. Long-term management of gastroesophageal reflux disease. *Scand J Gastroenterol Suppl*. 1995;213:25.

24. DeMeester TR. Indications for surgery in gastroesophageal reflux disease. In: Society for Surgery of the Alimentary Tract: Reflux Esophagitis and Other Disorders of the Foregut. *Dig Week*. May 14, 1995, San Diego, California.

25. Lundell L, Dalenback J, Hattlebakk J, et al. Outcome of open antireflux surgery as assessed in a Nordic multicentre prospective clinical trial. Nordic Gord study group. *Eur J Surg*. 1998;164:751.

26. Hinder RA. Gastroesophageal reflux disease: surgical options, choice of operations and outcomes. American Gastroenterological Association Postgraduate Course, May 1999. Atlanta, Georgia.

27. Chae FH, Stiegmann GV. Current laparoscopic gastrointestinal surgery. A review. *Gastrointest Endosc*. 1998;47:500.

28. Katkhouda N. Laparoscopic treatment of gastroesophageal reflux disease—Defining a gold standard. *Surg Endosc*. 1995;9:765.

29. Behar J, Shcahan DG, Brancani P, et al. Medical and surgical management of reflux esophagitis. A 38-month report on a prospective clinical trial. *N Engl J Med*. 1975;6:263.

30. Spechler SJ. Gastroesophageal reflux disease study group: Comparison of medical and surgical therapy for complicated gastroesophageal reflux disease in veterans. *N Engl J Med*. 1992;326:786.

31. Peters JH, DeMeester TR, Crookes P, et al. The treatment of gastroesophageal reflux disease with laparoscopic Nissen fundoplication. Prospective evaluation of 100 patients with "typical" symptoms. *Ann Surg*. 1998;228:40.

32. Hunter JG, Trus TL, Branum GD, et al. A physiologic approach to laparoscopic fundoplication for gastroesophageal reflux disease. *Ann Surg*. 1996;223:673.

33. Cueto-GJ, Weber-Sánchez A. Cirugía del esófago Procedimientos antirreflujo. *Cirugia Laparoscópica*, segunda edicion. McGraw-Hill Interamericana Healthcare Group, 1997.

34. Bell RC, Hanna P, Powers B, et al. Clinical and manometrical results of laparoscopic partial (Toupet) and complete (Rosetti-Nissen) fundoplications. *Surg Endosc*. 1999;10:724.

35. Collet D, FDCL Group. Conversions & complications of laparoscopic treatment of gastroesophageal reflux disease. *Am J Surg*. 1995;169:622.

36. Watson A, Jenkinson LR, Ball CS, et al. A more physiologic alternative to total fundoplication for the surgical correction of resistant gastro-esophageal reflux. *Br J Surg*. 1991;78:1088.

37. McKernan JB. Laparoscopic repair of gastroesophageal reflux disease: Toupet partial fundoplication versus Nissen fundoplication. *Surg Endosc*. 1994;8:851.

38. Cuschieri A, Hunter J, Wolfe E, et al. Multicenter prospective evaluation of laparoscopic antireflux surgery: Preliminary report. *Surg Endosc*. 1993;7:505.

39. Lundell L. Management of G.E.R.D. in 1995; The role of semifundoplication in the long-term management of gastro-esophageal reflux disease. In: *Diseases of the Esophagus*. Longman Group, Ltd.:1994;7: 245.

40. Thor KA, Silander T. A long-term randomized prospective trial of the Nissen procedure versus a modified Toupet technique. *Ann Surg*. 1989;210:719.

41. Guarner V, Martinez N, Gaviño JF. Ten year evaluation of posterior fundoplasty in the treatment of gastroesophageal reflux: long-term and comparative study of 13.5 patients. *Am J Surg*. 1980;2:139.

42. Guarner V. Trente ans d'expérience avec la fundoplastie postérieure dans le traitement du reflux gastro-aesophagien (analyse de 1499 cas). *Chirurgie* 1997;122:443.

43. Walker SJ, Sanderson CJ, Stoddard CJ. Comparison of Nissen total and Lind partial transabdominal fundoplication in the treatment of gastro-oesophageal reflux. *Br J Surg*. 1992;79:410.

44. Watson DI, Jamieson GG, Pike GK, et al. Prospective randomized double-blind trial between laparoscopic Nissen fundoplication and anterior partial fundoplication. *Br J Surg*. 1999;86:123.

45. McKernan JB, Champion JK. Minimally invasive antireflux surgery. *Am J Surg*. 1988;175:271.

46. Cueto GJ, Serrano BF, Weber SA, et al. El tratamiento quirúrgico del reflujo gastroesofágico por el método laparoscópico. *Rev Cirujano Gen*. 1993;15:103.

47. Laws BL, Clements RH, Swillie CM. A randomized, prospective comparison of Nissen fundoplication and Toupet fundoplication for gastroesophageal reflux disease. *Ann Surg*. 1997;225:647.

48. DeMeester TR. Complete and partial laparoscopic fundoplication for gastroesophageal reflux disease. *Surg Endosc*. 1991;11:613.

49. Trus T, Laycock W, Bramm G, et al. Follow-up of laparoscopic antireflux surgery. *Am J Surg.* 1996;171:32.

50. Dallemagne BC, Weerts JM, Lombard S. Laparoscopic Nissen fundoplication: Preliminary report. *Surg Laparosc.* 1991;1:141.

51. Jamieson CG, Watson DJ, Britten-Jones R, et al. Laparoscopic Nissen fundoplication. *Ann Surg.* 1994;220:137.

52. DeMeester TR, Bonavina I, Albertucci N. Nissen fundoplication for gastroesophageal disease: evaluation of primary repair in 100 consecutive patients. *Ann Surg.* 1986;204:9.

53. Hill LD, Kraemer SJM, Aye RW, et al. Laparoscopic Hill repair. *Contemp Surg.* 1994;44:13.

54. Nguyen NT, Schauer PR, Hutson W, et al. Preliminary results of thoracoscopic Belsey Mark IV antireflux procedure. *Surg Laparosc Endosc.* 1998;8:185.

55. Dunnington GL, De Meester T, et al. Outcome effect of adherence to operative principles of Nissen fundoplication by multiple surgeons. *Am J Surg.* 1993;166:654.

56. Hinder RA, Filippi C. The technique of laparoscopic Nissen fundoplication. *Surg Laparosc Endosc.* 1992;2:265.

57. Weber A, Muñoz J, Garteiz D, et al. Use of subdiaphragmatic bupivacaine instillation to control postoperative pain after laparoscopic surgery. *Surg Laparosc Endosc.* 1997;7:6.

58. Cueto J, Melgoza C, et al. A simple and safe technique for closure of trocar wounds using a new instrument. *Surg Laparosc Endosc.* 1996;6:392.

59. Cueto GJ, Rodriguez DM, Salas J, et al. Postoperative ulcer and hemorrhage: an uncommon complication of laparoscopic Nissen fundoplication. *Surg Laparosc Endosc.* 1998;8:219.

60. Johnson AB, Oddsdottir M, Hunter JG. Laparoscopic Collis gastroplasty and Nissen fundoplication: A new technique for the management of esophageal foreshortening. *Surg Endosc.* 1998;12:1055.

61. Swanstrom LL, Marcus DR, Calloway EQ. Laparoscopic Collis gastroplasty is the treatment of choice for the shortened esophagus. *Am J Surg.* 1996;171:477.

62. Polk HC, Zeppa R. Hiatal hernia and esophagitis. *Ann Surg.* 1971;173:775.

63. Patrick WJ. Management of post-fundoplication complications. American Gastroenterological Association Postgraduate Course, May 1999, Atlanta, Georgia.

64. Stein HJ, Brennner RK, Jamieson J, et al. Effect of Nissen fundoplication on esophageal motor function. *Arch Surg.* 1992;127:788.

65. Coley CM, Barry MJ, Spechler SJ, et al. Initial medical vs surgical therapy for complicated or chronic gastroesophageal reflux disease (G.E.R.D.): A cost-effectiveness analysis. *Gastroenterology* 1993;104:SupplA5.

66. Viljakka M, Nevalainen J, Isolauri J. Lifetime costs of surgical versus medical treatment of severe gastro-oesophageal reflux disease in Finland. *Scand J Gastroenterol.* 1997;32:766.

67. Hogan WH. Endoscopic treatment modalities for GERD: technologic score or scare? *Gastrointes Endosc.* 2001;53:541.

68. Filipi CJ, Lehman G, Rothstein RI, et al. Transoral flexible endoscopic suturing for treatment of gastroesophageal reflux disease: a multicenter trial. *Gastrointes Endosc.* 2001;53:416.

69. Feretis C, Benakis P, Dimopoulos C, et al. Endoscopic implantation of Plexiglas (PMMA) microspheres for the treatment of GERD. *Gastrointes Endosc.* 2001;53:423.

Chapter Twelve (Part Two) ▪ ▪ ▪ ▪ ▪ ▪ ▪

Laparoscopic Collis Gastroplasty

LEE SWANSTROM

THE SHORT ESOPHAGUS

One complicating factor in antireflux surgery is the shortened esophagus, which is thought to be the result of a vicious cycle of repetitive esophagitis, submucosal fibrosis, and subsequent axial shortening. While the true incidence of this problem is somewhat controversial, there is little doubt in the minds of most esophageal surgeons that this clinical finding exists.[1] The decreased morbidity of the laparoscopic approach has increased the overall number of antireflux procedures performed and has thereby made the identification and treatment of these patients more relevant.[2]

The success of a given antireflux procedure depends on the creation of a tension-free fundoplication. A fundopli-cation done around an intrinsically shortened esophagus will have a high failure rate due to mediastinal wrap herniation, disruption, or misplacement ("slipped Nissen"). An esophageal lengthening procedure is therefore indicated when, after extensive mediastinal esophageal mobilization, it is not possible to deliver the gastroesophageal junction 2.5 cm below the hiatus. The combination of a Collis gastroplasty and fundoplication has long been considered the treatment of choice for esophageal shortening secondary to complicated gastroesophageal reflux and/or paraesophageal hernia. Several studies have established the short- and long-term clinical success of this procedure using the open technique.[3–10]

LAPAROSCOPIC APPROACH

We developed a technique of performing a Collis gastroplasty in laparoscopic patients undergoing antireflux surgery who were found to have a truly shortened esophagus.[11] Once it is determined that the gastroesophageal junction is unable to be delivered at least 2.5 cm below the hiatus without undue tension despite extensive transhiatal mediastinal dissection (up to the carina), an endoscopic Collis gastroplasty is performed.

A 12-mm sealed thoracic port is placed into the right side of the chest at the fourth intercostal space in the anterior axillary line, and a pneumothorax using carbon dioxide at a pressure of 10 mm Hg is created. An 0° telescope is inserted and advanced to the mediastinal pleura at the posteroinferior pulmonary sulcus. This allows for transillumination and visualization from the abdominal cavity. Once the proper trajectory has been selected, the thoracic port is stabilized, the telescope is withdrawn, and a 3.5-cm endoscopic linear stapler is inserted. A small incision is made in the mediastinal pleura laparoscopically to allow passage of the stapling device into the abdominal cavity. A 40F bougie is inserted while gentle axial traction is placed on the distal esophagus. The fundus is then grasped along the greater curvature and rotated into the anteroposterior position. This allows the stapler to be placed parallel to the distal esophagus beginning at the angle of His. The stapler is fired, creating a 3-cm neoesophagus with a 56F lumen and a new angle of His. Additional firings can be done if more length is required. A chest tube is not routinely placed at the completion of the operation; the thoracic port is vented as the patient is given positive-pressure ventilation. Any residual carbon dioxide is rapidly reabsorbed from the thoracic cavity.

A fundoplication is then created around the neoesophagus. The fundus is passed through the posterior window and used to retract the esophagus to the left. This provides exposure for a loose hiatal closure with nonabsorbable sutures.

Once the appropriate placement of the wrap is determined, a 2- to 2.5-cm Nissen fundoplication can be created around a 56F bougie. The standard two to three wrap sutures are augmented by additional sutures to the posterior hiatus and anterior diaphragm and two sutures from the lateral neoesophagus to the insides of the fundoplication. All sutures are tied intracorporeally to minimize tissue trauma. A Toupet fundoplication is performed if the patient has significantly impaired esophageal peristalsis. The Toupet repair follows the same sequence as the Nissen except for the final sutures. These are placed from the fundus to the esophagus at the 10 and 2 o'clock positions to create a 3- to 4-cm long, 270°, partial fundoplication.

RESULTS

In our experience, the endoscopic Collis gastroplasty is safe and has resulted in no conversions to open surgery and no postoperative leakage in over 38 cases. To date, all patients have had improvement of their preoperative symptoms and none has required reoperation for wrap herniation or disruption. On postoperative follow-up studies, however, we have found a high occurrence of abnormal 24-hour pH tests (50%).[12] This has also been described in the open experience and is presumed to be due to functioning gastric mucosa above the wrap.[13]

Regarding the etiology of this acid production, several explanations have been advanced. First, all patients were noted on biopsy to have oxyntic mucosa proximal to their fundoplications regardless of the results of postoperative testing. This indicates that in the patients with normal 24-hour pH studies and negative Congo red tests, the parietal cells have become nonfunctional. Whether this is the result of a regional vagotomy during esophageal mobilization, or is secondary to the placement of a staple line across the fundus at the angle of His is unknown. Second, the amount of functional gastric mucosa above the midpoint of the distal high pressure zone relates to the amount of distal esophageal acid exposure. We found several patients with normal 24-hour pH tests who had black staining only inside the wrap on postoperative Congo red testing. We therefore recommend that the esophagus be mobilized as much as possible prior to Collis gastroplasty in an attempt to make the squamocolumnar junction as low as possible.

CONCLUSION

Although potential complications from neoesophageal acid production are cause for concern, the laparoscopic Collis gastroplasty with fundoplication provides excellent long-term protection from duodenogastroesophageal reflux, a condition thought to play a primary role in the progression of Barrett's esophagus to esophageal adenocarcinoma.[9,10] We have shown that the Collis gastroplasty with fundoplication abolishes gastroesophageal reflux.[12] We believe this to be the reason that the majority of patients are asymptomatic postoperatively. It is important to remember that only 20% (2/7) of the patients with abnormal 24-hour pH studies were experiencing heartburn

at 14 months. Because of this, we recommend rigorous objective follow-up that includes esophageal manometry, upper endoscopy, and 24-hour pH testing. Medical treatment for patients with abnormal 24-hour pH tests should be initiated regardless of symptoms.

REFERENCES

1. Raiser F, Hinder R, Mobride P, et al. Laparoscopic anti-reflux surgery in complicated gastroesophageal reflux disease. *Semin Laparosc Surg.* 1995;2:45.
2. Peters JH, Heimbucher J, Kauer WKH, et al. Clinical and physiologic comparison of laparoscopic and open Nissen fundoplication. *J Am Coll Surg.* 1995;4:385.
3. Orringer MG, Sloan H. Collis-Belsey reconstruction of the esophagogastric junction: indications, physiology and technical considerations. *J Thorac Cardiovasc Surg.* 1976;71:295.
4. Pearson FG, Henderson RD. Long term follow-up of peptic strictures managed by dilatation, modified Collis gastroplasty and Belsey hiatus hernia repair. *Surgery* 1976;80:396.
5. Ellis FH, Leonardi HK, Dabuzhsky L, et al. Surgery for short esophagus with stricture: An experimental and clinical manometric study. *Ann Surg.* 1978;188:341.
6. Orringer MB, Orringer JS. The combined Collis-Nissen operation; Early assessment of reflux control. *Ann Thorac Surg.* 1982;33:584.
7. Henderson RD, Marryatt GV. Total fundoplication gastroplasty (Nissen gastroplasty): Five year review. *Ann Thorac Surg.* 1985;39:74.
8. Stirling MC, Orringer MB. Continued assessment of the combined Collis-Nissen operation. *Ann Thorac Surg.* 1989;47:224.
9. Attwood SE, Smyrk TC, DeMeester TR, et al. Duodeno-esophageal reflux and the development of esophageal adenocarcinoma in rats. *Surgery* 1992;111:503.
10. Fein M, Ireland A, Manfred PR. Duodenogastric reflux potentiates the injurious effects of gastroesophageal reflux. *J Gastrointest Surg.* 1997;1:27.
11. Swanstrom LL, Marcus DM, Galloway GQ. Laparoscopic Collis gastroplasty is the treatment of choice for the shortened esophagus. *Am J Surg.* 1996;171:477.
12. Jobe BA, Horvath KD, Swanstrom LL. Postoperative function following laparoscopic Collis gastroplasty for the shortened esophagus. *Arch Surg.* 1998;133:867.
13. Martin CJ, Cox MR, Cade RJ. Collis-Nissen gastroplasty fundoplication for complicated gastro-oesophageal reflux disease. *Aust N Z J Surg.* 1992;62:126.

Chapter Twelve (Part Three) ∙ ∙ ∙ ∙ ∙ ∙ ∙

Antireflux Surgery: The Gastroenterologist's View

LUIS LANDA-VERDUGO and ROBERTO NEVAREZ-BERNAL

Gastroesophageal reflux is one of the most challenging and frequent clinical disorders confronting the gastroenterologist. In most cases, the treatment of choice is medical, but occasionally surgery is necessary. The surgical criteria for the gastroesophageal reflux (GER) patient has been evolving over the years. In this section, the guidelines for selection of either treatment will be discussed.

The treatment of GER requires an individualized approach, and aims to relieve the symptoms, to heal the esophagitis, and to prevent the recurrence of symptoms. These objectives can be attained by reducing the amount of damaging reflux into the esophagus by improving the antireflux barrier, decreasing the gastric acid component, and enhancing esophageal clearance.

MEDICAL TREATMENT

The medical therapy should be tailored to the severity of symptoms, the degree of esophagitis present, and the presence of other acid reflux complications. Lifestyle changes should be the basis of any therapeutic approach. Pharmacologic therapy with a combination of H_2 blockers, prokinetic agents, proton pump inhibitors, and cytoprotective agents is also regarded as the mainstay of medical treatment.[1-4]

DIET

The esophagus is not built to withstand repeated exposure to gastric fluids and their characteristically low pH. Once esophagitis is initiated, intolerance to irritating foods follows. For this reason, the diet of the GER patient should restrict the consumption of spicy foods, pepper, mustard, raw onion, garlic, and vinegar, as well as particularly tangy or salty dishes.

Patients are encouraged to avoid foods that have produced symptoms of heartburn or reflux in the past. If the patient is overweight, a return to a more normal body weight and BMI is of major importance. Patients should also teach themselves, with or without the help of a nutritionist, to avoid large meals and to restrict the ingestion of liquids with meals, particularly at night.

PHARMACOLOGIC THERAPY

Because gastric acid is one of the principal components that cause damage to the esophagus during reflux, antacids are useful in the immediate treatment of the symptoms of the disease.

Many types of antacids, such as sodium bicarbonate, calcium carbonate, bismuth, and aluminum hydroxides with or without magnesium, have been used in the treatment of the symptoms of gastroesophageal reflux. The advent of cimetidine marked an extraordinary shift in the reduction of acid production and gastric secretion. The development of its derivatives (H_2 antagonists) has created more potent drugs with fewer secondary effects, but these drugs also cost more. H_2 antagonists were the most commonly used antisecretory drugs, and in the past 20 years had been the cornerstone of therapy for the treatment of this disease. Their usefulness has been widely proven in the symptomatic relief of mild or nonerosive GER, but their efficacy is limited in more severe forms of the disease, such as erosive esophagitis,[1,3,6] for which other treatment options such as proton pump inhibitors (omeprazole, lansoprazole) are more effective.[4,6] Newer and more potent drugs, such as esomeprazole,[8] rabeprazole,[9] etc., are being introduced and now form the mainstay of medical treatment everywhere.

Medications that improve intestinal peristalsis are helpful for accelerating gastric emptying and diminishing the period that the gastric and esophageal mucosa are in contact with irritating juices.

OTHER RECOMMENDATIONS

Substances that lower the tone of the lower esophageal sphincter, such as nicotine, alcohol, and caffeine, should be avoided, as well as those that increase intra-abdominal pressure. All these lifestyle modifications should be accompanied by consultation with the clinician, who should educate and encourage the patient to apply these lifestyle changes.

Possible causes of poor response to GER treatment include a noncompliant patient, lack of adequate therapy or insufficient dosage, or an incorrect diagnosis.[6,7]

SURGICAL TREATMENT

Surgical treatment has come a long way since the 1950s, when GER, with or without a hiatal hernia, was treated with a laparotomy and suturing of the diaphragm. This procedure had recurrence rates of over 30%, even for the most talented surgeons. The abdominal approach, in which the diaphragmatic crura and phrenoesophageal ligament are sutured and a complete or posterior fundoplication is performed, has completely changed the feasibility of the operation, making its recommendation more plausible.

Today, with the spread of laparoscopic surgery, this surgery has become an even more viable option, if the surgeon has the necessary experience and is equipped with the necessary equipment. Surgery should be considered in several situations. All patients, especially the young, who have an inadequate response to medical management, present with a mechanically defective lower esophageal sphincter, or those with more serious complications are candidates for surgery.[1,5]

For effective patient selection, diagnostic tools such as endoscopy, imagenology, esophageal body and sphincter manometry, 24-hour pH monitoring, and occasionally 24-hour bile exposure monitoring and gastric emptying studies are necessary.[2]

In our opinion, GER surgery should be considered when the patient:

- Cannot or does not wish to follow the dietary recommendations, cannot eat without irritation, or is morbidly obese and unable to lose weight.
- Lives in a location without access to medication, adequate health care services, or is unable to afford the cost of long-term medication.
- Has insurance coverage for the operation and associated expenses that may expire after a short time.

- Has followed the medical treatment prescribed, but continues to have complications of the disease, such as esophageal stenosis, hemorrhage, or laryngeal or pulmonary complications due to nocturnal reflux.

The treatment of GER is a perfect example of the coordination that exists—and must always be maintained—between the clinical gastroenterologist and the surgeon. One must always keep in mind the economic burden of long-term medical treatment, as well as that of hospitalization and surgery. Although the surgical approach to treatment of GER is rarely used as the principal therapeutic option, the suc-cess rate is in the range of 80 to 90%, especially with laparoscopic procedures, which also have the advantages of significantly reduced cost, shorter hospital stay, and more rapid recovery.[6,7]

REFERENCES

1. De Meester TR, Peters JH, Bremner CG, et al. Biology of gastroesophageal reflux disease: pathophysiology relating to medical and surgical treatment. *Annu Rev Med*. 1999;50:469.
2. Scwab GP, Blum AL, Bodner E, et al. Gastro-oesophageal reflux disease: medical or surgical treatment? Report of an interactive workshop. *J Gastroenterol Hepatol*. 1997;12:785.
3. Tougas G, Armstrong D. Efficacy of H_2 receptor antagonists in the treatment of gastroesophageal reflux disease and its symptoms. *Can J Gastroenterol*. 1997;11(Suppl B):51B.
4. Klinkenberg-Knol EC, Nelis F, Debt J, et al. Long-term omeprazole treatment in resistant gastroesophageal reflux disease: Efficacy, safety and influence on gastric mucosa. *Gastroenterology* 2000;118:661.
5. Balint A, Mate M, Szabo K, et al. Surgical aspects of gastro-esophageal reflux disease—indication for surgery. An Update. *Acta Chir Hung*. 1999;38:123.
6. Fass R, Hixson LJ, Ciccolo ML, et al. Contemporary medical therapy for gastroesophageal reflux disease. *Am Fam Physician*. 1997;55:205, 217.
7. Castell D. My approach to the difficult GERD patient. *Eur J Gastroenterol Hepatol*. 1999;11(Suppl 1):S17.
8. Rohss K, Lundin C, et al. Esomeprazole 40 mg provides more effective acid control than omeprazole 40 mg. *Am J Gastroenterol*. 2000;98:2432.
9. Amitabh P. Rabeprazole. *Drugs* 1998;5:261.

Chapter Thirteen • • • • • •

Results of Laparoscopic Antireflux Surgery

BERNARD DALLEMAGNE

INTRODUCTION

Since the first report of laparoscopic fundoplication using Nissen's technique in 1991, the treatment of gastroesophageal reflux disease (GERD) has changed considerably all over the world.[1] The 1990s saw a resurgence of interest in these operations, which had practically fallen into disuse in the 1980s following the introduction of increasingly effective antacid drugs. If the number of antireflux operations increased, it was not due to a change in the indications, but rather to a reduction of contraindications, which during the era of open surgery were often dependent on the need for the procedure.

The advent of laparoscopic surgery of the gallbladder and the advantages it quickly showed spurred the development of other applications of laparoscopic procedures of the digestive tract, particularly antireflux surgery to treat GERD. This was an area of particular interest, due to its increasing frequency and the socioeconomic implications of its management. Many feasibility studies of laparoscopic fundoplication were published, and they showed the short-term effectiveness of the technique.[2–8]

The aim of this chapter is to review the long-term results of laparoscopic fundoplication and to estimate the outcome of antireflux surgery after more than 5 years of follow-up. In order to avoid skewing, a consecutive series of 100 patients operated on by a single surgeon in his third year of experience with the procedure was studied.

PATIENTS AND METHODS

Between January 1991 and December 1998, 994 patients underwent primary laparoscopic fundoplication at the Department of Digestive Surgery at the Clinics Saint Joseph, Liege, Belgium. Clinical data were prospectively recorded. In the year 1993, 165 patients were operated on. The population studied consisted of 100 consecutive patients operated on by a single surgeon. Before their surgery, all of the patients presented with typical symptoms of GERD (heartburn and regurgitation) that required uninterrupted medical treatment. In 43 patients extraesophageal symptoms (cough,

dyspnea, asthma, or ENT symptoms) were also present. All the patients had had continuous medical therapy, and all had received proton pump inhibitors (PPI). Twenty patients reported only partial control of their symptoms with PPIs.

Diagnostic Studies

Upper endoscopy was performed in all patients preoperatively. Esophagitis was graded based on the Savary-Miller system. Any length of intestinal metaplastic columnar epithelium on biopsy defined Barrett's esophagus. Seventeen patients presented with grade 1 esophagitis, 61 patients with grade 2, 8 patients with grade 3, 1 patient with grade 4, and 13 patients had Barrett's esophagus.

Twenty-four-hour ambulatory pH testing was performed in 54 patients. Esophageal acid exposure was quantitated by DeMeester's scoring system.[9] Abnormal esoph-ageal acid exposure was detected in 51 patients. Three patients had normal pH monitoring results.

Esophageal motility testing was also performed in all patients. An inefficient lower esophageal sphincter (LES) was defined by one or more of the following parameters: resting pressure <6 mm Hg, an overall length <2 cm, or an abdominal length <1 cm.[10] On the basis of these criteria, 91% of the patients had a defective LES: loss of basal tone, and insufficient length, both abdominal and total. Nine percent had a reduction of total and abdominal length of a normotonic LES. Esophageal motility disorders were observed in 18 patients.

Barium esophagograms were obtained in all patients: a hiatal hernia was observed in 71 patients (reducible in 81%), and gastroesophageal reflux was observed in 58 patients.

Operative Procedures

Two types of surgical procedures were performed: total fundoplication according to Nissen's technique, and posterior partial fundoplication. The choice of technique was based on the preoperative motility study of the esophagus and LES. In patients with deterioration of esophageal peristalsis and those having normal basal tone of the LES, a partial fundoplication was carried out. All the operations were performed laparoscopically, and there were no conversions to laparotomy.

The Nissen fundoplication consists of the construction of a 360° valve using the upper part of the gastric fundus, which was mobilized beforehand by division of two or three short gastric vessels and the gastrophrenic ligament. This valve, made up after the retroesophageal passage of the anterior and posterior walls of the fundus, measures 1.5 cm in length in its pre-esophageal portion and links the posterior gastric wall on the right of the esophagus and the anterior fundic wall on the left of the esophagus, according to the technique described by DeMeester.[11] A crural repair is performed systematically.

The posterior partial fundoplication uses the same principles of mobilization of the upper part of the gastric fundus, but the valve is attached to the left and right anterolateral borders of the esophagus, covering its posterior portion by approximately 270°. This valve is attached to the diaphragmatic crura. It is inspired by the technique described by Guarner.[12]

EVALUATION

Symptomatic, clinical, and radiological measures were used to analyze the outcome of the procedure. The 100 patients were examined directly and asked to fill out a questionnaire. At the time of the interview with the patient, a clinical examination was carried out, and the patient was invited to undergo a barium esophagogram. This study seems to be more acceptable to the patients, is easier than endoscopy or pH monitoring, and allows a precise delineation of the architecture and position of the antireflux valve. The questionnaire included 15 questions to assess the preoperative and postoperative severity of the symptoms of GERD (heartburn, chest pain, regurgitation, asthma, dysphagia, odynophagia, abdominal pain, nausea and vomiting, belching, abdominal distension, increased flatulence, indigestion, lack of appetite, bloating, and food intolerance). In this study heartburn, which was present preoperatively in all patients, was the key indicator of the success of the operation. For the postfundoplication symptoms severity of dysphagia, flatulence, and abdominal distension were selected as criteria for success (Table 13–1).

The symptomatic outcome was considered *excellent* if the patient was asymptomatic, *good* if the symptoms of GERD were relieved but minor gastroenterologic complaints (flatulence, abdominal distension) persisted, *fair* if the symptoms of GERD were improved but required medical therapy for complete relief, and *poor* if the symptoms remained unchanged or in the presence of severe side effects.

RESULTS

One hundred patients were contacted more than 5 years after surgery. Two patients had died (auto accident, infarction), 1 patient had a total gastrectomy for cancer, and 10 patients did not respond. The studied series included 37 women and 50 men (87 patients); 57 patients had a Nissen fundoplication (Group A) and 30 a partial posterior fundoplication (Group B). The mean age was 52 years (range: 32 to 78 years) and the duration of the follow-up was longer than 5 years in all patients, except for 2 patients who were

TABLE 13–1. CRITERIA FOR ASSESSING SEVERITY OF PRE- AND POSTOPERATIVE SYMPTOMS OF GERD

Heartburn:	None
	Grade 1: Minimal, occasional
	Grade 2: Moderate, requiring medical treatment
	Grade 3: Severe, constant; marked disability in activities of daily living
Dysphagia:	None
	Grade 1: Occasional, with coarse foods, lasts for seconds
	Grade 2: Requires clearing with liquids
	Grade 3: Severe, semiliquid diet required
	Grade 4: Liquids only
Flatulence:	None
	Grade 1: Occasionally
	Grade 2: Frequently
	Grade 3: Continuously
Abdominal distension:	None
	Grade 1: Occasionally
	Grade 2: Frequently
	Grade 3: Continuously

reoperated for complications and recurrence within the first 2 years of follow-up. These patients were excluded from the clinical and radiological studies. Fifty-three patients answered the questionnaire and presented for clinical and radiological examinations (34/56 Nissen, 19/29 partial); 34 patients answered the questionnaire. All the radiological and clinical data and responses to the questionnaires were integrated in the final database.

In Group A, the results were good to excellent in 94.8% of patients and fair in 2 (3.4%) patients. One patient had a poor result (1.7%) and required fundoplication revision and conversion to a partial posterior valve in the first 2 years of follow-up for persisting postoperative dysphagia. This patient had preoperative primary esophageal motility disorders. The heartburn disappeared without any additional treatment in 54/56 patients (96.4%; Table 13–2).

Thirty-four patients underwent a barium esophagogram, which demonstrated a well-positioned and continent valve in all of them. Four patients mentioned occasional heart-burn that did not require treatment. Moderate heartburn requiring PPI therapy was mentioned by two patients presenting with gastric ulcers found by endoscopy, but they had no esophageal lesion and the fundoplications were intact.

Among the patients not having had radiological evaluation (n = 22), 8 mentioned occasional heartburn that did not require treatment. No patient required postoperative endoscopic dilation for dysphagia. Eighteen patients (32%) mentioned occasional dysphagia with coarse food, and 3 patients rarely required clearing with liquids (5%). No patient reported chronic dysphagia. Increased flatulence was reported as being frequent to continuous in 58% of patients, and frequent to continuous abdominal distension was mentioned by 27% of patients. Forty-two percent of patients were asymptomatic when all gastrointestinal symptoms were considered (an excellent result).

In Group B, results were good to excellent in 83.4% and fair in 13.3% of the patients. One patient had a poor result and had to undergo reoperation for recurrent symptoms related to intrathoracic migration of the valve. This patient is excluded from the study of the long-term results. Heartburn disappeared without any therapy in 86% of patients (Table 13–3). Nineteen patients underwent a

TABLE 13–2. RESULTS OF NISSEN FUNDOPLICATION (GROUP A)

Symptom		Nissen		
		%	n	RX[1]
Heartburn	None	75	(42)	32/32 OK
	Grade 1	21.4	(12)	6/6 OK
	Grade 2	3.5	(2)	1/1 OK
	Grade 3	0		
Dysphagia	None	62.5	(35)	19/19 OK
	Grade 1	32.1	(18)	14/14 OK
	Grade 2	5.3	(3)	2/2 OK
	Grade 3	0		
	Grade 4	0		
Abdominal distension	None	30.3	(17)	
	Grade 1	42.8	(24)	
	Grade 2	14.2	(8)	
	Grade 3	12.5	(7)	
Flatulence	None	5.3	(3)	
	Grade 1	32.1	(18)	
	Grade 2	44.6	(25)	
	Grade 3	14.2	(8)	
Revisions	Heartburn			
	Dysphagia	1.7	(1)	

[1]Number of occurrences/number of controlled patients in the category;
OK = valve well positioned and competent.

barium esophagogram. An intact but herniated wrap was discovered in 7 patients (36.8%; Figure 13–1). Three of them were asymptomatic, 2 patients mentioned occasional heartburn not requiring treatment, and 2 patients mentioned disabling heartburn requiring PPI therapy. Among the patients having a satisfactory radiologic result (n = 12), 2 patients mentioned occasional heartburn. In the group of uncontrolled patients, 4 patients used antacids. No patient required postoperative endoscopic dilation for dysphagia.

Occasional dysphagia was mentioned by 9 patients (27%), 1 of whom had a migrated valve and 3 presenting with a normal

TABLE 13–3. RESULTS OF PARTIAL POSTERIOR FUNDOPLICATION (GROUP B)

Symptom		Partial		
		%	n	X-rays[1]
Heartburn	None	62	(18)	3/13 sus
	Grade 1	24.3	(7)	2/4 sus
	Grade 2	13.7	(4)	2/2 sus
	Grade 3	0		
Dysphagia	None	68.9	(20)	6/16 sus
	Grade 1	27.5	(8)	2/3 sus
	Grade 2	3.4	(1)	
	Grade 3	0		
	Grade 4	0		
Abdominal distension	None	24.1	(7)	
	Grade 1	44.8	(13)	
	Grade 2	20.6	(6)	
	Grade 3	10.3	(3)	
Flatulence	None	0		
	Grade 1	37.9	(11)	
	Grade 2	51.7	(15)	
	Grade 3	10.3	(3)	
Revisions	Heartburn	3.3	(1)	
	Dysphagia			

[1]Number of occurrences/number of controlled patients in the category;
sus = intrathoracic valve.

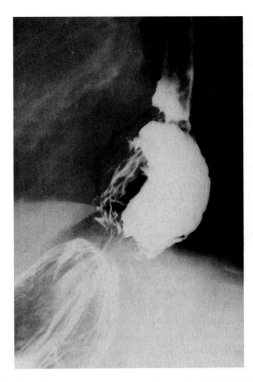

Figure 13–1. Barium esophagogram of a patient with a herniated partial posterior fundoplication.

valve. No dysphagia of Grade 3 was reported. Increased flatulence was mentioned as being frequent to continuous in 61% of the patients, and frequent to continuous abdominal distension was mentioned by 31% of the patients. No patient was totally free of all the symptoms we studied.

DISCUSSION

Fundoplication is effective in controlling symptomatic gastroesophageal reflux associated with an incompetent LES, either due to loss of resting tonicity or length and/or position.[13] The goal of surgical treatment for GERD is to relieve the symptoms of reflux by reestablishing the gastro-esophageal barrier. The challenge is to accomplish this without inducing dysphagia or other untoward side effects.

Published surgical series since the original description of the Nissen procedure in 1955 confirm that the open fundoplication allows the reconstruction of an effective antireflux barrier and controls symptoms of GERD in approximately 85 to 90% of patients with follow-up periods of about 10 to 15 years.[14] The incidence of side effects, dysphagia, flatulence, and abdominal bloating, was reduced by the modifications brought to the original valve of Nissen.[11] Laparoscopic fundoplication was introduced into clinical practice in 1991.[1] Evidence is rapidly accumulating to indicate that the procedure is highly effective in controlling symptomatic gastroesophageal reflux.[15] Peters et al[6] showed that laparoscopic fundoplication relieved the "typical" symptoms of heartburn, regurgitation, and dysphagia in 95% of patients for up to 4 years. Erosive esophagitis was healed in 90% of patients returning for follow-up endoscopy, and 24-hour ambulatory esophageal pH profiles returned to normal in 92% of patients tested >1 year after surgery. Hunter et[4] al also reported >90% improvement in symptoms and a similar reduction in esophageal acid exposure measured by 24-hour pH monitoring.

These studies had short postoperative follow-up periods and it appeared that study of the outcome of laparoscopically-constructed antireflux valves for a longer follow-up would be fruitful.

Despite the somewhat low rate of acceptance of radiologic evaluation (only 60% of patients consented), and the return rate of 87% for the questionnaires, this study confirms the effectiveness of the laparoscopic Nissen's fundoplication, modified according to the principles described by DeMeester: Important technical elements included crural and hiatal dissection, crural closure, and fundic mobilization by division of the short gastric vessels in all patients. A short (1 to 2 cm), loose fundoplication was constructed by enveloping the distal esophagus with the anterior and posterior wall of the gastric fundus.

This study has shown that laparoscopic fundoplication relieved the "typical" symptoms of heartburn and regurgitation in 96% of patients for more than 5 years.

One patient in the Nissen group underwent fundoplication revision for persistent dysphagia due to a primary esophageal dysmotility disorder which was unaffected by the transformation into a partial posterior valve.

No significant dysphagia was reported by 93% of the patients, and 4 patients mentioned the occasional need to clear food with liquids; endoscopic postoperative dilation was never necessary.

Radiologic evaluation was very satisfactory among all patients who accepted the examination, and the findings correlated well with the symptomatic outcome. On the other hand, the results of the partial fundoplications were disappointing, which were performed on patients presenting with esophageal motility disorders or normotonic LES. Control of symptoms was obtained in 86% of patients and the incidence of side effects is comparable to those found after total fundoplication.

In the entire series, 4 patients required continuing PPI therapy—2 with the Nissen procedure (for gastroduodenal ulcers) and 2 after partial fundoplication (for recurrent symptoms and endoscopic esophagitis; 3.5%).

We were also surprised by the significant incidence of intrathoracic migration, as this type of valve is attached to the diaphragm (but there is no fixation for the Nissen valve) and a diaphragmatic repair was carried out systematically. The study of preoperative esophagograms did not show signs of esophageal shortening in these patients. These migrations most likely explain the occasional or continuous recurrence of symptoms, which required medical therapy: Of 5 patients with recurrence, 4 had a subdiaphragmatic valve. Our concern also comes from the fact that 3 of 11 of the controlled asymptomatic patients had a migration, which may expose them to recurrence. Our results are in accordance with those presented by some laparoscopic surgeons, but do not compare with some of the experience with open procedures.[16,17]

Our treatment regimen has changed, and we now use posterior partial fundoplications only in patients presenting with very severe disorders of esophageal motility, such as that seen in scleroderma (waves of very low amplitude, with a very low percentage of propulsive waves). The construction of short and very floppy Nissen valves allows us to use them in the vast majority of patients, including those who present with "current" motility disorders related to esophageal irritation by gastric reflux, without a need for postoperative dilation for persistent dysphagia. The cut-off point is wave amplitude lower than 15 mm Hg with less than 35% propulsive waves, as measured by 24-hour esophageal manometric study.

The only alarming side effect unconnected to the type of procedure is the appearance or aggravation of flatulence and abdominal distension, symptoms described by about 50% of patients, with equal distribution between the total and partial fundoplication groups. More women complain of abdominal distension than men. No painful gas bloating was observed in the series. The patients mentioned a tendency toward reduction (or acclimatization) to these minor problems over the years, and these side effects caused no regrets about the surgery in the affected patients.

CONCLUSIONS

We conclude that the laparoscopic Nissen fundoplication is effective in treating gastroesophageal reflux and relieves most symptoms in >90% of patients. Symptomatic relief has persisted for more than 5 years after surgery, and there is every reason to expect that the effect will persist for the lifetime of these patients.

Even if statistical significance cannot be demonstrated from these unmatched groups, the technique of posterior partial fundoplication seems less effective in our hands, with an incidence of side effects comparable to that of the Nissen technique, but with a greater incidence of displacement of the valves. It is currently reserved for a very few selected patients who present with major esophageal motility disorders.

REFERENCES

1. Dallemagne B, Weerts JM, Jehaes C, et al. Laparoscopic Nissen fundoplication: preliminary report. *Surg Laparosc Endosc.* 1991;1:138.
2. Dallemagne B, Weerts JM, Jeahes C, et al. Results of laparoscopic Nissen fundoplication. *Hepatogastroenterology* 1998;45:1338.
3. Hinder RA, Filipi CJ, Wetscher G, et al. Laparoscopic Nissen fundoplication is an effective treatment for gastroesophageal reflux disease. *Ann Surg.* 1994;220:472.
4. Hunter JG, Trus TL, Branum GD, et al. A physiologic approach to laparoscopic fundoplication for gastroesophageal reflux disease. *Ann Surg.* 1996;223:673.
5. Jamieson GG, Watson DI, Britten-Jones R, et al. Laparoscopic Nissen fundoplication. *Ann Surg.* 1994;220:137.
6. Peters JH, DeMeester TR, Crookes P, et al. The treatment of gastroesophageal reflux disease with laparoscopic Nissen fundoplication: prospective evaluation of 100 patients with "typical" symptoms. *Ann Surg.* 1998;228:40.
7. Watson DI, Jamieson GG, Baigrie RJ, et al. Laparoscopic surgery for gastro-oesophageal reflux: beyond the learning curve. *Br J Surg.* 1996;83:1284.
8. Weerts JM, Dallemagne B, Hamoir E, et al. Laparoscopic Nissen fundoplication: detailed analysis of 132 patients. *Surg Laparosc Endosc.* 1993;3:359.
9. DeMeester TR, Wang CI, Wernly JA, et al. Technique, indications, and clinical use of 24 hour esophageal pH monitoring. *J Thorac Cardiovasc Surg.* 1980;79:656.

10. Zaninotto G, DeMeester TR, Schwizer W, et al. The lower esophageal sphincter in health and disease. *Am J Surg.* 1988;155:104.

11. DeMeester TR, Bonavina L, Albertucci M. Nissen fundoplication for gastroesophageal reflux disease. Evaluation of primary repair in 100 consecutive patients. *Ann Surg* 1986;204:9.

12. Guarner V. 30 years' experience with posterior fundoplasty in the treatment of gastroesophageal reflux (analysis of 1499 cases). *Chirurgie* 1997;122:443.

13. Spechler SJ GRSG. Comparison of medical and surgical therapy for complicated gastroesophageal reflux disease in veterans. *N Engl J Med.* 1992;326:786.

14. Luostarinen M, Isolauri J, Laitinen J, et al. Fate of Nissen fundoplication after 20 years. A clinical, endoscopical, and functional analysis. *Gut* 1993;34:1015.

15. Perdikis G, Hinder RA, Lund RJ, et al. Laparoscopic Nissen fundoplication: where do we stand? *Surg Laparosc Endosc.* 1997; 7:17.

16. Lundell L, Abrahamsson H, Ruth M, et al. Long-term results of a prospective randomized comparison of total fundic wrap (Nissen-Rossetti) or semifundoplication (Toupet) for gastro-oesophageal reflux [see comments]. *Br J Surg.* 1996;83:830.

17. Horvath KD, Jobe BA, Herron DM, et al. Laparoscopic Toupet fundoplication is an inadequate procedure for patients with severe reflux disease. *J Gastrointest Surg* 1999;3:583.

Chapter Fourteen ● ● ● ● ● ●

Use, Indications, and Results of Intraoperative Esophageal Manometry

ALBERTO DEL GENIO, GIUSEPPE IZZO, VINCENZO MAFFETTONE, VINCENZO NAPOLITANO, LUIGI BRUSCIANO, GIANLUCA RUSSO, and DANILO CUTTITTA

INTRODUCTION

Intraoperative esophageal manometry (IEM) was employed for the first time on human subjects in 1972 by Lanzara and Del Genio.[1,2] This first application was the result of many years of experimental studies on the surgical therapy of esophageal motile disorders. Their purpose was to quantitatively evaluate the surgical correction and the consequent long-term functional outcome in the surgical treatment of functional diseases of the esophagus. This depends on many variables, such as the surgeon's personal experience, the chosen procedure, and the anatomic configuration and functional situation of the patient. The intraoperative assessment of all these factors represents a very difficult task even for the most experienced surgeon.

The experimental studies[3,4] that preceded this first experience demonstrated the following points:

- Surgical manipulation and anesthetic gases and opiates (fentanyl) do not significantly alter lower esophageal sphincter (LES) pressure values.
- The technique was able to demonstrate the pressure drop and/or the ablation of the LES pressure values produced by the myotomy on the LES.
- In the Nissen fundoplication there is a positive correlation between the length and the tightness of the wrap, as well as the length and the pressure of the new high pressure zone.
- IEM is currently being employed by several authors either to demonstrate the complete ablation of the LES pressure during Heller's myotomies[5–19] or for the calibration of the antireflux procedures.[20,21] Nevertheless, many authors deny the validity of the technique and do not recommend its use.[22–26,34,35] Moreover, the growing success of laparoscopic esophageal surgery has given rise to more controversy. Many authors affirm that the intra-abdominal pressure created by the pneumoperitoneum significantly alters the results of the intraoperative manometric evaluation.

PATIENTS AND METHODS

From 1985 to date, intraoperative manometric recording has been employed in the course of 397 surgical procedures on the gastroesophageal (GE) junction, all performed by the same surgeon.

IEM has been employed to demonstrate the ablation of LES pressure during 209 Heller's extramucosal cardiomyotomies: 186 for achalasia (among which 6 were reoperations on patients with a recurrence; these patients had had the original procedure elsewhere), 18 for epiphrenic diverticulum, 3 for leiomyoma of the GE junction, and 2 for diffuse esophageal spasm (DES) (1 being a recurrence in a patient operated on elsewhere). The access route was via laparotomy in 107 patients and via laparoscopy in 102 patients (93 for achalasia, 3 for leiomyoma, and 6 for epiphrenic diverticula). IEM has also been employed to calibrate 397 Nissen-Rossetti fundoplications: 209 after Heller's myotomy, 159 in patients with gastroesophageal reflux disease (GERD) (including 3 reoperations on patients operated on elsewhere), 15 on patients with hiatal hernia without evidence of gastroesophageal reflux (GER) on 24-hour pH monitoring, and 14 for pathologic acid GER on patients with esophageal diverticula (7 pharyngoesophageal, 3 thoracic, and 4 epiphrenic). These procedures were performed via laparotomy in 202 cases and via laparoscopy in 195 (102 post-Heller, 86 for GER, and 7 for hiatal hernia).

For intraoperative manometric recordings, we em-ployed a 3-lumen catheter assembly. Each tube had an internal diameter of 1.1 mm and was closed at the tip. Radially-placed side openings were spaced at 5-cm intervals from the distal margin of the catheter. Each tube was perfused with distilled water at a constant rate of 0.6 mL/min by a low compliance perfusion system (Andorfer Medical Specialties). Pressure transducers incorporated into each perfusion line were connected to an amplifier and polygraph (Ote Biomedica, EP 12; Sensor Medics in the course of last year). Intragastric pressure was referred to as zero. We used the rapid pull-through technique during IEM and a station pull-through during standard manometry. In our opinion, a Heller myotomy has been correctly performed only when IEM documents the ablation of the lower esophageal sphincter high-pressure zone (LES-HPZ) or the persistence of only minimal residual pressure (<3 mm Hg).

Regarding the calibration of the fundoplasty, in our initial experience we performed a "normocalibrated" Nissen (nHPZ = 10 to 20 mm Hg; length 2 to 4 cm). However, with these figures we later saw a high recurrence rate (28.5%) in the first 12 months after surgery. This finding, and the observation that 6 to 12 months after surgery the nHPZ pressure values tended to decrease by half, led us to modify the intraoperative calibration of the fundoplication. In fact, during the last 15 years we have routinely calibrated the wrap to higher pressure values (20 to 40 mm Hg; length 2 to 4 cm; a "hypercalibrated Nissen"). We do not believe that it is appropriate to obtain nHPZ pressure values exceeding 40 mm Hg because a value more than twice that of a normal sphincter seemed enough to guarantee sufficient control of reflux.

The idea of a "hypercalibrated Nissen" is in contrast to the concept of a "floppy Nissen" supported by Donahue.[27] Also, our wrap is loose around the esophagus. A "hypercalibrated Nissen" does not necessarily mean a tight Nissen. We named our procedure the modified Nissen-Rossetti (N-R) hypercalibrated Nissen due to the higher pressure values obtained intraoperatively, which are twice those of a normal sphincter.

In 45 patients (24 with GER, 19 with achalasia, and 1 with epiphrenic diverticulum) we also measured the intraoperative LES pressure both during anesthetic induction (before opening the abdomen), and during anesthetic maintenance when the abdomen was open. This latter recording was performed before and after the mobilization of the GE junction.

During induction and before laparotomy, 42 of the 45 patients subjected to manometric recording showed a marked decrease in the LES pressure (40% of the resting tone) that lasted about 20 minutes (18.74 ± 4.03 min). After this period the LES pressure returned to values similar to those measured preoperatively. The remaining 3 patients did not show pressure modifications. Intraoperative measurements before and after the mobilization of the GE junction did not record significant pressure variations when compared with the preoperative findings.

Regarding the reliability of IEM in the course of laparoscopy, we did not find significant differences (i.e., pressure variations with respect to the gastric pressure, which is referred to as zero) between the LES or the nHPZ pressure values recorded with and without pneumoperitoneum (12 mm Hg). According to other authors,[28] this is because the pneumoperitoneum produces a homogeneous pressure increase (about 10 mm Hg) both in the stomach and in the GE junction. The intraoperative manometric recording took 5 to 15 minutes.

IEM documented the ablation of the LES pressure in 133 out of the 209 cardiomyotomies (63.6%) all performed with the aid of intraoperative endoscopy. In the remaining 76 patients the persistence of a HPZ (>3 mm Hg) was due to the pressure of the diaphragmatic pillars in 41 (19.6%) (7.3 ± 2.4 mm Hg), and in 35 (16.7%) was due to the incompleteness of the myotomy (9.5 ± 4.1 mm Hg residual pressure). In the majority of the cases (69.4%) the site of residual fibers was in the distal portion of the myotomy (i.e., on the stomach). In all patients the ablation of the LES pressure (<3 mm Hg) was finally demonstrated after the localization and section of the residual fibers.

After the fundoplication, IEM showed adequate pressure values (20 to 40 mm Hg) in 309 out of 397 N-R procedures (77.8%). In 80 patients (20.1%), the nHPZ pressure was lower than 20 mm Hg and it was necessary to tighten the wrap with one or two stitches. In the remaining 8 patients (2.0%) the wrap had to be dismantled and reconstructed because the nHPZ values exceeded 40 mm Hg. The nHPZ pressure values recorded after cardiomyotomy and N-R fundoplication were 26.04 ± 4.78 mm Hg with a length of 2.93 ± 0.7 cm in the laparotomy group and 24.82 ± 3.96 mm Hg with a length of 2.58 ± 0.8 cm in the laparoscopy group. The nHPZ pressure values after the N-R procedure in patients with GER and/or hiatal hernia were 25.32 ± 4.84 mm Hg with a length of 2.66 ± 0.8 cm in the laparotomy group and 26.54 ± 4.82 mm Hg with a length of 2.41 ± 0.5 cm in the laparoscopy group.[29]

There were two deaths in this series. Both patients were achalasic and had been treated by laparotomy. The deaths were caused by Boerhaave syndrome in a patient who spontaneously resumed oral solid feeding the day after surgery, and by acute pylephlebitis in a patient with severe cirrhosis.

After surgery, 395 patients were followed up by clinical examination (53.4 ± 15.2 months for the laparotomy group; 34.12 ± 11.1 months for the laparoscopy group). Two hundred and seven patients had a Heller's cardiomyotomy and N-R procedure (H + N − R: first group) while 188 patients had undergone a Nissen-Rossetti (N-R: second group). In the first group, 33 patients (15.9%) experienced transitory symptoms (dysphagia or gas bloating syndrome), which resolved spontaneously after 3 months, while 35 patients (16.9%) complained of persistent dysphagia. The symptom, however, occurred once or twice a week and did not impair adequate feeding.

The clinical follow-up of the 188 patients in the N-R group showed that GER-related symptoms such as heartburn and regurgitation were successfully cured by the procedure in all patients but one (0.5%). In this patient pH-monitoring demonstrated the persistence of GER that was found to be caused by the Nissen disruption. The patient was reoperated and his symptoms promptly resolved after the procedure. Twenty-five patients (13.2%) (20 with dysphagia and 5 with gas bloating syndrome) complained of transitory postoperative symptoms (dysphagia and gas bloating syndrome). Fifteen patients (7.9%) showed occasional dysphagia (Visick II) once or twice a week, and 5 patients (2.6%) had a persistent dysphagia. Among these 20 patients, as many as 11 showed the persistence after surgery of nonspecific esophageal motor disorders (NEMD), but only 3 had showed first-degree esophagitis at the preoperative evaluation. In the remaining 4 patients with persistent postoperative dysphagia, 3 patients had a nHPZ pressure >20 mm Hg. The patients with preoperative thoracic pain reported the resolution of the symptom in 77.2% of the cases (17/22 patients). Another patient developed the symptom only after surgery. A diagnostic laparoscopy showed that the fundal wrap had herniated into the thorax. A posterior hiatoplasty was performed through the same route. One patient with severe dysphagia and gas bloating syndrome was also submitted to reoperation. The symptoms were due to a "lazy resident repair" and resolved after the reoperation.

One hundred and forty-eight patients were also followed up by 24-hours esophagogastric pH monitoring and standard manometry. The duration of follow-up was 43.9 ± 11.7 months for the 87 patients in the laparotomy group and 34.84 ± 8.22 months for the 61 patients of the laparoscopy group. Among the 148 followed-up patients, 76 had undergone a H + N − R procedure while 72 only had N-R. At pH monitoring all 76 patients who had undergone the H + N − R procedure and 47 (65.2%) out of the 72 patients submitted to N-R showed the complete absence of reflux episodes (hypercompetent Nissen), while 23 patients (31.9%) had moderate nonpathologic GER (percentage of time the pH was <4 was <1%). In the remaining 2 patients (2.7%) of the N-R group, pH monitoring showed GER recurrence (only one of the patients was symptomatic). At standard manometry both had a new HPZ pressure of <8 mm Hg.

The comparison of the nHPZ pressure values found at standard manometry in the two followed-up groups did not show significant differences. In fact, in the patients submitted to Heller + Nissen-Rossetti the nHPZ values were 14.1 ± 3.97 mm Hg for the laparotomy group and 15.8 ± 2.68 mm Hg for the laparoscopy group, while the patients who underwent Nissen-Rossetti showed nHPZ values of 15.65 ± 4.61 mm Hg for the laparotomy group and 14.85 ± 6.44 mm Hg for the laparoscopy group. These values were significantly lower than those measured intraoperatively ($p <$ 0.01) but similar to those obtained from the control group of healthy subjects (14.6 ± 3.9 mm Hg). This marked pressure decrease occurred in the first 6 to 12 months after surgery. The percentage of postdeglutitive relaxations after surgery was 75.3 ± 3.44% in the H + N − R group and 79.4 ± 6.08% in the N-R group. These values were significantly lower when compared with the control group (>95%) ($p <$ 0.05).

The postoperative assessment of esophageal body motility showed the restoration of peristaltic contractions (40% of the postdeglutitive motor sequences) in 8 (11.4%) out of the 70 followed-up achalasic patients.

DISCUSSION

The results of our experience with IEM show that neither anesthesia nor surgical manipulations significantly alter intraoperative LES pressure values. This finding is consistent with the reports of several authors,[21,28–32] but in conflict with the opinion of others.[23] A moderate pressure decrease in the LES-HPZ can only be seen during induction. This pharmacologic interference, however, does not call into question the validity of the technique. In fact, the hypotonic effect lasts only 20 minutes, which is about the time the surgeon needs to reach the GE junction.

In our experience the pneumoperitoneum does not seem to significantly alter the LES-HPZ pressure values. This is because the intra-abdominal insufflation of carbon dioxide produces a homogeneous pressure increase of about 10 mm Hg both in the stomach (whose pressure is referred to as zero) and in the gastroesophageal junction.

Regarding the use of IEM in the course of Heller's procedure, our results suggest that the objective demonstration of the ablation of the LES-HPZ (residual pressure <3 mm Hg) could play an important role in the good outcome of the operation, even when the procedure has been performed with the aid of the intraoperative endoscopy. In this series, in fact, the intraoperative manometric recording demonstrated the persistence of a high pressure zone (9.5 ± 4.1 mm Hg) in 16.7% of apparently complete myotomies. In most cases the residual fibers were localized in the distal tract of the myotomy (69.4%) This finding confirms our opinion that no better means of controlling the ablation of the LES pressure are available to date. The functional ablation of the LES-HPZ, in fact,

is a necessary requisite for the resolution of the achalasia- and/or dyschalasia-related symptoms. As a matter of fact in this series we did not observe relapses in our patients treated for achalasia and esophageal diverticuli.

Regarding the role of IEM in the adequate calibration of the fundoplication, the results of this series show that the pressure of the fundic wrap was insufficient in 20.1% of the cases and exceedingly high in 2.01%. Yet all the procedures had been performed by the same surgeon and with the same technique. In fact we had to modify the fundic wrap in as many as 22.1% of the procedures. This suggests that both the tightness of the wrap and the functional activity of the fundal muscle fibers, which is highly subjective, contribute to the new high pressure zone values. In view of this, the reliability of the mechanical calibrations (balloons and bougies) proposed by several authors could be seriously questioned.

Regarding the correlation between intraoperative pressure values and long-term outcome, several observations seem to confirm our theory.[33,36,37]

First of all, our results show that the hypercalibrated Nissen-Rossetti procedure successfully cures and/or prevents GER and GER-related symptoms in a high percentage of cases (98.6%; 146/148 patients).

On the other hand, in a former experience with a normocalibrated fundoplication (10 to 20 mm Hg) we had observed a high recurrence rate (28.5%). In that same report we found two gastroesophageal recurrences at pH monitoring follow-up (only 1 symptomatic). In these two patients postoperative standard manometry showed a hypotonic nHPZ (8 and 6 mm Hg). On the other hand, 4 patients had postoperative persistent dysphagia, and in 3 of these nHPZ values exceeding 20 mm Hg were found by manometric follow-up. In spite of all our efforts, we did not manage to clearly define the cause of these marked differences between these nHPZ values and the expected ones.

In our opinion the high rate of success in this series must be ascribed to the hypercalibration of the fundoplasty. This is a technical modification we made about 15 years ago in order to reduce the high incidence of GER relapse we had observed after an earlier experience with a normocalibrated fundoplication. The follow-up manometric examinations showed that in the first 6 to 12 months after surgery, there was a significant ($p <$ 0.01) decrease of the nHPZ pressure values that could account for the high recurrence rate. We believe that the higher antireflux function of the hypercalibrated Nissen is due to the long-term persistence of adequate nHPZ pressure values (>10 mm Hg), which are similar to those found in healthy subjects. Moreover, a tighter wrap produces a more effective mechanical barrier. The hypercalibrated N-R, in fact, creates a residual postdeglutitive pressure gradient of 4.05 ± 2.94 mm Hg (vs. 1.02 ± 0.8 mm Hg for the normocalibrated procedure), which seems able to control reflux even in the case of inappropriate or spontaneous LES relaxations. With the term "hypercalibrated Nissen" we do not mean tight fundoplication; this definition is only related to the intraoperative pressure values we try to obtain, which are higher than those of the normal sphincter. In fact, our wrap is loose around the esophagus, consistent with the concept of the "floppy Nissen" supported by Donahue.[27]

The other important feature of the Nissen (hyper)calibrated with IEM is its ability to control reflux without impairing esophagogastric transit. This is a necessary requisite for the success of any antireflux procedure. Among the 15 patients in this series with postoperative dysphagia, only 3 showed a nHPZ pressure <20 mm Hg. Moreover, none of these 15 patients had a percentage of postdeglutitive relaxations <70%, a level similar to that of patients without dysphagia.

In our patients, postoperative dysphagia could be ascribed to the persistence of NEMD (11 patients), rather than to the tightness of the fundoplication and/or the preoperative chronic esophageal inflammation. Another possible cause of postoperative dysphagia yet to be verified could be the torsion of the distal esophagus. This may occur when the distance between the gastroesophageal junction and the portion of the anterior wall of the gastric fundus employed for the fundoplication is too short. Furthermore, the finding of moderate nonpathologic postoperative GER (percentage of time the pH was <4 was <1%) in 23 out of 72 followed-up patients (31.9%) who had the Nissen procedure also suggests that the total fundoplication does not impair esophageal clearing. The postoperative restoration of peristaltic activity of the esophageal body shown in 11.4% (8/70 patients) of our achalasic patients further confirms our theories about the validity both of IEM and of the hypercalibration of the N-R fundoplication.

REFERENCES

1. Del Genio A. L'elettromanometria esofagea intraoperatoria. In: *Manometria e pH-metria esofagea. Confronto sulle metodiche e sulle applicazioni cliniche*. Atti dei V Cong Ital sulla motilità esofagea. Piccin Ed. Padova:1979;219.
2. Lanzara A, Dei Genio A. La fundoplicatio sec. Nissen. In: *Archivio ed Atti della Soc Ital Chir*, 81° Congr. 1979;1:813.
3. Di Martino N, Amato G, Maffettone V, et al. Effetti della Dtubocurarina sullo sfintere esofageo inferiore (LES): studio elettromanometrico intraoperatorio. *Min Chir*. 1986;141:1.
4. Marcialis A, Caracò A, Pignatelli C, et al. In tema di fisiopatologia dei giunto gastroesofageo: comportamento manometrico dopo stimolazione farmacologica (ricerche sperimentali). *Giorn Ital Chir*. 1973; 29:119.
5. Hill LD. Intraoperative measurement of lower esophageal sphincter pressure. *J Thorac Cardiovasc Surg*. 1978;75:375.
6. Romeo G, Beneventano G, Migliore M, et al. Manometria esofagea intraoperatoria. *Min Chir*. 1995;46:211.
7. Mattioli S, Pilotti V, Felice V, et al. Intraoperative study on the relationship between the lower esophageal sphincter pressure and the muscular components of the gastroesophageal junction in achalasic patients. *Ann Surg*. 1993;218:635.
8. Di Martino N, Van Der Hoeven CW, Bemelman W, et al. Experimental study with three-dimensional manometric technique of the effects of Heller myotomy. *Comunic al Forth International Polydisciplinary Congress of OESO*. 1993;82:095.
9. Puglionisi A, Asole F, Clemente G, et al. Effectiveness of intraoperative LES pressure measurement during Nissen-Rossetti fundoplication. *It J Surg Sciences*. 1984;14:91.
10. Gozzetti G, Mattioli S, Di Simone MP, et al. La manometria esofagea intraoperatoria. *Min Chir*. 1991;46:195.
11. Del Genio A, Maffettone V, Izzo G. Intraoperatory esophageal manometry (IEM). Relazione al "Symposium International sur la chirurgie de l'oesophage," Bruxelles 4–5 dicembre 1993.
12. Bonavina L, Anseimino M, Baessato M, et al. Nissen fundoplication: intraoperative manometry or mechanical calibration? *Dig Surg*. 1990; 7:196.
13. Del Genio A, Maffettone V, Landolfi V, et al. Surgical treatment of achalasia: laparotomic versus laparoscopic approach. *Int J Surg Sciences*. 1994;1:45.
14. Del Genio A, Collard JM, Landolfi V, et al. Treatment of Zencker's diverticulum and associated hiatal hernia by means of mini-invasive
15. Peracchia A, Bonavina L, Nosadini A, et al. Management of recurrent symptoms after esophagomyotomy for achalasia. *Dis Esoph*. 1990;3:25.
16. Del Genio A, Landolfi V, Maffettone V, et al. Laparoscopic treatment of esophageal achalasia. Bit Surgery. Multimedia Surgical Monographs:1996;1:21.
17. Del Genio A, Maffettone V, Landolfi V, et al. Our experience in the laparoscopic treatment of oesophageal achalasia (first 66 consecutive cases). *Ital J Gastroenterol*. 1996;28:106.
18. Clemente G, D'Ugo D, Granone P, et al. Intraoperative esophageal manometry in surgical treatment of achalasia: a reappraisal. *Hepatogastroenterology* 1996;43:1532.
19. Morino M, Rebecchi F, Festa V, et al. Laparoscopic Heller cardiomyotomy with intra-operative manometry in the management of oesophageal achalasia. *Int Surg*. 1995;80:332.
20. Del Genio A, Maffettone V, Landolfi V, et al. Risultati long-term della chirurgia laparoscopica del reflusso gastro-esofageo (m.RGE). In: Bianchi Porro G, Pace F, eds. "Argomenti di patologia esofagea 1997" Vol. II Springer Verlag Milano Ed.:1997;185.
21. Slim K, Boulant J, Pezet D, et al. Intraoperative esophageal manometry and fundoplications: prospective study. *World J Surg*. 1996;20:55.
22. Orringer MB, Scheider R, Williams GW, et al. Intraoperative esophageal manometry: is it valid? *Ann Thorac Surg*. 1980;30:13.
23. Johnsson F, Ireland AC, Jarnieson GG, et al. Effect of intraoperative manipulation and anaesthesia on lower oesophageal sphincter function during fundoplication. *Br J Surg*. 1994;81:866.
24. Jamieson GG, Scheneider R, Williams GW, et al. Intraoperative esophageal manometry and clinical outcome in patients operated for gastroesophageal reflux disease. *World J Surg*. 1992;16:337.
25. Pandolfo N, Torre GC, Spigno L, et al. La manometria intraoperatoria nella chirurgia funzionale dell'esofago. *Min Chir*. 1991;46:221.
26. DeMeester TR. What is the role of intraoperative manometry? *Ann Chir*. 1980;30:1.
27. Donahue PE, Semelson S, Nyhus LM, et al. The floppy Nissen fundoplication. *Arch Surg*. 1985;120:663.
28. Kamiike W, Taniguchi E, lwase K, et al. Intraoperative manometry during laparoscopic operation for esophageal achalasia: does pneumoperitoneum affect manometry? *World J Surg*. 1996;20:973.
29. Di Martino N, Maffettone V, Landolfi V, et al. Comparison between traditional and miniinvasive approach in the treatment of esophageal achalasia. In: Peracchia A, et al. eds. *Recent Advances in Diseases of the Esophagus*. Monduzzi Eds., Bologna:1996;889.
30. Cooper JD, Gill FS, Nelems JM, et al. Intraoperative and postoperative esophageal manometric findings with Collins gastroplasty and Belsey hiatal hernia repair for gastroesophageal reflux. *J Thorac Cardiovasc Surg*. 1977;74:744.
31. Kim KC, Patdu R, Kim HW. The relationship between intragastric and lower esophageal sphincteric pressures during general anaesthesia. *Anesthesiology* 1977;46;424.
32. Torre GC, Pandolfo N, Parodi AG, et al. La manometria intraoperatoria. Esperienza personale. In: *Manometria e pH-metria esofagea* di Mattioli FP, Torre GC, Pandolfo N, Piccin Ed. Padova:1981;219.
33. Del Genio A, Izzo G, Di Martino N, et al. Intraoperative esophageal manometry (IEM): twenty years experience. *Dis Esoph*. 1997;10:253.
34. Rakik Š, Stein HJ, De Meester TR, et al. Role of esophageal body function in gastroesophageal reflux disease: implications for surgical management. *J Am Coll Surg*. 1997;185:380.
35. Szwerc MF, Wiechmann RJ, Maley RH, et al. Reoperative laparoscopic antireflux surgery. *Surgery*. 1999;126:723.
36. Gadenstatter M, Klinger A, Prommegger R, et al. Laparoscopic partial posterior fundoplication provides excellent intermediate results in GERD patients with impaired esophageal peristalsis. *Surgery*. 1999;126:548.
37. Swanstrom LL, Jobe BA, Kinzie LR, et al. Esophageal motility and outcomes following laparoscopic paraesophageal hernia repair and fundoplication. *Am J Surg*. 1999;177:359.

Chapter Fifteen ·······

Gastroesophageal Reflux Disease, Barrett's Esophagus, and Adenocarcinoma

ATTILA CSENDES and OWEN KORN

GASTROESOPHAGEAL REFLUX DISEASE

First described during the early decades of the 20th century, gastroesophageal reflux disease (GERD) has become the most common upper digestive tract disease in the Western Hemisphere, representing 75% of all esophageal diseases. GERD can be defined as the excessive exposure of the esophagus to reflux of gastric juices (acids and/or bile), usually symptomatic, that may provoke histopathologic lesions in the esophagus. There is sufficient evidence to support the fact that GERD is the beginning of a physiopathological process that, as it progresses to Barrett's esophagus, may lead to the formation of adenocarcinoma in the esophagus.

In practice, GERD should be considered an acquired disease, generally chronic or recurring in nature, that exposes a percentage of patients to a series of complications that affect their quality of life and may even pose a mortal threat.

Although epidemiological studies are scarce, they show GERD to be a disease that affects the population of the Western Hemisphere and is rarely found in Asian or African subjects. It is estimated that 10% of the adult population of the United States has heartburn daily and that 40% have it occasionally. In Chile the prevalence of pyrosis has reached the level of 60% of the adult population. Although it can affect adolescents, it more commonly appears during the third and fourth decades. GERD and esophagitis are more frequently found in women than men in a ratio of 2:1.

Its etiology has not yet to be clearly established, but it is generally linked to changes in dietary habits, aerophagy, alcohol abuse, and smoking. With respect to its pathophysiology, many related factors have been pinpointed, such as motility disturbances of the esophagus, the existence of a hiatal hernia, acid and/or bile reflux, delayed emptying of the stomach, and obesity, among others. However, all of these factors are more closely related to the consequences of the reflux than to its cause. However, the key point

from a mechanical point of view is that in order for stomach fluid to reflux up the esophagus, the walls at the esophagogastric union must be open to allow passage of the material. This means that the lower esophageal sphincter (LES) must be relaxed or incompetent.

The transitory relaxation of the sphincter not mediated by deglutition, apparently a physiological phenomenon that allows for the release of gases from the stomach, has been cited as a factor in the majority of cases of normal reflux, as well as in pathologic cases.[1] However, based on manometric evaluation, there is strong evidence that shows severe mechanical compromise of the LES in patients with GERD.[2]

Although the causes of this malfunction are not clear, recently our group surmised that the anatomic dilation of the cardia seen in these patients could explain it as an alteration in the arrangement of the muscle fibers that form the sphincter.[3] Based on these considerations, the goal of all therapy should be centered on restoring normal competence to the sphincter.

Clinically, GERD is manifested by heartburn and regurgitation and is sometimes linked to dysphagia. Although these symptoms characterize the syndrome, they should be carefully studied, and the reflux itself must be quantified and analyzed in patients being considered for surgery.

In our protocols, the upper endoscopy together with a biopsy from above and from below the squamocolumnar junction are the initial studies conducted on these patients. Though endoscopy cannot diagnose GERD, it nevertheless helps to evaluate mucosal damage to the esophagus (esophagitis is not found on the first endoscopy in 40% of GERD patients). It also helps to look for Barrett's esophagus, ulcer, or stenosis, at the same time ruling out other pathologies. This is fundamental in our country where gastric cancer is highly prevalent.

In general, when faced with a GERD patient without Barrett's esophagus, with or without esophagitis, we begin medical treatment using proton pump inhibitors and peristalsis stimulants. Six to twelve months later we clinically evaluate the patient and carry out an endoscopy. At this time we can clearly separate patients that do not respond to treatment and whose condition worsens from those that grow to depend on the medications. These two types of patients are usually candidates for surgery as they are considered high-risk patients. The gastroenterologists that deal with a large number of these patients do not always share this view.

Other indications that favor surgery are young age, severe mechanical incompetence of LES coupled with severe esophagitis, symptoms in the larynx and respiratory tract, the existence of a true hiatal hernia, and mixed reflux (acid/bile).

Once surgery has been specified, our rule is to complete the study with manometric testing of the esophagus, 24-hour pH monitoring, and stomach and esophageal x-ray studies. The study of the duodenal reflux using biliary monitoring is done only if mixed reflux is suspected.

The procedure for open surgery is the same as for laparoscopic surgery, and consists of (1) closure of the diaphragmatic crura; (2) proximal superselective vagotomy (to get a clear view of the gastroesophageal junction); (3) a Nissen fundoplication or calibration of the cardias (Hill-Larraín); and (4) anterior fundophrenopexia (to avoid a paraesophagic hernia) (Fig. 15–1).

Results observed in 215 patients with GERD without Barrett's esophagus that had open antireflux surgery had a morbidity rate of 5% with zero mortality. Follow-up after 5 years showed 85% of patients in Visick I and II.[4]

A recent study of 108 patients who had laparoscopic surgery showed a morbidity rate of 1% with zero mortality.[5] Follow-up after 4 years showed 85% of patients in Visick I and II. As detailed below, we deem it very important to separate the results of GERD patients from those of Barrett's esophagus patients who have undergone classic antireflux surgery.

BARRETT'S ESOPHAGUS

This condition is the result of severe and longstanding reflux of gastric fluid into the esophagus that erodes or causes metaplasia of the distal squamous epithelium of the esophagus. Also, there is fundic columnar epithelium, and sometimes cardial columnar epithelium below the Z line. Both types of epithelium can take the place of the normal distal esophageal epithelium. However, the term Barrett's esophagus (BE) is reserved for instances in which the replacement or metaplasia is of the specialized columnar or intestinal-type epithelium. Thus the current definition of BE includes endoscopic evidence of ascent of the Z line in the distal esophagus, as it spreads in a tongue-shaped lesion on any extension that biopsy shows to contain intestinal metaplasia.[6]

Clinical diagnosis is not possible. It is most frequent in male patients 45 years of age and older, with more than 5 years of reflux symptoms. It is found in 20% of the cases subjected to endoscopy due to symptoms that suggest GERD.

Pathophysiologically, it shares common features with GERD, although in the case of BE the type of refluxed material is of greater importance. The growth of intestinal metaplasia is attributed to the corrosive action of bile salts found in the duodenal reflux, whether they also contain acid or not.[7]

BE is characteristically associated with a mechanically incompetent lower esophageal sphincter, motility disorders of the esophagus, mixed reflux (acid/duodenal-bile), and a large dilation of the gastroesophageal junction or cardia that is often mistaken for a hiatal hernia.

BE can occur without complications or may cause ulcers and sometimes severe stenosis, especially in patients with extensive BE that has seriously affected the patient's quality of life. Generally, the metaplastic epithelium does not recede despite effective control of reflux. This keeps patients at risk because BE is a premalignant lesion due to its tendency to worsen and evolve into dysplasia, and finally into adenocarcinoma.

Diagnosis and treatment of these patients includes endoscopy and biopsy to confirm the diagnosis, and radiologic contrast studies of the stomach, esophagus, and duodenum to detect possible stenosis or true hiatal hernia. Also required are esophageal manometry to evaluate esophageal motility and the competence of the sphincter, 24-hour pH monitoring, and testing of the duodenal reflux for bilirubin using a 24-hour test.

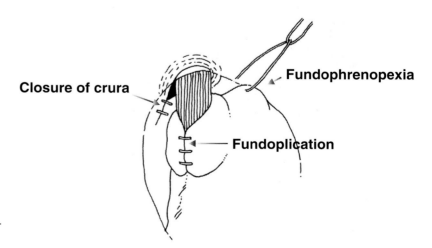

Figure 15–1. Surgical procedure to treat gastroesophageal reflux disease.

The treatment of patients with early BE consists of 6 to 12 months of intensive medical treatment (changes in eating and drinking habits, proton pumps inhibitors, and peristalsis stimulants). This is followed by another evaluation (to seek lessening of symptoms and response to medication) and an endoscopy (to eliminate dysplasia). The treatment is lifelong and the patient should undergo an endoscopy every 1 to 2 years. If the patient does not respond to medical treatment and in those with ulcer or stenosis, surgery is recommended.

By examining studies of surgery in patients with Barrett's esophagus, we noticed two trends:

- The majority of surgeons perform a fundoplication and include all reflux esophagitis patients submitted to surgery in a single group, without separating the results in patients with and without BE.
- In the majority of the surgical reports there is no late follow-up.

The importance of separating patients with BE from those without is based on the hypothesis that if all patients are grouped together, the worse results of patients with BE will be "buffered" by the better results of the non-BE patients. For example, if 100 cases are operated on and followed up, careful preoperative analysis may show that 80 patients had reflux esophagitis only, and 20 patients had BE. The 80 non-BE cases might have a 90% rate of favorable results at 8 to 10 years of follow-up, which means that 72 are well and 8 had failure of the antireflux procedure. For the 20 BE cases, 50% of them might have good results, meaning that 10 are well and 10 had a recurrence. Thus the final results of the entire group of 100 cases will be 82% with a good outcome and 18% with a bad outcome, but among the BE cases alone the rate with a poor outcome was 50%.

We have performed a prospective study in patients with BE submitted to classic open antireflux surgery. The study included 152 patients with extensive BE who had classic antireflux surgery and were followed for more than 8 years. The final late results were poor, with a rate of recurrence (Visick III or IV) of 60%, with appearance of dysplasia (10%) or adenocarcinoma (2.8%) at a mean time of 8 years after surgery.[8]

Therefore, based on these poor late results of classic antireflux surgery in patients with BE, and knowing that the presence of duodenal reflux is an important factor in the pathogenesis of BE, our group proposed to perform a different operation in patients with BE with intestinal metaplasia, one based on bile diversion. In patients with BE in whom significant gastroesophageal reflux has been documented, we proposed not only to perform antireflux surgery, but we also tried to improve some of the other pathological findings in these patients by performing the procedure outlined in Figure 15–2. This procedure consists of:

- Closure of the diaphragmatic crura
- Truncal or selective vagotomy
- Nissen's fundoplication or calibration of cardias (Hill-Larraín)
- Anterior fundophrenopexia (to avoid paraesophageal hernia)
- Partial distal gastrectomy
- a Roux-en-Y gastrojejunal anastomosis

Using this technique on a group of 195 patients with BE who were then followed for 94 months, yielded these results: surgical morbidity 8% and mortality 1%; Visick I or II 97% and Visick III or IV 3%. No cases of dysplasia or adenocarcinoma were seen during follow-up.[9]

As is generally known, no solid proof exists that the metaplastic epithelium of BE is ever reversed after medical or surgical treatment. This means that these patients must undergo endoscopies every 1 to 2 years for the rest of their lives in case foci of dysplasia or adenocarcinoma should appear.

DYSPLASIA AND ADENOCARCINOMA IN BARRETT'S ESOPHAGUS

Over the past 2 decades the incidence of adenocarcinoma of the esophagus has increased at a rate exceeding that of any other cancer. The risk of developing adenocarcinoma after BE is about 1% annually. The risk is also estimated to be 500 per 100,000 population, which is about the same as the risk for developing lung cancer.

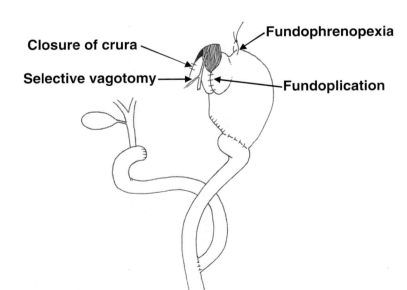

Figure 15–2. Partial gastrectomy with gastrojejunal Roux-en-Y anastomosis proposed by the authors for use in patients with Barrett's esophagus or acid/duodenal reflux.

Although the natural history of BE has not been clearly established, there is general consensus that it is a premalignant lesion. It is also generally agreed that the chain of events leading to BE begins with intestinal metaplasia, followed by low-grade dysplasia and then high-grade dysplasia, finally ending in a adenocarcinoma, all within a span of 20 years. There is no general consensus on the risk of developing cancer when BE develops, and the risk ratio varies from 1:40 to 1:125. This aspect is relevant because it fosters differing views on the seriousness of this disease for doctors treating BE, which results in a difference in therapeutic approaches.

Current evidence shows that older patients, those with a greater extent of BE, and those with mucosal irregularities or ulcers as well as stenosis, all have an increased risk of developing neoplasia. Diagnosis of dysplasia in BE is not simple; if the mucosa are very irritated, the patient must receive intensive treatment followed by reevaluation with new biopsies. Only two stages are currently defined: low-grade and high-grade dysplasia. However, for some groups, high-grade dysplasia is not synonymous with cancer, and for others the difference between high-grade dysplasia and intraepithelial cancer is subtle.

In general, when faced with low-grade dysplasia, the patient must receive intensive medical treatment or undergo antireflux surgery that includes bile diversion. Whichever the case may be, the patient must remain under strict endoscopic supervision and have an endoscopy at least once a year, including biopsies in quadrants 1 to 2 cm apart.

Treatment of high-grade dysplasia currently consists of the following three alternatives:

- Intensive endoscopic supervision and biopsies
- Ablative therapy (thermal, chemical, or mechanical)
- Esophagectomy

Those who advocate endoscopic follow-ups only base this treatment on the suppositions that high-grade dysplasia is not cancer, not all patients develop cancer, and the dysplasia can be kept stable over time.[10] Also, should cancer appear, it can take years to develop; therefore a strict protocol can detect neoplasia in time to allow the patient to keep his or her esophagus. Opponents of this protocol believe it is difficult to be 100% accurate when diagnosing high-grade dysplasia because traces of adenocarcinoma are sometimes found in dysplastic areas. Moreover, the rigorous and strict nature of the follow-up protocol is thought to vary with respect to the resolve of the medical team and the patient.

The goal of ablative therapies is to remove the metaplastic epithelium and allow the restoration of the squamous epithelium. There are three types of ablative therapies: thermal, chemical, and mechanical.[11]

Thermal ablative therapy is carried out with a multipolar electrocoagulator (MPEC), via argon beam plasma coagulation (ABPC), argon and potassium titanium phosphate lasers (KTP), or neodymium:yttrium-aluminum-garnet lasers (Nd:YAG). These types of therapy have drawbacks, including perforation of the esophagus, the fact that their effectiveness is highly operator-dependent, they require many sessions that are costly, and the pseudoregressive phenomenon sometimes seen in the underlying squamous mucosa of BE. Results obtained from these techniques to date have not been satisfactory.

The photochemical ablation of BE has centered on photodynamic therapy (PDT). This technique is based on the administration of porphyrins that photosensitize the epithelial tissues. The drug acts as a photosensitizer because it absorbs light energy and transfers it to oxygen molecules. This high-energy oxygen, termed singlet oxygen, can in turn interact with the tissue, causing necrosis. This type of therapy produces more uniform destruction of tissues, and less Barrett's mucosa is found in the underlying squamous tissues. The overall response of high-grade dysplasia to a single session is close to 90%, whereas total elimination of Barrett's mucosa occurs in about a third of patients. The most significant complications are cutaneous photosensitivity and esophageal stricture.

Mechanical ablative therapy consists of the endoscopic resection of mucosa. To date, few data about its use on high-grade dysplasia are found in the literature.

The use of esophagectomy in the treatment of high-grade dysplasia is currently the most commonly recommended strategy, but before this surgery is done, histologic confirmation must be obtained from two independent pathologists. This strategy is based on the fact that half of resected dysplastic esophagi also show foci of adenocarcinoma. Also, some patients have tumors that remain occult within the mucosa, even with positive lymph nodes.[12]

In cases of high-grade dysplasia, the need for esophagectomy is questioned by some, because it has high morbidity and mortality rates.

Based on current data, adenocarcinoma of the esophagus is the final stage in the physiopathologic events that begin with gastroesophageal reflux disease (GERD). GERD's natural history has not been clearly established, but some estimates suggest that 1 to 2% of GERD patients will develop adenocarcinoma after 15 to 20 years of reflux (Fig. 15–3). However, others estimate that 5 to 20% of patients with BE may develop adenocarcinoma. It is for this reason that BE must be considered a preneoplastic condition.

Adenocarcinoma of the gastroesophageal junction constitutes the type of cancer with the fastest growing incidence, and the number of cases tripled during the 1970s and 1980s. In the last decade alone, the incidence has doubled.

Some theories state that proto-oncogenes and the inertness of tumor-suppressing genes take part in dysplastic and carcinogenic changes in BE, which in turn results in the growth of metaplastic cells and thus adenocarcinoma. In patients with BE many alterations can be found, including abnormalities in the cell cycle, aneuploidy, cytogenetic alterations, microcell instability, alterations in linking molecules, and a wide spectrum of abnormalities of the cell phenotype.

Adenocarcinoma of the esophagus is predominant in white males older than 60, those in medium to high socio-economic groups, and those with a longstanding history of reflux, although it is not always symptomatic. It is found more frequently in BE cases that are more than 3 cm in size, and even more so if an ulcer and/or stenosis is present. However, it has also been seen in less serious cases of short duration without complications.

BE is diagnosed using endoscopy and biopsies. In addition to the progressive biopsies done by quadrants, all irregularities or ulcerated lesions must be biopsied. In the case of stenosis, it must be dilated in order to examine and take samples from the narrowed area and below it.

Once adenocarcinoma has been diagnosed, the aims of these studies must be to establish the staging and resectability of the

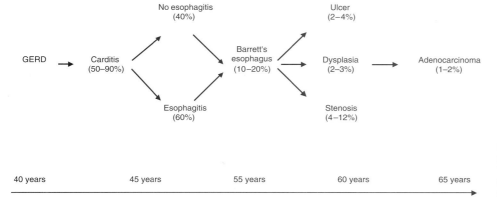

Figure 15–3. Estimated natural history of gastroesophageal reflux disease (GERD). The patient age line at bottom and percentages are approximate and based on recent data.

lesion and to determine if surgery is appropriate. The clinical examinations should include upper endoscopy; chest x-ray; double contrast radiographic study of the esophagus, stomach, and duodenum; computed tomography and/or magnetic resonance imaging of the chest cavity and abdomen; and endosonography. These studies enable the clinician to establish the stages of the lesions and evaluate their resectability. In spite of all the progress made during recent years, the rate of resection continues to be low, with no more than 30 to 40% of the patients having resectable lesions. An evaluation of heart, lung, liver, and kidney function, as well as the patient's nutritional and immunologic status, can help to determine the risk faced by the patient and his or her chances to survive surgery.

The rate of recovery from cancer of the esophagus is extremely low. However, in spite of the therapeutic alternatives, there is consensus that surgery is the procedure that offers the best chances of 5-year survival.

The technique suggested for tumors that affect the cardia or the distal portion of the esophagus includes a total esophagectomy coupled with a total gastrectomy if the lesion extends to the stomach, or the resection of the cardia alone if the lesion is limited. There is debate about whether the approach should be transthoracic with en-bloc resection of the lymph nodes and mediastinal fat, or transhiatal with videoscopic assistance. The latter is thought to be less radical, and though it might not seem to be as effective as the transthoracic approach, studies show that the survival rates are comparable.

The reconstruction is usually done with a segment of colon, but it is preferable to use the stomach whenever possible. Some groups advocate cervical anastomosis, avoiding the intrathoracic anastomosis because of the latter's greater risk of becoming fatally fistulous.

The morbidity of this type of surgery is high, approximately 30 to 40%, and the mortality rate seen in some groups is as high as 15 to 20%. However, mortality is much lower in medical centers with more experience, where rates as low as 2 to 4% can be attained. According to some studies, the 5-year survival rate is about 60% for stage I, 40% for stage IIa, 25% for stage IIb, 15% for stage III, and 2% for stage IV tumors. The Japanese series show better rates of survival than do health centers in Western countries, as is the case with other types of cancer.

REFERENCES

1. Dent J, Holloway RH, Toouli J, et al. Mechanisms of lower oesophageal sphincter incompetence in patients with symptomatic gastroesophageal reflux. *Gut* 1988;29:1020.
2. Zaninotto G, DeMeester TR, Schwiser W, et al. The lower esophageal sphincter in health and disease. *Am J Surg.* 1988;155:104.
3. Korn O, Csendes A, Burdiles P, et al: Anatomic dilatation of the cardia and competence of the lower esophageal sphincter: A clinical and experimental study. *J Gastrointest Surg.* 2000;4:398.
4. Csendes A, Braghetto I, Korn O, et al. Late results and objective evaluations of antireflux surgery in patients with reflux esophagitis. Analysis of 215 patients. *Surgery* 1989;105:374.
5. Csendes A, Burdiles P, Díaz JC, et al. Results of laparoscopic antireflux surgery in 108 patients. *Rev Chil Cir.* 2002 (in press).
6. Sampliner RE. Practice guidelines on the diagnosis, surveillance, and therapy of Barrett's esophagus. The Practice Parameters Committee of the American College of Gastroenterology. *Am J Gastroenterol* 1998;93:1028.
7. DeMeester SR, DeMeester TR. Columnar mucosa and intestinal metaplasia of the esophagus. Fifty years of controversy. *Ann Surg.* 2000; 231:303.
8. Csendes A, Braghetto I, Burdiles P, et al. Long-term results of classic antireflux surgery in 152 patients with Barrett's esophagus: Clinical, radiologic, endoscopic, manometric, and acid reflux test analysis before and late after operation. *Surgery* 1998;123:645.
9. Csendes A, Braghetto I, Burdiles P, et al. Results of the surgical treatment in 362 patients with Barrett's esophagus. *Rev Chil Cir.* 1998; 50:175.
10. Schnell T, Sontag SJ, Chejfec G. High-grade dysplasia still is not an indication for surgery in patients with Barrett's esophagus: An update. *Gastroenterology* 1998;114:AG 1149.
11. Van den Boogert J, Van Hillegersberg R, Siersema PD, et al. Endoscopic ablation therapy for Barrett's esophagus with high-grade dysplasia: A review. *Am J Gastroenterol.* 1999;94:1153.
12. Nigro JJ, Hagen JA, DeMeester TR, et al. Occult esophageal adenocarcinoma: Extent of disease and implication for effective therapy. *Ann Surg.* 1999;230:433.

Chapter Sixteen ......

Paraesophageal Hiatal Hernia

JEFFREY H. PETERS

Herniation of a portion of the stomach through the esophageal hiatus into the posterior mediastinum is a common affliction of modern man. The incidence of hiatal hernia is difficult to determine because of the absence of symptoms in a large number of patients. Upper gastrointestinal barium examinations in symptomatic patients identify some type of hiatal hernia in up to 15% of patients.

Hiatal hernias are classified according to their anatomic characteristics as sliding (type I, Fig. 16–1), characterized by a dome-shaped upward migration of the gastroesophageal junction into the posterior mediastinum; or paraesophageal (type II), characterized by an upward dislocation of the gastric fundus alongside a normally positioned gastro-esophageal junction. In addition, both types may occur together, resulting in a mixed hernia (type III, Fig. 16–2), characterized by an upward dislocation of both the cardia and the gastric fundus. In fact, over 90% of so-called paraesophageal hernias are actually of the mixed type. The end stage of a type I or II hernia occurs when the whole stomach migrates up into the chest by rotating 180 degrees around its longitudinal axis with the cardia and pylorus as fixed points. In this situation the abnormality is usually referred to as an intrathoracic stomach.

Paraesophageal hernias represent a small proportion of all hiatal hernias. In a review of 7310 hernias, 1047 (14.3%) were judged to be paraesophageal.[1] Sliding hiatal hernias are approximately seven times more common than para-esophageal hernias, which are found in an older population, than sliding hiatal hernias (Fig. 16–3). The clinical significance of paraesophageal hiatal herniation lies in its propensity to cause obstruction and strangulation of the stomach.

PATHOPHYSIOLOGY

Most adult hiatal hernias are acquired. A pure para-esophageal hernia rather than a sliding hernia develops when there is a defect, perhaps partly congenital, in the esophageal hiatus anterior to the esophagus. Structural deterioration of the phrenoesophageal membrane occurs over time, leading to thinning of the upper fascial layer of the membrane (the supradiaphragmatic continuation of the

endothoracic fascia) and loss of elasticity in the lower fascial layer (the infradiaphragmatic continuation of the transversalis fascia). The upper fascial layer is formed only by loose connective tissue and is of little importance. The lower fascial layer is thicker and stronger and is itself divided into an upper and lower leaf about 1 cm before attaching intimately with the esophageal adventitia. The attachment of the lower leaf of the lower layer protrudes upwards and can often be identified within the thoracic cavity during a thoracotomy. These observations suggest that the development of a para-esophageal hernia is a phenomenon largely related to age, and is secondary to upward stretching of the phreno-esophageal membrane with repetitive up and down movements of the esophagus during swallowing and the high pressures generated by the upward push of intra-abdominal pressure. The persistent posterior fixation of the gastric cardia to the preaortic fascia and to the median arcuate ligament is the only essential difference between a sliding and paraesophageal hernia. These fibers are described by Hill as acting as posterior tethers to the "bare area" of the stomach. Thus, with stepwise deterioration of key structures, an anterior defect in the hiatus occurs in association with a loss of fixation of the cardia, and a mixed or type III hernia develops. Most paraesophageal hernias are the end result of an ordinary sliding hernia.

Paraesophageal hernias are commonly associated with 180-degree rotation of the stomach around its longitudinal axis (mesoaxial rotation), resulting in a swap in orientation of the posterior and anterior walls of the gastric body. Less commonly, a volvulus occurs with upward displacement of the cardia as well (mesentericoaxial). Herniation of viscera other than stomach also occurs and has been referred to by some as a type IV hernia. *Parahiatal* hernias are characterized by herniation through a small defect adjacent to the esophageal hiatus. They are rarely seen and may be associated with previous trauma.

CLINICAL PRESENTATION

The clinical presentation of a paraesophageal hiatal hernia differs from that of a sliding-type hernia. Many patients with

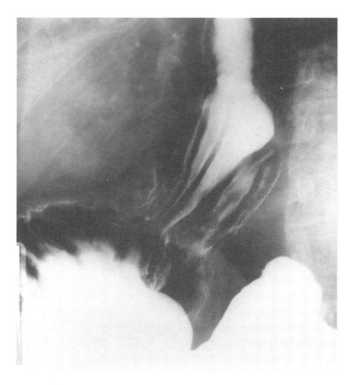

Figure 16–1. Radiograph of a type I or sliding hiatal hernia.

paraesophageal hiatal hernia are asymptomatic or complain of minor symptoms. When present, symptoms are generally related to either partial or complete gastric obstruction or the presence of gastroesophageal reflux disease.[2–6]

Obstructive symptoms range from mild nausea, bloating, or postprandial fullness to acute distress with dysphagia and retching. Vomiting is often intermittent, and if persistent, may herald an incarceration. Dysphagia and postprandial fullness occur secondary to compression of the adjacent esophagus by a progressively expanding herniated stomach by angulation of the gastroesophageal junction as the stomach becomes progressively displaced in the chest, and by volvulus of the stomach as the organ migrates progressively into the chest. Postprandial discomfort including epigastric and chest pain, shortness of breath, and bloating are common.

About one third of patients with a paraesophageal hernia complain of hematemesis due to recurrent bleeding from ulceration or ischemia of the gastric mucosa.[7] Bleeding may originate from riding ulcers, occurring in any part of the stomach due to compression from crura. It may be further exacerbated by stasis and congestion in the herniated portion of the stomach. Some patients develop nonulcer erosions, resembling a gastritis. Healing of these ulcers and erosions can be expected after hernia reduction, with reports of 100% resolution of anemia following repair.

Respiratory complications are frequently associated with a paraesophageal hernia and consist of dyspnea from mechanical compression and recurrent pneumonia from aspiration. Intermittent esophageal obstruction can develop in patients with an in-

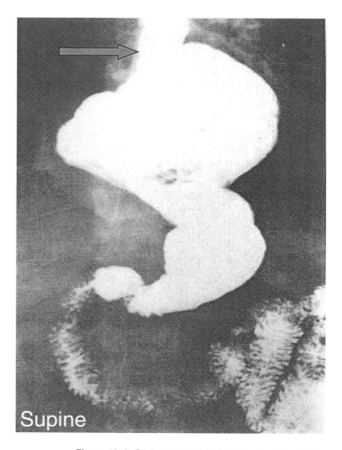

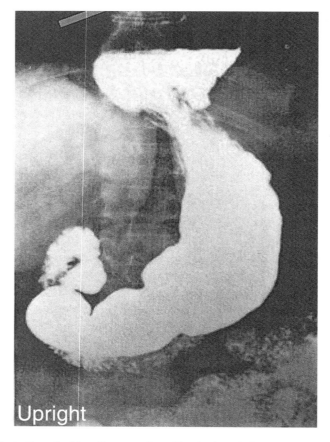

Figure 16–2. Supine and upright barium upper GI study in a patient with a mixed type III paraesophageal hernia. Arrow indicates the position of the gastroesophageal junction.

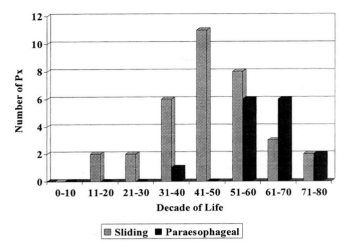

Figure 16–3. Age distribution of 18 patients with paraesophageal hernia compared to that of 34 patients with sliding hiatal hernia.

trathoracic stomach due to the rotation that has occurred as the organ migrates into the chest. Conversely, many patients with paraesophageal hiatal hernia are asymptomatic or complain of very minor symptoms.

The condition is life threatening in one fifth of patients in that the hernia can lead to sudden catastrophic events, such as excessive bleeding or volvulus with acute gastric obstruction or infarction. With mild dilatation of the stomach, the gastric blood supply can be markedly reduced, causing gastric ischemia, ulceration, perforation, and sepsis. Epigastric pain, the inability to vomit, and the inability to pass a nasogastric tube has been described as a triad of symptoms heralding incipient gangrene, and should prompt immediate intervention.

DIAGNOSIS

Clinical signs are uncommon but striking when present. Decreased breath sounds and dull percussion result from the migrating abdominal viscera that lie in the chest. Colonic or small-bowel herniation may result in bowel sounds over the left lower chest. A roentgenogram of the chest with the patient in the upright position can diagnose a hiatal hernia if it shows an air–fluid level behind the cardiac shadow (Fig. 16–4). This is usually caused by a paraesophageal hernia or an intrathoracic stomach. The accuracy of the upper gastrointestinal barium study in detecting a paraesophageal hiatal hernia is greater than for a sliding hernia, because the latter can often spontaneously reduce. The paraesophageal hiatal hernia is a permanent herniation of the stomach into the thoracic cavity, so that a barium swallow provides the diagnosis in virtually every case. When seen, attention should be focused on the position of the gastroesophageal junction to differentiate it from a type II hernia.

Fiber-optic esophagoscopy is very useful in the diagnosis and classification of a hiatal hernia because of the ability to retroflex the scope. In this position, a sliding hiatal hernia can be identified by noting a gastric pouch lined with rugal folds extending above the impression caused by the crura of the diaphragm, or measuring at least 2 cm between the crura, identified by having the patient sniff, and the squamous columnar junction on withdrawal of

the scope. A para-esophageal hernia is identified on retroversion of the scope by noting a separate orifice adjacent to the gastroesophageal junction into which gastric rugal folds ascend. A sliding-rolling or mixed hernia can be identified by noting a gastric pouch lined with rugal folds above the diaphragm with the gastroesophageal junction entering about midway up the side of the pouch.

TREATMENT

The treatment of paraesophageal hiatal hernia is largely surgical. Controversial aspects include indications for repair, surgical approach, and the role of fundoplication.

Indications

The presence of a paraesophageal hiatal hernia has traditionally been considered an indication for surgical repair. This recommendation is largely based upon two clinical observations. First, retrospective studies have shown a significant incidence of catastrophic, life-threatening complications of bleeding, infarction, and perforation in patients being followed with known paraesophageal herniation. Second, emergency repair carries a high mortality. In the classical report of Skinner and Belsey, 6 of 21 patients with a para-esophageal hernia treated medically because of minimal symptoms died from the complications of strangulation, perforation, exsanguinating hemorrhage, or acute dilatation of the herniated intrathoracic stomach.[8] These catastrophes occurred for the most part without warning. Others have reported similar findings.[3,5]

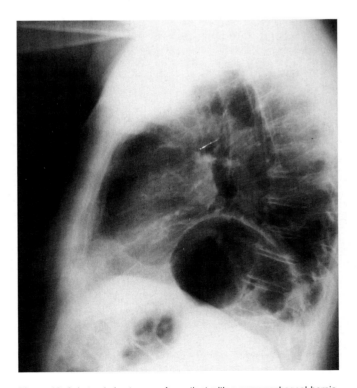

Figure 16–4. Lateral chest x-ray of a patient with a paraesophageal hernia. An air–fluid level can be seen posterior to the cardiac silhouette.

Recent studies suggest that catastrophic complications may be somewhat less common. Allen et al followed 23 patients for a median of 78 months with only four patients progressively worsening.[5] There was a single mortality secondary to aspiration that occurred during a barium swallow examination to investigate progressive symptoms. Although emergency repairs had a median hospital stay of 48 days compared to a stay of 9 days in those having elective repair, there were only 3 cases of gastric strangulation in 735 patient-years of follow-up.

If surgery is delayed and repair is done on an emergency basis, operative mortality is high,[9] compared to less than 1% for an elective repair (Table 16–1).[3,5,10] With this in mind, patients with a paraesophageal hernia are counseled to have elective repair of the hernia regardless of the severity of symptoms or size of the hernia.

Surgical Approach

The surgical approach to repair of a paraesophageal hiatal hernia may be either transabdominal or transthoracic. Each has its advantages and disadvantages. A transthoracic approach facilitates complete esophageal mobilization and removal of the hernia sac. Thoracotomy also allows for the occasional gastroplasty that may be required for esophageal lengthening to achieve a tension-free repair.[11] We have recently reviewed our experience with 54 patients treated between 1985 and 1997. Six of the 54 were thought to have some degree of shortening at surgery, and one required additional lengthening via a Collis gastroplasty. Swanstrom et al suggested that 30% of patients with paraesophageal hernias could be easily reduced following minimal esophageal dissection, 50% required extensive mediastinal dissection, and 20% required an additional lengthening procedure.[12]

The transabdominal approach facilitates reduction of the volvulus that is often associated with paraesophageal hernias. Although some degree of esophageal mobilization can be accomplished transhiatally, complete mobilization to the aortic arch is difficult or impossible without risk of injury to the vagal nerves.

Laparoscopic Repair. Several authors have reported the successful repair of paraesophageal hernias using a laparoscopic approach. Laparoscopic repair of a pure type II, or mixed type III, paraesophageal hernia is an order of magnitude more difficult than a standard laparoscopic Nissen fundoplication. Most would recommend that these procedures are best avoided until the surgeon has accumulated considerable experience with laparoscopic antireflux surgery. There are several reasons for this. First, the vertical and horizontal volvulus of the stomach often associated with para-esophageal hernias makes identification of the anatomy—in particular the location of the esophagus—difficult. Second, dissection of a large paraesophageal hernia sac usually results in significant bleeding, obscuring the operative field. Finally, redundant

tissue present at the gastroesophageal junction following dissection of the sac frustrates the creation of a fundoplication, which we believe should accompany the repair of all paraesophageal hernias. Mindful of these difficulties, and given appropriate experience, patients with paraesophageal hernia may be approached laparoscopically with expectation of success in the majority.

Role of Fundoplication

Controversy remains as to whether to perform an antireflux procedure at all, in selective cases only, or in all patients. The case against an antireflux procedure rests on the frequency of significant postoperative complications secondary to the fundoplication, as well as the slightly longer operative time and increased cost that additional surgery entails. Williamson et al reported the results of 115 patients, of whom only 19 (15%) had an antireflux procedure.[13] Eighty-four percent had symptomatic improvement at a median of 61 months after surgery, although no objective tests were carried out to document the absence of gastro-esophageal reflux or recurrent herniation. They concluded that there was little need for fundoplication unless there was documented reflux. Others have advocated adding a fundoplication in the presence of endoscopic esophagitis, in a reoperative setting, or when a significant sliding element is seen at surgery.[2]

Most, however, advocate the routine addition of an antireflux procedure following repair of the hernia defect. There are several reasons for this. Physiologic testing with 24-hour esophageal pH monitoring has shown increased esophageal exposure to acid gastric juice in 60 to 70% of patients with a paraesophageal hiatal hernia, nearly identical to the observed 71% incidence in patients with a sliding hiatal hernia.[13] Furthermore, there is no relation between the symptoms experienced by the patient with a paraesophageal hernia and the competency of the cardia. Selective testing in symptomatic patients would fail to detect a large proportion of patients with pathologic reflux. Routine pH testing may also support the decision to avoid a fundoplication in those with no increased acid exposure and normal lower esophageal pressure and geometry. Finally, dissection of the gastroesophageal esophagus may lead to postoperative reflux despite a negative preoperative pH score.

RESULTS

Most outcome studies report relief of symptoms following surgical repair of paraesophageal hernias in over 90% of patients. Table 16–2 shows the long-term results of open para-esophageal hernia repair.[10,11,14,15] Pearson et al reported that of 53 patients with very large paraesophageal hernias, most had an intrathoracic stomach.[11] All had a concomitant antireflux procedure and 36 a Collis gastroplasty. Ninety-one percent of patients were symptom free at a mean follow-up of 6 years.

The current literature states that laparoscopic repair of para-esophageal hiatal hernias is highly successful (Table 16–3).[16–23] Most authors report symptomatic improvement in 80 to 90% of patients and less than 10 to 15% prevalence of recurrent hernia. The problem of recurrent hernia following laparoscopic repair of *any* hiatal hernia is becoming increasingly appreciated. Recurrent hernia is now the most common cause of anatomic failure following laparoscopic Nissen fundoplication done for gastroesophageal reflux disease (GERD). Cornwell et al[24] compared the reasons for failure in patients following laparoscopic and open Nissen

TABLE 16–1. PREVALENCE OF ACUTE COMPLICATIONS

Author	Year	N	Acute Presentation
Wichterman et al[10]	1979	6/22	27%
Menguy[3]	1988	13/30	43%
Allen et al[5]	1993	5/147	3.4%

TABLE 16–2. SYMPTOMATIC RECURRENCE FOLLOWING OPEN PARAESOPHAGEAL HERNIA REPAIR

Author	Year	N	Follow-Up (yrs)	Symptomatic Recurrence
Orringer et al[14]	1972	62	>5	14.5%
Wichterman et al[10]	1979	22	5.2	0
Pearson et al[11]	1983	53	6.2	17%
Ellis et al[15]	1986	51	4.5	8%

fundoplication for GERD. The reasons for failure were significantly different. Failures following laparoscopic fundoplication were largely due to recurrent hernia (11 of 16), while failures following open fundoplication were due to wrap disruption/slippage or too long or tight a fundoplication (9 of 10). Soper et al[25] likewise found recurrent hernia to be the most common cause of anatomic fundoplication failure in an unselected group of patients undergoing laparoscopic fundoplication. Why this is so is unclear. It may be due to the selection of a laparoscopic approach in patients with a shortened esophagus; lack of, or breakdown of, the crural closure; less extensive esophageal mobilization; and/or a reduced tendency for adhesion formation after laparoscopic compared to open surgery. Horgan et al[26] have concluded that the most important technical factors preventing recurrence in the setting of reflux disease were effective crural closure, transhiatal esophageal mobilization, attention to the geometry of the fundoplication, and anchoring the wrap to the esophagus and surrounding tissues.

The problem of recurrent hernia following repair of large type III hiatal hernias has received less attention. Outcome following repair of these hernias is usually based upon symptomatic assessment alone. Although recurrence rates of 6 to 13% have been reported, they have largely been based upon the need for reoperation or investigations that are performed on a selective basis.[27] It is problematic that most studies include pure type II hernias, which may have a significantly different propensity for reherniation given the unaltered location of the gastroesophageal junction. Wu et al[23] recently reported on 38 patients who underwent repair for type II and type III hernias, 35 of whom had postoperative endoscopic or radiographic examinations. At a follow-up of 3 months or more postoperatively, some degree of anatomic recurrence was noted in 23% of patients who underwent laparoscopic repair of the hernia. The investigators also found no relationship of operative variables to the prevalence of hernia recurrence.

We have examined the outcome in 54 patients who underwent repair of a large type III hiatal hernia between 1985 and 1998.[24] The surgical approach was laparotomy in 13, thoracotomy in 14, and laparoscopy in 27. An antireflux procedure was included in all patients. Symptomatic outcome was assessed using a structured questionnaire at a median of 24 months and was complete in 51 of 54 patients (94%). A single radiologist, without knowledge of the operative procedure, assessed the integrity of the repair using video esophagrams. Videos were performed at a median of 27 months (35 months for the open repair group and 17 months for the laparoscopic group), and were completed in 41 of 54 patients (75%). Symptomatic outcome was similar in both groups, with an excellent/good outcome in 76% of patients after laparoscopic repair and 88% after an open repair. Reherniation was present in 12 patients and was asymptomatic in 7. A recurrent hernia was present in 12 (29%) of the 41 patients who returned for a follow-up video esophagram. Forty-two percent (9 of 21 patients) of the laparoscopic group had a recurrent hernia compared to 15% (3 of 20) of the open group ($P < 0.001$; Fig. 16–5).

The principles of laparoscopic repair of a large intrathoracic hernia are the same as for an open procedure, namely reduction of the hernia, excision of the peritoneal sac, crural repair, and fundoplication. However, there are several factors that make the laparoscopic repair of these large hernias complex. First, volvulus of the stomach is often associated with these hernias and makes identification of the anatomy, in particular the location of the esophagus, difficult. Second, type III hernias tend to be large, as shown by the measurements reported in this study, and the laparoscopic dissection of a large hernia sac frequently results in sufficient bleeding to obscure the field of view, impairing the recognition of the anatomy. Third, the hiatal opening in a patient with a large hernia is wide, with the right and left muscular crura often separated by 4 cm or more. This can make closure problematic due to the tension required to bring the crura together. Fourth, the right crus may be devoid of stout tissue, and sutures may pull through it easily. Finally, redundant tissue present at the gastroesophageal junction following dissection of the sac retards the creation of the fundoplication.

The use of prosthetic mesh as an adjunct to repair has been advocated for both open[28] and laparoscopic[29] repair of large hiatal hernias. Whether its use is beneficial or not remains controversial; we prefer to avoid prosthetic material if possible. In contrast to groin hernias, the esophageal hiatus is a very dynamic area with constant movement of the diaphragm, esophagus, stomach, and

TABLE 16–3. REVIEW OF REPORTED OUTCOME OF LAPAROSCOPIC REPAIR OF PARAESOPHAGEAL HERNIAS

Author	Year	N	Fundoplication (%)	Mean Follow-Up (months)	Morbidity (%)	Excellent/good Symptomatic Outcome (%)	Hernia Recurrence (%)
Oddsdottir et al[16]	1995	10	90	9	20	80	0
Pitcher et al[17]	1995	12	60	8	25	83	0
Willekes et al[18]	1997	30	76	—	27	—	0
Casabella et al[19]	1996	15	100	—	20	100	—
Trus et al[20]	1997	76	95	—	28	—	5
Perdikis et al[21]	1997	65	100	18	14	92	3
Gantert et al[22]	1998	55	73	10	16	—	3
Wu et al[23]	1999	38	100	12	16	79	23[1]

[1]On videos conducted at 3 to 5 months.

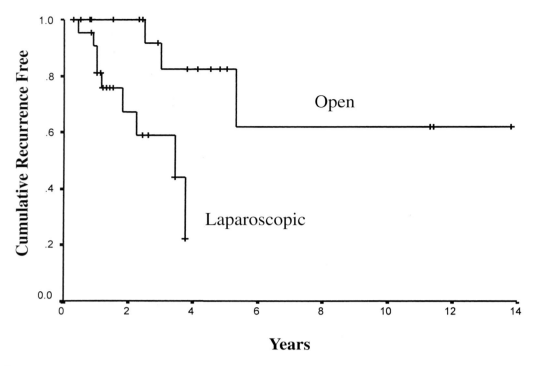

Figure 16–5. Kaplan–Meier plot of the cumulative proportion of patients who were recurrence free on follow-up of open and laparoscopic paraesophageal hernia repair. *(From Hashemi M, Peters JH, DeMeester TR, et al. Laparoscopic repair of large type III hiatal hernia: Objective follow-up reveals high recurrence rate. J Am Coll Surg. 2000;190:553.)*

pericardium. Erosion of prosthetic material placed in this area into the gastrointestinal tract will occur; the only question is how often. The short-term follow-up of most studies is insufficient to provide insight into this problem. In one of the largest and longest-term studies reported, Carlson et al followed 43 patients with mesh repair of large hiatal hernias for a mean of 52 months. Mesh erosion into the fundus of the stomach occurred in one (2.3%) patient.[28] In practice, the issue boils down to the risk of hernia recurrence given repair without the use of prosthetic mesh and that of mesh erosion and/or recurrent hernia in patients with prosthetic repairs; neither is well known. The 15% prevalence of recurrent hernia in patients following open repair is, we believe, not high enough to warrant placement of prosthetic mesh. On the other hand, the disturbingly high recurrence in the laparoscopic group may warrant its consideration in those undergoing laparoscopic repair.

The ideal management of the patient with reherniation with minimal or no symptoms is unknown. The decision is complicated by the fact that reoperation has greater morbidity and mortality and a higher chance of esophageal or gastric perforation, vagal injury, and gastroparesis.

Morbidity and Mortality

Mortality following elective repair should be less than 5%, and in centers with a large volume of esophageal surgery is less than 1%. Complications occur in 20 to 30% of patients. This is more common than elective repair of a sliding hiatal hernia associated with gastroesophageal reflux, largely due to the elderly, often debilitated population in which paraesophageal hernias are found. The report of Trus et al underscores the potential for complications in this elderly

population, even with laparoscopic repair.[20] Operating time was significantly longer than standard laparoscopic fundoplication (3.3 versus 2.5 hours). Of 64 patients, 13% suffered a visceral injury, 2 patients had severe pulmonary complications, and one patient died.

SUMMARY

Pure paraesophageal hernias are relatively uncommon. Most occur as mixed-type hernias in association with a sliding hiatal hernia. They represent an acquired defect and present in the elderly with postprandial fullness, chest pain, and dysphagia. Both esophageal manometry and preoperative endoscopic assessment can be difficult owing to distortions in the anatomy. Reflux symptoms occur in one third and 60% have evidence of reflux on objective testing. Life-threatening complications occur and require a high degree of suspicion for early diagnosis. Urgent intervention is indicated in the emergency situation once incarceration has taken place. Surgical repair following incarceration carries a high mortality. For this reason, given a relatively fit patient, elective repair should be offered as the treatment of choice. Surgical technique should include hernia reduction, crural closure, and fundoplication.

REFERENCES

1. Postlewaite RW. *Surgery of the Esophagus.* Appleton Century-Crofts: 1979;195.
2. Landreneau RJ, Johnson JA, Marshall JB, et al. Clinical spectrum of paraesophageal herniation. *Dig Dis Sci.* 1992;37:537.

3. Menguy R. Surgical management of large paraesophageal hernia with complete intrathoracic stomach. *World J Surg.* 1988;12:415.

4. Altorki NK, Yankelevitz D, Skinner DB. Massive hiatal hernias: The anatomic basis of repair. *J Thorac Cardiovasc Surg.* 1998;115:828.

5. Allen MS, Trastek VF, Deschamps C, et al. Intrathoracic stomach. Presentation and results of operation. *J Thorac Cardiovasc Surg.* 1993;105:253.

6. Wo JM, Branum GD, Hunter JG, et al. Clinical features of type III (mixed) paraesophageal hernia. *Am J Gastroenterol.* 1996;91:914.

7. Cameron AJ. Linear gastric erosion: A lesion associated with large diaphragmatic hernia and chronic blood loss anaemia. *Gastroenterology.* 1986;91:338.

8. Skinner DB, Belsey RH. Surgical management of esophageal reflux and hiatus hernia. Long-term results with 1030 patients. *J Thorac Cardiovasc Surg.* 1967;53:33.

9. Hill LD. Incarcerated paraesophageal hernia. A surgical emergency. *Am J Surg.* 1973;126:286.

10. Wichterman K, Geha AS, Cahow CE, et al. Giant paraesophageal hiatus hernia with intrathoracic stomach and colon: The case for early repair. *Surgery.* 1979;86:497.

11. Pearson FG, Cooper JD, Ilves R, et al. Massive hiatal hernia with incarceration: A report of 53 cases. *Ann Thorac Surg.* 1983;35:45.

12. Swanstrom LL, Marcus DR, Galloway GQ. Laparoscopic Collis gastroplasty is the treatment of choice for the shortened esophagus. *Am J Surg.* 1996;171:477.

13. Williamson WA, Ellis FHJ, Streitz JMJ, et al. Paraesophageal hiatal hernia: Is an antireflux procedure necessary? *Ann Thorac Surg.* 1993;56:447.

14. Orringer MB, Skinner DB, Belsey RHR. Long term results of the Mark IV operation for hiatal hernia and analyses of recurrences and their treatment. *J Thorac Cardiovasc Surg.* 1972;63:25.

15. Ellis FH, Crozier RE, Shea JA. Paraesophageal hiatus hernia. *Arch Surg.* 1986;121:416.

16. Oddsdottir M, Franco AL, Laycock WS, et al. Laparoscopic repair of paraesophageal hernia. New access, old technique. *Surg Endosc.* 1995;9:164.

17. Pitcher DE, Curet MJ, Martin DT, et al. Successful laparoscopic repair of paraesophageal hernia. *Arch Surg.* 1995;130:590.

18. Willekes CL, Edoga JK, Frezza EE. Laparoscopic repair of paraesophageal hernia. *Ann Surg.* 1997;225:31.

19. Casabella F, Sinanan M, Horgan S, et al. Systematic use of gastric fundoplication in laparoscopic repair of paraesophageal hernias. *Am J Surg.* 1996;171:485.

20. Trus TL, Bax T, Richardson WS, et al. Complications of laparoscopic paraesophageal hernia repair. *J Gastrointest Surg.* 1997;1:221.

21. Perdikis G, Hinder RA, Filipi CJ, et al. Laparoscopic paraesophageal hernia repair. *Arch Surg.* 1997;132:586.

22. Gantert WA, Patti MG, Arcerito M, et al. Laparoscopic repair of paraesophageal hiatal hernias. *J Am Coll Surg.* 1998;186:428.

23. Wu JS, Dunnegan DL, Soper NJ. Clinical and radiological assessment of laparoscopic paraesophageal hernia repair. *Surg Endosc.* 1999; 13:497.

24. Cornwell M, Trus T, Waring JP, et al. Patterns of failure and results of re-do fundoplication. *Surg Endosc.* 1997;11:171.

25. Soper NJ, Dunnegan D. Anatomic fundoplication failure after laparoscopic antireflux surgery. *Ann Surg.* 1999;229:669.

26. Horgan S, Pohl D, Bogetti D, et al. Failed antireflux surgery: What have we learned from re-operations? *Arch Surg.* 1999;134:809.

27. Hashemi M, Peters JH, DeMeester TR, et al. Laparoscopic repair of large type III hiatal hernia: Objective follow-up reveals high recurrence rate. *J Am Coll Surg.* 2000;190:553.

28. Carlson MA, Condon RE, Ludwig KA, et al. Management of intrathoracic stomach with polypropylene mesh prosthesis reinforced transabdominal hiatus hernia repair. *J Am Coll Surg.* 1998;187:227.

29. Frantzides CT, Richards CG, Carlson MA. Laparoscopic repair of large hiatal hernia with polytetrafluorethylene. *Surg Endosc.* 1999;13:906.

Chapter Seventeen ■ ■ ■ ■ ■ ■

Cardiomyotomy in the Treatment of Achalasia by Mini-Invasive Surgery

SANTIAGO HORGAN, DANIEL G. VANUNO, and CARLOS A. PELLEGRINI

Achalasia of the esophagus is a disease characterized by a long history of dysphagia, regurgitation of undigested food, and weight loss. These symptoms are caused by inadequate lower esophageal sphincter (LES) relaxation in response to swallowing, absence of peristalsis, and high basal pressure at the LES. As a result of poor esophageal emptying, the esophagus progressively dilates to accommodate the food that has not been transferred to the stomach, and it eventually becomes a large inert sac with a tight distal orifice.

The etiology of achalasia is not known; patients with achalasia have anomalies both of the muscle and the innervation of the esophagus. Of these, the neural component is generally considered to be the most important; indeed, Auerbach's plexus is absent in many patients. In most patients with achalasia, there are no ganglion cells in the body or in the LES.

The neural alterations described are thought to create an imbalance between cholinergic and noncholinergic stimuli. Indeed, it appears that the lack of relaxation of the LES and the presence of high basal tone are the consequences of an alteration in the mediation of the LES relaxation normally produced by nitric oxide (NO) and vasoactive intestinal peptide (VIP).[1,2] These studies have shown that in patients with achalasia there is a selective loss of postganglionic inhibitory neurons that contain NO and VIP.

DIAGNOSIS

The diagnosis of achalasia is established by a history of dysphagia and weight loss, and confirmed by typical findings in diagnostic studies.[3] All patients with symptoms of achalasia should be evaluated with an esophagogram, manometry, 24-hour pH monitoring, and upper endoscopy. Ultrasound is helpful in some patients.

An esophagogram is important to evaluate the anatomy of the esophagus. In patients with achalasia it will show a smooth tapering of the distal esophagus (bird's-beak shape) with dilation of the body (Fig. 17–1). As the disease progresses, the esophagus elongates, eventually acquiring the sigmoid shape typical of patients with end-stage disease. Esophagograms are also valuable in ruling out other diseases known to cause dysphagia, in particular, cancer of the esophagus. The study is particularly helpful to the surgeon when planning therapy, as the width, length, and overall shape of the esophagus will determine the kind of procedure to be used.

Manometry provides information about the relaxation of the LES in terms of pressure, and the motility of the body of the esophagus. The typical findings are absence of relaxation of the LES in response to swallowing, with increased basal tone, usually around 30 to 40 mm Hg, and absent or minimal evidence of peristalsis. Thus in order to make a diagnosis of achalasia on manometry, one has to find absence of peristalsis and either absence of or some evidence of defective relaxation. The total pressure or the basal tone of the LES is less important. In fact, it has been found that LES pressure is normal in 40% of patients with achalasia. The study of the relaxation of the LES and the determination of "complete" relaxation is difficult; thus, either absent or obviously impaired relaxation is clear in only 70 to 80% of patients. While manometry is the diagnostic gold standard for achalasia, diagnosis also rests in some of these patients on the clinical findings and on findings from upper gastrointestinal series. In addition, it is important to remember that achalasia is not just a disease, but is a spectrum of diseases, and that over time, many motility disorders can evolve into the more typical form of achalasia. Thus, in early stages achalasia patients may have only minimally impaired (and therefore difficult to detect) relaxation of the LES, which will become evident in time.

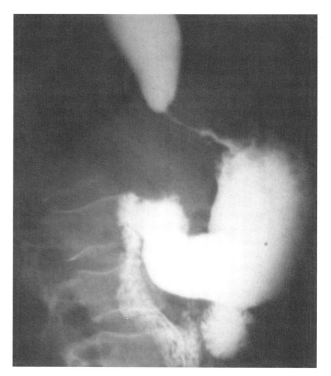 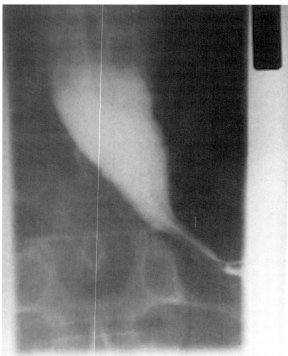

Figure 17–1. Esophagograms of a patient with achalasia.

Some other studies are helpful in the diagnosis of achalasia. The 24-hour pH study helps to determine the concomitant presence of gastroesophageal reflux disease, and rule out an acid reflux–induced stricture. Endoscopy should be performed in these patients to rule out cancer or other causes of distal esophageal obstruction. Typical findings are dilation and atony of the esophagus. The mucosa can be affected by esophagitis that results from fermentation of retained food. Endoscopic ultrasound is used to evaluate the thickening of the esophageal wall in patients in whom the diagnosis of achalasia is in question. In addition, radionuclide measurement of esophageal emptying may be useful to determine transit time through the esophagus. This transit is markedly delayed in patients with achalasia. If a good barium swallow is performed, this study is not needed.

TREATMENT

The treatment of achalasia has been the subject of controversy for many years. Since there is no treatment that can modify the poor peristalsis of the body of the esophagus, all therapeutic maneuvers have been directed at decreasing the pressure of the LES. There are several options available today to achieve this goal: medical treatment (including drugs and botulinum toxin injections), balloon dilation, and surgery.

Medical treatment with calcium channel blockers (nifedipine, verapamil)[4] and nitrates has been used with very little positive effect. This line of treatment should be reserved for patients who are poor candidates for surgery. Botulinum toxin has been used since 1993 when Pasricha et al[5] showed that botulinum toxin injection in the lower esophageal sphincter of piglets resulted in significant reduction of basal pressure. Shortly thereafter the same group reported their initial experience using botulinum toxin in patients with achalasia.[6] Their report showed that when injected into the LES, botulinum toxin caused a substantial and sustained reduction of LES pressure and improved emptying of the esophagus. This sparked considerable enthusiasm in the gastroenterology community and several groups started to use it as their first choice to treat achalasia.[7–9] This form of treatment is effective in about two thirds of patients initially, but symptoms recur in two thirds of the responders within the first 2 years,[8] so injections need to be repeated frequently. In addition to the recurrence rate, the botulinum injections induce changes that make the identification of the dissection planes between the mucosal and muscular layer more difficult during the performance of a subsequent myotomy.[18] This form of therapy should be used primarily in elderly patients who will not be treated with surgery.

Pneumatic dilation has been commonly used in the last two decades as the initial treatment for achalasia. In this procedure, the muscle fibers of the gastroesophageal (GE) junction are disrupted by pressure exerted by an inflated balloon. In 1980 Vantrappen and Hellemans from Belgium reported the largest series of pneumatic dilations.[10] Excellent results (no dysphagia) were obtained in 37.5% of 537 patients, and good results (occasional dysphagia of short duration) in 39.5%, thus achieving a 77% success rate. Perforation of the esophagus occurred in 2.6% of patients with a 0.2% mortality rate. Ferguson[11] reviewed the results of pneumatic dilation in many centers in the United States, Europe, and South America between 1980 and 1990, confirming Vantrappen's data. This review included almost 900 patients who were treated with different types of dilators; the overall improvement rate was 71%. More than 16% of patients required subsequent dilations, and 8% required a Heller myotomy. Gastroesophageal reflux disease (GERD) occurred in 27% of patients and the mortality rate was 0.3%. In the same review, Ferguson also analyzed the results of esophagomyotomy for achalasia performed in centers in the United States and abroad during the same decade. The overall success rate in 1199 patients was 89%. Fewer than 3% of patients required a second operation and the incidence of GERD was 10%. The mortality rate was 0.3%.

Only one prospective, randomized study has been performed to date to compare pneumatic dilation to Heller myotomy. In 1989, Csendes et al[12] from Chile published the results of their trial (mean follow-up, 62 months) which included 81 patients, 39 treated by dilation by a Mosher bag and 41 by surgery. Overall results were good in 65% of patients after one or more dilations and in 95% of patients after myotomy, thus showing a major difference in outcome in favor of surgery. Birgisson and Richter[13] reported that in their experience only one dilation is needed to relieve symptoms in 58% of patients with achalasia, two in 26% of the patients, and three in 16%. In their 9-year experience using Rigiflex dilators, 8 perforations (7%) occurred in over 115 dilations. Six of the perforations occurred with the 3.5 cm dilator, one with the 3.0 cm dilator and one with the 4.0 cm dilator.

These results suggest that surgical treatment has an advantage over dilation; a myotomy performed under direct vision is able to relieve the obstruction more precisely and more often than the blind rupture of the muscle fibers obtained with dilation, and with fewer complications. However, in spite of its better results, surgical treatment has been generally considered a second-line treatment to be used only in patients who failed or suffered complications of dilation. The pain of the surgical incision, the postoperative disability associated with a long recovery time, and the cost of the hospitalization have been the arguments commonly used in favor of pneumatic dilation as the initial treatment for achalasia. However, minimally invasive techniques make it possible today to obtain the results of surgery with much less discomfort, as well as a shorter hospital stay and recovery period.

MINIMALLY INVASIVE TECHNIQUES FOR ESOPHAGEAL MYOTOMY

In 1991, stimulated by the excellent results obtained with laparoscopic cholecystectomy, we decided to apply minimally invasive techniques to the treatment of achalasia and started performing the Heller myotomy thoracoscopically with good results, minimal postoperative pain, and shorter hospital stay.[14,15]

After observing that a large number of patients treated thoracoscopically were developing symptoms of reflux after the myotomy, we decided to approach these patients through the abdomen. The laparoscopic myotomy, first described by Cuschieri in 1991,[16] has several advantages over the thoracoscopic technique. First, the anesthesia is easier, as no double lumen tube is needed; second, the myotomy can be performed more easily through the abdomen; third, the myotomy can clearly be extended into the stomach (this decreases the chances of ending with an incomplete myotomy); fourth, a partial fundoplication can be added to avoid postoperative reflux; and finally, the absence of a chest tube decreases postoperative pain.

Currently our indications for thoracoscopic myotomies are in patients with a recurrence after a previous laparoscopic myotomy, patients with diffuse esophageal motor disorders, and patients with

nutcracker esophagus. The laparoscopic approach is our treatment of choice in patients with achalasia.

Thoracoscopic Approach

Our current operative technique is similar to that originally reported by us in 1991 with small modifications. After induction of general endotracheal anesthesia and double-lumen tracheal intubation, a 52F lighted bougie is placed inside the esophagus transorally. This bougie plays a key role during the thoracoscopic Heller myotomy; at the beginning of the procedure it facilitates identification of the esophagus by transillumination. Subsequently it helps gauge the depth of penetration of instruments and manipulation of the esophagus. An endoscope is used once the myotomy has been performed to allow an accurate assessment of the length to which the myotomy should be performed. If the myotomy is too short, dysphagia will persist; if it is too long (more than 0.5 to 1.0 cm into the gastric wall), gastroesophageal reflux will occur.

The patient is placed in the right lateral decubitus position, and five 10-mm ports are introduced in the left chest, as shown in Fig. 17–2. After upward retraction of the left lung, the inferior pulmonary ligament is divided. Aided by the transillumination from the endoscope or the lighted bougie, the esophagus is easily identified in the groove between the pericardium and the aorta (Fig. 17–3). Once the esophagus has been identified and exposed, the myotomy is subsequently carried down through the longitudinal and circular layers using a 90° angled hook. Once the submucosal plane is reached, the myotomy is extended upwards and downwards using hook cautery or bipolar scissors (Fig. 17–4), opening the muscle by applying gentle traction on the longitudinal muscle.

The lowest part of the myotomy represents the most delicate part of the procedure. It is crucial to the outcome and it is also the most difficult part of the operation because it is at this level that the muscle layers are less clearly identified and the mucosa is thinner, making the risk of perforation higher. In our original series,

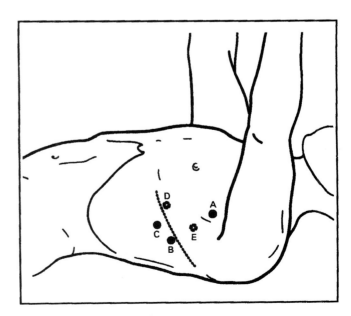

Figure 17–2. Approximate trocar placement for the thoracic approach.

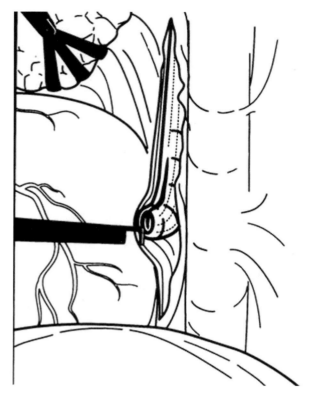

Figure 17–3. Thorascopic myotomy—technique.

we had three such perforations among 24 patients; two were repaired by an open technique and one by thoracoscopic suturing. After the myotomy is completed, the edges of the muscle layers are separated by blunt dissection, so that about 40% of the circumference of the mucosa becomes visible. The operation is completed by inserting a chest tube through the lowest trocar site. This operation is usually accomplished in 2 to 3 hours, the blood loss is minimal, and the recovery rapid.[21]

Laparoscopic Myotomy

The operation is performed under general anesthesia with the patient placed in the semilithotomy and reverse Trendelenburg position. A bean bag is used to safely maintain the reverse Trendelenburg position. Sequential pneumatic stockings are placed on the legs to diminish the risk of venous thrombosis, a risk which is increased by the position and the use of positive intraperitoneal pressure for several hours. An orogastric tube is used to deflate the stomach (the tube is pulled after the stomach is inspected and it is not reinserted) and a Foley catheter is inserted to empty the bladder and monitor urine output through the operation. The Foley catheter is left in place postoperatively only in patients who are going to use epidural analgesia after the operation; otherwise it is removed in the recovery room. The video monitor is placed over the patient's head. The surgeon stands between the legs of the patient with the first assistant on the right side. We use a camera holder to hold the liver retractor, thus avoiding the need for a second assistant. If the camera holder is not used, the second assistant stands on the left side of the patient.

Pneumoperitoneum is achieved using a Veress needle in the area where the first trocar will be placed. Open technique to establish pneumoperitoneum is rarely required. Once insufflation is established, the ports are positioned as shown in Fig. 17–5. The first port (5/11 mm, used for the camera) is placed using the Visiport™ (U.S. Surgical, Norwalk, CT), as we believe this decreases the chance of major vessel or bowel injury. The camera port is usually positioned 2 cm to the left of the umbilicus and about 10 cm below the costal margin. Once a routine laparoscopy of the abdomen is performed, and depending on the anatomy of the patient, the remaining ports are placed. A 5/11-mm port to provide access to instruments held by the surgeon's right hand is placed in the left midclavicular line 1 cm below the costal margin to avoid subcostal nerve injury, at a 45° angle with the camera port. A 5-mm port is then inserted in the epigastrium, near the midline, directly above the anterior edge of the left lobe of the liver, to provide access to instruments held by the surgeon's left hand. Unless the patient has a very large liver (in which case a 10-mm liver retractor is needed), we prefer to use a 5-mm liver retractor which is placed through a port positioned where the right anterior axillary line crosses the camera port line. A 5/11-mm port placed at the level of the camera port in the left anterior axillary line provides access to instruments held by the first assistant's right hand.

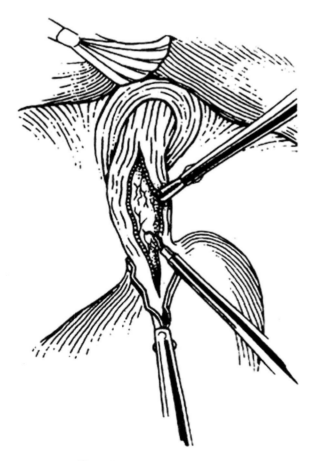

Figure 17–4. Laparoscopic myotomy.

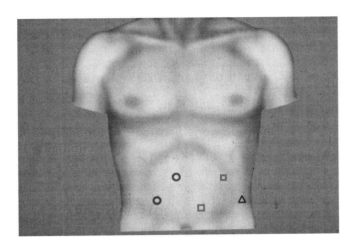

Figure 17–5. Approximate trocar placement for the abdominal approach.

In the original version of the laparoscopic technique, after adequate exposure of the hiatus was gained by retracting the left lobe of the liver anteriorly, the gastrohepatic ligament was opened and the right crus of the diaphragm dissected. Misidentification of the structures in this area can, however, lead to inferior vena cava injury or transection of the nerve of Latarjet (important for the preservation of adequate gastric emptying). We found that the left crus could always be easily identified by downward traction on the gastric fundus, so we start by dissecting the left crus and dividing the gastrohepatic ligament.

To that end the first assistant is asked to grasp the top of the fundus (or the greater curvature at a convenient point if a large hiatal hernia is present) with a Babcock clamp and pull downward. The peritoneum overlying the left crus of the diaphragm is then opened sharply. The division of the peritoneum continues to the left until the phrenogastric ligament is completely divided. Occasional use of electrocautery may be needed during this step. Dissection is carried down along the left crus and towards the upper pole of the spleen as far as possible. At this point it is usually easier to choose a point in the greater curvature several centimeters down from the divided phrenogastric attachments and to divide all short gastrics going upwards until one reaches the previously divided phrenogastric ligament.

We routinely divide all short gastric vessels to fully mobilize the fundus of the stomach. Although we prefer to use the harmonic scalpel (Ethicon, Inc., Somerville, NJ) to take down the short gastric vessels, clips can also be employed. In the latter case, we recommend that all the vessels be double clipped, to avoid the potential bleeding that can result from dislodging a clip when manipulating the stomach. Once the left crus has been completely dissected and with the greater curvature of the stomach free, the mediastinum may be entered and the "inner" side of the left crus can be separated from the left side of the esophagus. Conversely, one may decide to continue the division of the peritoneum that overlies the anterior aspect of the hiatus and the phreno-esophageal membrane towards the right until the right crus (at its top) has been exposed. The gastrohepatic ligament, a continuation of the peritoneum that overlies the right crus, is divided now from the top of the right crus. The division is extended downward as needed to expose the bottom of the right crus.

Esophageal Mobilization. The esophagus can now be approached from the right (with the assistant maintaining downward traction at the cardioesophageal junction), or from the left (with the assistant grasping the fundus and pulling down and to the patient's right). We use the tip of the electrocautery device (having previously retracted the wire) to bluntly dissect the esophagus, pushing it to the right or the left.

A 52F lighted bougie placed transorally into the esophagus provides a surface over which the esophageal wall can be dissected and a platform over which the myotomy can be carried out. At this time the fat pad from the esophageal junction is removed. The anterior vagus is identified, and carefully dissected from the esophagus. The myotomy is performed with an L-shaped hook electrocautery mounted at the tip of a suction-irrigation device (Surgiwand,™ U.S. Surgical, Norwalk, CT).

After marking the area of the muscularis externa to be divided with the heel of the electrocautery, the circular layer is identified. Initially, one or two circular fibers are lifted away from the mucosa by placing the tip of the hook electrocautery in the submucosal plane. These fibers are dissected away from the mucosa and divided. The rest of the myotomy is performed following this plane and the edges are then dissected away from each other also following this plane (Fig. 17–6).

Bleeding can occur close to the mucosa. Gentle pressure instead of coagulation should be applied over the mucosa, and these bleeding points will usually stop without any other treatment. We have found that in patients treated with botulinum toxin, the mucosa is difficult to separate from the muscularis propria as the submucosal plane has been lost. Consequently it is difficult to separate the muscle edges away from each other. This difficulty makes the operation longer and the risk of lacerating the mucosa greater.

A Dor fundoplication is routinely added to the myotomy to avoid postoperative reflux.[17] In principle, this operation is the reverse of a Toupet, with the wrap covering the anterior aspect of the distal esophagus and the wrap fixed to the edges of the diaphragm (Fig. 17–7). Its main advantage, under these circumstances, is that the fundus of the stomach covers the exposed mucosa of the esophagus.[19]

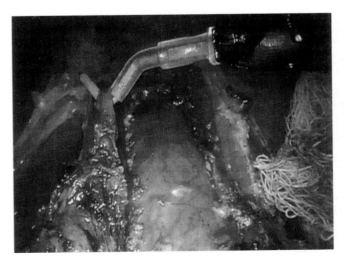

Figure 17–6. Esophageal myotomy with the Da Vinci Robotic System (Intuitive Surgical, Mountview, CA). See Color Section.

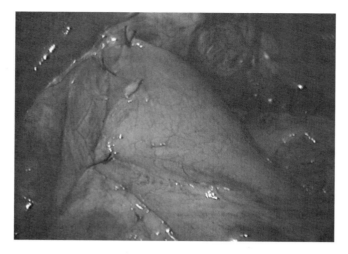

Figure 17–7. Dor anterior fundoplication. See Color Section.

Robotic-Assisted Myotomy

The Da Vinci Robotic System (Intuitive Surgical, Mountview, CA) was approved in the U.S. for use in general surgery in July 2000. This system became available at our Minimally Invasive Center at the University of Illinois at Chicago in September 2000, and since then we have used the system to perform Heller myotomies in all patients (Fig. 17–8). The Da Vinci surgical robot has a console where the surgeon sits that is connected to the three robotic arms. From this console all surgeon movements are transmitted without any delay to the tips of the robotic arms. This advanced system offers the following advantages: a magnified three-dimensional view of the operative field, 360° of freedom of movement at the articulated arms of the robot, and tremor elimination and control of the camera by the surgeon at the console, which eliminates the need for a camera holder. This permits the performance of the operation with more comfort and significantly less stress on the surgeon. Since the first case was performed in October 2000, we have performed 8 Heller myotomies with Dor fundoplication, including two redo myotomies.

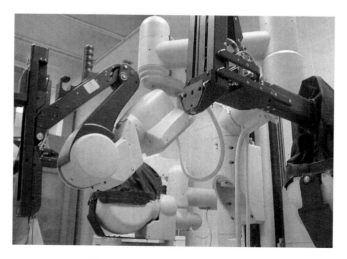

Figure 17–8. Da Vinci Robotic System.

We utilized the same technique as described in the laparoscopic approach; after dividing the short gastric vessels with the ultrasonic scalpel, the robotic arms are placed in the abdominal cavity through the upper 2 trocar ports, and the myotomy portion and the Dor fundoplication are performed entirely with the robotic system.

When we compare this initial experience with our standard laparoscopic myotomies, the total length of the operation, the length of stay, and the outcomes were very similar. The myotomy portion of the operation took significantly less time in the robotic group, and there were no mucosal perforations in this group. As technology continues to evolve, this will become an attractive alternative for the performance of Heller myotomies.

RESULTS

Our initial report showed that thoracoscopic myotomy yielded excellent results in terms of resolution of dysphagia.[14] Because of the high incidence of postoperative reflux in these patients, and because the laparoscopic route had become widely used in the treatment of reflux disease, in 1993 we started using the laparoscopic approach in a routine fashion. The results obtained in our first 57 patients treated by the laparoscopic approach showed that dysphagia was markedly reduced in the great majority of patients, with an average decrease from a 3.8 (on a scale of 0 to 4) preoperatively to a score of 0.7 postoperatively. Regurgitation, the other main symptom in patients with achalasia, decreased from a 2.7 (on the same scale) to a 0.9 score postoperatively. These results appear to be maintained over time. Analysis of our patients who have gone beyond 5 years suggests that dysphagia and regurgitation continue to be under control.[18] Our experience with the laparoscopic approach since 1995 has convinced us and others of its advantages: simplicity of anesthesia, no need for a chest tube, greater ease of performing the antireflux procedure, and relative ease in extending the myotomy into the stomach. In October 1999, our group published in the *Annals of Surgery* the combined results from the University of Washington in Seattle and the University of California–San Francisco. Our experience showed a median length of hospital stay of 72 hours for the thoracoscopic and 48 hours for the laparoscopic group. Eight patients required a second operation for recurrent or persistent dysphagia, and two patients required esophagectomy. There were no deaths. Good or excellent relief of dysphagia was obtained in 90% of patients (85% after thoracoscopic and 93% after laparoscopic myotomy). Abnormal gastroesophageal reflux developed in 60% of tested patients after thoracoscopic myotomy, and in 17% after laparoscopic myotomy. Laparoscopic myotomy and partial fundoplication corrected abnormal reflux present preoperatively in 4 of 7 patients. Patients with dilated esophagus had excellent relief of dysphagia after laparoscopic myotomy, and none required esophagectomy. We concluded that laparoscopic Heller myotomy has emerged as the preferred approach because: (1) it is more effective in the relief of dysphagia (particularly in patients with dilated esophagus); (2) it is associated with a shorter hospital stay; and (3) it is associated with less postoperative reflux.[22]

Our experience is echoed in the current literature. In 1997, Hunter et al[19] reported on 40 patients, of whom 90% had excellent to good results after laparoscopic myotomy. Of the 6 perforations, all occurred at the gastric end of the myotomy, and all were repaired laparoscopically. The Toupet fundoplication was used in these patients as an antireflux procedure.

In a recent study, Rosati et al[20] reported on 61 patients treated laparoscopically with excellent to good results in over 98%, with a mean follow-up period of 21 months (range, 1 to 62 months). Of 7 patients in whom perforation occurred, 5 were repaired laparoscopically; 3 patients were converted to open surgery, and 1 needed a postoperative dilation to relieve persistent dysphagia. Overall, LES pressure dropped from 52 to 27 mm Hg, and barium swallow showed a decrease in esophageal diameter from 52 mm before surgery to 27 mm postoperatively.

COMPLICATIONS

Laceration of the mucosa is the most common complication of laparoscopic myotomy. We have found that perforations occur more frequently in patients treated with botulinum toxin. These perforations usually occur at the GE junction, are very small, and can be closed laparoscopically using 5-0 silk sutures. The Dor fundoplication provides additional support to the repair.

Residual dysphagia is often the consequence of an incomplete myotomy, and can be avoided by extending the myotomy well into the stomach. We have found that when examined endoscopically, the LES is at least 1 to 2 cm below what the surgeon observes externally as the junction of the stomach and esophagus. For this reason it is important to extend the myotomy at least 2 cm beyond the point where the GE junction is identified. Intraoperative endoscopy is used to evaluate the completion of the myotomy.

CONCLUSIONS

Achalasia is a disorder characterized by the lack of peristalsis in the body of the esophagus and by the absence of relaxation of the LES. The goal of treatment is to decrease the basal tone of the LES, since the motility cannot be recovered. Medical treatment has very little or no effect in decreasing the LES pressure, and should therefore be used only in patients in whom balloon dilation or surgical treatment are not valid options.

The use of botulinum toxin has shown good results only in the short term, but has the potential to make a subsequent operation more difficult.

Pneumatic dilation is an appropriate treatment for patients with achalasia. On the other hand, when perforations occur during dilation, patients usually have to be treated surgically, and if not, a stricture can be the final result.

Surgery results in excellent improvement in a high percentage of patients, with a rate of complications similar to that with pneumatic dilation. In cases where perforations occur during the surgical myotomy, they can almost always be repaired during the same procedure with no change in outcome. Robotic surgery is emerging as an attractive alternative for the performance of a Heller myotomy.

REFERENCES

1. Aggestrup S, Uddman R, Sundler F, et al. Lack of vasoactive intestinal polypeptide nerves in esophageal achalasia. *Gastroenterology* 1983;84:924.
2. Guelrud M, Rossiter A, Souney PF, et al. The effect of vasoactive intestinal polypeptide on the lower esophageal sphincter in achalasia. *Gastroenterology* 1992;103:377.
3. Couturier D, Samama J. Clinical aspects and manometric criteria in achalasia. *Hepatogastroenterology* 1991;38:481.
4. Traube M, Dubovik S, Lange RC, et al. The role of nifedipine therapy in achalasia: results of a randomized, double-blind, placebo-controlled study. *Am J Gastroenterol.* 1989;84:1259.
5. Pasricha PJ, Ravich WJ, Kalloo AN. Effects of intrasphincteric botulinum toxin on the lower esophageal sphincter in piglets. *Gastroenterology* 1993;105:1045.
6. Pasricha PJ, Ravich WJ, Hendrix TR, et al. Treatment of achalasia with intrasphincteric injection of botulinum toxin. A pilot trial. *Ann Intern Med.* 1994;121:590.
7. Pasricha PJ, Ravich WJ, Hendrix TR, et al. Intrasphincteric botulinum toxin for the treatment of achalasia [see comments] [published erratum appears in *N Engl J Med.* 1995;333:75]. *N Engl J Med.* 1995;332:774.
8. Pasricha PJ, Rai R, Ravich WJ, et al. Botulinum toxin for achalasia: long-term outcome and predictors of response [see comments]. *Gastroenterology* 1996;110:1410.
9. Fishman VM, Parkman HP, Schiano TD, et al. Symptomatic improvement in achalasia after botulinum toxin injection of the lower esophageal sphincter. *Am J Gastroenterol.* 1996;91:17240.
10. Vantrappen G, Hellemans J. Treatment of achalasia and related motor disorders. *Gastroenterology* 1980;79:144.
11. Ferguson MK. Achalasia: current evaluation and therapy. *Ann Thorac Surg* 1991;52:336.
12. Csendes A, Braghetto I, Henriquez A, et al. Late results of a prospective randomised study comparing forceful dilatation and oesophagomyotomy in patients with achalasia [see comments]. *Gut* 1989;30:299.
13. Birgisson S, Richter JE. Achalasia: what's new in diagnosis and treatment? *Dig Dis* 1997;15(Suppl 1):1.
14. Pellegrini C, Wetter LA, Patti M, et al. Thoracoscopic esophagomyotomy. Initial experience with a new approach for the treatment of achalasia. *Ann Surg.* 1992;216:291; discussion 296.
15. Pellegrini CA, Leichter R, Patti M, et al. Thoracoscopic esophageal myotomy in the treatment of achalasia. *Ann Thorac Surg.* 1993;56:680.
16. Shimi S, Nathanson LK, Cuschieri A. Laparoscopic cardiomyotomy for achalasia. *J Roy Coll Surg Edinb.* 1991;36:152.
17. Dor J, et al. L'Interet de la technique midifiee la prevention du reflux apres cardiomyotomie extra muquese de Heller. *Mem Acad Chir.* 1962;88:881.
18. Horgan S, Hudda K, Eubanks T, et al. Does botulinum toxin injection make esophagomyotomy a more difficult operation? *Surg Endosc.* 1999;13:576.
19. Hunter JG, Trus TL, Branum GD, et al. Laparoscopic Heller myotomy and fundoplication for achalasia. *Ann Surg.* 1997;225:655; discussion, 664.
20. Rosati R, Fumagalli U, Bona S, et al. Evaluating results of laparoscopic surgery for esophageal achalasia. *Surg Endosc.* 1998;12:270.
21. Horgan S, Pellegrini C. Achalasia. In: Yim A, Hazelrigg S, Izzat WB, et al, eds. *Minimal Access Cardiothoracic Surgery.* WB Saunders:2000;253.
22. Patti MG, Pellegrini CA, Horgan S. Minimally invasive surgery for achalasia: an 8-year experience with 168 patients. *Ann Surg.* 1999;230:587.

Chapter Eighteen ▪ ▪ ▪ ▪ ▪ ▪

Laparoscopic Reoperations in the Esophageal Hiatus

JORGE CUETO-GARCÍA, MOUNIR GAZAYERLI, ROBERTO NEVAREZ-BERNAL, A. RASCHKE, and JOSÉ ANTONIO VÁZQUEZ-FRÍAS

INTRODUCTION

Although there is enough clinical evidence to justify that laparoscopic antireflux surgery is the new gold standard in the treatment of gastroesophageal reflux disease (GERD),[1,2] there is still scant information as to the feasibility and safety of reoperations of the esophageal hiatus with minimally invasive surgery. This is of importance because there is considerable evidence that the number of laparoscopic antireflux procedures being done around the world has increased considerably. Many such patients suffer from complications related to an incorrect clinical evaluation and incorrect selection of the operation, and complications related to the surgical procedure itself, and these patients will seek specialized medical attention and many of them will require reoperation.[3–6]

CAUSES OF FAILURE AND PREVENTION

If the patient has been carefully evaluated and a total wrap is the procedure selected initially, there is general agreement that the Nissen operation should be done with the modifications described by DeMeester et al[6,7]: a short wrap 2 to 3 cm long[2–4] above the gastroesophageal (GE) junction; the sutures must include the esophageal and gastric wall to avoid displacement of the plication with the hourglass-type of deformity; the fundus should be adequately mobilized and the short gastric vessels should be divided (a maneuver—though still controversial—now facilitated by the use of harmonic scissors); the fundus should be the area selected for the plication to avoid twisting the body of the stomach,[4] and that once the fundus is passed around the esophagus, it should remain there without tension. If these maneuvers are not done, the 360° wrap will be too tight and will produce stenosis and severe dysphagia that in many cases will not respond to dilatation, and a reoperation will be needed (Fig. 18–1). Trus et al,[8] among others,

has presented evidence that if the fundus is not mobilized adequately, there will be persistent unpleasant side effects such as dysphagia and gas-bloating years after the operation. Using a thorough postoperative evaluation, these workers as well as D'Allemagne et al[4] demonstrated better intermediate and long-term results with the DeMeester-Nissen type of fundoplication as compared to the Nissen-Rossetti type of operation, in which the short gastric vessels are not divided.

It is generally agreed by most (but not all[1,9,10]) surgical groups that, if possible, a short, floppy Nissen operation with the DeMeester modifications[6,7] is the procedure of choice for most patients with gastroesophageal reflux disease (GERD). Some patients with longstanding disease, severe chronic periesophagitis, Barrett's esophagus, or scleroderma may suffer from severe hypoperistalsis and could benefit from a well-constructed partial wrap, and may experience severe refractory dysphagia with a total wrap. This would also apply to elderly patients who suffer from frequent bronchial aspiration and other respiratory complications of GERD that cannot be controlled with medical therapy and require antireflux surgery. If the patient has an acquired short esophagus as discussed elsewhere, the surgical treatment is different and a fundoplication alone may not help these patients with end-stage disease. The proper treatment may be a Collis gastroplasty that can be done via laparoscopy and/or thoracotomy.[11]

If a partial fundoplication has been selected for a patient with GERD, it is our impression that some groups do not perform as adequate a mobilization of the gastric fundus as they routinely do for a total Nissen-DeMeester type of procedure. In fact, Laws et al,[12] in a randomized prospective study comparing total and partial fundoplication with patients operated on in a similar manner and with the same type of dissection and adequate mobilization of the gastric fundus that included division of the short gastric vessels, randomly received a total or a partial wrap, and there were no differences postoperatively. On the other hand, it has been

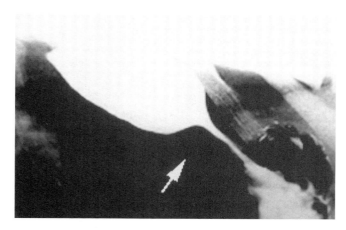

Figure 18–1. Postoperative esophagogram of a young female patient that had a Nissen-Rossetti operation with stenosis refractory to dilatation. She required a laparoscopic reoperation with dismantling of the entire wrap and reconstruction with a Toupet fundoplication.

shown in some studies that partial wraps have a higher rate of disruption and failure compared to total wraps.[6] In our experience there have been 3 patients (1 of our own initial experience) with disruption of the posterior lip of the partial fundoplication, probably due to tension related to incomplete mobilization of the gastric fundus. All were repaired by laparoscopy, and since 1993 the Toupet-type partial fundoplications have been made longer (4 cm) and a greater mobilization of the gastric fundus is achieved.

The hiatal defect(s) should be sutured with nonabsorbable material to prevent postoperative paraesophageal herniation,[13] which may in any case occur occasionally, even with adequate hiatal closure (e.g., in one of our own patients, 8 weeks postoperatively in an elderly male patient with chronic obstructive pulmonary disease).

Patients with achalasia with an incomplete cardiomyotomy had persistence of the symptomatology of obstruction, and those

with an adequate myotomy did not have a complementary antireflux operation and now present with gastrointestinal or respiratory symptoms of GERD. Our group has reoperated 2 patients who complained of severe dysphagia postoperatively and had achalasia with incomplete myotomies. In one instance a very tight, long 360° fundoplication produced an almost complete obstruction with a weight loss of 17 kg in 1 year (Figs. 18–2 and 18–3). A total wrap is not required—even if is constructed in an adequate manner—in these patients, who may continue to live with a severe motility disorder all their lives. There is general agreement that following an adequate cardiomyotomy, the required complementary antireflux procedure should be an anterior hemifundoplication (Dor type) or a posterior hemifundoplication.[14]

Reoperations may also be needed in the immediate postoperative period for perforations or lacerations, although these complications are now less frequent. If there is a gastroesophageal per-

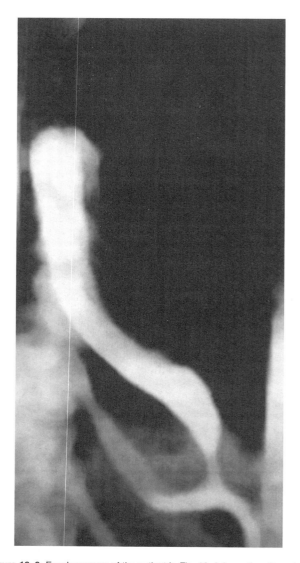

Figure 18–3. Esophagogram of the patient in Fig. 18–2 2 months after a laparoscopic reoperation when a redo-cardiomyotomy was done with dismantling of the 360° wrap and reconstruction with a Dor-type of hemifundoplication. The esophagus is of normal size and there is no obstruction at the GE junction.

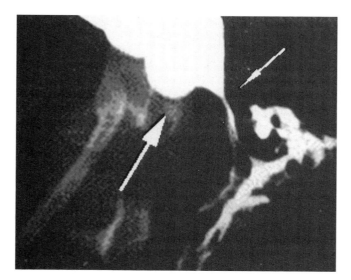

Figure 18–2. Postoperative esophagogram of a 17-year-old female 1 year after a cardiomiotomy for achalasia. The esophagus is very dilated and the cardiomyotomy is incomplete (*small arrow*); also, there is a deformity produced by a long Nissen-type fundoplication (*large arrow*).

foration, mediastinitis may ensue that demands emergency medical and surgical treatment and intensive care, and carries very high mortality and morbidity rates. In our experience a delayed perforation with a periesophageal abscess was drained by laparoscopy on the 12th postoperative day.

Since bariatric procedures are now being done by laparoscopy, among them gastric banding, vertical banded gastroplasty, and gastric bypass, it is anticipated that some of these patients may present with complications related to the procedure, and some may require laparoscopic reoperation. Such has been our experience, and 2 patients with adjustable gastric bands have been reoperated by laparoscopy, one due to early rupture of the band and one patient that voluntarily requested removal of the band.

In addition, from 8 to 10% of patients with well-documented GERD may require another surgical procedure such as a cholecystectomy or some type of vagotomy with or without a drainage procedure for associated peptic ulcer disease that can be performed most times during the same operation. Failure to perform these procedures may produce postoperative symptomatology not relieved by the antireflux valve.

PREOPERATIVE EVALUATION AND CLINICAL PICTURE

The patient with a postoperative complication of the esophageal hiatus requires a very precise preoperative evaluation. Most have had an antireflux procedure (open or laparoscopic), some a cardiomyotomy with or without an antireflux procedure, and in our experience a few others have undergone an operation for complicated peptic ulcer disease or a bariatric procedure such as gastric banding and/or a bypass operation.

As stated above, there might be an undesirable outcome due to an inadequate preoperative evaluation, such as in the case of a patient with complicated peptic ulcer and/or gallbladder disease that had undergone an ill-advised antireflux procedure. This sometimes occurs when patients have the so-called "atypical" symptoms of GERD, and fail to have an adequate endoscopic, manometric, and 24-hour pH evaluation before they undergo surgery. In fact, it has been shown that patients who benefit the most from antireflux procedures are those with "typical" gastrointestinal symptoms and with a satisfactory response to an adequate trial of medical therapy.[15]

The patient with a failed antireflux operation may complain of the "typical" gastrointestinal symptoms of GERD such as pyrosis, regurgitation, or dysphagia, that may or may not be controlled with dilatation, or respiratory types of symptomatology, or chest pain or a combination of any of these.[16,17]

Preoperative endoscopy, manometry, and imaging studies, as well as pH monitoring should be done in every patient. Additional studies such as assessment of gastric emptying may also be required.

SURGICAL TREATMENT

In the recent reports of Hunter et al[16] and Soper and Dunnegan,[17] the types of failures of laparoscopic antireflux surgery are thoroughly analyzed. The most common types of failures are a displaced or disrupted fundoplication; a tight, long 360° wrap that produces dysphagia and paraesophageal herniation, or a combination of these.[16–26] Some of these patients suffered from complicated chronic disease such as Barrett's esophagus and stenosis, and these patients should be carefully evaluated before surgery is performed.[16] Manometric evaluation is considered by several groups—ours included—to be a very useful tool in screening these patients preoperatively.

A careful review of the videotape of the previous procedure (if it was done laparoscopically) may provide information about the type of complication present.

Before the operation, the surgeon must have a thorough and complete discussion of the problem with the patient—and relatives if indicated—given the magnitude of the operation and the possibility of serious complications.

SURGICAL TECHNIQUE

As in open surgery, reoperations of the esophageal hiatus via the laparoscopic approach (as in open surgery) are very complicated, technically demanding, and require extensive surgical experience, special skills, and modern equipment and instruments. The technical problems are considerable due to the fact that in many instances there is considerable fibrosis and scarring, the anatomic planes of surgical dissection are lost, and the esophageal wall can be lacerated easily. The following are some important guidelines to follow when a laparoscopic reoperation is to be performed:

- The problem of adhesions. To establish the pneumoperitoneum, one has to be careful to avoid visceral injury due to adhesions, particularly when the previous operation was a laparotomy. In general, after a previous laparoscopic procedure, the adhesions are few and localized to the trocar entry sites. It is recommended that a left upper quadrant initial puncture be made, and if this is unsuccessful, to proceed using an open (Hasson) technique. After the initial trocar has been placed, using an angled scope, the location and extent of adhesions must be assessed and the rest of trocars inserted after enough room has been created using sharp and blunt dissection, harmonic scissors, or bipolar electrocautery. Once the adhesions in the surgical area have been taken down, one to three of the trocar punctures may be placed in the previous laparotomy scar. Next, the adhesions between the liver's edge and the stomach are taken down, and in the area of the hiatus one must avoid causing bleeding from the left gastric artery in the area of the lesser curvature and from the phrenic vessels in the upper lateral aspect of the left crus.
- Intraoperative endoscopy. Our group routinely uses the help of an endoscopist, who can provide assistance if needed in locating the GE junction, and when the light source of the video camera is dimmed, the light of the endoscope can help locate the surgical planes for dissection. The endoscopist can also perform dilatation if needed, and help rule out lacerations, angulations, or obstructions when the redo plication has been completed. In redo cardiomyotomies, if extensive fibrosis is present, the esophagoscopy can also help assess the adequacy of the myotomy and rule out any laceration or perforation.
- The dissection should be very careful and meticulous in both the crura and away from the esophageal wall, and irrigation (with air and fluid) by the anesthesiologist and/or endoscopist may help identify lacerations or perforations. Our group has repaired 2 lac-

erations, one in the distal esophagus and one in the posterior gastric wall, that were repaired with interrupted stitches of 000 polydioxanone. The fundoplication later acted as a serosal patch on top of this repair with no postoperative complications.

- Once the GE junction and both crura have been identified and cleared of adhesions, the dissection of the retro-esophageal area is patiently done, it is recommended that the nasogastric tube or a dilator be removed during this part of the procedure. A Penrose drainage tube may be passed to provide traction and help in the dissection and the creation of a wide retroesophageal window.
- If a paraesophageal hernia is present, more extensive dissection is required to identify all the hiatal defects that will require repair. This complication occurs more frequently in obese patients.
- In the greater curvature one has to be mindful of adhesions between the spleen and the stomach to avoid lacerating the former. If the short gastric vessels were not divided, it is frequently necessary to carry out this maneuver even for a partial fundoplication to achieve a very loose wrap.
- When suturing the fundoplication, one must keep in mind that the esophageal wall is more friable in redo operations. One patient referred to us sustained a laceration when the surgeon was tying an extracorporeal knot (seen on videotape review) and went on to develop a paraesophageal abscess.
- When the situation demands it because of extensive fibrosis and scarring, a hand-assisted procedure is a very useful option before conversion to formal laparotomy.

As to the type of reconstruction to be done, this must be individualized. In a young patient with disruption or displacement of the wrap with good esophageal peristalsis, a 360° Nissen-DeMeester procedure may be the option of choice.[16–18] In a patient with a detached partial wrap with poor peristaltic function, a long floppy partial fundoplication may be indicated.[18–21,23–25] The latter antireflux valve or an anterior hemifundoplication (Dor type) is also indicated after a redo cardiomyotomy for achalasia.[14]

RESULTS

The morbidity and mortality of laparoscopic antireflux surgery must be compared with the results obtained with decades of open conventional surgery, although it appears that there are some similarities. In the largest series reported by Hunter et al[16] the most important cause of failure of laparoscopic operations was transdiaphragmatic migration of the fundoplication (84%), which could be explained at least in part by the extensive dissection and mobilization done in this type of approach. Similarly, it appears that unless adequate repair of the hiatal defect is done, the prevalence of postoperative paraesophageal hernia is much higher than in open conventional surgery.[13] The same explanation could apply to the well-known fact that splenectomy for intraoperative lacerations is much more rare in laparoscopic than open surgery.

In the series of Hunter et al,[16] Soper et al,[17] and Floch et al,[18] most patients had had previous laparoscopic procedures, a trend that no doubt will continue as more and more antireflux procedures are done with this approach, although in our experience (Table 18–1) and that of De Paula et al,[26] most patients had had a previous laparotomy.

TABLE 18–1. RESULTS OF LAPAROSCOPIC REOPERATIONS IN 20 PATIENTS SINCE JUNE 1991

- 20 patients total: 12 males and 8 females
- Age range: 21–76 (average, 42)
- 13 had previous laparotomies (1 patient had 3) and 7 laparoscopies
- 8 patients had a displaced or disrupted Nissen-type of fundoplication
- 4 patients had a long, tight Nissen-Rossetti fundoplication
- 3 patients had a disrupted partial fundoplication
- 2 patients had a previous complete vagotomy, 1 with an anterior hemifundoplication
- 1 patient had a periesophageal abscess
- 2 patients had adjustable gastric bands: 1 replacement, 1 removal

Although the clinical experience with laparoscopic reoperations is limited, an analysis of the reports published thus far reveals surprisingly good results. The mortality rate is close to zero, and good or excellent results are obtained in 82 to 89% of patients. The morbidity ranges from 8 to 12% and the conversion rate to laparotomy 8 to 20%. The duration of the procedure ranged from 85 to 370 minutes (average, 220 min) with more time required for patients with previous laparotomies.

CONCLUSIONS

Although the number of patients operated on is small, it appears that reoperations of the esophageal hiatus by laparoscopy are feasible and safe, and since the total number of antireflux procedures by both approaches has increased sharply, it is anticipated that this method will be the option of choice for patients that have complications due to an inadequate preoperative evaluation and/or intraoperative complications.

A precise preoperative evaluation with clinical, endoscopic, and manometric means, as well as imaging and pH monitoring, should be done routinely, and other studies may be needed as well.

Reoperation done laparoscopically, just as in open surgery, can be a formidable technical challenge, and extensive previous clinical experience is required, as are advanced skills and modern equipment. However, if a careful dissection is patiently done, with assistance by intraoperative endoscopy, irrigation, and by other means, and several key methods of surgical technique are followed, the outcome can be satisfactory. The results so far obtained are quite good and do not differ substantially from those obtained with the standard laparoscopic antireflux surgery that is now the gold standard in the surgical treatment of GERD.

REFERENCES

1. Eypasch E, Neugebauer E. Laparoscopic antireflux surgery for gastroesophageal reflux disease (GERD). Results of a Consensus Development Conference of the European Association of Endoscopic Surgery (EAES). *Surg Endosc.* 1997;11:413.
2. Guidelines for surgical treatment of gastroesophageal reflux disease (GERD). Approved by the Board of Governors of the Society of American Gastrointestinal Surgeons (SAGES), 1996.
3. Stein HJ, Feussner H, Siewert JR. Failure of antireflux surgery: causes and management strategies. *Am J Surg.* 1996;171:36.
4. D'Allemagne B, Weerts JM, Jehaes C, et al. Causes of failures of lap-

aroscopic antireflux operations. Department de Chirurgie, Centre Hospitalier Saint Joseph-Esperance, Liege, Belgium. *Surg Endosc.* 1996;10:305.

5. Cueto J, Weber A. Laparoscopic reoperations in the esophageal hiatus. Proceedings of the Euro-Asian Congress of Endoscopic Surgery, Istanbul Turkey 17–21 June 1997. Monduzzi Editors;133.

6. De Meester TR. Surgical management of gastroesophageal reflux. In: Castell DO ed. *Gastroesophageal Reflux Disease, Pathophysiology, Diagnosis, Therapy.* Futura:1985;265.

7. Dunnington GL, De Meester T, et al. Outcome effect of adherence to operative principles of Nissen fundoplication by multiple surgeons. *Am J Surg* 1993;166:654.

8. Trus T, Laycock W, Bramm G, et al. Follow-up of laparoscopic antireflux surgery. *Am J Surg* 1996;171:32.

9. Thor KB, Silander T. A long-term randomized prospective trial of the Nissen procedure versus a modified Toupet Technique. *Ann Surg.* 1990;210:719.

10. Lundell L. Management of GERD in 1995. The role of semifundoplication in the long-term management of gastroesophageal reflux disease. In: Lundell L, ed. *Diseases of the Esophagus.* Longman Group, Ltd.:1994;Chap. 7:245.

11. Johnson AB, Oddsdottir M, Hunter JG. Laparoscopic Collis gastroplasty and Nissen fundoplication. A new technique for the management of foreshortening of the esophagus. *Surg Endosc.* 1998;12:1055.

12. Laws HL, Clements RH, Swillie CM. A randomized prospective comparison of Nissen fundoplication and Toupet fundoplication for gastroesophageal reflux disease. *Ann Surg.* 1997;225:647.

13. Watson DI, Jamieson GG, Devitt PG, et al. Paraesophageal hiatus hernia: an important complication of laparoscopic Nissen fundoplication. *Br J Surg.* 1995;82:521.

14. Patti MG, Pellegrini CA, Horgan S, et al. Minimally invasive surgery for achalasia. An 8-year experience with 168 patients. *Ann Surg.* 1999;230:587.

15. Peters JH, DeMeester TR, Crookes P, et al. The treatment of gastroesophageal reflux disease with laparoscopic Nissen fundoplication.

Prospective evaluation of 100 patients with "typical" symptoms. *Ann Surg.* 1998;228:40.

16. Hunter JG, Smith D, Branum GD, et al. Laparoscopic fundoplication failures. Patterns of failure and response to fundoplication revision. *Ann Surg.* 1999;230:595.

17. Soper NJ, Dunnegan D. Anatomic fundoplication failure after laparoscopic antireflux surgery. *Ann Surg.* 1999;229:669.

18. Floch NR, Hinder RA, Kingler PJ, et al. Is laparoscopic reoperation for failed antireflux surgery feasible? *Arch Surg.* 1999;134:733.

19. Horgan S, Pohl D, Bogetti D, et al. Failed antireflux surgery: what have we learned from reoperations? Department of Surgery, University of Washington Medical Center, Seattle, USA. *Arch Surg.* 1999; 134:809; discussion 815.

20. Bonavina L, Chella B, Segalin A, et al. Surgical therapy in patients with failed antireflux repairs. Department of Surgery University of Milan, Ospedale maggiore Policlinico I.R.C.C.S., Milano, Italy. *Hepatogastroenterology* 1998;45:1344.

21. Curet MJ, Josloff RK, Schoeb O, et al. Laparoscopic reoperations for failed antireflux procedure. Department of Surgery, University of New Mexico School of Medicine, Albuquerque, USA. *Arch Surg.* 1999; 134:559.

22. Lim JK, Moisidis E, Munro WS, et al. Re-operation for failed antireflux surgery. Department of Surgery, Concord, Strathfield Adventist Hospital, New South Wales Australia. *Aust NZ J Surg.* 1996; 66:731.

23. Cueto GJ, Weber A. Reoperaciones en la cirugia del hiato esofagico, en Cirugia Laparoscopica 1997. In: Cueto J, Weber A, eds. McGraw-Hill Interamericana:1997;92.

24. Reilly MG, Mullins S, Reddick EJ. Laparoscopic management of failed antireflux surgery. *Surg Laparosc Endosc.* 1997;7:90.

25. Watson DI, Jamieson GG, Game RS, et al. Laparoscopic reoperations following failed antireflux surgery. *Br J Surg.* 1999;86:98.

26. DePaula AL, Hashiba K, Bafutto M, et al. Laparoscopic reoperations after failed and complicated antireflux operations. *Surg Endosc.* 1995;9:681.

Chapter Nineteen • • • • • • •

*E*ndoscopic Esophagectomy: Subtotal Esophagectomy with a Videolaparoscopic Approach

CARLOS EDUARDO DOMENE

The improvement in video surgery in the past few decades has gradually led to an increase in the number of procedures that utilize this minimally invasive technique, while the progressive development of optical equipment and micro cameras, insufflators, and appropriate instruments has led to the rapid expansion of its application. Initially, during the 1960s, it was restricted to investigative procedures, especially diagnostic laparoscopy, but its use gradually spread to gynecologic procedures in a few medical centers, a situation that persisted until the end of the 1980s. Not even the description of a laparoscopic appendectomy in 1983 was sufficient to mobilize the general interest of surgeons in the new technique. The cholecystectomy performed by Mouret in 1987 was the cornerstone for the spread of the laparoscopic procedure.

The recent explosion of video surgery as a therapeutic method has not met with widespread acceptance. In fact numerous practitioners oppose its use, and only a few of them have constructive ideas that have actually contributed to its development. There has been a flood of surgeons operating without adequate training, using of video surgery in procedures where it is of dubious value, and the adaptation of various techniques to utilize this type of access even when the results were known to be inadequate.

After 10 years, some controversial aspects persist:

- The need for changes in technique and type of anesthesia used for operations such as hernioplasty and the correction of varicocele
- Its use in the treatment of cancer, for determining its extension, and the possible contamination of trocar entry sites
- Its use in major surgical interventions, such as esophagectomies and duodenopancreatectomies

In general, two major aspects tend to determine the severity of postoperative symptoms or complications: incisional trauma and operative trauma.

In video surgery, incisional trauma is minimized, as few symptoms of pain and a low incidence of complications are observed. When operative trauma is limited or localized, the benefits of video surgery are greatest, including rapid recuperation, less pain, a rapid return to normal activities, a low incidence of complications, and a more favorable aesthetic result. When operative trauma is extensive, however, complications inherent to the surgery itself occur, and a prolonged period of recovery and abdominal wall pain are inevitable consequences. This minimizes the benefits resulting from the lack of a large incision; moreover, difficulties introduced by the use of laparoscopic operative technique can actually contribute to the development of further complications.

Given these observations, operations using video surgery can be divided into three major types:

- *Type 1* (operative trauma is less than incisional trauma): In these cases, great advantages can be gained by the use of video surgery (for procedures such as cholecystectomy, fundoplication, and cardiomyotomy).
- *Type 2* (operative trauma and incisional trauma are equivalent): In such cases, video surgery is of dubious value (for procedures such as uncomplicated appendectomy).
- *Type 3* (operative trauma exceeds incisional trauma): In these cases, the disadvantages outweigh the advantages of the use of the technique instead of more conventional methods (for extensive procedures such as esophagectomy and duodenopancreatectomy).

Video surgery can be used in esophagectomies in various ways; video-assisted combined thoracoscopy and laparotomy, standard thoracoscopy and laparoscopy, and laparoscopy with transdiaphragmatic dissection. In this study, the entirely endoscopic techniques described below were used.

ESOPHAGECTOMY BY THORACOSCOPY, LAPAROSCOPY, AND CERVICOTOMY

This is a procedure indicated to facilitate the dissection of the thoracic and abdominal ganglia and prepare the gastric tube for manual cervical gastroesophageal anastomosis, for radical treatment of esophageal cancer.

Patients must be under general anesthesia, selectively intubated, and placed in left lateral decubitus position with ventral inclination.

The surgeon stands facing the patient with the monitor on his right. Five trocars are placed between the anterior and posterior axillary lines; the optic lens is inserted through a trocar in the eighth intercostal space along the midaxillary line, and the instruments for dissection are inserted in the fifth intercostal space along both anterior and posterior axillary lines; in the fourth space, the lung retractor is placed anteriorly and the aspirator posteriorly.

The lung is pushed aside, a maneuver that is facilitated by the anteriorized position of the patient; after total collapse of the organ, this traction may be unnecessary. The pleura is opened near the esophagus and the azygos vein is dissected and tied off with stitches and clips or vascular staples. From the cervical cupola to the hiatus of the diaphragm, the esophagus is dissected and the ganglia are removed with scissors and monopolar or bipolar coagulation or clips. A thoracic drain is inserted and the incisions are closed.

The patient is then moved to the horizontal dorsal decubitus position, with the surgeon standing between the patient's legs. One monitor and an assistant stands on his right side, with the other monitor on his left. Five trocars are placed: a 5-mm trocar on the right midclavicular line along the costal margin, and the other four, 10-mm trocars, one at the xiphoid process along the midline, one between the xiphoid process and the umbilicus, one along the midclavicular line at the left costal margin, and the final one in the lower part of left upper quadrant. The stomach is then released and the greater curvature is tied off with a bipolar forceps outside the gastroepiploic vessels. The left gastric vessels are divided and tied at the origin, and the ganglia of the celiac axis are removed. The gastric tube is prepared using a linear stapler from the gastric fundus to the fifth vessel of the lesser gastric curvature. The surgical specimen (the esophagus and the smaller gastric curvature) is attached to the gastric tube using two cotton stitches.

A left cervicotomy is conducted by dissection from the cervical esophagus, removal of the surgical specimen, and traction of the gastric tube, which is then removed from the cervical region, followed by the gastroesophageal anastomosis, performed manually or with the use of a circular stapler.

A tape drain is placed in the abdomen, followed by a video-assisted jejunostomy.[11] The incisions are then closed.

ESOPHAGECTOMY WITH TRANSDIAPHRAGMATIC DISSECTION AND CERVICOTOMY USING LAPAROSCOPY

This treatment is indicated for benign esophageal disease or palliative resections for cancer.

The patient is placed in the lithotomy position, with the surgeon standing between the patient's legs. One assistant stands on the left and another on the right of the patient. Five trocars are placed in the abdomen, in an arrangement similar to that described above.

The stomach is dissected, releasing the greater curvature from the gastroepiploic vessels; the lesser gastric curvature is freed and the left gastric vessels taken down. The entire stomach can be used for reconstruction. When the stomach is short or when a neoplastic lesion is present, the gastric tube is prepared as outlined above. The entire stomach and gastric tube continue to be perfused by the right gastric and gastroepiploic arteries.

The esophageal hiatus of the diaphragm is dissected, and the diaphragm is then cut from the hiatal ring to the level of the xiphoid process, separating it from the pleura and the pericardium. The posterior mediastinum is thus wide open, making a more complete dissection of the inferior and medial esophagus possible. The esophagus is pulled through the abdomen, and progressively dissected up towards its cervical portion.

Along with this procedure, left cervicotomy and digital dissection of the cervical esophagus is performed until the previously released portion of the organ is reached. Traction is applied to the esophagus and stomach through the cervical incision, the surgical specimen is removed and the cervical esophagogastric anastomosis is performed.

In cases of achalasia, pyloroplasty or extramucous pyloromyotomy is then performed, along with a video-assisted jejunostomy and the drainage of the abdominal cavity. The incisions are then closed.

RESULTS

Ten patients, five with esophageal neoplasia and five with achalasia in which esophagectomy was indicated, were operated on between 1995 and 1997. The patients with benign disorders[4] were treated using combined laparoscopic/cervicotomic access, and all of those with neoplasia underwent esophageal dissection using thoracoscopy and laparoscopy. All had some sort of contraindication to the performance of a thoracotomy (cirrhosis of the liver, malnutrition, advanced age, or heart or lung disease).

No complications were observed in the patients operated on for benign disorders using only laparoscopic access. In those patients operated on for cancer there were two complications: in the patient with cirrhosis, large quantities of ascitic fluid drained through the chest that required the placement of a drainage catheter for 9 days (the flow ceased with clinical measures). The patient with malnutrition presented with one partial dehiscence of the gastric tube, and was also treated in a conservative manner, with fasting and total parenteral feeding. No deaths were observed.

For the patients not requiring thoracoscopy and thoracic drainage, the recuperation time was short, physical activity was resumed early, and feeding was soon initiated by jejunostomy; few complaints of pain were received. The patients were fed orally starting on the seventh postoperative day, according to the healing of the cervical anastomosis as assessed by radiologic evaluation, and patients were released from the hospital in 7 to 10 days. Those who underwent thoracoscopy and thoracic draining complained of pain and difficulty in motion. These patients benefited less from the advantages of the use of a minimally invasive surgical procedure.

DISCUSSION

At present, numerous controversial aspects surrounding cancer of the esophagus remain. There have been clear modifications in the profile of the disease, as recent studies of molecular biology have shown, with an increased incidence of adenocarcinoma and its link to Barrett's esophagus.[3] Improved diagnosis and staging have made it possible to establish clearer diagnostic criteria, which allow better evaluation and comparison of the results of treatment.[2] Neoadjuvant chemotherapy, sometimes in conjunction with radiotherapy, has brought new possibilities for the improvement of surgical results.[15] The extent of removal of ganglia required in curative esophagectomy has not yet been clearly established,[10] nor has the palliative treatment appropriate for advanced forms of the disease.[36] Continuing multicentered studies are fundamental for the evaluation of treatment protocols, so a significant number of cases can be collected, despite the difficulty in controlling the multiple variables present in such studies.[20]

In this vast and constantly developing field of study, video surgery has contributed in various ways to the staging of tumors using thoracoscopy and laparoscopy,[17,28] as well as being useful in various kinds of treatment. The treatments conducted completely by video surgery include various types of resection such as:

- Radical, using thoracoscopy and laparotomy[34]
- Radical, using thoracoscopy and laparotomy[11]
- Palliative, using thoracoscopy and laparotomy[7]
- Palliative, using laparoscopy and transdiaphragmatic dissection[11]

It has also been used in association with conventional invasive surgery to improve the visualization and ability to teach such procedures as:

- Video-assisted thoracotomy[21,30,12]
- Laparotomy and cervicoscopy/thoracoscopy[36]
- Laparotomy with transhiatal access[36,41]

In the staging of cancer of the esophagus, no method or combination of methods has yet been determined to be the best, due to the involvement of lymph nodes and even metastases.[27] Endoscopic ultrasound has shown promise of greater accuracy than computed tomography in the staging of these patients, but frequent blockage of the passageway through the substenotic area due to the neoplasm has been observed.[26]

In 45 patients studied, the correlation of the staging established by the surgical specimen with that previously determined by thoracoscopy was 93%, and the stage as determined by laparoscopy was 94%.[16–19] Of the 26 patients staged with thoracoscopy and laparoscopy,[25] in 6 the presence of metastases not detected radiologically was revealed, which required a radical change in the treatment (i.e., staging by video surgery revealed the need for a change in the treatment in 23% of the patients).[22] The use of thoracoscopy in the staging of cancer of the esophagus is thought to be as accurate as the use of mediastinoscopy to stage lung cancer,[13,16,18] and it is routinely used to determine treatment and establish prognosis. The development of new instruments with "touch" sensors for use in video surgery should further increase the accuracy of the method.[32] A multicenter study[16] has shown thoracoscopy to be a valuable tool in the staging of intrathoracic tumors, and in the preoperative staging of esophageal cancer it allows better tailoring of accompanying therapy, as well as more accuracy in determining the presence of involvement of lymph nodes

and the degree of invasion of the esophageal wall by a tumor. The morbidity of the procedure is practically zero, and no complications or fatalities have been described. However, one must consider the cost of the operating room and the general anesthesia, as well as the instruments and equipment necessary for this method.[42]

Esophageal tumors limited to the mucosa (invasion of the muscular layer of the mucosa, the muscularis mucosae) can be treated using endoscopic resection with satisfactory results and a low rate of recurrence.[1,29] The involvement of the submucosa by the tumor may require radical resection of the esophagus with lymphadenectomy to cure the disease.[10] The en bloc removal of the esophagus along with the mediastinal lymph nodes and the celiac trunk has increased the number of cures of superficial tumors and has also led to good results for transmural forms of the disease.[39,24] In analyzing the risk factors for mortality after treatment of esophageal cancer, Saito et al[38] found that the immune status and age of the patient, as well as use of chemotherapy and three-field lymphadenectomy, were important factors. Video surgery can be used in both the curative and palliative treatment of esophageal cancer, making dissection and freeing of the esophagus and stomach possible by thoracoscopy and laparoscopy, using a technique similar to that adopted in thoracotomy and laparotomy. These concepts make it possible to consider video surgery as a valid option for these indications, with a decrease in morbidity and mortality versus that of the extensive dissection involved in radical esophagectomy.

Video-assisted surgery does not require significant modifications of surgical technique or instruments, yet several benefits, including better illumination of the operative field, a magnified view of structures, use of smaller incisions,[21] better lymph node removal,[30,12] and safer transdiaphragmatic release,[36,41] have been reported.

The implementation of complete operations performed via video surgery, especially in thoracoscopic removal, may lead to certain risks. Wu et al[40] performed 22 esophagectomies for cancer with no complications or recurrences within 11.2 months. Collard[6,7] operated on 14 patients (11 of whom had cancer) using thoracoscopy, laparotomy, and cervicotomy, with two conversions (for bleeding and loss of selectivity in pulmonary insufflation) and one death. An average of 21 to 51 ganglia were removed in each surgical specimen, a result similar to that obtained with traditional thoracotomy. Peracchia et al[34,35] performed 18 esophagectomies, with 5.5% mortality and 33.3% morbidity. After an average follow-up time of 17 months, only 14 of the patients were still free of disease, although one tumor occurred at the site of a trocar incision after 6 months, and three others died 14, 20, and 28 months after surgery from recurrence of cancer. Cuschieri[9] treated 34 patients, 6 with metastases and 2 with severe pleural adhesions; 26 underwent esophageal resection via thoracoscopy with one conversion (due to aortic bleeding) and no fatalities. Three cases of pneumectomy, two recurrent nerve lesions, and one esophagogastric anastomotic fistula were observed. A Belgian multicenter study[8] demonstrated that only 20 esophagectomies had been conducted in 296 cases of thoracoscopy, illustrating the fact that the percentage of esophagectomies performed via this route is still very low. Esophagectomy using thoracoscopy associated with either laparoscopy or laparotomy is an operation in which operative trauma is greater than incisional trauma. Therefore in these cases there may be no benefit for the patient when this technique is used. O'Brien[31] emphasized that the benefits of less invasive surgery may be outweighed by the potential for greater complications in some situa-tions, because some difficult procedures become even more problematic with video surgery. In such cases the tech-nique brings no apparent advantages for the patient or the institution.

Loscertales[23] points out numerous technical and tactical problems presented by esophagectomies via thoracoscopy, such as adequate positioning of the patient on the operating table, safe release of pleuropulmonary adhesions, and the dissection and division of the azygos vein, as well as the separation of the esophagus from the descending aorta, the aortic arch, and the posterior wall of the trachea. Immediate thoracotomy is indicated whenever critical hemorrhage is encountered, as it is difficult to contain via thoracoscopy. This also applies to cases in which invasion of the tracheobronchial tree and/or the aorta are found, or when dissection of the aortic arch is difficult due to the risk of massive bleeding. This author suggests thoracoscopic surgery for selected tumors of the middle third of the esophagus (stage T1 to T2 and N0 to N1).

If there are greater risks and difficulties with this surgery, other doubts are raised: Is there an advantage in seeing ganglia better and dissecting more thoroughly, and does this make the operation more radical? Are there fewer pulmonary complications? Does it cost less? Does the patient receive the benefits of less pain and faster recuperation?

Even in thoracoscopic operations for benign afflictions with no need for resection of the esophagus (such as in the treatment of leiomyomas and diverticuli), important complications not seen when thoracotomy was used have been published. The difficulty in performing procedures exactly as they are done with traditional techniques has also been pointed out, and this also makes the widespread acceptance of video surgery difficult.

In answering questions about the safety of the operation, the reduced risk of postoperative complications, and radical nature of some oncologic cases, Collard[6,7] declared that esophagectomy via video surgery does not bring any greater benefits for the patient. He describes serious complications and extensive bleeding due to the procedure itself, making it unsafe because it can lead to more serious problems, and can make it hard to regain control of the situation. The morbidity and mortality are similar to or higher than that of conventional procedures, and the survival rates to date lead to the supposition that the operation is merely palliative. The same author concluded that although radical esophagectomies were possible in selected patients, a more radical procedure performed through small parietal incisions would still be an invasive procedure due to the magnitude of internal dissection and the precarious clinical condition of these patients. He does, however, emphasize that thoracoscopy and laparoscopy are excellent alternatives to classical methods for diagnosing and staging tumors.

In a recent review of the literature on esophagectomy using thoracoscopy, Peracchia et al[34,35] identified 107 cases (99 malignant tumors), with 49.2% morbidity, 12 conversions (11.2%), 4 laryngeal recurrent nerve lesions (3.8%), and two deaths (1.9%). Between 9 and 51 ganglia were removed in each surgical specimen. There were blood losses of from 200 to 1500 mL, and the operative time of the thoracoscopy varied from 120 to 360 minutes. Due to the great difficulties and potential risks of thoracoscopy, these authors recommend that the procedure, although feasible in some cases, should be performed only by surgeons highly experienced in esophageal surgery with thoracic access, as well as in advanced laparoscopic surgery. Mortality, as in conventional surgery, was due to factors common to both procedures, and not complications due to the thoracoscopic method as such. The extensive procedure required can be performed using video surgery, but it takes longer and there is greater pulmonary exclusion. Moreover, for these authors, total mediastinal lymphadenectomy is impossible due to the difficulties of access to the paratracheal and infra-aortic ganglia. On the other hand, early tumoral recurrence in parietal incisions can compromise long-term results. Postoperative complications are similar to those of traditional surgery, and do not seem to be lessened by the minimally invasive nature of thoracoscopy. For these reasons, esophagectomy through thoracoscopy, although technically possible, does not seem to offer any clear advantages over traditional surgery, and its use should be reserved for special studies in selected centers.

REFERENCES

1. Adachi Y, Sasaki Y, Kiwano H, et al. Curative local excision for mucosal esophageal carcinoma. *Int Surg.* 1993;78:141.
2. Akiyama S, Sekiguchi H, Fujiwara M, et al. Intra-aortic ultrasonography in advanced esophageal cancer. *Semin Surg Oncol.* 1997;13:234.
3. Altorki NK, Oliveria S, Schrump DS. Epidemiology and molecular biology of Barrett's adenocarcinoma. *Semin Surg Oncol.* 1997;13:270.
4. Bardini R, Asolati M. Thoracoscopic resection of benign tumors of the esophagus. *Int Surg.* 1997;82:5.
5. Carreño JR, Cicero RS. Esophageal fistulas. Results of conservative treatment. *Int Surg.* 1995;80:251.
6. Collard JM. Chirurgie vidéo-endoscopique et cancer de l'oesophage: réflexions. *Chirurgie* 1994;120:426.
7. Collard JM. Role of videoassisted surgery in the treatment of oesophageal cancer. *Ann Chir Gynaecol.* 1995;84:209.
8. Coosemans W, Lerut TE, Van-Raemdonck DE. Thoracoscopic surgery: the Belgian experience. *Ann Thorac Surg.* 1993;56:721.
9. Cuschieri A. Thoracoscopic subtotal oesophagectomy. *Endosc Surg Allied Technol.* 1994;2:21.
10. DeMeester TR. Esophageal carcinoma: current controversies. *Semin Surg Oncol.* 1997;13:217.
11. Domene CE, Santo MA, Pinotti HW. Tratamento laparoscópico do megaesôfago. Anais do III Congresso Brasileiro de Cirurgia Video Endoscópica, Salvador, Brazil, 1997.
12. Endo M. Combined thoracoscopy in transthoracic esophagectomy. Abstracts of IV International Symposium of Thoracoscopy and Video Assisted Thoracic Surgery, Sao Paulo, Brazil, 1997.
13. Fiocco M, Krasna MJ. Thoracoscopic lymph node dissection in the staging of esophageal carcinoma. *J Laparoendosc Surg.* 1992;2:111.
14. Gayet B. Vidéo-chirurgie et oesophage. *Chirurgie* 1994;120:153.
15. Ide H, Nakamura T, Hayashi K, et al. Neoadjuvant chemotherapy with cisplatinum/5-fluorouracil/low-dose leucovorin for advanced squamous cell carcinoma of the esophagus. *Semin Surg Oncol.* 1997; 13:253.
16. Krasna MJ. Role of thoracoscopic lymph node staging for lung and esophageal cancer. *Oncology Huntingt.* 1996;10:793.
17. Krasna MJ. The role of thoracoscopic lymph node staging in esophageal cancer. *Int Surg.* 1997;82:7.
18. Krasna MJ, Flowers JL, Attar S, et al. Combined thoracoscopic/laparoscopic staging of esophageal cancer. *J Thorac Cardiovasc Surg.* 1996;111:800.
19. Krasna MJ, Reed CE, Jaklistsch MT, et al. Thoracoscopic staging of esophageal cancer: a prospective, multiinstitutional trial. *Ann Thorac Surg.* 1995;60:1337.
20. Law SY, Wong J. Esophageal cancer surgery: the value of controlled clinical trials. *Semin Surg Oncol.* 1997;13:281.
21. Liu HP, Chang CH, Lin PJ, et al. Video-assisted endoscopic esophagec-

tomy with stapled intrathoracic esophagogastric anastomosis. *World J Surg* 1995;19:745.

22. Locicero J. Laparoscopy/thoracoscopy for staging. II. Pretherapy nodal evaluation in carcinoma of the esophagus. *Semin Surg Oncol.* 1993;9:56.

23. Loscertales J. Problemas técnicos en la resección esofágica por tora-coscopia. Abstracts of IV International Symposium of Thoracoscopy and Video Assisted Thoracic Surgery, Sao Paulo, Brazil, 1997.

24. Lozac HP, Topart P, Perramant M. Ivor Lewis procedure for epider-moid carcinoma of the esophagus. A series of 264 patients. *Semin Surg Oncol.* 1997;13:238.

25. Luketich JD, Schauer PR, Landreneau RJ, et al. Pre-treatment mini-mally invasive staging of esophageal cancer to assess response rates to a chemotherapeutic regimen. Abstracts of IV International Sympo-sium of Thoracoscopy and Video Assisted Thoracic Surgery, Sao Paulo, Brazil, 1997.

26. Massari M, Cioffi U, Desimone M, et al. Endoscopic ultrasonography for preoperative staging of esophageal carcinoma. *Surg Laparosc En-dosc.* 1997;7:162.

27. Mattioli FP, Cagnazzo A, Razzetta F. Chirurgia miniinvasiva dell'e-sofago. Nostra esperienza. *Minerva Chir.* 1994;49:33.

28. McCarthy JF, Wood AE. The evolution of thoracoscopic assisted sur-gery. *Int Surg.* 1997;82:18.

29. Moreira LF, Kamikawa Y, Naomoto Y, et al. Endoscopic mucosal re-section for superficial carcinoma and high-grade dysplasia of the esophagus. *Surg Laparosc Endosc.* 1995;5:171.

30. Nakaghama T, Inoue H, Yoshida T, et al. Thoracoscopy assisted esophageal surgery. Abstracts of IV International Symposium of Tho-racoscopy and Video Assisted Thoracic Surgery, Sao Paulo, Brazil, 1997.

31. O'Brien PE. The endosurgical revolution: is it under control? *Aust NZ J Surg.* 1994;64:588.

32. Ohtsuka T, Furuse A, Kohno T, et al. New tactile sensor techniques for localization of pulmonary nodules. *Int Surg.* 1997;82:12.

33. Pellegrini CA. The role of minimal access surgery in esophageal dis-ease. *Curr Opin Gen Surg.* 1994;117:9.

34. Peracchia A, Rosati R, Fumagalli U, et al. Thoracoscopic esophagec-tomy: are there benefits? *Semin Surg Oncol.* 1997;13:259.

35. Peracchia A, Rosati R, Fumagalli U, et al. Thoracoscopic dissection of the esophagus for cancer. *Int Surg.* 1997;82:1.

36. Pinotti HW, Cecconello I, Oliveira MA. Transhiatal esophagectomy for esophageal cancer. *Semin Surg Oncol.* 1997;13:253.

37. Rosati R, Bona S, Fumagalli U, et al. The role of thoracoscopy in benign esophageal disease. Abstracts of IV International Symposium of Thora-coscopy and Video Assisted Thoracic Surgery, Sao Paulo, Brazil, 1997.

38. Saito T, Kinoshita T, Shigemitsuly Y, et al. Risk factors associated with postoperative mortality in patients with esophageal cancer. *Int Surg.* 1993;78:93.

39. Siewert JR, Stein HJ. Barrett's cancer: indications, extent, and results of surgical resection. *Semin Surg Oncol.* 1997;13:245.

40. Wu YC, Liu HP, Lin PJ, et al. Preoperative concurrent chemoradio-therapy followed by thoracoscopic esophagectomy in patients with esophageal cancer. Preliminary surgical results. Abstracts of IV Inter-national Symposium of Thoracoscopy and Video Assisted Thoracic Surgery, Sao Paulo, Brazil, 1997.

41. Yahata H, Sugino K, Takiguchi T, et al. Laparoscopic transhiatal esophagectomy for advanced thoracic esophageal cancer. *Surg Lap-arosc Endosc.* 1997;7:13.

42. Yim APC. Cost-effectiveness of thoracoscopy. The Asian perspective. *Int Surg.* 1997;82:32.

*G*astric Surgery

Chapter Twenty ● ● ● ● ● ●

Surgical Treatment of Peptic Ulcer Disease

NAMIR KATKHOUDA, MELANIE H. FRIEDLANDER, STEVEN W. GRANT, KRANTHI K. ACHANTA, RAHILA ESSANI, and JEAN MOUIEL

INTRODUCTION

Laparoscopic surgical treatment of duodenal ulcers is directed at patients who are refractory to medical treatment with H_2-receptor antagonists or to a medical regimen designed to eradicate *Helicobacter pylori*.[1] In the absence of *H. pylori*, patients with persistent peptic ulcer disease may benefit from vagotomy. Those with early recurrence of ulcer disease or a contraindication to medical therapy are also candidates for vagotomy. Complications of peptic ulcer disease, such as bleeding and gastric outlet obstruction secondary to scarring of the duodenal bulb, are valid indications for primary surgical treatment.

Since most of these complications are life-threatening and usually require surgical intervention, good judgment must be exercised by the surgeon when choosing the laparoscopic approach. Laparoscopy is not recommended in unstable patients, such as those presenting with diffuse peritonitis and septic shock or life-threatening hemorrhage. Laparoscopic surgery is also contraindicated in patients who are considered at high risk for anesthetic complications and need an operation that can be done as quickly and as simply as possible.[2–4] Nevertheless, some complications, such as perforated duodenal ulcers with chemical peritonitis, gastric outlet obstruction, recurrences, and moderate bleeding, can be addressed laparoscopically.

Laparoscopic Treatment of Gastric Outlet Obstruction

Two laparoscopic surgical options have been described: (1) laparoscopic total truncal vagotomy and gastrojejunostomy, and (2) laparoscopic total truncal vagotomy and antrectomy with a Billroth II reconstruction.

The first operation is simpler and is known to have a lower morbidity and mortality in open surgery. It is, however, associated with a higher recurrence rate and is probably physiologically less satisfying when the stomach is chronically distended, because in such patients an element of gastric atony can contribute to poor gastric emptying.

Laparoscopic vagotomy and antrectomy, on the other hand, is a more radical approach; it not only denervates the stomach but also removes the gastrin-secreting part of the stomach and the non-functional antrum and probably speeds gastric emptying. This is a more technically challenging procedure and should be reserved for the experienced surgeon with advanced laparoscopic skills. The procedure can be performed either intra-abdominally or in a laparoscopically-assisted fashion, which may decrease the morbidity rate.

LAPAROSCOPIC TOTAL TRUNCAL VAGOTOMY

The patient is placed in a supine position with the legs spread apart (a modified dorsal lithotomy position). The surgeon stands between the patient's legs in the so-called French position. The monitor should be placed in front of the surgeon so that he may operate comfortably with two hands.

Pneumoperitoneum is created by insufflation of carbon dioxide at a pressure of 14 mm Hg. Five trocars are then introduced into the upper part of the abdomen. The introduction of the trocars is very important because a misplaced trocar renders the procedure very difficult to perform. Trocar positioning is the same as for any laparoscopic foregut operation except that the video laparoscope is inserted at the level of the umbilicus in order to gain good access not only to the hiatus, but also to the different parts of the stomach. Mobilization of the greater curvature is more easily accomplished if the laparoscope is located at the level of the umbilicus. Two trocars are inserted, one for the right hand of the surgeon for the operating instruments, and the second for the left hand of the surgeon to hold the grasping forceps (assuming the surgeon is right-handed). These two trocars are triangulated with the umbilical video laparoscope. Then the next trocar is placed for the grasping forceps of the first assistant, and finally the last trocar is the xiphoid trocar, inserted at the left side of the falciform ligament for retraction of the left lobe of the liver, as in a laparoscopic antireflux procedure (Fig. 20–1). This retraction can be performed with an irrigation suction device that can serve both purposes: irrigation of the hiatus and gentle retraction of the left lobe (American Hydrosurgical Instruments, Inc.). Upon entering the abdomen, a thorough exploration of the peritoneal cavity is undertaken to exclude intra-abdominal lesions that might have been missed by the preoperative work-up. The liver is then retracted and the procedure is begun.[5,6]

Access to the hiatus is straightforward with recognition of the following landmarks: The avascular aspect of the lesser sac, the caudate lobe, and the right crus of the diaphragm. The avascular aspect of the lesser sac is opened using electric scissors to allow recognition of the caudate lobe and the right crus of the diaphragm. A gastric vein may be encountered in the upper part of the lesser omentum; if so, it should be divided between clips. A meticulous dissection will prevent bleeding, minimizing trauma and blood loss and allowing easier identification of anatomic structures. The right crus is then grasped with the left hand while the patient is placed in a reverse Trendelenburg position. This allows the stomach and the greater omentum to move inferiorly in the abdominal cavity, providing greater access to the hiatus, even in obese patients.

The avascular plane between the esophagus and the right crus is entered, and care should be taken not to dissect within the fibers of the esophagus. The right trunk is usually recognized easily because it lies on the left crus near the junction of the right and left crural fibers (Fig. 20–2). The right vagus nerve is divided between clips, and a portion can be sent for pathologic evaluation. Although it is a rare finding, a second right vagal trunk may be present. The phrenoesophageal membrane is then divided, allowing division of all small branches of the left vagal trunk.

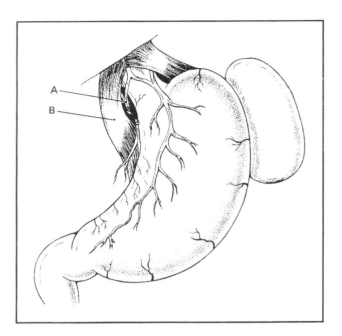

Figure 20–2. Posterior vagotomy. **A.** Right vagus nerve. **B.** Right diaphragmatic crus.

The fat pad is removed, allowing identification of the inconstant left trunk of the vagus nerve. At this point, dissection behind the esophagus and under the left crus allows identification of other branches of the vagus nerve (e.g., criminal nerve of Grassi). Division of these nerves and the nerve trunks completes the bilateral truncal vagotomy. At the end of this step, the esophagus is cleared of all the fatty tissues and the nerve fibers, using a hook dissector coagulator if necessary.

The harmonic scalpel (Ethicon Endosurgery, Cincinnati, OH) and/or scissors greatly facilitates this dissection by dividing tissue and providing hemostasis in one step with minimal trauma to the surrounding tissue. This instrument has an oscillating blade that moves at 55,000 cycles per second, producing heat and coagulation of small vessels, thereby reducing the number of clips required during this step of the procedure. This instrument can also serve as an atraumatic grasper.

LAPAROSCOPIC GASTROJEJUNOSTOMY

This procedure is straightforward; only a minor dissection of the gastric pouch is required. The key to performing an efficient gastrojejunostomy is positioning the anastomosis on the posterior aspect of the stomach about 8 cm proximal to the pylorus. Mobilization of the greater curvature of the stomach begins at the level of the entrance of the left gastric gastroepiploic artery in the gastrocolic ligament. It is not necessary to divide the gastroepiploic artery because dissection can be performed distal to the gastroepiploic arcade, thereby preserving it. The gastrocolic ligament is then opened using electrical scissors, and again the harmonic scissors may allow a safe and fast dissection of this plane. Superior retraction of the stomach allows exposure of the posterior aspect of the stomach. Division of any adhesions between the stomach and the anterior surface of the body of the pancreas allows better mobilization of the gastric pouch.

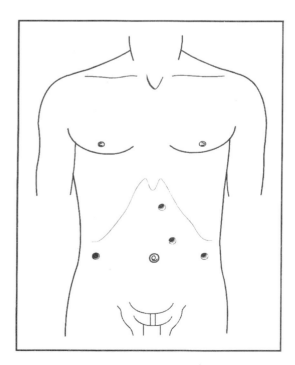

Figure 20–1. Trocar position for total truncal vagotomy.

The portion of jejunum to be used for the gastrojejunostomy is then chosen; this step is easily done with the surgeon standing on the patient's right side. Tilting the patient into a Trendelenburg position facilitates exposure of the small bowel. The jejunum is identified by following the small bowel toward the angle of Treitz, which can be recognized by its tension and attachment to the transverse mesocolon. It is important at this point not to exert too much traction on the angle of Treitz because a mesenteric tear could result. In this event, the tear may be repaired using intracorporeal suturing techniques and 3-0 polypropylene threaded on a SH needle. When the second jejunal loop is identified, it is mobilized and approximated to the stomach using two Babcock clamps. At this point the left lateral trocar is removed and replaced by an 18-mm trocar, which allows an endolinear cutter (ELC) 60 or 35 (Ethicon Endosurgery, Cincinnati, OH) to be introduced with the tip of the cutter pointing toward the liver. A 35 cutter is smaller and may be easier to manipulate. A gastrotomy and enterotomy are then performed, the stapler is introduced, and two shots of the ELC 35 or one shot of the ELC 60 is fired, creating a side-to-side communication between stomach and jejunum (Fig. 20–3). The lumen of the anastomosis must be checked carefully for hemostasis, and one suture is placed at the end of the staple line, as in open surgery, to prevent tension. This stitch is placed intracorporeally using nylon. Finally, the two enterotomies are closed, using either two more triangulated firings of the ELC 35 or, even simpler, a running suture of 3-0 polypropylene with intracorporeal ties. The operation is then completed by carefully introducing a nasogastric tube in the efferent loop of the jejunum, enabling decompression of the efferent loop in the immediate postoperative period. This nasogastric tube is removed the following day.

The postoperative management is straightforward. The diet should not be resumed immediately postoperatively because gastric atony complicated by stasis may occur in the presence of a chronic gastric outlet obstruction. The patient is usually fed on the third day after a gastrograffin swallow shows the integrity of the anastomosis and emptying of the stomach.

DISTAL GASTRECTOMY OR ANTRECTOMY

The first step is opening of the gastrocolic ligament inferior to the right gastroepiploic vessel as previously described for the gastrojejunostomy. The harmonic scissors are ideal for this, but clips can be used to secure any large vessels. This mobilization allows anterior retraction of the stomach using Babcock clamps, which exposes the duodenum in its posterior aspect. The posterior aspect of the first portion of the duodenum is carefully dissected, as in open surgery, using an atraumatic right-angle dissector. At this point, it is usually necessary to ligate the right gastroepiploic vessel near its origin at the gastroduodenal artery. The upper limit of the duodenum is dissected and the right gastric artery is identified and ligated between two clips to secure hemostasis. The next step is the transection and closure of the duodenum using an endolinear cutter 60. Once the stapler has been fired, the line of sutures is inspected, and hemostasis is confirmed. This maneuver allows exposure and retraction of the distal part of the antrum with one grasper, and dissection along the lesser curve using the harmonic scissors or the clip-applier as needed. The 30° telescope is essential for visualization of the posterior aspect of the stomach and the lesser sac. Any large vessel encountered is dissected and cut between two clips. From this point the anastomosis can be completed using an intra-abdominal or extra-abdominal method.

The intra-abdominal technique involves firing the ELC 60 between the stomach and the jejunum, which allows creation of a Billroth II gastrojejunostomy. The specimen can then be resected with several shots of the ELC 60 with green staples, which are specifically for thicker tissue such as the stomach (Fig. 20–4). Another possibility is to first resect the specimen and use the staple

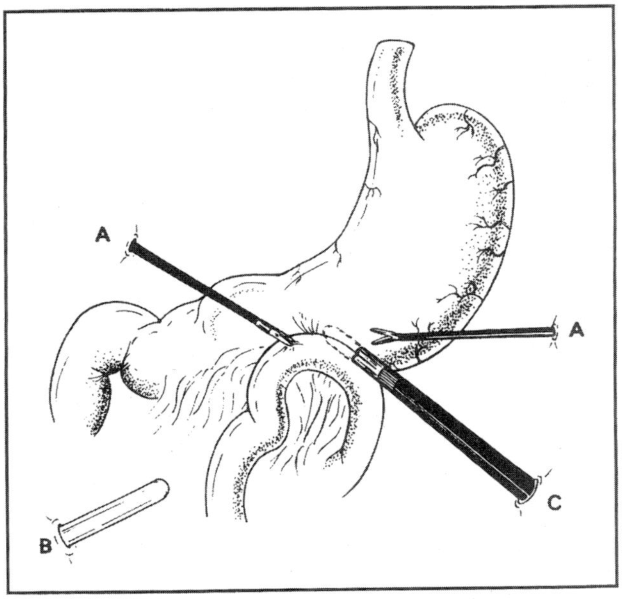

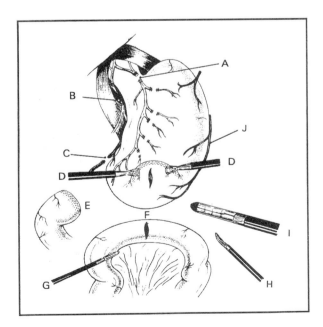

Figure 20–3. Laparoscopic gastrojejunostomy. **A.** Traction clamps. **B.** Laparoscope. **C.** Endoscopic stapler.

Figure 20–4. Laparoscopic bilateral vagotomy with antrectomy. **A.** Left vagotomy. **B.** Right vagotomy. **C.** Left gastric artery. **D.** 10-mm Babcock grasper. **E.** Duodenal stump. **F.** Jejunum. **G.** 5-mm Dissector. **H.** 5-mm Scissors. **I.** Stapler. **J.** Right gastroepiploic artery.

line to introduce the cutter between the jejunum and the posterior aspect of the stomach (Fig. 20–5). The enterotomies and the gastrotomies are then closed with running sutures.

The extra-abdominal technique consists of a lap-aroscopically assisted antrectomy and a small abdominal incision (4 cm). The stomach and jejunum are exteriorized, permitting completion of the resection and anastomosis outside the abdomen. This technique is probably quicker, easier, and safer and can be performed by most surgeons. This method is therefore recommended in order to minimize the length of the operation. No drains are needed after vigorous irrigation of the abdomen, and care should be taken to close all fascial defects to prevent hernias at the trocar sites.

TREATMENT OF HEMORRHAGIC PEPTIC ULCERS

When upper gastrointestinal bleeding is due to a visibly bleeding gastroduodenal artery, the choice of laparoscopic treatment remains controversial. Except in the hands of a few experts, laparoscopic application of laser energy, electrocautery, or even clips is not ideal because there is a significant risk of recurrent bleeding. A definitive and reliable option is open surgical treatment using the Weinberg procedure. This consists of opening the duodenum, suturing the bleeder, closing the duodenum, and then performing a truncal vagotomy if the patient's condition will tolerate the extra time needed for this procedure.

This procedure may be possible laparoscopically (Fig. 20–6), but usually the patient is not hemodynamically stable enough for a lengthy laparoscopic procedure, and the open approach is preferable in most cases. If the patient is hemodynamically stable, the procedure can be attempted laparoscopically. The principles of obtaining hemostasis are identical to those for open surgery for a bleeding peptic ulcer.

The laparoscopic endo-organ concept has not yet gained wide acceptance, but it could prove to be of great use in the future for the control of bleeding duodenal ulcers. The laparoscope is inserted into the abdomen with simultaneous introduction of trocars into the gastric pouch. A grasper can then be advanced into the stomach itself to isolate and control the bleeding vessel with the assistance of pyloric dilation. Definitive hemostasis could then be achieved using a specially-devised clip, an intragastric suture, or even an external suture placed through the wall of the duodenum, incorporating the bleeding vessel. The concept of endo-organ surgery is still experimental but is currently in development.

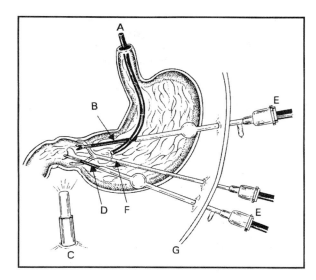

Figure 20–6. Laparoscopic endo-organ repair of a hemorrhagic peptic ulcer. **A.** Gastroscope. **B.** Dissector. **C.** Laparoscope. **D.** Sutures. **E.** Percutaneous balloons. **F.** Apparatus used for dissection of the pylorus. **G.** Abdominal wall.

REFERENCES

1. Bardhan KD, Cust G, Hinchiffle RC, et al. Changing patterns of admission and operations for duodenal ulcer. *Br J Surg.* 1989;76:230.
2. Katkhouda N, Mouiel J. A new technique of treatment of chronic duodenal ulcer without laparotomy by videocoelioscopy. *Am J Surg.* 1991;161:361.
3. Katkhouda N, Mouiel J. Laparoscopic treatment of peptic ulcer disease. In: Hunter JG, Sackier JM, eds. *Minimally Invasive Surgery.* McGraw Hill:1993;123.
4. Katkhouda N, Mouiel J. Laparoscopic treatment of peritonitis. In: Zucker K, ed. *Surgical Laparoscopy Update.* Quality Medical Publishers:1993;287.
5. McDermott EWM, Murphy JJ. Laparoscopic truncal vagotomy without drainage. *Br J Surg.* 1993;90:236.
6. Pringle R, Inweing AD, Longrigg JN, et al. Randomized trial of truncal vagotomy with either pyloroplasty or pyloric dilatation in the surgical management of chronic duodenal ulcer. *Br J Surg.* 1983;70:482.

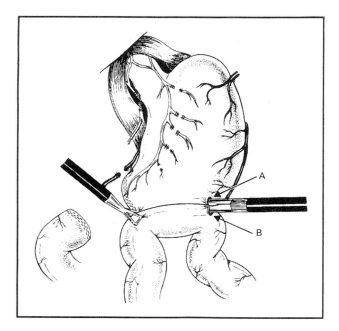

Figure 20–5. Variation on the procedure shown in Figure 20–4. **A.** Gastrotomy. **B.** Enterotomy.

Chapter Twenty-One ■ ■ ■ ■ ■ ■ ■

*T*he Laparoscopic Treatment of a Perforated Peptic Ulcer

JORGE CUETO-GARCÍA and JOSÉ ANTONIO VÁZQUEZ-FRIAS

INTRODUCTION

The first report of a perforated peptic ulcer was documented in the year 167 BC.[1] Though there are some reports of nonsurgical management of this entity,[2–4] the treatment is essentially surgical. The sooner the diagnosis is made, preoperative resuscitation achieved, and the surgical treatment performed, the better the prognosis. A delayed diagnosis might carry a mortality of 90% or greater as opposed to 0 to 10% with early treatment.[5]

DIAGNOSIS

In most cases the diagnosis is made based on clinical and roentgenographic findings. Symptoms and signs of perforated peptic ulcer have been extensively described in the medical and surgical literature. The diagnosis may be confirmed in the x-ray department by insufflating air into the stomach through a nasogastric tube or by swallowing a water-soluble contrast medium.

As pointed out elsewhere in this volume, in patients with an acute abdomen with uncertain diagnosis, laparoscopy is a very valuable diagnostic tool, and in some cases the treatment can be carried out at the same time.[5–8] Differential diagnosis should be made with acute cholecystitis, pancreatitis, bowel obstruction, dissecting aortic aneurysm, acute appendicitis, and acute diverticular disease.[9,10] It should be kept in mind that 5 to 20% of patients have no previous peptic ulcer history and that elderly people and patients that have received steroids, analgesics, or broad-spectrum antibiotics may present with atypical signs and symptoms that obscure the diagnosis. In this group of elderly or debilitated patients, it is most important to establish the diagnosis and to proceed rapidly with the surgical treatment, both of which can be done at the same time with laparoscopic surgery.[11]

PREOPERATIVE TREATMENT

As soon as the patient arrives at the ER a prompt and thorough clinical evaluation must be done, nasogastric suction applied, emergency laboratory and imaging work-up done, fluid and electrolyte losses replaced, and the vascular volume and visceral perfusion monitored constantly with the use of a bladder catheter and a central venous line if needed. Broad-spectrum antibiotics must be given intravenously, and an anesthesiologist on duty in the operating room. Cardiopulmonary assessment is of great value, particularly in aged patients and those with concomitant diseases, before surgery is begun.

SURGICAL TREATMENT

Once the diagnosis is established and vigorous resuscitation has been achieved, the basic principles of surgical treatment are: closure of the perforation with an extensive, thorough abdominal irrigation and lavage, and drainage and/or debridement of septic foci if needed. When indicated and depending on the patient's condition, age, and duration and extent of the peritonitis, a definitive peptic ulcer laparoscopic procedure can be performed just as in conventional open surgery.[11–15] Repair of a perforated ulcer can be done by a simple suture,[16,17] with an omental (Graham) patch,[18–21] with fibrin glue,[22] by use of ligamentum teres[23,24] or falciform ligament,[25] or with oxidized cellulose sponge,[26] among other methods. Combined laparoscopic and endoscopic procedures have also been used in which the endoscopist introduces a grasping instrument through the perforation, and once in the peritoneal cavity, the omentum is delivered, grasped, and pulled into the lumen of the gastrointestinal tract and fixed.[1,27] In France in 1990 Mouret et al[18] reported the first successful laparoscopic treatment of a perforated peptic ulcer. Since then, large series of patients treated successfully with mini-invasive surgery have been reported.[28–36]

SURGICAL TECHNIQUE

Pneumoperitoneum is established via the umbilicus as in any other mini-invasive procedure, and maintained at 15 mm Hg during port insertion (Fig. 21–1), after which it may be lowered to 10 mm Hg. When abdominal distention is a problem, a semi-open or open technique using a Hasson trocar is used in order to avoid damage to the abdominal contents. A complete exploration of the peritoneal cavity is made to rule out other pathology. Usually a Graham omentopexy is performed in a fashion similar to the conventional technique once the perforation is found. Nonabsorbable monofilament 00 or 000 suture material is recommended since some gastrointestinal secretions can digest absorbable suture. When suturing the perforation one must avoid undue tension in the already inflamed and damaged borders of the ulcer. Intra- or extracorporeal knots can be used, the latter being the preference of the authors.

Once the perforation has been closed, thorough lavage of the entire abdominal cavity under direct vision using pressure-irrigation is performed. Here lies one of the greatest advantages of mini-invasive surgery: the opportunity to perform an extensive and careful lavage of the entire peritoneal cavity under direct vision.

When subphrenic abscesses are found, they can be completely aspirated, debrided, and drained. Closed-system semiflexible constant suction drains are placed in the abscess cavity and brought out through one of the trocar incisions.

As in open surgery, definitive treatment should be individualized, discussed with the patient and family if possible, and the anesthesiologist consulted, if the patient is stable, if there is evidence of chronic ulcer, if the perforation has occurred recently, and if the patient's condition allows. Management consists of some form of vagotomy with or without pyloroplasty. Recent studies have demonstrated that the mini-invasive approach does not increase surgical time and that postoperative pain is considerably less.[28–32] In this regard it must be mentioned that the harmonic scalpel has helped shorten surgical time in as many as 30% of our surgeries of this type, and has also made them safer. On the other hand, it is well known that as many as two thirds of patients that recover from the suture-patch procedure for perforated duodenal ulcer will relapse, and one half of these will eventually require a definitive operation.[37–40] However, when the pa-tient is unstable, aged, septic, or has a complicating or life-threatening condition, it is preferable to close the defect with an omental patch, drain any collections of fluid, perform lavage, and complete the procedure as soon and as safely as possible. A recent randomized controlled trial[41] revealed that *Helicobacter pylori* infection rates in patients with perforated duodenal ulcers exceed 80%, that eradication of the organism prevents ulcer recurrence in these patients, and that immediate acid-reducing surgery in the presence of generalized peritonitis is unnecessary because the remission rate after eradication of *H. pylori* is comparable to that achieved by immediate proximal gastric vagotomy during emergency laparotomy.

DISCUSSION

There are many recent reports of successful management of patients with perforated peptic ulcers by means of laparoscopy (Fig. 21–2), and it is apparent that urgent treatment via mini-invasive surgery is effective;[6,11,16,18–26,28,29,31,34] it also has acceptable morbidity and mortality rates compared with conventional surgery as reported by several studies (all but one randomized).[28,42–44] One of the most important advantages of the procedure is the ability to confirm the diagnosis and perform the operation at the same time.

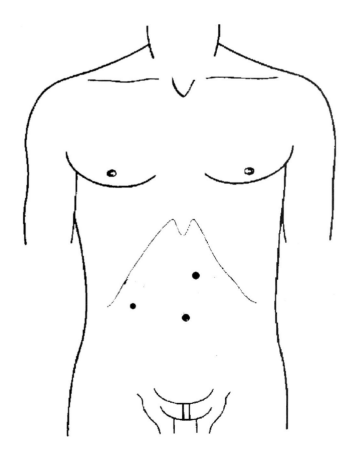

Figure 21–1. Trocar position for the treatment of perforated duodenal ulcer. One 5-mm and two 10-mm trocars are used.

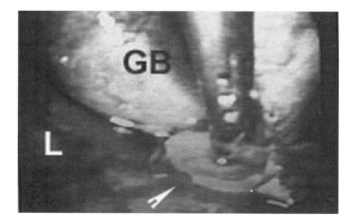

Figure 21–2. Perforated duodenal ulcer. Arrow is pointing to the perforated ulcer. GB, gallbladder, L liver.

In elderly patients and those with chronic lung disease or obesity, a long vertical incision can restrict breathing due to postoperative pain. This is minimal with the small incisions used in laparoscopic surgery, and pain is considerably diminished, thus there are few ventilatory problems postoperatively.[28,42–44] The same can be said about the ileus that complicates peritonitis; it is more prolonged in open surgery. There is objective evidence that bowel motility returns faster after mini-invasive surgery.[45,46]

One of the most frequent complications in open surgery in these patients is wound infection and dehiscence, particularly in elderly, debilitated, or malnourished patients; this is also much rarer with laparoscopy. It should also be mentioned that laparoscopy produces less immunosuppression and inflammatory response compared to open surgery, an important fact that could affect the outcome for some patients with sepsis.[47,48]

The disadvantages of mini-invasive surgery, such as prolonged surgical time, limited availability of equipment, higher cost, and the shortage of skillful laparoscopic teams, must be taken into account, but as with many other advanced laparoscopic procedures, these obstacles can and will be overcome, by adequate training and as surgeons gain experience with these procedures. Also, technological advances continue to be made in the field, and this will also alleviate some problems with mini-invasive surgery. The possibility that pneumoperitoneum may aggravate long-standing peritonitis is still controversial, and while some experimental findings support this theory,[49–51] other authors have found contrary results.[52–54] Further studies will be required to clarify this matter, but currently it does not appear to have any clinical significance.

REFERENCES

1. Lau WY, Leow CK. History of perforated duodenal and gastric ulcers. *World J Surg.* 1997;21:890.
2. Crofts TJ, Park KG, Steele RJ, et al. A randomized trial of nonoperative treatment for perforated peptic ulcer. *N Engl J Med.* 1989;320:970.
3. Cocks JR, Kernutt RH, Sinclair GW, et al. Perforated peptic ulcer: a deliberate approach. *Aust NZ J Surg.* 1989;59:379.
4. Cocks JR. Perforated peptic ulcer—the changing scene. *Dig Dis.* 1992;10:10.
5. Memon MA, Fitzgibbons RJ Jr. The role of minimal access surgery in the acute abdomen. *Surg Clin North Am.* 1997;77:1333.
6. Cueto J, Diaz O, Garteiz D, et al. The efficacy of laparoscopic surgery in the diagnosis and treatment of peritonitis. Experience with 107 cases in Mexico City. *Surg Endosc.* 1997;11:366.
7. Chung RS, Diaz JJ, Chari V. Efficacy of routine laparoscopy for the acute abdomen. *Surg Endosc.* 1998;12:219.
8. Salky BA, Edye MB. The role of laparoscopy in the diagnosis and treatment of abdominal pain syndromes. *Surg Endosc.* 1998;12:911.
9. De Dombal FT. Perforated peptic ulcer and acute pancreatitis. In: De Dombal FT. *Diagnosis of Acute Abdominal Pain,* 1st ed. Churchill-Livingstone:1980.
10. Cope Z. Perforation of a gastric or duodenal ulcer, and acute pancreatitis. In: Cope Z, ed. *The Early Diagnosis of the Acute Abdomen,* 14th ed. Oxford University Press:1972;79.
11. Cueto GJ, Weber AS, Serrano BF. Laparoscopic treatment of perforated duodenal ulcer. *Surg Laparosc Endosc.* 1993;3:216.
12. Casas AT, Gadacz TR. Laparoscopic management of peptic ulcer disease. *Surg Clin North Am.* 1996;76:515.
13. Katkhouda N, Offerman S, Waldrup D, et al. Tratamiento quirúrgico de la enfermedad ulcerosa péptica. In: Cueto J, Weber A, eds. *Cirugía Laparoscópica,* 2nd ed. McGraw Hill Interamericana:1997;97.
14. Uyama I, Ogiwara H, Takahara T, et al. Laparoscopic Billroth I gastrectomy for gastric ulcer: Technique and case report. *Surg Laparosc Endosc.* 1995;5:209.
15. Goh P, Tekant Y, Isaac J, et al. The technique of laparoscopic Billroth II gastrectomy. *Surg Laparosc Endosc.* 1992;2:258.
16. Memon MA, Brow G. Laparoscopic closure of acutely perforated duodenal ulcer—an early experience. *Br Med J.* 1993;86:106.
17. Perissat J, Collet D, Edye M. Therapeutic laparoscopy. *Endoscopy* 1992;24:138.
18. Mouret P, Francois Y, Vignal J, et al. Laparoscopic treatment of perforated peptic ulcer. *Br J Surg.* 1990;77:1006.
19. Kavic MS. Laparoscopic repair of ruptured duodenal peptic ulcer: a case report. *J Laparoendosc Surg* 1993;3:41.
20. Oshima I, Ozaki M, Ariga T, et al. A case of perforated duodenal ulcer treated with laparoscopic closure and anchoring omentum. Asian Pacific Congress of Endoscopic Surgery. "Minimally Invasive Surgery—2000." Singapore, August 3, 1993.
21. Arillaga A, Sosa JL, Najjar R. Laparoscopic patching of crack cocaine-induced perforated ulcers. *Am Surg.* 1996;62:1007.
22. Takeuchi A, Kawano T, Toda T, et al. Laparoscopic repair for perforation of duodenal ulcer with omental patch: report of initial 6 cases. *Surg Laparosc Endosc.* 1998;8:153.
23. Costalat G, Alquier Y. Combined laparoscopic and endoscopic treatment of perforated gastroduodenal ulcer using the ligamentum teres hepatis (LTH). *Surg Endosc.* 1995;9:677.
24. Costalat G, Dravet F, Noel P, et al. Coelioscopic treatment of perforated gastroduodenal ulcer using the ligamentum teres hepatis. *Surg Endosc.* 1991;5:154.
25. Munro WS, Bajwa F, Menzies D. Laparoscopic repair of perforated duodenal ulcers with a falciform ligament patch. *Ann Roy Coll Surg Engl.* 1996;78:390.
26. Tate JJ, Dawson JW, Lau WY, et al. Sutureless laparoscopic treatment of perforated duodenal ulcer. *Br J Surg.* 1993;80:235.
27. Branicki FJ, Nathanson LK. Minimal access gastroduodenal surgery. *Aust NZ J Surg.* 1994;64:589.
28. Lau WY, Leung KL, Zhu XL, et al. Laparoscopic repair of perforated peptic ulcer. *Br J Surg.* 1995;82:814.
29. Matsuda M, Nishiyama M, Harai T, et al. Laparoscopic omental patch repair for perforated peptic ulcer. *Ann Surg.* 1995;221:236.
30. Thompson AR, Hall TJ, Anglin BA, et al. Laparoscopic application of perforated ulcer: results of a selective approach. *South Med J.* 1995;88:185.
31. Champault GG. Laparoscopic treatment of perforated peptic ulcer. *Endosc Surg Allied Technol.* 1994;2:117.
32. Robertson GS, Wemyss-Holden SA, Maddern GJ. Laparoscopic repair of perforated peptic ulcers. The role of laparoscopy in generalised peritonitis. *Ann Roy Coll Surg Engl.* 2000;82:6.
33. Khoursheed M, Fuad M, Safar H, et al. Laparoscopic closure of perforated duodenal ulcer. *Surg Endosc.* 2000;14:56.
34. Druart ML, Van Hee R, Etienne J, et al. Laparoscopic repair of perforated duodenal ulcer. A prospective multicenter trial. *Surg Endosc* 1997;11:1017.
35. Katkhouda N, Mavor E, Mason RJ, et al. Laparoscopic repair of perforated duodenal ulcers: outcome and efficacy in 30 consecutive patients. *Arch Surg.* 1999;134:845.
36. Naesgaard JM, Edwin B, Reiertsen O, et al. Laparoscopic and open operation in patients with perforated peptic ulcer. *Eur J Surg.* 1999;65:209.
37. Chassin JL. Perforated peptic ulcer. In: Chassin JL, ed. *Operative Strategy in General Surgery,* 2nd ed. Springer-Verlag:1994;228.
38. Griffin GE, Organ CH. The natural history of the perforated duodenal ulcer treated by suture plication. *Ann Surg.* 1976;183:382.
39. Drury JK, McKay AJ, Hutchinson JS, et al. Natural history of perforated duodenal ulcers treated by suture closure. *Lancet* 1978;2:749.
40. Boey J, Wong J. Perforated duodenal ulcers. *World J Surg.* 1987; 11:319.

41. Enders KW, Lam YH, Joseph JY, et al. Eradication of *Helicobacter pylori* prevents recurrence of ulcer after simple closure of duodenal ulcer perforation. *Ann Surg.* 2000;231:153.

42. So JB, Kum CK, Fernandes ML, et al. Comparison between laparoscopic and conventional omental patch repair for perforated duodenal ulcer. *Surg Endosc.* 1996;10:1060.

43. Miserez E, Eypasch E, Spangenberger W, et al. Laparoscopic and conventional closure of perforated peptic ulcer. A comparison. *Surg Endosc.* 1996;10:831.

44. Lau WY, Leung KL, Kwong KH, et al. A randomized study comparing laparoscopic versus open repair of perforated peptic ulcer using suture or sutureless technique. *Ann Surg.* 1996;224:131.

45. Tittel A, Schippers E, Anurou M, et al. Minor abdominal trauma by laparoscopic surgery? Comparison of adhesion formation and intestinal motility after laparoscopic and conventional operations in the dog. *Zentralbl Chir.* 1996;121:329.

46. Bohm B, Milsom JW, Fazio VW. Postoperative intestinal motility following conventional and laparoscopic intestinal surgery. *Arch Surg.* 1995;130:415.

47. Vittimberga FJ Jr., Foley DP, Meyers WC, et al. Laparoscopic surgery and the systemic immune response. *Ann Surg.* 1998;227:326.

48. Jacobi CA, Ordemann J, Zieren HU, et al. Increased systemic inflammation after laparotomy vs laparoscopy in an animal model of peritonitis. *Arch Surg.* 1998;133:258.

49. Bloechle C, Emmermann A, Zornig C. Effect of carbon dioxide pneumoperitoneum on bacteraemia and endotoxaemia in an animal model of peritonitis (letter). *Br J Surg.* 1995;82:1702.

50. Bloechle C, Emmermann A, Strate T, et al. Laparoscopic vs open repair of gastric perforation and abdominal lavage of associated peritonitis in pigs. *Surg Endosc.* 1998;12:212.

51. Ozman MM, Col C, Askoy AM, et al. Effect of CO_2 on bacteremia and bacterial translocation in an animal model of peritonitis. *Surg Endosc.* 1999;13:801.

52. Benoit S, Cruaud P, Lauroy J, et al. Does laparoscopic treatment of abdominal infections generate bacteremia? Prospective study: 75 patients. *J Chir.* 1995;132:472.

53. Jacobi Ordemann J, Bohm B, et al. Does laparoscopy increase bacteremia and endotoxemia in a peritonitis model? *Surg Endosc.* 1997;11:235.

54. Balague C, Targarona EM, Pujol M, et al. Peritoneal response to a septic challenge. Comparison between open laparotomy, pneumo-peritoneum laparoscopy, and wall lift laparoscopy. *Surg Endosc.* 1999;13:792.

Chapter Twenty-Two • • • • • • •

Anterior Lineal Gastrotomy with Posterior Truncal Vagotomy

FERNANDO GÓMEZ-FERRER BAYO, J.G. BALIQUE, S. AZAGRA,
I.N. BICHA-CASTELO, F. CASTRO-SOUSA, P. ESPALIEU, D. RODERO,
and E. ESTOUR

Between January 1991 and February 1995 data were gathered on 136 patients operated on in 14 surgical centers. All patients underwent posterior truncal vagotomy (PTV) and anterior linear gastrectomy (ALG) for chronic duodenal ulcer. Recurrence and repeated bleeding were the main indications for surgery. An antireflux procedure was simulta-neously carried out in 17 patients, and 13 underwent cholecystectomy. There were no preoperative complications or deaths, and the mean duration of operation was 65 minutes (range, 25 to 180 min) and the immediate postoperative morbidity rate was 2 to 9% with a mean hospital stay of 3.1 (range 2-13) days. A total of 131 patients were evaluated between 6 and 33 (mean 25) months after operation. Of these, 126 (96.2%) were graded as Visick I or II, 4 (3.9%) were Visick III, and 1 patient (0.8%) was considered Visick IV. Gastric function studies were performed in 45 patients before and after operation, with a maximum acid output reduction of 83% 3 months after the operation. Laparoscopic PTV with ALG is a simple, efficient, rapid, and safe method of treating patients with chronic duodenal ulcer.

The efficacy of laparoscopic surgery in the treatment of chronic duodenal ulcer has been demonstrated in the short and medium term by a number of authors employing different methods. Conventional techniques have been applied using minimally invasive approaches, including transthoracic truncal vagotomy;[1] transabdominal truncal vagotomy[2] alone or in association with pneumatic dilatation of the pylorus, pyloromyotomy or pyloroplasty; truncal vagotomy and antrectomy; anterior and posterior supraselective vagotomy;[3] posterior truncal vagotomy (PTV) and supraselective anterior vagotomy, PTV, and anterior seromyotomy;[4–6] and PTV with anterior linear gastrectomy (ALG).[7–9]

Based on the hypothesis that gastrostomy with eversion sutures would be more effective than seromyotomy, in 1986 Gómez-Ferrer et al[10–12] began removing a fold of the anterior wall of the stomach in close proximity to the lesser curve, using a mechanical stapler. This technique was called anterior linear gastrectomy (ALG). This procedure was in turn supported by the results obtained in two experimental studies,[13,14] and a recent report from Belgium confirms the value of the techniques at open operation.[19]

The aim of the present study was to report early results in 136 patients with chronic duodenal ulcer subjected to PTV and ALG. The limited number of patients involved ruled out a prospective randomized study.

PATIENTS AND METHODS

A simple protocol was issued to all participating centers, comprising the measures described below.

A total of 236 patients (111 men) from 14 surgical centers were studied. Mean age was 48.1 (range, 23 to 69) years. The mean duration of disease was 9.5 (range, 3 to 19) years. Associated pathology in the form of gastroesophageal and biliary reflux was observed in 17 and 13 patients, respectively. Sixty-five patients had suffered one of more episodes of bleeding in the past. The remainder failed to respond to or comply with medication.

PREOPERATIVE EVALUATION

Eighty patients underwent gastroduodenal transit evaluation. Eighty-six patients were subject to esophagogastroduodenal endoscopy to confirm the diagnosis of duodenal ulcer and exclude pyloric stenosis, gastric ulcer, gastro-esophageal reflux, esophagitis, and/or hiatal hernia. All patients consulted the surgical services directly, and as a result no routine evaluation or treatment of possible *Helicobacter pylori* infection was carried out from 1991 to 1993. Possible *H. pylori* infection was evaluated by biopsy whenever it was performed. H$_1$ blockers, omeprazole, and amoxicillin were administered when *H. pylori* was found.

Hepatobiliopancreatic echography was performed in 35 patients, and basal acid output (BAO), maximum acid output (MAO), and peak acid output (PAO) were determined along with gastrinemia in 57. Esophageal manometry was carried out in 14 patients, and esophageal pH monitoring in 13.

Smokers were required to have ceased tobacco consumption entirely, with no oral intake of food for 8 hours before surgery. Sodium cephamycin (single dose of 1 g) was given for antibiotic coverage 1 hour before operation.

SURGICAL TECHNIQUE

Under general anesthesia, the patient is positioned lying face up with the legs separated (20° anti-Trendelenburg position). The surgeon stands between the open legs. The first assistant stands to the left of the patient, with the second to the right.

Five trocars are required for the same number of ports, their uses varying according to the surgical stage (detailed below): supraumbilical (12-mm optics), below the right costal margin (10 mm, liver fan retractor), below the left costal margin (5 mm, grasping forceps), midpoint between the supraumbilical and left ribcage ports (15 mm, scissors, hook, endoclip, stapler), and subxiphoid (5 mm, grasping forceps, irrigation, aspiration) (Fig. 22–1).

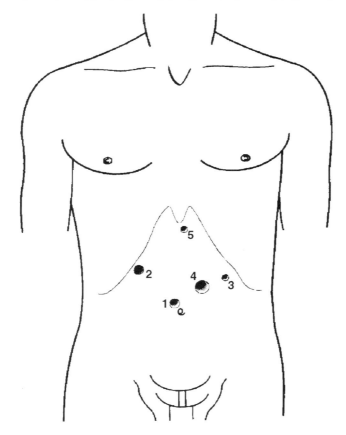

Figure 22–1. Ports used for positioning cannulas: 1. Supraumbilical (12 mm); 2. Below right costal margin (10 mm); 3. Below left costal margin (5 mm); 4. Midpoint between supraumbilical and left costal port (15 mm); and 5. Subxiphoid port (5 mm).

Posterior Truncal Vagotomy

After inspecting the entire abdominal cavity, the liver retractor is introduced through the right subcostal port. The first assistant holds the laparoscope with the left hand (umbilical port) and pulls slightly on the stomach to the left to move the lesser omentum away from the left subcostal port.

The surgeon manipulates forceps through the sub-xiphoid port with the left hand, and coagulating scissors through the left transrectal port with the right hand.

The lesser omentum is sectioned together with the phrenoesophageal membrane, preserving the nerves. The right diaphragmatic crus is identified and separated from the esophagus to the left. An intra-abdominal pressure of 13 to 14 mm Hg makes dissection easier. The posterior vagus nerve is identified, together with the Grassi criminal nerve (present in 9% of patients).[18] Whenever located, the celiac branch is always preserved. About 1 to 2 cm of the posterior vagus nerve is removed and sent for histopathological study.

Anterior Linear Gastrectomy

The surgeon identifies the crow's foot and grasps it with the right hand through the left subcostal port using Babcock forceps. This is then held in the first assistant's right hand, while the second assistant pulls on the anterior wall of the stomach 1 to 2 cm from the cardia towards the diaphragm, through the subxiphoid port. A vertical fold is created as a result. A number of sutures may be placed through the abdominal wall to hold the gastric wall 1 to 5 cm from the lesser curve, thus contributing to forming the fold.

An Endo-GIA 30 stapler (Autosuture, Ascot, UK) is introduced through the port situated midway between the supraumbilical and left costal ports, and closed to include the first branch of the crow's foot. The instrument is then fired, until a closed gastric tube 1 to 1.5 cm in diameter is finally created. An Endo-GIA 60 is then introduced and fired two or three times until the cardia is reached. The fundus is freed and retracted, and the linear gastrectomy completed (avoiding displacement to the left) to the uppermost part of the fundus and beyond, 1 to 5 cm above the cardia. The surgeon holds the suture-section line open with the left hand and positions the stapler at the angle formed by the stapled lines. It is important to stay 1 to 1.5 cm away from the lesser curve and to pass 1 to 5 cm from the cardia, to avoid displacement towards the left side of the stomach (Figs. 22–2 and 22–3).

White vascular cartridges are used to improve hemostasis. Gastric sealing may be tested by introducing methylene blue through the nasogastric tube. The specimen is then removed and sent for histopathological study and a simple radiograph is taken to verify that all staples are correctly positioned. The aponeurotic flaps are closed with absorbable sutures, and the nasogastric tube is left in place for 24 hours. On the second day oral fluid intake is restarted.

This procedure was combined with laparoscopic cholecystectomy in 16 patients and with laparoscopic Nissen fundoplication in 12.

RESULTS

The mean duration of surgery was 65 min (range, 25 to 180) and the laparoscopic approach proved feasible in all patients. In all

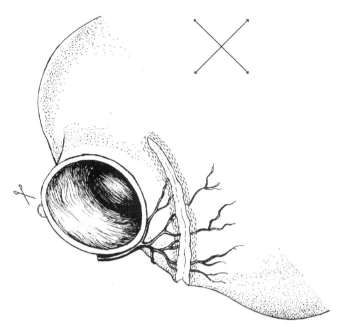

Figure 22–2. Oblique view of the stomach, showing the sectioned posterior vagus nerve. Traction sutures are positioned instead of grasping forceps for clarity. Gastric fundus displacement is also shown.

patients undergoing cholecystectomy, and in those subjected to the Nissen operation, the mean surgical time was prolonged by 25 and 40 min, respectively. No conversion to open surgery was required, and no serious preoperative complications occurred. Esophagogastric transit was evaluated in 128 patients, and no contrast leakage was recorded in any patient. In the immediate postoperative period the morbidity rate was 2 to 9% (one case each of atelectasis, thrombophlebitis, omphalitis, and parietal hematoma). The mortality rate was zero and the mean hospital stay was 3.1 (range, 2 to 13) days.

A total of 131 patients were evaluated at 25 months (mean 6.3). Of these, 126 (96.2%) were rated as Visick I or II, 4 (3.0%) as Visick III, and 1 patient (0.8%) as Visick IV, due to asymptomatic ulcer recurrence 4 months after surgery. pH studies were performed in 45 patients before and after surgery, with mean BAO and MAO reductions of 78% and 83% respectively, 3 months after the operation. Only 40 of the 86 patients subjected to preoperative endoscopy underwent repeat endoscopy 3 to 6 months after surgery (many refused postoperative endoscopy or gastric secretion tests) and, in all but one patient, ulcer healing was demonstrated. In this single patient, however, pain had disappeared and the condition was under medical control.

DISCUSSION

The efficacy of the medical treatment of duodenal ulcer has been clearly demonstrated. Omeprazole achieves healing in 90% of patients, although recurrences develop in 50 to 99% when medication is suspended.

Two decades ago most elective surgery in patients with duodenal ulcer was performed to provide relief from drug-resistant pain. Today, with the development of effective antisecretory and antibiotic agents, nonemergent indications for surgery are few, and include refractory ulcers and recurrences when medication is interrupted.

In 1986 Gómez-Ferrer believed that the surgical literature was lacking experimental studies on the possible nerve regeneration of the anterior gastric wall following seromyotomy of the lesser curve (Taylor's operation). As a result, his group used 28 rats (including 4 controls) to compare PTV with anterior seromyotomy (12 animals) and gastrotomy from the crow's foot to the uppermost part of the fundus, followed by eversion suturing (12 animals).[10,11] Both methods proved effective, although gastrotomy involved sectioning the two intramural gastric plexuses. Moreover, on extending section to the uppermost part of the fundus, the branches descending from the intramural esophageal plexuses were also divided. It was concluded that a fast and safe method for performing gastrotomy with eversion sutures would be to remove a fold from the anterior wall of the stomach, in close proximity to the lesser curve, using a mechanical stapler. Gómez-Ferrer called this

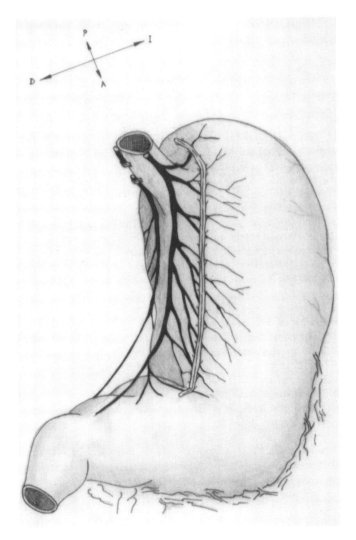

Figure 22–3. View of the stomach after resection of the anterior gastric wall. Note the medial displacement of the upper section trajectory, to avoid any mistaken displacement to the left that might leave the innervation partially intact.

procedure anterior linear gastrectomy (ALG),[7,11,16,18] and it has been applied in humans during conventional surgery since 1986.

With the aim of establishing the efficacy of the above technique, a second experimental study was carried out in 31 rats to evaluate the pH of gastric secretions on a weekly basis for 3 months after PTV and ALG. Gastric pH was found to be significantly higher after PTV with seromyotomy. Moreover, there was no wound infection, mortality, diarrhea, or gastric stasis, and all animals increased body weight normally.[12,13] With the availability of endo-staplers, PTV was performed with ALG in humans, via a laparoscopic approach.[7–9]

Conventional bilateral truncal vagotomy with pyloroplasty (0.5 to 0.9% mortality rate, 6 to 7% recurrence rate, 75 to 85% Visick I) entails major morbidity in 15% of patients undergoing conventional surgery.[17] In this sense, gastric emptying disorders due to antral hypomotility, absence of the third phase of the interdigestive motor complex with acceleration of the early phase of liquid emptying, and delayed emptying of solids (phytobezoars) are well-documented problems.[18] No extensive studies have been published on the results of laparoscopic surgery.

Supraselective vagotomy, when performed by means of open surgery, has a 0.1% mortality rate and offers good results in the immediate postoperative period. However, after 5 years the rate of recurrence reaches 17%, and increases to 27 to 30% after 10 years, depending on the surgeon's experience.[19] In addition, excellent experimental studies have demonstrated reinnervation after this type of surgery.[19,20] When performed laparoscopically, the procedure becomes tedious and time consuming, except when carried out by a highly expert surgeon, and its reproducibility is consequently low. Ischemic necrosis of the lesser curve occurs in 1% of patients, and Cadiere et al[21] have occasionally observed clip migration towards the stomach interior and had two cases of giant ischemic ulcers affecting the lesser curve. The technique reportedly may also damage Latarget's nerve, and dysphagia frequently results from the dissection of the last 6 cm of esophagus. Destruction of anatomic cardial retention mechanisms in turn leads to gastroesophageal reflux in 15% of patients, necessitating fundoplication, with its attendant risk of morbidity.[3,21]

PTV and anterior seromyotomy performed laparoscopically is a difficult and time-consuming operation that causes significant bleeding and is poorly reproducible, it carries a risk of preoperative or late perforation of the gastric mucosa, along with nerve regeneration if the sectioned seromuscular component is sutured. In the experimental setting ALG has been found to be more effective than seromyotomy. Despite the good results reported by Katkhouda and Mouiel,[6] a number of surgeons no longer perform this operation.[22,23]

PTV and ALG, as proposed in the present study, is a simple and rapid technique as dissection is limited to identifying the posterior vagus nerve, and this does not usually pose a problem. As is well known, Grassi's criminal nerve is present in a number of patients and it must be sought.[22] Before this, the crow's foot is identified, working 1 to 2 cm from the cardias and reaching the uppermost part of the fundus. The technique is safe, as the endostapler can achieve perfect sealing and hemostasis, and no problems have been encountered with leakage or bleeding. Moreover, there is no risk of subjecting the lesser curve to ischemia or of damaging Latarget's nerve. The results of the multicenter study, with 96.2% of patients scoring Visick I or II, were favorable. The

data are similar to those already published on seromyotomy and supraselective vagotomy.[3,6]

Finally, the method is easy to perform laparoscopically, as demonstrated by the fact that though it is costly, it is being adopted by a growing number of surgeons.[23,24] In any case, experience with a greater number of patients must be accumulated, with longer follow-up, to make a definitive evaluation.

In the authors' opinion, surgery for chronic duodenal ulcer should be performed laparoscopically. Bilateral truncal vagotomy with drainage and gastrectomy should be avoided as definitive procedures because they are associated with an unacceptably high incidence of side effects. Proximal gastric vagotomy and seromyotomy are limited by morbidity and surgeon experience, and both are difficult to perform laparoscopically. PTV and ALG constitute a good alternative, considering that recurrences are easier to manage than severe complications.

Acknowledgments. The following surgeons and institutions contributed patients to the study: Gómez-Ferrer: Hospital Clínico Universitario (Valencia, Spain), Clínica Quirón (Valencia, Spain), Hospital Erasmus (Brussels, Belgium), Hospital Severo Ochoa (Mostoles, Spain) (27 patients); Balique: Centro Hospitalaire Regional universitaire Bellevue (St. Etienne, France) (25 patients); Azagra: C.H.U. Vesale (Montigny-le-Tilleul, Belgium) (23 patients); Bicha-Castelo: Hospital Clínico Universitario (Lisbon, Portugal) (14 patients); Castro-Sousa: Hospital Universitario (Coimbra, Portugal) (12 patients); Espalieu: Clique de la Jomayére (St. Etienne, France) (9 patients); Rodero: Hospital La Fé (Valencia, Spain) (6 patients); Estour: Clique Saint Joseph (Valence, France) (6 patients); Múgica: Hospital San Eloy (Baracaldo, Spain) (5 patients); Ornelas: Hospital de Funchal (Madeira, Portugal) (5 patients); Sbih: Hospital Birtraria C.H.U. Ouest Lager (Algeria) (6 patients). Total: 136 patients.

REFERENCES

1. Dubois F. Laparoscopic vagotomy problems. *Gen Surg.* 1991;8:348.
2. Champault G, Belbassen N, Rink P, et al. Ulcere duodenal: interet la vagotomie tronculaire par thoracoscopic. *Ann Chir.* 1993;47:340.
3. Dallemagne B, Weerts JM, Jehuet C, et al. Laparoscopic highly selective vagotomy. *Br Surg.* 1994;81:554.
4. Taylor TV, MacLoed DA, Gunn A, et al. Anterior lesser curve seromyotomy and posterior truncal vagotomy in the treatment of chronic duodenal ulcer. *Lancet* 1982;2:846.
5. Mouiel J, Katkhouda N. Laparoscopic truncal and selective vagotomy. In: Zucker KA, Bailey RW, Reddick EJ, eds. *Surgical Laparoscopy.* Quality Medical Publishing:1991;263.
6. Katkhouda N, Mouiel J. A new technique of surgical treatment of chronic duodenal ulcer without laparotomy by videocelioscopy. *Am J Surg.* 1991;161:361.
7. Gómez-Ferrer F, Arenas J, Pardo J, et al. Gastrectomía lineal anterior mas vagotomía troncular posterior laparoscópica, nueva técnica para el tratamiento de la úlcera duodenal crónica. *Acta Chirurgica Catalonlae* 1992;13:117.
8. Gómez-Ferrer F. Gastrectomie linéaire antérieur et vagotomie tronculaire posterieur. *J Coelio-chirurgie.* 1992;4:35.
9. Gómez-Ferrer F. Ulcera duodenal crónica y cirugía: nueva técnica laparoscópica. *Cirugía Española* 1992;52:464.
10. Gómez-Ferrer F, Antón V, Liomburt A. Regeneración nerviosa en la pared anterior Del. estómago después de gastrotomía y vagotomía tron-

cular posterior en la rata. *Revista Española de Enfermedades Digestivas.* 1993;84:85.

11. Gómez-Ferrer F. Experimental study of vagal regeneration on the anterior gastric wall : seromyotomy versus gastrotomy and suture. *Br J Surg.* 1992;79(Suppl):S125 (Abstract).

12. Gómez-Ferrer F, María M, Antón V, et al. Gastrectomie linéaire antérieur, une alternative a la denervation gastrique antérieur otude expérimentale. *Lyon Chirurgical* 1992;88:359.

13. Gómez-Ferrer F. Minimal linear gastrectomy: a new experimental method to denervate the anterior gastric wall. *Br J Surg.* 1992;79(Suppl):S123 (Abstract).

14. Gómez-Ferrer F. Posterior truncal vagotomy and denervating anterior linear strip gastrectomy: a new laparoscopic technique for treating chronic duodenal ulcers. In: Stelchen FM, Welter R, eds. *Minimally Invasive Surgery.* Quality Medical Publications:1994;609.

15. van Ilee R, Mistaen W, Hendricks L, et al. Anterior gastric wall stapling combined with posterior truncal vagotomy in the treatment of duodenal ulcer. *Br J Surg.* 1995;82:934.

16. Pietri P, Alagni G. La vagotomia Oggi. Padova, Italy. *Piectri Ed.* 1975;37.

17. Fourtanier G. Traitement chirurgicale des ulcéres du duodenum et de l'estomac, simples et compliqués. In: *Editions Techniques—Encyclopédia Medico Chirurgicale.* Estomac Intestin:1990;9024A10,5.

18. Jtan R. Troubles de la vidange gastrique. *Presse Med.* 1992;21:1072.

19. Joffe SN, Crocket A, Doyle D. Morphologic and functional evidence of reinnervation of the gastric parietal cell mass after parietal cell vagotomy. *Am J Surg.* 1982;143:80.

20. Cuesta MA, Dominguez MD, Alonso MR, et al. Vagal regeneration after parietal cell vagotomy: an experimental study in dogs. *World J Surg.* 1987;11:94.

21. Cadiere GB, Bruyns H, Himpens J, et al. Vagotomie supraselective par coelioscopic. *J Coelio-chirurgie.* 1993;6:8.

22. Balique JG, Chabert M, Payan B, et al. Vagotomie tronculaire droite et gastrectomie linéaire entérieur pour ulcére duodénal: opération de Gómez-Ferrer. Technique et premiers résultats. *Lyon Chirurgical* 1993;89:5.

23. Azagra JS, Alle JL, Guergen M, et al. Seromyotomie fundique: once ans d'expérience. Une série Franco-Belge continue de 172 USA. *Lyon Chirurgical* 1994;90:165.

24. Estour E. Opération de Gómez-Ferrer. Technique. *J Coelio-Chirurgie.* 1994;12:38.

Chapter Twenty-Three ▪ ▪ ▪ ▪ ▪ ▪

Billroth II Laparoscopic Gastrectomy

PETER M. Y. GOH and AHMET ALPONAT

Laparoscopic gastric resection was originally an operation for the treatment of benign gastric ulcers.[1–3] With the widespread practice of *Helicobacter pylori* eradication for the management of peptic ulcer disease, which offers the patient the prospect of a permanent cure, the role of ulcer surgery has decreased dramatically.

The laparoscopic surgeon who is interested in stomach resections will now have to turn to resection for cancer or benign tumors of the stomach. As benign tumors of the stomach are rare, the focus is on surgery for cancer of the stomach.[4]

INDICATIONS FOR LAPAROSCOPIC INTERVENTION IN CANCER OF THE STOMACH

Laparoscopy has an important diagnostic role before radical gastrectomy for cancer of the stomach. A diagnostic laparoscopy affects the management in 15 to 20% of cases. Discovery of peritoneal, omental, or liver metastases that were missed on computed tomography (CT) scan can lead the surgeon to abandon a radical resection in favor of more conservative approaches or expectant management. It has never been shown that palliative resection actually benefits the patient in terms of length of survival. Only in patients who are actively bleeding or obstructed is a palliative resection ever beneficial.

Early gastric cancer provides the widest scope for the application of laparoscopic techniques. Small superficial lesions[5] can be excised intraluminally by endoscopic mucosal resection.[6] Types I to IIb can be resected by the Japanese wall lifting laparoscopic wedge resection technique.[7] In more difficult situations, such as near the cardia or the pylorus, transgastric surgery can be used.[8,9] Types IIc and III are lesions that require laparoscopic gastrectomy with a D1 lymph node dissection.[10,11,12] This also applies to early cancers with submucosal involvement.

More advanced lesions up to stage T3N1 are amenable to laparoscopic radical D2 gastrectomy and this will be the main topic of discussion in this chapter.

The indication for laparoscopic radical gastrectomy is tumors of Union International Contre de Cancer (UICC) stage T1N0M0 to stage T3N1M0. Preoperative staging is done by CT scan, endoscopic ultrasound, and diagnostic laparoscopy. It is imperative to have as much information as possible about the stage of the disease before embarking on laparoscopic surgery with intent to cure.

The patient should be fit for general anesthesia and medically able to withstand a major resection. A relatively thin patient is preferable as obesity does make the operation more difficult. Previous abdominal surgery may result in dense adhesions that will certainly make the procedure more difficult and time consuming. In this regard previous operations to the upper abdomen pose more of a problem than those in the lower abdomen.

The operation is quite feasible even after a previous laparoscopic cholecystectomy. Patients with tumors in the antrum or prepyloric region require a radical subtotal gastrectomy. Where the tumor is in the body, fundus, or cardia, a total radical gastrectomy with or without splenectomy is required.

PREOPERATIVE PREPARATION

Necessary investigations include an endoscopy and biopsy, CT scan, chest x-ray, electrocardiogram, complete blood count, electrolytes and creatinine, liver function tests, coagulation profile, and blood group and cross-match. In addition, we perform endoscopic ultrasound and diagnostic laparoscopy on all patients.

Patients with a history of heart or lung disease and those older than 55 years of age should have a lung function test, including spirometry and estimations of functional vital ca-pacity and FEV_1. In addition, these patients should have a comprehensive cardiac assessment, including exercise treadmill test and cardiac ultrasound. It is important to ensure that the time and effort put into performing a curative resection does not result in patient demise from cardiac or lung complications.

All patients should have a week of high-protein and high-calorie enteric nutrition, as well as preoperative chest physiotherapy, prior to surgery. Patients should receive bowel preparation the night before the operation to empty the colon in case colonic or vascular involvement makes colonic resection necessary. Antibiotics covering a wide spectrum of aerobic and anaerobic bacteria are started the morning of the surgery. If the patient has any gastric outlet obstruction, the stomach is emptied by nasogastric tube at this time.

OPERATING ROOM SETUP

The operation is done under general anesthesia with the patient intubated and paralyzed. Use of nitric oxide is discouraged as this may cause bowel distension. The patient is fitted with a nasogastric tube and urinary catheter.

Positioning of the patient (Fig. 23–1) is supine with legs parted on arm boards in the same plane. The surgeon stands between the legs and the each of the two assistants on either side. Two 20-inch high-resolution monitors are positioned on either side of the patient. Subsidiary screens or monitors may be positioned around the patient.

TROCAR POSITIONS AND CHOICE OF LAPAROSCOPE AND CAMERA

Five trocars are used. For maximum flexibility and stapler access, all ports should be 12 mm in diameter. The ports are positioned as shown in the diagram in Fig. 23–2. The central umbilical port is for the laparoscope, and the operator's instruments are inserted through the lower ports. The upper two ports are for the assistants to retract the liver or hold up the stomach. A 30° laparoscope is the optical device of choice, and it should be connected to a 3-chip CCD camera.

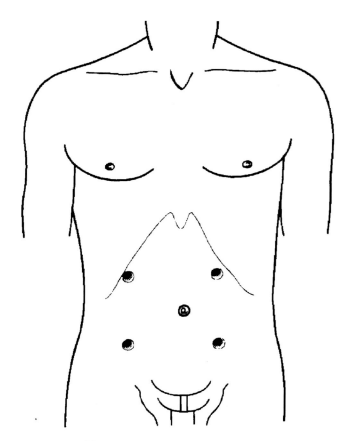

Figure 23–2. Diagram of the port positions.

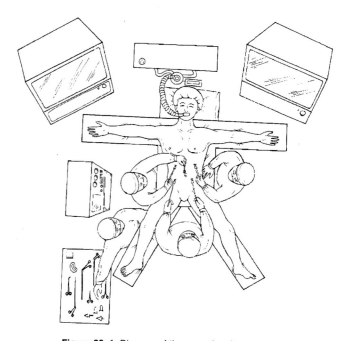

Figure 23–1. Diagram of the operation theatre setup.

DISSECTION OF THE GREATER OMENTUM

The first task is to take the greater omentum off the transverse colon. The two assistants hold up the greater omentum with atraumatic bowel clamps, letting the transverse colon hang down by gravity. The surgeon provides countertraction on the colon with bowel forceps in the left hand and divides the omentum with the right hand using a pair of coagulating scissors. The plane of dissection is along the avascular window between the colon and the omentum (Fig. 23–3). Several vascular strands may have to be coagulated before division. It is important to locate the cavity of the lesser sac as the omentum has several layers and this may cause confusion. To avoid thermal injury to the colon, it is best to keep the line of resection about 0.5 to 1 cm away from the colon. The dissection is begun in the midtransverse colon and extended to the right (of the operator) to the lower tip of the spleen. At this point the dissection changes direction and the omentum is divided just off the spleen, in a cephalad direction towards the greater curvature of the stomach, stopping at its edge at the level of the intended proximal resection line of the stomach. This point is usually either just proximal or just distal to the lowest short gastric vessel. This dissection is best done with a pair of 5-mm ultrasonic or harmonic scissors (U.S. Surgical, Norwalk, CT) which results in little bleeding and saves on the use of clips. To the left (of the operator), the dissection extends to the hepatic flexure of the colon.

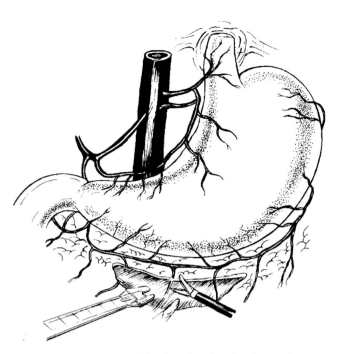

Figure 23–3. Diagram of the dissection at gastrocolic omentum.

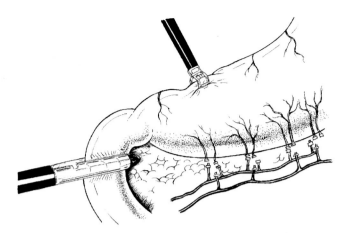

Figure 23–4. Diagram of duodenal transection with the Endo-GIA stapler.

DISSECTION OF THE DUODENUM AND GROUP 6 LYMPH NODES

The greater omentum around the hepatic flexure is divided away from the mesocolon. This can usually be done along an avascular plane, but some small vessels may have to be divided either with the coagulating or ultrasonic scissors. The omentum in this area merges with the group 6 (subpyloric) lymph nodes, which must be included in the resected specimen. The right gastroepiploic vessels also reside with-in this group of nodes and must be isolated, clipped, and transected.

The best plane to follow is the fairly avascular plane just above the head of the pancreas. Just before coming to the lower edge of the first part of the duodenum one reaches the superior pancreaticoduodenal branches, a leash of tiny vessels that must be dealt with meticulously and precisely, one strand at a time. Smaller vessels may be coagulated and then divided. Large vessels must by ligated or clipped. Beware of putting too many clips in this area as it will interfere with the duodenal transection when using the Endo-GIA stapler (U.S. Surgical, Norwalk, CT). Dissection of this area is complete when one reaches the lower edge of the duodenum at the intended margin of resection and have cleared a minimum 1-cm length of the duodenal stump. The duodenum is cleared of all tissue circumferentially to facilitate transection with the Endo-GIA stapler.

DISSECTION OF THE GROUP 12 LYMPH NODES AND THE HEPATIC HILUM

For a radical subtotal gastrectomy, the regional lymph nodes are removed. This includes the group 12 nodes, which are located along the hepatic hilum and adjacent to the common hepatic artery. The dissection usually starts at the hepatic hilum. Hook diathermy is used to break the peritoneal layer, after which all the fat and lymph node tissue along the hepatic hilar structures are slowly dissected off in a downward and medial direction. Small vessels and lymphatics can usually be coagulated by fine cautery graspers. It is important to apply coagulation very precisely to avoid injury to the hepatic artery and bile duct. The proper technique is to interpose the jaws of curved dissecting forceps below the tissue to be transected, lift the tissue away from the biliary and vascular structures, apply cautery to the tissue, and then cut it precisely with scissors. The tissue and nodes are gently reflected medially, to be included later in the gastric specimen.

LOCATING THE SUPERIOR EDGE OF THE DUODENUM AND TRANSECTION

The first part of the duodenum can usually be identified by the location of the vein of Mayo, which runs across the pylorus. If any difficulties are encountered, gastroscopic localization should be done. The superior edge of the duodenum is cleared of tissue, which will include the group 5 lymph nodes. The right gastric vessels need to be clipped and cut. To create a plane under the duodenum, small fragile vessels may need to be diathermied and cut. Once the margin around the duodenum is clear of tissue, the Endo-GIA stapler is introduced through the right upper port and positioned transversely across the duodenum so that both blades of the stapler protrude beyond the superior border (Fig. 23–4). The duodenum is then transected. Usually the resected margin on the duodenum is hemostatic because of the triple row of titanium clips deployed across the anastomotic line.

TAKING THE LESSER OMENTUM OFF THE LIVER AND DEALING WITH THE LESSER CURVE VESSELS

The pylorus is grasped and pulled downwards to apply traction to the lesser omentum, thus facilitating its division by diathermy or ultrasonic scissors. The dissection starts towards the inferior surface of the liver, is continued along the surface, and then curved downward to the lesser curvature of the stomach, to the intended line of resection. This whole area is relatively avascular. Close to the resection margin, branches of the left gastric vessels will need to be divided, but again, avoid placing any clips here as they will interfere with the stapler. Preferably, the thick bunch of tissue can be divided with the Endo-GIA stapler during transection of the stomach.

TRANSECTION OF THE STOMACH

The partially transected stomach is pushed upwards to the left upper quadrant with endo-Babcocks, exposing its posterior surface. Membranous attachments to the pancreas are divided with the ultrasonic scissors, uncovering the left gastric pedicle which is seen entering the stomach. It is seldom necessary to divide it, except for a near-total gastrectomy, in which case the use of a vascular Endo-GIA is necessary for its transection. The stomach is repositioned and the anterior surface is brought into view. The resection should aim to leave about one third of the stomach behind. To transect the stomach, we use multiple applications of the 30-mm Endo-GIA stapler. The stapler is inserted through the left upper port to simplify maneuvering. The transection is started at the greater curvature, and subsequent applications are made at the apex of the previous staple line, aiming towards the lesser curvature (Fig. 23–5). Depending on the thickness of the stomach, up to five or more staples may be needed. The resection margin is usually hemostatic, but occasionally there may be bleeding, which can easily be controlled by intracorporeal suturing. Following complete transection, the stomach specimen is placed in the right upper quadrant for removal at the end of the operation. Staplers that are 60 mm long and 12 mm in diameter are now available (U.S. Surgical, Norwalk, CT) and these are good alternatives to the Endo-GIA 30.

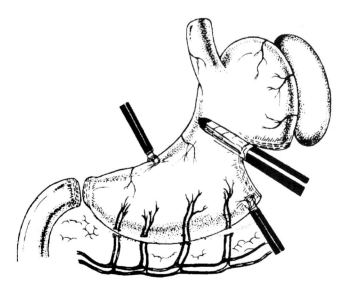

Figure 23–5. Diagram of subtotal gastrectomy using the Endo-GIA stapler.

DISSECTING THE GROUP 7, 8, 9, AND 11 LYMPH NODES

These lymph nodes are situated along the main proximal branches of the celiac axis, namely the splenic, hepatic, and left gastric arteries. The upper border of the pancreas is identified with the laparoscope, and with careful dissection using diathermy, tissue is cleared off the pancreas in the direction of the tail. In the vicinity of the mid-pancreas, the coronary vein is visualized. Avoid damage to it as there may be troublesome bleeding. Upon further dissection lateral to the vein, the surgeon will encounter the splenic artery, identifiable by its pulsation and tortuous course. Tissue and nodes (group 11) are cleared off the artery and retrieved for labeling and pathologic analysis. The dissection is traced back along the artery towards the celiac axis, where more tissue and nodes are carefully removed from around the hepatic artery (group 8), left gastric artery (group 7), and the celiac axis itself (group 9). The use of the ultrasonic scissors here is helpful. The latest generation of scissors are 5 mm in diameter and give better hemostasis and visualization of fine structures than the older 10-mm variety.

PERFORMING THE BILLROTH II ANASTOMOSIS

The initial step is to identify the duodenojejunal junction by lifting the transverse colon cephalad and tilting the operating table to a head-down position.[13,14] Once identified, the proximal jejunum is followed distally until a suitable length of jejunum can be brought up, in an antecolic fashion, to the stomach remnant without undue tension. Two seromuscular sutures (2-0 polyglactin) are intracorporeally knotted to anchor the jejunum to the anterior portion of the stomach (some surgeons prefer a posterior anastomosis for more dependent drainage), one near the greater curvature and the other about 2 cm from the resection margin, along the proposed anastomotic line. Two stab incisions are made with the diathermy on the stomach and the jejunum, halfway along the anastomotic line. On the stomach side, its thickness and propensity to bleed from submucosal vessels may cause some difficulties, but careful diathermy will overcome this. The stab incisions are enlarged with forceps, and the Endo-GIA stapler, which is inserted through the right upper port, is positioned with its one blade in the stomach and the other in the jejunum. Endo-Babcocks are used to approximate the wound margins against the hilt of the stapler to strengthen the anastomosis (Fig. 23–6). The stapler is closed and fired. Another Endo-GIA stapler is placed through the left upper port and the blades are positioned in the opposite direction to complete the anastomosis. This method is preferred because closure of the gastrojejunostomy has less chance of narrowing the anastomosis and causing an outlet obstruction. A single-layer, continuous suture is used to close the common stab wound, running perpendicular to the anastomosis (Fig. 23–7). The suture line is made using 2-0 polyglactin with a curved atraumatic needle. Intracorporeal sutures are placed using the Szabo Berci (Storz, Tuttlingen, Germany) needle-holder and flamingo assisting device. We now routinely perform an entero-enterostomy joining the afferent to the efferent loop about 30 cm down from the gastrojejunostomy. This is done to avoid problems caused by kinking of either the afferent or efferent loop, or temporary

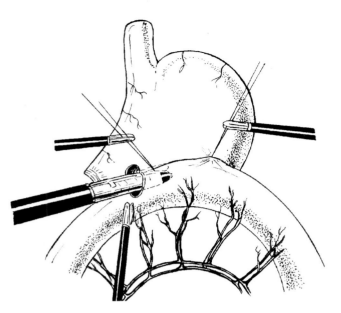

Figure 23–6. Diagram of gastrojejunostomy with the Endo-GIA stapler.

obstruction of one of the loops due to edema. The anastomosis may also be done side-to-side with the Endo-GIA 30 stapler (2 shots) or Endo-GIA 60 stapler (1 shot). The common stab wound is closed by continuous intracorporeal suturing with 3-0 polydiaxanone or polyglactin.

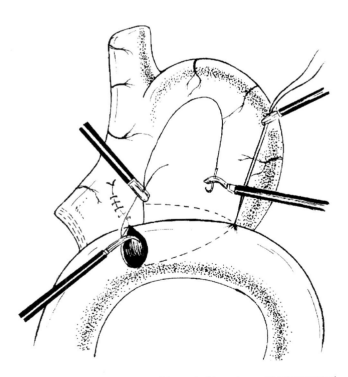

Figure 23–7. Diagram of closure of the gastrojejunostomy with intracorporeal suturing.

CHECKING THE ANASTOMOSIS AND REMOVAL OF THE SPECIMEN

The anastomosis is checked for leakage as well as patency by passing a gastroscope into the stomach and distending it by filling it with air. The patient is tilted head-down and the area around the anastomosis is flooded with saline. Any leakage is confirmed by bubbling. The patency of both the afferent and efferent jejunal loops is determined by gently passing the scope into the loops. The fluid is suctioned and hemostasis is secured, particularly in the retroperitoneal area and the celiac axis. Suction drains are placed through the right and left upper ports and positioned under the right and left lobes of the liver. The stomach specimen is grasped with the lower forceps and brought to the midline. The umbilical incision is extended vertically, usually not more than 3 cm, to retrieve the specimen. We prefer to place the specimen in a large plastic bag, which is then pulled through the incision with a twisting action. The bag will prevent spillage of gastric contents and cancer tissue into the peritoneal cavity. Finally, the wounds are closed and infiltrated with bupivacaine for postoperative pain relief.

DRAINAGE AND CLOSURE

Suction drains are positioned, one in the vicinity of the duodenal stump and one under the left lobe of the liver in the vicinity of the anastomosis. All 12-mm wounds are closed with a single interrupted stitch of 2-0 polyglactin to attach to the fascial layer. The skin can be closed with subcuticular poliglecaprone sutures. Infiltration of bupivacaine into the trocar wounds will give relief from wound pain for several hours.

POSTOPERATIVE CARE

The patient should have routine postoperative monitoring of parameters and adequate analgesia with narcotics for the first day. The pain from the operation should diminish rapidly after that if there are no complications, and the patient can begin to ambulate on the second postoperative day. The patient should not be fed and should have intermittent or continuous nasogastric suction for at least 3 days. Adequate hydration with IV fluids is imperative as is chest physiotherapy. On the third day after the operation, patients with subtotal gastrectomy may be given fluids orally if there are no signs of complications, and gradually moved to a solid diet.

COMPLICATIONS

The most common complications of this operation are bleeding, anastomotic inadequacy, and anastomotic leak.

Bleeding is mainly an intraoperative problem as most surgeons would ensure a reasonably dry field before exiting the abdominal cavity. The best strategy is to try and avoid causing bleeding in the first place. All small vessels below 1 mm is size should be coagulated before transection. This can be done with electrocautery or with the harmonic scissors. Larger vessels between 1 and 2 mm in size such as the short gastric vessels need a reasonably long application of the harmonic scissors in the coagulation mode before transection. For vessels larger than 2 mm a clip is usually required. Key vessels like the right gastroepiploic artery should be isolated and clipped securely with at least two metal clips or an absolock PDS clip before transection. The left gastric artery may require a vascular Endo-GIA stapler or may need to be ligated. It is best to avoid using the Endo-GIA to transect large sections of omentum in an attempt to speed the resection as the stapler is not hemostatic on omentum and troublesome bleeding may result. Suture lines closed with the Endo-GIA stapler seldom bleed significantly. If bleeding is troublesome, intracorporeal sutures over the bleeding point will often achieve control. The harmonic scissors have proven to be a great time-saving device for this operation. It allows one to cut through omentum with impunity and is especially useful when performing lymph node dissection. There is very little bleeding when it is used properly and all but the largest vessels can be sealed by the device.

Anastomotic inadequacy is one of the major problems in a laparoscopically-stapled gastrojejunostomy anastomosis. This is the main reason why we now advocate a hand-sutured closure of the common stab wound. The stapled anastomosis must be at least 6 cm long. The common stab wound can be created in the middle of the anastomotic line (Italian style) or at one end. If the latter technique is used, it is best to have the common stab wound on the afferent side as efferent limb obstruction is the more disastrous consequence. The afferent limb is a conduit for bile and pancreatic juices and there need not be a large communication. The patency of the anastomosis must be checked by endoscopy after the operation. If there is any doubt about patency of one of the loops during this procedure, an enteroenterostomy joining the afferent and efferent loops side to side is a worthwhile precaution. Some workers advocate doing this routinely. The anastomosis is done laparoscopically with the Endo-GIA and the common stab wound again closed by suture. Alternatively, the anastomosis can be done open after the umbilical wound is extended to retrieve the specimen. In Japan, a Billroth I–type anastomosis is usually performed via the extraction wound. When relative obstruction is discovered in the postoperative period, an endoscopy or contrast study should be performed to estimate the severity of the problem. When due to edema, a period of nasogastric suction and parenteral nutrition may suffice to resolve the problem. If there is kinking or narrowing of either limb that is not due to edema, a laparoscopic enteroenterostomy should be immediately performed.

Anastomotic leaks have seldom been reported in laparoscopic gastric surgery, but the same precautions must be taken to ensure a leak-proof anastomosis as in open surgery. Most important, the anastomotic line must be well vascularized and not under tension. Stapling must be done carefully to ensure no breaks in the staple line. A hand-sewn anastomosis must be done precisely and all anastomotic lines should be tested by the underwater insufflation test. Anastomotic dehiscence should be treated by open surgery as the patient is usually too much at risk to benefit from the advantages of laparoscopic surgery.

IS LAPAROSCOPIC GASTRECTOMY ADEQUATE AS A CANCER OPERATION?

The adequacy of laparoscopic radical gastrectomy in terms of cancer clearance unfortunately cannot currently be addressed as there are no controlled data and the number of centers doing the procedure remains small. From an anatomic viewpoint it is possible to

perform the same procedure as in open surgery. It is not known, however, whether the pneumoperitoneum itself produces any inherent disadvantages in terms of its effect on tumor biology. This area is being researched extensively and the answer will soon become apparent. Perhaps it will prove to be necessary to use helium or argon as the inflationary gas of choice or a gasless technique may be necessary. Up to this time, however, there have been no reports indicating a proliferation of port site recurrences in stomach cancer patients. Nevertheless it is always necessary to observe the basic cancer surgery principles of minimum handling of the tumor and protection of normal tissues from contamination by tumor cells. Any inherent disadvantages in the long term will be revealed in time.

BENEFITS OF THE LAPAROSCOPIC APPROACH

The procedure holds the promise of less pain, quicker mobilization, faster gut recovery, and a shorter hospital stay. The procedure produces a better cosmetic result and a lower possibility of keloid scar formation. There is also the possibility of a reduction in troublesome adhesions.[15]

The disadvantages are higher cost, greater technical difficulty, a need for specialized equipment, longer operating time, and unknown effects on cancer biology.

Although most progressive surgeons feel that open gastrectomy for benign disease is obsolete, the role of laparoscopic surgery in cancer remains controversial and will be the subject of intensive study in the next decade. At present, laparoscopic gastric resection is being increasingly used in the management of early gastric cancers, especially in patients in whom the size of the lesion and the possibility of lymph node metastasis make endoscopic mucosal resection or laparoscopic wedge resection inadequate.

REFERENCES

1. Goh PMY, Tekant Y, Kum CK, et al. Totally intraabdominal laparoscopic Billroth II gastrectomy. *Surg Endosc.* 1992;6:160.
2. Goh PMY, Tekant Y, Isaac J, et al. The technique of laparoscopic Billroth II gastrectomy. *Surg Laparosc Endosc.* 1992;2:258.
3. Goh PMY, Kum CK. Laparoscopic Billroth II gastrectomy: a review. *Surg Oncol.* 1993;2(Suppl):13.
4. Goh PMY, Alponat A, Mak K, et al. Early international results of laparoscopic gastrectomies. *Surg Endosc.* 1997;11:650.
5. Japanese Gastric Cancer Association. Japanese classification of gastric carcinoma, 2nd ed. *Gastric Cancer.* 1998;1:24.
6. Hiki Y. Endoscopic treatment of early gastric cancer. In: Nishi M, Ichikawa H, Nakajima T, et al, eds. *Gastric Cancer.* Springer-Verlag:1994;392.
7. Ohgami M, Kumai K, Katajima M, et al. Laparoscopic wedge resection of stomach for early gastric cancer using a lesion lifting method. *Dig Surg.* 1994;11:64.
8. Ohashi S. Laparoscopic intraluminal (intragastric) surgery for early gastric cancer. *Surg Endosc.* 1995;9:169.
9. Ohashi S. Laparoscopic intragastric surgery and its modification for early gastric cancer: a new technique in laparoscopic surgery. Proceedings of Second International Gastric Cancer Congress, Munich, 1997;1789.
10. Kitano S, Shimoda K, Miyahara M, et al. Laparoscopic approaches in the management of patients with early gastric carcinomas. *Surg Laparosc Endosc.* 1995;5:359.

11. Matsuda M, Terayama H, Asama T, et al. Laparoscopic distal gastrectomy using the combination of pneumoperitoneum and an abdominal wall lifting technique for early gastric cancer. Proceedings of Sixth World Congress of Endoscopic Surgery, Rome, 1998;597.

12. Melotti G, Meinero M, Tamborrino E. Laparoscopic gastric surgery, gastric resection for cancer. In: *Laparoscopic Surgery in the Nineties.* Meinero M, Melotti G, Mouret P, eds. Masson:1994;273.

13. Goh P, Kum CK. Laparoscopic Billroth II gastrectomy. In: *Operative Strategies in Laparoscopic Surgery.* Phillips E, Rosenthal RJ, eds. Springer:1995;155.

14. Goh P, Alexander DJ. Laparoscopic gastroenterostomy and Billroth II gastrectomy. In: *Laparo-Endoscopic Surgery*, 2nd ed. Brune IB, ed. Blackwell Science Ltd.:1996;199.

15. Goh P, Kum CK. Gastrectomy. In: *Operative Laparoscopy and Thoracoscopy.* MacFayden BV, Ponsky JL, eds. Lippincott, Raven:1996;523.

Chapter Twenty-Four • • • • • • •

R2 Level Resections for Gastric Cancer

CARLOS BALLESTA-LÓPEZ, X. BASTIDA-VILA, and C. BETTONICA-LARRAÑAGA

Laparoscopic surgery for gastric resection should fulfill the basic principles already established in conventional surgery.

In benign pathology, the most common entities that are treated by resection are gastric and duodenal recurring ulcers; benign tumors (the most common being leiomyomas); ectopic pancreas; and gastric APUDomas. The most common malignant pathologies are low malignancy tumors of muscular origin (leiomyoblastoma, or neuromyoblastoma) and carcinomas of various histologic types.

The surgical technique to be employed will vary depending on each specific disease, and can range from gastric resection with vagotomy for gastric and duodenal recurring ulcers, local or atypical resections via gastrotomy for benign tumors of the posterior gastric wall, or oncologic gastrectomy with lymphadenectomy (R2), according to a group of Japanese surgeons.[1]

DIAGNOSTIC TESTS

Diagnostic tests should be used to confirm the presence or absence of disease and determine its possible etiology. Some useful tests include endoscopic examination, functional tests (such as gastric secretion and gastrin level) in cases of recurring ulcer disease, and histologic examination and determination of tumoral extension in cases of malignant disease. We will not analyze the different tests and diagnostic procedures here. For this information, consult one of the many books available on surgical pathology.

SURGICAL TECHNIQUE

The setup of the surgical team and laparoscopic equipment, and placement of ports are the same as that used for most other laparoscopic procedures.[2] The patient is placed in the French position with a slight inclination to either side as needed. The surgeon stands between the patient's legs, with an assistant on either side and the surgical nurse on the surgeon's right side. One or two monitors are placed on either side of the patient's head so that the surgeon and the assistants can each have a clear view of the procedure (Fig. 24–1).

Port Placement

Five trocars are needed to perform laparoscopic gastric surgery.

Once abdominal insufflation to a pressure of 12 mm Hg is accomplished through the use of a Veress needle placed in the periumbilical zone, an 11-mm trocar is placed there for the laparoscope. In obese patients, the port is placed in the linea alba 2 or 3 cm above the umbilicus. A second 12-mm trocar is placed in the middle right upper quadrant midclavicular line, through which clamps and the Endo-GIA 30 are introduced.

A third 15-mm trocar is placed on the left midclavicular line, through which the surgeon can control clamps, scissors, and the Endo-GIA 60 to section the stomach for gastrectomies or to perform gastroenteroanastomosis. A 10-mm trocar is placed in the left subcostal region to be used by the second assistant to introduce instruments to help in the exposure of the stomach. Finally, a 10-mm trocar is placed in the subxiphoid region for the liver retractor, or in some cases a clamp, to improve exposure (Fig. 24–2).

Laparoscopic Instruments

A 0° or 30° laparoscope can be used (introduced in through the first port), three 5-mm grasping clamps (through port numbers 2, 3, and 4), a liver retractor/grasping clamp (through port number 5), two pairs of monopolar scissors, a needle-holder, a blunt coagulator, and a clipper (through port number 3), and a 60-mm Endo-GIA with three loads is prepared for gastrectomies, or with a single load for gastroenteroanastomosis. Also, 2-0 silk sutures to close the Endo-GIA entry ports and do other suturing are needed, as are two Penrose drains that are placed at the end of the procedure.

Goals of Surgical Technique

The basic goals of oncologic surgical resection are:

- A resection whose border is tumor-free and free of lymphatic and vascular permeability with a margin of at least 2 cm.
- Complete resection of the tumoral mass.

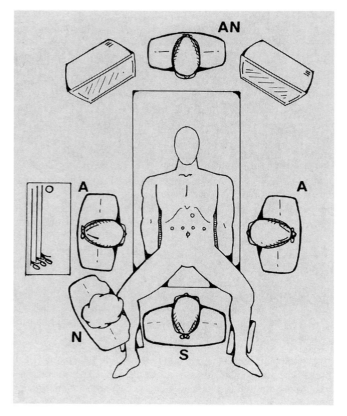

Figure 24–1. Setup of the surgical team and equipment.

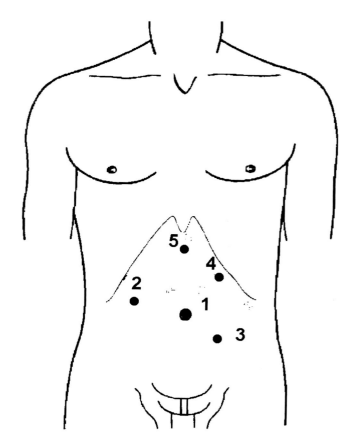

Figure 24–2. Placement of the trocars for gastric resection.

- Lymphadenectomy of all the regional lymphatic ganglia to the first level (L1), and if possible to the second level (L2). The issue of lymphadenectomy to the first or second level has been controversial. Maruyama et al[3] have proven the superiority of lymphadenectomy to L2 over that of L1; these results have been confirmed by Siewert et al in Germany,[4] but not by Roder et al[5] or other groups.[6–8]

Since all the authors agree that dissection to a minimum of L1 is necessary to perform curative surgery for gastric cancer, and this is possible laparoscopically, then it is possible to perform successful laparoscopic surgery for gastric cancer.[2] To accomplish these goals it is necessary to ligate the vessels at their bases and perform ample resections with lymphadenectomy.

In 1994 we established a laparoscopic protocol for staging and treatment, both radical and palliative, for gastric cancer, using the algorithm shown in Fig. 24–3.

Notes on the Surgical Technique

Visual Examination. Once the first trocar is placed and the laparoscope is introduced, an examination of the peritoneal cavity is performed to determine if ascites is present, and if there are

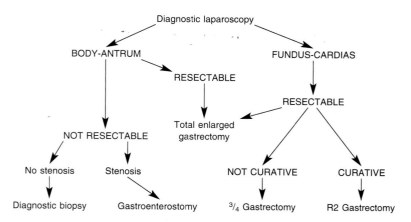

Figure 24–3. Algorithm for the treatment of gastric cancer.

peritoneal or hepatic metastases. After the second and third trocars are placed, samples of the ascitic fluid and biopsies of possible metastases are obtained.

Determination of the Resectability of the Tumor. With the clamps placed through the second and third ports, the stomach is mobilized to evaluate the degree of fixation to other organs, specifically the pancreas and mesocolon. For this purpose a window is created in the gastrocolic omentum approximately 2 cm outside of the gastroepiploic vessels. The number and characteristics of the adenopathies are observed. Samples are taken from the subpyloric ganglia and the left gastric artery to allow TNM staging and determine resectability of the tumor.

Palliative Surgery. This is used largely in cases of nonresectable cancer of the distal third of the stomach, which commonly produces stenosis. A laparoscopic antecolic gastroenteroanastomosis can be performed to solve this problem.

Five trocars are placed (Fig. 24–2); the fifth trocar allows the liver retractor to be introduced for evaluation of gastric resectability, and can then be changed to a clamp to expose the colon.

The surgeon introduces clamps through the second and third trocars to grasp the colon at the transverse level and approximately 15 cm from the splenic angle. The colon is lifted towards the anterior abdominal wall, exposing the angle of Treitz. The assistant's clamp placed in the fourth trocar replaces the surgeon's (in port 3), leaving his right hand free and the fifth trocar (subxiphoid) in his left hand.

By lifting the colon, the surgeon locates angle of Treitz and with the aid of two clamps (trocars 2 and 3) marks the distal 30 to 40 cm. Once this point is marked, the colon is left in its normal position and the jejunum is passed in front of it with no tension; the loop is secured in an isoperistaltic fashion.

The ascended loop is fixed to the anterior gastric surface at the level of the greater curvature at least 4 cm from the tumoral infiltration zone, and secured by two silk stitches 4 cm apart. Once the loop is secured without tension to the anterior gastric surface, a hole is made with the electrocautery on the antimesenteric border at the left limit of the fixed loop. Another hole is made parallel to the first one, but on the anterior gastric surface.

The stapler is introduced through the third trocar and one side is placed on the stomach and the other on the loop, assisted by the surgeon's second clamp and the assistant's fourth clamp. Then the endostapler is activated, performing the anastomosis. Once a wide gastro-jejunal anastomotic mouth and its patency are assured, the hole used to introduce the endostapler is closed with intracorporeal 2-0 silk stitches. Once the airtightness of the suture is demonstrated by intragastric pressurized methylene blue, the trocars are removed and the procedure is finished.

Resective Surgery. When performed to effect a cure, oncologic surgery with lymphadenectomy are customarily done according to a well-known technique.[2,9]

Laparoscopy is performed under general anesthesia administered via an endotracheal tube; a nasogastric tube is then placed. The patient is placed in decubitus position with the legs separated, and a table with equipment for laparotomy must be set up next to the laparoscopic equipment for use if necessary.

The surgeon stands between the legs of the patient with an assistant on either side. Pneumoperitoneum is established (12 mm Hg) and the trocars are placed as outlined above. Diagnostic

peritoneal lavage is performed with 100 mL of saline at 37°C to detect neoplastic cells. The fluid is then recovered from Douglas' space and the subphrenic spaces.

During this stage an examination of the abdominal cavity is performed to detect infiltration of the gastric serosa, peritoneal implants, and hepatic metastases.

Once the tumor's resectability is confirmed, the greater omentum is detached from the transverse colon to obtain an avascular plane. Once the lesser sac has been entered, an examination of the posterior gastric surface and the anterior pancreatic aspect is performed. An intraoperative lymph node biopsy is performed of the subpyloric group and the left gastric vessels. The left gastric vessels are dissected, clipped, and sectioned (assuring that two titanium clips are left in the proximal end of the vessels). Dissection of the gastrocolic omentum is extended until it is completely dissected from the splenic to the hepatic angles.

The right gastroepiploic vessels are ligated at their origin next to the pancreas and the gastrosplenic ligament is dissected to the third or fourth short vessel. Sometimes adhesions between the spleen and the omentum require electrocoagulation.

The gastrohepatic omentum is completely dissected from the cardias to the pylorus including all lymph nodes of the lesser curvature (from the pyloric group up to the right pericardial group). Once this dissection is completed, the distal three-quarters of the stomach are free.

The proximal line of section is performed with two consecutive shots from the 30-mm Endo-GIA through the second trocar. The gastric section is performed with two consecutive shots from the 60-mm Endo-GIA and a single shot from the 30-mm Endo-GIA through the third trocar. (Fig. 24–4) The specimen is placed in a plastic bag over the right hepatic lobe. At this time, the celiac trunk, and hepatic and splenic artery lymphadenectomies are

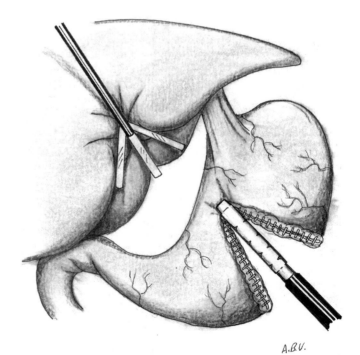

A.B.V.

Figure 24–4. Line of section for the gastrectomy.

performed along the pancreas, obtaining between 10 and 15 nodes which are extracted in a bag through the 15-mm trocar port. Once the lymphadenectomy is completed, two silk stitches are placed, suspending the gastric stump from the anterior abdominal wall to allow the gastrojejunal anastomosis to be performed with the posterior surface of the stomach.

The assistant's clamps raise the transverse colon with the surgeon identifying the duodenojejunal union and the first jejunal loop, which is brought up to the supramesocolic space through a 10-mm incision in the transverse mesocolon.

The loop is secured to the posterior gastric surface by way of its antimesenteric border with two seromuscular 2-0 silk stitches, approximately 2 cm above the line of gastric section (Fig. 24–4).

A small enterotomy and gastrotomy is performed with the electrocautery at the end of the fixed loop, and in the gastric stump. A 30-mm Endo-GIA is inserted through it to perform a laterolateral transmesocolic gastroenteroanastomosis (Fig. 24–5). The Endo-GIA's entry port is sutured with 4 or 5 intracorporeal sutures. Once the anastomosis is completed, saline solution with methylene blue is introduced through the nasogastric tube to test the integrity of the anastomoses. Two aspiration drains are placed; one in the right subhepatic space near the duodenal stump and the other in the left subphrenic space. The gastrectomy specimen is extracted in its bag through a subxiphoid incision of about 4 cm, being careful to avoid leakage and contamination of the peritoneal space with neoplastic cells. After desufflating the abdominal cavity the trocars are removed and the entry ports are closed.

DATA ANALYSIS

Gastric cancer is widespread in the Western world and presents a resectability index of around 60 to 80% at the time of diagnosis.[10–12]

The methods of clinical staging (TNM) have a diagnostic precision of about 83% for echography and 85% for CT,[13] and misdiagnosis results in unnecessary laparotomies for advanced disease which increase hospital stay and cost.[19,20] The use of laparoscopy has increased the diagnostic precision in digestive tract neoplasms to around 96%.[3,4,14] Laparoscopy can be used as a diagnostic or therapeutic method by performing palliative gastroenteroanastomosis or gastric resections, depending on oncologic criteria.[2,5–18]

Using the criteria and surgical technique described here, we prospectively analyzed the effectiveness of surgical staging compared with clinical staging using the pathologic criteria. The index of resectability, palliative surgery, and oncologic radicality of subtotal laparoscopic gastrectomy were also analyzed.[19,20]

In order to evaluate the contribution of laparoscopy to the treatment of gastric cancer, we performed a prospective study of 76 patients in whom gastric cancer had been diagnosed and treated between January 1994 and January 2000, with ages ranging from 43 to 84 years. We analyzed the accuracy of diagnoses, comparing the clinical TNM (by endoscopy with biopsy, radiology, and CT), laparoscopic TNM (determined by the degree of infiltration of the gastric wall and other organs), lymph node infiltration via intraoperative biopsy taken from the subpyloric and the left gastric nodes, resectability of the tumor and the presence of hepatic or peritoneal metastases by performing a peritoneal lavage for neoplastic cells at the beginning of the laparoscopic procedure, and finally the pathologic TNM as determined by analysis of the re-

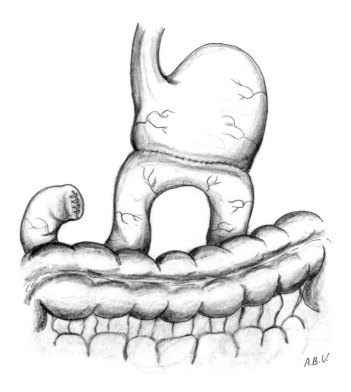

Figure 24–5. Final result of the gastric resection and gastroenterostomy

sected specimens. The type of surgery performed was evaluated as well as the surgical time, the intra- and postoperative complications, and the radicality of the gastric resection (number of nodes and resection borders).

From the prospective analysis of these parameters, 18 patients were ASA 1, 21 were ASA 2, 28 were ASA 3, and 9 were ASA 4, and we obtained the following results: Clinical staging coincided with pathologic staging in 37 of the 76 patients (48.68%), whereas surgical staging coincided with pathologic staging in 73 of the 76 patients (96.05%). The three patients in whom the surgical TNM did not coincide with the pathologic TNM were as follows: One was a lymph node biopsy from the subpyloric group, which was reported as negative preoperatively and proven positive in the definitive study; another patient who was reported as serosa negative and later proven positive in the definitive study; and a third patient in whom the surgeon reported a tumor-free resected border and the surgical specimen had less than 1 cm between the tumor and the gastric section border.

Surgical Procedures

In 24 patients without pyloric stenosis a diagnostic laparoscopy with biopsy was performed, confirming the unresectability of the tumor, and found peritoneal carcinomatosis not detected by the cTNM in 16 cases, and multiple hepatic metastases in 8 cases. The lavage cytology was positive in all cases.

Sixteen patients presented with pyloroantral stenosis. In 7 cases fixation to the pancreas was found associated with peritoneal carcinomatosis. In 9 cases not detected by TNM a 30-mm antecolic laterolateral gastroenteroanastomosis was performed with an endostapler. Average surgical time was 47 minutes (range,

TABLE 24–1. SURVIVAL OF PATIENTS UNDERGOING
GASTROENTEROANASTOMOSIS

Survival	No. of Patients
Less than 1 month	2
1–3 months	3
3–6 months	2
6–12 months	7
12–17 months	2

27 to 58). Thirty-six patients had a subtotal Billroth II transmesocolic gastrectomy performed.[2]

In patients who had diagnostic laparoscopy, oral intake was resumed after 12 hours, and they were discharged between the second and the fifth day without incident. Maximum survival was 17 months, with 43.75% surviving <6 months (Table 24–1).

Of the 36 subtotal gastrectomies performed via laparoscopy, the histologic type, the distance between the tumor and the free border, the number of nodes extracted, the duration of the surgery, the rate and causes of conversion to laparotomy, number of intraoperative incidents and postoperative complications, and the rate of recurrences or peritoneal implants found with endoscopy, CT, or autopsy, were all evaluated every 3 months during the first year and every 6 months thereafter.

RESULTS

- The borders of resection varied for the distal border from 2 to 6.5 cm and for the proximal border from 6 to 17 cm, not including a single case of conversion to laparotomy due to an inferior proximal border of less than 1 cm.
- The number of extracted nodes was between 13 and 41 (median, 23).
- The surgical time was directly related to the patient's body habitus (obese patients having longer times), technical problems, and surgical experience. It ranged from 75 minutes to 390 minutes (median, 196 minutes); the first gastrectomy took 270 minutes.
- Conversion to laparotomy was necessary in 7 patients (19.44%), with 3 due to hemorrhage and 2 due to an incorrectly performed gastric section (in one case the free border was less than 1 cm from the tumor).

The most common postoperative complications were: two fistulas (5.55%) that were managed with parenteral nutrition; and one case of anastomotic dehiscence, which forced a laparotomy on three occasions for successive dehiscence of the sutures (2.7% mortality).

Among intraoperative incidents, we should point out that the nasogastric tube was sectioned on three occasions with the endostapler, which required removing the suture and performing it again. On one occasion the anastomotic line was perforated by the nasogastric tube that the anesthesiologist introduced at the end of the procedure; this was repaired with a 2-0 silk suture. In all four cases the problem was managed laparoscopically.

Maximum follow-up was 72 months with CT and endoscopy every 3 months during the first year and every 6 months thereafter. We have had 2 deaths. One was in a 73-year-old patient operated for a gastric lymphoma who presented with retroperitoneal lymph node enlargement 3 months after the intervention and did not respond to chemotherapy. No implants at the trocar sites were seen. The other was a 56-year-old patient with an adenocarcinoma

(T3N1M0) who presented with a retropancreatic and periportal nodal recurrence 14 months postsurgery. A cephalic duodenopancreatectomy with retroperitoneal lymph node extraction was performed by laparotomy, and there were no hepatic metastases or implants at the trocar sites. Death occurred at 26 months after the initial intervention. The remaining patients are clinically free of disease.

The histologic type of tumor was adenocarcinoma (30 cases), lymphoma (5 cases) and 1 neuromyoblastoma in a cirrhotic patient (Child C).

CONCLUSIONS

There is a significant difference between clinical and laparoscopic TNM staging, with laparoscopic staging being more precise and consistent. It is possible that in the near future diagnostic laparoscopy will supplant other preoperative tests, such as CT. Laparoscopy allows evaluation of the resectability of some gastric cancers by determining their fixation to other organs, and evaluating the presence of pyloric stenosis and carcinomatosis.

Specially-trained surgical teams can perform gastric oncologic surgery by laparoscopy with oncologic results similar to those obtained by laparotomy, but with the clear advantages that laparoscopic surgery offers over open surgery (i.e., shorter hospital stay and less morbidity and mortality, among others).

The surgical time for gastric oncologic surgery by laparoscopy is acceptable, with less time needed for diagnostic laparoscopy and palliative surgery (gastroenteroanastomosis), and in all cases laparoscopic times are shorter than those for laparotomy.

In the follow-up of our patients we have shown that the risk of neoplastic implants in the trocar entry sites is zero.

Oncologic gastrectomy is not a simple procedure, and it requires teams that are specially trained in laparoscopic surgery. When exclusively laparoscopic surgeons perform laparoscopic surgery, the number of complications and risks for the patient is reduced.

REFERENCES

1. Japanese Research Society for Gastric Cancer. *Japanese Classification of Gastric Carcinoma* (first English edition). Kanehara & Co. Ltd.: 1995;19.
2. Ballesta López C, Bastida Vila X, Catarci M, et al. Laparoscopic Billroth II distal subtotal gastrectomy with gastric stump suspension for gastric malignancies. *Am J Surg.* 1996;171:289.
3. Maruyama K, Sasako M, Kinoshita T, et al. Effectiveness of systematic lymph node dissection in gastric cancer surgery. In: *Gastric Cancer*, Nishi M, Ichikawa H, Nakajuma T, Maruyama K, Tahara E, eds. Springer-Verlag:1994;293.
4. Siewert RJ, Böttcher K, Roder JD, et al. Prognostic relevance of systematic lymph node dissection in gastric carcinoma. *Br J Surg.* 1993; 80:1015.
5. Roder JD, Bonenkamp JJ, Craven J, et al. Lymphadenectomy for gastric cancer in clinical trials: update. *World J Surg.* 1995;19:546.
6. Kockerling F, Reck T, Gall FP. Extended gastrectomy: Who benefits? *World J Surg.* 1995;19:541.
7. Wanebo HJ, Kennedy BJ, Chmiel J, et al. Cancer of the stomach: a patient care study by the American College of Surgeons. *Ann Surg.* 1993;218:583.

8. Bonenkamp JJ, Van de Velde CJH, Sasako M, et al. R2 compared with R1 resection for gastric cancer: morbidity and mortality in a prospective, randomized trial. *Eur J Surg.* 1992;158:413.

9. Ballesta López C, Bastida Vila X, Betonica Larrañaga C, et al. Contribution of laparoscopy to the treatment of gastric cancer: oncological gastrectomy (D2) by laparoscopy. *Video-Revista de Cirugía* 1995;XII(5):7.

10. Ballesta López C, Bastida Vila X. Laparoscopic D2 gastrectomy. The First International Gastric Cancer Congress in Kyoto, Japan, March 29–April 1, 1995.

11. Kriplani AK, Brij M, Kapur L. Laparoscopy for preoperative staging and assessment of operability in gastric carcinoma. *Gastrointest Endosc.* 1991;37:441.

12. Catarci M, Zaraca F, Gossetti F, et al. Laparoscopía diagnóstica: indicaciones y técnica. In: Ballesta-López C. ed. *Laparoscopía Quirúrgica.* Video Médica:1992;40.

13. Cuesta MA, Nagy A. *Minimally Invasive Surgery in Gastrointestinal Cancer.* Churchill Livingstone:1993.

14. Possik RA, Franco EL, Pires DR. Sensitivity, specificity, and predictive value of laparoscopy for the staging of gastric cancer and for the detection of liver metastases. *Cancer* 1986;58:1.

15. Goh P, Tekant Y, Isaac J, et al. The technique of laparoscopic Billroth II gastrectomy. *Surg Laparosc Endosc.* 1992;2:258.

16. Lointier P, Leroux S, Ferrier C, et al. A technique of laparoscopic gastrectomy and Billroth II gastrojejunostomy. *J Laparoendosc Surg.* 1993;4:353.

17. Kitano S, Iso Y, Moriyama M, et al. Laparoscopy-assisted Billroth I gastrectomy. *Surg Laparosc Endosc.* 1994;4:146.

18. Goh P, Tekant Y, Kum CK, et al. Totally intra-abdominal laparoscopic Billroth II gastrectomy. *Surg Endosc.* 1992;6:160 (Letter).

19. Bouvet M, Mansfield PF, Skibber JM, et al. Clinical, pathologic and economic parameters of laparoscopic colon resection for cancer. *Am J Surg.* 1998;176:554.

20. Bhalla R, Formella L, Kerrigan DD. Need for staging laparoscopy in patients with gastric cancer. *Br J Surg.* 2000;87:362.

Chapter Twenty-Five ● ● ● ● ● ● ●

*L*aparoscopic Adjustable Gastric Banding for the Treatment of Morbid Obesity

RODOLFO SÁNCHEZ, JOSÉ ANTONIO VÁZQUEZ-FRÍAS,
MARTÍN SALVADOR VALENCIA-REYES, and JORGE CUETO-GARCÍA

INTRODUCTION

Today obesity is a major health problem. It is defined by the National Institutes of Health as weight greater than 20% above the desirable body weight.[1,2] Thus, about one third of the adult population of the U.S. is overweight. Morbid obesity is defined as a body mass index (BMI) of 40 kg/m² or more, or 35 kg/m² plus a comorbid condition. Prevalence estimates for U.S. adults are 8% with a BMI ≥35 kg/m² and 2.8% with a BMI ≥40 kg/m², and the relative risk for all-cause mortality is increased at BMIs ≥30 kg/m².[3–5] The long-term results of medical therapy to achieve a sustained weight loss in these patients has resulted in a high rate of recidivism, and it is generally agreed that surgical treatment may be the only effective therapy for control of obesity. Surgery can only be successful if three steps are followed meticulously: a detailed preoperative evaluation must be done, an appropriate surgical procedure performed, and a close follow-up by a multidisciplinary team.[6,7]

The emergence of mini-invasive surgical procedures has had a widespread effect in the field of bariatrics. Operations such as the placement of the Swedish adjustable gastric band (SAGB),[8–10] the vertical banded gastroplasty,[11] and the Roux-en-Y gastric by-pass[12] are being done laparoscopically with results that compare favorably with those obtained with open surgery. Laparoscopic implantation of the SAGB has several important advantages over the other bariatric procedures, include the lack of stapling and reduced risk of contamination or resection. Moreover, it is a completely reversible procedure that can be adjusted to meet patient needs.

MATERIAL AND METHODS

From March 1998 to February 2000, patients with BMIs greater than 40 kg/m² or 35 kg/m² with one or more comorbidities were considered candidates for laparoscopic placement of the SAGB. Surgical procedures were performed in hospitals in Monterrey, Leon, Guadalajara, and Mexico City, all in Mexico. All of the patients were submitted to a thorough preoperative evaluation including laboratory tests, radiographic studies, cardiopulmonary examination, nutritional counseling, and in most cases a psychiatric consultation. Detailed information about the surgery as well as the postoperative recovery period was given preoperatively in several sessions. Exclusion criteria were: patients with incomplete follow-up; operations performed with another type of adjustable gastric band; and patients with drug and alcohol abuse, pregnancy, systemic infection, esophageal or gastric varices, autoimmune diseases, or unwillingness to change his or her eating habits. Patients with known reflux esophagitis (with or without a hiatal hernia) were not excluded; instead they were sent for additional studies, including endoscopy, manometry, and 24-hour pH monitoring.

RESULTS

A total of 678 patients had the procedure, including 454 females and 224 males aged 12 to 72 years (average, 44 years). Their BMIs ranged from 32 kg/m² to 93 kg/m² (mean, 44.5 kg/m²). There were 6 (0.8%) early and 9 (1.3%) late complications. Among the early ones were one patient with bleeding that required reoperation, one conversion to laparotomy due to severe adhesions, three port site infections, and one brachial plexus injury that spontaneously resolved in 4 weeks. The late complications included five with esophagitis and three with "pouchitis" that required medical treatment (liquid-based diet, proton pump inhibitors, and antacids); and there was one with upper gastrointestinal bleeding that required hospitalization and conservative treatment. Band-related complications occurred in 6 patients, including one band that ruptured a year postoperatively (it was removed and replaced with a new one via laparoscopy) and four disconnections or fractures of the valve tube (which were replaced with new ones). There was one patient with superficial cellulitis at the injection port site that was managed with antibiotics and wound care. It did not require band removal. There was no mortality in this series.

The average BMI decrease was 17.2 kg/m^2 (range, 12.3 to 28.7 kg/m^2) during the first year. The number of patients available for medium-term follow-up is small at this time. There were 3 patients who declined to have additional SAGB adjustments after a 40-, 43- and 45-pound weight loss. Of those patients, one decided to have his band removed by laparoscopy, stating that he was pleased with the result he had attained (11 months after SAGB placement).

Most frequent comorbidities were: type II diabetes (84 patients), hypertension (57 patients), cholelithiasis (32 patients), venous insufficiency (26 patients), knee and/or spine articular disease (24 patients), and sleep apnea (17 patients).

SURGICAL TECHNIQUE

All patients received general anesthesia, and surgery was performed on a surgical table that allows a steep Fowler position and separation of the patient's legs (the surgeon stands between them). A single dose of IV cephalotin was administered 1 hour before the operation. The placement of the trocars (5 to 6 total, 10 to 11 mm in size) is shown in Fig. 25–1. If the situation demands it, a sixth trocar is placed in the left lower costal area for a 10-mm Babcock forceps to retract the fatty tissue of the gastrosplenic ligament and allow for better exposure. A 30° laparoscope is always used and placed in the subxiphoid trocar. Careful and adequate liver retraction is of utmost importance.

Once adequate exposure is obtained, the anesthesiologist introduces a gastric catheter with a 50-mL balloon tip that is inflated within the stomach and then pulled back to identify the gastroesophageal (GE) junction; then the surgeon marks its equator with a bipolar forceps. Sponges with radiological markers are placed in each side of the hiatal area for blunt dissection and hemostasis. Dissection is usually begun in the left side of the esophageal hiatus, at the angle of His (which is sometimes lost if there is a hiatal hernia). An assistant applies traction in the GE junction towards the right of the patient and inferiorly, as the surgeon identifies the left crus and the left posterior aspect of the GE junction with sharp and blunt dissection. The short gastric vessels should be left undisturbed. Once the left crus is identified, gauze is placed in this area which is the exit of the retrogastric tunnel that is dissected from the right side of the hiatus.

Traction on the GE junction is now provided to the left of the patient and inferiorly. The gastrohepatic omentum is entered in its avascular plane to locate the right crus. If necessary, branches of the left gastric artery are divided. It is important when performing this procedure to avoid dissection in the area of any previous antireflux procedures. Dissection in this case is 1.5 to 2 cm below the GE junction, just above the left gastric artery. The right crus is grasped and pulled to the right of the patient by an assistant. Another assistant provides upward traction of the stomach and to the left of the patient. If the dissection plane is too low, the obvious finding will be the free posterior gastric wall; SAGB placement in this area leads to band migration. The posterior dissection must be performed in the retrogastric area and not in the lesser sac.[8,15]

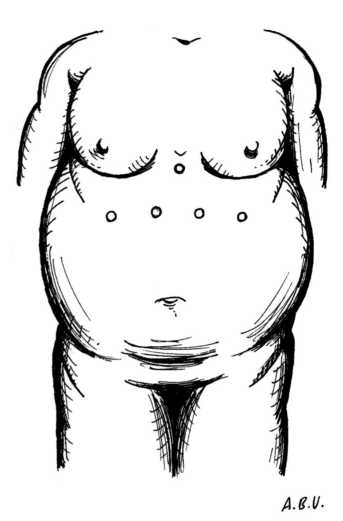

A.B.V.

Figure 25–1. Trocar placement for laparoscopic SAGB surgery.

Periodically the surgeon, particularly if inexperienced, should pause to look for the gauze located in the angle of His to verify the correct direction of dissection and to avoid entering the mediastinum. A blunt dissector passes without difficulty and one can identify the gauze in the angle of His. In patients with a large hiatal hernia and/or chronic esophagitis, dissection can be very difficult, so caution is appropriate. The lateral and upward traction provided by one of the assistants *must* be gentle; we believe that traumatic traction or dissection and careless use of the monopolar electrocautery during this part of the procedure may result in band erosion.

The SAGB (Fig. 25–2) is carefully introduced through one of the left trocars (which has been enlarged to 18 mm) and its end is grasped with a forceps placed in the retrogastric tunnel to pull it through gently. Once the band is in place, it is secured (Figs. 25–3 and 25–4) and then fixed with 4 to 6 2-0 nonabsorbable gastrogastric sutures (Fig. 25–5). This fixation will prevent band migration and pouch enlargement. By using pre-, intra- and postoperative manometry, our group has shown that the length and pressure of the so-called neosphincter increases after the placement and fixation of the band (Fig. 25–6).[16] No liquid should be left inside the band at this time since this may also contribute to band erosion.

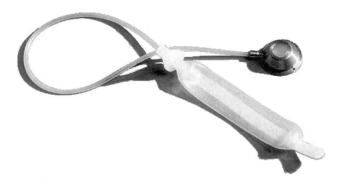

Figure 25–2. The Swedish adjustable gastric band.

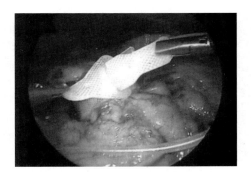

Figure 25–4. The properly secured band.

Finally, the anesthesiologist irrigates the GE junction in order to detect any laceration; hemostasis is done and 30 to 40 mL of bupivacaine is instilled in the subdiaphragmatic space to decrease postoperative shoulder pain.[17] The secured end of the band is extracted in the area chosen for placement of the reservoir (our group usually prefers the lower-most left subcostal trocar site that was also used to introduce the band). The reservoir is sutured to the fascial plane with 4 stitches of 2-0 polydioxanone. This surgical ("pouchless") technique should produce a reservoir with a capacity between 10 and 15 mL; otherwise the patient will not lose weight.[8–14,18]

Subcutaneous nadroparin is administered for 7 days. The patient is offered crushed ice and allowed to walk the evening of the procedure. Usually the patient is discharged between the first and second postoperative day and put on a liquid diet for the next 3 to 4 weeks and given nutritional guidance.

DISCUSSION

Obesity likely results from a genetically predetermined body mass set point that exerts control over body weight through alterations in the basal metabolic rate. This set point may be further influenced by learned eating behavior, perception of body image, socioeconomic status, and the availability of food.[19] The risks of morbid obesity are well known and do not require further discussion.[7,9,20] In a recent report,[21] data were examined from several prospective studies and the researchers concluded that 280,000 annual deaths attributable to obesity occur in the U.S. In addition, the lack of sustained long-term results and the expense of years of trying different types of medical treatment add to the frustration of the obese patient. It is generally accepted that surgical treatment offers the only means of long-term control of the disease and its comorbidities.[7]

The adjustable gastric band was developed in 1981 by Kuzmak.[22] Since then, substantial laparoscopic experience has been obtained, mainly in Europe, where results have been very encouraging.[8,10,23–26] In the U.S., initial evaluation is being carried out in a few centers; initial reports are not as encouraging as those mentioned above, but they appear promising. The learning curve must always be kept in mind.[9,27]

Early reports showed a very low operative mortality rate but a high complication rate (higher than 15%), mainly due to band migration.[11,16,20,23] Initially, band misplacement, malfunction, erosion, and infectious complications resulted in a reoperation rate that reached 18%; with time, morbidity and reoperation rates have dropped to acceptable levels.[24–27] The most frequent complication, migration of the band with enlargement of the pouch, has been practically eliminated by creating a smaller pouch (15 mL), fixing the band with gastrogastric stitches, and never overfilling the balloon (9 mL should be the limit). Larger volumes may also cause gastric wall ischemia, resulting in band erosion into the stomach lumen. If an infection from the injection port reaches the band, erosion may ensue.[28] Band leakage has also been described, and in most cases the band was punctured during surgery, but the authors

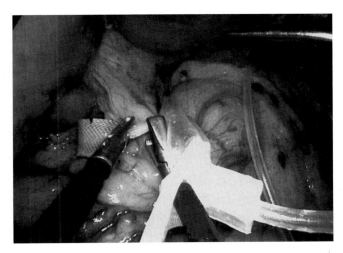

Figure 25–3. The band is secured with its locking mechanism.

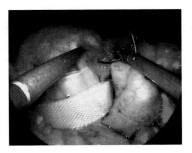

Figure 25–5. The gastrogastric seromuscular sutures prevent migration of the band and produce a plication-like effect.

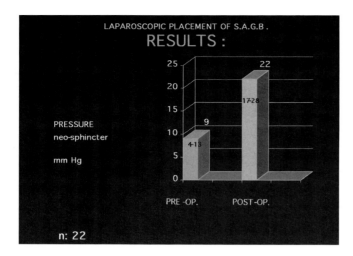

Figure 25–6. Increase in resting pressure of the neosphincter following placement of the SAGB and gastrogastric plication.

had one patient in whom a leak in the balloon was detected more than a year after the operation (at least three adjustments had been previously performed).[29] This was discussed with the manufacturer. Forsell et al[18] described some similar cases.

Patient positioning is very important and adequate padding is essential. One of our patients developed paresthesia in the right arm due to compression of the brachial nerve plexus. A recent report by Fielding et al[2] that followed 335 patients from 1 to 18 months, indicated no mortality, an overall morbidity of 7.4% and an excellent sustained weight loss. Other groups[8,10,13,23–27] have reported similar results.

In patients with previous surgery or chronic esophagitis, dissection could be extremely difficult, and adequate exposure is required to accomplish surgery. If a conversion to laparotomy is to be done, a hand-assisted procedure[30] may be considered first. Our group has used it successfully three times by enlarging the preferred trocar site only 5 to 6 cm.

The most important advantages of the SAGB are the lack of need for stapling, resection, or bypass, and the fact that it is completely reversible. Adjustments are performed on an outpatient basis with local anesthesia.

Some doubts still exist as to the efficacy of the procedure in the extremely obese (BMI >50), although Belachew et al,[10] among others, state that in their experience results are satisfactory (50 to 60% estimated weight loss [EWL] at 2 to 3 years of follow-up). The main disadvantage of the SAGB is the inability to maintain a sustained weight loss in the so-called "sweet-eaters," as in other restrictive operations such as vertical-banded gastroplasty (VBG). In our initial experience, an important issue has been the lack of ability of some patients to abstain from drinking liquids rich in calories after surgery; in fact, surgeons agree that a useful preoperative screening method needs to be found to avoid performing this procedure in these patients.

Another aspect that deserves attention is gastroesophageal reflux disease (GERD), which has a higher prevalence in the obese (37 to 72%).[31] Deitel et al[32] demonstrated that the VBG produced an effective antireflux valve that controlled the symptoms of the disease before a substantial weight loss was achieved. Our group and others have presented evidence gathered by clinical and manometric testing and pH monitoring that by using SAGB, an effective antireflux valve is constructed and the symptoms of GERD are controlled.[14–16] In the 22 patients with GERD symptoms, the resting pressure of the neosphincter increased from 4 to 13 mm Hg (average, 9) to 17 to 28 mm Hg (average, 22), and the intraabdominal esophageal length from 0 to 2.5 cm (average, 1.2) to 2 to 3.2 cm (average, 2.9) (Fig. 25–6). The most likely explanation for those findings probably is the high and snug positioning of the band, and the gastrogastric fixation achieved by placing several seromuscular sutures that produces the plication-like effect responsible for these changes. In the two patients in which the band was removed, manometric studies postoperatively (after band removal) showed resting pressures similar to those obtained after the initial postoperative (after band placement) evaluation, although both patients had significant weight loss. Patients with symptoms of GERD noticed immediate improvement of their symptoms (particularly those related to the respiratory tract). In this regard, it is interesting to mention that Dixon et al[31] reported a significant improvement in asthmatic symptoms in patients who have undergone this procedure.

CONCLUSIONS

Laparoscopic placement of the SAGB is not only feasible, safe, and effective, but it also improves quality of life.[33] The advantages of this approach are its lack of the need for stapling or resection, the fact that it is totally reversible and can be adjusted to the needs of each patient. The well-known advantages of minimally invasive surgery also apply. In short- and intermediate-term follow-up, it has produced adequate and sustained weight loss with very low morbidity and mortality rates. In order to achieve these results, patients must be evaluated carefully, the surgery performed meticulously to avoid preventable complications, and patients closely followed. A properly performed operation will also produce an effective antireflux valve that works independently of the ensuing weight loss. Long-term carefully controlled studies are necessary to establish the efficacy and limitations of the procedure.

REFERENCES

1. Abraham S, Johnson CL. Prevalence of severe obesity in adults in the United States. *Am J Clin Nutr.* 1988;33(2 Suppl):364.
2. Fielding GA, Rhodes M, Nathanson LK. Laparoscopic gastric banding for morbid obesity. *Surg Endosc.* 1999;13:550.
3. Kuczmarski RJ, Carroll MD, Flegal KK, et al. Varying body mass index cutoff points to describe overweight prevalence among U.S. adults: NHANES 11 (1988 to 1994). *Obes Res.* 1997;5:542.
4. Calle EE, Thun MJ, Petrelli JM, et al. Body-mass index and mortality in a prospective cohort of U.S. adults. *N Engl J Med.* 1999;341:1097.
5. Monteforte MJ, Turkelson Ch M. Bariatric surgery for morbid obesity. *Obes Surg.* 2000;10:391.
6. Danford D, Fletcher SW. Methods for voluntary weight loss and control: National Institutes of Health technology assessment. Conference. *Ann Intern Med.* 1993;119;641.
7. National Institutes of Health Consensus Development Conference Panel. Gastrointestinal surgery for severe obesity: Consensus Development Conference Statement. *Ann Intern Med.* 1991;115:956.
8. Forsell P, Hallberg D, Hellers G. A gastric band with adjustable inner diameter for obesity surgery. *Obes Surg.* 1993;3:303.
9. Chae FH. Laparoscopic bariatric surgery. *Surg Endosc.* 1999;513:547.

10. Belachew M, Legrand M, Defechereux T, et al. Laparoscopic adjustable silicone gastric banding in the treatment of morbid obesity: A preliminary report. *Surg Endosc.* 1994;8:1354.
11. Lonroth H, Dalcoback J, Haglind E, et al. Vertical banded gastroplasty by laparoscopic technique in the treatment of morbid obesity. *Surg Laparosc Endosc.* 1996;61:102.
12. Gagner M, Garcia-Ruiz, Area MI, et al. Laparoscopic isolated gastric bypass for morbid obesity. *Surg Endosc.* 1999;13:SI9.
13. Sánchez R, Cueto J, Weber A. Gastroplastía laparoscópica en el tratamiento de la obesidad-mórbida. In: Cueto J, Weber A, eds. *Cirugía Laparoscópica,* 2nd ed. McGraw-Hill Interamericana:1997;131.
14. Cueto J, Sánchez R. The use of the adjustable gastric band in morbid obesity. Second International Symposium, Advanced Laparoscopic Surgery. Baptist Hospital of Miami, July 30, 1998.
15. Cueto J, Sánchez R. Selected problems in minimally invasive surgery for general surgeons. Placement of the Swedish adjustable gastric band in the treatment of morbid obesity. Eighth International Meeting of the Society of Laparoendoscopic Surgeons, New York, December 11, 1999.
16. Cueto J, Vázquez J, Sánchez R. The adjustable gastric band is an effective antireflux valve. Presented at the EAES Meeting in Linz, Austria, July 23–26, 1999.
17. Weber A, Muñoz J, Garteiz D, et al. Use of subdiaphragmatic bupivacaine instillation to control postoperative pain after laparoscopic surgery. *Surg Laparosc Endosc.* 1997;7:6.
18. Forsell P, Hallerback B, Glise H, et al. Complications following Swedish adjustable gastric banding: a long-term follow-up. *Obes Surg.* 1999,9:11.
19. Hacker DC, Deitel M. The etiology of obesity. *Obes Surg.* 1991;1:21.
20. Lee IM, Manson JE, Henneckens CH, et al. Body weight and mortality: A 27 year follow-up of middle-aged men. *JAMA.* 1993;270:2823.
21. Allison DB, Fontaine KR, Manson JE, et al. Annual deaths attributable to obesity in the United States. *JAMA.* 1999;1282:1530.
22. Kuzmak LI. A preliminary report on silicone gastric banding for morbid obesity. *Clin Nutr* 1986;5:73.
23. Angrisani L, Lorenzo M, Esposito G, et al. Laparoscopic adjustable silicone gastric banding: preliminary results of the University of Naples. *Obes Surg.* 1997;7:19.
24. O'Brien PE, Brown WA, Smith A, et al. Prospective study of a laparoscopically placed adjustable gastric band in the treatment of morbid obesity. *Br J Surg.* 1999;86:113.
25. Abu-Abeid S, Szold A. Results and complications of laparoscopic adjustable gastric banding an early and intermediate experience. *Obes Surg.* 1999;9:188.
26. Miller K, Hell E. Laparoscopic adjustable gastric banding; a prospective 4-year follow-up study. *Obes Surg.* 1999;9:183.
27. Greenstein W, Martin L, MacDonald MD, et al. The USA Lap-Band study group. The Lap-band system as surgical therapy for morbid obesity: intermediate results of the USA multicenter, prospective study. *Surg Endosc.* 1999;13:S1.
28. Catona, A, La Manna L, Forsell P. The Swedish adjustable gastric band: Laparoscopic technique and preliminary results. *Obes Surg.* 2000;10:15.
29. Ponson AP, Janssen MI, Klinkenbijl JH. Leakage of adjustable gastric bands. *Obes Surg.* 1999;9:258.
30. Naitoh T, Gagner M, Garcia Ruiz A, et al. Hand-assisted laparoscopic digestive surgery provides safety and tactile sensation for malignancy or obesity. *Surg Endosc.* 1999;13:157.
31. Dixon JB, Chapman L, O'Brien P. Marked improvement in asthma after Lap-Band surgery for morbid obesity. *Obes Surg.* 1999;9:385.
32. Deitel M, Khanna RK, Hagen J, et al. Vertical banded gastroplasty as an antireflux procedure. *Am J Surg.* 1988;155:512.
33. Weiner R, Datz M, Wagner D, et al. Quality-of-life outcome after laparoscopic adjustable gastric banding for morbid obesity. *Obes Surg.* 1999;9:539.

Chapter Twenty-Six ● ● ● ● ● ●

Laparoscopic Roux-En-Y Gastric Bypass for Morbid Obesity

PAOLO GENTILESCHI and MICHEL GAGNER

INTRODUCTION

From 1960 to 1990, the incidence of obesity in American adults increased from 13 to 35%.[1] At present, approximately 4 million people in the United States are severely obese, and 1.5 million are morbidly obese.[2] Morbid obesity is defined as having a BMI (body mass index, determined by dividing body weight expressed in kg by height expressed in meters squared) greater than 40 or a BMI greater than 35 with concomitant obesity-related morbidity. The comorbid conditions that affect the health risks of morbidly obese patients were outlined in a 1985 National Institutes of Health Consensus Conference.[3] These comorbidities include hypertension, diabetes, hypertrophic cardiomyopathy, hyperlipidemia, obstructive sleep apnea, cholelithiasis, venous stasis and thromboembolic disease, degenerative arthritis, certain cancers, and psychosocial consequences. The relationship between BMI and mortality was recently described by the American Cancer Society.[4] In this large, prospective study, the lowest rates of death from all causes were found at BMIs between 22.0 kg/m^2 and 23.4 kg/m^2 in women and 23.5 kg/m^2 and 24.9 kg/m^2 in men. Among healthy patients who had never smoked, the relative risk for all-cause mortality increased with BMIs of approximately 30 kg/m^2 or more.

Nonsurgical methods fail to maintain clinically significant weight loss more than 5 years in morbidly obese patients.[5] Therefore, for the past 30 years, morbidly obese patients have been referred for surgical therapy in order to provide both significant and durable weight loss. Surgery has been shown to be the only effective treatment for morbid obesity on a long-term basis.[6–8] Table 26–1 shows a modification of the Reinhold classification, which can be used to document results of surgical therapy.[9] The excess body weight is the difference between the preoperative weight and ideal body weight.

Many surgical techniques have been described for treating obesity. Operative procedures can be categorized as restrictive or malabsorptive. In the U.S., the two most commonly performed procedures are vertical-banded gastroplasty (VBG), which is a restrictive operation, and Roux-en-Y gastric bypass (RYGB), which is considered a hybrid procedure.

The gastric bypass operation was first described by Mason in 1969,[10] and initially consisted of a loop gastrojejunostomy and a stapled pouch of 10% of gastric volume. Numerous investigators have since introduced modifications, including Roux-en-Y gastrojejunostomy, a reinforced staple line or an isolated gastric pouch (stapled and divided), a smaller pouch (15 to 30 mL), different lengths of Roux limb segments, and various types of banded pouch outlets. Roux-en-Y gastric bypass produces significant weight loss in patients with morbid obesity. Most studies report a weight loss of 60 to 70% of excess body weight (Table 26–2).[6,7,11–13] Long-term weight loss extends to 10 years or longer.[6] In the U.S., Roux-en-Y gastric bypass is the standard by which other bariatric operations are judged.[14]

A laparoscopic approach to RYGB was first described by Wittgrove in 1994.[15] Since then, other investigators have described various techniques of laparoscopic Roux-en-Y gastric bypass (LRYGB), with promising results but relatively short follow-up.[16–20]

In this chapter, we have analyzed in detail the outcomes of RYGB and LRYGB, and discuss both weight loss results and postoperative complications. Our technique for performing LRYGB is also described.

OUTCOMES OF OPEN RYGB FOR MORBID OBESITY

In 1987, Sugerman et al[21] reported the results of a randomized prospective trial comparing RYGB with VBG for morbid obesity. The trial included preoperative dietary separation of "sweet eaters" versus "non-sweet eaters." Randomization was stopped at 9 months because a greater weight loss ($p < 0.05$) was noted after RYGB than VBG. After 3 years, VBG patients had lost 37 ± 20% of

TABLE 26–1. MODIFIED REINHOLD CLASSIFICATION

Result	BMI	Excess Body Weight (%)
Excellent	<30	0–25
Good	30–35	26–50
Failure	>35	>50

excess weight compared with 64 ± 19% of RYGB patients. No significant difference between the loss of excess weight in sweet eaters (69 ± 17%) or non-sweet eaters (67 ± 17%) after RYGB was noted at 1 year. Conversely, sweet eaters who had a VBG lost significantly less excess weight (36 ± 13%) than did non-sweet eaters, who had a VBG (57 ± 18%) (*p* < 0.02), or sweet eaters who had RYGB (*p* < 0.0001). RYGB was therefore clearly superior to VBG for sweet eaters, probably because of the development of symptoms of dumping syndrome.

An interesting prospective randomized study called the Adelaide Study was published in 1990.[22] The results of three bariatric operations, gastrogastrostomy, VBG, and RYGB, were compared in 310 morbidly obese patients. Mean preoperative weight was 198% of the ideal weight (range, 160 to 318%). Patients were randomly submitted to one of the three procedures, with no postoperative deaths. Compliance with follow-up at 3 years was 91%. When success was defined as a loss of more than 50% of excess weight, the success rates at 3 years were 17% for gastrogastrostomy, 48% for VBG, and 67% for RYGB (*p* < 0.001).

In 1994, Brolin et al[8] reported the results of weight loss and dietary intake after VBG and RYGB. Over a 5-year period, 138 patients were prospectively selected for either VBG or RYGB, based on their preoperative eating habits. "Sweet eaters" and "snackers" received RYGB (108 patients), and the remaining 30 underwent VBG. Mean follow-up was 39 ± 11 months after VBG and 38 ± 14 months after RYGB. Mean weight loss peaked at 74 ± 23 lb at 12 months after VBG and 99 ± 24 lb at 16 months after RYGB (*p* < 0.001). Twelve of 30 VBG patients lost >50% of their excess weight versus 100 of 108 RYGB patients (*p* < 0.0001). According to the authors, the results of the study showed that VBG adversely alters postoperative eating behavior toward soft, high-calorie foods, resulting in poor weight loss. Conversely, RYGB caused greater weight loss despite inferior preoperative eating habits.

Pories and colleagues[6] have thoroughly detailed long-term results of Roux-en-Y gastric bypass. Outcomes on weight loss and improvement in comorbidities were extensively analyzed. Over a 14-year period with a 97% follow-up in 608 patients, mean weight loss was 49.2% of preoperative excess body weight. Of 298 glucose-intolerant patients, 271 (91%) maintained normal fasting

glucose levels. In 353 patients with hypertension, only 85 (14%) remained hypertensive. Significant reductions in blood pressure, plasma levels of glucose, triglycerides, and low-density lipoproteins, with an increase in the plasma levels of high-density lipoproteins, were also reported by other investigators.[23]

Recently, MacLean et al[7] reported their experience with 274 RYGB patients, with 243 of them (89%) being followed up for 5.5 ± 1.5 years. Before surgery, 13 patients were obese (BMI 36 to 39 kg/m^2), 134 were morbidly obese (BMI 40 to 49 kg/m^2), and 96 were super-obese (BMI >50 kg/m^2). In the obese and morbidly obese group, the BMI declined from 44 ± 3 kg/m^2 to 26 ± 4 kg/m^2 at 2.1 ± 1.4 years after RYGB. The super-obese group fell from 56 ± 6 kg/m^2 to 31 ± 5 kg/m^2 at 2.3 ± 1.5 years. The final mean BMI was 29 ± 4 kg/m^2 for the obese and morbidly obese group and 35 ± 7 kg/m^2 for the super-obese group. These results revealed a success rate of 93% in obese or morbidly obese patients and 57% in super-obese patients.

Also for super-super-obese patients (BMI >60), RYGB has been shown to produce effective weight loss.[12] In particular, long-limb RYGB resulted in significantly greater weight loss than conventional RYGB, without causing additional metabolic sequelae or diarrhea. Over a 7-year period, Brolin et al[8] prospectively compared two modifications of RYGB in 45 super-super-obese patients (BMI >60): RYGB-1, in which the length of defunctionalized jejunum measured 75 cm, and RYGB-2, in which the defunctionalized jejunum measured 150 cm. Respective mean preoperative BMI was 63.4 for 22 RYGB-1 patients, and 61.6 for 23 RYGB-2 patients. Mean follow-up was 43 ± 17 months. Weight loss stabilized by 24 months at a mean 50% excess weight loss in RYGB-1 patients and 64% excess weight loss in RYGB-2 patients. Nineteen of 23 RYGB-2 patients achieved at least 50% excess weight loss versus 11 of 22 RYGB-1 patients (*p* < 0.03). Weight loss was significantly greater at 24 through 36 months in RYGB-2 patients versus RYGB-1 patients (*p* < 0.02). The authors concluded that the long-limb modification of RYGB is a safe and effective operation in super-super-obese patients.

Early major complications of open RYGB include anastomotic leaks (1.2 to 3.0%), splenic injuries (0.7 to 2.5%), deep venous thrombosis or pulmonary embolism (0.6 to 2.0%), and seromas or wound infections (14.4 to 18.9%).[6–8] Thirty-day mortality ranges from 0.4% to 1.5%.[6–8] The most common late complications of RYGB are gastric outlet stenosis and obstruction (3.4 to 14.6%), marginal ulcer (0.2 to 13.3%), small bowel obstruction (4.7%), incisional hernia (4.7 to 23.9%), and symptomatic gallbladder disease (10 to 11.4%).[24,25] Nutritional deficiencies of iron, vitamins B$_{12}$, A, D, and E, folate, and calcium can occur without supplementation.[24,25] Finally, the revision rate of RYGB ranges from 2 to 15%

TABLE 26–2. OUTCOMES FOR OPEN RYGB

Author	No. Pts.	BMI	ECR (%)	Mortality (%)	Follow-up (mo)	Wt. Loss
Sugerman	182	213% IBW	—	1	12	67% EWL
Brolin[8]	90	62	5	0	43	64% EWL
Poires[6]	608	50	25.5	1.5	168	49% EWL
Fobi[13]	944	46	2.7	0.4	24	80% EWL
MacLean[7]	243	49	—	0.4	66	BMI 29

ECR, early complication rate; EWL, excess weight loss.

of cases, most commonly because of staple line dehiscence, marginal ulcer, outlet stenosis, and insufficient weight loss.[26]

OUR TECHNIQUE FOR LRYGB

This is a detailed description of our surgical technique for LRYGB (Fig. 26–1).

The patient is placed in a supine and reverse Trendelenburg position with the arms extended. The legs are abducted. After placement of intravenous catheters, monitoring devices, and venodyne boots, the patient is endotracheally intubated and general anesthesia is induced. A Foley catheter is inserted. The abdomen is prepped and draped in a standard sterile fashion.

During the first part of the procedure (gastrojejunostomy), the surgeon stands between the patient's legs. The first assistant stands to the right of the patient and the second assistant stands to the left of the patient (Fig. 26–2). During the second part of the operation (jejunojejunostomy) the surgeon stands to the right of the patient, the first assistant stands on the surgeon's left side and the second assistant remains in the same position as in the first part. Two video monitors are placed above the patient's shoulders.

An umbilical incision is made in the skin and brought down through the subcutaneous tissue and fascia. The peritoneum is entered under direct vision and a 10-mm trocar is introduced into the abdomen. Pneumoperitoneum with carbon dioxide insufflation to 15 mm Hg is initiated. A 30° scope is introduced into the peritoneal cavity and initial evaluation is performed. Five additional trocars are inserted under endoscopic visualization. A 10- to 12-mm epigastric port, a 10-mm trocar placed in the midline between the epigastric port and the umbilical port, a 10-mm port in the right subcostal region, a 10- to 12-mm port in the left subcostal region, and a 5-mm port in the left lateral flank are used (Fig. 26–3).

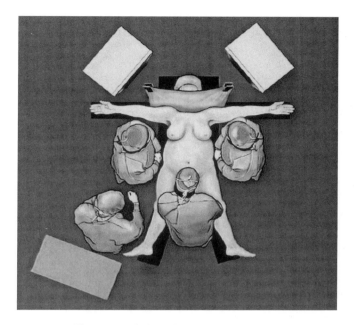

Figure 26–2. Position of surgeon and assistants.

The scope is moved to the trocar in the midline between the umbilicus and epigastrium and the right subcostal port is used for liver retraction with a closed fan retractor. A soft bowel clamp is introduced in the left flank port and used to grasp and pull the stomach laterally. The remaining two trocars, the one in the left subcostal area and the epigastric one, are used for dissection and stapling during the creation of the gastric pouch. The harmonic scalpel (Ethicon Endo-Surgery, Cincinnati, OH) is used to dissect and coagulate.

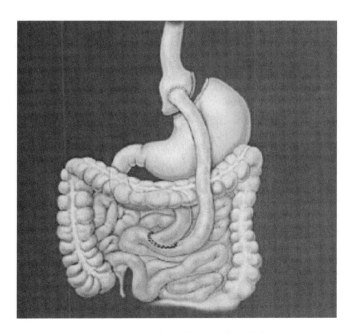

Figure 26–1. The completed Roux-en-Y gastric bypass.

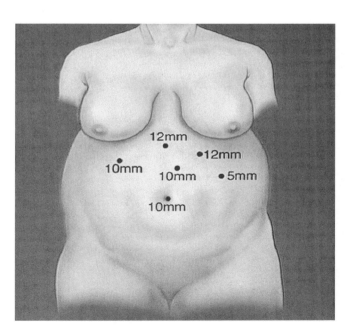

Figure 26–3. Trocar size and positioning.

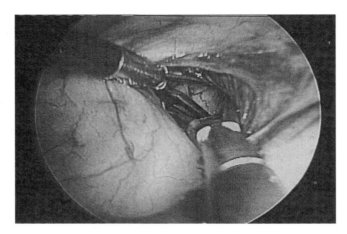

Figure 26–4. Dissection between the gastric branches of the anterior vagus nerve and gastric wall. See Color Section.

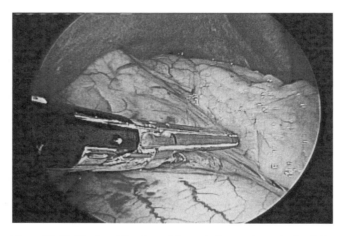

Figure 26–5A. Stapling of the stomach to create the gastric pouch. See Color Section.

With the liver retracted superiorly and the stomach retracted laterally, the dissection starts approximately 3 cm distal of the gastroesophageal junction along the lesser curvature. An opening in the avascular window (usually just distal to the second vein) of the gastrohepatic omentum is created and the dissection is carried out inside the gastric branches of the anterior vagus nerve and branches of the left gastric artery (Fig. 26–4). Particular care must be taken to dissect the retrogastric tunnel between the gastric serosa and vagus nerves, avoiding injuries to vagus nerves and their branches. The dissection is continued posteriorly and superiorly up to the angle of His. The gastric pouch (volume, 10 to 20 mL) is created with sequential firings of a 45-mm 3.5 cutting stapler (Endo-GIA, U.S. Surgical Corp., Norwalk, CT), starting from the anterior opening along the lesser curvature (Fig. 26–5A,B). Exposure is improved by alternating dissection with transection. A small, short posterior gastric artery is usually seen and preserved for the blood supply to the pouch. The first firings are performed with the stapler introduced through the epigastric port, and the last are performed with the stapler moved to the left trocar port for an improved gastric transection towards the angle of His. In this way a small gastric pouch is created, with a volume ranging from 10 to 20 mL (Fig. 26–6). When performing the last firings, care must be taken to avoid injury to the spleen.

At this point, the anvil of a 25-mm circular end-to-end stapler (U.S. Surgical Corp., Norwalk, CT) is prepared for placement by removing the spring (by depressing the base plate). The anvil is flipped, inserted in the open end of a nasogastric tube, and secured with a 2-0 polypropylene stitch that is passed between the holes of the anvil and the tube (Fig. 26–7).

The nasogastric tube is coated with lubricating jelly and inserted per os by the anesthesiologist with blunt end first (with the anvil attached to the other end as described above). The nasogastric tube is advanced into the gastric pouch by the anesthesiologist under laparoscopic visualization. A small hole is created at the staple line of the pouch and the nasogastric tube is gently grasped and pulled out (Fig. 26–8, 26–9, and 26–10). The tube is pulled through the left operating port, clamped extracorporeally, and cut. The harmonic scalpel is used to detach the tube from the anvil and the last portion of the tube is finally removed.

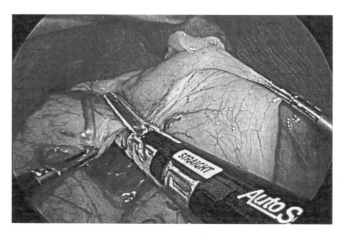

Figure 26–5B. Further stapling of the stomach to create the gastric pouch. See Color Section.

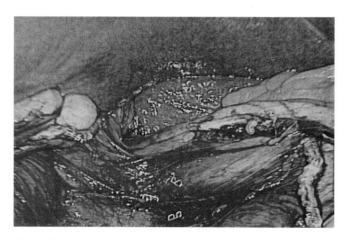

Figure 26–6. Completed separation of the proximal gastric pouch from the distal portion. See Color Section.

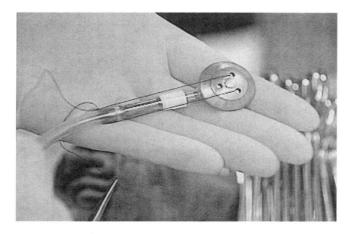

Figure 26–7. The anvil is flipped and secured to the nasogastric tube.

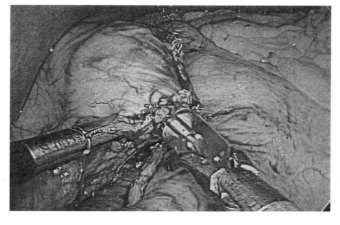

Figure 26–9. The nasogastric tube is grasped and pulled into the abdominal cavity. See Color Section.

The greater omentum is then transected in order to create a window for the Roux limb down to the transverse colon.

Attention then turns to the ligament of Treitz, which is reached by superiorly retracting the transverse colon. A precut 50-cm umbilical tape is used to measure the desired length of small bowel from the ligament of Treitz (Fig. 26–11). A 50-cm segment is chosen in patients with BMI <50, and a 100-cm tract is chosen in patients with BMI >50. Care must be taken to stretch the bowel along the umbilical tape when performing the measurements in order to avoid longer limbs. The small bowel is divided with a linear stapler (Endo-GIA, U.S. Surgical Corp., Norwalk, CT) (Fig. 26–12). The mesentery is also divided at the stapling point to allow better movement of the jejunum. The staple line of the distal limb is resected with the harmonic scalpel. The left operating trocar site is enlarged to allow the introduction of the stapler. The 25-mm circular stapler is first prepared by taping a plastic camera drape around the distal shaft and then introduced into the abdomen (Fig. 26–13). The stapler is passed into the lumen of the distal bowel and advanced to a point approximately 5 cm from the end of the bowel (Fig. 26–14). The spike is advanced through the intestinal wall and the sharp end is detached and re-

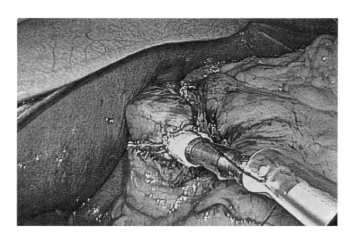

Figure 26–10. The nasogastric tube is pulled until the anvil appears through the staple line. See Color Section.

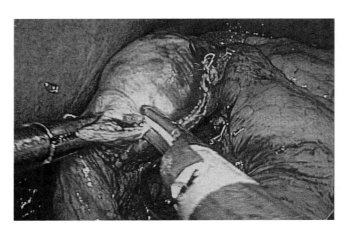

Figure 26–8. The staple line is opened with the harmonic scalpel. See Color Section.

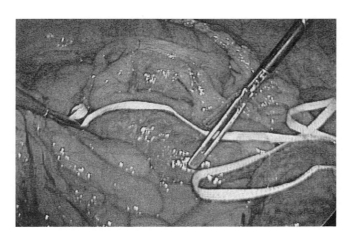

Figure 26–11. Roux limbs are measured with a precut umbilical tape. See Color Section.

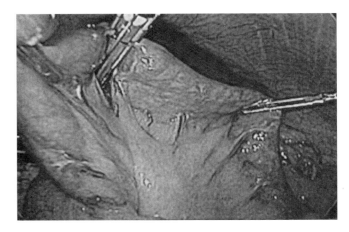

Figure 26–12. The bowel is transected with a stapler. See Color Section.

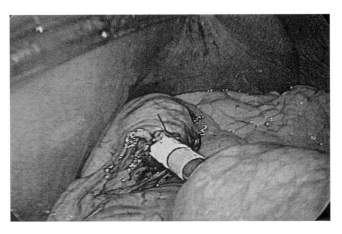

Figure 26–15. The stapler is brought up to the staple line to perform the gastrojejunostomy. See Color Section.

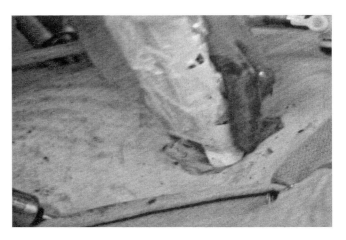

Figure 26–13. The circular stapler is introduced into the abdominal cavity.

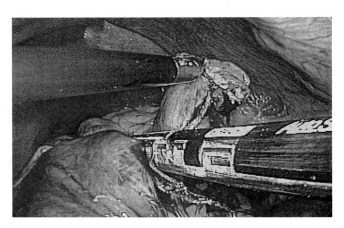

Figure 26–16. The remaining jejunal loop is transected with a stapler. See Color Section.

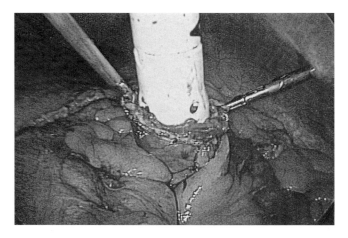

Figure 26–14. The circular stapler is introduced into the jejunal loop. See Color Section.

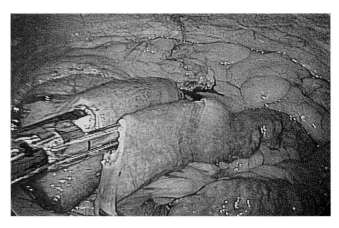

Figure 26–17. A side-to-side jejunojejunostomy is performed with a stapler. See Color Section.

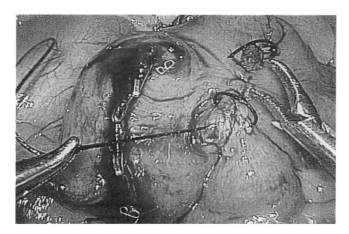

Figure 26–18. The enterotomies are closed with a running suture. See Color Section.

moved. The stapler and the bowel are moved toward the anvil in an antecolic end-to-side fashion and the stapler is attached to the anvil and fired (Fig. 26–15). The circular stapler is removed together with the plastic drape to prevent contamination of the wound. The end of the bowel is closed with an Endo-GIA stapler and the remaining intestine is removed with an endobag (U.S. Surgical Corp., Norwalk, CT) (Fig. 26–16). The integrity of the gastrojejunostomy is tested by injecting 50 mL of methylene blue through an orogastric tube while closing the distal efferent limb with a bowel clamp. If an anastomotic leak is observed, additional stitches using 2-0 silk and intracorporeal suturing and knot-tying technique are mandatory. Once the integrity of the gastrojejunostomy has been confirmed, the methylene blue is aspirated and the orogastric tube removed.

The remaining steps of the procedure are performed with the surgeon standing on the right side of the patient and the first assistant standing on the left. Again, the umbilical tape is used to measure the desired length of the Roux-en-Y limb (100 cm in patients with BMI <50, 150 cm in patients with BMI >50). An enterotomy is performed at the desired point as well as in the proximally divided bowel. A side-to-side jejunojejunostomy is created with the stapler (Fig. 26–17). The small enterotomies are hand-sewn intracorporeally with a 2-0 silk running suture (Fig. 26–18). The abdomen is irrigated and careful inspection made for signs of bleeding. Two 7-mm Jackson-Pratt drains are placed, one on the right overlying the gastrojejunostomy, and one on the left overlying the jejunojejunostomy. All trocar sites are closed with the use of a suture-passer (Karl Storz Endoscopy, Tuttlingen, Germany) except the umbilical one, which is closed with an open technique.

DISCUSSION

Long-term weight loss outcomes of open RYGB are quite satisfactory.[6] Also the early and late postoperative complication rates after open RYGB are acceptable, although not ideal.[6–8] Morbidly obese patients have significant comorbidity, increasing the risks of postoperative complications. Many of the complications occurring after open RYGB are related to the long abdominal incisions required for access and to the subsequent period of bedrest. Pulmonary, thromboembolic, and wound-related complications are common and can be extremely severe. Extensive laparotomies are also associated with postoperative pain and prolonged ileus, increasing hospital stay.

Since the introduction and development of laparoscopic techniques, many abdominal procedures have been performed laparoscopically, with the positive impact of reducing perioperative complications and improving postoperative recovery.[27] Proven benefits of laparoscopic surgery include shorter hospital stay, quicker return to normal activity, less pain, and better cosmesis. The incidence of incisional hernia is also clearly diminished. Other advantages include less systemic and immunologic stress, reduced adhesion formation, and reduced incidence of ileus.[28] Because morbidly obese patients are at high risk for cardiopulmonary and wound-related complications, the idea of a laparoscopic approach to bariatric surgery came from the need to offer such patients the important benefits derived from a less invasive approach.

Wittgrove first described a laparoscopic approach to RYGB.[15] As shown in Table 26–3, LRYGB has now been performed by various surgeons from many institutions, using different techniques. Briefly, the main differences are in the method of creation of the gastrojejunostomy (hand-sewn, mechanical side-to-side, and mechanical end-to-side), in the position of the gastrojejunostomy (antecolic or retrocolic), and in the length of the Roux limbs.

Early major complications after LRYGB include gastrointestinal leaks, bowel obstruction, intra-abdominal and gastrointestinal bleeding, pneumonia, and pulmonary embolism. In the reported largest series (Table 26–3), gastrointestinal leaks most commonly occurred at the gastrojejunostomy and incidence ranged from 0 to 3%.[16–20] The occurrence of this severe complication seems to be related mainly to the learning curve period rather than to the surgical technique used. Wittgrove et al[15] had a leak rate of 3% in the first 300 patients, and a leak rate of 1% in the last 200 patients. Incidence of bowel obstruction ranged from 0 to 1.5%.[16–20] Bowel obstruction can occur in the early postoperative period, or later because of adhesions. In this case, the surgical technique may have influenced the reported varying rates. In the retrocolic technique, where the jejunal loop is brought up to the gastric pouch through a mesenteric window, small bowel obstruction can result from an internal hernia. The incidence of postoperative

TABLE 26–3. OUTCOMES OF LRYGB FOR MORBID OBESITY

Author	No. Pts.	Complications (%)	LOS	Follow-Up (mo)	Wt. Loss (Mean)
Gagner[16]	52	15.0	4 d	1–36	BMI: preop, 55.5; postop, 34
Lonroth[17]	67	31.0	—	6–24	40.5 kg
Schauer[18]	275	3.3	2 d	1–33	EWL: 77% at 30 mo
Higa[20]	400	15.2	1.6 d	1–22	EWL: 69% at 12 mo
Wittgrove[19]	500	7.8	2.5 d	10–72	EWL: 80% at 60 mo

EWL, excess weight loss; LOS, length of hospital stay (median); preop, preoperatively; postop, postoperatively.

intra-abdominal and gastrointestinal bleeding ranged from 0.25 to 5.9%,[16–20] in most cases coming from the gastric staple line. Pulmonary complications have rarely followed LRYGB. They have ranged from minor and transient problems to severe pulmonary embolism. Only one case of mortality occurred in the series listed in Table 26–3, and it was due to a fatal pulmonary embolus that occurred in a patient whose postoperative period was already complicated by small bowel obstruction, pneumonia, and venous thrombosis, which ultimately caused the embolism.

Incidence of early minor complications after LRYGB has been reported up to 27%,[18] These include pulmonary atelectasis, ileus, genitourinary retention and infection, and wound infection. Late complications and side effects of LRYGB are similar to those after open RYGB. In particular, gastrojejunostomy stenosis has ranged from 4.7 to 5.25% in the largest series, but it is well controlled with endoscopic dilation.[16–20] Other common late complications include marginal ulcers, symptomatic cholelithiasis, and trocar site hernia. Nutritional side effects are similar to the ones after open RYGB, and most frequently include iron deficiency, anemia, and hypokalemia, all of which can be treated by supplementation.

The overall reported morbidity and mortality rates after LRYGB seem to be comparable to those in the open series. Some postoperative complications seem to be associated with the approach used. Early bowel obstruction was not clearly reported in the open series; cardiopulmonary and wound-related early and late complications are very rare after LRYGB, while in the open series they were frequent. For example, in one study of open RYGB that carefully evaluated for wound complications, the incidence was 15%, and the rate of incisional hernia was 16.9%.[24]

In the studies listed in Table 26–3, hospital stay ranged from 1.6 to 4 days. Although average postoperative stay is rarely reported in the open RYGB studies, the laparoscopic approach appears to be associated with faster recovery and quicker return to full activity.

The surgical principles of open and laparoscopic RYGB are essentially the same; therefore long-term weight loss results were expected to be similar. The long-term results shown in Table 26–3 demonstrate successful weight loss outcomes in all the studies. Wittgrove et al,[19] who carried out the longer follow-up (10 to 72 months), reported an average 80% excess weight loss (EWL) at 60 months. As for the comorbidities after LRYGB, Wittgrove reported that the total number of comorbidities was reduced overall by 96%, from 1752 preoperatively to 71 postoperatively.[19] Gastro-esophageal reflux disease, type 2 diabetes mellitus, sleep apnea, hypertension, hypercholesterolemia, hypertriglyceridemia, stress incontinence, and arthritis either disappeared or were ameliorated in most patients.[18,19]

In conclusion, LRYGB seems to be a safer and better alternative to open RYGB. Nevertheless, LRYGB is a challenging operation that takes time to master. As recommended by the American Society of Bariatric Surgeons,[29] "laparoscopic obesity operations should be undertaken only by surgeons who are experienced both in video-laparoscopic techniques and in the complexities of open bariatric operations and the field of morbid obesity."

REFERENCES

1. Alverez-Cordero R. Treatment of clinically severe obesity, a public health problem: Introduction. *World J Surg.* 1998;22:905.

2. Kucamarski RJ. Prevalence of overweight and weight gain in the United States. *Am J Clin Nutr.* 1992;55:495S.

3. Health Implications of Obesity. National Institutes of Health Consensus Development Conference Statement. *Natl Inst Health Consens Dev Conf Consens Statement.* 1985;5:1.

4. Calle EE, Thun MJ, Petrelli JM, et al. Body-mass index and mortality in a prospective cohort of U.S. adults. *N Engl J Med.* 1999;341:1097.

5. Gastrointestinal surgery for severe obesity: National Institutes of Health Consensus Development Conference Statement. *Am J Clin Nutr.* 1992;55:615S.

6. Pories WJ, Swanson MS, Mac Donald KG, et al. Who would have thought it? An operation proves to be the most effective therapy for adult-onset diabetes mellitus. *Ann Surg.* 1995;222:339.

7. MacLean LD, Rhode BM, Nohr CW. Late outcome of isolated gastric bypass. *Ann Surg.* 2000;231:524.

8. Brolin RE, Robertson LB, Kenler HA. Weight loss and dietary intake after vertical banded gastroplasty and Roux-en-Y gastric bypass. *Ann Surg.* 1994;220:782.

9. Reinhold RB. Critical analysis of long-term weight loss following gastric bypass. *Surg Gynecol Obstet.* 1982;155:385.

10. Mason EE, Ito C. Gastric bypass. *Ann Surg.* 1969;170:329.

11. Sugerman HJ, Londrey GL, Kellum JM. Weight loss with vertical banded gastroplasty and Roux-Y gastric bypass for morbid obesity with selective versus random assignment. *Am J Surg.* 1989;157:93.

12. Brolin RE, Kenler HA, Gorman JH. Long-limb gastric bypass in the superobese: a prospective randomized trial. *Ann Surg.* 1991;215:387.

13. Fobi MAL, Lee K, Holness R, et al. Gastric bypass operation for obesity. *World J Surg.* 1998;22:925.

14. Mason EE, Tang S, Renquist KE, et al. National Bariatric Surgery Registry Contributors: A decade of change in obesity surgery. *Obes Surg.* 1997;7:189.

15. Wittgrove AC, Clark CW, Tremblay LJ. Laparoscopic gastric bypass, Roux-en-Y: preliminary report of 5 cases. *Obes Surg.* 1994;4:353.

16. Gagner M, Garcia-Ruiz A, Arca MJ, et al. Laparoscopic isolated gastric bypass for morbid obesity. *Surg Endosc.* 1999;13:S6.

17. Lonroth H. Laparoscopic gastric bypass. *Obes Surg.* 1998;8:563.

18. Schauer PR, Ikramuddin S, Gourash W, et al. Outcomes after laparoscopic Roux-en-Y gastric bypass for morbid obesity. *Ann Surg.* 2000;232:515.

19. Wittgrove AC, Clark CW. Laparoscopic gastric bypass, Roux-en-Y—500 Patients: technique and results, with 3–60 month follow-up. *Obes Surg.* 2000;10:233.

20. Higa KD, Boone KB, Ho T, et al. Laparoscopic Roux-en-Y gastric bypass for morbid obesity. *Arch Surg.* 2000;135:1029.

21. Sugerman HJ, Starkey JV, Birkenhauer R. A randomized prospective trial of gastric bypass versus vertical banded gastroplasty for morbid obesity and their effects on sweets versus non-sweets eaters. *Ann Surg.* 1987;205:613.

22. Hall JC, Watts JM, O'Brien PE, et al. Gastric surgery for morbid obesity. The Adelaide Study. *Ann Surg.* 1990;211:419.

23. Cowan GS, Buffington CK. Significant changes in blood pressure, glucose, and lipids with gastric bypass. *World J Surg.* 1998;22:987.

24. Kellum JM, De Maria EJ, Sugerman FU. The surgical treatment of morbid obesity. *Curr Prob Surg.* 1998;35:791.

25. Printen KJ, Scott D, Mason EE. Stomal ulcers after gastric bypass. *Arch Surg.* 1980;115:525.

26. Wittgrove AC, Clark GW. Laparoscopic gastric bypass, Roux-en-Y: Technique and results in 300 patients with 3–34 month follow-up. Scientific presentation, 6th World Congress of Endoscopic Surgery, Rome, Italy, June 3–6, 1998.

27. Buanes T, Mjaland O. Complications in laparoscopic and open cholecystectomy: a prospective comparative trial. *Surg Laparosc Endosc.* 1996;6:266.

28. Schauer PR, Sirinek KR. The laparoscopic approach reduces the endocrine response to elective cholecystectomy. *Am Surg.* 1995;61:106.

29. Deitel M. Laparoscopic bariatric surgery. *Surg Endosc.* 1997;11:965.

Chapter Twenty-Seven ∙ ∙ ∙ ∙ ∙ ∙

*L*aparoscopic Biliopancreatic Diversion With Duodenal Switch for Morbid Obesity

SUBHASH KINI and MICHEL GAGNER

Morbid obesity has become a health crisis in the United States.[1] The incidence of obesity is rising in the West. The prevalence of obesity in the United States increased from 12% in 1991 to 17.9% in 1998.[2]

Life-threatening comorbidities include coronary artery disease, hypertension, diabetes mellitus, and hyperlipidemia.[3] Other problems include gastroesophageal reflux, biliary lithiasis, degenerative osteoarthritis, hernia, sleep apnea, venous stasis, skin infections, urinary stress incontinence, and socioeconomic and psychiatric problems.[4,5] An increased risk of uterine, breast, and colon cancer is seen with morbid obesity.[6] Data from cohort studies and national statistics suggest that the number of annual deaths attributable to obesity among U.S. adults is approximately 280,000.[2]

Calorie-restriction programs lead to temporary weight loss with return to preprogram weight within 1 to 5 years. An exercise plan should be initiated as long as there is no contraindication. Weight loss through exercise results in weight loss of 2 to 3 kg, but it decreases the chance of rapid postprogram weight gain. Appetite suppressants have been used with limited success. However, there are no pharmacologic agents that have been proven to give a long-term and sustained weight loss.

Vertical banded gastroplasty and Roux-en-Y gastric bypass and biliopancreatic diversion are probably the most popular surgical options in the United States. Gastric banding was recently approved by the FDA. The Roux-en-Y gastric bypass (RYGB) has become the gold-standard obesity surgery in North America, with a percent excess weight loss (EWL) ranging between 50 and 74%.[7–9] Interestingly, this success rate falls short for a subpopulation of patients who are classified as superobese, or those patients with a body mass index (BMI) above 50 kg/m^2 or 225% above ideal body weight (IBW).[10,11] Sugerman et al[12] found that when using less than 40% EWL as the definition for failure, Roux-

en-Y gastric bypass was ineffective in up to 19% of superobese patients, and in fact 31% remained more than 200% above IBW.

The biliopancreatic diversion (BPD) achieves a greater weight loss than RYGB (Table 27–1), and this weight loss is durable.

Scopinaro et al[13] performed the first biliopancreatic diversion in 1976, which was a hybrid of gastric restriction and intestinal malabsorption. The mechanism of initial weight loss relied on gastric restriction (partial gastrectomy, resulting in a 200 to 300-mL pouch), and the weight loss was maintained by selective malabsorption of fat and starch due to diversion of biliary and pancreatic secretions into the distal ileum.

BPD has been found to be an efficient surgical treatment of morbid obesity that allows normal eating habits and despite malabsorption is well tolerated by the great majority of patients.[14,15] This operation appears to result in very satisfactory weight loss, improved quality of life, and a low incidence of complications.[15,16] The average percentage excess body weight (EBW) loss with BPD is more than 75 to 80%.[14,15,17] This weight reduction after BPD is maintained even on long-term follow-up. In a large series, there was a 78% loss of the initial EBW at 12 years follow-up.[13]

Since the first operation many modifications in the technique have taken place. In an effort to reduce the side effects of BPD—such as marginal ulceration and malabsorption of iron, protein, and calcium—the procedure was modified by both Hess and Hess[18] and Marceau et al.[19] These modifications included the addition of a duodenal switch procedure as well as lengthening the common absorptive channel, to create what is now known as the biliopancreatic diversion with duodenal switch (BPD-DS).

The BPD-DS operation consists of a sleeve gastrectomy (restrictive component) followed by division of the ileum 250 cm proximal to the ileocecal valve. The distal end of the small bowel is anastomosed to the duodenum, and the proximal end

179

TABLE 27–1. COMPARISON OF RYGB AND BPD-DS

	RYGB	BDD-DS
No. patients	243	457
Follow up (months)	66 ± 18	51 ± 25
Preoperative BMI	49 ± 7	47 ± 9
Current BMI	31 ± 6	30 ± 7
Weight loss	48 ± 18	46 ± 20
BMI <35 kg/m²	79%	81%

From Marceau P, Hould FS, Potvin M, et al. Biliopancreatic diversion (duodenal switch procedure). *Eur J Gastroenterol Hepatol.* 1999;11:99.

("biliopancreatic limb") anastomosed end-to-side to the distal ileum 50 to 100 cm proximal to the ileocecal junction (Fig. 27–1).

In a series of 440 patients undergoing BPD-DS, Hess and Hess reported 80% EWL at 2 years and 70% EWL at 8 years, with a 0.5% perioperative mortality and 9% morbidity.[18] Similarly, Marceau et al reported 73% EWL at 4 years in a series of 465 patients with a mortality of 1.9%.[19] Because of the consistent results of maintained weight loss between 70 and 80% EBW, and acceptable long-term nutritional complications, BPD-DS has become more widely accepted as a surgical treatment for morbid obesity. Despite its success, patients undergoing BPD or BPD-DS are at higher risk for developing certain metabolic complications such as iron deficiency anemia,[18] protein malnutrition,[20,21] metabolic bone disease,[22,23] and fat-soluble vitamin deficiency.[22,24] These complications can almost always be prevented with supplementation, which has been documented to be inconsistent among practicing bariatric surgeons.[25] Patient compliance plays a significant role in the development of metabolic complications in both BPD and Roux-en-Y gastric bypass[26] and should be assessed through preoperative screening and reinforced on postoperative visits.

This operation has vastly improved the lives of seriously obese patients who have much comorbidity. In one study, all type II diabetics had essentially been cured of their disease.[18]

Despite the impressive results of open BPD-DS, laparotomy in morbidly obese patients continues to carry significant complications.[27] Laparoscopy has the advantage of permitting patients to ambulate early and perform respiratory physiotherapy. In fact, laparoscopy has its greatest impact on those morbidities that occur most frequently in morbidly obese patients: wound[28] and cardiopulmonary

complications. The late complication rate of incisional hernia in morbidly obese patients ranges from 10 to 25% in large series.[11,13,18,29,30] Laparoscopic access has been successfully applied to bariatric surgery and has resulted in effective and safe outcomes. Laparoscopic gastric banding, vertical banded gastroplasty, and gastric bypass have all proven to be beneficial over their open counterparts in reducing hospital stay and recovery time, while experiencing weight loss comparable to the open counterparts.[27,31–37]

Since we have a great number of superobese patients, we attempted to use an operation that would provide the superobese patient with enough maintained weight loss to achieve valid reduction in his or her actuarial mortality risk, and at the same time decrease the morbidities associated with laparotomy (cardiopulmonary insufficiency, thromboembolus, and incisional hernia). Therefore, we chose the BPD-DS as the procedure that could potentially benefit the superobese population, yet minimize wound and cardiopulmonary complications by applying a laparoscopic technique. After gaining significant experience in laparoscopic Roux-en-Y gastric bypass, laparoscopic BPD-DS was first carried out in pigs and then applied clinically. We reported our early results of the first series of morbidly obese patients who underwent laparoscopic BPD-DS.[38]

PATIENT SELECTION

Patient selection is extremely important in the surgical treatment of morbid obesity. This is even more important in the superobese. We follow the guidelines for bariatric surgery as outlined by the NIH Consensus Conference (Table 27–2).[39] All patients are considered for surgery who have a BMI of more than 40, or a BMI between 35 and 40 in the presence of associated disease that is subject to improvement by weight loss (hypertension, diabetes, radiologically proven arthritis, sleep apnea).

All patients fulfill the requirements for bariatric procedures as per the American Society of Bariatric Surgery Consensus:

- Age: 18 to 70 years old.
- Stable obesity for more than 5 years.
- Failure of dietary or drug therapy for more than 1 year.
- Absence of endocrine pathology.
- Comprehension and compliance by the patient.
- No dependency on drugs or alcohol.
- Acceptable operative risks.

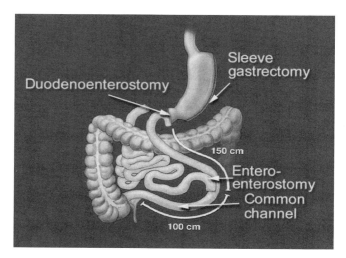

Figure 27–1. BPD-DS after completion of the procedure.

TABLE 27–2. RECOMMENDATIONS OF THE 1991 NIH CONSENSUS DEVELOPMENT CONFERENCE STATEMENT ON GASTROINTESTINAL SURGERY FOR SEVERE OBESITY

1. Patients seeking therapy for the first time should be considered for an integrated nonsurgical program with a dietary regimen, exercise, and behavior modification and support.
2. Well-informed and motivated patients with acceptable risks could be considered for gastric bypass or restrictive procedures.
3. Patients who are candidates should be evaluated by a multidisciplinary team with medical, surgical, psychiatric, and nutritional expertise.
4. A surgeon with substantial experience with the appropriate procedures should perform the surgery, working in a clinical setting capable of supporting all aspects of management and assessment.
5. Lifelong medical surveillance after the procedure is necessary.

From National Institutes of Health. Gastrointestinal surgery for severe obesity: NIH Consensus Development Conference statement. *Am J Clin Nutr.* 1992;55:6155.

Patients are selected for the laparoscopic BPD-DS procedure according to their BMI. All patients with a BMI above 60 kg/m² are offered this procedure with full knowledge of its novelty as performed laparoscopically. Several patients with a BMI below 60 kg/m² have presented to the authors requesting this specific operation.

Patients who are likely candidates for surgery are evaluated by a dedicated team of physicians, nutritionists, and psychiatrists or psychologists before being considered for surgery. Specialist consultations are obtained as indicated.

Esophagogastroduodenoscopy is performed to screen for *H. pylori* and incidental pathology. Pulmonary function tests, sleep apnea study, and cardiac work-up are individualized according to the comorbid conditions present.

Contraindications

The major contraindication is an unacceptable operative risk. The others include:

- Serious psychiatric disorder.
- Unwillingness to cooperate in the long-term follow-up.
- No commitment to accept significant long-term changes in eating habits.
- Inability to maintain a high level of protein intake.

Informed consent is obtained after a detailed explanation of the laparoscopic and open alternatives—their relative risks and benefits including short-term and long-term complications. Patient preparation consists of prophylaxis against deep venous thrombosis and pulmonary embolism by perioperative sequential compression devices; low-dose subcutaneous heparin is used in selected cases.

SURGICAL TECHNIQUE

Our technique of laparoscopic BPD-DS has been described earlier.[38] After placing appropriate monitoring devices and pneumatic compression stocking, patients undergo general anesthesia and endotracheal intubation. All procedures are performed using the French position (legs abducted with the surgeon standing between the patient's legs; Fig. 27–2). Entry into the peritoneal cavity is es-

tablished via the umbilicus using the open technique. A carbon dioxide pneumoperitoneum is created up to 15 mm Hg. Seven trocars are required for each procedure and up to nine have been used. Extralong trocars are occasionally needed in patients who have very thick abdominal walls. The positions of the trocars are shown in Figure 27–3.

The liver is retracted with an unopened nondisposable fan retractor through the most lateral port in the right upper quadrant. The stomach is grasped with a Dorsey bowel clamp, which has been through the most lateral port on the left upper quadrant, and pulled down.

The steps of laparoscopic BPD-DS are outlined in the following sections.

Devascularization of Greater Curve of the Stomach

The gastroepiploic branches and the short gastric vessels, along the greater curvature of the stomach, are divided using the 5-mm ultrasonic scalpel.

Transection of the Pylorus

An opening is created in the lesser sac just superior to the duodenum 1 to 2 cm beyond the pylorus using a right-angle instrument. The duodenum is transected using a 3.5/45-mm linear stapler.

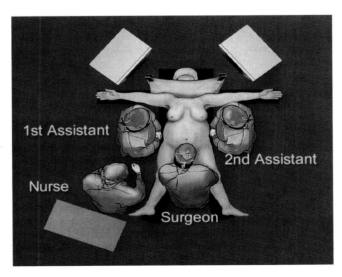

Figure 27–2. Position of patient.

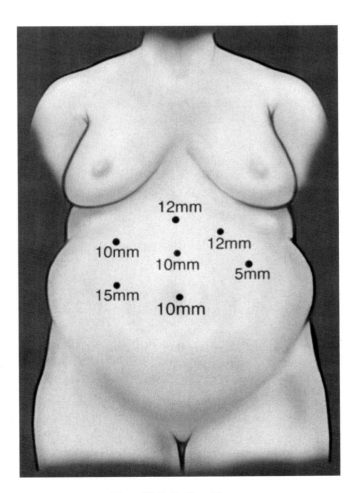

Figure 27–3. Position of trocars.

Sleeve Gastrectomy

A sleeve gastrectomy is performed by sequential firings of a linear stapler parallel to an intragastric 60 French bougie that is positioned along the lesser curvature of the stomach. A 15-mm retrieval bag, coated with mineral oil, is introduced to remove the sleeve gastrectomy specimen. Once the stomach is divided, it is introduced into a bag. The skin incision at the 15-mm port site is enlarged.

Transection of the Small Bowel

The patient is now placed in a Trendelenburg position and turned to the left. The surgeon and first assistant move to the left side of the patient (with the first assistant closer to the head end of the patient than the surgeon). The second assistant stands between the legs of the patient.

A precut 50-cm umbilical tape (with a mark at its midpoint) is used to measure 50 to 100 cm from the ileocecal junction, depending on the BMI of the patient; 75 cm for patients with a BMI below 50 and 100 cm for patients with a BMI of 50 or more (Fig. 27–4). All small bowel measurements are performed under medium-stretch, which we have found to correlate with measurements made by hand via laparotomy within ± 15 cm, using a porcine model. This point is tagged with a silk suture. Another 150 cm is then measured proximal to this silk tag and the small bowel is divided at this point with a linear stapler.

Anastomosis of Upper Segment of Roux Limb to Duodenum

The anvil of a 25-mm circular end-to-end stapler (CEEA®, U.S. Surgical Corporation, Norwalk, CT) is prepared for placement by removing the spring and by depressing the base plate and inserting the anvil in the open end of a nasogastric tube. The anvil is then secured to the nasogastric tube using a 2-0 polypropylene suture and is coated with mineral oil (Fig. 27–5). The nasogastric tube is coated with lubricating jelly and the anesthesiologist passes the nasogastric tube with blunt end first (the anvil is attached to the other end of the nasogastric tube). The jaw thrust maneuver is used to get the anvil through the pharynx.

Next, 5 cm of mesentery is removed with an ultrasonic scalpel. The proximal end of the Roux limb is opened.

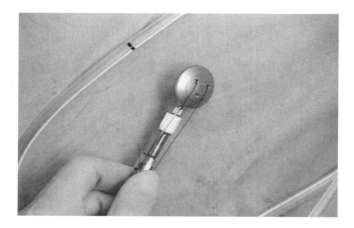

Figure 27–5. Anvil of circular stapler.

The 25-mm circular stapler is prepared by taping a plastic camera drape around the distal shaft and placing a looped 2-0 polypropylene suture through the pin. The drape acts as a wound protector during the removal of the "contaminated" device. The left upper quadrant port site is enlarged and the 25-mm circular stapler is passed transabdominally into the alimentary limb (Figs. 27–6 and 27–7). The alimentary limb is driven up the handle of the circular stapler. The pin is advanced at a point approximately 5 cm from the end of the bowel and the sharp end is detached. The circular stapler is attached to the anvil (Fig. 27–8) that is in the gastroduodenal pouch and the circular stapler is fired. An antecolic end-to-side duodenoenterostomy is thus created. The open end of the Roux limb is stapled close with a linear stapler. The small remnant of small bowel is removed in a bag. The tape is loosened from the sheath of the circular stapler and removed. The circular stapler is withdrawn through the drape.

Checking the Anastomosis

The doughnuts are checked to see that they are complete. A methylene blue test is performed after every duodenoenteric anastomosis to confirm the integrity of all staple lines. This is carried out by injecting 50 mL of methylene blue through an orogastric tube and occluding the alimentary limb with a bowel clamp. Once the

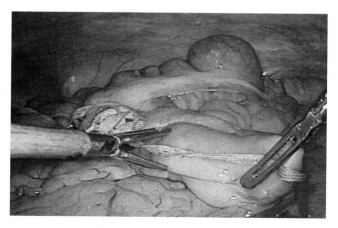

Figure 27–4. Measurement of small bowel. See Color Section.

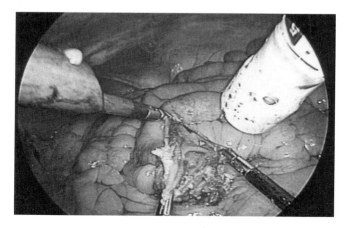

Figure 27–6. Insertion of circular stapler into bowel. See Color Section.

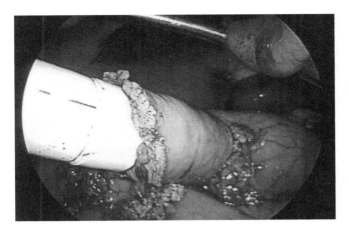

Figure 27–7. Insertion of circular stapler into bowel. See Color Section.

integrity is confirmed, the methylene blue is aspirated and the orogastric tube removed. The size of the gastric pouch is approximated by the volume of methylene blue required to distend the pouch.

Anastomosis of Biliopancreatic Limb to Lower Segment of Roux Limb to Form a 75- to 100-cm Absorptive Common Channel

Enterotomies are made with an ultrasonic scalpel in the side of the bowel of both the biliopancreatic and common limbs. A side-to-side anastomosis is performed with a linear stapler. The small enterotomies are hand sewn intracorporeally with 2-0 silk (Fig. 27–9). Cholecystectomy is performed selectively when stones or sludge are present.

Two soft closed-suction drains are placed at the gastrojejunostomy and enteroenterostomy sites and brought out through port sites: one over the proximal anastomosis and duodenal stump, and one over the distal anastomosis. All of the ports are closed with a fascial closure instrument (Karl Storz, Tuttlingen, Germany).

POSTOPERATIVE CARE

All patients receive a patient-controlled opioid analgesic postoperatively.

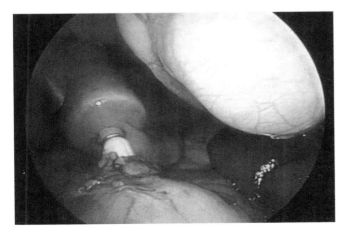

Figure 27–8. Joining the two ends of the stapler. See Color Section.

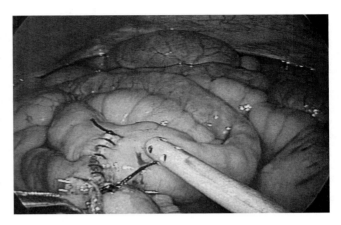

Figure 27–9. Intracorporeal side-to-side anastomosis of small bowel. See Color Section.

A water-soluble (Gastrografin) upper gastrointestinal contrast study is routinely performed on the first postoperative day in all patients. After confirming a normal contrast study, clear liquids and oral analgesics are instituted on the first postoperative day followed by a puree diet on the second postoperative day. Inpatient nutrition consultation, diet advancement, and drain removal are performed before discharge.

The patient is followed up at 3 weeks, 3 months, 6 months, and annually thereafter. All patients receive follow-up nutritional counseling for enriched diet and are given daily multivitamins, oral calcium supplements, iron, and fat-soluble vi-tamins (A, D, E, and K). Patients with an intact gallbladder are prescribed ursodiol (Actigall, Ciba, Summit, NJ) for gallstone prophylaxis.[40] Laboratory evaluation for nutritional deficiencies is performed at each visit beginning at 3 months. This includes iron, ferritin, vitamin B_{12}, folate, albumin, PTH, calcium, phosphorus, alkaline phosphatase, zinc, selenium, manganese, cholesterol profile, triglycerides, occasional vitamin D and A levels, as well as routine electrolyte and hematology panels. Patients are encouraged to attend a monthly support meeting that is attended by the surgeons, nutritional clinical nurse coordinator, and social worker.

OUR INITIAL EXPERIENCE

These are the results of our first 40 patients (Table 27–3). The patients included 12 men and 28 women with a median age of 43

TABLE 27–3. DEMOGRAPHIC PROFILE OF PATIENTS UNDERGOING LAPAROSCOPIC BPD-DS

Demographic	Median Number (Range)
Number	40
Male	12
Female	28
Age (years)	43 (20–67)
Weight (kg)	167 (104–273)
BMI (kg/m²)	60 (41–89)
Degree of obesity:	
BMI 40–49	8 (20%)
BMI 50–64	16 (40%)
BMI >65	16 (40%)

(range, 20 to 67). The median BMI was 60 kg/m² (range, 41 to 89). Of all patients, 75% were considered superobese (BMI above 50). Significant comorbid conditions were present in 75% of patients.

Thirty-nine out of 40 procedures (98%) were successfully completed laparoscopically. One operation was converted to laparotomy due to severe dense adhesions from a previous open cholecystectomy, and technical difficulties that resulted in an unsatisfactory duodenoenteric anastomosis. The operative time ranged from 110 to 360 minutes (median, 210 minutes). In addition to a downward trend in operative time with experience, there is a significant correlation between BMI and operative time.

There was some variation in the common channel length that was constructed: 28 patients had a 100-cm common channel, 11 patients had a 75-cm common channel, and one patient had a 125-cm common channel. Six patients underwent concomitant procedures. The mean blood loss was 150 mL.

The median length of hospital stay was 4 days; the range was 3 to 8 days if two outliers (15 and 210 days) are excluded. The median follow-up was 6 months (range, 1 to 12 months), with a mean weight loss (± SEM) of 33 ± 2 kg (32% ± 2% EWL) at 3 months, 48 ± 3 kg (46% ± 2% EWL) at 6 months, 62 ± 3 kg (58% ± 3% EWL) at 9 months, and 109 ± 0.5 kg (65% ± 1% EWL) at 12 months (Table 27–4).

Complications

Six patients developed seven major complications (15%) and 10 patients developed minor complications (22.5%; Table 27–5). Major morbidity in our series (15%) is comparable to that of other bariatric procedures including open BPD-DS.

Mortality. There was one 30-day mortality within the series (2.5%). One patient (male, BMI 66) died on the 10th postoperative day from respiratory arrest. His comorbidities included NIDDM and obstructive sleep apnea. His hospital course was uncomplicated and he was discharged on the fourth postoperative day. After being transported by ambulance to an outside hospital on the 10th postoperative day the patient suffered respiratory arrest, with several unsuccessful attempts at resuscitation. Autopsy revealed intact anastomoses, possible intra-abdominal infection, and no evidence of pulmonary emboli or infection.

There was one late death in this series. This patient (female, BMI 85) experienced a protracted hospital course after developing necrotizing fasciitis, multiorgan system failure, and sepsis following anastomotic leak, and finally succumbed 6 months after surgery. Her comorbidities included hypertension and obstructive sleep apnea for which she was CPAP-dependent (continuous positive airway pressure) when lying flat. In addition, the patient had been nonambulatory due to her body habitus and pulmonary status.

TABLE 27–4. EARLY WEIGHT LOSS AFTER LAPAROSCOPIC BPD-DS

	3 Months (n = 35)	6 Months (n = 19)	9 Months (n = 1)	12 Months (n = 3)
Mean weight lost (kg ± SEM)	33 ± 2	48 ± 3	62 ± 3	109 ± 0.5
Mean % excess weight loss (% EWL ± SEM)	32 ± 2%	46 ± 2%	58 ± 3%	65 ± 1%

TABLE 27–5. COMPLICATIONS

Major Morbidity	**15%**
Anastomotic leak rate	2.5%
Anastomotic leak	2.5%
Hemorrhage	10%
Abscess	2.5%
Minor Complications	**22.5%**
Abdominal with hematoma	2.5%
Wound infections	15%
Atelectasis	2.5%
Cholecystitis	2.5%
Trocar site hernia	2.5%

EWL, excess weight loss; SEM, standard error of the mean.

Anastomotic Leak. The methylene blue test was positive for intraoperative leak in 2 patients. One leak was repaired with intracorporeal sutures and a subsequent methylene blue test was negative. The second patient was converted to an open procedure in order to revise the proximal anastomosis after unsuccessful intracorporeal repair. The latter patient was a man with a BMI of 67 who had a previous laparotomy for cholecystectomy and was found to have exten-sive adhesions. Hand-assisted laparoscopy was attempted but exposure was inadequate for successful repair of the posterior anastomotic leak. This patient did well postoperatively except for the development of a wound infection.

All postoperative upper gastrointestinal studies were negative, with no evidence of leak at the proximal anastomosis.

Despite a negative Gastrografin study, there was one anastomotic leak, detected 1 week postoperatively secondary to suspicious drainage from a drain, which was surgically revised.

Thromboembolism. One patient with postoperative deep venous thrombosis (DVT) developed upper gastrointestinal bleeding after overanticoagulation. He was treated nonoperatively with endoscopy and a vena caval filter.

Hemorrhage. Three additional patients developed hemorrhage from the staple line. One patient was reexplored laparoscopically on the first postoperative day, and the only finding was a clot along the gastrectomy staple line. The second patient had active bleeding at the proximal anastomosis on postoperative day 7 that was controlled endoscopically with an epinephrine injection, and one patient had a gradual hematocrit drop from 32 to 22% over the course of 3 days, with blood in her drains. She was treated conservatively without blood transfusions and had an unremarkable course thereafter.

Subphrenic Abscess. One patient returned 3 weeks after surgery with fever and left shoulder pain. After a CT scan diagnosed a subphrenic abscess, it was successfully treated with percutaneous drainage and antibiotics.

Conversion. When looking at major morbidity and mortality in comparison to patient BMI, there was a higher complication rate in the patients with a BMI of 65 or more. In the 16 patients with a BMI of 65 or more, the complication rate was 38%. Conversely, the complication rate for patients with a BMI of 40 to 64 was 8.3% (Table 27–6).

Minor Complications. Table 27–5 lists minor complications. In our early experience, laparoscopic BPD-DS has proven to be

TABLE 27–6. MAJOR COMPLICATIONS ACCORDING TO PATIENT BMI

	BMI < 65	BMI ≥ 65
No. patients	24	16
Major morbidity	2	4[1]
Conversion	0	1
Mortality	0	2[2]
TOTAL	2 (8.3%)	

[1]One patient experienced two complications (DVT, hemorrhage), and therefore counted as one morbidity.

[2]Early anastomotic leak is counted under mortality.

feasible with successful completion in 39 of 40 patients. With experience, operative time quickly decreased from 330 minutes for the first case to a mean of 210 minutes, with a significant correlation between operative time and patient BMI.

Improvement in Comorbidity

Of the 9 patients who were diabetic (one insulin-dependent) requiring medication, all nine were normoglycemic and off all medications at 3 months (100%). There was an overall improvement in comorbidities at 3-month follow-up, with the majority of patients experiencing complete resolution of their problems such as hypertension (80%), hypercholesterolemia (55%), and sleep apnea (70%).

Anastomotic Leak

Our anastomotic leak rate of 2.5% is comparable to the open BPD-DS series, which ranges between 2 and 5%.[18,19,41] Despite attempts to diagnose leak with routine diagnostic examinations, our one anastomotic leak occurred 7 days after surgery in a patient who was bedridden and who had predominant truncal distribution of adipose tissue with a massive abdominal pannus extending below her knee. Due to the adverse outcome in this patient we now consider the bedridden patient to be contraindicated for laparoscopic BPD-DS.

Hemorrhage

Bleeding in 3 out of 4 patients occurred at a staple line while they were on some form of anticoagulation. We initially placed all patients on prophylactic subcutaneous or low-molecular-weight heparin. The first patient was over-anticoagulated for DVT, as mentioned previously. After the second patient was found to have bleeding along the gastric staple line, we changed the size of the stapler used on the sleeve gastrectomy. The distal thicker antrum was still divided with a 4.8 linear stapler; however, division of the thinner gastric body and fundus was felt to be more hemostatic using a 3.5 linear stapler. After the third patient had a bleeding complication at the proximal anastomotic line, heparin use was reevaluated. Only sequential compression devices (SCDs) and early ambulation were instituted as prophylaxis.

Thromboembolic Prophylaxis

The issue of thromboembolic prophylaxis is brought to the forefront once again and has proven its advantages and disadvantages in our small series, as it has in the experience of others. Although the incidence of postoperative thromboembolic events ranges from 1 to 3% in most recent bariatric series,[9,42,43] the incidence of thromboembolism does not seem to be altered by routine use of prophylaxis as documented by Eriksson et al.[43] A recent survey of members of the American Society for Bariatric Surgery (ASBS) showed that 95% of surgeons used prophylaxis: 65% used some form of anticoagulation and 33% used SCDs.[42] Unfortunately, this article is representative of only 31% (or 128 surgeons) of ASBS members surveyed, the majority of whom perform open bariatric procedures where patients may be at higher risk for thromboembolism. The effect of laparoscopy on the incidence of thromboembolic events is unclear. However, the incidence of thromboembolism has been observed to be reduced in laparoscopic cholecystectomy when compared to open cholecystectomy,[44] as is mortality.[45–47] Although there is increased venous stasis with the application of pneumoperitoneum and a potentially longer operative time, patients ambulate much earlier after laparoscopic surgery. In addition, although obese patients are at a higher risk for thromboembolism, they are still classified as a moderate risk group by the standards of the 1997 International Consensus Statement for the prevention of venous thromboembolism.[48] According to this statement, SCDs are recommended as a safe and effective antithrombotic measure. SCDs are also recommended for those higher-risk general surgery patients who are prone to bleeding, which may characterize the population undergoing laparoscopic BPD-DS. Alternatively, morbidly obese patients who are considered high risk (obesity-hypoventilation syndrome, previous thromboembolic event) may benefit from a vena cava filter. The emerging role of low-molecular weight heparin (LMWH) is controversial, but it may be advantageous due to its higher efficacy and lower rate of bleeding when compared to unfractionated heparin.[49,50] However, because of the increased incidence of bleeding in our series, we routinely use SCDs and early ambulation for patients undergoing laparoscopic BPD-DS, which we have found to be effective.

Wound Infection

The rate of wound infection was higher than expected. All patients were treated with opening of the infected trocar site, wound packing, and oral antibiotics. All resolved uneventfully, except one that developed into necrotizing fasciitis as described. One wound infection occurred at the laparotomy site in the converted patient. All other infections occurred in the right upper quadrant trocar site through which the circular stapler is passed. Infection rates of all classes of surgical wounds are higher in the morbidly obese patient.[51] In addition, pharmacokinetics of various antibiotics have been shown to be altered in obese patients as compared to controls.[11,12,29]

Therefore, increasing the frequency and dosage of preoperative and intraoperative prophylactic antibiotics is recommended. Forse et al[52] found that only by doubling the preoperative cefazolin dose to 2 g IV, would minimal inhibitory concentrations for gram-positive and gram-negative bacteria be reached in the serum and adipose tissue of morbidly obese patients. In fact, the cephalosporins should be redosed every 3 hours from time of skin incision to ensure maintenance of serum levels and even be continued for several doses postoperatively.[53] These pharmacokinetic studies were performed on patients with BMIs ranging between 40 and 50 kg/m². The 6 patients (15%) who developed wound infections had BMIs ranging from 50 to 80 kg/m². Although broad-spectrum antibiotics with dosage corrected for weight were administered pre-operatively, contamination from the enteric contents of the circular stapler is the most likely source of infection. The rate of wound infection subsequently decreased after we instituted the use of a plastic sleeve around the stapler to protect the wound from contamination.

High BMI Is Not an Absolute Contraindication

When looking at major morbidity, mortality, and conversion, there is a higher rate of complication in patients with a BMI of 65 or more when compared to those with a BMI below 65 (38% versus 8.3%). One must weigh the increased morbidity and mortality of superobese patients with associated comorbidities against the risk of surgery. We operated on several patients who were superobese with various comorbidities (4 of whom had a BMI above 80) who had no complications. Although there is no documentation in the bariatric literature correlating postoperative morbidity and BMI, it is recognized by bariatric surgeons that superobese patients carry a higher perioperative morbidity and mortality rate. In fact, the complication rate correlates with increased weight in nonbariatric surgery as well. Women weighing over 300 lbs were found to have a 20% mortality rate after surgery for uterine neoplasms, in comparison to women who weighed between 200 and 250 pounds, who had a 2% mortality rate.[54] Therefore, we cannot conclude that there is a specific maximum BMI above which surgery is contraindicated, but the existence of serious comorbidities in superobese patients certainly correlates with higher surgi-cal risk.

SUMMARY

In our short follow-up, weight loss has been significant and comparable to open data. The majority of patients have experienced complete resolution or improvement of their comorbid conditions, with 100% of diabetic patients and 80% of hypertensive patients off all medication. All patients are closely followed clinically and with laboratory studies. Thus far, 4 patients (10%) have had low iron levels that responded to increased supplementation and 5 patients (12.5%) were found to have elevated parathyroid hormone (PTH) levels with normal calcium levels.

Few studies report on laparoscopy in the superobese patient. Our preliminary results are acceptable, considering that the superobese patient carries a higher risk, the procedure is technically complex, and this initial experience includes familiarization with laparoscopic maneuvers specific to this operation, which have not been previously described. Caution still must be maintained with the superobese patient who has serious comorbidities. Patient selection (BMI below 65) or alternative preoperative strategies may be necessary to decrease major complications in advanced laparoscopic BPD-DS.

Laparoscopic BPD-DS appears to have many advantages in terms of quicker recovery time and shorter hospital stay, with comparable morbidity when compared to open BPD-DS. However, the procedure itself is technically complex and difficult. The longer operative time, in addition to the greater number of staplers required, may result in a more costly procedure than laparoscopic gastric bypass. Laparoscopic BPD-DS carries with it a greater risk of intra-operative and early postoperative bleeding, due to the extensive gastric staple line that is creased with the sleeve-

gastrectomy. The mortality and major morbidity rate is high and appears to be related more to the extent and morphology of obesity. In fact, it may be that the superobese patient with "android"-type (truncal obesity) morphology would fare better with an open technique, as compared to the "gynecoid"-type patient who would benefit from a laparoscopic technique.

REFERENCES

1. Balsiger BM, Murr MM, Poggio JL, et al. Bariatric surgery. Surgery for weight control in patients with morbid obesity. *Med Clin North Am.* 2000;84:477.
2. Allison DB, Fontaine KR, Manson JE, et al. Annual deaths attributable to obesity in the United States. *JAMA.* 1999;282:1530.
3. Mason EE, Doherty C, Cullen JJ, et al. Vertical gastroplasty: Evolution of vertical banded gastroplasty. *World J Surg.* 1998;22:919.
4. Doldi SB, Lattuada E, Zappa MA, et al. Biliointestinal bypass: Another surgical option. *Obes Surg.* 1998;8:566.
5. NIH Conference. Gastrointestinal surgery for severe obesity. Consensus Development Conference Panel. *Ann Intern Med.* 1991;115:956.
6. Sugerman HJ. Surgery for morbid obesity. *Surgery.* 1993;114:865.
7. Benotti PN, Forse RA. The role of gastric surgery in the multidisciplinary management of severe obesity. *Am J Surg.* 1995;169:361.
8. Brolin RE. Gastrointestinal surgery for obesity. *Semin Gastrointest Dis.* 1998;9:163.
9. Pories WJ, Swanson MS, MacDonald KG, et al. Who would have thought it? An operation proves to be the most effective therapy for adult-onset diabetes mellitus. *Ann Surg.* 1995;222:339.
10. MacLean LD, Rhode BM, Sampalis J, et al. Results of the surgical treatment of obesity. *Am J Surg.* 1993;165:155.
11. MacLean LD, Rhode BM, Nohr CW. Late outcome of isolated gastric bypass. *Ann Surg.* 2000;231:524.
12. Sugerman HJ, Londrey GL, Kellum JM, et al. Weight loss with vertical banded gastroplasty and Roux-Y gastric bypass for morbid obesity with selective versus random assignment. *Am J Surg.* 1989;157:93.
13. Scopinaro N, Adami GF, Marinari GM, et al. Biliopancreatic diversion. *World J Surg.* 1998;22:936.
14. Hell E, Miller KA, Moorehead MK, et al. Evaluation of health status and quality of life after bariatric surgery: Comparison of standard Roux-en-Y gastric bypass, vertical banded gastroplasty and laparoscopic adjustable silicone gastric banding. *Obes Surg.* 2000;10:214.
15. Totte E, Hendrickx L, van Hee R: Biliopancreatic diversion for treatment of morbid obesity: Experience in 180 consecutive cases. *Obes Surg.* 1999;9:161.
16. Baltasar M, Bou R, Cipagauta LA, et al. "Hybrid" bariatric surgery: Bilio-pancreatic diversion and duodenal switch. Preliminary experience. *Obes Surg.* 1995;5:419.
17. Cossu ML, Coppola M, Fais E, et al. Preliminary results of biliopancreatic diversion in the treatment of morbid obesity. Clinical considerations on 69 patients with a 3-year follow-up. *Minerva Chir.* 2000;55:211.
18. Hess DS, Hess DW. Biliopancreatic diversion with a duodenal switch. *Obes Surg.* 1998;8:267.
19. Marceau P, Hould FS, Simard S, et al. Biliopancreatic diversion with duodenal switch. *World J Surg.* 1998;22:947.
20. Gianetta E, Friedman D, Adami GF, et al. Etiological factors of protein malnutrition after biliopancreatic diversion. *Gastroenterol Clin North Am.* 1987;16:503.
21. Grimm IS, Schindler W, Haluszka O. Steatohepatitis and fatal hepatic failure after biliopancreatic diversion. *Am J Gastroenterol.* 1992;87:775.
22. Chapin BL, LeMar HJ, Knodel DH, et al. Secondary hyperparathyroidism following biliopancreatic diversion. *Arch Surg.* 1996;131:1048.

23. Compston JE, Vedi S, Gianetta E, et al. Bone histomorphometry and vitamin D status after biliopancreatic bypass for obesity. *Gastroenterology*. 1984;87:350.

24. Smets RM, Waeben M. Unusual combination of night blindness and optic neuropathy after biliopancreatic bypass. *Bull Soc Belge Ophtalmol*. 1999;271:93.

25. Brolin RE, Leung M. Survey of vitamin and mineral supplementation after gastric bypass and biliopancreatic diversion for morbid obesity. *Obes Surg*. 1999;9:150.

26. Brolin RE, Gorman JH, Gorman RC, et al. Are vitamin B_{12} and folate deficiency clinically important after roux-en-Y gastric bypass? *J Gastrointest Surg*. 1998;2:436.

27. Chae FH, McIntyre RC. Laparoscopic bariatric surgery. *Surg Endosc*. 1999;13:547.

28. Sugerman HJ, Kellum JM, Reines HD, et al. Greater risk of incisional hernia with morbidly obese than steroid-dependent patients and low recurrence with prefascial polypropylene mesh. *Am J Surg*. 1996;171:80.

29. MacLean LD, Rhode BM, Forse RA. Late results of vertical banded gastroplasty for morbid and super obesity. *Surgery*. 1990;107:20.

30. Brolin RE. Prospective, randomized evaluation of midline fascial closure in gastric bariatric operations. *Am J Surg*. 1996;172:328.

31. Belachew M, Legrand M, Vincent V, et al. Laparoscopic adjustable gastric banding. *World J Surg*. 1998;22:955.

32. De Wit LT, Mathus-Vliegen L, Hey C, et al. Open versus laparoscopic adjustable silicone gastric banding: A prospective randomized trial for treatment of morbid obesity. *Ann Surg*. 1999;230:800.

33. Fielding GA, Rhodes M, Nathanson LK. Laparoscopic gastric banding for morbid obesity. Surgical outcome in 335 cases. *Surg Endosc*. 1999;13:550.

34. Lonroth H, Dalenback J, Haglind E, et al. Vertical banded gastroplasty by laparoscopic technique in the treatment of morbid obesity. *Surg Laparosc Endosc*. 1996;6:102.

35. Wittgrove AC, Clark GW. Laparoscopic gastric bypass, Roux-en-Y-500 patients: Technique and results, with 3–60 month follow-up. *Obes Surg*. 2000;10:233.

36. Fried M, Peskova M, Kasalicky M. The role of laparoscopy in the treatment of morbid obesity. *Obes Surg*. 1998;8:520.

37. Schauer PR, Ikramuddin S, Gourash W, et al. Outcomes after laparoscopic roux-en-Y gastric bypass for morbid obesity. *Ann Surg*. 2000;232:515.

38. Ren CJ, Patterson E, Gagner M. Early results of laparoscopic biliopancreatic diversion with duodenal switch: A case series of 40 consecutive patients. *Obes Surg*. 2000;10:514.

39. National Institutes of Health. Gastrointestinal surgery for severe obesity: NIH Consensus Development Conference statement. *Am J Clin Nutr*. 1992;55:615S.

40. Broomfield PH, Chopra R, Sheinbaum RC, et al. Effects of ursodeoxycholic acid and aspirin on the formation of lithogenic bile and gallstones during loss of weight. *N Engl J Med*. 1988;319:1567.

41. Rabkin RA. Distal gastric bypass/duodenal switch procedure, Roux-en-Y gastric bypass and biliopancreatic diversion in a community practice. *Obes Surg*. 1998;8:53.

42. Wu EC, Barba CA. Current practices in the prophylaxis of venous thromboembolism in bariatric surgery. *Obes Surg*. 2000;10:7.

43. Eriksson S, Backman L, Ljungstrom KG. The incidence of clinical postoperative thrombosis after gastric surgery for obesity during 16 years. *Obes Surg*. 1997;7:332.

44. Sarli L, Pietra N, Sansebastiano G, et al. Reduced postoperative morbidity after elective laparoscopic cholecystectomy: Stratified matched case-control study. *World J Surg*. 1997;21:872.

45. Steiner CA, Bass EB, Talamini MA, et al. Surgical rates and operative mortality for open and laparoscopic cholecystectomy in Maryland. *N Engl J Med*. 1994;330:403.

46. Hannan EL, Imperato PJ, Nenner RP, et al. Laparoscopic and open cholecystectomy in New York State: Mortality, complications, and choice of procedure. *Surgery*. 1999;125:223.

47. Shea JA, Healey MJ, Berlin JA, et al. Mortality and complications associated with laparoscopic cholecystectomy. A meta-analysis. *Ann Surg*. 1996;224:609.

48. Nicolaides AN, Arcelus J, Belcaro G, et al. Prevention of venous thromboembolism. European Consensus Statement, 1–5 November 1991, developed at Oakley Court Hotel, Windsor, UK. *Int Angiol*. 1992;11:151.

49. Hull RD, Pineo GF. Prophylaxis of deep venous thrombosis and pulmonary embolism. Current recommendations. *Med Clin North Am*. 1998;82:477.

50. Kakkar VV, Boeckl O, Boneu B, et al. Efficacy and safety of a low-molecular-weight heparin and standard unfractionated heparin for prophylaxis of postoperative venous thromboembolism: European multicenter trial. *World J Surg*. 1997;21:2.

51. Bates T, Roberts JV, Smith K, et al. A randomized trial of one versus three doses of Augmentin as wound prophylaxis in at-risk abdominal surgery. *Postgrad Med J*. 1992;68:811.

52. Forse RA, Karam B, MacLean LD, et al. Antibiotic prophylaxis for surgery in morbidly obese patients. *Surgery*. 1989;106:750.

53. Mann HJ, Buchwald H. Cefamandole distribution in serum, adipose tissue, and wound drainage in morbidly obese patients. *Drug Intell Clin Pharm*. 1986;20:869.

54. Prem KA, Mensheha NM, McKelvey JL. Operative treatment of adenocarcinoma of the endometrium in obese women. *Am J Obstet Gynecol*. 1965;92:16.

55. Marceau P, Hould FS, Potvin M, et al. Biliopancreatic diversion (duodenal switch procedure). *Eur J Gastroenterol Hepatol*. 1999;11:99.

Liver and Biliary Tract Surgery

Chapter Twenty-Eight • • • • • •

*C*holecystectomy

JORGE CUETO-GARCÍA and MOISÉS JACOBS

Since its original description by Langenbuch in 1882, cholecystectomy has been one of the most frequent procedures in general surgery throughout the world. With the early attempts to perform laparoscopic cholecystectomy by Mühe in Germany in 1985, Kleiman's[5] experience in animals in 1987, and the first successful laparoscopic cholecystectomy in France by Mouret in 1987, interest was stimulated, although at first the procedures were received with hostility and skepticism.[1–4] Actually laparoscopic resection of the gallbladder is considered the procedure of choice in practically every case of cholecystectomy, including acute cholecystitis, cirrhotic patients, children, and other special cases.[7]

DIAGNOSIS AND PREOPERATIVE EVALUATION

There are many texts where the clinical basis of diagnosis and preoperative evaluation for these patients are described extensively. A candidate for laparoscopic cholecystectomy should be evaluated with the same standard protocol used in open surgery. For patients over 40 years of age, a complete cardiopulmonary evaluation should be performed. Ultrasonography is important not only to diagnose gallstones but because it allows detection of cases that could have special technical difficulties, like a thickened gallbladder wall due to edema in acute cholecystitis, or fibrosis suggesting a scleroatrophic gallbladder (which is a major challenge for laparoscopic cholecystectomy). The number and size of the stones, and the presence of intra or extrahepatic bile duct dilatation or stones, should be documented, and the presence of an inflammatory process or mass in the peripancreatic region should be verified. Hepatic function should be assessed, to seek for unsuspected bile duct stones, liver damage, pancreatitis, or other associated problems.[4–11]

In acute cholecystitis, principles similar to those for conventional surgery should be applied. Once the diagnosis is established, the patient is admitted to the hospital and left fasting, with intravenous solutions, parenteral antibiotics, and any hydroelectrolytic or metabolic imbalances corrected. Surgery can be done 8 to 12 hours later, which has been proven to be the most appropriate management for most of these cases.

Formal contraindications for laparoscopic procedures are the same as for conventional surgery: inability to tolerate general anesthesia and severe clotting disorders. It should be noted that most situations that were considered contraindications are today circumstances that require extreme care but do not contraindicate the laparoscopic procedure: for example, bile duct stones, peritonitis with gangrene or gallbladder perforation, biliary pancreatitis, and cholecystectomy in patients with heart or lung disease. Some patients at high risk of not tolerating pneumoperitoneum can be handled with a minimum pressure of 6 to 8 mm Hg or with devices designed to elevate the abdominal wall with external retraction to diminish the adverse effects of pneumoperitoneum, as described in Chapter 6. All patients who will be submitted to a laparoscopic procedure should be clearly informed that there is a possibility that this procedure could require conversion to open surgery, with a probability that varies between 1 and 3% in most series. The patient should be operated upon in a hospital that has all of the necessary facilities, including complete laparoscopic equipment, and transoperative monitoring and imaging equipment to perform an intraoperative cholangiography if necessary, and also invasive endoscopy if needed, as suggested by the endoscopic surgical associations and societies, such as the European (EAES), American (SAGES), and Mexican (AMCL) associations.

ANESTHESIA

Patients are fasted from midnight before the operation, and admitted to the hospital on the morning of the procedure. Usually a single dose of intravenous antibiotic, mainly a cephalosporin, is given, and compression stockings are placed. All patients are operated upon under general endotracheal anesthesia, with monitoring that should include electrocardiography, pulse oxymetry, and capnography. There are reports of successful laparoscopic cholecystectomies under epidural regional anesthesia, but the author's group has no experience with this. Anesthesiologists should be properly trained and familiarized with the indications, contraindications, and complications that can arise during a laparoscopic procedure, especially in high-risk patients and with prolonged procedures, and be prepared for a possible conversion to open surgery (Chapter 4).

PATIENT POSITION

There are two surgical techniques in which the patient is placed in a different position. They are known as the *European* and the *American* position. In the European position, which has been adopted by the author for all cases of cholecystectomy and practically all laparoscopic procedures (excepting appendectomies and inguinal repairs), the patient is placed on the operating table with the legs astride, and with the surgeon standing in between them, with the assistants on either side of the patient and the monitors at the head of the table. A variant places the surgeon on the left side of the patient with one assistant on the right side and the camera operator between the legs. Either way, this position has the advantage of allowing the surgical team to work with comfort and with less interference in their movements. As a special warning, remember to protect the legs, knees, and ankles.

In the American position, the patient is placed in the same way as for any other procedure, and the surgeon stands on the left of the patient with the camera operator at his or her side and another assistant on the right of the patient.

Initially a nasogastric tube was placed in all patients; however, the author only uses it when gastric distention is found upon introducing the laparoscope or when some other problem makes it necessary. Also, initially a Foley catheter was placed in all patients, but this is unnecessary and is only indicated in special situations.

TECHNIQUE

The first step is to create the pneumoperitoneum, with the patient in the Trendelenburg position. We accomplish this by the closed technique, using a Veress needle through the umbilicus, but in some special instances a semiopen or Hasson's technique can be performed, as is described in Chapter 6. A number of patients have had previous surgery, and special care must be taken in them to avoid bleeding and damage to internal structures. Once the first trocar is placed in the umbilical position, the 0-degree laparoscope is introduced and a complete examination of the abdominal cavity is performed. If a common bile duct stone or a complicated case is suspected, it is better to introduce a 30-degree laparoscope to have a wider range of vision. With the patient in the reverse Trendelenburg position, the second trocar is placed under direct laparoscopic vision, on the midline between the xiphoid and the umbilicus, ensuring that its entry into the abdominal cavity is on the right side of the falciform ligament, which avoids difficulties when the trocar is placed in the ligament or on its left because this makes the instrument's movements more difficult. Also the trocar is directed towards the gallbladder, so that there is no need to reposition it continuously throughout the procedure. Another two 5-mm trocars are placed, one near the midclavicular line for the grasper for the left hand of the surgeon, and another on the anterior axilar line for the assistant's grasper. In extremely obese patients, in some cases when bile duct exploration is required, or in some other difficult cases, an additional 5 or 10-mm trocar is placed in the upper left or right quadrant of the abdomen, through which other instruments such as

a suction cannula or an atraumatic liver retractor can be introduced to depress and separate the duodenum and other viscera, exposing the surgical area, similar to the way an assistant exposes the work area in conventional surgery, or it can be also used to move the liver's free border upward, in case adequate traction cannot be provided with the other instruments.

As for the surgical technique itself, many variants have been described. We should note, however, that it must be performed with all the necessary precautions, to avoid the most important complication, which at the beginning of the learning curve causes great concern, namely lesions to the common bile duct. It is also important to note, especially for the beginner, that anatomy under laparoscopic vision is quite different from that seen in conventional surgery, so it is necessary to become familiar with it by participating with experienced surgical groups, and later as a surgeon, to be assisted in the first procedures by surgeons experienced in laparoscopic procedures.

In the author's recommended technique, with the laparoscope through the umbilical trocar, a grasper is introduced through the lateral 5-mm trocar to take the fundus of the gallbladder. The assistant applies traction upward and backward, to establish optimal exposure. Another grasper is introduced through the midclavicular trocar. When the anatomy is evident, this grasper is used to take Hartmann's pouch and apply the necessary traction. However, in cases of doubtful anatomy or when adhesions are present, it is preferable to use an atraumatic instrument; there have been reports of biliary tree or even duodenal lacerations with serrated instruments. Working with both hands, and with the assistant's exposition, the surgeon takes the grasper that holds Hartmann's pouch in his or her left hand and applies upward and lateral traction to identify the structures in the cholecystoduodenal ligament and the common bile duct. A 5 or 10-mm instrument, generally an atraumatic curved dissector, is introduced through the subxiphoid trocar with the right hand, and blunt dissection is started in the cholecystoduodenal ligament, which is simple when there is no intense acute or chronic inflammation. This dissection allows identification of the cystic duct, bile duct, and cystic artery. Also a scissors can be used, to make a small cut on the peritoneum of the cholecystoduodenal ligament and to dissect in the Calot's triangle, taking care to avoid bleeding in these initial steps of the dissection. With either instrument, it is safer to begin dissection at Hartmann's pouch and then proceed downwards to find the cystic duct, to avoid damage to the bile duct. The use of monopolar electrocautery is contraindicated near the bile duct, duodenum, or colon, due to the well-known complications that this instrument may produce. Once the cystic duct is identified, the author recommends the following maneuvers:

1. Clearly identify the union of the cystic duct with the gallbladder (Hartmann's pouch).
2. Identify the "T," or junction of the cystic duct with the common bile duct.

Once these maneuvers have been performed, while traction on Hartmann's pouch is maintained upward and to the left of the patient, the surgeon continues to dissect or cut the right peritoneal attachments, which join the gallbladder at the level of the infundibulum to the hepatic bed. If hemorrhage is encountered, it is generally minimal, and does not require major maneuvers to be controlled. Once the right attachment is released, the cystic duct is dissected not only on its anterior and right lateral aspects but also on its posterior aspect, for which it is better to use a curved or mixter dissector. When performing this maneuver, one must take extreme measures to avoid bleeding, because often there is a branch from the cystic artery to the duct and sometimes these structures adhere strongly and may be lacerated if dissection is not cautious. Although bleeding at this point is seldom copious, it makes the procedure difficult.

Once the junctions of the cystic duct to the gallbladder and to the bile duct are identified, and the right peritoneal attachment of the gallbladder is dissected, traction is applied to Hartmann's pouch to the right side of the patient and slightly upwards, to enable dissection of the left peritoneal attachment. At this point care must be taken to avoid injury to the small arteries that accompany the cystic lymph node, located near the cystic artery's bifurcation. The dissection does not require electrosurgery, except for some exceptional cases, for which the authors strongly recommend the use of bipolar energy or, even better, the harmonic scalpel. The objective of dissecting both peritoneal attachments and the posterior aspect of the cystic duct is to accomplish a complete exposition of Calot's triangle, to verify that no other structure crosses in a vertical or diagonal direction (which could be the bile duct or the hepatic artery), and to have enough length of the cystic duct to have space to apply the staples away from the common bile duct.

In cases of acute inflammation, intense fibrosis, and particularly of sclerotrophic gallbladders, dissection can be troublesome, and as with conventional surgery, can be very difficult and time consuming. In these cases, various maneuvers can be performed. When the gallbladder is totally "buried" or surrounded by adhesions, initial traction can be applied on its fundus and countertraction to the omentum with atraumatic instruments, or an additional trocar can be placed to introduce a retractor to smoothly separate the liver, avoiding laceration, to enable dissection of the omental or visceral adhesions to the gallbladder's wall, using combined dissection. Another instrument useful for these difficult cases that can be introduced through the additional trocar is an aspiration cannula, which helps maintain a clean operative field to allow a safe and complete dissection. In case of hemorrhage, the bipolar electrocautery or harmonic scalpel should be used. In some instances the duodenum is found to be intimately adhered to the vesicular bed, and it must be very carefully separated, avoiding lacerations. In cases where the left lobe of the liver or the falciform ligament is falling into the operative field, a liver retractor can also be introduced through the additional port.

Once the three stages described are completed—identification of the cystic duct's junction with the gallbladder and with the biliary duct, and complete dissection of Calot's triangle—a decision on performing an intraoperative cholangiography should be made. The routine use of intraoperative cholangiography remains controversial, advocated for many years emphasizing its safety and value to identify ductal anomalies, unsuspected problems, or stones. If cholangiography is practiced on an elective basis according to surgeon experience, it is highly recommended that in the first 50 to 100 procedures it should be done, to acquire dexterity, reduce the possibility of damaging the main bile duct, and detect the presence of common duct stones. Intraoperative cholangiography can be performed with fluoroscopy or with plain radiographs. The author used to add 2 to 3 mL of 2% plain lidocaine to the contrast material to produce relaxation of the sphincter of Oddi. The indications and techniques for intraoperative cholangiography are described in Chapter 29.

In some cases, the common bile duct cannot be visualized, which requires a more extensive dissection; however, no structure should be clipped, ligated, electrocoagulated, or divided until all members of the surgical team are completely sure of the anatomy, because damage to the common bile duct is a tremendous accident with significant morbidity and morbidity. On some occasions it is possible to dissect the common bile duct with blunt dissectors with gauze, which exists in a commercial disposable form or can be made by the instrumentalist nurse, to allow cleaning and dissection of the duct in order to identify it with precision.

Once all the structures have been clearly identified, then the cystic duct and artery are divided. To perform this, two staples are placed in the cystic duct proximal to the main duct and as close as possible to the gallbladder to prevent spillage. There are staples that come in disposable 5 or 10-mm instruments and staples for reusable instruments. The best is the one with which the group has obtained the best results; also the security of each instrument should be taken into account, as well as the cost benefit for each particular case. Two staples are also placed distally and one proximally on the cystic artery, and both structures are divided with scissors. Again, a monopolar electrocoagulator should not be used to divide the structures because the heat can cause damage to the duct. If the cystic duct is wide or if staples are not available, an absorbable suture material of 00 or 000 caliber can be used. The dissection of both peritoneal attachments carried out earlier will greatly facilitate the rest of the procedure. To dissect and release the gallbladder from the rest of the hepatic bed, now far from the important structures described, a hook or spatula connected to the monopolar electrocautery device can be used, with the irrigation and aspiration device at the same time. Dissection is performed, ensuring careful hemostasia, while the graspers in the fundus and Hartmann's pouch move to give a good exposure.

Before removing the gallbladder completely, a careful examination of the hepatic bed is performed, to verify hemostasia; the bleeding points are cauterized, and the cystic duct and artery are revised. When there is contamination or perforation of the gallbladder wall, with escape of bile or calculi, abundant irrigation must be performed, with aspiration, avoiding the porta hepatis, because the aspiration cannula can dislodge the staples if done blindly. Before removing the gallbladder, the authors instill bupivacaine in both hemidiaphragms, which reduces the postoperative pain that sometimes appears in the shoulders, neck, or abdomen. No drains are left except in cases of severe infection or when an examination of the bile duct was performed; then a closed-system drain is introduced by the most lateral 5-mm trocar, placing it in the porta hepatis area under direct laparoscopic vision, once the gallbladder has been removed.

The author recommends extracting the gallbladder by the umbilical orifice, for which the laparoscope is changed to the subxyphoid port; a 10-mm toothed clamp is introduced through the umbilical trocar, to take the gallbladder by Hartmann's pouch and extract it with extreme care. A recent variant consists of introducing a 5-mm laparoscope when a 5-mm trocar is in the subxyphoid position, extracting the gallbladder through the umbilical port.

Extraction can be a tedious maneuver, with complications if it is not performed with extreme care, especially in obese patients, when the gallbladder is large, partially gangrened, or contains large calculi. For these cases it is better to enlarge the umbilical incision than to affront the gallbladder to the umbilicus, once the trocar is extracted, and take it with a Kocher clamp. A small cut is made in the neck, and the bile or stone contents are aspirated with a cannula, avoiding spillage into the peritoneal cavity. Many types of instruments can be introduced through the gallbladder's neck, to extract or fragment the stones until it can be removed, under laparoscopic vision. In some instances, the incision must be extended 5 to 7 mm, and with the aid of small retractors the gallbladder can be extracted. Postoperative complications have been reported, due to stones left in the abdominal cavity and the trocar's orifice, like abscess formation and intestinal obstruction, so it is desirable to avoid this situation. When the gallbladder is perforated or is infected it is better to place it in a plastic bag and avoid contamination or spillage.

All incisions of 10 mm or greater should be sutured to avoid herniations and postoperative complications.[12]

CHOLECYSTECTOMY FROM THE FUNDUS TO THE PORTA HEPATIS

Some cases complicated by acute or chronic inflammation do not allow dissection in the way described. In these cases, an additional 5 to 10-mm trocar is placed in the left superior quadrant to insert a retractor, and the cholecystectomy is performed from the fundus towards the porta hepatis, as is advised in conventional surgery, with very good results.

Careful retraction of the hepatic border allows dissection of the gallbladder from the hepatic bed downward, until the structures in the porta hepatis can be identified. In these cases, hemostasia is accomplished with bipolar electrocautery or harmonic scalpel. In some exceptional cases, when the posterior wall is intimately adhered to the hepatic bed or to the common bile duct, or when there is risk of hemorrhage, it is convenient to perform what is called a partial cholecystectomy, to avoid damage to other structures or conversion to a laparotomy. If the cystic duct and artery can be identified and divided, part or all of the posterior wall of the gallbladder can be left intact on the hepatic bed, the stones extracted, and the bile aspirated and washed. Other cases present a fusion of Hartmann's pouch to the common bile duct, making it dangerous to dissect between them; for these patients it is better to open the gallbladder at Hartmann's pouch and make the cholecystectomy upward, leaving in place a small portion of Hartmann's pouch. The stones and the rest of the gallbladder can be extracted within a sterile plastic bag. The gallbladder is divided using a harmonic scalpel, monopolar cautery, or scissors and bipolar cautery. The vesicular wall left in the hepatic bed is electrodesiccated or coagulated, to avoid formation of a mucocele. When part of Hartmann's pouch is left in place, one or two stitches of absorbable suture can close the opening and a closed drain is left.

CONVERSION TO LAPAROTOMY

Between 2 and 6% of patients subjected to laparoscopic cholecystectomy require conversion to laparotomy. Mostly this happens at the beginning of the surgical team's experience, when the equipment fails or because of severe bleeding. Once ability is acquired and experience is considerable, there are practically no indications to perform a conversion to laparotomy other than uncontrollable bleeding, unexpected malignant neoplasm, or when the common bile duct is injured and laparoscopic repair is not possible.

Conversion to laparotomy should not be interpreted as a complication, but rather good surgical judgment.

EVOLUTION AND POSTOPERATIVE CARE

Most patients are discharged within 24 hours. Some patients, operated on early in the morning, could be discharged the same day; however, when a group is beginning with the procedure, this is not a good practice, because time is required to detect possible complications and treat them quickly.

Intravenous solutions are discontinued 6 hours after surgery, clear liquids are given, the patient is encouraged to walk the same day, and is discharged next day with a regular diet. At that time most patients have had a bowel movement. In cases of acute, gangrened, or perforated cholecystitis or peritonitis, the intravenous solutions and antibiotics are maintained as long as required.

COMPLICATIONS

The possibility of complications due to pneumoperitoneum, bleeding, bile accumulations, lacerations, or sectioning of the common bile duct should be kept in mind. The most important aspect is prevention, but if they do present, then adequate treatment should be immediately given. The acceptance of laparoscopic cholecystectomy due to the initial results reported by pioneer groups gave the false impression of being a "simple and easy" procedure. However, morbidity and mortality were greater than for conventional surgery, owing to a number of factors that are analyzed in the corresponding section. The most important factors were, and in some places still are, the lack of sufficient training of surgeons and deficiencies in equipment and instruments. As the experience and dexterity with the procedure has grown, morbidity and mortality statistics are favorable over those for conventional surgery.[15,16] In cases where injury to the common bile duct is suspected, or biliary leakage is important, it is helpful to ask for an endoscopist, to establish the precise diagnosis, perform a papillotomy, or insert a splint. In some cases of biliary leakage without injury to the common bile duct, a laparoscopic reintervention to place a closed drain system can avoid a formal laparotomy. In general, all bile duct injuries should be evaluated and treated in an institution with ample experience.

REFERENCES

1. Mühe E. Die erste Cholecystektomie durch das Laparoskop. *Langenbecks Arch Klin Chir.* 1986;369:804.
2. Mühe E. Laparoskopische Cholecystektomie. Spätergebnisse. *Langenbecks Arch Chir.* 1991;suppl:416.
3. Mirrizzi PL. La Colangiograftía durante las operaciones de las vìas biliares. *Bol Doc Cir* (Buenos Aires). 1932;16:1133.
4. Postgraduate course in therapeutic laparoscopy. 76th Clinical Congress of the American College of Surgeons. San Francisco, California, October 12, 1990.
5. Kleiman A, García P. Colecistectomía laparoscópica en ovejas. *Rev Argent Cir.* 1987;52:317.
6. Dubois F, Berthelot G. Cholecystectomy under celioscopy. *Ann Chir.* 1990;44:205.

7. Cueto GJ, Serrano BF, Ramírez AG, et al. Colecistectomía por laparoscopia. *Cirujano General*. 1991;13:52.

8. Lui S, Leighton T, Davis I, et al. Prospective analysis of cardiopulmonary responses to laparoscopic cholecystectomy. *J Laparoendosc Surg*. 1991;1:241.

9. Shantha TR, Harden J. Laparoscopic cholecystectomy: Anesthesia-related complications and guidelines. *Endoscopy*. 1991;1:173.

10. Westerband A, Van de Water J, Amzallag M, et al. Cardiovascular changes during laparoscopic cholecystectomy. *Surg Gynecol Obstet*. 1992;173:535.

11. Reddick EA, Olsen DO. Laparoscopic laser cholecystectomy: A comparison with mini-lap cholecystectomy. *Surg Endosc*. 1989;3:131.

12. Cueto GJ, Garteiz D, Melgoza OC, et al. A simple and safe technique for closure of trocar wounds using a new instrument. *Surg Laparosc Endosc*. 1996;6:392.

Chapter Twenty-Nine • • • • • • •

*C*holangiography

MOISÉS JACOBS and JORGE CUETO-GARCÍA

Laparoscopic cholecystectomy is considered the first treatment option for cholelithiasis in the entire world, since the experiences of Mouret and Dubois in France were popularized, owing to the advantages of avoiding pain, reducing postoperative complications arising from the surgical wound, allowing the hospital stay to average one day, and allowing return to normal activity in a shorter time than with conventional surgery. It also offers the advantages of reducing the patient's fear of the surgery, has a better cosmetic result, and has lower hospital costs than open surgery.[1-3] However, a decade after its introduction, laparoscopic surgery is still unfamiliar to some surgeons.[4-5]

Ever since Mirizzi introduced transoperative cholangiography in 1932, it has been of great value in conventional surgery of the gallbladder and biliary tree, especially when their anatomy is not clear or the presence of choledocolithiasis is suspected. There are surgeons who perform it regularly, and others who according to their experience, only perform it when they consider it necessary. Surgeons who perform surgery of the bile ducts know that a transoperative cholangiography is an indispensable requisite to a proper surgical technique.[6-8]

Laparoscopic cholecystectomy should be the same careful procedure that has been performed by laparotomy, but by using a "minimal access" method.[9-12] This is why all surgeons should be trained to perform the procedure by laparoscopy, including the possibility of performing a "routine" or selective cholangiography, the same as for conventional surgery.

A report on the frequency of damaging the biliary tree in laparoscopic surgery[13] points out that in a series of 18 lesions produced in the main bile ducts, 15 did not have a cholangiography performed, and most of them were not recognized during the operation. This is why some authors, like Sackier et al, recommend cholangiography as a means of identifying the union of the cystic duct to the common bile duct, avoiding damaging the main bile ducts with this, and enabling identification of a lesion during surgery.[13] Deyo also emphasizes that in most cases of biliary lesion during laparoscopy, cholangiography was not obtained, and he recommends the use of transoperative cholangiography, because many complications would have been avoided with it.[14]

Aside from excluding the presence of choledocolithiasis, laparoscopic cholangiography is of great value in cases where the biliary anatomy is not clear due to adherences, inflammation, or congenital malformations. This is because the view obtained in laparoscopy is very different from traditional surgery. However, the surgeon can be unfamiliar with it, especially when performing his or her first cases. Iatrogenic damage to the biliary tree can be minimized with transoperative cholangiography, because it provides a clear definition of the anatomy. It is important to note the surprise that many surgeons express when they recognize, by way of a transoperative cholangiography, that what they thought to be the cystic duct was in reality the hepatic duct or the common bile duct. This is why one of the most valid recommendations for a safe cholecystectomy is the realization of a transoperative laparoscopic cholangiography.[16] However it must be noted that cholangiography is not a substitute for a meticulous and careful dissection of Calot's triangle, to define the structures in this area.

Some groups have chosen other options to substitute for translaparoscopic cholangiography. Endoscopic cholangiography can be an adequate option to preoperatively resolve choledocolithiasis, when the surgeon does not have the necessary equipment to resolve the problem operatively or prefers to perform the procedure without performing a bile duct exploration. This technique is effective in around 90% of cases, if an amply experienced endoscopist who obtains good results when handling the biliary tree, with a low incidence of complications, is available. On the other hand, this method does not show the biliary anatomy transoperatively, and in the mind of the author is unacceptable, if this is performed in the postoperative phase, knowing that if choledocolithiasis is found and the endoscopist is not able to extract the calculi, the patient is subject to another surgical procedure, increasing the morbidity and mortality. Endoscopic retrograde cholangiography performed in a systematic way preoperatively to rule out choledocolithiasis increases the cost and the morbidity and mortality unnecessarily, and should only be performed in selected cases.

Performing a preoperative intravenous cholangiography, in place of a transoperative one, is recommended by some groups, mainly in Europe; however, it is controversial and impractical, it does not define the operative anatomy of the bile ducts in an adequate way, and it is useless in cases where there is hyperbilirubinemia above 2 mg/dL. In spite of technologic advances, the use of fine tomographic images, and contrast mediums that produce greater opacity of the biliary tree, it does not make the anatomy clearer during the laparoscopic procedure, and is not superior to preoperative ultrasonography to rule out choledocolithiasis.[17,18]

The biliary tree should be adequately evaluated during laparoscopic cholecystectomy, by way of a transoperative cholangiography, with which high-quality diagnostic images are obtained that provide the surgeon with all the necessary information to take the pertinent decisions.

The indications for cholangiography with this method are not necessarily the same as for conventional surgery, because of other factors such as the surgeon's capacity for laparoscopic surgery, experience with the procedure, and the need to precisely define the length of the cystic duct and its relation to the right hepatic duct, common hepatic duct, and common bile duct, especially during the learning phase (Table 29–1).

There are many ways to perform cholangiography by laparoscopy:

• Cholangiography by continuous transoperative infusion.
• Cholecystocholangiography.
• Transcystic cholangiography.
• Cholangiography by direct piercing of the common bile duct.

The main techniques that allow the surgeon to perform translaparoscopic cholangiography in different situations are described in the following sections.

CHOLANGIOGRAPHY BY CONTINUOUS TRANSOPERATIVE INFUSION

Nagai et al[19] have pointed out that, due to the difficulties that arise when performing transcystic cholangiography, they have adopted cholangiography by continuous transoperative infusion as a method of visual confirmation, which has proven useful to rule out biliary lesions transoperatively. This method depends on hepatic function being normal, there being no interference with the metabolism of bilirrubin, the amount of radiopaque material used, and the time of exposition before taking the roentgenograms. In most cases, opacification is not clear, and it does not rule out the presence of choledocolithiasis.

Technique

There are two steps:

1. An infusion of iotroxic acid is started after endotracheal intubation is achieved or when starting the procedure.

TABLE 29–1. INDICATIONS FOR TRANSLAPAROSCOPIC CHOLANGIOGRAPHY

• Jaundice current or previous
• Dilated bile duct (> 1 cm)
• Small stones and extensive cysts
• Antecedents of pancreatitis
• Necessity of anatomic definition of the biliary via
• Teaching

2. After about 20 minutes, roentgenograms are taken, once the cystic duct is occluded with a clip (to observe the relations between the staples and the biliary tree).

CHOLECYSTOCHOLANGIOGRAPHY

One of the most simple forms of obtaining radiologic images of the biliary tree consists of performing a cholecistography by direct piercing of the gallbladder. This simple technique allows observation of the common bile duct in almost 80% of cases when the cystic duct is patent. It has the disadvantage, however, of not reaching a precise anatomic definition, when compared to conventional cholangiography. It has also been of great use for children with biliary atresia or when the biliary tree's anatomy has not been well defined due to adherences and the gallbladder's fundus is within sight.

Technique

Cholecystocholangiography consists of the following steps:

1. The gallbladder's fundus is grasped with a traction clamp.
2. If a laparoscopic needle is available, it is introduced through one of the 5-mm trocars and the vesicular contents are aspirated. Then without removing the same instrument, 20 mL of radiopaque material is injected. Films are taken 10 to 15 minutes later.

   Alternatively, the Veress needle or a no. 16 venous catheter can be used in a percutaneous manner to aspirate the vesicular contents. Then without removing the needle, the radiopaque material is injected. Films are taken 10 to 15 minutes later.

TRANSCYSTIC CHOLANGIOGRAPHY

The ideal method of performing a translaparoscopic cholangiography is still transcystic cholangiography. In recent years, various clamps and catheters have been designed for this test, with the catheters having the ability to be introduced by a 5-mm trocar or percutaneously by way of a needle; there are metal and flexible models available, and each one has advantages and disadvantages. It is important for the surgeon to know the techniques and adopt the most appropriate one.

Technique

The following variants exist:

• With clamps.
• With a metal catheter through a trocar.
• With a metal catheter by percutaneous insertion.
• With a soft catheter through a trocar.
• With a soft catheter by percutaneous insertion.

Transcystic Cholangiography With Clamps

Bayley and Zucker[21] point out that with the use of clamps that are specially designed for cholangiography, it is possible to obtain and maintain exposition of the gallbladder and the cystic duct. The clamp designed by Olsen has a central duct for the catheter to be passed, and two small atraumatic graspers in the distal portion to take the cystic duct. The catheter is introduced through the clamp and is guided into the cystic duct, which is held by the graspers.

The use of a cholangiography clamp that holds the cystic duct and allows passage of a catheter is not a practical technique, because the clamp complicates the introduction of the catheter into the cystic duct, and sometimes it can interfere with the radiologic vision. The clamp must be held in position during the entire procedure, and if it inadvertently moves, it frequently lies on the common bile duct, occluding the passage of radiopaque material. With the development of new catheters the use of clamps has become less frequent.

Technique. It consists of the following steps:

1. Dissection of the cystic duct and artery.
2. Flushing of the cystic duct.
3. Placement of staples on the cystic artery, without sectioning it (to have control in case of rupture and avoid retraction of the cystic duct due to an involuntary total section).
4. The clamp that applied traction to Hartmann's pouch is retired from the 5-mm trocar placed along the midclavicular line.
5. A clamp is introduced through the surgeon's trocar to hold Hartmann's pouch.
6. A pair of scissors (preferably microscissors) is introduced through the 5-mm trocar that is placed along the midclavicular line, and the anterior wall of the cystic duct is opened, just at the level where it unites with Hartmann's pouch, until bile is seen to escape.
7. The closed microscissors are inserted in the duct.
8. The microscissors are opened, enlarging the duct.
9. The cholangiography clamp with the catheter in place is inserted through the 5-mm midclavicular trocar, and it is opened to advance the catheter and place it in the cystic duct.
10. The clamp is secured with the cystic duct wall, and it must remain in that position throughout the cholangiography.
11. The clamp that holds the gallbladder fundus is removed, ensuring that the liver does not fall abruptly, and moves the cholangiography clamp or catheter.
12. ml of iodinated contrast material are injected, and two films are taken, one with the patient in a neutral position and one in Fowler's position. The laparoscope with the camera should be retired a couple of centimeters and directed leftwards, to avoid obstructing vision.
13. Once the films are taken, the clamp is opened, the catheter is retracted, and the entire instrument is removed.

Transcystic Cholangiography With a Metal Catheter Through a Trocar

In most cases the author prefers using a metal catheter for cholangiography inserted through the 5-mm trocar, because it can be easily guided towards the cystic duct, allows placement of a staple to avoid the escape of contrast medium during the injection without becoming occluded, and has a special olive at the tip to avoid accidentally coming out during the roentgenograms.

Technique. It consists of the following steps:

1. Dissection of the cystic artery and duct.
2. Flushing of the cystic duct.
3. Placement of staples on the cystic artery without sectioning it.
4. Placement of staples at the union of Hartmann's pouch and

the cystic duct, to avoid biliary escape from the gallbladder (optional).

5. Scissors are inserted through the 5-mm trocar placed along the anterior axillary line, to cut the anterior wall of the cystic duct, at the level of its union to Hartmann's pouch, until escape of bile is observed.
6. The closed microscissors are placed in the duct.
7. The microscissors are opened, enlarging the duct
8. The scissors are removed, and the metal catheter is inserted through the same trocar, with its plastic adapter, and it is placed under direct vision at the cystic duct's opening. Gentle irrigation is performed, until the olive at the tip of the catheter is completely inside the cystic duct.
9. Irrigation with saline solution is done, to visually verify that the cystic duct and the common bile duct are distended by the fluid, and a staple is gently placed above the olive to occlude the cystic duct's opening.
10. ml of iodinated contrast material are injected, and two films are taken, one with the patient in a neutral position and one in Fowler's position. The laparoscope with the camera should be retired a couple of centimeters and directed leftwards, to avoid obstructing vision.
11. The staple placed on the cystic duct is removed and the catheter is extracted.

Transcystic Cholangiography With a Metal Catheter by Percutaneous Insertion

Technique. Steps 1 through 7 from the previous technique are followed by:

8. A no. 14 needle is placed at the chosen spot, to insert the metal catheter.
9. The needle is removed, leaving the plastic oversheet in place, and the catheter is inserted, advancing it under direct vision to the open cystic duct. Gentle irrigation is performed until the olive at the tip of the catheter is completely inside the cystic duct.

Steps 10 and 11 are the same as for the previous technique.

Transcystic Cholangiography With a Soft Catheter Through a Trocar

Technique. Steps 1 through 7 from the previous technique are followed by:

8. The catheter is introduced through the same trocar, with its plastic adapter and its introductor, and it is placed under direct vision at the mouth of the cystic duct. The catheter is then advanced; if it has an inflatable balloon, then this is used to occlude reflux. Gentle irrigation is performed.

The remaining steps are the same as for the previous methods.

Transcystic Cholangiography With a Soft Catheter by Percutaneous Insertion

Technique. Steps 1 through 7 from the previous technique are followed by:

8. A no. 14 needle is placed in the chosen spot, to insert the catheter.

9. The needle is removed, leaving the plastic oversheet in place, and the catheter with its introducer is inserted. It is advanced under direct vision until the introducer is at the mouth of the cystic duct. The catheter is then pushed over the introducer, directing it into the cystic duct; if it has an inflatable balloon, then this is used to occlude reflux. Gentle irrigation is performed.

The remaining steps are the same as for the previous methods.

CHOLANGIOGRAPHY BY DIRECT PIERCING OF THE COMMON BILE DUCT

When the anatomy is not clear, as is the case with intense chronic cholecystitis, scleroatrophic gallbladders, or in cases where none of the previous techniques have been possible, cholangiography by direct injection with a fine needle of the common bile duct may be another useful alternative for radiologic observation of the biliary tree. In the author's experience, although used only on few occasions, it has avoided lesions to the common bile duct, which makes it worthwhile.

Technique

1. With the laparoscopic needle inserted through the 10-mm trocar with a reductor, a gentle piercing with rotating movements is performed until the duct is found, contrast material is injected, and the needle is removed to take the films.
2. If another film is necessary, the same procedure is repeated, using the previous orifice.
3. It is recommended to leave a drain connected to aspiration when the procedure has ended. The radiographic images should then be studied not only to rule out the presence of lithiasis, but also to perfectly identify the anatomy of the biliary tree.

To perform a successful laparoscopic cholangiography, adequate exposition and observation of the gallbladder and the cystic duct must be maintained throughout the procedure, and a careful opening of the duct is essential, or false entrances will be created with the catheter if multiple cuts are performed.

One should select a catheter with adequate capacity to perform a cholangiography, and choose the site on the abdominal wall that is most adequate for its introduction.

It is important to remember various points when performing radiologic studies:

- It is necessary to preoperatively take measures to ensure that the x-ray equipment can enter, and that the patient is in an adequate position, to avoid changing positions during the procedure.
- It is convenient to correct the table's position, dissection is performed with Fowler's and left rotation.
- If cholangiography is foreseen, it is recommended to use radiolucent trocars, which will not interfere with the radiological vision of structures.
- If metal trocars are employed, mobilization is necessary, especially of the surgeon's trocar, and the laparoscope must be partially removed so as to not interfere with radiologic vision.
- Laparoscopic vision of the catheter must be maintained, to avoid its inadvertently coming out of the cystic duct, and then retreat

or move the laparoscope to the left, just before the films are taken, to avoid obstructing radiological vision of the bile ducts.
- It is useful to add 2 mL of 1 or 2% lidocaine, without epinephrine, to relax the musculature of Oddi's sphincter, and allow an easier passage of the radiopaque material.
- When there is a doubt over a defect on fluoroscopy, one can move the syringe, and if the radiolucid images move synchronously, then they are probably bubbles.
- During laparoscopic cholangiography, special attention should be paid not only to the observation of the cystic duct and the common bile duct but also to the right hepatic and the common hepatic ducts, which are at a greater risk of lesion than during a conventional procedure.

The time a surgeon takes to perform a cholangiography is inversely proportional to his or her experience. In the first cases, the surgical team will take longer, but as ability is developed, the procedure's time will be reduced, and will probably improve on the time taken for a conventional procedure.

Fluoroscopy is a practical method of performing cholangiographies if the necessary equipment is available in the operating room. It is a method that allows dynamic and immediate observation of the anatomy, as well as performance of a biliary exploration under radiologic vision in cases of choledocolithiasis; the manipulation of the calculi is much easier with direct vision. Modern fluoroscopy equipment with digital subtraction offers much clearer and more precise definition and even allows close-ups and storage of images in the equipment's memory to be studied later, as well as other functions, all of this with a much lower exposure to radiation than traditional equipment and with a much faster developing time. According to a multicenter study performed by SAGES, ordinary fluorocholangiography is the most effective way to detect unsuspected lithiasis, and provides valuable information on the biliary anatomy, localization of the calculi, anomalies, and the extension of the lithiasic disease.[22]

It is likely that in the near future, this will be the preferred method for transoperative observation for the biliary tree. The author prefers fluoroscopy, because of these advantages, and at least in his workplace, the cost of this study is equivalent to the cost of cholangiography with conventional imaging. To preserve a graphic register of the fluoroscopy on the tape where the case is being recorded, the camera without the laparoscope can be focused on the monitor, registering the dynamic image. The author considers it to be the procedure of choice anyplace where the equipment is available.

The controversy on performing transoperative cholangiography in all cases, or only in those where it is deemed necessary, has resurged with laparoscopic cholecystectomy. In a prospective study with 500 cases, Voyles et al grouped patients as high risk or low risk for having choledocolithiasis, based on the ultrasonographic report on the common bile duct's caliber, liver function tests, and precedents of pancreatitis or jaundice. Of the 233 patients classified as low risk, subjected to laparoscopic cholecystectomy without cholangiography, none developed residual lithiasis.[23] A survey applied to SAGES affiliates, which accounted for 19,747 laparoscopic cholecystectomies, made clear that opinions on transoperative cholangiography were based on the surgeons' experience; 42% performed systematic cholangiography, and 59% performed it selectively when normal liver function tests were obtained. However, 80% recommend it when small multiple calculi are found or when a dilated cystic duct is present. The difference can be attributed to the technical difficulties that unfamiliarized surgeons face, when compared to those who generally perform the procedure without trouble. In this study, cholangiography was attempted in 51.2% of the cases, and completed successfully in 73%.[24]

There are now more reports on the utility of laparoscopic ultrasonography as another means of evaluating the biliary tree. Apparently, cholangiography is more sensitive than ultrasonography (92.8 versus 71.4%) but less specific (76.2 versus 100%). Ultrasonography requires surgical experience and in some cases, like obesity, can be difficult to evaluate; also it does not provide the anatomic definition that cholangiography provides. Both methods can be complementary; time and prospective randomized studies (with random group assignment) will place this new diagnostic modality in perspective.[24–27]

Transoperative cholangiography is a procedure that has proven its value in conventional cholecystectomy for the last 60 years. It should be performed during laparoscopic cholecystectomy in the cases in which the surgeon deems it necessary. It is a procedure that avoids iatrogenic lesions to the bile ducts and is necessary to detect the presence of choledocolithiasis in laparoscopy.

PERSONAL EXPERIENCE WITH TRANSLAPAROSCOPIC CHOLANGIOGRAPHY

The number of cases of laparoscopic cholecystectomy performed consecutively by my group, without selection, that in my judgment require cholangiography, is increasing. The type of cholangiography performed and the number of patients studied are shown in Table 29–2. The cannulation with a Ranfac catheter (Ranfac Corp., 635 Avon Industrial Park, Avon MA 023322) was performed with the technique described. In 3 cases of scleroatrophic gallbladder, the radiopaque material was injected directly into what was observed of the biliary tree by fluoroscopy. This was done because there was no clear definition of structures, and apparently the gallbladder was directly continuous with the common bile duct, which was corroborated on 3 occasions. This avoided a serious lesion to the bile ducts.

In 11 cases, cholecystocholangiography by direct piercing of the gallbladder was performed. One of them was a patient with a double gallbladder, in whom cholecystocholangiography was done by piercing the accessory gallbladder, and performing transcystic cholangiography in the main gallbladder. Two patients in whom severe necrohemorrhagic pancreatitis made dissection of the biliary pedicle and bile ducts necessary, had radiopaque material injected in the gallbladder. Observing its passage into the duodenum, allowed us to perform extraction of multiple vesicular lithiasis, cholecystectomy, and laparoscopic gastrostomy in one patient, and cholecystectomy with transcystic drainage of the biliary tree in the other. Three cases of cholecystitis and jaundice presented an enlarged gallbladder, in which the vesicular piercing was performed transcutaneously with a no. 16 catheter. In all of the cases, adequate imaging of the bile ducts was obtained.

The time to perform a cystic cannulation varied between 25 minutes for the first cases, to a 3-minute average in the last. Only 3 cases (1.06%, and mainly at the beginning of the series) could not have a transcystic cholangiography performed due to technical difficulties. The rest of the patients had a cholangiography obtained successfully. The results of cholangiography allowed greater understanding of doubtful anatomy in 94 cases (33.21%), ruled out the presence of suspected lithiasis in 102 cases (36.04%), and confirmed the presence of choledocolithiasis in 65 (22.9%). In all cases, an adequate view of the biliary tree was obtained, although in some cases, mainly when plain films were obtained, the studies had to be repeated due to defective technique.

REFERENCES

1. Cueto GJ, Serrano BF, Ramírez AG, et al. Colecistectomía por laparoscopia. *Cirujano General.* 1991;13:52.
2. Dubois F, Berthelot G, Leverth H. Cholecystectomie par cellioscopie. *Press M.* 1989;18:980.
3. Weber SA, Serrano BF, Cueto GJ. La cirugía laparoscópia: Evolución y perspectiva actual. *Cirujano General.* 1992;14.
4. Pérez Castro VJ. Colecistectomía por laparoscopia. *Cirujano General.* 1991;13:141.
5. Mirrizzi PL. La colangiografía durante las operaciones de las vías biliares. *Bol Soc Cir* (Buenos Aires). 1932;16:1133.
6. Hickens NF, Best RR, Hunt HB. Cholangiography. *Ann Surg.* 1936;103:210.
7. Berci G, Sackier JM, Paz-Partlow M. Routine or selected intraoperative cholangiography during laparoscopic cholecystectomy? *Am J Surg.* 1991;161:355.
8. Hermann RE. A plea for a safer technique of cholecystectomy. *Surgery.* 1976;79:609.
9. Andrén-Sanberg A, Alinder G. Accidental lesions of the common bile duct at cholecystectomy. *Ann Surg.* 1985;201:328.
10. Phillips EH, Berci G, Carroll B, et al. The importance of intraoperative cholangiography during laparoscopic cholecystectomy. *Am Surg.* 1990;56:792.
11. Bagnato JV, McGee GE, Hatten LE, et al. Justification for routine cholangiography during laparoscopic cholecystectomy. *Surg Laparosc Endosc.* 1991;1:89.
12. Davidoff AM, Pappas TN, Murray EA, et al. Mechanisms of major biliary injury during cholecystectomy. *Ann Surg* 1992;215:196.
13. Sackier JM, Berci G, Phillips E, et al. The role of cholangiography in laparoscopic cholecystectomy. *Arch Surg.* 1991;126:1021.
14. Deyo GA. Complications of laparoscopic cholecystectomy. *Surg Laparosc.* 1992;2:41.
15. Zucker KA, Bailey RW, Gadacz TR, et al. Laparoscopic cholecystectomy: A plea for cautious enthusiasm. *Am J Surg.* 1991;161:36.
16. Hunter JG. Avoidance of bile duct injury during laparoscopic cholecystectomy. *Am J Surg.* 1991;162:71.
17. Alinder G, Herling P, Holmin T. Routine operative cholangiography or pre-operative infusion cholangiography at elective cholecystectomy: A short effectiveness analysis. *Acta Chir Scand.* 1987;153:431.
18. García-Caballero M, Martin-Palanca A, Vara-Thorbeck C. Common bile duct stones after laparoscopic cholecystectomy and its treatment:

TABLE 29–2. CHOLANGIOGRAPHY: TYPE OF PROCEDURE AND NUMBER OF CASES

Cholangiography Type	Cases
Transcystic catheter (trocar)	195
Transcystic catheter (percutaneous)	6
Transcystic soft catheter by trocar	53
Transcystic soft catheter (percutaneous)	15
Translaparoscopic cholecystocolangiography	8
Percutaneous cholecystocolangiography	3
Cholangiography by direct injection of the common bile duct	3

The role of ultrasound and intravenous and intraoperative cholangiography. *Surg Endosc.* 1994;8:1182.

19. Nagai K, Matsumoto S, Taketo K, et al. The usefulness of intraoperative drip infusion cholangiography during laparoscopic cholecystectomy. *Surg Laprosc Endosc.* 1992;2:287.

20. Yamamoto H, Yoshida M, Ikeda S, et al. Laparoscopic cholecystcholangiography in a patient with biliary atresia. *Surg Laparosc Endosc.* 1994;4:370.

21. Bailey RW, Zucker KA. Laparoscopic cholangiography and management of choledocolithiasis. In: Zucker KA, ed. *Surgical Laparoscopy.* St. Louis, Quality Medical Publishing, 1991.

22. Berci G, Morgentern L. Laparoscopic management of common bile duct stones: A multi-institutional SAGES study. *Surg Endosc.* 1994;8:1168.

23. Voyles CR, Petro AB, Meena AL, et al. A practical approach to laparoscopic cholecystectomy. *Am J Surg.* 1991;161:365.

24. Brodish RJ, Fink AS. ERCP, cholangiography, and laparoscopic cholecystectomy. The Society of American Gastrointestinal Endoscopic Surgeons (SAGES): Opinion survey. *Surg Endosc.* 1993;7:3.

25. Barteau JA, Castro D, Arregui ME, et al. A comparison of intraoperative ultrasound versus cholangiography in the evaluation of the common bile duct during laparoscopic cholecystectomy. *Surg Endosc.* 1995;9:490.

26. John TG, Banting SW, Pye S, et al. Preliminary experience with intracorporeal laparoscopic ultrasonography using a sector scanning probe. A prospective comparison with intraoperative cholangiography in the detection of choledocolithiasis. *Surg Endosc.* 1994;8:1176.

27. Pietrtabissa A, Di Candio G, Giulianotti PC, et al. Comparative evaluation of contact ultrasonography and transcystic cholangiography during laparoscopic cholecystectomy: A prospective study. *Arch Surg.* 1995;130:1110.

28. Cueto GJ, Rojas DO, Serrano BF, et al. Laparoscopic surgery is safe alternative in the management of choledocolithiasis. *Int J Surg SCI.* 1994;1–2:60.

Chapter Thirty (Part One) ......

Endoscopic Common Bile Duct Exploration

MOISÉS JACOBS, JOSÉ ANTONIO VÁZQUEZ-FRÍAS, and JORGE CUETO-GARCÍA

INTRODUCTION

Between 8 and 15% of patients undergoing laparoscopic cholecystectomy present with choledocholithiasis. Such prevalence increases with age, and it is logical to think that the number of patients with this complication will increase. Since life expectancy is continuously increasing and these patients harbor other associated pathologies, the importance of early diagnosis and rapid and efficient treatment are clear.[1,2,3]

Since Curvoisier et al performed the first common bile duct exploration (CBDE) in 1899, this procedure has been considered a very important step in the training of every surgeon. However, in the 1960s and 1970s, after the introduction of endoscopic retrograde cholangiopancreatography (ERCP) was demonstrated to be efficient and safe, it became the treatment of choice of choledocholithiasis, both pre- and postoperatively, although its morbidity, mortality, and costs are not insignificant.[1,3,5]

Since 1992 laparoscopic cholecystectomy has become the new gold standard in the treatment of gallbladder disease,[2,6] and as a logical consequence the use of intraoperative cholangiography (IOC) flourished, and due to the pioneering work of Jacobs, Franklin, and others, along with the technological advances in equipment and instruments, laparoscopic common bile duct exploration (LCBDE) has demonstrated its safety and efficacy in the treatment of choledocholithiasis.[7–10]

DIAGNOSIS OF CHOLEDOCHOLITHIASIS

The most important component in the diagnosis of choledocholithiasis is a thorough clinical evaluation. There are many regimens to aid in the diagnosis of choledocholithiasis, but in general one must always consider the age of the patient, history of recent painful episodes, presence of jaundice, choluria, and pancreatitis, the size and number of stones, and diameter of the common bile duct (CBD).[11–13] Laboratory tests are very important (bilirubin, alkaline phosphatase, and amylase, among others) as are radiological studies such as ultrasound, computed tomography (CT) scans, and magnetic resonance (MR) cholangiography. Ultrasound has an advantage in that it can be repeated as often as needed, but its efficacy and sensitivity are directly dependent on the experience and the skill of the operator. Intravenous cholangiography is still used in some institutions, but it is no longer in wide use. Studies such as MR cholangiopancreatography and spiral CT have shown excellent results compared to ERCP, and they will become more widely used in the future.[14–17] At present, their main disadvantages are lack of availability and cost.

There is evidence that some patients with choledocholithiasis may remain asymptomatic for long periods of time,[18] but in those with pain, obstructive jaundice, pancreatitis, or cholangitis, it is important to make an early diagnosis and provide adequate treatment to avoid complications that may be serious or even lethal.

PREOPERATIVE TREATMENT OF CHOLEDOCHOLITHIASIS

As mentioned above, there is controversy over the best method to use to treat the patient with documented or suspected choledocholithiasis before laparoscopic cholecystectomy. For many groups, the preferred method is to perform an ERCP followed by a laparoscopic cholecystectomy, and there are many reports that show the success of this approach.[1,3,4,5] However, ERCP has significant morbidity and mortality, particularly when performed by an inexperienced endoscopist. Even in expert hands the procedure has a mortality of up to 2% and a morbidity of 5 to 8% with a success rate of 85 to 95%.[1,3,5] Additionally, in a recent report by Taylor et al,[19] up to 33% of patients subjected to a "successful" preoperative ERCP had residual lithiasis at the time of laparoscopic cholecystectomy. The procedure is also not indicated in very young patients. Finally, in some cases, jaundiced patients or those with dilated CBDs submitted to a preoperative ERCP had normal findings. Such patients are exposed to the risks related to the procedure, and yet need to have it repeated, with its associated risks and expense. For all these reasons and because it is able to diagnose both cholelithiasis and choledocholithiasis in a single procedure, it is recommended that if the surgical group has the experience, equipment, and training, a laparoscopic exploration of the common bile duct should be employed.[20–25]

LAPAROSCOPIC COMMON BILE DUCT EXPLORATION (LCBDE)

After a careful preoperative clinical evaluation has been performed, we recommend that an IOC be done to detect choledocholithiasis. IOC can be completed in 65 to 98% of cases with a less than 5% false positive and negative rate.[26] An IV injection of 1 mg of glucagon is given to relax the smooth muscle fibers; intraductal injection of 3 to 4 mL of 2% lidocaine (without epinephrine) can be mixed with the contrast material to perform the same function.[24] It should be pointed out that becoming experienced in performing IOC facilitates some maneuvers required in laparoscopic cystic duct exploration (LCDE). There is still controversy about whether IOC should be done on a routine or more selective basis.[6,26,27] Our group believes that IOC should be performed selectively on a liberal basis, and we fully agree with Vezakis et al[28] that one of the most important reasons to do it— aside from detecting stones—is that ". . . it minimizes the extent of the [CBD] injury so that it can be repaired easily without any consequences for the patient. The prevention of a major bile duct injury makes IOC cost-effective."

The image obtained, whether by fluoroscopy or still radiograph, must be of high quality in order to allow selection of the proper method for performing the LCBDE. The operating room must have all the necessary imaging equipment to perform these studies, which have been used for decades in conventional surgery. Newer imaging equipment with digital subtraction and amplification ability greatly facilitates this.

Several reports have shown that although both IOC and intraoperative ultrasound are very precise, the latter can be more sensitive and specific in detecting choledocholithiasis (97 vs. 99%, and 89 vs. 94%, respectively) although some anatomic abnormalities may not be detected.[26,29–31] These methods can also be used in a complementary manner. Occasionally a cholecystocholangiogram can be very useful.

During the operation is important to maintain adequate exposure by applying traction to the gallbladder fundus, and for this reason the laparoscopic cholecystectomy must not be completed until the LCBDE has been done.

Generally, transcystic LCDE is more popular, but if the cystic duct is very small, if the stones are large, or the cystic duct is not dilated, a transcholedochal route must be chosen. The most important factor is whether the CBD is dilated. One word of caution: When the diameter of the CBD is very small, the morbidity and risks from transcholedochal CBDE may be extremely high, regardless of the method (open or endoscopic) employed. The finding of a small, asymptomatic stone without any other clinical, laboratory, or radiological abnormality may not require any additional treatment since most of these stones will pass spontaneously to the duodenum. Finally, there are patients that require CBD exploration for causes other than choledocholithiasis.[32]

LAPAROSCOPIC CYSTIC DUCT EXPLORATION (LCDE)

This is by far the most popular method employed today, but the cystic duct must have a minimum diameter to allow the introduction of the instruments. If necessary, the cystic duct can be carefully dilated using a flexible guidewire and an angioplasty balloon.[32–34] This must be done gently to avoid tearing or lacerating the CBD. Usually the small incision used for the IOC (Fig. 30–1) can be used for the introduction of the endoscope and the other instruments.

LCDE can usually be done with a small cholangioscope (2.7 to 3.2 mm in diameter with a 1-mm working channel) or under direct fluoroscopic guidance, although in some patients both methods can be used in a complementary manner. Both methods require the use of Fogarty catheters, Dormia-Segura wire baskets, and lithotriptor probes (Figs. 30–2 and 30–3).

In order to introduce the cholangioscope and the other instruments, atraumatic instruments must be used to avoid damage to the equipment. When stones are being retrieved care must be taken to avoid lacerations of the CBD. As recommended by Fitzgibbons and others, ureteral catheters are very useful to verify the patency of the ampulla of Vater (Figs. 30–4, 30–5, and 30–6).

The method is safe and effective, but requires experience and familiarity with the endoscope. LCDE is successful 85 to 90% of the time,[32–34] but it is almost impossible to advance it proximally due to the sharp angle at which the cystic duct enters the CBD. Swanstrom's[32] maneuver, namely applying inferior traction on the infundibulum of the gallbladder to negotiate the angle of entrance into the CBD, has been used with some success.

LCDE can be performed with special equipment and technique.[24,32] To introduce the scope and/or instruments, it is best to use the right lateral trocar, and in some instances an additional trocar must be placed or a specialized introductory device used. Some catheters have a double lumen that is useful to inject additional contrast medium. The authors prefer to use a 14 gauge angiocath

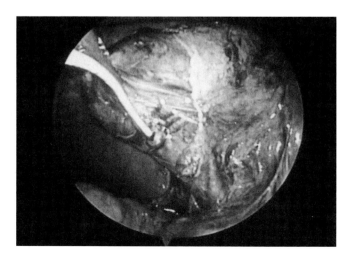

Figure 30–1. Cholangiocatheter passed through cystic duct.

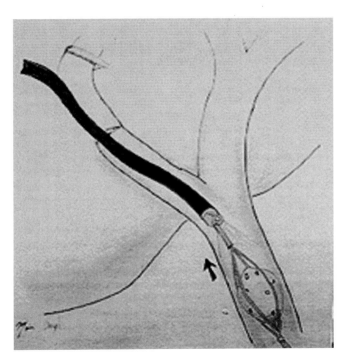

Figure 30–2. Illustration of an LCDE. A wire basket is used to remove a common bile duct stone using a 3-mm cholangioscope.

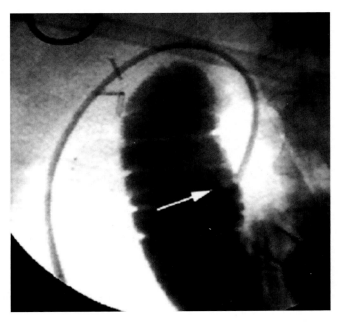

Figure 30–4. A ureteral catheter has been advanced to the duodenum.

placed percutaneously, through which a no. 4 Fogarty embolectomy catheter can easily pass, obviating the need for another trocar and allowing the surgical team full use of all the trocars.

On four occasions, with assistance from an experienced urologist, lithotripsy under direct vision was initially carried out for impacted stones in the ampulla of Vater. In such cases special precautions must be taken to avoid damage to the CBD wall.

Once the stones are extracted, a complete IOC must be done. If postoperative drainage is necessary, a flexible 2- to 3-mm catheter can be introduced through the cystic duct. This catheter can be extremely useful for three reasons: it achieves decompression of the biliary tract; additional cholangiograms can be done if

needed after the fifth or sixth week; and the radiologist can use it to introduce a flexible guidewire to remove any residual stones.[35]

TRANSCHOLEDOCAL LAPAROSCOPIC COMMON BILE DUCT EXPLORATION

When the cystic duct is very small or friable, when the stones are very large and the CBD is dilated and/or the transcystic LCBDE has failed, or if the surgeons are more comfortable doing one, a transcholedochal LCBDE should be done.[24,32,36]

The CBD is carefully dissected using atraumatic instruments, and gauze and a Kuttner can be useful as in conventional surgery. Hemostasis is usually achieved with gauze if the electrocautery is used carefully. An angled scope (30° or 45°) is preferred by many

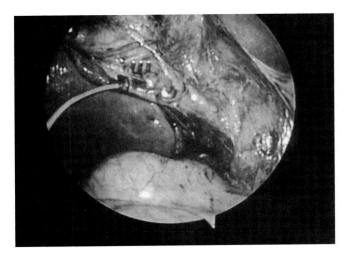

Figure 30–3. Transcystic duct passage of a no. 4 Fogarty embolectomy catheter. See Color Section.

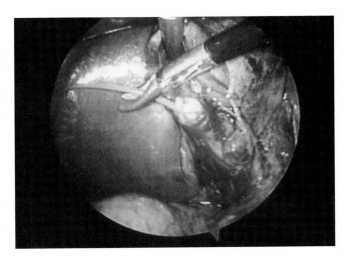

Figure 30–5. Transcystic stone extraction using a Fogarty embolectomy catheter. See Color Section.

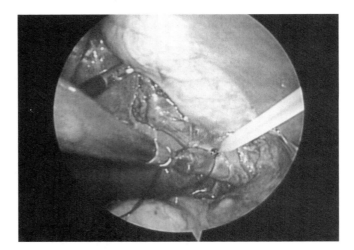

Figure 30–6. Closure of dilated cystic duct using an endoloop. See Color Section.

surgeons. The choledochotomy is usually less than 1 cm, and a cholangioscope and Fogarty catheters as well as the Dormia-Segura wire baskets are used and can be advanced proximally and distally without difficulty. If the patient is obese or if technical difficulties arise, an additional trocar can be placed in the left side of the abdomen and a 5- or 10-mm liver retractor can be introduced to provide the necessary exposure. Intraductal lithotripsy can also be performed using the same precautions.

Once the stones have been removed, an IOC is done, and if no abnormalities are found, some groups prefer to insert a T-tube before the choledochotomy, whereas others prefer to do a primary suture as in conventional surgery if the common bile duct is dilated.[25,32,34] The choledochotomy should be done with 000 or 0000 absorbable suture with noncutting needles using intra- or extracorporeal knots. Martin et al[20] recently published a report of a large successful experience with primary suture of the CBD.

Occasionally, a residual stone can be left behind if external biliary drainage is provided. This should be done for prolonged or complicated procedures (Figs. 30–7 and 30–8). These stones can be removed later by an interventional radiologist when a tract has formed (Fig. 30–9).

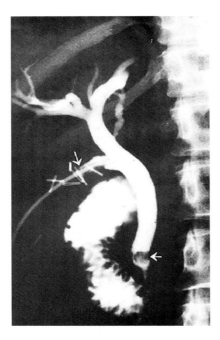

Figure 30–8. Completion cholangiogram after LCDE in a 32-year-old female with a recent history of biliary pancreatitis and jaundice. After removal of several CBD stones, another one is seen distally (*left arrow*) and left in place due to the long, difficult procedure, along with an external cystic duct drainage catheter (*center arrow*).

In complicated biliary tract operations (e.g., perforated piocholecysto or severe pericholecystitis in obese or elderly patients), intraoperative ERCP can be done and is being used more frequently for these indications.[37–40] With the assistance of an

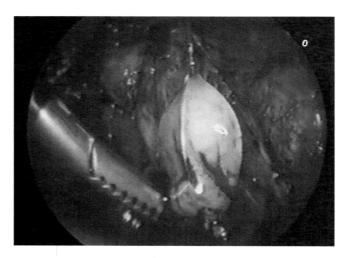

Figure 30–7. Laparoscopic common bile duct extraction of a 1-cm stone with purulent secretion in a 68-year-old male with jaundice and acute cholangitis.

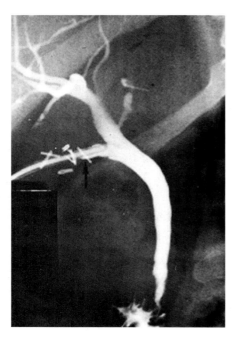

Figure 30–9. Six weeks later the same patient as in Fig. 30–8 underwent a cystic duct cholangiogram, at which time the 6–7 mm stone spontaneously had passed to the duodenum. The CBD is not dilated and the cystic duct catheter was removed 4 days later.

experienced invasive endoscopist, its use allows identification of the CBD and confirmation of the presence of CBD stones. A sphincterotomy can be performed, and if needed, stents can be placed to ensure adequate postoperative internal drainage with negligible prolongation of the procedure and minimal morbidity. Some groups have documented the cost effectiveness of this procedure.

RESIDUAL CHOLEDOCHOLITHIASIS

In a small number of cases, as sometimes occurs in conventional surgery, the surgeon faces the complication of residual stones in the CBD. As mentioned above, in some cases our group has elected to leave behind one or more stones and provide external biliary drainage. In case of an acute complication, an immediate ERCP should be done, and rarely a laparotomy has to be done.

Otherwise, on an elective basis the patient is carefully followed, a cholangiogram performed, and residual stones extracted by an experienced radiologist with the aid of a cholangioscope and/or special wire baskets. This procedure has been done suc-

cessfully for a number of years, carries a low risk of complications, and is less expensive than other endoscopic procedures.[35]

Some groups have documented the advantages of employing transhepatic CBD stone extraction when ERCP has failed.[41] The use of intraductal infusion of stone solvents is another option. Finally, the use of extracorporeal shock wave lithotripsy is another alternative that has been used successfully, the main disadvantage being the limited availability of the necessary equipment.[42,43]

DISCUSSION

The exploration of the common bile duct can be carried out by different methods, with three being most popular today: (1) conventional open surgical exploration, still the gold standard which for obvious reasons will be remain popular in many hospitals worldwide; (2) ERCP, which in the hands of experts has proven to be a safe and effective procedure with acceptable morbidity and mortality rates; and (3) LCBDE, which since 1991 has been performed by both the transcystic and transcholedochal routes.[1,3,5,7,25,32] To select the best method, the patient must be thoroughly evaluated and the method

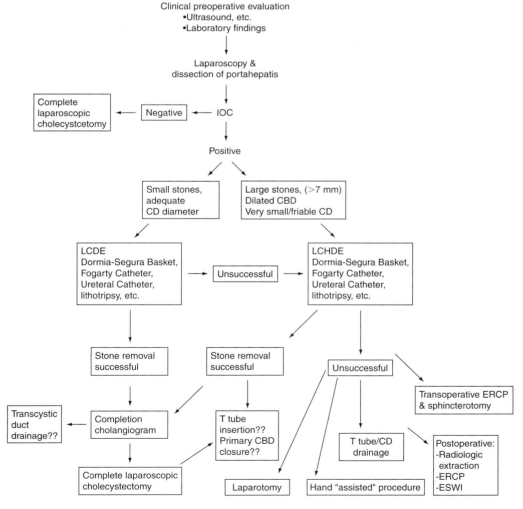

Figure 30–10. Algorithm for the laparoscopic treatment of choledocholithiasis. CD = cystic duct; CBD, common bile duct; ESWL, electroshock-wave lithotripsy.

chosen based on surgeon experience and preference, as well as the equipment available in the operating room and the experience and dexterity of the invasive endoscopist, among other factors.

Several large prospective studies, but particularly the one by the European Association of Endoscopic Surgery (EAES) published in 1999,[25] as well as the work of Jacobs et al,[7] Franklin,[8] Phillips,[33] Martin et al,[20] and Millat et al[44] and many others have objectively shown the advantages of LCBDE.[21,22,24,36,45,46]

If the surgical group has the training and experience, and if the operating room is well equipped, many surgical groups—ours included—suggest the method of choice be LCBDE and that ERCP should not be done preoperatively unless there are special circumstances, such as an elderly patient with suppurative cholangitis,[24,32,46,47] or patients presumed to have choledocholithiasis by preoperative work-up, including dilated CBD by ultrasound or elevated liver function tests. Many groups prefer to perform a preoperative ERCP if there is an expert endoscopist available.

Other groups have shown that the policy using ERCP only in certain circumstances (e.g., when CBD stones become symptomatic) has resulted in considerable savings and a substantial reduction in the number of ERCPs.[48] This is an important consideration, because the patient with a recent history of elevated liver function tests or a dilated CBD may show no abnormalities on IOC, and by selective use of ERCP one can avoid the risk of complications and the added expense to the patient and family. The recent work by Urbach et al[49] confirms the advantages of this policy, particularly with regard to savings and cost efficiency.

The prospective and well-controlled study of the EAES clearly shows that both methods (preoperative ERCP and LCBDE) produce similar results, the difference being that the latter involves a shorter hospital stay and is less expensive.[25] However, we again emphasize that a group carrying out these procedures must have the necessary experience and training, as well as the needed equipment and instruments, in order to avoid the undesirable results produced by inexperienced or ill-equipped practitioners.[45] LCBDE is still a relatively new procedure, and many surgical groups have just recently begun to perform it. Thus the results, costs, and morbidity and mortality will improve when these groups acquire more experience and become more familiar with the approach.

Many groups have documented a high success rate with LCBDE. In the report by Martin et al,[20] successful exploration was done in 98% of cases, with a morbidity of 7% and a mortality of 0.3%. These and other reports have shown that LCBDE is becoming more popular. Based on these findings, the preferred approach is to attempt an LCBDE except in unstable, high-risk patients until experience with the technique is gained.[50]

LCBDE with IOC used to select suitable patients and procedures has also been successfully applied to cases of mild to moderate acute biliary pancreatitis, without the need for an preoperative ERCP and its attendant risks.[51–53]

In patients with severe CBD dilatation and multiple stones, several groups have successfully used choledocoduodenolaterolateral anastomosis with carefully defined indications as in conventional surgery.[54,55]

Other procedures that require more complete evaluation are anterograde sphincterotomy, a procedure that has yet become popular, and the direct approach of the papilla through an endoscopic duodenotomy as recently described by Fowler.[56]

CONCLUSIONS

It is clear that LCBDE is an evolving technique that is still being perfected, but the results have seen steady improvement, and as with other endoscopic operations, the advancing technology (including improved optical systems, cholangioscopes, and lithotriptors, and perhaps the capability to perform transoperative lithotripsy) will allow surgeons to perform better, quicker, and safer operations. There is abundant proof in the recent literature that confirms that surgical groups with adequate training and experience working in well-equipped surgical suites can carry out LCBDE in a safe, efficient, and cost-effective manner. (See Fig. 30–10.)

REFERENCES

1. Paul A, Millat B, Holthausen U, et al. Diagnosis and treatment of common bile duct stones (CBDS). Results of a consensus development conference of the EAES. *Surg Endosc.* 1998;12:856.
2. NIH Consensus Conference. Gallstones and Laparoscopic Cholecystectomy. *JAMA.* 1992;269:1018.
3. Society of American Gastrointestinal Endoscopic Surgeons (SAGES) Committee on Standards of Practice. Guidelines for the clinical application of laparoscopic biliary tract surgery. Reviewed and approved by the Board of Governors, October 1999.
4. Neoptolemos JP, Carr-Locke DL, Fossard DP. Prospective randomized study of preoperative endoscopic sphincterotomy versus surgery alone for common duct stones. *Br J Surg.* 1987;294:470.
5. Perissat J, Huibregtse K, Keane FB, et al. Management of bile duct stones in the era of laparoscopic cholecystectomy. *Br J Surg.* 1994;81:799.
6. Neugebauer E, Troidl H, Kum K, et al. The European Association for Endoscopic Surgery (EAES) Consensus Development Conferences on laparoscopic cholecystectomy, appendectomy, and hernia repair. Consensus statements, September 1994. *Surg Endosc.* 1995;9:550.
7. Jacobs M, Verdeja J, Goldstein H. Laparoscopic choledocolithotomy. *Surg Laparosc Endosc.* 1991;1:79.
8. Franklin ME. Laparoscopic common bile duct exploration by choledochotomy. *Prob Gen Surg.* 1995;12:55.
9. Berci G, Cuschieri A, eds. *Bile Ducts and Bile Duct Stones.* WB Saunders:1997.
10. Berci G, Morgenstern L. Laparoscopic management of common bile duct stones: a multi-institutional Society of American Gastrointestinal Endoscopic Surgeons (SAGES) study. *Surg Endosc.* 1994;8:1168.
11. Haner-Jensen M, Karesan R, Nygard K, et al. Predictive ability of choledocholithiasis indicators: A prospective evaluation. *Ann Surg.* 1984;202:64.
12. Huguier M, Bornet P, Charpak Y, et al. Selective contraindications based on multivariate analysis for operative cholangiography in biliary lithiasis. *Surg Gynecol Obstet.* 1991;172:170.
13. Menezes N, Marson LP, Debeaux AC, et al. Prospective analysis of a scoring system to predict choledocholithiasis. *Br J Surg.* 2000;87:1176.
14. Pickth D. Radiologic diagnosis of common bile duct stones. *Abdom Imaging.* 2000;25:618.
15. Soto JA, Alvarez O, Munera F, et al. Diagnosing bile duct stones: comparison of unenhanced helical CT, oral contrast-enhanced CT cholangiography, and MR cholangiography. *AJR.* 2000;175:1127.
16. Stiris MG, Tennoe B, Aadland E, et al. MR cholangiopancreaticography and endoscopic retrograde cholangiopancreaticography in patients with suspected common bile duct stones. *Acta Radiol.* 2000;41:269.
17. Pickuth D, Spielmann RP. Detection of choledocholithiasis: comparison of unenhanced spiral CT, US. *Hepatogastroenterology* 2000;47:1514.
18. Rosseland AR, Glomsaker TB. Asymptomatic common bile duct stones. *Eur J Gastroenterol Hepatol.* 2000;12:1171.

19. Taylor EW, Rajgopal U, Festekjian J. The efficacy of preoperative endoscopic retrograde cholangiopancreatography in the detection and clearance of choledocholithiasis. *JSLS.* 2000;4:109.

20. Martin IJ, Bailey IS, Rhodes M, et al. Towards T-tube free laparoscopic bile duct exploration. A methodologic evolution during 300 consecutive procedures. *Ann Surg.* 1998;228:29.

21. Slim K, Pezet D, Chipponi J. Laparoscopy versus endoscopy for bileduct stones. *Lancet* 1998;351:984.

22. Lauter DM, Froines EJ. Laparoscopic common duct exploration in the management of choledocholithiasis. *Am J Surg.* 2000;179:372.

23. Cueto J, Rojas O, Serrano F, et al. Laparoscopic surgery is a safe alternative in the management of choledocholithiasis. *Int J Surg Sci.* 1994;1–2:60.

24. Cueto J, Rojas O, Rodríguez M, et al. Tratamiento de la coledocolitiasis. *Cirugía Laparoscópica*, 2nd ed. McGraw-Hill Interamericana:1997;159.

25. Cuschieri A, Lezoche E, Morino M, et al. The European Association for Endoscopic Surgery (EAES) multicenter prospective randomized trial comparing two-stage vs. single-stage management of patients with gallstone disease and ductal calculi. *Surg Endosc.* 1999;13:952.

26. Soper NJ. Intraoperative screening for common bile duct stones: Ultrasound or cholangiography? Journal of Laparoendoscopic & Advanced Surgical Techniques, Symposium Summaries. *J Laparoendosc Adv Surg Tech.* 1998;8:169.

27. Sackier JM, Berci G, Phillips E, et al. The role of cholangiography in laparoscopic cholecystectomy. *Arch Surg.* 1991;126:1021.

28. Vezakis A, Davides D, Ammori BJ, et al. Intraoperative cholangiography during laparoscopic cholecystectomy. *Surg Endosc.* 2000;14:1118.

29. Catheline JM, Capelluto E, Turner R, et al. Comparison of laparoscopic ultrasound and cholangiography during laparoscopic cholecystectomies. Results of a prospective study. *Gastroenterol Clin Biol.* 2000;24:619.

30. Barteau JA, Castro D, Arregui ME, et al. A comparison of intraoperative ultrasound versus cholangiography in the evaluation of the common bile duct during laparoscopic cholecystectomy. *Surg Endosc.* 1995;9:490.

31. Pietrtabissa A, Di Candio G, Giulianotti PC, et al. Comparative evaluation of contact ultrasonography and transcystic cholangiography during laparoscopic cholecystectomy: A prospective study. *Arch Surg.* 1995;130:1110.

32. Swanstrom LL. Common bile duct exploration. In: *Minimally Invasive Surgery*, Hunter JG, Sackier JG, eds. McGraw-Hill:1993;231.

33. Phillips EH. Laparoscopic transcystic duct common bile duct exploration. *J Laparoendosc Adv Surg Tech.* 1998;8:169.

34. Memon MA, Hassaballa H, Memon MI. Laparoscopic common bile duct exploration: The past, the present, and the future. *Am J Surg.* 2000;179:309.

35. Castañeda WR, Maynar M, DiSegni R, et al, Interventional radiology in biliary tract. In: Cueto J, Weber A, eds. *Laparoscopic Surgery*, 2nd ed. McGraw Hill Interamericana:1997;188.

36. Dorman JP, Franklin ME Jr., Glass JL. Laparoscopic common bile duct exploration by choledochotomy. *Surg Endosc.* 1998;12:926.

37. Rijna H, Kemps WG, Eijsbouths Q, et al. Preoperative approach to common bile duct stones: results of a selective policy. *Dig Surg.* 2000;17:229.

38. Cemachovic I, Letard JC, Begin GF, et al. Intraoperative endoscopic sphincterotomy is a reasonable option for complete single-stage minimally invasive biliary stones treatment: short-term experience with 57 patients. *Endoscopy* 2000;32:956.

39. Filauro M, Comes P, De Conca V, et al. Combined laparoendoscopic approach for biliary lithiasis treatment. *Hepatogastroenterology* 2000;47:922.

40. Kalimi R, Cosgrove JM, Marini C, et al. Combined intraoperative laparoscopic cholecystectomy and endoscopic retrograde cholangiopancreatography: Lessons from 29 cases. *Surg Endosc.* 2000;14:232.

41. Van Der Velden JJ, Berger MY, Bonjer HJ, et al. Percutaneous treatment of bile duct stones in patients treated unsuccessfully with endoscopic retrograde procedures. *Gastrointest Endosc.* 2000;51(4 pt 1):418.

42. Cipolletta L, Costamagna G, Blanco MA, et al. Endoscopic mechanical lithotripsy of difficult common bile duct stones. *Br J Surg.* 1997;84:1407.

43. Ragheb S, Choong CK, Gowland S, et al. Extracorporeal shock wave lithotripsy for difficult common bile duct stones: *N Z Med J.* 2000;113:377.

44. Millat B, Atger J, Deleuze A, et al. Laparoscopic treatment of choledocholithiasis: a prospective evaluation in 274 consecutive unselected patients. *Hepatogastroenterology* 1997;44:28.

45. Keeling NJ, Mensiez D, Motson RW. Laparoscopic exploration of the common bile duct: beyond the learning curve. *Surg Endosc.* 1999;13:109.

46. Hawasli A, Lloyd L, Cacucci B. Management of choledocholithiasis in the era of laparoscopic surgery. *Am Surg.* 2000;66:425; discussion 430.

47. Fanning NF, Horgan PG, Keane FB. Evolving management of common bile duct stones in the laparoscopic era. *J R Coll Edinb.* 1997;42:389.

48. Ammori BJ, Birbas K, Davides D, et al. Routine vs. "on demand" postoperative ERCP for small bile duct calculi detected and intraoperative cholangiography. Clinical evaluation and cost analysis. *Surg Endosc.* 2000;14:1123.

49. Urbach DR, Khajanchee YS, Jobe BA, et al. Cost-effective management of common bile duct stones: a decision analysis of the use of endoscopic retrograde cholangiopancreatography (ERCP), intraoperative cholangiography, and laparoscopic bile duct exploration. *Surg Endosc.* 2001;15:4.

50. Sharma VK, Howden CW. Metaanalysis of randomized controlled trials of endoscopic retrograde cholangiography and endoscopic sphincterotomy for the treatment of acute biliary pancreatitis. *Am J Gastroenterol.* 1999;94:3211.

51. Soper NJ, Brunt LM, Callery MP, et al. Role of laparoscopic cholecystectomy in the management of acute gallstone pancreatitis. *Am J Surg.* 1994;167:42.

52. Cueto J, Nevarez R, Vázquez-Frias JA. The laparoscopic treatment of acute biliary pancreatitis (ABP). 7th World Congress of Endoscopic Surgery. Monduzzi editore. Singapore, June 2000:171.

53. Chang L, Lo S, Stabile BE, et al. Preoperative versus postoperative endoscopic retrograde cholangiopancreatography in mild to moderate gallstone pancreatitis. A prospective randomized trial. *Ann Surg.* 2000;231:82.

54. Cueto J, Pérez-Fernández L, Cervantes C. La colédocoduodeno anastomosis latero-lateral en la obstrucción de las vías biliares. *Rev Gastroent Mex, Enero-Febrero.* 1972;37:4.

55. Delgado FG, Blannes FM, Delgado JM. Choledocoduodenoanastomosis. In: Cueto J, Weber A, eds. *Laparoscopic Surgery*, 2nd ed. McGraw Hill Interamericana:1997;167.

56. Fowler D. Transduodenal Sphincterotomy: 2000 Society of American Gastrointestinal Endoscopic Surgeons (SAGES) Clinical Congress. Atlanta, Georgia.

Chapter Thirty (Part Two) ● ● ● ● ● ■

Magnetic Resonance Cholangiopancreatiography

CARLOS ROBERTO GIMÉNEZ, RAÚL MARTINEZ, ENRIQUE PALACIOS, and W. RICARDO CASTAÑEDA

INTRODUCTION

In the evaluation of obstructive jaundice and pancreaticobiliary disorders, different noninvasive diagnostic imaging modalities have been used: helical computed tomography (CT), nuclear medicine, abdominal magnetic resonance imaging (MRI), and MR cholangiopancreatography (MRCP). All of these procedures depict the biliary tree and pancreatic duct without instrumentation.[1] In addition, endoscopic ultrasound (EUS) or intraductal pancreatic ultrasound, percutaneous transhepatic cholangiography (PTC), and endoscopic retrograde cholangiopancreatography (ERCP) are used to evaluate the biliary tree and pancreatic duct; however, these require the use of endoscopic instrumentation or percutaneous access to the biliary tree.

Obstructive jaundice has varied etiologies such as benign lithiasis, postsurgical or posttrauma stenosis, pancreatic pseudocyst, choledocal cyst (Caroli's disease), benign inflammatory stenosis, primary sclerosing cholangitis, biliary tree ascaridiasis, hydatid cyst with communication with the biliary tree, aortic aneurysms, and hepatic artery aneurysms. Malignant diseases that can affect the biliary tree are pancreatic carcinoma, cholangiocarcinoma, gallbladder carcinoma, ampullary carcinoma, lymphomas, duodenal carcinoma, hilar lymphadenopathy from gastrointestinal cancer metastasis (gastric carcinoma, colonic carcinoma, pancreatic carcinoma), and nongastrointestinal carcinoma (lung cancer and breast cancer). Before the introduction of MRCP, the imaging methods used to determine the exact site of obstruction and the etiology were ERCP and PTC. CT cholangiography has not seen wide use because it requires the use of iodinated contrast medium that may produce side effects.

Ultrasound and CT offer important information about the presence of obstruction and ductal dilatation, but these methods do not demonstrate intraductal anatomy or the precise site of obstruction. Ultrasound permits good visualization of the biliary tree, but is less sensitive than the invasive techniques to detect the site and cause of obstruction.[3]

MR is proving valuable in the evaluation of the biliary tree, main pancreatic duct, and surrounding structures. MRCP is a relatively new application of MR used for depicting biliary tract anatomy without instrumentation or contrast media. The image quality of MRCP is similar to that of ERCP and PTC and may reduce the risk of complications of invasive procedures in selected patients.

The accuracy of MRCP has improved with the use of the new pulse sequences, but more experience in the interpretation of the images and recognition of its limitations are still needed.

TECHNIQUES

MRCP is based on the principle that static fluids have long T2 weighted (T2W) relaxation times. Static fluids, including bile and pancreatic fluids, have high signal intensities on heavily T2W MR images, producing strong tissue differentiation between bright bile and solid organs, such as the liver and pancreas, which have low signal intensity. Differentiation between bile and its surroundings is possible because bile and pancreatic fluid are simple fluids consisting largely of water (97%), acting like intrinsic contrast and giving us an image similar to ERCP or PTC. Initially, this principle was applied in MR myelography and MR urography. MRCP is a noninvasive tool that does not require the administration of oral or intravenous contrast media, and is thus without biological side effects. MRCP can be used in pregnancy after the second trimester; however, ultrasound is still the first diagnostic method of choice in these patients.

These techniques can be divided between two-dimensional acquisitions versus three-dimensional acquisitions, respiratory triggering versus breath-holding scanning, studies with or without fat suppression, and single- versus multi-sectional acquisitions.

In conjunction with the techniques previously mentioned, numerous sequences have been used: steady state free precession (SSFP), two-dimensional fast spin echo (2D-FSE), three-dimensional fast spin echo (3D-FSE), and half-Fourier rapid acquisition with relaxation enhancement (RARE), or half-Fourier acquisition single-shot turbo spin echo (HASTE). Comparison studies were made between the first four sequences and it was concluded that half-Fourier RARE offered the highest contrast image and the best spatial resolution.[23] The image quality in this sequence is similar to ERCP. It has also been demonstrated that the breath-holding technique is better than the non–breath-holding technique, because it eliminates movement artifacts.[23] This new sequence demonstrates ducts as small as 1 mm in diameter and reduces the possibility of artifacts simulating or masking various pathologic conditions. The most common artifacts are surgical clips, vascular and biliary metallic stents, biliary drainage catheters, gastrointestinal gas, and spinal metallic bars.[2,19,22]

Multislice sequence images should be analyzed one at a time to avoid the masking of small filling defects in the hyperintense bile, reconstruction should be done with maximal intensity projection (MIP) and single section or shaded surface display. Small stones can be demonstrated in T2W images as they differ from the air bubbles that float and adhere to the anterior wall of the duct and from clots that have certain T1W and T2W characteristics.

INDICATIONS

MRCP can be useful in the evaluation of a wide range of biliopancreatic illnesses such as choledocholithiasis, prelaparoscopic cholecystectomy and postcholecystectomy evaluation (Fig. 30–10), anatomical variants of the biliary tree and pancreatic ducts, acute pancreatitis, benign stenosis of the biliary tract, and evaluation of biliodigestive derivations. In the evaluation of malignant disease, conventional MR and MRCP evaluates the biliary tree, and allows the assessment of extension and staging with one imaging method, without the need to use iodinated contrast medium, important in patients with a history of allergy to contrast media.

MRCP can also play an important role in patients in whom ERCP could not be performed or failed to provide a good demonstration of the biliary tree.[14]

CONTRAINDICATIONS

MRCP is absolutely contraindicated in patients with a heart pacemaker, cranial surgical clips, cochlear or valvular prostheses, or intraocular foreign bodies.

There is a relative contraindication in patients with neurostimulators, metallic prostheses, or penile implants. In 1 to 4% percent of patients, claustrophobia can also be a contraindication.

CLINICAL APPLICATIONS

Before MRCP, the only noninvasive imaging methods available to evaluate pancreaticobiliary disorders were ultrasound and CT. However, these procedures cannot effectively demonstrate the anatomy in the coronal planes. ERCP and PTC are effective in diagnosing these disorders, but are invasive and carry the risk of complications. With further improvements and refinements it is possible that MRCP could replace those invasive procedures.

Experience and technical dexterity are required by the radiologist and endoscopist to perform ERCP and PTC procedures. The risk of complications is between 3 and 8% for ERCP[2] and 3 to 5%

for PTC.[3] The most common complication related to PTC is hepatic artery injury that can cause pain, hemorrhage, and hemobilia. Other complications include sepsis, bile peritonitis, and pneumothorax.[2] ERCP morbidity is 7% and the most frequent complications are pancreatitis (1 to 5%),[4,10] aspiration pneumonia,[2,4] cholan-

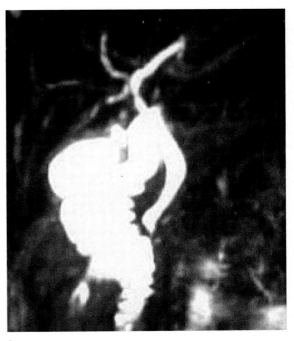

A

B

Figure 30–10. A. Normal MRCP. **B.** MRCP postcholecystectomy. Image shows dilatation of both intra- and extrahepatic bile ducts with mild dilatation of the duct of Wirsung. There is no clear evidence of obstruction; this is a typical finding in patients following cholecystectomy.

gitis (0.8%), bleeding, perforations, drug side effects (0.6%), pancreatic abscesses (0.3%), and transient hyperamylasemia (40% to 70%) that is usually asymptomatic. The mortality rate of ERCP is 0.2 to 1%.[11] In patients with complete obstruction or who have had previous surgery, cannulation failure can occur or can cause incomplete filling of the biliary tree.[4,5] ERCP is an invasive procedure that is operator-dependent, requiring sedation in most cases. In 3 to 9% of patients, the papilla cannot be catheterized.[20] Another disadvantage of ERCP is the false-positive cases of biliary lithiasis produced by small air bubbles that may be injected inadvertently during the procedure. False-negatives can also occur in microlithiasis or when there is distention or dilatation of the biliary ducts.

The principal advantages of ERCP are the direct visualization of lesions with the ability to do a biopsy. The second most important advantage is the ability to do treatment of lithiasis and of benign and malignant stenosis by stent placement.

Ultrasound is the most common diagnostic imaging method used in the evaluation of obstructive jaundice, with an 80% sensitivity for choledocholithiasis and a specificity of 98%.[6] Some conditions that can decrease its sensitivity are obesity, abdominal distention, and obstructive process in the intrapancreatic portion of the common bile duct. However, ultrasound does provide information to help decide if other imaging modality is necessary for further evaluation (CT, PTC, or ERCP).

MRCP has superior image quality, multiplanar and three-dimensional capabilities, and provides a significant diagnostic advantage.

BILIARY TREE

Normal Anatomy

Excellent correlation exists between MRCP and ERCP in the evaluation of the biliary ducts and pancreatic duct.[4] There is commonly a discrepancy on the size of the bile ducts between ERCP and MRCP. THe reason for this is that during MRCP the ducts are in their physiologic state and the true diameter of the duct is represented, while during ERCP, the injection of contrast media under pressure artificially increases the diameter of the duct. ERCP can demonstrate subtle stenoses and filling defects in the secondary branches better than MRCP.[12]

Congenital Anomalies

MRCP is 98% accurate in demonstrating aberrant bile ducts and is 95% accurate in demonstrating cystic duct variants. This information is valuable before performing laparoscopic cholecystectomy.[26] Iatrogenic lesions of the biliary tree due to laparoscopic cholecystectomy occur in 0.6%, an incidence twice as high as that for open conventional cholecystectomies (Fig. 30–11).[30]

MRCP can also provide precise information for the diagnosis and classification of choledochal cysts in the preoperative and postoperative period (Fig. 30–12).[28,29]

Intrahepatic Bile Duct Alterations

MRCP is an important tool in the diagnosis of primary sclerosing cholangitis, oriental cholangitis, cholangitis with microabscesses, cholangitis in acquired immune deficiency syndrome (AIDS), and in patients with hydatidosis.

In primary sclerosing cholangitis (PSC), alterations can be observed in the intrahepatic and extrahepatic biliary ducts. PSC is characterized by dilated segments of the biliary tree interspersed with narrowed segments, resulting in the appearance of beaded and stenotic segments (Fig. 30–13).[22,27]

Secondary sclerosing cholangitis (SSC) can be present in patients with biliary-enteric anastomosis. The etiology is reflux into the biliary tree causing an inflammatory response with edema of the biliary tract and surrounding parenchyma with the development of typical microabscesses (Fig. 30–14).

In oriental cholangitis, there is decrease in the size of liver segments two and three with dilatation of the corresponding biliary ducts (Fig. 30–15).

Multiple strictures and mural irregularities of the biliary ducts characterize the biliary tract changes in AIDS.

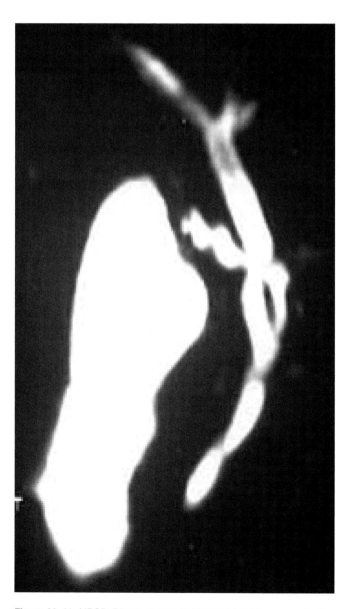

Figure 30–11. MRCP. Biloma, a case of postcholecystectomy complication and double barrel cystic duct.

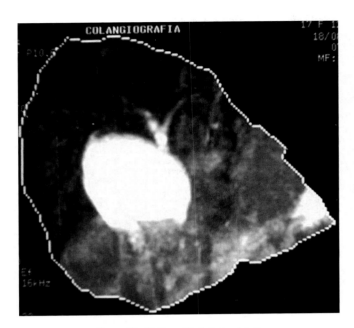

Figure 30–12. Type IV choledocal cyst.

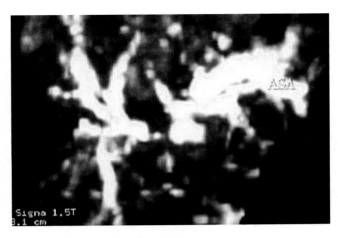

Figure 30–14. Choledocholenteric anastomosis. Patient with severe cholangitis with multiple microabscesses appearing as round fluid collections hanging from the bile ducts.

In complicated hepatic hydatidosis that opens into the biliary tree, membranes can be observed as linear filling defects. These membranes can produce obstruction and dilatation of the common bile duct (Fig. 30–16).

Choledocholithiasis

MRCP depicts stones as rounded or faceted low-signal-intensity filling defects in the high-signal-intensity bile. The stones can be free or impacted in the biliary tract (Fig. 30–17). Sometimes the small stones are demonstrated only in the axial scans, giving the

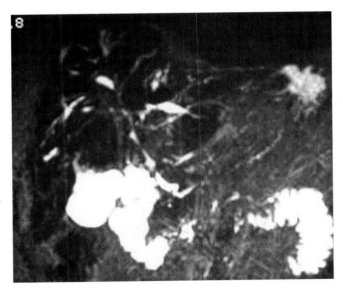

Figure 30–13. Primary sclerosing cholangitis in a patient with ulcerative colitis. Observe the diffuse areas of bile duct narrowing with areas of dilatation in both the intra- and extrahepatic bile ducts.

meniscus effect. The differential diagnosis of these filling defects includes air bubbles, clots, parasites, biliary sludge, debris, and intraductal tumors.

The sensitivity of MRCP for choledocholithiasis using all MR sequences and postprocessing images is high and is diagnostic in almost all patients (Fig. 30–18).[6] MRCP can demonstrate stones as small as 2 mm.[13,19] With the use of the newer sequences, MRCP has a sensitivity that ranges from 81 to 100% and a specificity that ranges from 85 to 100% in the diagnosis of choledocholithiasis. The positive predictive value ranges from 82 to 100% and the negative predictive value ranges from 94 to 100%. The primary utility of MRCP may lie not in the detection of stones, but in their exclusion. With MRCP the use of ERCP can be limited to those patients with pathology in the biliary tree that can be treated endoscopically, thus eliminating the morbidity of this procedure when used as a diagnostic tool.[22,17]

Bile Duct Stenosis

MRCP can visualize the common bile duct, either normal or dilated, in 96 to 100% of cases.[24] Stenoses are visualized as a narrowing or interruption of the bile duct with prestenotic dilatation. In some cases, total absence of signal can be a sign of stenosis, preventing evaluation of the contour and symmetry and of the transition between the normal and the diseased segments (Fig. 30–19).

Benign stenoses can be due to extrahepatic primary sclerosing cholangitis, anastomotic strictures of the bile ducts, iatrogenic occlusion of the bile duct, and chronic pancreatitis (Fig. 30–20).

Malignant stenosis can appear as abrupt obstructions, asymmetry of the bile duct wall, mural irregularities, and eccentric stenosis (Fig. 30–21).

The use of MRCP allows us to classify a Klatzkin tumor using the Bismuth classification. MRCP can provide important preoperative information. The conventional study of the upper abdomen, with the acquisition of T1W and T2W images, provides a complete evaluation of this disease for diagnosis and staging. This has a great impact on planning the different therapeutic options,

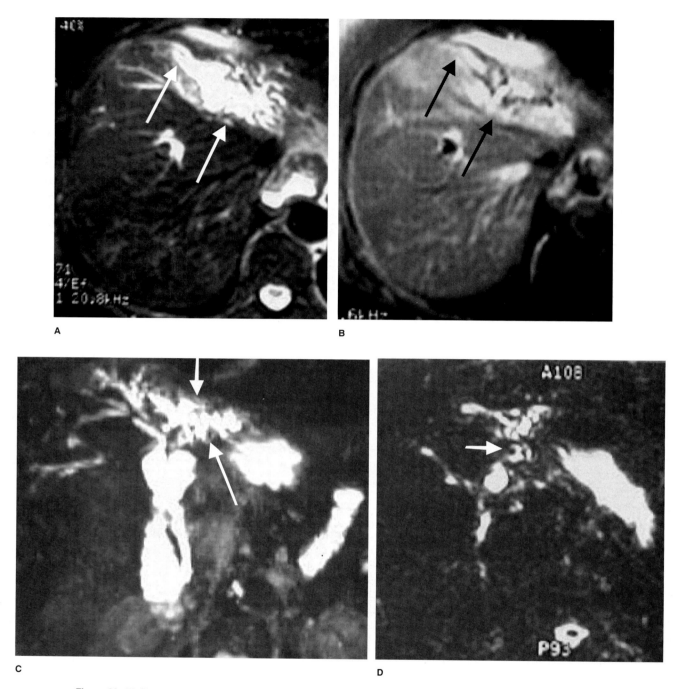

A

B

C

D

Figure 30–15. Recurrent pyogenic cholangitis/oriental cholangitis. **A.** 2D-FSE T2. Note the atrophy and increased signal intensity of the lateral segment of the left lobe secondary to the infection (*arrows*). **B.** Axial FSE T1 FS. Following the administration of gadolinium, observe the enhanced appearance of the parenchyma and the dilated hypointense ducts (*arrows*). **C.** MRCP. Observe the dilatation of the bile ducts on the lateral segment of the left lobe and of the common hepatic duct (*arrows*). **D.** 2D-FSE T2 axial images demonstrate filling defects in the left hepatic duct (*arrow*). Similar filling defects were observed in the common hepatic duct. When evaluating MRCP images it is important to look at the source images as well as the reconstructed MRCP.

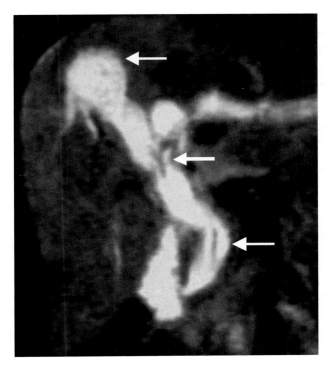

Figure 30–16. A round collection can be seen on the superior and lateral aspect of the right lobe of the liver. This collection is connected with the biliary radicals. The common hepatic duct and the common bile duct are dilated, with hypointense linear defects corresponding to residue of the hidatic membranes (*arrows*).

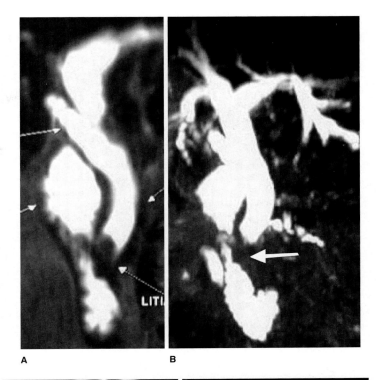

A   B

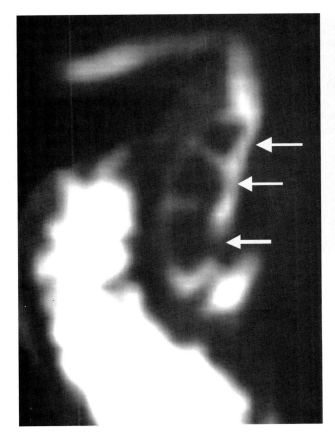

Figure 30–17. Multiple faceted stones in the common bile duct (*arrows*).

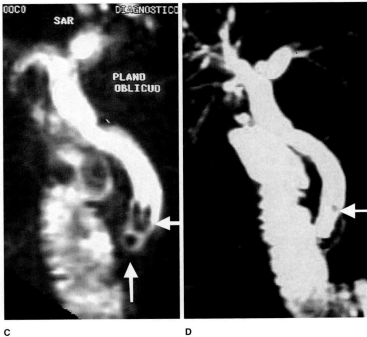

C   D

Figure 30–18. A. Source image; observe dilatation of the intra- and extrahepatic bile ducts. A large stone is impacted at the level of the papilla causing a meniscus sign (*arrow*). **B.** MIP fails to show the presence of the impacted stone (*arrow*). **C.** Source image showing two stones in the distal common bile duct (*arrows*). **D.** Only a small filling defect is seen in the MIP image (*arrow*).

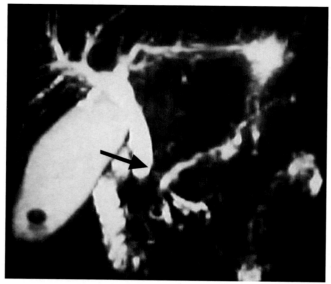

A

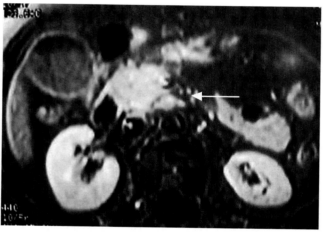

B

Figure 30–19. A. Dilatation of the common bile duct and the duct of Wirsung with irregular and asymmetric stricture secondary to a malignant obstruction (*arrow*). **B.** FSE T1 FS with gadolinium. A large mass in the head of the pancreas with marked enhancement is present (*arrow*).

such as surgery, or palliative procedures such as endoscopic drainage or PTC (Fig. 30–22).

Patients with liver transplants can show anastomotic and nonanastomotic strictures involving the hepatic duct bifurcation, the peripheral ducts, or both. Hepatic artery occlusion, rejection, and cytomegalovirus infection have been cited as causes of nonanastomotic strictures. MR can also demonstrate the presence of a neoplasm such as lymphoma in patients with liver transplant (Fig. 30–23).

Gallbladder carcinoma can affect the biliary tree due to tumoral invasion through the liver and the biliary ducts or by extrinsic compression caused by hilar lymphadenopathy (Fig. 30–24).

Complete obstruction of the biliary tree can be caused by benign processes such as postcholecystectomy dilatation without obstruction, choledocholithiasis, edema or fibrosis of the ampulla of Vater, dyskinesia of the sphincter of Oddi, or by malignant processes

such as carcinoma of the ampulla of Vater, pancreatic carcinoma, duodenal carcinoma, and cancer of the gallbladder (Fig. 30–25).

With MRCP, the exact site of the obstruction can be identified in patients with obstructive jaundice.[2] It also allows the differentiation between choledocholithiasis and tumor. MRCP does not allow the identification of the type of tumor and a precise diagnosis was made in only 30% of patients.[2] Also, MRCP cannot differentiate between a complete obstruction and a severe stenosis.[1]

Comparisons between MRCP and ERCP have been made. The obstruction site was demonstrated in from 91 to 100% of cases with MRCP and in 83% of cases with ERCP.[33] The sensitivity, specificity, and accuracy of MRCP to distinguish between benign and malignant lesions were 81, 92, and 87%, respectively, and for ERCP 71, 92, and 83%; however, the differences were not significant. The diagnostic accuracy was 72% for MRCP and 61% for ERCP. It was reported that MRCP appears to provide fast and accurate diagnosis of extrahepatic obstruction of the biliary tract, similar to that of ERCP.[16]

In our experience, a good correlation between MRCP and ERCP/PTC was found, with a correlation coefficient of 0.96, while the correlation coefficient between ultrasound and ERCP was 0.88. The diagnostic information obtained with MRCP was similar to that obtained with ERCP or PTC. Our results are similar to those of other researchers.[5,9,10] Some authors believe that MRCP techniques need to be improved to compete with ERCP, and it should only be used in patients in whom ERCP or PTC cannot be carried out.[1,7]

ERCP should not be used in patients with choledocholithiasis, pancreatitis, or abdominal pain, or in patients with sclerosing cholangitis and AIDS cholangiopathy if MRCP is available.[19]

DUCT OF WIRSUNG

The normal diameter of the duct of Wirsung is 2 to 3 mm, and its diameter increases from the tail toward the head.[33] The lateral branches are not usually seen unless they are dilated. With the half-Fourier RARE sequence, a normal duct can be visualized in the head and the body in 97% of cases and in the tail in 83% of cases. Dilated ducts are seen in 100% of cases. The duct of Wirsung can show a descending or a vertical course.

Matos et al[31] improved pancreatic duct visualization with the intravenous injection of secretin. They also demonstrated that there was a marked reduction in duodenal filling in patients with decreased pancreatic exocrine function. Therefore this technique could be useful for the diagnosis of ampullary dysfunction or stenosis and to detect failure in pancreatic exocrine function, as well as to evaluate pancreatic exocrine function postduodenopancreatectomy.[32]

Congenital Anomalies

The current resolution of MRCP allows identification of ducts as small as 1 mm in diameter without risk of developing pancreatitis.[19] The incidence of pancreas divisum is 12% and MRCP can demonstrate it with an accuracy of 100%.[18] The patients are usually young and present with recurrent bouts of pancreatitis. To demonstrate drainage of both papillae and the independent course of each duct, both MR and MRCP should be utilized (Fig. 30–26).[15]

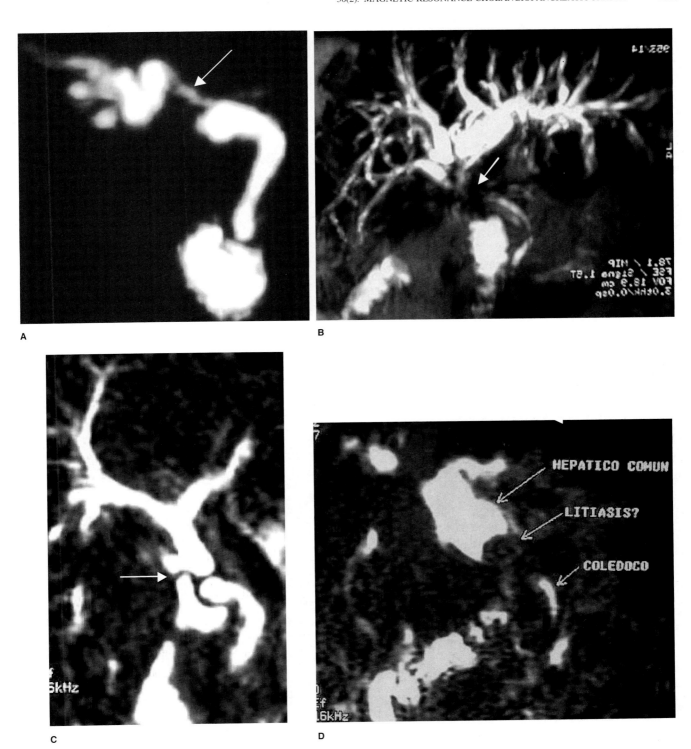

Figure 30–20. A. Postsurgical stricture on the posterior branch of the right hepatic duct (*arrow*). **B.** Partial obstruction of the common hepatic duct produced by clipping during surgery (*arrow*). **C.** Stricture of a choledochojejunoanastomosis (*arrow*). **D.** Obstruction of a hepatojejunoanastomosis by a large stone (*arrows*). Hepatico commun = common hepatic duct; litiasis, lithiasis; coledoco = common bile duct.

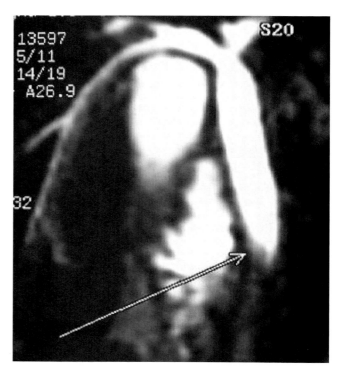

Figure 30–21. (left) Pancreatic carcinoma. Note the irregular eccentric narrowing of the distal common bile duct (*arrow*).

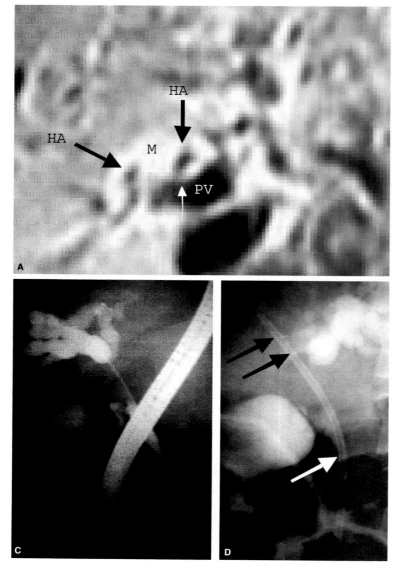

Figure 30–22. (below) Cholangiocarcinoma. **A.** FSE T1 FS with gadolinium. An enhancing hilar mass is seen encasing the branches of the hepatic artery (*black arrows*) and causing compression of the portal vein (*white arrow*). M, mass; HA, hepatic artery; PV, portal vein. **B.** MRCP showing the dilatation of the intrahepatic radicals due to obstruction at the level of the porta hepatis (*arrow*). **C.** ERCP demonstrates a long segment of narrowing (*arrow*). **D.** Endoscopically-placed stent across the segment of narrowing in the proximal common bile duct and common hepatic duct (*white arrow*). Note the persistent dilatation of the left biliary radicals, which were not drained by the endoscopic stent (*black arrows*).

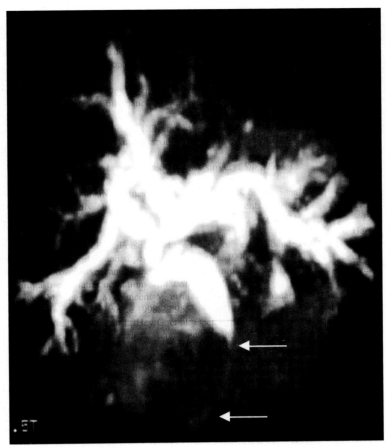

A

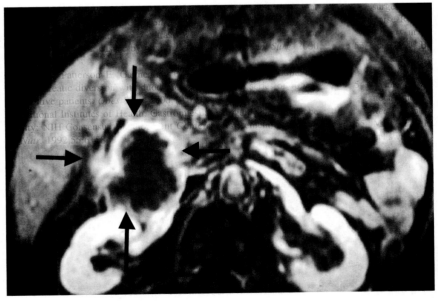

B

Figure 30–23. Lymphoma post hepatic transplantation.
A. MRCP. Extrinsic compression of the distal common
bile duct with proximal dilatation (*arrows*). **B.** FSE T1
FS with gadolinium. Note the peripheral enhancement
of the necrotic mass (*arrows*).

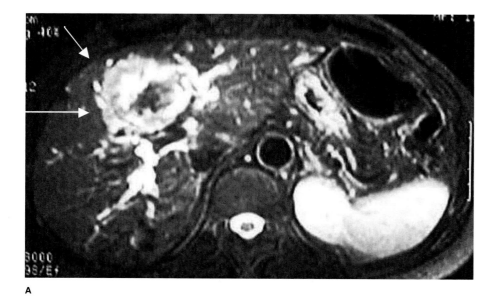

A

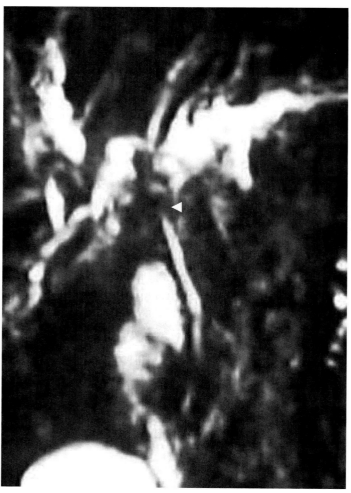

Figure 30–24. FSE T2 FS of cancer of the gallbladder. **A.** Tumor of the gallbladder with invasion of the hepatic hilum is seen (*arrows*). **B.** MRCP showing dilatation of the intrahepatic radicals secondary to obstruction at the level of the porta hepatis (*arrow*).

B

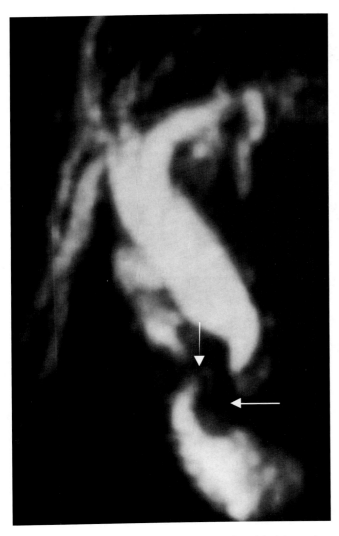

Figure 30–25. Ampullary carcinoma. Observe dilatation of the intra- and extrahepatic bile ducts and a segment of narrowing of the distal common bile duct with a round mass protruding into the duodenum (*arrows*).

Annular pancreas can appear in a complete or an incomplete form and it can be diagnosed at birth or later in life. On MRCP the pancreatic duct can be seen surrounding the duodenum (Fig. 30–27).

Acute Pancreatitis

MRCP is very sensitive for detecting or for ruling out choledocholithiasis. This concept is important to avoid the use of ERCP or surgery in patients in whom choledocholithiasis has not been proved. In the future, MR will become the method of choice for the evaluation of acute pancreatitis, because it provides significant information about ductal dilatation and ductal disruption and permits the evaluation of complications without the use of contrast media or invasive procedures (Fig. 30–28).

Chronic Pancreatitis

In chronic pancreatitis MRCP can detect ductal abnormalities, including luminal narrowing, dilatation, and irregularities in the duc-

tal system, and lithiasis in the main and secondary ducts. In severe cases, dilation of the ducts gives a beaded appearance. MRCP can also demonstrate stones as small as 2 mm. In focal chronic pancreatitis in the pancreatic head, MRCP can demonstrate stenosis in the biliary tract and main pancreatic duct, giving the appearance of a funnel (Fig. 30–29).[12,33]

A pseudocyst can be demonstrated, as well as compression of the biliary and pancreatic ducts. In some cases, communication between the main pancreatic duct and the pseudocyst can be demonstrated (Fig. 30–30).

In cystic fibrosis, pancreatic atrophy with diffuse calcification and dilation of the main pancreatic duct can also be seen. It is common for the biliary tree to be affected and its appearance is similar to that seen in primary sclerosing cholangitis (Fig. 30–31).

Pancreatic Trauma

MRCP may be useful in pancreatic trauma in patients with severe lesions and when there is suspicion of a lesion in the main pancreatic duct either after surgery for pancreatic trauma or in patients with a long-standing fistula.[21]

Pancreatic Carcinoma

MRCP, along with abdominal MR and MR angiography can provide the necessary information for the complete evaluation of pancreatic carcinoma by characterizing and staging lesions. MRCP is also helpful in planning adequate treatment or surgical intervention. Intraductal mucin-producing tumors can be accurately identified with MR (Figs. 30–32 and 30–33). MR also provides important postsurgical information, allowing the detection of abnormal fluid collections and fistulas.[25]

Limitations

Complications of MR and MRCP have not been reported. However, these examinations do have certain disadvantages: there is less resolution than with ERCP and PTC and they are not indicated for patients with claustrophobia. These disadvantages reduce their diagnostic accuracy for early chronic pancreatitis (stage 1) and in detecting small dilatations of the biliary tree.[7] The presence of debris, clots, hemobilia, and/or air in the biliary tree can simulate lithiasis or endoluminal lesions.[1,8] The presence of metallic clips and metallic stents reduces the resolution and quality of the images.[1] Ascites or fluid collections in the upper abdomen reduce the quality of the digital reconstruction. Patient movement, peristalsis, and breathing cause artifacts that can mask stones or small polyps in MIP reconstructions, and can also overestimate the degree of ductal stenosis, thereby diminishing the diagnostic yield of MRCP.[9,34]

CONCLUSION

MR and MRCP are proving to be valuable diagnostic tools in the evaluation of the pancreaticobiliary tree and surrounding tissues. These examinations permit the diagnosis of neoplastic processes and their extension. They are also sensitive in the diagnosis of biliary lithiasis to select the appropriate management.

In the diagnosis of malignant biliary obstruction and staging, CT and ERCP are generally the first examinations of choice, particularly when palliative therapy such as stent or decompression

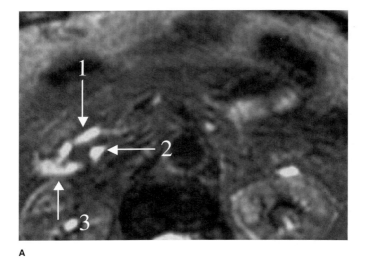

A

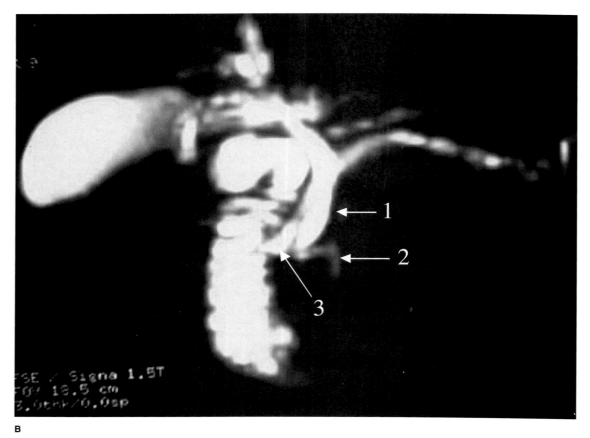

B

Figure 30–26. Pancreas divisum. **A.** Axial FSE TE FS. 1, duct of Santorini; 2, common bile duct; 3, duodenum. **B.** MRCP. 1, common bile duct; 2, a small Wirsung duct draining into the distal common bile duct. 3, duodenum. The duct of Santorini is of a larger caliber with a beaded appearance, and is seen draining into the lesser papilla.

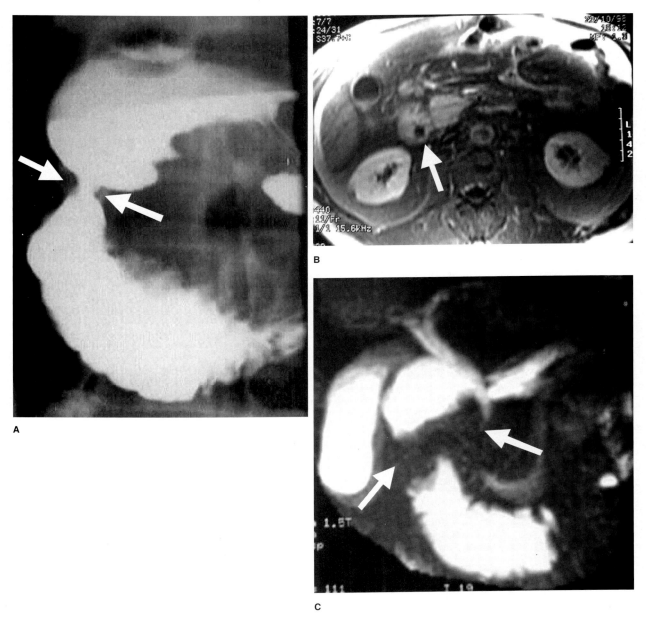

Figure 30–27. Annular pancreas. **A.** Upper GI series showing stenosis of the second portion of duodenum (*arrows*). **B.** FSE T1 FS with gadolinium. Note the abnormal pancreatic tissue surrounding the duodenum in the area of narrowing (*arrow*). **C.** Cholangio MRI. Note the dilatation of the bile ducts secondary to distal stenosis due to chronic pancreatitis, which also causes narrowing of the second portion of the duodenum (*arrows*).

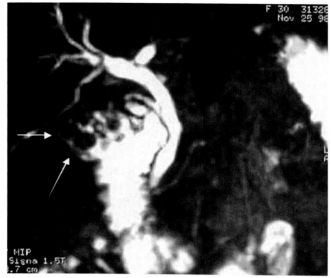

A

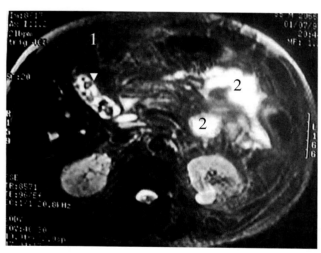

B

Figure 30–28. Acute pancreatitis in a 30-year-old woman with a 20-week pregnancy. **A.** MRCP. Gallbladder stones (*arrows*) and dilated biliary radicals without apparent stones. It is likely that a stone has spontaneously passed across the papilla into the duodenum and that residual dilatation is present in the bile ducts. The duct of Wirsung is also dilated. **B.** FSE T2 FS. 1, gallbladder stones; 2, small peripheral peripancreatic fluid collections.

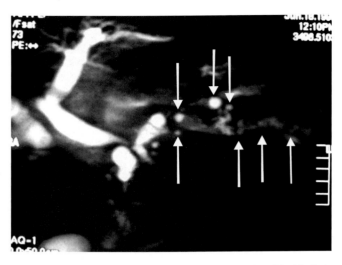

Figure 30–29. Chronic pancreatitis. MRCP. Note the dilatation of the bile ducts secondary to narrowing of the distal common bile duct. A dilated, beaded duct of Wirsung is seen with retention cysts (*arrows*). *(Courtesy of Dr. Julio Loureiro, Argentina.)*

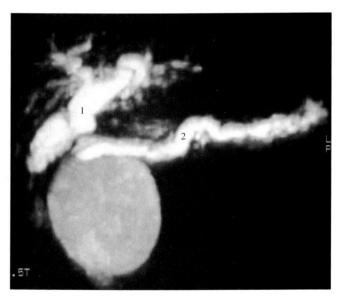

Figure 30–30. MRCP. Pseudocyst of the head of the pancreas causing displacement, obstruction, and dilatation of the bile duct (1) and the duct of Wirsung (2).

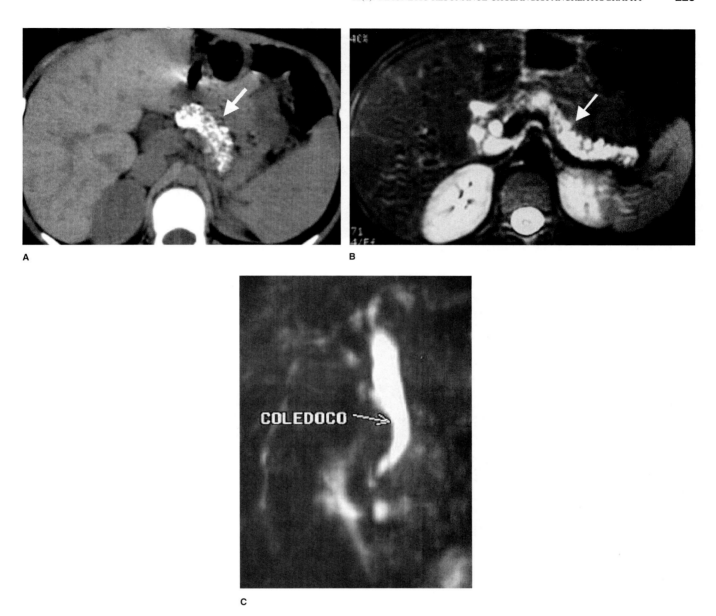

Figure 30–31. Cystic fibrosis in a 15-year-old female. **A.** CT shows diffuse calcifications of the pancreas (*arrow*). **B.** MRI, FSE T2 FS. Innumerable retention cysts are seen with stones within their lumens (*arrow*). **C.** MRCP, distal common bile duct with proximal dilatation. Coledoco = common bile duct (CBD).

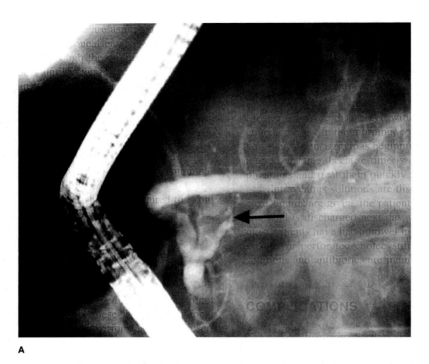

A

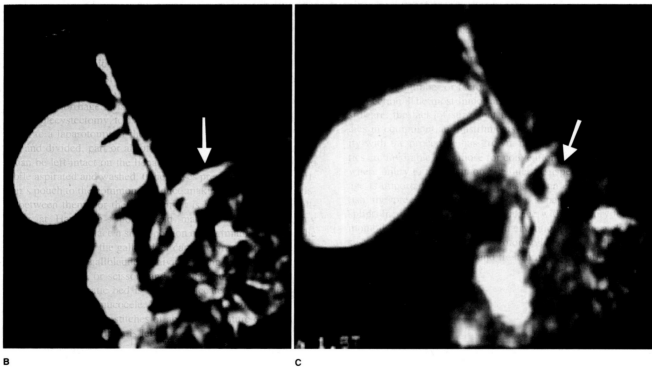

B   **C**

Figure 30–32. Benign tumor of the bile duct causing ectasia in a 30-year-old male presenting with acute pancreatitis. **A.** ERCP showing normal biliary ducts and a dilated duct of Wirsung. Filling defects are seen within the duct of Wirsung and the secondary pancreatic duct (*arrow*). **B.** MRCP showing decreased dilatation of the duct of Wirsung (*arrow*). **C.** An oblique MRCP reconstruction more clearly showing the dilatation of the secondary pancreatic duct and the filling defect (*arrow*).

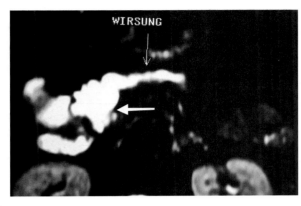

A

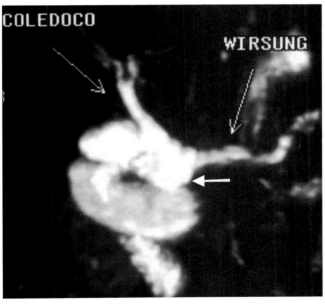

B

Figure 30–33. Benign ductal tumor causing ectasia in a 62-year-old male with recurrent episodes of pancreatitis. **A.** FSE T2 FS image showing cystic dilatations of the pancreatic duct within the uncinate process with dilatation of the duct of Wirsung (*arrow*). **B.** MRCP. Note the moderate dilatation of the common bile and the duct of Wirsung with cystic dilatations at the level of the uncinate process. Coledoco = common bile duct (CBD).

drainage catheter placement are contemplated. Otherwise, MRCP should be the method of choice. MR technology and pulse sequences are constantly being refined and improved, resulting in higher-quality MRCP images similar to those seen in ERCP.

REFERENCES

1. Wallner BK, Schumacher KA, Weidenmaier W, et al. Dilated biliary tract: Evaluation with MR cholangiography with a T$_2$-weighted contrast-enhanced fast sequence. *Radiology* 1991;181:805.
2. Ishizaki Y, Wakayama T, Okada Y, Kobayashi T. Magnetic resonance cholangiography for the evaluation of obstructive jaundice. *Am J Gastroenterol.* 1993;88:2072.
3. Pasanen PA, Partanen K, Pikkarainen P, et al. Diagnostic accuracy of ultrasound, computed tomography and endoscopic retrograde cholangiopancreatography in the detection of obstructive jaundice. *Scand J Gastroenterol.* 1991;26:1157.
4. Soto J, Barish MA, Yucel EK, et al. Pancreatic duct MR cholangiopancreatography with a three-dimensional fast spin-echo technique. *Radiology* 1995;196:459.
5. Hall-Craggs MA, Allen CM, Owens CM, et al. MR cholangiography: Clinical evaluation in 40 cases. *Radiology* 1993;189:423.
6. Guibaud L, Bret PM, Reinhold C, et al. Diagnosis of choledocholithiasis: Value of MR cholangiography. *AJR.* 1994;163:847.
7. McDermott VG, Nelson RC. MR cholangiopancreatography: Efficacy of three-dimensional turbo spin-echo technique. *AJR.*1995;165:301.
8. Outwater EK, Gordon SJ. Imaging the pancreatic and biliary ducts with MR. *Radiology.* 1994;192:19.
9. Barish M, Yucel EK, Soto JA, et al. MR cholangiopancreatography efficacy of three-dimensional turbo spin echo technique. *AJR.* 1995;165:295.
10. Morimoto K, Shimoi M, Shirakawa T, et al. Biliary obstruction: Evaluation with three-dimensional MR cholangiography. *Radiology* 1992;183:578.
11. Bilbao MK, Dotter CT, Lee TG, et al. Complications of endoscopic retrograde cholangiopancreatography (ERCP). A study of 10,000 cases. *Gastroenterology* 1976;70:314.
12. Takehara Y, Ichijo K, Tooyama N, et al. Breath-hold MR cholangiopancreatography with a long-echo-train fast spin-echo sequence and a surface coil in chronic pancreatitis. *Radiology* 1994;192:73.
13. Becker CD, Grossholz M, Mentha G, et al. MR cholangiopancreatography: technique, potential indications and diagnostic features of benign, postoperative and malignant conditions. *Eur Radiol.* 1997;7:865.
14. Soto JA, Yucel EK, Barish MA, et al. MR cholangiopancreatography after unsuccessful or incomplete ERCP. *Radiology* 1996;199:91.
15. Hirohashi S, Hirohashi R, Uchida H, et al. Pancreatitis: evaluation with MR cholangiopancreatography in children. *Radiology* 1997;203:411.
16. Lee MG, Lee HJ, Kim MH, et al. Extrahepatic biliary diseases: 3D MR cholangiopancreatography compared with endoscopic retrograde cholangiopancreatography. *Radiology* 1997;202:663.
17. Reuther G, Kiefer B, Tuchmann A, et al. MR-Cholangiopancreatography as a single-shot projection: techniques and results of 200 examinations. *Rofo-Fortschr-Geb-Rontgenstr-Neuen-Bildgeb-Verfahr.* 1996;165:535.
18. Bret PM, Reinhold C, Taourel P, et al. Pancreas divisum: evaluation with MR cholangiopancreatography. *Radiology* 1996;199:99.
19. Fulcher AS, Turner MA, Capps GW, et al. Half-Fourier RARE MR cholangiopancreatography: experience in 300 subjects. *Radiology* 1998;207:21.
20. Calvo MM, Calderon A, Heras I, et al. Magnetic resonance study of the pancreatic duct. *Rev Esp Enferm Dig.* 1999;91:287.
21. Nirula R, Velmahos GC, Demetriades D. Magnetic resonance cholangiopancreatography in pancreatic trauma: a new diagnostic modality? *J Trauma.* 1999;47:585.
22. Fulcher AS, Turner MA, Capps GW. MR Cholangiography technical advances and clinical applications. *Radiographics* 1999;19:25.
23. Irie H, Honda H, Tajima T, et al. Optimal MR cholangiopancreatographic sequence and its clinical application. *Radiology* 1998;206:379.
24. Barish MA, Yucel EK, Ferrucci JT. Magnetic resonance cholangiopancreatography. *N Engl J Med.* 1999;341:258.
25. Takeyoshi I, Ohwada S, Nakamura S, et al. Segmental pancreatectomy for mucin-producing pancreatic tumors. *Hepatogastroenterology* 1999;46:2585.
26. Taourel P, Bret PM, Reinhold C, et al. Anatomic variants of the biliary tree: diagnosis with MR cholangiopancreatography. *Radiology* 1996;199:521.
27. Ernst O, Asselah T, Talbodec N, et al. MR cholangiopancreatography: a promising new tool for diagnosing primary sclerosing cholangitis [letter. *AJR.* 1997;168:1115.

28. Folsing C, Helmberger T, Sittek H, et al. [Caroli syndrome: diagnostic possibilities of magnetic resonance tomography and MR cholangiopancreaticography.] Das Caroli-Syndrom: Diagnostische Moglichkeiten von Magnetresonanztomographie und MR-Cholangiopankreatikographie. *Rontgenpraxis* 1996;49:226.

29. Pavone P, Laghi A, Catalano C, et al. Caroli's disease: evaluation with MR cholangiopancreatography (MRCP). *Abdom Imaging*. 1996; 21:117.

30. Deziel DJ, Millikan KW, Economou SG, et al. Complications of laparoscopic cholecystectomy: a national survey of 4,292 hospitals and an analysis of 77,604 cases. *Am J Surg*. 1993;165:9.

31. Matos C, Metens T, Deviere J, et al. Pancreatic duct: morphologic and functional evaluation with dynamic MR pancreatography after secretin stimulation. *Radiology* 1997;203:435.

32. Sho M, NakajimaY, Kanehiro H, et al. A new evaluation of pancreatic function after pancreatoduodenectomy using secretin magnetic resonance cholangiopancreatography. *Am J Surg*. 1998;176:279.

33. Fulcher AS, Turner MA. MR Pancreatography a useful tool for evaluating pancreatic disorders. *Radiographics* 1999;19:5.

34. Watanabe Y, Dohke M, Ishimori T, et al. Diagnostic pitfalls of MR cholangiopancreatography of the biliary tract and gallbladder. *Radiographics* 1999;19:415.

Chapter Thirty (Part Three) . . . . . .

Extracorporeal Shock Wave Lithotripsy in the Treatment of Gallbladder and Biliary Tree Gallstones

JULIÁN SÁNCHEZ-CORTÁZAR and ARMANDO LÓPEZ-ORTIZ

INTRODUCTION

Before the 1970s, open cholecystectomy was the procedure most commonly used for gallstone disease. In the last decade, due to improvements in medical imaging technology and other advancements, laparoscopic surgery has become the gold standard for management of gallbladder disease,[1] and endoscopic retrograde cholangiopancreatography (ERCP) and open as well as laparoscopic exploration of the common bile duct system are accepted alternatives in the management of calculous disease of the biliary tract.

In the 1970s, the advent of treatment with chemical solvents and the development of interventional techniques for treating the gallbladder and biliary tract increased the options for treatment of these entities. Soon thereafter, extracorporeal shock wave lithotripsy (ESWL) offered an alternative treatment to open surgery. Today, all these treatments are still being used, and each has its own place in the management of selected patients for whom standard treatments are not suitable.

During the first half of the 1980s, ESWL had great success in the treatment of urinary tract calculi, with first-generation devices that produced shock waves to shatter stones. In this type of machine, the patient is submerged in a water bath in a supine position while focused shock waves are used to break up the stones. Careful anesthetic management and constant monitoring are necessary when using this technique.[3,4] This machine uses fluoroscopy to locate the stones.

In the mid 1980s, fragmentation systems were diversified with the arrival of second-generation devices. Instead of using a water bath, these devices used a water cushion that obviated the need for immersion.

There was also development of ESWL devices that used a different strategy. These devices were piezoelectric and electromag-netic machines, and they caused less pain to the patient, making anesthetic management unnecessary. Some of these devices used ultrasound (US) or a combination of US and fluoroscopy to locate stones.

CHOLELITHIASIS

Gallstone formation is caused by precipitation of bilirubin pigments and cholesterol salts; they can also be formed by precipitation of calcium in the form of palmitate, carbonate, aragonite, and apatite. In most reports the gallstones are of a mixed type.[5] Recent reports confirm that bile duct ectasia and stasis are contributing factors in stone formation.[6]

The criteria for use of ESWL to treat gallbladder stones with ESWL are:[7]

- History of colicky gallbladder pain.
- Radiolucid stones visible with cholecystography (Fig. 30–34).
- One to three radiolucid stones, each with a volume of less than 3 mL.
- Gallstones visible with US (Fig. 30–35).

The exclusion criteria are:

- Acute cholecystitis (Fig. 30–36).
- Gastroduodenal ulcer.
- Acute pancreatitis.
- Bleeding diatheses or anticoagulation therapy.
- Pregnancy.
- More than 3 gallstones, or gallstones larger than 3 mL.
- Radiopaque gallstones.

ESWL requires presurgical evaluation that should include coagulation and liver function tests, complete blood count, and sometimes a cardiologic evaluation.

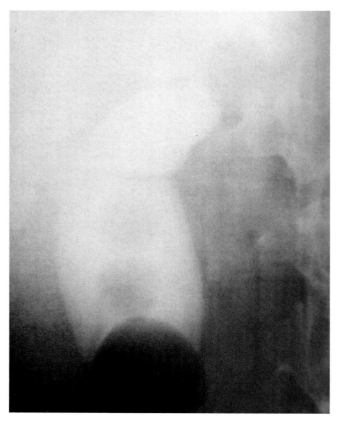

Figure 30–34. Cholecystogram showing two radiolucid stones.

The treatment is carried out with the patient in either a supine or prone position. Localization of the gallstones is done via US, cholecystography, or fluoroscopy. We deliver nearly 1600 shock waves to the targets and radiographic verification of stone fracture is obtained. Rabenstein defines successful treatment as pulverization of stones to a size smaller than 4 mm. Fragmentation refers to stone particles that are larger than 4 mm (Fig. 30–37).[8]

Results vary from author to author, but adequate fragmentation of the calculi was obtained in about 80% of the reported cases.[9] In cases in which pulverization is obtained, the outcome is favorable in 87.5%, and in those in which fragmentation occurs, the favorable outcome is nearly 72.2%.[8] The use of computed tomography (CT)

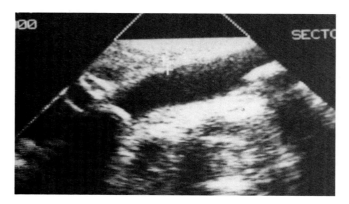

Figure 30–35. Gallbladder US. Two echogenic stones are visible.

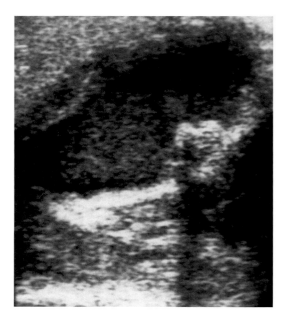

Figure 30–36. Gallbladder US of gallbladder with acute cholecystitis. Note the narrowing of the gallbladder wall.

has shown that calculi with attenuation under 50 Hounsefield units (HU) have better fragmentation and elimination than calculi with attenuation of more than 100 HU.[10] These results were confirmed by Uchiyama et al.[11] Koshiyama described another favorable prognostic factor. He found in 67 gallbladder scintigraphies that patients who had a large uptake of radioisotope and rapid evacuation showed quicker elimination of fragments than patients with small gallbladders, poor uptake, and slow evacuation. These findings suggest that coordination between the sphincter of Oddi and gallbladder contraction is an important factor for successful treatment.[12]

This treatment has been used in conjunction with the oral administration of chemical solvents such as quenodeoxycolic acid and

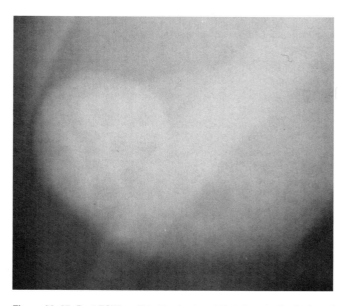

Figure 30–37. Post ESWL gallbladder treatment that shows pulverization of the stones after application of 2000 shock waves.

urodesoxycolic acid, which can be administered alone or combined,[3] for at least 3 to 18 months. The use of these agents reduces the amount of time needed for elimination of the fragments. Unfortunately, these agents have well-known side effects, such as diarrhea and transitory hypercholesterolemia, which sometimes require discontinuation of treatment.[13] Dion and Morin[14] reported in their 1995 article that treatment with ESWL is not usually recommended because of these side effects. The East-Danish Gallstone Study Group reports that there are inconsistent results with the use of oral bile acid treatment with ESWL.[15]

Other reports have found that sphincterectomy is a secure and safe procedure for the elimination of fragments after ESWL and is an important adjuvant treatment for gallbladder hypomotility and also helps to diminish the formation of new stones.

Immediate complications secondary to ESWL include transitory elevation of hepatic enzymes[16] and a reduction of hepatic blood flow on scintigraphy, which is seen in nearly 70% of patients within 3 days after treatment but tends to improve in the following week.[17] Other complications are petechiae at the site of shock wave application and hematuria.[16] Pain is sometimes also a problem and is associated with the evacuation of small particles; this complication occurs in up to 30% of patients.[18] Rarely, pancreatitis[3] and acute obstruction of the extrahepatic biliary tract may occur. Some patients also present with hemobilia, which resolves spontaneously.

There are a few reports of isolated bacteremia[19] and suprarenal malfunction[20] in some patients after ESWL. The recurrence of pain after successful treatment with ESWL occurs in up to one-third of patients and is due to reformation of calculi in 40 to 60% of patients.[21] Cesmeli et al[22] report that this recurrence is associated with the use of hormonal therapy. It presents in 5.5% of patients after 1 year, 12% after more than 2 years, and 30.5% within 3 years or more.[23] The recurrence after 5 and 6 years is up to 50 to 60%.[22,23] This is why Rabenstein et al recommend more rigorous treatment with ESWL, and the use of more shock waves and more frequent sessions to obtain complete pulverization, lessening the need for oral agents to help dissolve calculi. Those patients with pain and no evidence of gallbladder lithiasis, but with unexplained common bile duct dilatation as seen on US may have microlithiasis of the biliary tract and dysfunction of the sphincter of Oddi, a condition Wehrman et al[21] called postlithotripsy syndrome.

Recent reports have shown the advantages of using a minilithotripter, including reduced treatment costs.[24]

GALLSTONES OF THE INTRA- AND EXTRAHEPATIC BILIARY TREE

Gallstones of the biliary tree may be intrahepatic or extrahepatic in location. Most of these are residual or recurrent gallstones of the common hepatic and common bile ducts. Most intrahepatic gallstones are primarily associated with changes in the integrity of the biliary tree,[25] and almost 50% of them are related to congenital malformations.[26] A small number are thought to be a complication of conservative treatment of hepatocellular carcinoma, as suggested by the report from Koda et al.[27]

Cases requiring management that is different from or complementary to ERCP are usually due to the presence of single or multiple stones that are larger than 2 cm in diameter, as such stones are hard to capture, fragment, or extract by endoscopic methods. These cases usually pose other problems, such as stenosis of the biliary ducts with or without cholangitis. Such cases are known

collectively as difficult gallstones of the biliary duct (Fig. 30–38).[2,28,29]

Conservative management of these calculi by a multidisciplinary team has been suggested to allow the use of two or more procedures for the resolution of such stones. Success rates of over 80% have been achieved by Masci et al[30] with such treatment.

Extrahepatic gallstones are treated successfully with endoscopic methods in 80% of cases;[2,28] the remaining cases failed to respond due to impaction (56%), presence of large gallstones (>2 cm in isolated or mixed forms) (38%), and the presence of stenosis (6%).[31] Patients with calculi inaccessible to the Dormia basket and the impacted basket[32] can be treated with alternative methods, such as the use of deflectors, baskets, balloons, flexible endoscopic devices, insertion of photoelectrohydraulic (laser) or electrohydraulic devices through percutaneous tracts or a T-tube fistulous tract.[33] These patients can also be subjected to ESWL alone[2,3] or combined with other treatments.

Successful common bile duct treatments using fragmentation have been achieved in up to 80 to 92% of reported cases (Fig. 30–39),[2,28,29,34] with a 43 to 90% rate of spontaneous elimination, while the remaining 10 to 40% require the use of adjuvant therapy along with endoscopic maneuvers.[2,28,29,35] Failure may be related to nonvisualized calculi in 5 to 10% of cases[34,36] or with stenosis in up to 6% of cases.[29]

Partial hepatic resection,[25,37] endoscopic extraction, intervention with a Dormia basket, stent placement,[30] and endocorporeal lithotripsy with pulsed laser[33] are therapeutic modalities used in the treatment of intrahepatic gallstones. Adamek et al[37] mentioned the benefits of combined treatment, reporting up to a 90% success rate. They also noted the lack of benefit of the use of ESWL compared to the high benefit of pulsed laser when used as monotherapy. The use of ESWL in the intrahepatic bile ducts has had success rates of 19 to 33%[13,37] as monotherapy, with mortality reported to be 0.3%.[38]

Contraindications to ESWL are the same as for other regimens, and the laboratory studies required prior to ESWL are those used to detect clotting problems and alterations in hepatic function.

The treatment can be applied with the patient in supine or prone decubitus position, depending on the mobility of the water cushion. Gallstone localization is carried out using real time US and fluoroscopy systems with water-based contrast media passed

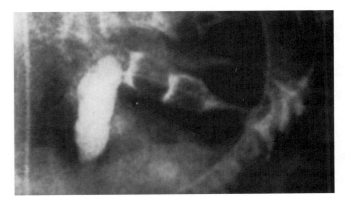

Figure 30–38. Patient with large gallstones inside the common bile duct for which attempts at extraction failed. The patient had opacification of the biliary tree seen upon administration of contrast media through a nasobiliary catheter during ESWL.

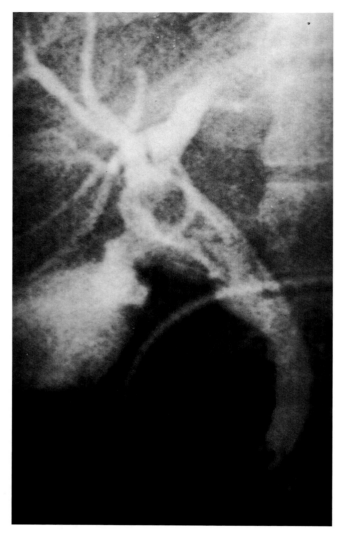

Figure 30–39. The same patient seen in Fig. 30–38 after ESWL.

through a nasobiliary catheter previously placed by endoscopy, through a T-tube tract, or percutaneously.

Most third-generation machines come equipped with or can be used in conjunction with US and fluoroscopic devices.[4] The number of shock waves applied varies according to the size of the gallstones and their localization, and may range from 750 to 2100 shots of 14 to 17 Kw.[39]

The complications of this type of treatment are the same as for as gallbladder ESWL, among them pain related to the expulsion of fragments, hemobilia, hematuria, ecchymosis at the site of contact with the water cushion, and pancreatitis.[29,36]

SUMMARY

For calculous disease of the gallbladder and biliary ducts, ESWL has an important complementary role for the treatment of patients that require or prefer an alternative conservative treatment to lap-

aroscopic surgery. ESWL can be used as monotherapy for gallbladder stones or as an adjuvant treatment for endoscopic or interventional modalities. ESWL costs are high, primarily for those cases that require many treatments to completely fragment the stones. However, ESWL can benefit 75% of patients with gallbladder stones and 60% of patients with stones of the common bile duct and common hepatic duct when used as monotherapy, and its efficacy increases to 90% when it is used concomitantly with endoscopic procedures. ESWL shows little benefit when used as monotherapy in patients with in-trahepatic stones, but it has an important role in combined treatment. It has been demonstrated that oral bile acid solvents do not have an important role when used concomitantly with ESWL.

REFERENCES

1. Seibold F. Conservative therapy of gallstones (abstract). *Fortschr Med.* 1998;116:26.
2. Merret ??, AUTHOR, AUTHOR, et al. Extracorporeal shock wave lithotripsy for bile duct stones: An Australian experience. *J Gastroeneterol Hepatol.* 1990;5:537.
3. Hernández-Graulau JM, Castañeda-Zúñiga WR. *Interventional Radiology*, 3rd ed. Williams & Wilkins:1997;1350.
4. Rassweiler J, Henkel TO, Körmann KU, et al. Lithotripter technology: Present and future. *J Endourol.* 1992;6:1.
5. Sutor DJ, Wooley SE. A statistical survey of the composition of gallstones in eight countries. *Gut* 1971;12:55.
6. Dhiman RK, Phanish MK, Chawla YK, et al. Gallbladder motility and lithogenicity of bile in patients with choledocholithiasis after endoscopic sphincterotomy. *J Hepatol.* 1997;26:1300.
7. Paumgartner G. Fragmentation of gallstones by extracorporeal shock waves. *Semin Liver Dis.* 1987;7:317.
8. Rabenstein T, Benninger J, Farnbacher M, et al. Optimized extracorporeal shockwave lithotripsy of gallbladder calculi: a prospective randomized therapy comparison (abs). *Z Gastroenterol.* 1999;37:209.
9. Uchiyama K, Tanimura H, Ishimoto K, et al. Extracorporeal shock wave lithotripsy (ESWL) for biliary stones. *Nippon Geka Hokan* 1994;63:199.
10. Kratzer W, Mason RA, Vogel J, et al. Low pretreatment gallbladder stone densities at computed tomography predict rapid stone clearance following extracorporeal shock wave lithotripsy (abs). *Ital J Gastoenterol.* 1995;27:484.
11. Uchiyama F, Otsuka K, Maeda Y, et al. Extracorporeal shock wave lithotripsy: elimination of densely calcified gallstones and gallstones with calcified rims. *Eur J Gastroenterol Hepatol.* 2000;12:305.
12. Koshiyama H. Evaluation of factors in fragment disappearance after extracorporeal shockwave lithotripsy for gallstones (abs). *Nippon Shokakibyo Gakkai Zasshi* 1996;93:338.
13. Griffith DP, Gleeson MJ. Gallstones: advantages and disadvantages of five treatment alternatives. *J Lithotripsy Stone Dis.* 1990;2:184.
14. Dion YM, Morin J. The role of extracorporeal shock wave lithotripsy in the treatment of symptomatic cholelithiasis. *Can J Surg.* 1995;38:162.
15. The East-Danish Gallstone Study Group. Bile acid therapy vs. placebo before and after extracorporeal shock wave lithotripsy of gallbladder stones (abs). *Ugeskr Laeger* 1998;160:408.
16. Adwers JR. Gallstone lithotripsy: Early American results and the new reality. *J Lithotripsy Stone Dis.* 1990;2:199.
17. Oztür KE, Günalp B, Mas R, et al. Evaluation of hepatocyte function after extracorporeal shockwave lithotripsy with hepatobiliary scintigraphy. *Am J Gastroenterol.* 1998;93:1905.
18. Sackmann M, Delius M, Sauerbuch T, et al. Shock wave lithotripsy of gallbladder stones. First 175 patients. *N Engl J Med.* 1988;318:393.

19. Kullman E, Jönsson KA, Lindström E, et al. Bacteremia associated with extracorporeal shockwave lithotripsy of gallbladder stones. *Hepatogastroenterology* 1995;42:816.

20. Saydam S, Bora S, Bakir H, et al. The effects of lithotripsy on adrenocortical hormones. *Int Surg.* 1995;8:271.

21. Wehrmann T, Lembcke B, Caspary WF, et al. Sphincter of Oddi dysfunction after successful gallstone lithotripsy (postlithotripsy syndrome): manometric data and results of endoscopic sphincterotomy. *Dig Dis Sci.* 1999;44:2244.

22. Cesmeli E, Elewaut AE, Kerre T, et al. Gallstone recurrence after successful shockwave therapy: the magnitude of the problem and the predictive factors. *Am J Gastroenterol.* 1999;94:474.

23. Adamek HE, Sorg S, Bachor OA, et al. Symptoms of post-000extracorporeal shock wave lithotripsy: Long term analysis of gallstone patients before and after successful SWL. *Am J Gastroenterol.* 1995;90:1125.

24. Wehrmann T, Scmitt T, Braden B, et al. Extracorporeal shockwave lithotripsy in cholecystolithiasis using a new type of minilithotripter. *Dtsch Med Wochenschr.* 1999;124:1158.

25. Ker CG, Kuo KK, Chen HJ, et al. Morphology duct in surgical treatment of hepatolithiasis. *Hepatogastroenterology* 1997;44:317.

26. Nuzzo G, Clemente G, Giuliante F, et al. Intrahepatic calculosis. *Ann Ital Chir.* 1998;69:765.

27. Koda M, Murawaki Y, Horie Y, et al. Is choledocholithiasis a late complication of nonresectional therapy for hepatocellular carcinoma? *Hepatogastroenterology* 1999;46:3091.

28. Harz C. Extracorporeal shock wave lithotripsy and endoscopy: combined therapy for problematic bile duct stones. *Surg Endosc.* 1991; 5:196.

29. Eckhauser FE, Raper SE, Knol JA, et al. Extracorporeal lithotripsy. An important adjunct in nonoperative management of retained or recurrent bile duct stones. *Arch Surg.* 1991;126:829.

30. Masci E, Farti L, Mariani A, et al. Multidisciplinary conservative treatment of difficult bile duct stones: a real alternative to surgery. *HPB Surg.* 1997;10:229.

31. White DM, Correa RJ, Gibbons RP, et al. Extracorporeal shockwave lithotripsy for bile duct calculi. *Am J Surg.* 1998;175:10.

32. Kratzer W, Mason RA, Grammer S, et al. Difficult bile duct stone recurrence after endoscopy and extracorporeal shockwave lithotripsy. *Hepatogastroenterology* 1998;45:910.

33. Jackobs R, Adamek HE, Maier M, et al. Fluoroscopically guided laser lithotripsy versus extracorporeal shock wave lithotripsy for retained bile duct stones: a prospective randomized study. *Gut* 1997;40:679.

34. Weber J, Adamek HE, Reimann JF. Extracorporeal piezoelectric lithotripsy for retained bile duct stones. *Endoscopy* 1992;24:239.

35. Lomanto D, Fiocca F, Nardovino M, et al. ESWL experience in the therapy of difficult bile duct stones. *Dig Dis Sci.* 1996;41:2397.

36. Cervera SJ, Barinagarrementeria R, Rodriguez JJ. Treatment of bile duct calculi with extracorporeal lithotripsy. *Rev Gastroenterol Mex.* 1991;56:183.

37. Adamek HE, Schneider AR, Adamek MU, et al. Treatment of difficult intrahepatic stones by using extracorporeal and intracorporeal lithotripsy techniques: 10 years' experience in 55 patients. *Scand J Gastroenterol.* 1999;34:1157.

38. Dagenais M, Lapointe R, Déry R. Role of extracorporeal shock wave lithotripsy in the treatment of common bile duct and intrahepatic calculi. *Ann Chir.* 1995;49:659.

39. Ihse I. Extracorporeal shock wave lithotripsy of bile duct stones. Initial Swedish experience. *Acta Chir Scand.* 1990;156:87.

Chapter Thirty-One ● ● ● ● ● ●

Choledocoduodenostomy

**FERNANDO DELGADO-GOMIS, FRANCISCO BLANES-MASSON,
and JAVIER MARTÍN-DELGADO**

HISTORY

In 1875, Loreta in Bologna attempted the first surgery to cure biliary lithiasis, a procedure consisting of emptying and cleaning the gallbladder and a subsequent cholecystorraphy. The modern era of biliary surgery is said to have begun when Lagenbuch performed the first cholecystectomy in 1882.

Two years later, Kummel, following Lagenbuch's lead, performed the first choledocotomy with calculi extraction. Thus even at the beginning, biliary surgery was found to be a successful treatment for biliary lithiasis. Exploration and sometimes surgery of the common bile duct should also be performed, because it often contains calculi.

The logical next step was the development of methods to diagnose common bile duct pathology, to reduce diagnostic failures due to manual instrumented exploration of the biliary tract. Three nonoperative methods became popular over the years:

- Direct choledocoscopy, performed for the first time in 1923 by Bakes[1]
- Preoperative cholangiography, introduced by Mirizzi in 1937[2]
- Biliary manometry, developed by Caroli in 1945[3]

Using these techniques, the status of the bile ducts can be ascertained, and many patients have benefited from them. Closure over a T-tube increases the effectiveness of choledocotomy, and Flörchen[4] standardized supraduodenal choledocoduodenoanastomosis, which was performed for the first time by Riedel in 1891.[5] English practitioners showed some resistance to this last technique, until Madden et al,[6] Degenshein,[7] and Hurwitz[8] defended it as a simple and effective technique. The development of transduodenal sphincterplasty completed the surgeon's armamentarium for the treatment of common bile duct stones.[9] At the same time, endoscopic retrograde cholangiopancreatography (ERCP) with sphincterotomy and biliary tract cleansing was also developed.[10]

During the 1960s, the discussion of biliary surgery centered on the efficacy of biliary bypass or transduodenal papillotomy as a method of treatment for choledocolithiasis,[11–13] and ERCP was promoted for cholecystectomized patients and for those who had contraindications for surgery. This technique has been perfected over the years, and morbidity and mortality have been drastically reduced, which has increased its usefulness even more. Conventional surgery for biliary lithiasis with ERCP is also effective and safe, with a morbidity of 5%, due mainly to respiratory and wound complications, with a mortality rate near 0.5%, which increases with patient age and the severity of the disease (acute cholecystitis, suppurative cholangitis, etc.).[14]

The situation did not improve until laparoscopic biliary surgery was developed by Mouret[15] and Dubois et al[16] in France, and Reddick and Olsen[17] in the United States, establishing laparoscopic cholecystectomy as the procedure of choice for the treatment of cholecystitis, and modifying the new technique for the treatment of choledocolithiasis. Since calculi in the main biliary tract are present in about 4 to 15% of patients operated on for cholecystitis (increasing with the age of the patient),[18,19] it is important to decide which therapy should be employed.

In the beginning of the laparoscopic era, methods of preoperative evaluation of the biliary treat vigorously sought to select only patients without choledocolithiasis for laparoscopic procedures, and to perform an ERCP with retrieval of CBD calculi before laparoscopic cholecystectomy in patients in whom this complication was suspected. This is the reason that led to the increase in the number of ERCPs performed preoperatively, a situation that has been changed in recent years. At the present time, transcystic and/or transcholedocal exploration and extraction of calculi within the common bile duct and trans and/or postoperative ERCP are methods accepted for the treatment of choledocolithiasis.[20] With the advent of advanced techniques in laparoscopic surgery that allow more precise dissection, hemostasia and bimanual suturing, latero-lateral choledocoduodenoanastomosis (CDA) is being reevaluated.[21,22]

In this chapter we will not discuss the controversy surrounding these different options for the treatment of CBD lithiasis, Instead, we will detail the indications for CDA, and describe our laparoscopic technique and the results obtained.

INDICATIONS

There is agreement among all researchers[23–25] that the primary indication for the performance of a CDA is a threshold diameter of the common bile duct, which we have established as 14 mm or greater, as measured by echography. If this condition is present, we perform a CDA when the patient presents with:

- Common bile duct diameter over 20 mm
- Presence of multiple stones
- Juxtapapillary diverticulum
- ERCP failure

There remains a number of patients who present with a common bile duct diameter between 14 and 20 mm, as measured by echography, in which we must decide between ERCP and CDA as a therapeutic modality. To make the right decision, we take into account the availability of expert endoscopists and laparoscopic surgeons in our center, as well as the rate of choledocolithiasis in our patient population. We should add that CDA is performed at the same time as cholecystectomy, which reduces the risk and the costs to the patient.

Just as transduodenal sphincterotomy had to find its niche when derivation appeared, in today's laparoscopic era, it is biliary performed by this modality, which must find its place next to ERCP, since it appeared later and there are few surgeons capable of performing it. We believe that in time CDA will also find its proper set of indications.

SURGICAL TECHNIQUE

We usually place the patient in supine position with the legs astride and a slight anti-Trendelenburg, as for laparoscopic biliary surgery.[26] We also use the same ports for the surgery, with a 10-mm port in the right umbilical margin through which we introduce the laparoscope, and a 5-mm subxiphoid port through which the liver retractor, the aspirator, and a clamp to hold the CDA traction suture are inserted. Another 5-mm port is placed in the right iliac fossa for the instruments the surgeon manipulates with the left hand, and a 10-mm port is placed in the left hypochondrium, taking care not to damage the vessels of the anterior rectus abdominalis muscle, to introduce the instruments the surgeon manipulates with the right hand. The exact position of these last two ports depends in part on the characteristics of the patient's abdomen, because they must allow firm grasping and handling of the gallbladder, and all instruments must reach the entire hepatic bed without difficulty from both ports.

Once the cholecystectomy is performed, which is generally difficult due to long-standing lithiasis, the procedure continues as follows:

- Closure of the cystic stem with extracorporeal knots to avoid the staples normally used to close the cystic duct.
- The duodenum is taken by its upper curvature with an Allis clamp inserted through the right iliac fossa port, and with curved scissors inserted through the left hypo-chondrium port; the peritoneum is severed at the level of the external border of the second duodenal portion (Kocher's maneuver), until enough duodenum is free to be mobilized to approximate it without tension on the biliary tract.

- The peritoneum covering the common bile duct is dissected longitudinally, ensuring that the selected point of entry into the main biliary tract is correct. At this point care must be take not to damage the veins in the choledocal wall, which would cause a hemorrhage that is difficult to manage.
- Pierce the common bile duct at the point nearest the duodenum with the tip of a scalpel, and using microscissors, open the bile duct to the imaginary line of section chosen in an ascending longitudinal fashion to a distance of approximately 20 mm. At this point, the contents (bile, detritus, calculi) of the common bile duct will escape, and they should be aspirated as much as possible, though spillage into the subhepatic space has never created morbidity in our patients (Fig. 31–1).

We use a specially designed scalpel, because one of proper design is not yet commercially available. We construct a new one for each procedure like this: A small, fine-point scalpel blade is broken in half, and the sharp piece is grasped with a needle-holder. Then both are placed in a metallic converter from 10 to 5 mm, which enters the abdomen through the 10-mm trocar site in the left hypochondrium. With the tip of the scalpel protected, the converter can be brought near to the anterior wall of the common bile duct without danger; then by advancing the needle-holder, the tip of the scalpel is exposed and the incision made. The scalpel should not be moved without reinserting the tip into the converter, to avoid damage to the abdominal viscera.

1. Piercing the abdominal wall with a venous puncture trocar with the needle removed and the plastic oversheet in place in a location verified laparoscopically to be directly over the common bile duct allows insertion of a double-lumen catheter (one to inflate the balloon, and another one that is used for washing the common bile duct and cholangiography). The diameter of the venous puncture trocar should be large enough to allow passage of the balloon catheter, the width of which is chosen according to the diameter of the common bile duct. The catheter is inserted through the choledocotomy, and manipulated so the calculi that it contains are extracted, and it is

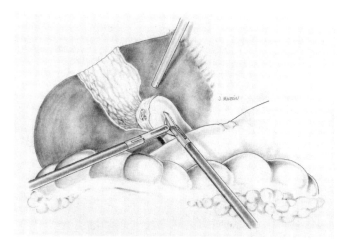

Figure 31–1. At the point nearest to the duodenum at the imaginary line of section chosen, the common bile duct is opened in an ascending longitudinal fashion.

handled with a dissector inserted through the left hypochondrium (Fig. 31–2).

2. A completion cholangiography of the complete extraction of calculi from the common bile duct, in both the ascending and descending portions, should be done before suturing the choledocotomy. Another way to verify the patency of the CBD is introducing a choledoscope.

3. Using a 0-0 polyglycolic acid suture with a curved needle and with an extracorporeal knot, the apex of the common bile duct incision is aligned with the inferior aspect of the duodenum. This stitch is tied and cut, leaving the free end long for traction, and the other end is cut short so the stitch will not become loose.

4. The duodenum is entered and incised with scalpel or microscissors, from an area most proximal to the pylorus to the point where the previous stitch was placed, and in the rest of the incision is done with a hook-shaped electrocautery to cauterize the edges of the mucosa.

5. Several interrupted stitches of 2-0 polyglycolic are placed to join the right edge of the choledocotomy (next to the stitch described above), with the superior edge of the duodenotomy until the inferior angle of the choledocotomy is reached, joining it to the most proximal part of the duodenal incision (posterior aspect of the choledocoduodenostomy). These sutures should include all layers of the common bile duct wall and the seromuscular layer of the duodenum, and the knot should be tied intraluminally. The last stitch is also left with a long end, also for traction and this knot is tied extraluminally.

6. Using the two long strands as reference of the ends of the anastomosis, the anterior aspect is sutured with simple extracorporeal stitches, completing the choledocoduodenal anastomosis. We recommend that these stitches be placed alternatively at each end of the anastomosis, to facilitate placement of the last suture.

7. To simplify the placement of these stitches, the subxiphoid clamp should tetract the liver, and at the same time traction should be applied at the long end of the distal stitch, while the dissector, which enters through the right iliac fossa trochar site, is maintaining tension on the end of the stitch that was placed

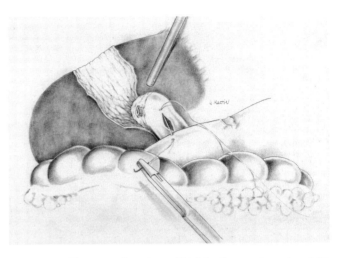

Figure 31–3. Placement of a suture, which joins the superior vertex of the common bile duct to the inferior vertex of the duodenal section line.

immediately before. The long end is cut once the current stitch is tied (Figs. 31–3, 31–4, 31–5, and 31–6).

8. These anastomosis can also be performed with two running hemostatic sutures, stitching the posterior aspect first, and then the anterior one, with 3-0 polyglycolic acid sutures, These may be tied with intracorporeal knots or fixed at both ends with absorbable staples (which reduces operative time).

9. Once the anastomosis is complete, the bag with the collected calculi is tied and removed from the subhepatic space along with the gallbladder. They are both extracted through the umbilical port in the usual fashion.

10. At the conclusion of the procedure, gentle lavage and aspiration of the subhepatic space with warm saline is performed until the space is satisfactorily clean. A Penrose drain is placed near the anastomosis through an appropriate stab wound, confirmed laparaoscopically. We do not advise using one of the trocar ports as the point of exit for the subhepatic drain.

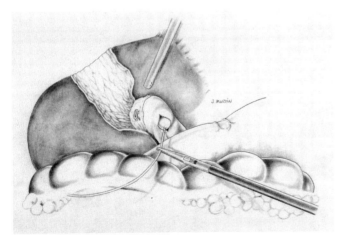

Figure 31–2. Extraction of the Fogarty probe with the inflatable balloon from the common bile duct, this procedure can be done in ascending or descending fashion.

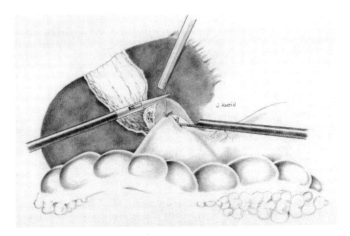

Figure 31–4. The loose end of the first knot has been left long and tension applied, so it can be used for traction when cutting the muscular layers of the duodenum from the most proximal point of the theoretical section line selected, coagulating with the hook-shaped electroscalpel.

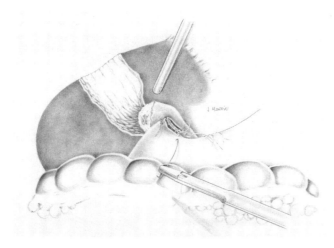

Figure 31–5. Placement of loose stitches joining the right edge of the chole-docotomy at its most distal with the superior edge of the duodenotomy. These stitches penetrate the entire common bile duct wall and the seromuscular layer of the duodenum.

RESULTS

The mean age for these patients—10 women and 4 men—was 74.3 years (range, 61 to 84). Their symptoms are shown in Table 31–1. Pain in the right hypochondrium was present in all patients, and obvious jaundice was seen in 10 patients (71.4%). Bilirubin elevation was present in 8 patients, but alkaline phosphatase and gamma-glutamyl transferase levels were abnormal in all. The diagnosis was established by ultrasonography, with a mean common bile duct diameter of 18.4 mm (range, 14 to 26). Trans-cystic cholangiography was performed during all of the procedures, making the dilatation of the CBD obvious in all patients, which coincided with the echographic findings and the existence of multiple stones in 12 of the 14 patients.

The duration of the surgical procedure was 226 minutes (mean). The first patient was converted to laparotomy after the

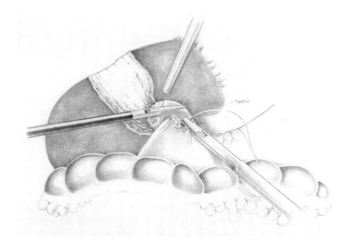

Figure 31–6. Using the two long ends of the sutures at the ends of the anastomosis as reference points, the anterior aspect of the CDA is sutured with stitches alternatively placed at each end of the anastomosis, to facilitate tying the last part of the suture line.

TABLE 31–1. PREOPERATIVE SYMPTOMATOLOGY

Sign	No. of Patients	%
Abdominal pain	14	100
Fever	5	41
Obvious jaundice	10	71
Nausea and vomiting	5	41

anastomosis was completed to verify its patency; there were no other instances of conversion in the other procedures. Recovery of intestinal peristalsis was quite rapid, averaging 36 hours. Regarding postoperative complications, there was only one—an incisional abscess—that formed in the patient who required conversion. One patient had a urinary infection. There was no mortality.

In the follow-up of these patients (up to 2 years), we have found no digestive symptoms that were due to the procedure itself, such as the pain or cholangitis reported by Madded, Lygidakis, and Parrilla in open surgery. These complications are very likely directly related to the size of the anastomosis, which should be no less than 20 mm in diameter.

We should point out that although the surgical time was quite long, these patients had complicated lithiasic biliary tract disease, and in such cases the cholecystectomy is difficult to perform and requires longer operative times. In fact, in three patients, the time required to perform the cholecystectomy was longer than the one needed for the CDA.

In December of 1993 we performed the first supraduodenal latero-lateral choledocoduodenostomy, after performing many common laparoscopic procedures. Since then we have had 14 patients in whom this procedure has been indicated as treatment for complicated main biliary tract lithiasis.

CONCLUSIONS

Latero-lateral choledocoduodenoanastomosis (CDA) is a useful technique for treatment of complicated main biliary tract lithiasis, as long as it is performed for a precise type of indication. Performing laparoscopically lowers the morbidity and mortality, and provides the patient with the well-known benefits offered by this type of minimaly invasive surgery.[7]

In the elderly patient with a dilated common bile duct and multiple stones, all that is required to make the diagnosis preoperatively is echography, an operation which is well tolerated by the patient. The procedure that combines cholesystectomy and cholechoduodenostomy in a single procedure makes this surgery more comfortable for the patient and more economical for the health care system.

REFERENCES

1. Bakes J. Die cholledochopaapilloskopie. *Archiv fuer Klinische Chirugie* 1923;126:473.
2. Mirizzi PL. Operative cholangiography. *Surg Gynecol Obstet.* 1937;65:702.
3. Caroli J. La radiomanometria biliare. Etudes techniques. *Sem Hop Paris.* 1945;21:1278.

4. Flörchen H, Steden E. Die nachun Fenergebuire der Choledocoduo-denostomie. *Archiv for Klinische Chirurgie* 1923;124:49.

5. Riedel H. Uber den zungenfoermigen fortastz des rechten lebberlap-pens und seine pathognostiche bedentung fur die erkrankungen der gal-lenblose nebst bemerkungen gallenstein-operationen. *Berl Klin Wschr.* 1988;25:577.

6. Madden JL, Chun JY, Kandalaft S, et al. Choledochoduodenostomy: an unjustly malignant surgical procedure. *Am J Surg.* 1979;119:45.

7. Degenshein GA. Choledochodudenostomy: an 18-year study of 175 consecutive cases. *Surgery* 1974;76:319.

8. Hurwitz AL, Degenshein GA. The role of choledochoduodenostomy in common duct surgery reappraisal. *Surgery* 1964;56:1147.

9. Jones SA. Sphincteroplasty (not sphincterotomy) in treatment of bili-ary tract disease. *Surg Clin North Am.* 1973;53:1123.

10. Classen M, Demling L. Endoscopische Shinkterotomie der papilla Vater. *Deutsche Medizinische Wochenschritt* 1974;99:496.

11. Rutledge RH. Sphincteroplasty and choledochoduodenostomy for be-nign biliary obstructions. *Ann Surg.* 1976;183:476.

12. Stuart M, Hoerr SO. Late results of side-to-side choledochoduodenos-tomy and of transduodenal sphincteroplasty for benign disorders. *Am J Surg.* 1972;123:67.

13. Parrilla P, Ramirez P, Sanchez Bueno F, et al. Long-term results of choledochoduodenostomy in the treatment of choledocholithiasis: as-sessment of 225 cases. *Br J Surg.* 1991;78:470.

14. McSherry CK, Glenn F. The incidence and causes of death following surgery for non-malignant biliary tract disease. *Ann Surg.* 1980; 191:271.

15. Mouret P. La cholecystectomie endoscopique a 4 ans. La coelio-chirugie tient une solide tète de pont. *Lyon Chir.* 1991;87/2 bis:179.

16. Dubois F, Berthelot G, Levard H. Cholecystectomie par coelioscopie. *Presse Med.* 1989;18:980.

17. Reddick EJ, Olsen DO. Laparoscopic laser cholecystectomy: a compar-ison with mini-lap cholecystectomy. *Surg Endosc.* 1989;3:131.

18. Glenn F. A 26 year experience; the treatment of 5037 patients with non-malignant biliary tract disease. *Surg Gynecol Obstet.* 1959;Nov, 109:591.

19. Coelho JCV, Buffara M, Pozzobon CE, et al. Incidence of common bile duct stones in patients with acute and chronic cholecystitis. *Surg Gynecol Obstet* 1984;158:76.

20. Petelin JB. Laparoscopic approach to common duct pathology. *Am J Surg.* 1993;165:487.

21. Rhodes M, Nathanson L. Laparoscopic choledochoduodenostomy. *Surg Laparosc Endosc.* 1996;6:318.

22. Prudkov MI. Minilaparotomy and open laparoscopic surgeries in treat-ment of patients with cholelithiasis. *Khirurgiia Mosk.* 1997;1:32.

23. Lygidakis NJ. Choledochoduodenostomy in calculous biliary tract dis-ease. *Br J Surg.* 1981;68:752.

24. Lygidakis NJ. Choledochoduodenostomy versus T tube drain-age af-ter choledochotomy. *Am J Surg.* 1983;145:639.

25. Denbesten L, Berci G. The current status of biliary tract surgery; an in-ternational study of 1072 consecutive patients. *World J Surg.* 1986;10:116.

26. Delgado F. Cirugía laparoscópica para cirujanos generales. Ed. Acirhospe. Madrid 1995. ISBN: 84-605-2259-8.

27. Aretxabe S, Bahamondes JC. Choledocoduodenostomy for common bile duct stones. *World J Surg.* 1998;22:1171.

Chapter Thirty-Two • • • • • •

*L*aparoscopic Surgery and Cancer of the Gallbladder

LUIS POGGI

Cancer of the gallbladder can be difficult to diagnose due to its nonspecific presentation. Symptoms become evident when the process is in an advanced stage, but when the tumor is small it can only be discovered by the pathologist. The gastroenterologist and/or surgeon may not suspect the diagnosis.[1,2] However, diagnostic tests have improved with sophisticated echotomographic procedures and aspiration cytology,[3] allowing an accurate preoperative diagnosis and more conservative surgery; some surgeons agree that laparoscopic cholecystectomy offers adequate margins of safety. Ultrasonography allows evaluation of polyps in the gallbladder wall that constitute an important element, their size being indicative of the possibility and risk of being a neoplasm.[4]

The incidence of the disease is highest in Japan and South America (specially in the southern region), and it is the most common malignant tumor found in women and the second most frequent among digestive tumors in Chile.[2,5,6] Gallbladder cancer is a highly malignant tumor with a poor 5-year survival rate.[7]

PATHOLOGIC CONSIDERATIONS

The incidence of gallbladder cancer has increased in recent years. Small lesions can be detected when the entire gallbladder is scanned using the technique described by the Japanese. The procedure consists of extending the gallbladder and using a stereoscope to determine the nature of suspicious lesions. Most gallbladders are fragmented, making the pathologist's work difficult. Given that a preoperative diagnosis is made in less than 10% of cases,[1,8,9] it is understandable why a poor result can be expected.

Roa et al[6] favor the hypothesis of progression from dysplasia to cancer in an estimated time span of 15 years. In most cases (over 90%), the histologic type is an adenocarcinoma[10] and 80% affect the muscular zone. Prognosis is directly proportional to the depth of invasion of the gallbladder wall and staging is as follows: in situ tumor (pTis), tumor invading mucosa (pT1a), tumor invading muscular layer (pT1b), tumor invading the subserosa (pT2), and tumor invading serosa or adjacent organ (pT3).[11] Another important prognostic factor is the involvement of deep layers of the wall, lymphatic involvement, or invasion of adipose tissue.

The presence of polyps is considered high risk, with the risk increasing with polyp size; a diameter over 20 mm carries a greater probability of cancer. The number of polyps is also important, with the risk increasing with a greater number of lesions. Less than three polyps, each under 5 mm, implies a lower risk of cancer;[12] however, rapid growth of a small polyp should suggest malignancy.[13] The presence of cholelithiasis is also related to the disease, and there is an 80 to 95% incidence of cholelithiasis with gallbladder cancer.[14,15] The greater the number of calculi and the time of evolution, the greater the risk.

DIAGNOSIS

The typical clinical presentation is only seen in advanced disease. Jaundice, pain, and weight loss are the most frequent symptoms, but as mentioned, they are generally associated with advanced and inoperable stages.

Ultrasonography can demonstrate suspicious lesions like polyps, irregular thickening of the wall, or cholelithiasis; however, it has limitations for establishing diagnosis of the primary lesion as well as node or hepatic involvement. Quantification of tumor markers like CA 19-9 is also important. The presence of multiple calculi, three or more polyps over 10 mm, or rapid growth are indications for surgery.[8]

A cytologic examination of bile—which is difficult to obtain preoperatively—is of great value owing to its high sensitivity; however, the micropunctures required to aspirate bile contribute to tumor dissemination.[3,16,17]

SURGERY FOR CANCER OF THE GALLBLADDER

Resectability is related to the size and the amount of dissemination of the primary tumor. The prognosis is related to the invasion of the different layers of the gallbladder wall, as well as node and adipose tissue involvement. A simple cholecystectomy is sufficient for early stages of the disease (pTis and pT1a). Wedge excisions and more extensive excisions are reserved for more advanced stages.[18]

With the advent of laparoscopic cholecystectomy, complications such as tumor seeding in the umbilicus or any other port of entry is associated with cancer that infiltrates the entire gallbladder wall.[19]

In our series of over 4500 laparoscopic cholecystectomies since 1991 at the Guillermo Almenara Hospital, which is part of the Peruvian Institute of Social Security, we have only seen one case of seeding to the umbilicus in a total of 67 adenocarcinomas of the gallbladder. The presence of tumor invasion into the liver and hepatic hilum with node or adipose tissue involvement forced a conversion in 46 cases, and the others were inadvertent, found only as an incidental discovery by the pathologist.

We recommend extracting all gallbladders in polyethylene bags to eliminate seeding in the trocar site.[15] The possibility of extracting gallbladders with unsuspected cancer is reportedly around 3%, and the tumors are generally found to be localized in the wall or with multiple polyps.[9]

If the lesion is small and there is no escape of neoplastic cells, the chance of dissemination is low, but if the wall is damaged and there is microscopic leakage in the zones of traction, then the instruments will be contaminated.[17] A fragmented extraction of the gallbladder, common in this laparoscopic age, makes the pathologist's job even more difficult.

Vaporization has been described, and consists of dissemination when extracting the contaminated instruments through the insufflation trocar, producing a spray of tumor cells that can seed the abdomen. The presence of tumor cells in the CO_2 filters proves this phenomenon.

When cancer of the gallbladder is found during a laparoscopic procedure, a conversion to laparotomy should be done to allow a more extensive or radical resection according to the stage.[20,21] If an advanced or disseminated cancer is found, then a biopsy should be taken to confirm diagnosis, laparoscopy should be suspended, and iodine solution should be applied to the trocar sites to reduce contamination.

LAPAROSCOPY AND CANCER OF THE GALLBLADDER

Very few surgeons favor the use laparoscopic cholecystectomy for cancer of the gallbladder. Conventional oncologic surgery indicates a wedge resection for cases limited to the mucosa, and a more ample hepatic resection when there is node or adipose tissue involvement.

When polyps are found, laparoscopy can have an important role, because certain characteristics are more likely to be produced in malignant pathology. For polyps of more than 5 mm, rapid growth, association with longstanding multiple lithiasis, thickening of the wall, or the presence of more than 3 polyps are factors suggestive of ma-

lignancy; in other cases a laparoscopic cholecystectomy might be considered, although this is not universally accepted.[11] Shinkai et al[12] relate the size and number of polyps to the rate of malignancy.

Some recommendations have been made as prophylactic measures:

- In all laparoscopic cholecystectomies, the gallbladder should be extracted in a polyethylene bag.
- Damage to the gallbladder wall (33% incidence) should be avoided to reduce the possibility of dissemination.
- If cancer of the gallbladder is found during a laparoscopy, an immediate conversion should be done to perform a resection that is determined by the stage.
- If cancer is found incidentally, then a reintervention should be considered to perform complementary surgery according to the stage.
- If a pTis or pT1a stage tumor is found, then no other procedure is required.
- If a pT2 or pT3 stage tumor is found, then more extensive surgery should be performed. The precise indication for surgery is related to the diagnosis and the extension of the tumor.

In spite of new technology, laparoscopic surgery is still not safe enough to be considered as the procedure of choice for cancer of the gallbladder; however, if we can make an earlier diagnosis and reduce the risk of dissemination, then the technique and possibly the indication may be modified in the future.

REFERENCES

1. Aretxabala X, Burgos L, Roa I, et al. Cáncer de vesícula biliar. Evaluación prospectiva de 100 casos potencialmente curativos. *Rev Chilena de Cirugía* 1994;46.
2. Klinger J, De la Fuente H, Olivares P. Cáncer de la vesícula biliar Hospital Gustavo Fricke 1980–1990. *Rev Chil Cir.* 1993;45:145.
3. Dodd L, Moffat E, Hudson E, et al. Fine-needle aspiration of primary gallbladder carcinoma. *Diagnostic Cytopathol.* 1996;15:151.
4. Haribhakti S, Kapoor V, Gujral R, et al. Staging of carcinoma of the gallbladder—Ultrasonography evaluation. *Hepatogastroenterology* 1997;44:1240.
5. Arancibia H, Carvajal C, Reyes J, et al. Cáncer de vesícula un estudio de 6,823 biopsias.
6. Roa I, Araya W, Witsuba I, et al. Cáncer de Vesícula en la IX Región de Chile. Impacto en el estudio anatomo-patológico en 474 casos. *Rev Med Chil.* 1994;122:1248.
7. Sheth S, Bedford A, Chopra S. Primary gallbladder cancer recognition of risk factors and the role of prophylactic cholecystectomy. *Am J Gastroenterol.* 2000;95:1402.
8. Aretxabala X, Burgos L, Roa I. Cáncer de vesícula biliar. Algunas consideraciones. *Rev Med Chile* 1996;732.
9. Mori T, Souda S, Hashimoto J, et al. Unsuspected gallbladder cancer diagnosed by laparoscopic cholecystectomy: a clinicopathological study. *Surg Today.* 1997;27:710.
10. Levin B. Gallbladder carcinoma. *Ann Oncol.* 1999;10(Suppl 4):129.
11. Yamaguchi K, Chijiwa K, Ichimiya H, et al. Gallbladder carcinoma in the era of laparoscopic cholecystectomy. *Arch Surg.* 1996;131:981.
12. Shinkai H, Kimura W, Muto T. Surgical indications for small polypoid lesions of the gallbladder. *Am J Surg.* 1998;175:114.
13. Mangel A. Management of gallbladder polyps. *South Med J.* 1997;90:438.
14. Adson M. Carcinoma de la vesícula biliar. *Surg Clin North Am.* 1973;53:1203.

15. Zapata C, Valdivia M. Neoplasias malignas de vesícula y vías biliares extrahepáticas. Revisión clínico patológica de 81 casos. *Rev Gastroent Del Perú.* 1992;12:71.

16. Poggi L, Miyasato C, Alzamora N, et al. La Cirugía biliar y el papel de la citología en el diagnóstico y detección de neoplasias de la vía biliar. Revista del Cuerpo Médico del Hospital Guillermo Almenara, Lima Perú 1988;XII:Núm 1.

17. Doudle M, King G, Thomas W, et al. The movement of mucosal cells of the gallbladder within the peritoneal cavity during laparoscopic cholecystectomy. *Surg Endosc.* 1996;10:1092.

18. Ruckert J, Ruckert R, Gellert K, et al. Surgery of the carcinoma of the gallbladder. *Hepatogastroenterology* 1996;43:527.

19. Cotlar A, Mueller C, Pettit J, et al. Trocar site seeding of inapparent gallbladder carcinoma during laparoscopic cholecystectomy. *J Laparoendosc Surg.* 1996;6:35.

20. Wysocki A, Bobrzynki A, Krzywon J, et al. Laparoscopic cholecystectomy and gallbladder cancer. *Surg Endosc.* 1999;13:899.

21. Pearlstone DB, Curley SA, Feig BW. The management of gallbladder cancer: before, during and after laparoscopic cholecystectomy. *Semin Laparosc Surg.* 1998;5:121.

Chapter Thirty-Three • • • • • •

*H*ydatid Liver Disease: An Update

MIGUEL A. STATTI and RICARDO PETTINARI

DEFINITION

Hydatid liver disease is caused by two echinococcus species of flatworms of the order Cestoda. *Echinococcus granulosus* is more often found than *Echinococcus multilocularis* and produces cystic lesions. The liver is frequently affected, but cysts are also seen in lungs and may grow in almost any organ.

ETIOLOGY

The cyst is the larval stage of the flatworm's life cycle. The cyst consists of a hydatid layer and a pericystic layer. The hydatid layer has an external laminar membrane and an internal or germinal layer. This layer creates the hydatid fluid, the brood capsules, and the daughter cysts. The hydatid fluid is transparent and has antigenic material that may cause dangerous allergic reactions. This fluid contains hydatid sand. The hydatid sand is the sediment of hydatid fluid, and consists of brood capsules that originate in the germinal layer. Brood capsules are special structures that create new protoscolices. The pericystic layer is part of the host reaction to the cyst and consists of a fibrous membrane. Cysts are prone to grow and complications are frequent, causing the symptoms of disease.

EPIDEMIOLOGY

The life cycle of the parasite begins with ova shed in dog feces. Cows, sheep, and other livestock are the intermediate hosts, and they ingest the ova. The ova hatch and the larva penetrate the intestinal wall and migrate to different organs, where they form cysts. When these animals are butchered, the infected viscera are used to feed dogs. The scolex then attaches to the small bowel of the dog (the primary host) where the adult taenia develops, completing the life cycle.

Man is an accidental intermediate host and gets infected by close contact with infected dogs or by eating vegetables contami-

nated by dogs feces. Turkana in Kenya has the highest documented frequency of infection, 9%.[1] The disease is also common in other countries, such as Uruguay, Cyprus, Greece, Chile, Iran, and Spain. In Argentina there are 1.42 new cases per 100,000 inhabitants per year, for an annual incidence in the southern part of the country of up to 41 new cases.

CLINICAL PRESENTATION

Rural life and contact with dogs are common findings in those affected,[5] and up to 30% of patients have had previous surgery for hydatid disease. The liver is affected in 60% of cases. Patients may harbor nonsymptomatic cysts for long periods, and the cysts are sometimes found in a routine scan carried out to diagnose vague symptoms. In other cases, the cyst causes compression and elicits pain in the right upper quadrant, and palpation reveals a liver mass or an enlarged liver. Sometimes the cyst ruptures, migrates, or becomes infected. Rupture into the bile duct can cause icterus with or without cholangitis or pancreatitis. Rarely, the cyst can open into the abdominal cavity, causing a hydatid acute abdomen, hydatid ascites, or an anaphylactic reaction. The cyst can also migrate to the thorax and open into the pleura or bronchi, causing hydatid "vomica." The cyst can also migrate to the peritoneum and implant in the peritoneal cavity or in any abdominal organ. If infected, the cyst can cause a serious septic disease.

DIAGNOSIS

Any liver mass in a patient from an endemic area must raise suspicion about hydatid disease. Immunophoresis shows the 5th arc of Capron in 60% of cases. Enzyme-linked immunosorbent assay (ELISA) is also a sensitive tool for detecting hydatid disease. Sonography is the most important aid in diagnosis and can reveal the cyst and its characteristics. A computed tomography (CT) scan is more expensive but it offers better localization of the cysts and establishes their exact number. The differential diagnosis includes nonparasitic liver cysts, biliary cystadenoma, liver abscess, and solid tumors. The peripheral calcification is nearly pathognomonic of hydatid disease.

TREATMENT

Living cysts that are less than 5 cm in diameter and calcified (dead) cysts, if asymptomatic, may warrant watchful waiting and probably will not cause symptoms. The cysts do not always grow and sometimes they die spontaneously. A treatment plan must be considered for cysts bigger than 5 to 10 cm or when a complication is present, regardless of cyst size. Today there are many treatment modalities.

Medical

Some centers have used mebendazole in the past,[2] but now albendazole is more commonly used. In one center[3] 68 patients were followed for 3 to 7 years; 41% of the patients were cured, 17% showed significant amelioration, 24% showed slight amelioration, and 15% did not show any change. The treatment regimen is albendazole 10 mg/kg/d (800 mg/d) for 28 days, followed by 2 weeks with no medication, and this cycle is repeated four times. Cure is not guaranteed, but results are encouraging, indicating that albendazole is an important aid in the treatment of the disease. We support the use of albendazole for 1 month preoperatively and 1 month postoperatively to lower the possibility of relapse in surgical patients. In generalized peritoneal disease or in patients not suitable for surgery, we recommend three to six drug cycles.

Radiologic

In some centers,[4–6] for high-risk patients or those with repeated surgery, cyst puncture and evacuation is carried out. This treatment proved useful in Saremi and McNamara's[4] experience. They treated 32 patients with a procedure involving percutaneous cutting and aspiration. The patients were tested for 25 months with periodic sonography and CT scans. By 6 months the cavities disappeared in 66% of cases. No anaphylactic reaction was recorded, and no dissemination occurred. Odriozola and Pettinari[7] treated 15 patients, and in their series the cavity took 60 days to close. This treatment is used in cases of relapse or in patients who are not good surgical candidates.

Endoscopic

If the cyst ruptures into the biliary tract, papillotomy can effectively clean the bile duct, allowing the resolution of icterus and cholangitis. We saw also an occasional patient whose cyst was drained completely through the ampulla, resulting in cure. Endoscopic stenting has proven to be a safe method to treat postoperative benign biliary strictures secondary to hydatid liver disease, especially for patients who have been surgically treated on one or more occasions.[8]

Surgical

The goals in surgical treatment of hydatid disease are: (1) Scolices should not be shed by surgical manipulation, (2) anaphylaxis must be minimized through careful handling of the cyst fluid, (3) the germinal layer and the cyst contents must be completely eliminated, and (4) any biliary communication needs to be treated. Surgical mortality is around 2%.[9] The procedures in use range from simple marsupialization, resection of the emerging portion of the cyst (unroofing) and drainage, and pericystectomy, to hepatectomy. Odriozola and Pettinari,[7] presented their experience with 804 cases, with morbidity of 25.7% and mortality of 3.6%.

Laparoscopic

Some reports have shown that cystostomy and pericystectomy can safely be performed laparoscopically.[10–19] There are concerns about seeding of protoscolices and the occurrence of more anaphylactic reactions than are usually seen with open surgery; however, this is a recent development. Nevertheless Khoury et al[20] recently reported a case of anaphylactic shock that complicated the laparoscopic treatment of hydatid cysts of the liver.

Techniques

Cystectomy. Cystectomy can be done in small, peripheral cysts with direct vision, with electrocautery used for bilistasis and hemostasis. The Nd:YAG laser or clips can be used if necessary. The cyst is placed in a bag to effect intact removal or morcellated.

Cystostomy. The cyst is punctured in the upper portion to avoid fluid leakage and the contents drained completely by aspiration. The fluid is sent to the laboratory to confirm the presence of parasites and the wall of the cyst is sent for pathologic study. Adequate aspiration equipment is absolutely necessary and a sterile second set must be ready to be used if needed. The use of scolicidal solutions is under debate; formalin is no longer used, peroxidized water may produce gas embolism, and saline solution may cause electrolytic imbalance. The least concentration-dependent agent is 1.5% cetrimide/0.15% chlorhexidine.[20] We routinely use saline. Some authors use physiologic solution only to wash the cavity.[21]

Next, complete aspiration of the cavity is performed. The dome of the cyst can be extirpated to make aspiration easier. Daughter cysts, if present, can be placed in a bag for safe extraction. Once the germinal layer is extracted, a careful search for open small biliary ducts must be made, and if present they must be sutured or clipped. Methylene blue must be instilled through the cystic duct to reveal small leaks into the cavity. Hemostasis of the tissues near the edge of the cyst must be thoroughly performed with electrocautery or by means of sutures. The omentum can be introduced in the residual cavity (omentoplasty), to avoid leaving an empty space that would be prone to infection.

In Argentina, Pettinari et al[22] conducted a multicentric study of laparoscopic treatment of hydatid disease, studying 42 patients in all. There was a 9.5% conversion rate. Operative time was longer than 2 hours in 58% of the cases. Conservative procedures were frequently used. The postoperative stay was 1 to 4 days in 76% of the patients. Infection of the residual cavity was the complication most frequently observed and it was treated by percutaneous drainage. There were no recurrences in 29 patients over 3 to 12 months of follow-up.

This technique has apparent advantages over the conventional procedures: the patient experiences less postoperative pain and has a faster recovery and minimal adhesions are produced (this is important in case open surgery in the right upper quadrant such as cholecystectomy is needed later, or in cases of reinfection, which occurs in up to 30% of patients). Theoretical disadvantages include: seeding of the scolices during the manipulation of the cyst, though to date none has been reported, and exacerbation of anaphylactic reactions, with a single case reported to date.[20] Reports in the literature[10–19] are encouraging, but the number of patients treated and reported on is small and more data are needed to make a definitive judgment. More experience in centers that treat large numbers of patients will be necessary to determine the exact role of this procedure.

FOLLOW-UP

All patients with hydatid disease must have periodic testing done. If surgery is done, reinfection must be carefully sought. If serological markers were positive before surgery, they should be checked 1 year after surgery, and if they are negative the test should be repeated in 5 years. If they are positive, reinfection should be suspected.

Sonography must be performed 3 months after surgery to establish postoperative status. It must be repeated 1 year after surgery, and if negative, in 5 years. We also recommend that patients should not eat raw home-grown vegetables.

PREVENTION

In endemic areas, control of the disease must attempted using these guidelines:

- Parasiticidal treatment of dogs with praziquantel
- Slaughterhouses should practice good sanitation
- Education of the population about the etiology of hydatid disease
- Registration of dogs and monitoring of dog echinococcosis
- Serologic surveys should be made in the population at risk

REFERENCES

1. MacPherson C, Romig T, Rees P. Portable ultrasound-scanner versus serology in screening for hydatid cysts in a nomadic population. *Lancet* 1987;2:259.
2. Gocmen A, Toppare MF, Kiper N. Treatment of hydatid disease in childhood with mebendazole. *Eur Respir J.* 1993;6;253.
3. Nahmias J, Goldsmith R, Soibelman M, et al. Three to seven year follow-up after albendazole treatment of 68 patients with cystic echinococcosis. *Ann Trop Med Parasitol.* 1994;88:295.
4. Saremi F, McNamara TO. Hydatid cysts of the liver: long term results of percutaneous treatment using a cutting instrument. *AJR.* 1995;165:1163.
5. Giorgio A, Tarantino L, Francica G, et al. Unilocular hydatid liver cysts: treatment with US-guided, double percutaneous aspiration and alcohol injection. *Radiology* 1992;184:705.
6. Khuro MS, Wani NA, Javid G, et al. Percutaneous drainage compared with surgery for hepatic hydatid cysts. *N Engl J Med.* 1997;337:881.
7. Odriozola M, Pettinari R. Abdominal hidatidosis. Extraordinary number. *Relatos Rev Arg Cir.* 1998;32:256.
8. Yilmaz U, Sakin B, Boyacioglu S, et al. Management of postoperative biliary strictures secondary to hepatic hydatid disease by endoscopic stenting. *Hepatogastroenterology* 1998;45):65.
9. Loi A, Mannu B, Montisci R, et al. Surgical treatment of hydatidosis. *Ann Chir Gynaecol.* 1991;80:59.
10. Katkhouda N, Fabiani P, Benizri F, et al. Laser resection of a liver hydatid cyst under videocoelioscopy. *Br J Surg.* 1992;79;560.
11. Lujan Mompean JA, Parrilla Paricio P, Robles Campos R, et al. Laparoscopic treatment of a liver hydatid cyst. *Br J Surg.* 1993;80:907.
12. Rogiers X, Bloechle C, Broelsch CE. Safe decompression of hepatic hydatid cyst with a laparoscopic surgiport. *Br J Surg.* 1995;82:111.
13. Sonzini Astudillo P, Sarria Allende F, Duret L, et al. Liver hidatidosis: laparoscopic treatment. *Rev Argent Cirug.* 1995;69:132.
14. Sever M, Skapin S. Laparoscopic pericystectomy of liver hydatid cyst. *Surg Endosc.* 1995;9:1125.
15. Guibert L, Gayral F. Laparoscopic pericystectomy of a liver hydatid cyst. *Surg Endosc.* 1995;9:442.
16. Yucel O, Talu M, Unalmiser S, et al. Videolaparoscopic treatment of liver hydatid cysts with partial cystectomy and omentoplasty. A report of two cases. *Surg Endosc.* 1996;10:434.
17. Diez J, Decoud J, Gutierrez L, et al. Laparoscopic treatment of symptomatic cysts of the liver. *Br J Surg.* 1998;85:25.
18. Saglam A. Laparoscopic treatment of liver hydatid cysts. *Surg Laparosc Endosc.* 1996;6:16.
19. Alper A, Emre A, Acarli K, et al. Laparoscopic treatment of hepatic hydatid disease. *J Laparoendosc Surg.* 1996;6:29.
20. Khoury G, Jabbour-Khoury S, Soueidi A, et al. Anaphylactic shock complicating laparoscopic treatment of hydatid cysts of the liver. *Surg Endosc.* 1998;12:452.
21. Besim H, Karayalcin K, Hamamci O, et al. Scolicidal agents in hydatid cyst surgery. *HPB Surg.* 1998;10:347.
22. Pettinari R, Antozzi M, Sonzini P, et al. Hepatic hidatidosis, videolaparoscopic surgery, multicentric study, 1992–1997. 1998 World Congress in Hydatidosis, Portugal.

Chapter Thirty-Four • • • • • •

Laparoscopic Hepatectomy

LAURENT BIERTHO AND MICHEL GAGNER

The indications for laparoscopy have rapidly increased since its first use for cholecystectomy in 1987. Shorter hospitalization, less postoperative pain and ileus, a faster return to normal life, and more cosmetic scars explain the success of laparoscopy. However, laparoscopic liver surgery has been slow to develop, due to the complexity of the procedure, lack of correct instrumentation, and fear of gas embolism.

Increased experience in laparoscopic surgery and development of new instruments led to the application of laparoscopy to solid organs. Splenectomy, adrenalectomy, and nephrectomy are now performed by laparoscopy in many centers. But laparoscopic liver surgery is a technical challenge, and presents specific difficulties in localizing nonvisible lesions, controlling hemorrhage from large intrahepatic vessels, achieving hemostasis of the plane of transection, and avoiding gas embolism.

Liver biopsy, fenestration of solitary cysts and polycystic liver, and management of hydatid cysts have been attempted first.[1,2] Development of new instruments and techniques, allowing a correct isolation and closure of vessels and bile ducts, has allowed resection of benign and malignant liver tumors under laroscopy.[3]

In this chapter we will review the indications, techniques, and results of laparoscopic hepatectomy.

PREOPERATIVE WORKUP

Laparoscopic liver resection must be used for selected cases. Liver function (one of the main prognostic factor in hepatic surgery) and coagulating factor synthesis (I, II, V, VII, IX, X) are assessed.

Preoperative Imaging Studies

Liver tumors are rare lesions, but are discovered more frequently because of the improvement in imaging studies and widespread use of ultrasonography as a screening exam. All imaging techniques have a sensitivity of 100% for focal hepatic masses larger than 2.0 cm.[4]

Ultrasonography is usually the first examination for patients with liver-related complaints. Combined with Doppler sonography, it can assess the patency of the inferior vena cava, portal and hepatic veins, and portal hypertension. In the case of end-stage cirrhosis, its sensitivity is greatly decreased (detection of hepatomas in only 45% of cases).[5] Moreover, tumors located immediately under the right hemidiaphragm can be difficult to detect.

Computed tomography (CT) is helpful in evaluating patients with known or suspected liver tumor (Fig. 34–1). CT and MRI are relatively unreliable for the detection of lesions smaller than 1 cm in diameter. A way to increase the sensitivity of conventional CT is to use contrast material (intravenously or into the hepatic artery), or to inject Lipiodol into the hepatic artery and perform a scan 7 to 10 days later.[6] Most hepatic neoplasms are hypointense, when the normal parenchyma is brightly enhanced, but hepatocellular carcinoma and some hepatic metastases (renal-cell carcinoma, breast cancer) are considered hypervascular because they are hyperintense early after the contrast bolus.[7]

The combination of helical CT and advanced software technology has made possible the reconstruction of three-dimensional CT images. This technique provides more precise diagnostic information and a realistic virtual image of a tumor's location in the liver. It has allowed maximal liver sparing, by precise localization of the segment to resect, in patients with poor liver reserve.[8]

CT portography is considered the most sensitive exam for surgical planning. An angiographic catheter is placed in the superior mesenteric artery or splenic artery and a CT is performed during the injection of contrast. This exam is essential to evaluate the hepatic arterial anatomy when planning surgical resection, transplantation, or chemoembolization of the tumor.[7,9] It has also shown a very high sensitivity for hepatic metastases (92 to 94%),[10] and can detect hepatomas as small as 1 cm in diameter.[9]

Magnetic resonance imaging is less commonly used for liver tumors, due to its limited availability and cost. MRI appears to be slightly more sensitive and specific in the diagnosis of focal lesions than CT, and it can be useful when CT findings are equivocal (Fig. 34–2). MRI also has a distinct advantage over CT in the setting of fatty liver.

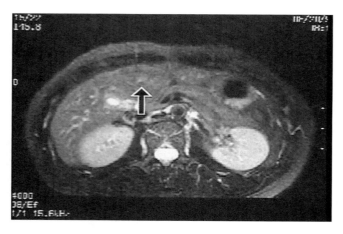

Figure 34–1. CT scan of focal nodular hyperplasia.

INDICATIONS

Tumor Location

Tumors must be easily accessed by laparoscopy. Tumors located in the anterolateral segments (segments II to VI, following Couinaud's classification[11]) are the usual indications (Fig. 34–3).[12–14]

Tumor Type

Benign Tumors. *Hemangioma* is the most common benign liver tumor. It has been found in up to 7.3% of the population.[12] Hemangioma rarely causes symptoms and is usually found incidentally. Some may grow to 10 cm or more in diameter. Indications for open surgical resection are hemangiomas of more than 10 cm (risk of hemorrhage), symptomatic lesions, doubtful lesions, or complicated hemangiomas (ruptured). Laparoscopic resection of hemangiomas should be reserved for doubtful or symptomatic lesions, of small or medium size, favorably located.[13,14]

Hormone-Dependent Tumors. Hormone-dependent tumors (liver cell adenoma and focal nodular hyperplasia) are usually found in young, healthy women, and can be related to the use of

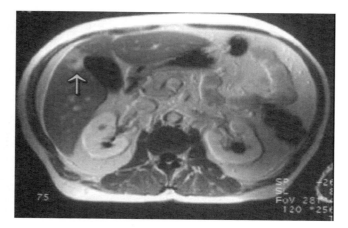

Figure 34–2. MRI of hepatocellular cholangiocarcinoma.

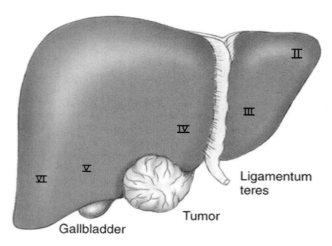

Figure 34–3. Favorable segments.

contraceptive pills. Indications for open surgical resection are bleeding, unexplained pain, planning of pregnancy, or doubtful diagnosis (malignant degeneration of liver cell adenomas). Those large, hypervascularized tumors are associated with a high risk of bleeding. Indications for laparoscopic resection should be limited to small or medium-size lesions, located on the edges or surfaces of easily accessible segments (II–VI).

Malignant Tumors. The potential risk of neoplastic dissemination associated with laparoscopy necessitates the highest degree of caution. *Hepatoma* is the most frequent primary liver tumor. The ideal treatment of hepatoma in the cirrhotic liver is transplantation, solving the problems of both carcinoma and cirrhosis. Some authors[12,15–18] have described laparoscopic resection of hepatocellular carcinoma (HCC) with a morbidity and morality comparable to classical surgery. Their indications were (1) primary liver tumors for definitive diagnosis in a cirrhotic liver and (2) focal and lateral tumors less than 4 cm in diameter with a resection margin of at least 1 cm.[17,18] Liver cirrhosis was not considered a contraindication.[12,17,18]

Liver metastasis is a common cause of death from cancer. Carcinoma of the colon and rectum frequently presents with solitary or a few metastases only to the liver.[14,15] Thus the most frequent metastasectomy relates to carcinoma of the large bowel. The second most frequent cause of liver metastases is breast carcinoma. Laparoscopic treatment of these is controversial. On one hand, the presence of a cancer, with a previous major abdominal operation, and the still unclear carcinologic risk of laparoscopy, make minimally inva-sive access unsuitable for liver resection.[19] On the other hand, isolated, easily accessible metastasis, or doubtful lesions arising in an oncologic context, may constitute a good indication for laparoscopic resection.[15,16,19–23]

CONTRAINDICATIONS

In addition to the usual contraindications to liver surgery, extensive adhesions from previous surgery, and invasive, deep-seated, or giant lesions, either with a close relationship to the main vascular structures or located in posterior/posterosuperior segments (segments I, VII, VIII), are also considered contraindications.[20–23]

TECHNIQUES

Operating Room Setup

The patient is positioned in the inverted-Y position with the surgeon standing between the patient's legs, the first assistant on the left side and the second assistant on the right (Fig. 34–4). Some authors prefer to place the patient in a supine position, and to stand on the patient's right side, for resection of segments II to IV, while for resection of segments IV and V they place the patient in a left-side semidecubitus position with the surgeon standing on the left side.

Constant monitoring of hemodynamic status, end-tidal carbon dioxide, and oxygen saturation are essential for early diagnosis and correction of gas embolism. A 30- and/or 45-degree laparoscope is introduced just above or at the level of the umbilicus by a 10-mm trocar. Two 10-mm ports surround the umbilicus (their position depending on the location of the tumor), and a subxiphoid trocar is used for the liver retractor, irrigation, or suction device. Four to seven trocars are usually necessary to allow proper manipulations, depending on the complexity of the procedure (Fig. 34–5).

Laparoscopic Exploration

Laparoscopic ultrasound exploration of liver tumors is mandatory to confirm the preoperative diagnosis, to give precise localization of the lesion and its relationship to the main vascular and biliary structures, and to determine the feasibility of the surgical procedure.[14] If necessary, a needle biopsy or aspiration may be performed directly or under echo guidance.

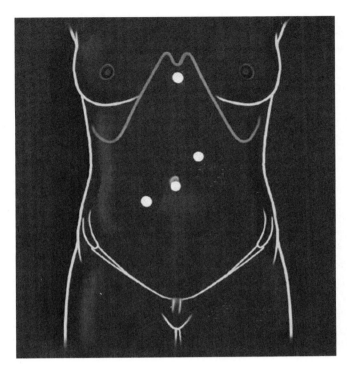

Figure 34–5. Trocar placement.

Four-Hand Approach

The "four-hands" approach, in which two additional trocars allow two surgeons to work simultaneously, has been described by Katkhouda et al.[24] It is used for major hepatic resections. Using the laparoscopic ultrasonic dissector, the first surgeon performs an instrumental fracture of the liver parenchyma, exposing all bile ducts and vessels, while the second surgeon controls all the vasculobiliary pedicles with clips or other hemostatic tools. This approach speeds up surgery and reduces the risk of hemorrhage and gas embolism.

Instruments

An *ultrasonic dissector* is very important for liver resection. The cavitational ultrasonic suction aspirator (CUSA) is tissue specific, with rapid disruption of liver parenchymal cells. Biliovascular structures are more resistant to disruption, and are controlled with clips. The laparoscopic coagulation shears (LCS) differs in that it causes denaturation of proteins and thus allows coagulation of small vessels of up to 2 to 3 mm in size. The main advantages of these devices are the very limited heat generation, the lack of smoke production, and the absence of current flow through the patient. An *argon beam coagulator* (Fig. 34–6) can be used with the ultrasonic dissector, to decrease bleeding and prevent bile leakage. It is associated with an increase in pneumoperitoneum pressure.[25] The *Nd:YAG laser* allows a deeper hemostatic layer than that achieved with the CO_2 laser or argon beam coagulator; furthermore, in comparison with electrosurgery it produces less tissue necrosis.[14] On the other hand, it is an expensive device and not easy to use. The *water jet dissector*[26,27] seems to be very interesting in liver surgery. It creates a high-pressure water jet, disintegrating liver cells with a relative sparing of more

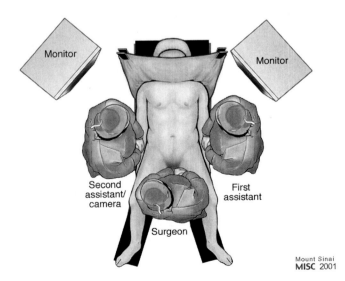

Figure 34–4. Operating room setup.

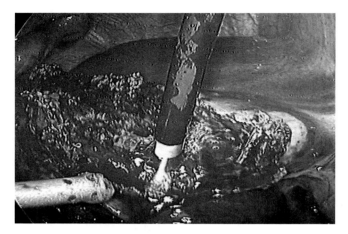

Figure 34–6. Argon beam coagulator.

fibrous tissues. In a prospective study of 60 open liver resections comparing the ultrasonic dissector with the water jet dissector, Rau et al[26,27] have shown a faster dissection with less blood loss for the water jet dissector. Concerns with this technique include poorer visibility and the possible dissemination of cancer cells.

Gasless Laparoscopy

Gas embolism is one of the most important complications of laparoscopic liver surgery. Gasless laparoscopy is used to avoid the risk of gas embolism.[15,28] This technique seems to be feasible and safe, to prevent the risk of gas embolism. When visibility is insufficient with gasless laparoscopy, some authors[29] have used a low-pressure pneumoperitoneum of 4 mm Hg (for cirrhotic patients in which portal pressure is about 10 mm Hg). Other ways to avoid this complication are careful localization of vessels using ultrasound, use of a vascular stapler, creation of positive pressure pulmonary insufflation when approaching the vessels, and probably by diminishing pneumoperitoneum pressure.

Hand-Assisted Liver Resection

A hand-assisting device (Fig. 34–7) has been used to perform laparoscopic hepatectomy.[23,30] The hand port can be made in the

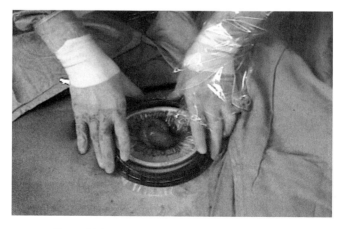

Figure 34–7. Hand-assisting device. See Color Section.

left flank or in the suprapubic area. A 10-mm trocar is introduced above the umbilicus for the laparoscope. Two other 10-mm ports are placed to allow access to the tumor (Fig. 34–8). This technique could increase safety by providing better control of bleeding vessels and allowing access to uneasily accessible lesions, while restoring a tactile sense and reducing operative time.

Nonanatomic Liver Resection

Nonanatomic liver resection consists of resection close to the tumor margin for benign lesions, and with a margin of 1 to 2 cm for malignant tumors. The limit of resection is marked, using electrocautery (Fig. 34–9). Liver resection can be performed with an endoscopic ultrasonic dissector (Fig. 34–10). Biliary and vascular structures are divided between clips. Clamping of the hilum (Pringle maneuver) or selective vascular clamping can also be useful. Hemostasis and prevention of bile leakage from raw liver surface is achieved by application of fibrin sealant or with the argon beam coagulator. Linear endovascular staplers are used for hepatic veins. The specimen is resected in an endobag through an enlarged trocar site.

Segmentectomy or Subsegmentectomy

A segmentectomy or subsegmentectomy is the anatomic resection of one segment. For Mouiel et al,[14] it should replace the "wedge resection"[31] to avoid residual ischemia or necrosis and to reduce the rate of biliary leakage complications. Segments II to VI are usually involved.

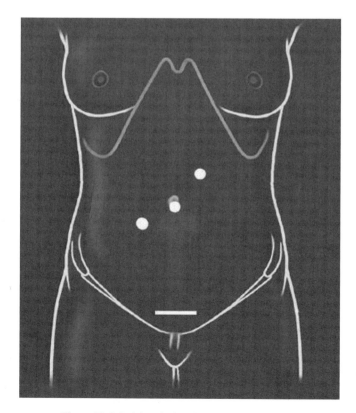

Figure 34–8. Incisions for hand-assisted liver resection.

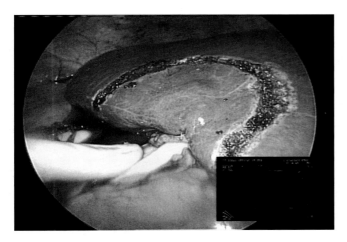

Figure 34–9. Tumor margins are marked with electrocautery. See Color Section.

Left Lobectomy

A left lobectomy consists of the resection of liver segments II and III. The falciform and left triangular ligaments are divided, to allow access to the left liver, and the inferior vena cava (IVC) is identified. The liver is displaced inferiorly, and the junction between the left hepatic vein and the IVC is exposed to gain extrahepatic control of the vein. This maneuver should not be attempted if the retrohepatic course of the hepatic vein is too short. The hepato-duodenal ligament is dissected, and the porta hepatis is also controlled. The liver capsule is then scored on the anterior and inferior surface 1 cm to the left of the falciform ligament. Using the four-hand approach, the liver parenchyma is fractured with long atraumatic forceps, an endoscopic "Lucane" clamp,[19] or the ultrasonic dissector. Intermittent clampage of the porta hepatis and/or left hepatic vein can be useful to allow a careful dissection and to control bleeding. The vasculobiliary structures of segments II and III are divided between clips. The left hepatic vein is divided using a vascular endostapler. Drains can be placed in the residual space and subphrenic space. The specimen is placed in an endobag, fragmented, and extracted through an enlarged port.

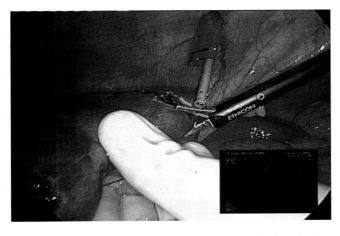

Figure 34–10. Liver resection using an ultrasonic dissector. See Color Section.

Right Lobectomy

The patient is placed in a left hemilateral position and the surgeon stands on the patient's left.[19] The right lobe is mobilized to expose the inferior vena cava. The hepatic pedicle is controlled. The most dangerous part of the dissection is to control the right hepatic vein. During parenchymal transection, intermittent portal triad clamping is used. The liver is transected with the ultrasonic harmonic scalpel, and the right hepatic vein and portal structures are divided by a vascular endostapler at the end of the transection. The raw surface of the liver is sealed with fibrin sealant and the specimen is extracted as before. Most of the right lobectomies have been performed using an "assisted laparoscopy" approach: Liberation of the liver is done under laparoscopy, and then a midline supraumbilical incision is made to introduce an abdominal wall lifter, with liver resection continuing using a "laparoscopic-assisted" gasless technique.

RESULTS

In 1993, Azagra et al[3] performed the first "anatomic" laparoscopic left lateral segmentectomy, for a liver cell adenoma. Operative time was 6 hours 30 minutes, and the blood loss was 600 mL. The postoperative course was uncomplicated, with the patient discharged on the eighth postoperative day. More recently, laparoscopic wedge resections, nonanatomic resections, and other anatomic resections have been performed. We will now review the indications, procedures (Table 34–1), and main outcomes (Table 34–2) of laparoscopic hepatectomies found in the literature.

Laparoscopic resection of benign tumors was performed first.[13–15,19,21,22,24,27,32–37] Lesions were usually located on segments II to VI. The most frequent indications were liver cell adenomas, focal nodular hyperplasia, and hemangiomas. Laparoscopy has also been used for malignant tumors[15,22,33,34,36,38] and metastasis.[14,15,21,22,27,30,32,34]

The main indications for malignant tumors were hepatocellular carcinoma (HCC). Presence of cirrhosis was not a contraindication. The most often operated metastases were from colorectal carcinomas, followed by breast carcinomas. Abdel-Atty et al[38] have also reported three laparoscopic resections for perforated HCC. All three patients had an ascites leakage lasting less than 7 days.

To decrease the incidence of gas embolism, some authors have successfully used gasless laparoscopy[22,28,29] or low-pressure laparoscopy.[15,18] For Hashizume et al,[15] an airless lifting wall device was used when a larger hepatic vein was included in the tissue to be resected. They nevertheless experienced two cases of gas embolism (one of which was documented by echocardiography). Ker et al[18] main-tained an abdominal pressure of 4 to 6 mm Hg using an abdominal wall lifting device, and 8 mm Hg without it (considering that portal pressure in cirrhotic patients is about 10 mm Hg).

Right lobe resection has been performed using a laparoscopy-assisted approach.[12,15] When liberation of the liver is complete, a midline supraumbilical incision is created, and an abdominal wall lifter is introduced. The procedure is then completed in the same way as for a gasless laparoscopy.

A hand-assisting device has been used to perform laparoscopic hepatectomy.[23,30] It allows access to uneasily accessible lesions,

TABLE 34–1. INDICATIONS AND PROCEDURES

Authors	Cases	Indications		Operation Type	
Azagra	1	Liver cell adenoma	1	Left lateral segmentectomy	1
Descottes	16	Hemangioma	6	Right lobectomy	1
		Focal nodular hyperplasia	6	One or two-segment resection	5
		Liver cell adenoma	2	Subsegmentectomy	2
		Metastasis	1	Nonanatomic resection	8
		Hepatocellular carcinoma	1		
Katkhouda	12	Focal nodular hyperplasia	3	Left lateral segmentectomy	3
		Liver cell adenoma	9	Nonanatomic resection	9
Mouiel	10	Benign tumors	8	Tumorectomies	7
		Chronic abscess	1	Left lobectomies	3
		Metastasis	1		
Hashizume	70	Malignant (colon and breast metastasis, hepatocellular ca)	47	Wedge resection	5
				Segmentectomy	30
				Bisegmentectomy	5
		Benign (hemangioma, focal nodular hyperplasia, hydatid cyst, biliary cyst)	23	Left formal hepatectomy	16
				Extended left hepatectomy	1
				Right formal hepatectomy	12
				Extended right hepatectomy	1
Fong	11	Hepatocellular carcinoma	4	One-segment resection	4
		Cystic carcinoma	1	Left lateral segmentectomy	1
		Metastasis	6		
Samama	4	Colon cancer metastasis	2	Left lobectomy	4
		Focal nodular hyperplasia	2		
Cuschieri	5	Metastasis	5	Left lobectomy	1
				Left lateral segmentectomy	1
				Bisegmentectomy	2
				Segmentectomy	1
Ker	9	Hepatocellular carcinoma	9	Subsegmentectomy	9
Huscher	20	Hepatocellular carcinoma	12	Segmentectomy	5
		Cholangiocarcinoma	1	Left formal hepatectomy	6
		Cholangioadenoma	1	Bisegmentectomy	1
		Regenerative nodule metastasis	1	Right formal hepatectomy	4
			5	Extended right hepatectomy	1
				Mesohepatectomy	3
Yamanaka	3	Hepatocellular carcinoma	3	Partial hepatectomy	3
Watanabe	1	Hepatocellular carcinoma	1	Left lateral segmentectomy	1
Kaneko	11	Metastasis	3	Left lateral segmentectomy	3
		Hepatocellular carcinoma	4	Partial hepatectomy	8
		Hemangioma	2		
		Wilson's disease	1		
		Hemochromatosis	1		
Rau	17	Hemangioma	7	Left lateral segmentectomy	8
		Focal nodular hyperplasia	5	One-segment resection	9
		Hydatid cyst	2		
		Biliary cyst	1		
		Metastasis	2		
Cunningham	2	Hemangioma	2	Nonanatomic resection	2
Mizoe	1	Hepatocellular carcinoma	1	Left lateral segmentectomy	1
Abdel-Atty	3	Hepatocellular carcinoma	3	Nonanatomic resection	3
Cherqui	30	Focal nodular hyperplasia	9	Left lateral segmentectomy	1
		Liver cell adenoma	3	Bisegmentectomies	8
		Other benign tumors	6	Segmentectomies	9
		Hepatocellular carcinoma	8	Nonanatomic resection	11
		Breast metastases	2		
		Cholangiocarcinoma	1		
		Lymphoma	1		
Hamy	7	Focal nodular hyperplasia	7	Left lateral segmentectomy	4
				Nonanatomic resection	3
Crocco	4	Hepatocellular carcinoma	1	Nonanatomic resection	4
		Focal nodular hyperplasia	3		
Cuesta	2	Liver cell adenoma	1	Nonanatomical resection	2
		Focal nodular hyperplasia	1		
TOTAL	239	Benign tumor	113	Nonanatomic resection	70
				Subsegmentectomy	11
		Malignant tumor	121	One or two-segment resection	79
				Left lateral segmentectomy	41
				Left lobectomy	9
				Right lobectomy	18

TABLE 34–2. OPERATIVE AND POSTOPERATIVE DATA

	Cases	Op Time (min)	Conversion (%)	Blood Loss	Hospital Stay (days)	Morbidity (%)	Mortality (%)
Azagra	1	330	0	600	8	0	0
Descottes	16	232 ± 130	6.2	NA	5.2 ± 3.2	6.25	0
Katkhouda	12	173 (91–325)	8.33	173 (91–325)	NA	0	0
Mouiel	10	NA	10	NA	NA	NA	0
Hashizume	70	NA	4.2	NA	NA	5.7	1.4
Fong	11	248 (158–358)	55	260 (100–500)	5	18	0
Samama	4	240 (180–300)	0	NA	6.25 (4–10)	25	0
Cuschieri	5	NA	0	NA	NA	0	0
Ker	9	NA	0	NA	NA	11	0
Huscher	20	193 (120–270)	0	398 (100–1200)	11 (5–25)	45	5
Yamanaka	3	NA	0	NA	NA	33	0
Watanabe	1	NA	0	120	13	0	0
Kaneko	11	198 (60–415)	9	478 (40–2500)	NA	0	0
Rau	17	183.5 ± 55.1	5.9	458 ± 343	7.8 ± 8.2	5.9	0
Cunningham	2	NA	0	200	3 (2–4)	0	0
Mizoe	1	660	0	NA	14	0	0
Abdel-Atty	3	170 (120–210)	0	233 (100–400)	8.3 (6–10)	100	0
Cherqui	29	214 ± 87	6.6	300 (0–1500)	9.6 (3–40)	20	0
Hamy	7	NA	0	NA	NA	0	0
Crocco	4	NA	25	NA	NA	25	0
Cuesta	2	NA	0	NA	2.5 (2–3)	0	0
TOTAL	238	205 (out of 143)	7.11%	349 (out of 125)	9 (out of 107)	14.04%	0.840%

restores a tactile sense, provides better control of bleeding vessels, and reduces operative time. Nevertheless, in the first study using that technique,[23] 6 of 11 patients needed a conversion (because of adhesions in 4 cases and difficulty in identifying tumor margins in 2 cases). The number of patients having been operated upon using this technique is too small to draw conclusions, but the hand-assisted technique could be promising.

Rau et al[27,32] have performed a prospective control study comparing 17 patients operated upon by laparoscopy with 17 operated upon by laparotomy, using a water jet dissector for liver resection. They conclude that operative time is longer by laparoscopy, there is no difference in blood loss, and hospital stay is shorter (when excluding the one converted patient).

SUMMARY

We have found 239 laparoscopic hepatectomies in the literature, from 21 studies performed between 1993 and 2001. There is no prospective, randomized trial comparing liver tumor resection under laparotomy versus laparoscopy.

For malignant tumors, 121 operations were performed, and 113 were performed for benign tumors. Less than one segment was resected in 81 cases, 120 were one or two-segment resections, and 27 were major hepatectomies (more than two segments resected). Only a few right lobectomies were performed completely under laparoscopy. Most of the procedures required a midline supra-umbilical incision, and an abdominal wall retractor, to perform a gasless laparoscopy.

The conversion rate was 7.11% (17 of 239; Table 34–3). Causes of conversion were insufficient resection margins (one

case), tumors localized too close to a large vessel (2 cases), probable gas embolism (3 cases), bleeding (2 cases), insufficient exposure (3 cases), difficulty in identifying tumor margins (2 cases), and adhesions (4 cases, one due to carcinoma).

The mean blood loss (a predictive factor of postoperative complications) was 349 mL (data available for 125 patients). Mean hospital stay was 9 days (data from 107 patients).

Morbidity was 14.04% (32 of 228; Table 34–4). It consisted of biliary leakage (4 cases), pleural effusion (6 cases), prolonged ascites discharge (one case), ascites discharges lasting 7 days (3 cases), postoperative ascites (one case), *Clostridium difficile* colitis (one case), *Pyoderma gangrenosum* infection (one case), pulmonary infection (4 cases), pulmonary insufficiency (one case), hematomas in trocar sites (4 cases), incisional hernia (3 cases, one requiring bowel resection), and coagulopathy with severe thrombopenia (one case). One patient had both pulmonary infection and bile leakage.

There were three probable cases of gas embolism of the 239 cases (1.26%).[15,36] Only one was documented by cardiac echog-

TABLE 34–3. CAUSES OF CONVERSION

Cause of Conversion	No. Patients	Percentage
Adhesions	4	1.67
Gas embolism	3	1.26
Insufficient exposure	3	1.26
Proximity to vessels	2	0.84
Bleeding	2	0.84
Difficulty identifying tumor margins	2	0.84
Insufficient resection margins	1	0.42
TOTAL	17/239	7.11

TABLE 34–4. MORBIDITY

Morbidities	Cases (datas from 228 pts)	Percentage
Pleural effusion	6	2.63
Ascites discharges	5	2.19
Biliary leakage	4	1.75
Pulmonary infection	4	1.75
Hematomas	4	1.75
Incisional hernias	3	1.32
Coagulopathies	2	0.88
Ascites	1	0.44
Pulmonary insufficiency	1	0.44
Pyoderma gangrenosum	1	0.44
Clostridium colitis	1	0.44
	32	14.04

raphy. One of them[36] appeared while using an argon-beam coagulator, which is known to increase abdominal pressure, and led to a cardiac arrest. Operations were converted, and were finished uneventfully. Gas embolisms are exceedingly rare events in laparoscopic liver surgery, with one study reporting 15 probable events in 113,253 cases (0.013%). We suppose that gas embolism could be reduced using gasless or low-pressure laparoscopy.

Mortality was 0.84%. One case was due to a coagulopathy with severe thrombopenia, and the other case was due to liver failure and coagulopathy.

CONCLUSION

Laparoscopic hepatectomy is feasible, with mortality and morbidity rates comparable to open procedures, according to an extremely careful selection of patients. The size of the lesions seems to be less important than the anatomic location in anterolateral regions (segments II to VI).

Resection of benign tumors is safe and should offer the usual advantages of minimally invasive techniques (reduced hospitalization, faster return to normal life, more cosmetic scars), but requires solid experience with both laparoscopic and hepatic surgery.

Resection of hepatocarcinoma is feasible, but we lack prospective randomized trials, of large cohorts, to compare the outcomes of laparoscopic resection with those of open surgery. Those patients should be included in prospective studies.

Laparoscopic resection of isolated and accessible colo-rectal liver metastasis could be a good alternative to open resection, if carcinologic rules can be respected, and if the current prospective randomized trials show the safety of laparoscopy for carcinomas. No recurrence in a trocar site has yet been reported after laparoscopic hepatectomy.

For the resection of lesions located in less-accessible segments (I, VII, VIII), hand-assisted techniques may be useful for the exposition, but advances in laparoscopic hepatic surgery will probably depend upon development of new instrumentation.

REFERENCES

1. Katkhouda N, Mavor E. Laparoscopic management of benign tumors. *Surg Clin North Am.* 2000;80:4.
2. Katkhouda N. Laparoscopic management of benign cystic lesions of the liver. *J Hepatobiliary Pancreat Surg.* 2000;7:212.
3. Azagra JS, Goergen M, Gilbart E, et al. Laparoscopic anatomical (hepatic) left lateral segmentectomy: Technical aspects. *Surg Endosc.* 1996;10:758.
4. Wernecke K, Rummeny E, Bongartz G, et al. Detection of hepatic masses in patients with carcinoma. *AJR Am J Roentgenol.* 1991;157:731.
5. Dodd GI, Miller W, Baron R, et al. Detection of malignant tumors in end-stage cirrhotic livers: Efficacy of sonography as a screening technique. *AJR Am J Roentgenol.* 1992;159:727.
6. Lipiodol-computed tomography in the diagnosis of small hepatocellular carcinoma. *Lancet.* 1990;337:143. Editorial.
7. Kido C, Sasaki, T, Kaneko M. Angiography of primary liver cancer. *Am J Radiol.* 1971;113:70.
8. Togo S, Shimada H, Kanemura E, et al. Usefulness of three-dimensional computed tomography for anatomic liver resection: Sub-subsegmentectomy. *Surgery.* 1998;123:73.
9. Marks WM, Jacobs RP, Goodman PC, et al. Hepatocellular carcinoma: Clinical and angiographic findings and predictability for surgical resection. *Am J Radiol.* 1979;13:7.
10. Seneterre E, Taourel P, Bouvier Y, et al. Detection of hepatic metastases: Ferumoxides-enhanced MR imaging versus unenhanced MR imaging and CT during arterial portography. *Radiology.* 1996;200:785.
11. Couinaud C. *Le foie: études anatomiques et chirurgicales.* Paris, Masson: 1957.
12. Huscher CG, Lirici M, Chiodini S, et al. Laparsocopic surgery section. Current position on advanced laparoscopic surgery of the liver. *J R Coll Surg Edinb.* 1997;42:219.
13. Cunningham J, Katz L, Brower S, et al. Laparoscopic resection of two hemangiomata. *Surg Laparosc Endosc.* 1995;5:277.
14. Mouiel J, Katkhouda N, Gugenheim J, et al. Topics: Laparoscopic surgery for hepatobiliry pancreatic disease. Possibilities of laparoscopic liver resection. J Hepatobiliary Pancreatic Surg 7:1–8, 2000.
15. Hashizume M, Shimada M, Sugimachi K. Laparoscopic hepatectomy: new approach for hepatocellular carcinoma. J Hepatobiliary Pancreat Surg. 2000;7:270.
16. Huscher CGS, Lirici MM, Chiodini S. Laparoscopic liver resections. *Semin Laparosc Surg.* 1998;5:204.
17. Hashizume M, Takaneka K, Yanaga K, et al. Laparoscopic hepatic resection for hepatocellular carcinoma. *Surg Endosc.* 1995;9:1289.
18. Ker CG, Chen HY, Juan CC, et al. Laparoscopic subsegmentectomy for hepatocellular carcinoma with cirrhosis. *Hepatogastroenterology.* 2000;47:1260.
19. Descottes B, Lachachi F, Sodji M, et al. Early experience with laparoscopic approach for solid liver tumors: Initial 16 cases. *Ann Surg.* 2000;232:5.
20. Mouiel J. Possibilities of laparoscopic liver resection. *J Hepatobiliary Pancreat Surg.* 2000;7:1.
21. Samama G, Chiche L, Brefort JL, et al. Laparoscopic anatomical hepatic resection. Report of four left lobectomies for solid tumors. *Surg Endosc.* 1998;12:76.
22. Kaneko H, Takagi S, Shiba T. Laparoscopic partial hepatectomy and left lateral segmentectomy: technique and results of a clinical series. *Surgery.* 1996;120:468.
23. Fong Y, Jarnagin W, Conlon KC, et al. Hand-assisted laparoscopic liver resection: lessons from an initial experience. *Arch Surg.* 2000;135:854.

24. Katkhouda N, Hurwitz M, Gugenheim J, et al. Laparoscopic management of benign solid and cystic lesions of the liver. *Ann* Surg. 1999;229:4.

25. Crocco B, Azzola M, Russo R, et al. Laparoscopic liver tumor resection with the argon beam. *Endosc Surg.* 1994:2:186.

26. Rau HG, Meyer G, Jauch KW, et al. Liver resection with the water jet: Conventional and laparoscopic surgery. *Chirurg.* 1996;67:546.

27. Rau HG, Meyer G, Cohnert TU, et al. Laparoscopic liver resection with the waterjet dissector. *Surg Endosc.* 1995;9:1009.

28. Watanabe Y, Sato M, Ueda S, et al. Laparoscopic hepatic resection: A new and safe procedure by abdominal wall lifting method. *Hepatogastroenterology.* 1997;44:143.

29. Yamanaka N, Tanaka T, Tanaka W, et al. Laparoscopic partial hepatectomy. *Hepatogastroenterology.* 1998;45:29.

30. Cuschieri A. Laparoscopic hand-assisted surgery for hepatic and pancreatic disease. *Surg Endosc.* 2000;14:991.

31. Lefor AT, Flowers JL. Laparoscopic wedge biopsy of the liver. *Am Coll Surg.* 1994;178:307.

32. Rau HG, Buttler E, Meyer G, et al. Laparoscopic liver resection compared with conventional partial hepatectomy—a prospective analysis. *Hepatogastroenterology.* 1998;45:2333.

33. Mizoe A, Tomioka T, Inoue K, et al. Systematic laparoscopic left lateral segmentectomy of the liver for hepatocellular carcinoma. *J Hepatobiliary Pancreat Surg.* 1998;5:173.

34. Cherqui D, Husson E, Hammoud R, et al. Laparoscopic liver resections: A feasibility study in 30 patients. *Ann Surg.* 2000;232:753.

35. Hamy A, Paineau J, Savigny L, et al. Laparoscopic hepatic surgery. Report of a clinical series of 11 patients. *Int Surg.* 1998;83:33.

36. Croce E, Azzola M, Russo R, et al. Laparoscopic liver resection with the argon beam. *Endosc Surg Allied Technol.* 1994;2:186.

37. Cuesta M, Meijer S, Paul A, et al. Limited laparoscopic liver resection of benign tumors guided by laparoscopic ultrasonography: Report of two cases. *Surg Laparosc Endosc.* 1995;5:396.

38. Abdel-Atty M, Farges O, Jagot P, et al. Laparoscopy extends the indications for liver resection in patients with cirrhosis. *Br J Surg.* 1999;86:1397.

Chapter Thirty-Five ● ● ● ● ● ●

*L*aparoscopic Cryotherapy for Hepatic Tumors

GREGG H. JOSSART and MICHEL GAGNER

Cryotherapy of the liver, a method of destroying hepatic tumors by freezing, can be used to treat a variety of hepatic pathologies. The results of open hepatic cryotherapy are now available for almost 900 patients,[1] the majority having received cryotherapy for liver metastases from colorectal carcinoma and primary hepatocellular carcinoma.

The United States reports approximately 150,000 new cases of colorectal cancer per year, and 75,000 of these will ultimately develop liver metastases.[1,2] About 20% of these patients with liver metastases (15,000 cases/year) have disease confined to the liver, but only 4000 (25%) are eligible for hepatic resection.[1,2] This leaves approximately 11,000 patients/year in the United States to be treated with alternative therapies. Hepatic cryotherapy has been proven to be a useful treatment option for these patients.

Hepatocellular carcinoma (HCC) is a prevalent problem on a worldwide basis, with approximately 250,000 deaths per year attributed to this tumor.[2,3] Patients with HCC generally have a poor survival rate, which can be improved with resection; however, most patients present with advanced disease and surgical resection is usually not an option. Hepatic cryotherapy has also been shown to be a useful form of therapy for these patients.

Hepatic cryotherapy, using intraoperative ultrasound monitoring, was introduced in the 1980s by Onik et al,[4] who combined the freezing process with intraoperative ultrasound for monitoring the extent of freezing. Presently cryotherapy is used to treat tumors in the brain, oropharynx, lung, breast, uterus, prostate, kidney, and liver.[5]

The methods of tissue destruction by freezing include protein denaturation, osmotic driven shifts of intracellular and extracellular water, membrane destabilization, cellular rupture, and tissue ischemia.[6,7] In vitro studies have revealed that the most efficacious tumor killing occurs with a rapid freeze–slow thaw cycle done more than once.[8–11]

While data on the long-term outcome of patients treated with cryotherapy are limited, some have reported impressive results. For example, Zhou et al[12] reported a 5-year survival rate of 49% following cryotherapy in patients with unresectable hepatocellular carcinoma less than 5 cm in size. Others[1] have noted a 2-year disease-free survival rate of 65%. Experience with cryotherapy for hepatic metastases from colorectal tumors has been more variable. Ravikumar et al[13] reported a 2-year survival rate of 78% and a disease-free survival rate of 39%. In contrast to these reports, Adam and colleagues[14] have noted a 44% local recurrence despite adequate cryotherapy. The problems with most studies for unresectable hepatocellular carcinoma and for metastatic disease include the lack of appropriate controls; small sample size; limited follow-up; and variability in size, number, and etiology of hepatic lesions. Thus, meaningful comparisons between studies are difficult.

Complications related to hepatic cryotherapy are infrequent and include fever, thrombocytopenia, bile leak, hepatic abscess, pleural effusion, myoglobinuria, and reversible acute renal failure.[1,2]

The recent parallel developments of laparoscopic ultrasound probes and long, small-diameter cryoprobes that can be passed through laparoscopic ports have led to the technique of laparoscopic hepatic cryotherapy.

The standard laparoscopic equipment needed to perform laparoscopic cryotherapy includes a variety of trochar sizes to accommodate instruments ranging from 3 to 11 mm in diameter. A variety of graspers, dissectors, soft bowel clamps, scissors, and cautery are needed to take down adhesions and mobilize the liver. Laparoscopic needle drivers and sutures may be needed for intracorporeal suturing of the liver or other structures. A laparoscopic liver retractor may be needed to manipulate the liver for mobilization, inspection, and probe placement. Two video towers are preferable. Ideally a video image splitter (Twin Video System, model 20201120, Karl Storz, Culver, CA) that produces a picture-in-picture image is particularly helpful during the combined ultrasound and cryotherapy portions of the procedure.

There are two types of cryosurgical systems we have used clinically. Systems such as the CMS AccuProbe® 450 System (CryoMedical Sciences, Rockville, MD) use liquid nitrogen as the cryogen and nitrogen gas as the warming agent. We have adopted a more recent system that uses argon gas as the cryogen and helium as the warming agent. This system (Cryocare®, EndoCare, Irvine, CA) runs up to 8 cryoprobes simultaneously and relies on the rapid expansion of argon gas (the Joule-Thompson principle) in the tip of the cryoprobe to cool tissue rapidly. Differences between this system and devices using liquid nitrogen include no bulky insulation on cryoprobes, faster freezing rates, and increased portability due to a lack of heavy storage dewars in the unit. In our experience, iceballs created by this system are comparable or slightly larger than liquid nitrogen systems for identical-sized probes. Because the cryogenic effect is isolated to the cryoprobe tip, there is limited freezing of the probe shaft, which reduces the risk of injury to adjacent organs.

Laparoscopic ultrasound is used to identify and characterize the size, shape, and location of hepatic lesions. It is also essential for proper placement of the cryotherapy probe and monitoring the development and progression of the freeze ball. Current laparoscopic ultrasound probes fit through 10-mm ports and have flexible tips. One example is the Laparoscopic Ultrasound Transducer Type 8555 (B&K Medical Systems, Marlborough, MA). It has a 60-degree convex array capable of transducing at frequencies of 5, 6.5, and 7.5 MHz. The system has several modes of function including B-mode, M-mode, spectral Doppler, and color-flow monitoring. Dexterity with laparoscopic ultrasound and understanding ultrasonographic anatomy of the liver, particularly when viewing from a number of angles and positions, is essential when performing laparoscopic cryotherapy.

Patients undergoing cryotherapy of hepatic lesions should be prepared for surgery in the same manner that patients undergoing major abdominal procedures are prepared. CT and MRI scans are useful to determine unresectability and to characterize the lesions (Fig. 35–1). Positron emission tomography (PET) scanning is an additional imaging modality that may demonstrate otherwise unsuspected extrahepatic disease.[15]

Patient positioning is dependent on the location of the hepatic tumors to be treated. The supine position is most often adequate. Patients with lesions in the posterior sector of the right lobe of the liver (segments VI, VII) can be placed in an oblique position with the right side elevated up to 45 degrees and the right arm elevated and across the chest. This position provides added exposure to the flank and facilitates placement of cryotherapy probes posteriorly. Alternatively, the right posterior liver can be approached using the supine position and completely mobilizing the right liver off the diaphragm, as reported by Lezoche et al.[16] However, this may lead to an increased incidence of surface parenchymal splits and pleural effusion. The entire abdomen and chest are prepped and draped to provide access to these cavities.

Most patients undergoing laparoscopic cryoablation of hepatic tumors will have had previous abdominal surgery, and laparoscopic lysis of adhesions will be necessary. After extrahepatic recurrent disease is excluded, the liver is evaluated with a 7.5-MHz convex array laparoscopic ultrasound probe. Once the tumor to be ablated is characterized, the capsule of the liver overlying the tumor is scored using electrocautery. The cryotherapy probe is inserted through the capsule under ultrasound guidance into the tumor (Fig. 35–2). It is generally easier to place the probe having the ultrasound and cryotherapy probes in parallel. This will provide a longitudinal image of the cryotherapy probe by ultrasound (Fig. 35–3). The tip of the cryotherapy probe should be positioned at the distal or deep edge of the tumor. When proper placement of the probe is confirmed, the freezing process is begun. Tissue temperature is continuously monitored through the cryotherapy probe. Progressive development of the iceball is monitored by ultrasound. The iceball does not conduct sound waves; therefore it casts an ultrasonographic shadow behind its superficial surface and a hyperechoic rim. Because freeze progression cannot be completely monitored from a static ultrasound probe, it is continually repositioned on the liver surface. This may require temporary replacement of the ultrasound probe through other trochar sites. The deep progression of the freeze ball can be monitored by placing the ultrasound probe along the inferior edge or behind the posterior edge of the liver and transmitting the ultrasound waves anteriorly. Freezing is completed when the tissue temperature reaches −160°C and the iceball has obtained 1-cm margins beyond the tumor edge or

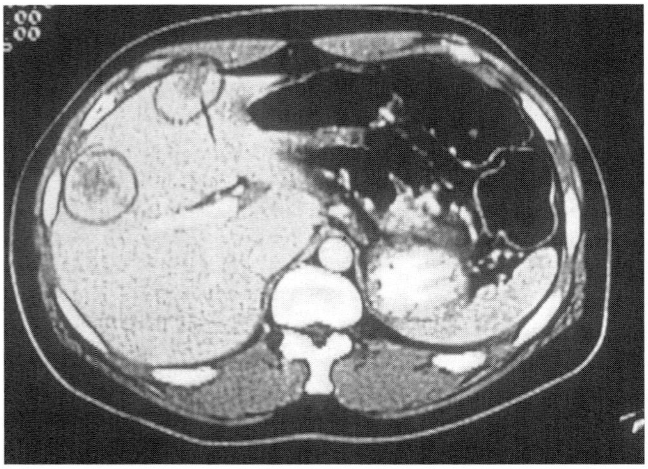

Figure 35–1. CT scan of a patient with colorectal liver metastasis to both lobes of the liver.

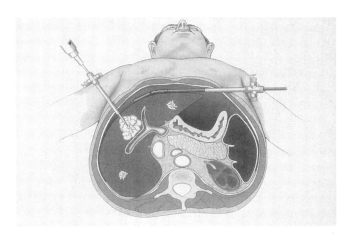

Figure 35–2. Cross-sectional illustration of ultrasound-guided placement of cryoprobe into liver metastasis.

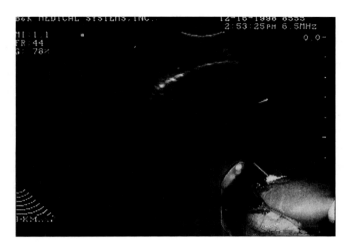

Figure 35–3. Picture within picture demonstrating ultrasound-guided placement of cryoprobe into liver metastasis.

reaches adjacent hepatic or vascular structures. A 40-cm, 4.9-mm diameter cryotherapy probe is usually suitable for most laparoscopic applications. Passive thawing follows the completed freeze phase, and when the temperature reaches −4°C a second freeze–thaw cycle can be performed. Removal of the cryotherapy probe can be accomplished by careful torquing of the probe. Excessive movement of the probe may result in shearing of the iceball–liver interface, cracking of the iceball, and increased risk of hemorrhage. The exit site of the probe should be inspected for bleeding and bile leakage. Hemostatic agents, electrocautery, or suturing of the hepatic capsule may be required.

Other liver lesions can be treated in a similar fashion. Larger tumors may require multiple passes of the cryotherapy probe in different positions to completely ablate the lesion with appropriate margins. Tumors up to 10 cm have been treated by cryotherapy, but the risk of bleeding increases with the size of the lesion.[3] Many separate lesions can be treated in this way in one session, although the number treated should be dictated by the patient's hemodynamic status, core temperature, and coagulation status, plus good clinical judgment.

Postoperatively, most patients do well and are discharged in 2 or 3 days. For patients who have had cryotherapy of large lesions or multiple lesions, it is reasonable to increase their intravenous fluids perioperatively to prevent cryotherapy-related acute renal failure. We usually obtain a CT or MRI scan about 6 weeks to 3 months postoperatively, which usually demonstrates central necrosis and a rim of fibrosis at the site of cryoablation.

To date, laparoscopic cryotherapy has been reported in approximately 60 patients.[16–19] We have reported the successful laparoscopic cryotherapy of 12 patients with primary and secondary hepatic tumors.[17] One patient was converted for hemorrhage from the frozen tumor. Disease-free survival at a mean follow-up of 10.8 months was 58% (7 of 12 patients). Lezoche et al[16] reported the successful laparoscopic cryotherapy of 18 patients with primary and secondary hepatic tumors. Two patients were converted to open cryotherapy for hemorrhage from surface parenchymal splits. Disease-free survival at a mean follow-up of 10.8 months was 78% (14 of 18 patients). Cuschieri et al reported a series of 22 patients of which 12 were treated with open cryotherapy, 6 with laparoscopic cryotherapy, and 4

with a laparoscopically assisted approach. While survival and recurrence in the laparoscopic group are not detailed, 3 patients with recurrence were treated with laparoscopic cryotherapy.[18]

These studies confirm that laparoscopic hepatic cryotherapy can be performed for primary and secondary hepatic tumors in all segments of the liver and sizes up to about 10 cm. It appears to be safe and has less wound-related morbidity than the open approach. Unfortunately, the current results of laparoscopic cryotherapy for hepatic tumors are limited. A larger patient group and longer follow-up are needed to better assess the utility of laparoscopic cryoablation of hepatic tumors.

Presently, laparoscopic cryotherapy for hepatic tumors can be offered to patients in selected clinical conditions. Indications for cryotherapy include patients with unresectable secondary or primary lesions of the liver, comorbid medical conditions precluding hepatic resection, or limited hepatic reserve. Patients with recurrent metastatic or primary tumors to the liver may also be good candidates for cryoablative treatment. Tumor histologies that are acceptably treated by hepatic cryotherapy include hepatocellular, colorectal, carcinoid, neuroendocrine, sarcoma, Wilm's, renal cell, and adrenocortical tumors.[5] There may be a role in treating unresectable intrahepatic cholangiocarcinoma, locally invasive gallbladder cancer, or a deeply located hepatic adenoma. Patients with metastases from melanoma, breast, esophagus, lung, stomach, pancreas, and gynecologic tumors have historically not demonstrated improved survival following hepatic resection.[5] The value of hepatic cryotherapy for metastases from these lesions remains undetermined. Resolving these issues and continued technical advancement are the current challenges in laparoscopic cryotherapy of hepatic tumors.

Other interstitial therapies and imaging modalities for the treatment of unresectable hepatic tumors are in development. Open real-time MRI and CT are being developed and may provide better intraoperative monitoring or even allow percutaneous ablation in the radiology suite. Indeed, Schuder et al,[20] using ultrasound guidance, reported a strictly percutaneous approach in 8 patients, and Lee et al[21] and Klotz et al[22] have reported using both CT and MRI for hepatic cryosurgery in an animal model. In addition, alternatives to cryotherapy, such as radiofrequency, microwave, and electrical ablative therapies, are all being developed and may offer the advantage of smaller-diameter probes and possibly more thorough ablation.

REFERENCES

1. Seifert JK, Junginger T, Morris DL. A collective review of the world literature on hepatic cryotherapy. *J R Coll Surg Edinb.* 1998;43:141.
2. McCarty TM, Kuhn JA. Cryotherapy for liver tumors. *Oncology.* 1998;July:979.
3. Iannitti DA, Heniford T, Hale J, et al. Laparoscopic cryoablation of hepatic metastases. *Arch Surg.* 1998;133:1011.
4. Onik GM, Atkinson D, Zemel R, et al. Cryosurgery for liver cancer. *Semin Surg Oncol.* 1993;9:309.
5. Ravikumar TS. Interstitial therapies for liver tumors. *Surg Oncol Clin North Am.* 1996;5:365.
6. Bayjoo P, Jacob G. Hepatic cryosurgery: Biological and clinical considerations. *J R Coll Surg Edinb.* 1992;37:369.
7. Rubinsky B, Lee CY, Bastacky J, et al. The process of freezing and mechanism of damage during hepatic cryosurgery. *Cryobiology.* 1990;27:85.

8. Ravikumar TS, Steele GD. Hepatic cryosurgery. *Surg Clin North Am.* 1989;69:433.

9. Ravikumar TS, King V, Steele GD. Cryosurgery for colorectal cancer liver metastases: An experimental study. *Surg Forum.* 1989; 40:419.

10. Stewart GJ, Preketes A, Horton M, et al. Hepatic cryotherapy: Double-freeze cycles achieve greater hepatocellular injury in man. *Cryobiology.* 1995;32:215.

11. Bischof J, Christov K, Rubinsky B. A morphological study of cooling rate response in normal and neoplastic human liver tissue: Cryosurgical implications. *Cryobiology.* 1993;30:482.

12. Zhou XD, Tang YU, Yu YQ, et al. The role of hepatic cryosurgery in the treatment of hepatic cancer: A report of 113 cases. *J Cancer Res Clin Oncol.* 1993;120:100.

13. Ravikumar TS, Kane R, Cady B, *et al.* A 5-year study of cryosurgery in the treatment of liver tumors. *Arch Surg.* 1991;126:1520.

14. Adam R, Akpinar E, Johann M. Place of cryotherapy in the treatment of malignant liver tumors. *Ann Surg.* 1997;225:39.

15. Abdel-Nabi H, Doerr R, et al. Staging of primary colorectal carcinomas with fluorine-18 fluorodeoxyglucose whole-body PET: Correlation with histopathologic and CT findings. *Radiology.* 1998; 206:755.

16. Lezoche E, Paganini AM, Feliciotti F, et al. Ultrasound-guided laparoscopic cryoablation of hepatic tumors: Preliminary report. *World J Surg.* 1998;22:829.

17. Heniford BT, Arca MJ, Iannitti DA, et al. Laparoscopic cryoablation of hepatic metastases. Semin Surg Oncol. 1998;15:1.

18. Cuschieri A, Crosthwaite G, Shimi S, et al. Hepatic cryotherapy for liver tumors. *Surg Endosc.* 1995;9:483.

19. Tandan VR, Litwin D, Asch M, et al. Laparoscopic cryosurgery for hepatic tumors. *Surg Endosc.* 1997;11:1115.

20. Schuder G, Pistorius G, Schneider G, et al. Preliminary experience with percutaneous cryotherapy of liver tumors. *Br J Surg.* 1990;85:1210.

21. Lee FT, Chosy SG, Warner TF, et al. Percutaneous hepatic tissue ablation with radiofrequency or cold temperature monitored by CT in real time: Radiologic–pathologic correlation. Presented at the Association of University Radiologists annual meeting, New Orleans, March 1998.

22. Klotz HP, Flury R, Schonenberger A, et al. Experimental cryosurgery of the liver under magnetic resonance guidance. *Comput Aided Surg.* 1997;2:340.

Chapter Thirty-Six ▪ ▪ ▪ ▪ ▪ ▪

Operative Laparoscopy for Portal Hypertension: Experimental and Clinical Studies

PAOLO GENTILESCHI and MICHEL GAGNER

The normal portal venous pressure is 5 to 10 mm Hg, which is sufficient pressure to maintain portal blood flow through the hepatic sinusoids in excess of 1 L/min. Portal hypertension is present when the portal venous pressure exceeds 10 mm Hg.

Liver cirrhosis is the most common cause of portal hypertension. Other causes such as portal vein thrombosis or hepatic vein outflow obstruction should be considered when the picture is not that of chronic liver disease. The consequences of portal hypertension are varices and bleeding, ascites, and liver failure with hepatic encephalopathy. Acute variceal bleeding is associated with a mortality rate between 20 and 50%, depending on the liver disease, and requires an intensive multidisciplinary approach.

Treatment modalities for portal hypertension include pharmacologic and endoscopic therapy, radiologic or surgical decompression, devascularization procedures, and liver transplantation. These methods are primarily used for the management of varices and variceal bleeding, but some of these treatments apply to the other complications of portal hypertension.

Patients with variceal bleeding are initially treated with endoscopic therapy, often in combination with pharmacologic therapy. Pharmacologic therapy is usually considered for the secondary prevention of variceal bleeding and for the treatment of acute variceal bleeding. Beta-adrenergic receptor antagonists and nitrates reduce the risk of rebleeding from 75 to 50%.[1] In the acute bleeding patient, vasopressin and nitroglycerin in combination with somatostatin are generally used.[2] These drugs reduce acute bleeding and may be used in combination with sclerotherapy.[3] A recent meta-analysis has shown that the use of octreotide for acute variceal bleeding is effective and associated with fewer major complications than vasopressin.[4]

Endoscopic therapy in secondary prevention of variceal bleeding uses both sclerotherapy and banding.[5,6] Randomized studies suggest that banding is more effective than sclerotherapy because earlier obliteration of varices can be obtained with fewer sessions and fewer side effects.[6] Endoscopic therapy is also the first line treatment of acute variceal bleeding, controlling 90% of such episodes.[6] Subsequently, the obliteration of esophageal varices is usually performed with a 6-week course of endoscopic therapy, with a success rate of 50%.[6] Nevertheless, 30 to 50% of varices will rebleed, either because of a failure of endoscopic therapy or because of their recurrence.[7]

Second-line treatment for variceal bleeding requires decompression of the varices, either radiologically or surgically.

The transjugular intrahepatic portosystemic shunt (TIPS) has been widely used in the last 5 years.[8] It is an effective and relatively safe method to treat patients who were not successfully managed by sclerotherapy or banding.[8] Unfortunately, shunt stenosis occurs in 50 to 70% of patients, leading to rebleeding episodes in 20% and reintervention in 30 to 40% of patients.[9] Controlled trials comparing TIPS with endoscopic therapy have demonstrated that man-agement of bleeding has initially been better with TIPS, but the benefit lessens by 1 year.[10] Furthermore, hepatic encephalopathy, a consequence of portal diversion, occurs in 25 to 30% of TIPS patients.[11] This rate is significantly higher when compared to endoscopic therapy.[6]

Surgical shunts may be total, partial, or selective, according to the degree of diversion of the portal flow. All surgical shunts are effective, controlling bleeding in approximately 90% of cases. The degree of diversion influences the rate of encephalopathy. This occurs in 30 to 50% of total shunts, in 10 to 15% of partial shunts (8 mm diameter), and in 10% of selective shunts.[12]

Recently, a prospective randomized trial has compared TIPS with a small-diameter (8-mm) prosthetic H-graft portacaval shunt as definitive treatment for variceal bleeding due to portal hypertension.[13] Of the 132 patients involved over a median follow-up period of 4 years, 66 underwent 8-mm prosthetic H-graft portacaval shunt placement and 66 underwent TIPS. Both shunts provided partial portal decompression, although the portal vein–inferior vena cava pressure gradient was lower after the H-graft portacaval shunt ($P < 0.01$). Shunt stenosis/occlusion was more frequent after TIPS. After TIPS, 42 patients failed (64%), whereas after H-graft portacaval shunt 23 failed (35%) ($P < 0.01$). Major variceal rehemorrhage, hepatic transplantation, and late death were significantly more frequent after TIPS ($P < 0.01$). The authors concluded that TIPS provides less optimal outcomes than H-graft portacaval shunt for patients with portal hypertension and variceal bleeding.

Also a retrospective case-control comparison between TIPS and the surgical (portacaval, distal splenorenal) shunt (PSS) has been recently reported.[9] Forty Child-Pugh class A or B cirrhotic patients were included in the study. Twenty patients who underwent TIPS were compared with 20 matched PSS patients. Thirty-day mortality was greater following TIPS than PSS (20% vs 0%; $P = .20$); long-term mortality did not differ. Significantly more rebleeding episodes ($P < .001$), rehospitalizations ($P < .05$), diagnostic studies of all types ($P < .001$), shunt revisions ($P < .001$), and hospital ($P < .005$), professional ($P < .05$), and total ($P < .005$) charges occurred following TIPS compared with the surgical shunt.

On the basis of this data, the enthusiasm and wide acceptance of TIPS in clinical practice may be revised. To date, good-risk patients with portal hypertension and variceal bleeding can still be referred for a surgical shunt. Further randomized trials are needed to demonstrate an evidence-based advantage of one therapy over the other.

Devascularization procedures include splenectomy, gastric and esophageal devascularization, and esophageal transection. Extensive procedures are associated with a rebleeding rate of less than 10%.[14] Reported higher rebleeding rates (30 to 40%) are thought to be related to less aggressive operations.[14]

The outcome of patients with advanced liver cirrhosis has been dramatically changed by liver transplantation.[15] Approximately 80% of Child-Pugh class C patients can now be cured if they are suitable candidates for transplantation.[15] On the other hand, because of the limitation in the donor supply, high cost of the procedure, and risks of immunosuppression, liver transplantation remains indicated for end-stage disease rather than portal hypertension.[15]

Each of the therapies mentioned may be indicated at different timepoints and for different patients. Advanced centers should have multidisciplinary expertise and specific treatment algorithms for the management of such high-risk patients.

The other major complication of portal hypertension is ascites. It is usually a more severe complication than bleeding because it indicates more advanced liver disease. Primary therapy includes diet, diuretics, and paracentesis. Intractable ascites is an indication for liver transplantation. Other methods are TIPS and side-to-side portosystemic shunting that decompress the liver and may control ascites.

The role of diagnostic laparoscopy and laparoscopic liver biopsy is well known in the diagnosis of liver diseases, although improvements in imaging studies and percutaneous bioptic techniques have rendered them often unnecessary.[16] On the other hand, there is an increasing interest in the future role of operative laparoscopy in patients with portal hypertension. Two experimental studies have investigated the feasibility of using the laparoscopic approach for two operations. Initial clinical experiences with different procedures have also been reported. Experimental and clinical studies on operative laparoscopy for portal hypertension are presented and discussed in this chapter.

EXPERIMENTAL STUDIES

In 1997, Tsimoyiannis and co-workers reported an experimental study on a laparoscopic modified Sugiura procedure in the pig.[17] Six pigs were used. The steps of the procedure were (1) mobilization of the lower esophagus and truncal vagotomy, (2) esophageal resection-anastomosis with an EEA stapler, (3) devascularization of the corpus and fundus of the stomach and the lower 10 cm of the esophagus, (4) splenectomy, (5) Nissen fundoplication, and (6) pyloroplasty.

Six trocars were used. The diaphragmatic hiatus was identified and dissected with the two crura. The lower esophagus was therefore mobilized completely. Truncal vagotomy was performed and all esophageal vessels were clipped. A polypropylene ligature no. 0/0 was then passed posteriorly to encircle the esophagus. A gastrotomy about 3 cm in length was performed on the anterior surface of the stomach, close to the gastroesophageal junction. A CEEA stapler was introduced intraperitoneally and then into the lower esophagus through the gastrotomy. The esophageal wall was li-gated to the axis of the stapler 2 cm above the gastro-esophageal junction by using the previously inserted ligature. The esophageal resection-anastomosis was then performed by firing the stapler. The gastrotomy was then sutured. Devascularization of the corpus and fundus of the stomach was performed by using clips or stapler. The coronary vein, diaphragmatic veins, and paraesophageal veins, as well as the vessels of the corpus and fundus of the stomach, were ligated and divided. At this point, a splenectomy and Nissen fundoplication were performed. The last step of the procedure was pyloroplasty. A necropsy was performed at the end of each procedure to evaluate and confirm technical success.

The mean operative time was 180 minutes, while the mean estimated blood loss was 260 mL. Necropsy revealed no leak from the staple lines and occlusion of all vessels at the end of each procedure. The experimental study confirmed the feasibility of the operation.

We investigated the technical feasibility of using a laparoscopic approach to direct side-to-side portacaval shunt in a porcine model. Another study on laparoscopic H-graft portacaval shunt is currently underway.

Laparoscopic side-to-side portacaval shunt was performed in 5 female 50-kg pigs. On the morning of surgery, each pig received intravenous fluids, was sedated with ketamine, received pentobarbital intravenously for induction of anesthesia, and an endotracheal tube was positioned. The animal was then placed on the ventilator and received isoflurane for anesthesia. The animal was then secured in a 30-degree left lateral decubitus position with a slight reverse Trendelenburg position. An open technique was used for the induction of pneumoperitoneum. Five trocars were used: one at the umbilicus for the laparoscope, one at the left subcostal area for the liver retractor, one at the right lower quadrant for the bowel retractor; the first operating port was placed at the midline, just below the xiphoid, and the second was placed laterally on the right

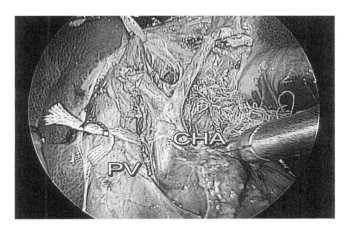

Figure 36–1. Dissection of the portal vein (PV), common hepatic artery (CHA), and common bile duct at the hepatic hilum. See Color Section.

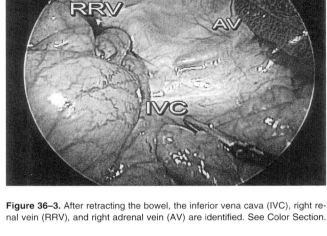

Figure 36–3. After retracting the bowel, the inferior vena cava (IVC), right renal vein (RRV), and right adrenal vein (AV) are identified. See Color Section.

of the umbilicus. With the liver and bowels well retracted, the procedure started with the isolation of the portal vein, common hepatic artery, and common bile duct at the hepatic hilum (Fig. 36–1). Careful dissection was performed. The portal vein was isolated for a 7 to 8-cm tract and encircled with a precut umbilical tape (Fig. 36–2). Then attention was turned towards the inferior vena cava (IVC; Fig. 36–3). To visualize the IVC, there is a need for extensive bowel retraction. Starting from the hilum of the right kidney, the peritoneum was opened and the right renal vein and right adrenal vein were identified (Fig. 36–3). The inferior vena cava was subsequently identified and isolated for a 7 to 8-cm tract. Also the IVC was encircled with a precut umbilical tape (Fig. 36–4). At this point of the procedure, heparin was administered intravenously (10,000 U). The portal vein and IVC were further dissected to be able to approximate the two veins without tension (Fig. 36–5). To perform a side-to-side anastomosis, both veins were cross-clamped together with two laparoscopic vascular clamps (Fig. 36–6). The phlebotomies were performed with a no. 11 blade, introduced into the abdomen through a laparoscopic grasper (Fig. 36–7). The direct anastomosis was performed using a 6-0 Goretex suture (CV-6, W.L. Gore & Associates, Flagstaff, AZ). A running posterior

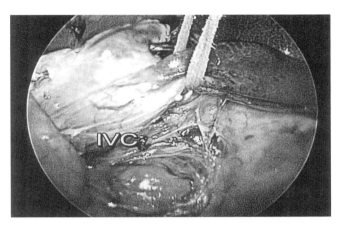

Figure 36–4. The inferior vena cava (IVC) is encircled with an umbilical tape. See Color Section.

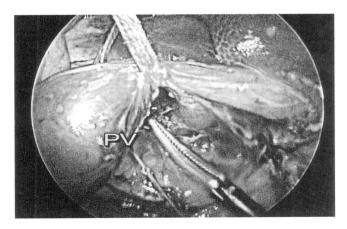

Figure 36–2. The portal vein is encircled with an umbilical tape. See Color Section.

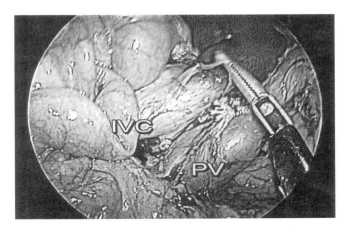

Figure 36–5. The portal vein (PV) and inferior vena cava (IVC) are approximated before clamping. See Color Section.

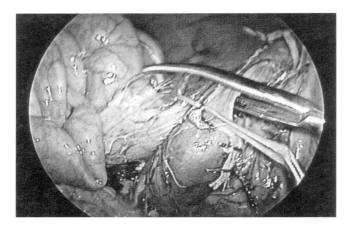

Figure 36–6. Cross-clamping of the portal vein (PV) and inferior vena cava (IVC). See Color Section.

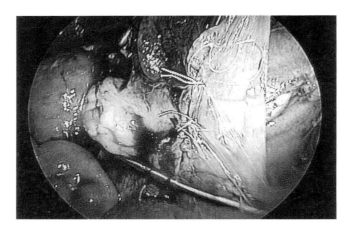

Figure 36–8. Final side-to-side portocaval shunt. See Color Section.

and running anterior vascular suture was performed. An intracorporeal laparoscopic knot-tying technique was used (Fig. 36–8). The clamps were released and the anastomosis was inspected for leakage. Additional suturing was placed in cases of bleeding from the anastomotic line. At the end of the procedure, euthanasia and necropsy were performed and the portacaval shunt was carefully evaluated. In all 5 cases, the anastomosis was found to be patent and intact. Mean operative time was 242 ± 48.1 minutes (range, 190 to 300 minutes). Mean anastomotic time was 41.4 ± 8.9 minutes (range, 30 to 55 minutes). The operation was found to be feasible, although technically challenging. Expertise in laparoscopic vascular suturing is required. A study on a laparoscopic H-graft (8-mm) portacaval shunt is currently underway. Also a new vascular clamp is currently under evaluation to perform a side-clamping of the IVC, thus avoiding IVC cross-clamping.

Both these operations (the modified Sugiura and the portacaval shunt) were found to be feasible using a laparoscopic approach. On the other hand, it must be emphasized that it is different to operate on healthy young animals and sick, portal hypertensive patients. However, it is also true that the laparoscopic approach to portal hypertensive patients has been successfully used in a clinical setting.

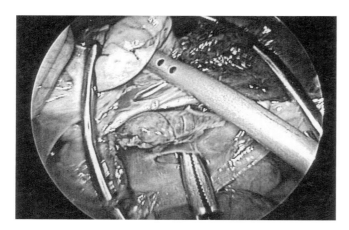

Figure 36–7. The phlebotomies are performed. See Color Section.

CLINICAL REPORTS

Clinical reports involving operative laparoscopy for portal hypertension include the following procedures: portacaval H-graft shunt, splenectomy, devascularization of the lower esophagus and upper stomach, esophagogastric devascularization and transection, gastric devascularization and splenectomy, azygoportal disconnection with splenic artery ligation, and transesophageal suturing of the gastric and esophageal varices.[18–24]

All of these procedures have been performed laparoscopically in humans, either as a single case report[21–24] or as initial series.[18–20] The first series of patients was reported in 1994.[18] Seven patients with esophagogastric varices were treated by laparoscopic-assisted devascularization of the lower esophagus and upper stomach. Three of the 7 patients had an episode of variceal bleeding, and the remaining 4 had moderate to large gastric varices with red color signs. The operative procedure was performed using an abdominal wall retractor without pneumoperitoneum. A 3 to 5-cm long midline skin incision was also performed. Through the midline incision, the lower part of the stomach was devascularized using standard surgical instruments. The upper stomach and lower esophagus were devascularized using laparoscopic instruments and suture devices. The procedure time ranged from 100 to 180 minutes with minimal blood loss (70 to 320 g). No complications were seen. Follow-up (mean 11.4 months) showed no recurrence of gastric varices although 2 patients were treated additionally by sclerotheraphy.

In 1997, Zilberstein et al described a minimally invasive approach to bleeding esophageal varices.[19] After failure of endoscopic sclerosis and balloon tamponade, 4 patients with persistent bleeding were treated by laparoscopic surgery. An azygoportal disconnection with splenic artery ligation and suturing of the gastroesophageal varices without opening the esophagus was performed laparoscopically. The procedure started with dissection of the diaphragmatic hiatus and isolation of the esophagus. Then, the gastric fundus was devascularized. The splenic artery was ligated between clips as well as the vessels of the gastric lesser curvature. Trans-orally, a 12-mm probe was then inserted into the esophagus and the varices were sutured transmurally with interrupted stitches. A floppy Nissen fundoplication was performed at the end of the procedure. The patients experienced a quick hospital stay (between 8 and 10 days) and recovery. No bleeding recurred. The evolution demonstrated stabilization of the hepatic function and regression of the varices from grades III and IV to grade I.

The last series of patients was reported in 1998.[20] Laparoscopic gastric devascularization and splenectomy (Hassab's operation) was performed to treat recurrent sclerotheraphy-resistant giant esophageal varices (n = 4) and recurrent rebleeding gastric varices (n = 6). After splenectomy, laparoscopic devascularization of the short gastric vessels was completed along the greater curvature of the upper stomach. First, the posterior wall of the fundus was devascularized. Next, the lesser omentum was opened and the esophageal branches of the left gastric vessels were cut along the lower esophagus. The left gastric artery and vein were then transected with a stapling device. Finally the upper stomach was freed from the posterior wall and the devascularization completed. Operative time ranged from 200 to 400 minutes (mean $\pm$ standard deviation, 287.5 ± 66.0 minutes). Blood loss ranged from 10 to 1500 mL (average, 515.5 ± 507.9 mL). Conversion to an open procedure was necessary in one patient because of bleeding from the splenic vein. No major complications were encountered. Postoperative endoscopy revealed that varices disappeared, and no patient had recurrence of the varices after operation during the mean follow-up period of 12.8 ± 4.1 months (range, 8 to 20 months).

Single case reports include a patient with gastric varices secondary to sinistral portal hypertension (left-sided, caused by splenic vein thrombosis) who was successfully treated by laparoscopic splenectomy[21]; an azygoportal disconnection with splenic artery ligation and transesophageal suturing of the varices performed laparoscopically in a patient with situs inversus totalis[22]; a laparoscopic portacaval H-graft shunt[23]; and a laparoscopic esophagogastric devascularization and transection in a patient with bleeding esophageal varices.[24]

All of these case reports showed a successful application of minimally invasive techniques to the treatment of high-risk conditions in sick, portal hypertensive patients, with acceptable length of hospital stay. The wide variety of pathologic conditions and treatments prevents us from drawing conclusions on such approaches, but they represent successful attempts to improve the management of patients with severe portal hypertension and poor open outcomes.

CONCLUSION

To date, surgery has a defined role in the treatment of bleeding portal hypertensive patients. Only low-risk patients undergoing elective surgery should be treated with a carefully selected portal blood flow-preserving operation. These surgical procedures do not affect the hepatic hilum and do not preclude the performance of a liver transplantation.

Versatility is important when selecting an operation. Not all patients are candidates for one type of operation and not all have a good postoperative course. Patient anatomy and medical history should guide to an appropriate selection of treatment. Thus, it is unwise to perform an esophageal transection in patients with a history of several sclerotherapy sessions. However, conventional open surgery is still associated with high rates of morbidity and mortality in these patients.[12]

The objective of the described procedures performed by laparoscopy is to reproduce the effectiveness of conventional surgery and to eliminate the complications and mortality of the latter. Although there are still few laparoscopic reported experiences with portal hypertension surgery, the absence of major complications and mortality in addition to the rapid patient recovery make laparoscopy a good alternative for these patients. However, it is necessary to evaluate a larger number of patients for a critical analysis and recommendation of this approach in the future.

REFERENCES

1. Gimson AES, Westaby D, Hegarty J, et al. A randomized trial of vasopressin plus nitroglycerin in the control of acute variceal hemorrhage. *Hepatology.* 1986;6:410.
2. Valenzuela JE, Schubert T, Fogel RM, et al. A multi-center, randomized, double-blind trial of somatostatin in the management of acute hemorrhage from esophageal varices. *Hepatology.* 1989;10:958.
3. Helmy A, Hayes PC. Current endoscopic therapeutic options in the management of variceal bleeding. *Aliment Pharmacol Ther.* 2001; 15:575.
4. Corley DA, Cello JP, Adkisson W. Octreotide for acute esophageal variceal bleeding: A meta-analysis. *Gastroenterology.* 2001;120:946.
5. De Franchis R, Primignani M, Arcidiacono R, et al. Prophylactic sclerotherapy (ST) in high risk cirrhotics selected by endoscopic criteria: A multicenter randomized controlled trial. *Gastroenterology.* 1991; 101:1087.
6. Steigman GV, Goff JS, Michaletz-Onody P, et al. Endoscopic sclerotheraphy as compared with endoscopic variceal ligation for bleeding esophageal varices. *N Engl J Med.* 1992;326:1527.
7. Krige JE, Bornman PC, Goldberg PA, et al. Variceal re-bleeding and recurrence after endoscopic injection sclerotheraphy: A prospective evaluation in 204 patients. *Arch Surg.* 2000;135:1315.
8. Bass NM, Yao FY. The role of the interventional radiologist. Transjugular procedures. *Gastrointest Endosc Clin North Am.* 2001;11:131.
9. Helton WS, Maves R, Wicks K, et al. Transjugular intrahepatic portasystemic shunt vs surgical shunt in good-risk cirrhotic patients. A case-control comparison. *Arch Surg.* 2001;136:17.
10. Kerlan RK, LaBerge JM, Gordon RL, et al. Transjugular intrahepatic portosystemic shunts: Current status. *Am J Roentgenol.* 1995;164:1059.
11. Freedman AM, Sanyal AJ, Risnado J, et al. Complications of transjugular intrahepatic portosystemic shunt: A comprehensive review. Radiographics. 1993;13:1185.
12. Sarfeh IJ, Rypins EB. Partial vs total portacaval H-graft diameters. *Ann Surg.* 1986;204:356.
13. Rosemurgy AS, Serafini FM, Zweibel BR, et al. Transjugular intrahepatic portosystemic shunt vs small-diameter prosthetic H-graft portacaval shunt: Extended follow-up of an expanded randomized prospective trial. *J Gastrointest Surg.* 2000;6:589.
14. Idezuki Y, Kokudo N, Sanjo K, et al. Sugiura procedure for management of variceal bleeding in Japan. *World J Surg.* 1994;18:216.
15. Bismuth H, Adams R, Mathur S, et al. Options for elective treatment of portal hypertension in cirrhotic patients in the transplantation era. *Am J Surg.* 1990;160:105.
16. Rossi P, Sileri P, Gentileschi P, et al. Percutaneous liver biopsy using an ultrasound-guided subcostal route. *Dig Dis Sci.* 2001;46:128.
17. Tsimoyiannis EC, Siakas P, Tassis A, et al. Laparoscopic modified Sugiura procedure: Experimental study on the pig. *Int Surg.* 1997; 82:312.
18. Kitano S, Tomikawa M, Iso Y, et al. Laparoscopy-assisted devascularization of the lower esophagus and upper stomach in the management of gastric varices. *Endoscopy.* 1994;26:470.

19. Zilberstein B, Sallet JA, Ramos A, et al. Video laparoscopy for the treatment of bleeding esophageal varices. *Surg Laparosc Endosc.* 1997;3:185.

20. Hashizume M, Tanoue K, Morita M, et al. Laparoscopic gastric devascularization and splenectomy for sclerotherapy-resistant esophagogastric varices with hypersplenism. *J Am Coll Surg.* 1998;187:263.

21. Jaroszewski DE, Schlinkert RT, Gray RJ. Laparoscopic splenectomy for the treatment of gastric varices secondary to sinistral portal hypertension. *Surg Endosc.* 2000;14:87.

22. Zilberstein B, Di Dio LJ, Eshkenazy R, et al. The treatment of portal hypertension by videolaparoscopy in situs inversus totalis. *Hepatogastroenterology.* 2000;47:678.

23. Desmaizieres FC, Bobbio A. The world's first laparoscopic portacaval H-graft shunt. *J Chir.* 1999;136:333.

24. Manzano-Trovamala FJR, Guttierrez RL, Marquez GM, et al. Esophagogastric devascularization and transection for bleeding esophageal varices: First case presentation. *Surg Laparosc Endosc.* 1996;4:300.

Chapter Thirty-Seven ■ ■ ■ ■ ■ ■

Current Status of Transjugular Intrahepatic Portosystemic Shunting

RICARDO DI SEGNI, BEATRIZ LOSCERTALES, W. RICARDO CASTAÑEDA, JORGE RAMIREZ, MARCOS HERRERA, and WILFRIDO R. CASTAÑEDA

INTRODUCTION

Interventional radiologists' involvement in the diagnosis of portal hypertension includes demonstration of portosystemic collaterals and by measurement of the portal-systemic gradients either by free and hepatic vein wedge venography and pressure measurements, or by detecting other associated abnormalities in the spleen, liver, or other organs by magnetic resonance imaging (MRI), computed tomography (CT), or ultrasound (US). In the past the only interventions performed by the interventional radiologist were the infusion of vasoconstrictors into the superior mesenteric artery or the transhepatic embolization of esophageal varices.[1,2]

In 1969 Rösch et al[3] published an innovative paper describing a percutaneous technique for the construction of a portosystemic shunt in dogs. However, the lack of a vascular stent delayed the application of this technique in patients with portal hypertension. In 1985 Abecassis et al[4] published the creation of the first successful percutaneous portosystemic shunt in humans by using an angioplasty balloon to dilate the transparenchymal tract. Since appropriate vascular stents were not available at the time, these shunts had a very short-term patency.

Transjugular intrahepatic portosystemic shunting (TIPS) resurfaced in 1985 when Palmaz et al[5] demonstrated the feasibility of keeping the transparenchymal tract open by the use of a balloon-expandable metallic stent in a canine model. Richter et al[6] reported successful portosystemic shunting with the Palmaz stent in humans in 1988. Since then, numerous researchers have demonstrated the clinical success of TIPS.

TIPS currently plays a major role in the management of the complications of portal hypertension. The procedure has been shown to be effective in controlling bleeding from esophageal varices in large clinical trials.[7]

The universal indication for TIPS is the treatment of the complications of portal hypertension, such as variceal bleeding and as-cites. In recent years other selected indications have been described; however, the treatment of variceal bleeding remains the main indication.

INDICATIONS

TIPS has been demonstrated to be as effective as sclerotherapy for controlling acute hemorrhage secondary to esophageal varices.[8] The primary treatment for esophageal varices is endoscopic sclerotherapy, the administration of vasoconstrictive drugs, and the placement of gastroesophageal balloons.[9] In a recent meta-analysis of 811 patients, comparing TIPS with the endoscopic treatment for the prevention of variceal rebleeding, TIPS proved to be more effective than sclerotherapy (19% vs. 47%) in preventing rebleeding from esophageal varices, although the incidence of encephalopathy was higher with TIPS than with sclerotherapy (34% vs. 19%).[10] In another meta-analysis of 11 published randomized clinical trials, Luca et al[11] reached the same conclusion.

In patients in whom sclerotherapy and other modalities of conservative management have failed, percutaneous portosystemic shunting is the treatment of choice.[12–14] Recurrent esophageal variceal bleeding is a strong indication for TIPS if the classic conservative treatment with beta blockers and sclerotherapy has failed.[12–14] Another less common indication for TIPS is the therapy of refractory ascites. This remains a less widely accepted indication and more clinical trials are necessary to settle the issue.[15]

TIPS has also been used in the management of portal hypertension complicating the Budd-Chiari syndrome,[16–18] in patients with malignant portal and hepatic vein obstruction, and in pediatric patients with recurrent gastrointestinal bleeding in extrahepatic biliary atresia.[19] In these latter cases, infants as young as 10 months old have benefited from TIPS, with adequate control of variceal bleeding prior to hepatic transplantation.[20] TIPS has also been used as a bridge prior to hepatic transplantation in patients with Budd-Chiari syndrome.[21]

TIPS has been used as a bridge to liver transplantation in adults, although this remains a controversial indication.[22] It has also been used as a palliative treatment to control variceal bleeding in patients following liver transplantation. Amesur et al[23] performed TIPS 6 months to 13 years following surgery, in 6 patients to manage recurrent variceal bleeding after sclerotherapy and in 6 patients to manage intractable ascites. Bleeding was controlled in 4 out of 6, with 2 of them undergoing subsequent second transplantation, while the other 2 maintained a patent shunt for 3 and 36 months, respectively. Of the patients with ascites, 3 died shortly thereafter, 2 of liver failure and 1 following splenectomy. Of the other 3, one achieved good control of the ascites and 2 underwent retransplantation.

TIPS is a very effective therapy for lowering the portocaval pressure gradients in patients bleeding from gastric varices.[22] TIPS has also been demonstrated to improve the thrombocytopenia associated with hypersplenism and appears to be promising in patients with complications from secondary hypersplenism.[24]

De la Rubia et al[25] reported a patient who underwent TIPS placement for severe hepatic veno-occlusive disease after bone marrow transplantation.

Aithal et al[26] reported two cases of portal hypertension secondary to arterioportal fistulae. One of those cases was successfully treated with a TIPS placement.

CONTRAINDICATIONS

Absolute contraindications are:

- Right-sided heart failure with elevated central venous pressure.
- Polycystic liver disease.
- Severe hepatic failure.
- Large hepatocellular carcinoma (HCC) infiltrating the porta hepatis that precludes the placement of the stent. Small peripheral HCC is not a contraindication for TIPS.

Relative contraindications include:

- Active intrahepatic or systemic infection.
- Severe hepatic encephalopathy poorly controlled by medical therapy.
- Portal vein thrombosis.
- Stenosis of the celiac axis, since shunt creation in this setting can cause liver necrosis.

PATIENT SELECTION

It is well documented that the early and long-term morbidity and mortality after an episode of variceal hemorrhage are closely related to the etiology and severity of the underlying hepatic disease.[27] The modified Child-Pugh score allows stratification of patients with portal hypertension who are candidates for TIPS. Recent studies suggest that early measurement of the hepatic venous pressure gradient (HVPG) during variceal bleeding may be used as a guide for making therapeutic decisions in the management of patients with acute variceal bleeding. Patients with a high HVPG have a very high risk and commonly have a poor clinical outcome, and are candidates for more aggressive therapy such as surgery or TIPS. Those with lower HVPG have a high probability of a good outcome, and thus may be managed more conservatively, using medical and endoscopic treatment.[28]

The use of endoscopic ultrasound to perform Doppler evaluation of the blood flow in portal hypertension is currently investigational, but it may have a role in selecting the optimal treatment approach for the patient.[9] It is also important to know the etiology of the liver disease; the number of episodes of bleeding and the therapy received; and the preprocedural laboratory parameters such as hemoglobin, prothrombin time, platelet count, bilirubin, albumin, alanine and aspartate aminotransferases, alkaline phosphatase, and ammonia levels. Evaluation of pre-TIPS imaging findings is helpful in planning the procedure, particularly the anatomy of the splenoportal venous system and the presence of malignancy. Some authors have advocated intravenous broad-spectrum antibiotic administration that is begun preoperatively and continued for 2 to 3 days after the procedure; however, there is no consensus on its utilization. The antibiotic therapy is aimed at gram-positive and gram-negative organisms. In a recent study using ceftriaxona, the incidence of infections was reduced from 20% to 2.6%.[29]

The practitioner must have a thorough understanding of hepatic venous anatomy. The size and shape of the liver and its vessels can be dramatically altered by cirrhosis. Additionally, the location and relationship between the hepatic veins (HV) and portal veins (PV) can vary significantly among patients. Anatomic variations of these venous systems occur in approximately 30% of cases. These variants can have a profound impact on the performance of TIPS and in the incidence of related complications.

TIPS is a technically demanding procedure and it is recommended that its performance be restricted to practitioners experienced in this technique.

THE TIPS PROCEDURE

TIPS involves a precise puncture in an anatomically difficult region, balloon dilation of the tract, use of carbon dioxide (CO_2) for portal vein visualization, and the use of a metallic endoprosthesis. Balloon occlusion combined with the use of CO_2 provides a better demonstration of the portal system than the wedge injection of contrast medium.[30] TIPS can be performed with a good outcome on an emergency basis in extremely ill patients who are considered poor surgical candidates. A significantly lower morbidity and mortality is associated with TIPS in comparison to the traditional surgical shunts.

The most critical and difficult part of the creation of TIPS is gaining access to the portal vein. A TIPS procedure in experienced hands can be performed in an average of 1 hour or less, most of this time being spent procuring access to the portal circulation. Most of the procedural complications occur secondary to the attempts to puncture the portal vein (PV). TIPS is a side-to-side portosystemic shunt created between the hepatic vein and the portal vein. By far the most suitable vessels to use to create the shunt are the right hepatic vein (RHV) and the right portal vein (RPV). Other vessels such as the middle and left hepatic veins can be used in cases in which the RHV is not suitable. It is essential to appropriately select the entrance point into the PV. Ideally the peripheral portion of the right portal vein (RPV) is chosen to create a successful shunt, although such precision is not always possible (Fig. 37–1A,B). Fluoroscopy continues to be the modality of choice for most steps of the procedure, particularly for the puncture of the PV. Ingenious and creative methods that employ different imaging modalities have been described for localization of the PV, such as real-time US guidance,[31] transhepatic percutaneous placement of either a target guidewire into the PV or a target coil in the parenchyma adjacent to the PV under US guidance,[32] and arterial portography and catheterization of the recanalized umbilical vein under US guidance.[33] Most centers have abandoned these techniques due to the associated complications and the time involved.

Excellent demonstration of the PV can be obtained by wedge or balloon occlusion hepatic venography using CO_2, which is considered by some authors the contrast material of choice. CO_2 can give adequate opacification in about 90% of cases.[30]

The two most commonly used transhepatic needle puncture sets are the Colapinto or a modification of the original Colapinto set by Ring,[34] and the Rösch-Uchida system.[35] The most commonly used access is through the right internal jugular vein (RIJV), although other vessels can be used. Puncture into the RIJV is made using anatomic landmarks or under US guidance. The authors prefer to use the Rösch-Uchida needle set. A long 10F angiographic sheath with a side port, hemostatic valve, and a radiopaque tip is first placed through the RIJV into the inferior vena cava. A 10F polytetrafluoroethylene (PTFE) catheter covering a blunt, long 14G metal stiffening cannula is introduced over the guidewire inside the sheath. A 5F catheter assembled with a 0.038" flexible needle that locks to the hub of the 10F PTFE catheter is then introduced through the metal cannula. This needle assembly is used to puncture from the HV to the RPV across the liver. It usually requires fewer than five passes with the needle through the liver to enter the RPV. When advancing the needle, puncture of the liver capsule should be avoided, because this can result in hemoperitoneum. An accurate puncture is aided by using the anatomic features gleaned from the hepatic wedge venograph and bone landmarks to guide needle placement. Each pass of the needle is made in a slightly different direction. In patients with massive ascites and a scarred liver, extra care should be taken when creating the tract. In these cases the RPV is closer to the liver capsule. Short needle passes of 2 to 3 cm are recommended in these situations. Once the RPV has been entered, a guidewire is advanced. When using a Bentson floppy guidewire, the floppy segment of the wire is made to bend in the distal RPV branches until cannulation of the main portal vein (MPV) occurs. Alternatively, an angled glidewire can be used to gain access. The PV is ideally entered approximately 2 to 3 cm distal to the bifurcation of the MPV on the main RPV trunk (Fig. 37–2). Puncture at the level of the MPV bifurcation must be avoided because at this level the portal vein can be located extrahepatically, increasing the risk of hemorrhage which can lead to exsanguination and death.

Once a guidewire is advanced into the portal system, the 5F catheter is advanced over it for venography and pressure measurements. Balloon dilation of the parenchymal tract with a high-pressure angioplasty balloon is then required. The tract is initially dilated with an 8-mm balloon catheter. The next step is the placement of the stent to cover the tract from the PV into the RHV.

The four most commonly used stents are the Palmaz (Johnson and Johnson), Wallstent (Boston-Scientific), Strecker

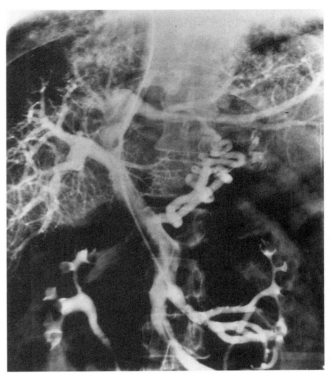

A

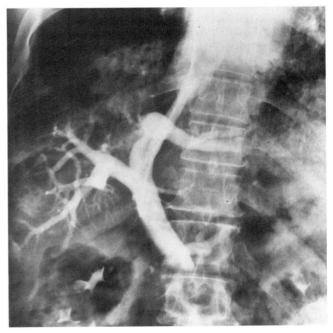

B

Figure 37–1. A. Portal venogram following transhepatic approach to the portal vein shows hepatopetal flow toward the liver and opacification of left gastric varices. **B.** Portal venogram post-TIPS shows antegrade flow through the TIPS into the inferior vena cava. Note the lack of opacification of the left gastric varices.

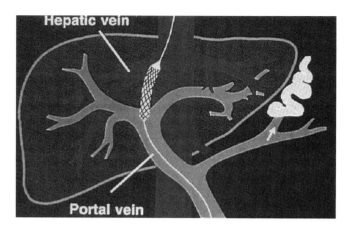

Figure 37–2. Diagram illustrating the placement of TIPS from the right hepatic vein to the right portal vein.

(MediTech), and the Gianturco-Rösch Z-stent (Cook). Most practitioners prefer to use the Wallstent, because of its flexibility, low profile, its retrievability up to a certain point, and the fact that it is self-expanding. These properties allow this stent to conform to the curvature of the tract. Its main disadvantage is its low radiopacity. This problem has been partially overcome by the manufacturer, who made the alloy more radiopaque. The major problem with the Wallstent is the somewhat unpredictable final position of the stent once it has expanded. Longer stents are now available, and this helps to compensate for errors in placement. A recent study using a longer Palmaz stent proved its efficacy, with a primary patency rate of 76% at 8 weeks and a secondary patency rate of 100%.[36,37]

The goal of the procedure is to bring the portosystemic gradient down to 10 to 12 mm Hg. In the majority of the series reported there was a decrease in the portal pressure of at least 50%. We know from surgical experience that complete elimination of the portosystemic gradient is counterproductive, since this will cause a high-volume flow through the shunt, thus increasing the risk of hepatic encephalopathy. Additionally, the shunt size needs to be adjusted such that it decreases the portosystemic gradient to below 15 mm Hg, while still maintaining sufficient hepatopetal circulation to preserve any remaining hepatic function. It has been proven that there is an inverse relationship between the degree to which the portal pressure is reduced and the incidence of encephalopathy. Use of shunts greater than 10 mm in diameter has resulted in a significant increase in the incidence of encephalopathy.[38]

After the stent has been placed, pressure measurements are taken to assess for residual pressure gradients. A portogram will demonstrate the position, patency, and good function of the shunt.

A study with color Doppler US is performed the next day to assess the results and to establish the baseline values for flow velocities through the shunt. Ultrasonographic studies are scheduled before discharge with a close follow-up for the first 3 months, and then testing at varying intervals for long-term shunt surveillance.

Some authors have successfully used alternative techniques to increase the overall safety of the procedure. The use of CO_2 as a contrast medium considerably decreases the amount of iodinated contrast material needed.[30] Hawkins et al[30] described a technique that uses CO_2 coupled with fine needle access for optimal visualization and location of the PV. Advantages of this method include accurate determination of the exact point of entrance into the PV and evaluation of the parenchymal tract by performing angiograms and tractograms in multiple projections, less needle-related trauma, and avoidance of complications from the use of iodinated contrast media. Hawkins et al,[30] Rees et al,[38] and Semba et al[39] reported less extravasation of contrast when using CO_2 during wedge injections.

Fontaine et al[40] described the use of CT localization and marking of the PV prior to the performance of 150 TIPS procedures and found this an extremely useful method. Under CT guidance, a 21G needle (Acoustic, MediTech-Boston Scientific, Watertown, MA) is placed at a point 1 to 2 cm lateral to the MPV on the RPV trunk, then a guidewire is advanced as a marker. After fixing the wire to the skin the patient is transported to the angiographic suite for the performance of the TIPS procedure. The additional time and cost needed can be justified by the resulting more precise puncture and lower number of complications. One of the disadvantages of this method is the manipulation of the needle and wire across the peritoneal cavity in patients with ascites, which increases the risk of infection, and a higher potential for bleeding complications in patients with coagulopathy. Recent studies in animals have described the use of MRI guidance during TIPS placements.[41,42]

COMPLICATIONS

TIPS is considered a minimally invasive technique when compared to surgery in these high-risk patients. It can, however, have serious procedural complications in approximately 10% of cases. However, with increasing experience, the complication rate has dropped markedly to less than 5%. Mortality is higher in institutions where fewer than 150 TIPS procedures have been performed. In institutions with larger numbers of cases, the complication rate is 1.4%.[43]

Complications associated with TIPS can be classified as early or late. Early complications are related to the technical procedure or to the underlying disease, namely the severity of liver failure. Late complications are related to shunt stenosis or occlusion and to a significant diversion of portal flow from the liver, causing encephalopathy. Technical complications are related to the access site, the transhepatic puncture, or the stent deployment.

Early medical complications include septicemia, intravascular hemolysis, coagulopathy, and bleeding. Sanyal and Reddy reported bacterial infection of shunts during the follow-up period, but all of the cases responded to administration of IV antibiotics. The clinical diagnosis was based on the presence of fever with positive blood culture.[44]

Hepatic encephalopathy, a late complication of TIPS, occurs with an incidence of 5 to 50%.[43] Papatheodoridis et al[10] found an incidence of encephalopathy of 34% post-TIPS versus 19% postsclerotherapy. On the basis of the higher incidence of encephalopathy, they advocated that sclerotherapy should be the first therapy used for variceal bleeding in spite of the higher incidence of rebleeding following sclerotherapy (47% vs. 19% for TIPS). Most of the cases of encephalopathy can be managed medically with diet and lactulose administration. Only about 4% of the encephalopathy associated with TIPS is refractory to medical management.[43]

TIPS have a rather poor primary patency rate, ranging from 20 to 80% at 12 months. The cause of this low patency is thought to be pseudointimal hyperplasia related to active inflammation. LaBerge et al[45] suggested a relationship between bile duct injury and development of pseudointimal hyperplasia.

The high incidence of stenosis following TIPS mandates a careful surveillance protocol with frequent US evaluations and early revision of stenotic or occluded shunts in asymptomatic patients. As a consequence of stent stenosis or occlusion, patients can have recurrence of bleeding in up to 15 to 25% of cases. Approximately 10% of these patients die as a consequence of recurrent bleeding.[43,45] Saxon et al[46] reported a small group of patients with a lower incidence of shunt stenosis when using stent grafts for shunt revision. A more recent study by Andrews et al[47] on the use of covered stents in de novo procedures reported a patency rate of 75%. Haskal[48] reported on 14 patients, 7 with stent-graft placement, and 7 post-TIPS failures. All stent-grafts were patent at a mean of 19 months with a maximum of 10% of stenosis within the graft stent. Sze et al[49] reported on the efficacy of covered stents in the management of the TIPS obstruction in patients with associated biliary fistulas; 4 out of 4 biliary fistulas disappeared following stent-graft placement.

Covered stents are the future of TIPS and will likely improve the long-term outcome of the procedure.[50] Several experimental studies with covered stents have shown variable patency rates.[51-54] The best results were obtained with encapsulated PTFE, which had a patency of 87.5% at 5 months, and with nonporous polycarbonate urethane-covered stents, which had 100% patency at 5 weeks, but with a 26% incidence of stenosis.[52,54]

FOLLOW-UP

One of the major problems with TIPS is the high incidence of stent failure due to stenosis or occlusion, with an incidence in the range of 20 to 80% within the first year.[43] It is for this reason that US surveillance is crucial to detect early signs of dysfunction. This is easily accomplished by color Doppler US. Ullerich et al[55] studied 147 Doppler ultrasonographic examinations and correlated them with the results of direct portal venography. They concluded that Doppler ultrasonography appears to be able to detect hemodynamically-significant TIPS stenoses. Fischer et al[56] also concluded that PV, HV, and TIPS patency could be unequivocally assessed with echo-enhanced Doppler in 90% of cases.

Rebleeding after TIPS occurs in 10 to 20% of patients and is usually associated with a shunt stenosis or thrombosis.[43,57] The rationale for the US surveillance is to avoid recurrence of the complications of portal hypertension.[57]

Rösch reported that stenosis within the parenchymal tract is secondary to proliferation of pseudointimal tissue and is more commonly seen with the use of Wallstents.[58,59] However, shunt stenosis and/or occlusion also occur with all the other stents that have been used for TIPS.

Stenosis and occlusion respond well to balloon dilatation, thrombectomy, thrombolysis, or restenting, with an overall 98% secondary shunt patency.[59,60]

In trying to solve the problem of shunt failure, use of devices such as covered stents or treatment of the stent site with radiation or antiproliferative drugs has been advocated. A recent experimental study using P^{32} irradiation in a swine model of TIPS failed to improve the patency rate.[61]

CONCLUSIONS

Since the introduction of TIPS into clinical practice in 1988, the initial enthusiasm has been tempered by a more critical appraisal of its role in the management of portal hypertension. TIPS undoubtedly plays a major role in the rescue of recurrent variceal hemorrhage following failed endoscopic sclerotherapy. Randomized trials comparing TIPS with endoscopic methods in the secondary prophylaxis of variceal hemorrhage have shown better control of bleeding after TIPS but no effect on survival.[60,61] Its exact role awaits further assessment. Experience with TIPS in patients with refractory ascites or hepatorenal syndrome has been disappointing in some series (62, 63). Very few reports exist now of randomized studies comparing TIPS with paracentesis for refractory ascites.

There are no published data comparing surgical shunts with TIPS in the management of complications of portal hypertension. There are currently trials underway that compare the use of TIPS with the creation of a splenorenal shunt in patients with cirrhosis and variceal bleeding, and their results are anxiously awaited. One of the major problems that has not been solved is the early shunt failure that occurs in approximately 50% of patients after 1 year. The need for continued shunt surveillance by Doppler sonography and direct portography is the major limitation of TIPS. It is hoped that with the refinement of the covered stent this problem will be overcome.

REFERENCES

1. Reuter SR, Redman HC. Cirrhosis and portal hypertension. In: *Gastrointestinal Angiography,* 2nd ed. Williams & Wilkins:1977;306.
2. Keller FS, Dotter CT, Rösch J. Percutaneous transhepatic obliteration of gastroesophageal varices: some technical aspects. *Radiology* 1978; 129:327.
3. Rösch J, Hanafee WN, Snow H. Transjugular portal venography and radiological portocaval shunt: an experimental study. *Radiology* 1969; 92:1112.
4. Abecassis M, Gordon JD, Colapinto RF, et al. The transjugular intrahepatic portosystemic shunt (TIPS): an alternative for the management of life-threatening variceal hemorrhage. *Hepatology* 1985;5:1032A.
5. Palmaz JC, Sibbit RR, Reuter SR, et al. Expandable intrahepatic portocaval shunt stents: early experience in the dog. *AJR.* 1985;145:821.
6. Richter GM, Noeldge G, Palmaz JC, et al. Transjugular intrahepatic stent shunt: preliminary clinical results. *Radiology* 1990;174:1027.
7. Coldwell DM, Ring EJ, Rees CR, et al. Multicenter investigation of the role of transjugular intrahepatic portosystemic shunts in the management of portal hypertension. *Radiology* 1995;196:335.
8. Sanyal AJ, Freedman AM, Shiffman ML, et al. Transjugular intrahepatic shunt (TIPS) vs. sclerotherapy for variceal hemorrhage: results of a randomized prospective trial (Abstr). *Hepatology* 1992;16:A88.
9. Binmoeller KF, Borsatto R. Variceal bleeding and portal hypertension. *Endoscopy* 2000;32:189.
10. Papatheodoridis GV, Goulis J, Leandro G, et al. Transjugular intrahepatic portosystemic shunt compared with endoscopic treatment for prevention of variceal rebleeding: a meta-analysis. *Hepatology* 1999; 30:612.
11. Luca A, D'Amico G, La Galla R, et al. TIPS for prevention of recurrent bleeding in patients with cirrhosis: meta-analysis of randomized clinical trials. *Radiology* 1999;212:411.
12. Zemel G, Katzen BT, Becker GJ, et al. Percutaneous transjugular portosystemic shunt. *JAMA.* 1991;266:390.

13. Rössle M, Haag K, Ocho A, et al. The transjugular intrahepatic portosystemic stent-shunt procedure for variceal bleeding. *N Engl J Med* 1994;330:165.

14. Martin M, Zajko AB, Orons PD, et al. Transjugular intrahepatic portosystemic shunt in the management of variceal bleeding: indications and clinical results. *Surgery* 1993;114:719.

15. Ferral H, Bjarnason H, Wegryn SA, et al. Refractory ascites: early experience in treatment with transjugular intrahepatic portosystemic shunt. *Radiology* 1993;189:795.

16. Yamada K, Nakamura K, Ogawa K, et al. A case of Budd-Chiari syndrome successfully treated by transcatheter recanalization of the right hepatic vein and transjugular intrahepatic portosystemic shunt. *Radiat Med.* 1999;17:85.

17. Nicoll A, Fitt G, Angus P, et al. Budd-Chiari syndrome: intractable ascites managed by a transhepatic portocaval shunt. *Austral Radiol.* 1997;41:169.

18. Bilbao JI, Pueyo JC, Longo JM, et al. Interventional therapeutic techniques in Budd-Chiari syndrome. *Cardiovasc Intervent Radiol.* 1997;20:112.

19. Astfalk W, Huppert PE, Schweizer P, et al. Recurrent intestinal bleeding from jejunostomy caused by portal hypertension following hepatoportojejunostomy in extrahepatic biliary atresia (EHBA)—successful treatment by transjugular intrahepatic portosystemic shunt (TIPS). *Eur J Pediatr Surg.* 1997;7:147.

20. Steventon DM, Kelly DA, McKiernan P, et al. Emergency transjugular intrahepatic portosystemic shunt prior to liver transplantation. *Pediatr Radiol.* 1997;27:84.

21. Ryu RK, Durham JD, Krysl J, et al. Role of TIPS as a bridge to hepatic transplantation in Budd-Chiari Syndrome. *J Vasc Interv Radiol.* 1999;10:799.

22. Trevillyan J, Carroll PJ. Management of portal hypertension and esophageal varices in alcoholic cirrhosis. *Am Fam Phys.* 1997;55:1851.

23. Amesur NV, Zajko AB, Orons PD, et al. Transjugular intrahepatic portosystemic shunt in patients who have undergone liver transplantation. *J Vasc Interv Radiol.* 1999;10:569.

24. Pursnani KG, Sillin LF, Kaplan DS. Effect of transjugular intrahepatic portosystemic shunt on secondary hypersplenism. *Am J Surg.* 1997;173:169.

25. de la Rubia J, Carral A, Montes H, et al. Successful treatment of hepatic veno-occlusive disease in a peripheral blood progenitor cell transplantation with a transjugular intrahepatic portosystemic stent-shunt (TIPS). *Hematologica* 1996;81:536.

26. Aithal GP, Alabdi BJ, Rose JD, et al. Portal hypertension secondary to arterio-portal fistulae: two unusual cases. *Liver* 1999;19:343.

27. Mahl TC, Groszmann RJ. Pathophysiology of portal hypertension and variceal bleeding. *Surg Clin North Am.* 1990;70:251.

28. Bosch J, Garcia-Pagan JC. Complications of cirrhosis I. Portal hypertension. *J Hepatol.* 2000;32(1 suppl):141.

29. Guberg V, Deibert P, Ochs A, et al. Prevention of infectious complications after transjugular intrahepatic portosystemic shunt in cirrhotic patients with a single dose of ceftriaxona. *Hepatogastroenterology* 1999;46:1126.

30. Hawkins IF, Johnson AW, Caridi JG, et al. CO_2 fine-needle TIPS. *J Vasc Interv Radiol.* 1997;8:235.

31. Longo JM, Bilbao JI, Rousseau HP, et al. Color Doppler US guidance in transjugular placement of intrahepatic portosystemic shunts. *Radiology* 1992;184:281.

32. Jarman JT, Reed JD, Kopecky KK, et al. Localization of the portal vein for transjugular catheterization: percutaneous placement of a metallic marker with real-time US guidance. *J Vasc Interv Radiol.* 1992;3:545.

33. Wenz F, Nemcek AA, Tischler HA, et al. Ultrasound-guided paraumbilical vein puncture: an adjunct to transjugular intrahepatic portosystemic shunt (TIPS) placement. *J Vasc Interv Radiol.* 1992;3:549.

34. LaBerge JM, Ring EJ, Gordon RI, et al. Creation of transjugular intrahepatic shunts with the Wallstent endoprosthesis: results in 100 patients. *Radiology* 1993;187:413.

35. Rösch J, Uchida BT, Barton RE, et al. Coaxial catheter-needle system for transjugular portal vein entrance. *J Vasc Interv Radiol.* 1993;4:145.

36. Borsa JJ, Fontaine AB, Hoffer EK, et al. Primary placement of Palmaz long medium stents in transjugular intrahepatic portosystemic shunts. *J Vasc Interv Radiol.* 2000;11:189.

37. Hayes PC, Readhead DN, Finlatson NDC. Transjugular intrahepatic portosystemic stent-shunt. *Gut* 1994;35:445.

38. Rees CR, Niblett RL, Lee SP, et al. Use of carbon dioxide as a contrast medium for transjugular intrahepatic portosystemic shunt procedures. *J Vasc Interv Radiol.* 1994;5:383.

39. Semba CP, Saperstein L, Nyman U, et al. Hepatic laceration from wedged venography performed before transjugular intrahepatic portosystemic shunt placement. *J Vasc Interv Radiol.* 1996;7:143.

40. Fontaine AB, Verschyl A, Hoffer E, et al. Use of CT-guided marking of the portal vein in creation of 150 transjugular intrahe-patic portosystemic shunts. *J Vasc Interv Radiol.* 1997;8:1073.

41. Solomon SB, Magee C, Acker DR, et al. TIPS placement in swine, guided by electromagnetic real-time needle tip localization displayed on previously acquired 3D-CT. *Cardiovasc Intervent Radiol.* 1999;22:411.

42. Kee ST, Rhee JS, Burrs K, et al. MR-guided transjugular intrahepatic portosystemic shunt placement in a swine model. *J Vasc Interv Radiol.* 1999;10:529.

43. Freedman A, Sanyal A, Tisnado J, et al. Complications of transjugular intrahepatic portosystemic shunts: a comprehensive review. *Radiographics* 1993;13:1185.

44. Sanyal AJ, Reddy KR. Vegetative infection of transjugular intrahepatic portosystemic shunts. *Gastroenterology* 1998;115:110.

45. LaBerge JM, Ferral D, Lind A, et al. Histopathologic study of stenosis and occluded transjugular intrahepatic portosystemic shunts. *J Vasc Interv Radiol.* 1993;4:779.

46. Saxon RR, Hans AT, Barry TV, et al. Stent-graft for revision of TIPS stenosis and occlusion: a clinical pilot study. *J Vasc Interv Radiol.* 1997;8:539.

47. Andrews RT, Saxon RR, Bloch RD, et al. Stent-grafts for de novo TIPS: technique and early results. *J Vasc Interv Radiol.* 1999;10:1371.

48. Haskal ZJ. Improved patency of transjugular intrahepatic portosystemic shunts in humans: creation and revision with PTFE stent-grafts. *Radiology* 1999;213:759.

49. Sze DY, Vestring T, Liddell RP, et al. Recurrent TIPS failure associated with biliary fistulae: treatment with PTFE-covered stent. *Cardiovasc Intervent Radiol.* 1999;22:298.

50. Haskal ZJ, Brennecke LH. TIPS formed with polyethylene terephthalate-covered stent: experimental evaluation in pigs. *Radiology* 1999;213:853.

51. Haskal ZJ, Brennecke LJ. Porous and non porous polycarbonate urethane stent-grafts for TIPS formation: biologic responses. *J Vasc Interv Radiol.* 1999;10:1255.

52. Bloch R, Pavcnik D, Uchida BT, et al. Polyurethane-coated Dacron-covered stent-grafts for TIPS: results in swine. *Cardiovasc Intervent Radiol.* 1998;21:497.

53. Cejna M, Thurnher S, Pidlich J, et al. Primary implantation of polyester-covered stent-graft for TIPS: a pilot study. *Cardiovasc Intervent Radiol.* 1999;22:305.

54. Haskal ZJ, Davis A, McAllister A, et al. PTFE-encapsulated endovascular stent-graft for TIPS: experimental evaluation. *Radiology* 1997;205:682.

55. Ullerich H, Menzel J, Kucharzik T, et al. Can the function of the transjugular intrahepatic portosystemic shunt be evaluated noninvasively by Doppler sonography? *Zeitschrift fur Gastroenterologie* 1999;37:771.

56. Fischer G, Rak R, Sackmann M. Improved investigation of portal-hepatic veins by echo-enhanced Doppler sonography. *Ultrasound Med Biol.* 1998;24:1345.

57. Gschwantler M, Gebauer A, Rohrmoser M, et al. Clinical outcome two years after implantation of a transjugular intrahepatic portosystemic shunt for recurrent variceal bleeding. *Eur J Gastroenterol Hepatol.* 1997;9:15.

58. Rösch J. Technical evolution of TIPS. Proceedings of the Fourth International Course on Vascular and Interventional Radiology as a Therapeutic Alternative. Las Palmas, Spain. February 1994:216.

59. Rösch J. TIPS: the present status (abstract 161). *Cardiovasc Intervent Radiol.* 1994;17(Suppl 1):S95.

60. Cabrera J, Maynar, M, Granados R, et al. Transjugular intrahepatic portosystemic shunt versus sclerotherapy in the elective treatment of variceal hemorrhage. [Clinical Trial. Journal Article. Randomized controlled trial]. *Gastroenterology* 1996;110:832.

61. Lessie T, Yoon HC, Nelson HA, et al. Intraluminal radiation for TIPS stenosis: preliminary results in swine model. *J Vasc Interv Radiol.* 1999;10:899.

62. Rossi P, Maccioni E, Salvatori FM, et al. Transjugular intrahepatic portosystemic shunt (TIPS): indications and results after 22 months of experience. *Radiologia Medica* 1994;87:585.

63. Nazarian GK, Bjarnason H, Dietz CA Jr., et al. Refractory ascites: midterm results of treatment with transjugular intrahepatic portosystemic shunt. *Radiology* 1997:205:173.

Chapter Thirty-Eight ・・・・・・ ■

*I*nterventional Radiology in the Biliary Tract

RICARDO DI SEGNI, BEATRIZ LOSCERTALES, W. RICARDO CASTAÑEDA,
MARCOS HERRERA, MARY BETH LOBRANO, and WILFRIDO R. CASTAÑEDA

HISTORY

Burkhardt and Muller originally described the technique of cholangiography in 1921. Using a needle through the liver, they accomplished opacification of the gallbladder.[1] Huard and Do-Xuan-Hop were able to visualize the biliary ducts injecting iodized oil (lipiodol). Despite these earlier efforts, cholangiography was not extensively used until 1969.[2]

The technique was initially used almost exclusively by surgeons for visualization of the biliary tract using a large needle to access the biliary radicles. The method was only used in those patients already scheduled to have surgery. The major complication was bile leakage and bile peritonitis. In 1966, Seldinger reported his experience with transhepatic cholangiography via a right subcostal approach using a sheathed needle technique to decompress the biliary system and lower the complication rate.[3] Ohto and Tsuchiya[2,4] described a technique in 1969 using a fine needle, which was almost harmless to the liver, eliminating the need for immediate surgical intervention, with a spectacular decrease in the number of complications. Fine-needle cholangiography became the cornerstone for the majority of intrahepatic biliary interventional procedures. The technique is readily available, inexpensive, easy to learn, and associated with lower morbidity and mortality rates.

PERCUTANEOUS FINE-NEEDLE TRANSHEPATIC CHOLANGIOGRAPHY

As originally designed, percutaneous fine-needle transhepatic cholangiography (PTC) is a safe and effective technique for the evaluation of biliary pathology. It accurately demonstrates abnormalities present and sometimes it can help to diagnose their etiology. The percutaneous transhepatic approach is effectively used for drainage as primary or palliative therapy for many biliary abnormalities demonstrated by cholangiography or other diagnostic methods. PTC is a diagnostic procedure, which could also be the first step for a wide spectrum of interventional procedures.

PTC involves the sterile placement of a small-gauge needle (21 to 22 G) into a peripheral biliary radicle with the use of imaging guidance, followed by the injection of contrast material to delineate the biliary anatomy. Percutaneous transhepatic biliary drainage is a therapeutic procedure that includes the sterile cannulation of a peripheral biliary duct after PTC, followed by the introduction of a guidewire and catheter manipulation. The procedure is completed when an internal or external stent is placed for drainage.

Indications

PTC is indicated for the definition of the level of obstruction in patients with dilated biliary ducts and it can modify the therapeutic approach after evaluation of the biliary anatomy.

In some cases the etiology of cholangitis can be defined, and the diagnosis of suspected bile duct inflammatory disorders such as sclerosing cholangitis could be confirmed. In cases of postsurgical complications, the site and magnitude of the bile leak can be assessed.[5-8] PTC has been proven to be 100% accurate in detecting the site of the lesion, and 88.5% accurate in detecting the nature of it.[9]

Percutaneous transhepatic biliary drainage (PTBD) is indicated for the decompression of the biliary tree regardless of the etiology. It is a simple way to remove bile duct stones that are otherwise inaccessible to the surgeon. The technique is also useful for the diversion of bile in patients with bile leaks or as a palliative treatment in patients with malignancy.[10-14]

Contraindications

Coagulopathy is a relative contraindication for PTC and PTBD. Every effort should be made to correct or improve the coagulation parameters before the procedure. Correction is done with the administration of vitamin K or blood products. If the bleeding disorder cannot be corrected, endoscopic retrograde cholangiopancreatography (ERCP) is the preferred procedure. A history of a life-threatening reaction to iodinated contrast medium is a relative contraindication. These patients can be prophylactically treated with steroids. The use of nonionic contrast medium has been proven to cause fewer allergic reactions. A recent study in rabbits compared the degree of hepatic damage caused by the injection of ionic, nonionic, and CO_2 contrast medium for identification of the biliary duct anatomy. The study showed that ionic contrast medium caused more severe hepatic damage, with severe scarring and the development of necrotic areas.[15] Because of the risk of uncontrollable hemorrhage, PTC is absolutely contraindicated in patients with known hepatic vascular tumors or vascular malformations.

Patient Preparation

A coagulation profile is obtained, and if abnormalities are found, correction is undertaken prior to the procedure. An intravenous (IV) line is inserted for the administration of fluids, antibiotics, and sedation. Administration of wide-spectrum antibiotics is used as prophylaxis of sepsis before and during the procedure.

Technique

With the patient in a supine position under IV sedation, (butorphanol in combination with Versed), and monitoring of EKG, pulse oxymetry, and blood pressure, anesthesia is infiltrated locally in the right subcostal space or in the subxyphoid region for access into the left biliary ducts. Alternatively, an intercostal block, and rarely, a peridural block can also be performed. Access into the ducts can be achieved using fluoroscopic or ultrasonographic (US) guidance. In many centers, initial access into the biliary system is accomplished with US guidance, and the rest of the procedure is completed under multidirectional fluoroscopy. The advantages of US are real-time visualization of the duct and needle at the time of the puncture, with a selection of second or third biliary branches. Ultrasound allows evaluation of the size, position, and direction of the ducts as well as the course of the guidewire. Color Doppler capabilities allow differentiation of bile ducts from vessels. The number of needle passes is reduced and the success rate of bile duct cannulation has been reported close to 100% with minimal or nonsevere complications.[16] Puncture of the left biliary duct is highly successful under the guidance of US when the diameter of the ducts is greater than 3 mm.[17] Advantages of this approach include less pain, better patient tolerance, avoidance of the pleura with decrease in the pneumothorax rate, and easier manipulation of catheters and wires across obstructions of the common bile duct. In many centers this is the preferred approach. An alternative to the use of PTC is magnetic resonance cholangiopancreatography (MRCP).

Despite some authors' opinion,[18] several studies have demonstrated the feasibility, safety, and accuracy of MRCP. The results of these studies have demonstrated that this technique has sensitivity, specificity, and diagnostic accuracy rates of 91 to 97%, 98 to 100% and 97 to 98%, respectively. The same studies have shown its efficacy in diagnosing the presence, location, and cause of stenoses and obstructions, in both benign and malignant disease, in both the intrahepatic and extrahepatic bile ducts. MRCP is also a useful method in the follow-up of liver transplant recipients. Because breath-hold MRCP is not invasive and does not use ionizing radiation and potentially toxic contrast agents, it is recommended as the imaging technique of choice in pediatric patients. MRCP is a useful diagnostic tool that provides important information for planning therapeutic procedures and makes it possible to limit the use of invasive procedures to interventional purposes. The use of MR as a guidance method is in evolution.[19–29]

The puncture site selected is usually between the seventh and the tenth intercostal space, slightly anterior to the midaxillary line and below the costophrenic angle. Under normal, shallow breathing the needle is advanced under fluoroscopic control parallel to the tabletop until the tip reaches the midline at the level of the twelfth thoracic vertebral body. The stylet is removed, and a small amount of diluted contrast medium is injected as the needle is slowly withdrawn, until a biliary duct is opacified. In patients with dilated bile ducts a 99 to 100% success rate can be achieved with 4 to 6 passages.[30] The entrance in other structures, such as veins, arteries, or lymphatics, needs to be recognized. Because contrast medium has a higher specific gravity than the bile, it flows to the most dependent posterior ducts. For better visualization of the anterior ducts, a simple technique described by Young et al is useful, using 30 to 50 mL of CO_2, can be used.[31] If obstruction is encountered, usually an indwelling catheter is left for drainage.

PERCUTANEOUS BILIARY DRAINAGE PROCEDURES

The technique of percutaneous drainage is simple to describe although sometimes difficult to perform. The first and most important step is duct visualization. The two types of biliary drainage techniques are external when the bile is collected in a bag, and internal when the bile is drained internally into the duodenum. Indwelling catheters can be placed for external or internal biliary drainage after the site of stenosis or obstruction has been crossed with specialized guidewires (Fig. 38–1). A recent experimental study in rats demonstrated that preoperative internal drainage could lead to better liver regeneration and hepatic function recovery after hepatectomy than external biliary drainage.[32] This technique offers the possibility of decompression of the bile ducts in either benign or malignant diseases and can also be used as a palliative therapy with low morbidity and mortality.

Surgical decompression is contraindicated in the presence of a high common hepatic duct obstruction or in cases of a mass extending into the hilum and causing a separate noncommunicating obstruction of the left and right ducts. An additional consideration is that up to 90% of patients with obstructive jaundice who undergo exploratory laparotomy are found to have inoperable tumors.[33–36]

The principal application of PTBD has been for the nonoperative drainage of malignant biliary obstruction. The net result of PTBD is improvement of the quality of life, and the length of survival has to be weighed against the possibility of complications. Numerous sets for drainage and different catheters have

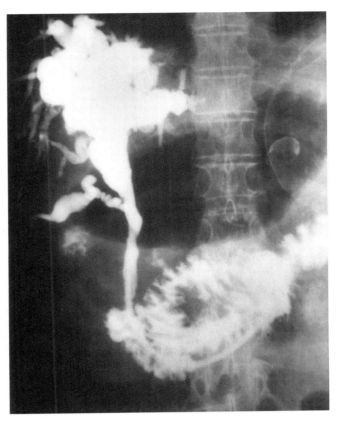

Figure 38–1. Cholangiogram shows a high-grade stenosis of the common bile duct. The catheter has been passed across the obstruction of the common bile duct and its tip is in the duodenum. Note lack of opacification of left bile duct.

been developed for specific conditions. The most popular and useful catheters are the self-retaining locking pigtail(s) (Boston Scientific), which can function as internal or external stents and range in diameter from 5 to 14 Fr. Several plastic materials have been used in the manufacturing of the stents procuring for better luminal patency and greater resistance to kinking and fragmentation.

When internal drainage is desired, several types of stents are available that can be placed via the percutaneous approach or endoscopically. Five of the most common types are the Teflon stent (Cook-Europe), Carey-Coons (MediTech), Temp-Tip design (MediTech), C-Flex stent (Cook Inc., Bloomington, IN), and silastic stent (USCI). The C-flex stent has an introducing system that makes placement easy and accurate. The silastic stent has a Malecot design that prevents migration and a radiopaque marker for better fluoroscopic placement.

Self-expandable metallic stents are currently used in the management of malignant biliary obstruction. Their design helps to overcome some of the problems associated with the conventional plastic endoprosthesis. Stent insertion is performed percutaneously with a technical success close to 100% in obstruction of the right and left biliary ducts (Fig. 38–2). Metallic stents have been implanted in patients with different types of malignancies such as bile duct, ampullary, or pancreatic carcinoma and in hepatic, hilar, and lymph node metastasis. The overall primary patency rates range

from 1 to 9 months (mean, 5.1 months), as effective or better than the plastic stents.[37,38]

For patients in whom there is a contraindication to the standard transhepatic drainage method, an unusual technique for stent placement was described by Amigdalos et al.[39] The insertion of the biliary wallstents is accomplished via a transjugular approach similar to the transjugular intrahepatic portosystemic shunt procedure. This approach has been specifically used in patients with ascites, underlying coagulopathy, and inaccessibility to endoscopic manipulation.[39]

BILIARY STRICTURES

Biliary strictures can be treated via a percutaneous approach. Most of the bile duct strictures are secondary to surgical trauma. Other types of strictures can be secondary to malignancy due to primary cancer of the bile ducts or metastatic involvement. Benign strictures can also be related to radiation fibrosis, congenital infections, or sclerosing cholangitis.

Strictures can be managed with balloon dilatation. Reports from several institutions indicate that the percutaneous dilatation of benign strictures generally yields good short-term results. Percutaneous balloon dilatation is offered to patients with high surgical risk secondary to medical problems, strictures not amenable to corrective operations, previous failed attempt at surgical correction, and advanced liver disease.[40,41]

PERCUTANEOUS EXTRACTION OF RETAINED BILIARY STONES

In the United States more than 500,000 operations are performed each year on the extrahepatic biliary system for stone removal. One of the most popular techniques involves the steerable catheter developed by Burhenne and a Dormia basket. In experienced hands it has a success rate of 95%.[42] Besides these devices, several other techniques are used for biliary stone removal including rigid and flexible forceps, a choledoscope associated with ultrasonic or electrohydraulic lithotripsy. Percutaneous transhepatic cholangioscopic lithotripsy has proven to be a safe and effective method for treating biliary stones inaccessible through the endoscopic retrograde method.[43] Two simple techniques to remove biliary stones with good results are the fluoroscopic pushing technique that places a balloon against the stone, and the flushing of fluids to mobilize the stone within the ductal system. If the stone is larger than 6 mm, a papillotomy is required. Smaller stones may be pushed after dilatation of the ampulla.[44]

CHOLECYSTOSTOMY

Recent studies have shown that percutaneous cholecystostomy should be the treatment of choice for those patients with acute calculous and acalculous cholecystitis classified as a high surgical risk. This technique has proved to be safe and effective and can be performed as a definitive or palliative treatment. Preoperative percutaneous cholecystostomy can also decrease postoperative morbidity and mortality.[45–53]

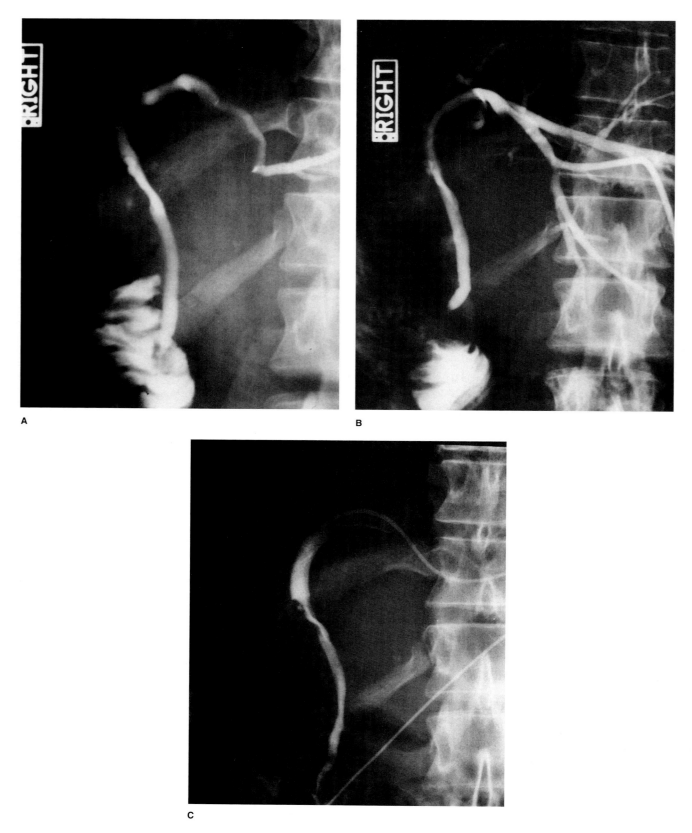

A

B

C

Figure 38–2. A. Cholangiogram in patient post-trisegmentectomy shows high-grade stenosis of proximal left bile duct. **B.** Cholangiogram postdilatation shows an increase in diameter at site of stenosis. **C.** Cholangiogram post-wallstent placement shows a widely patent lumen.

COMPLICATIONS

Complications can be considered acute or delayed. The acute complications occur in about 5 to 10% of patients. The most common are hemobilia, hemorrhage, and sepsis. Electrolyte imbalance occurs in almost all patients who have purely external drainage. Less common complications are pneumothorax, biliothorax, pancreatitis, subphrenic abscess, peritonitis, percutaneous tumor seeding, and death. Complications of biliary drainage procedures are more common in malignant obstructions than in benign obstructions. Of the acute complications, the most dramatic is death that occurs during or immediately after the procedure and is usually the result of a serious intrabdominal or intrahepatic hemorrhage or sepsis. Severe hemorrhage can occur after repeat puncture of the liver with a thin-gauge needle. Death can also occur as a complication of biliary-pleural fistula or sepsis. Pancreatitis is a rare occurrence and may be related to catheter occlusion of the pancreatic duct.[54] Pleural complications are infrequent and related to the technique itself, or in patients with hyperexpanded lungs such as in emphysema.

Obstruction of the catheter or dislodgment of the catheter occurs with distressing frequency (Fig. 38–3). The most common delayed complications include cholangitis, bile leakage, dislodgment of the catheter, and infection of the catheter site,[55] and usually are related to catheter malfunction. Less common delayed complications include peritoneal seeding of carcinoma[56] and tumor ingrowth through the interstices of metallic stents. Bile leakage into the peritoneal cavity or formation of a biloma is fortunately rare.

CONCLUSIONS

The percutaneous procedures in the biliary system originated in the 1920s in an attempt to obtain a better radiologic diagnosis. Percutaneous biliary drainage was developed in order to diminish the high morbidity and mortality rates of surgical interventions in malignant obstructions. However, due to the high incidence of bile leaks following cholangiograms, patients had to be taken directly to the operating room to avoid biliary peritonitis. Subsequent refinements in the technique of percutaneous transhepatic fine-needle cholangiography allowed the development of multiple techniques for the diagnosis and treatment of a variety of disease entities with minimal complications. Techniques include diagnostic cholangiography and biliary drainage, endoluminal endoscopy, biopsy, radiotherapy, and lithotripsy. In the 1990's the number of percutaneous biliary procedures dramatically diminished due to a marked improvement in endoscopic techniques. Endoscopic procedures are preferred because they are less invasive, have fewer complications, and are more comfortable for patients than the invasive techniques. The management of CBD dilatation secondary to calculi, malignancy, or other benign etiology is endoscopic as a first choice. The percutaneous approach is indicated in selected

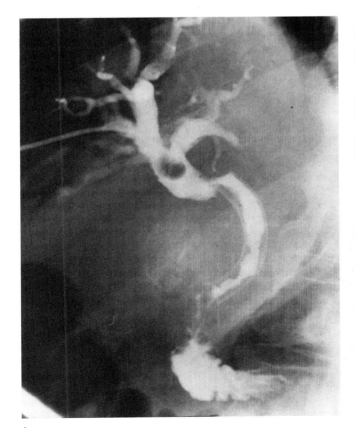
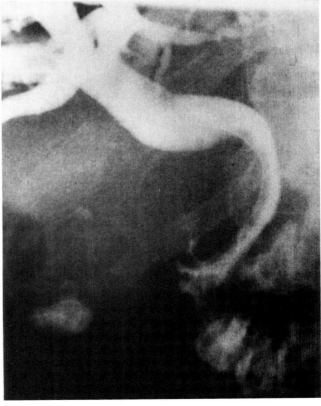

A

B

Figure 38–3. A. Cholangiogram 3 months post-wallstent placement due to recurrent jaundice shows narrowing of the lumen of the wallstent. **B.** Cholangiogram after cleaning-up and placing a second wallstent shows free flow into the duodenum.

cases where endoscopy or surgery cannot be used. Even with a partially limited rol, interventional radiology still has ample indications. Currently, for the interventional radiologists, biliary cases are more difficult and better skills are needed as well as different techniques. Other than drainage procedures in cases of achalculous cholecystitis, other procedures, which previously involved the gallbladder, have been abandoned with the advent of laparoscopic cholecystectomy.

REFERENCES

1. Burkhardt H, Muller W. Versuche uber die Punktion der Gallenblase und ihre Roentgendearstellung. *Dtsch Chiru.* 1921;161:168.
2. Ohto M, Tsuchiya Y. Medical cholangiography: Technique and cases. *Medicina* (Tokyo). 1969;6:735.
3. Seldinger SI. Percutaneous transhepatic cholangiography. *Acta Radiol.* 1966;253(suppl):1.
4. Tsuchiya Y. A new safer method of percutaneous transhepatic cholangiography. *Jpn J Gastroenterol.* 1969;66:438.
5. Kaufman Sl, Kadir S, Mitchell SE. Percutaneous transhepatic biliary drainage for bile leaks and fistulas. *AJR.* 1985;144:1055.
6. Vásquez JL, Thorsen MK, Dodds WJ, et al. Evaluation and treatment of intra-abdominal bilomas. *AJR.* 1985;144:933.
7. Mueller P, Ferruci JT Jr, Simeone JF, et al. Detection and drainage of bilomas: Special considerations. *AJR.* 1983;140:715.
8. Walker AT, Shapiro AW, Brooks DC, et al. Bile duct disruption and biloma after laparoscopic cholecystectomy: Imaging evaluation. *AJR.* 1992;158:785.
9. Yadav RK, Magu S, Sharma A, et al. Evaluation of various diagnostic signs on percutaneous transhepatic cholangiography in obstructive jaundice. *J Indian Med Assoc.* 1998;96:330.
10. Hoevels J, Lunderquist A, Ihse I. Percutaneous transhepatic intubation of the bile ducts for combined internal-external drainage in preoperative and palliative treatment jaundice. *Gastrointest Radiol.* 1978;3:23.
11. Hanson JA, Hoevels J, Simert G, et al. clinical aspects of non-surgical percutaneous transhepatic bile drainage in obstructive lesions of the extrahepatic bile duct. *Ann Surg.* 1979;189:58.
12. Ferruci JT Jr, Mueller PR, Harbin WP. Percutaneous transhepatic biliary drainage: Technique, results and applications. *Radiology.* 1980; 135:1.
13. Ferruci JT, Mueller PR. Interventional radiology of the biliary tract. *Gastroenterology.* 1982;82:974.
14. Neff RA, Frankuchen EI, Cooperman AM, et al. The radiological management of malignant biliary obstruction. *Clin Radiol.* 1983;34:143.
15. Culp WC, Mladinich CR, Hawkins IF Jr. Comparison of hepatic damage from direct injections of iodinated contrast agents and carbon dioxide. *JVIR.* 1999;10:1265.
16. Koito K, Namieno T, Nagakawa T, et al. Percutaneous transhepatic biliary drainage using color Doppler ultrasonography. *J Ultrasound Med.* 1996;15:203.
17. Hayashi N, Sakai T, Kitagawa M, et al. US-guided left-sided biliary drainage: Nine-year experience. *Radiology.* 1997;204:119.
18. Hatano S, Kondoh S, Akiyama T, et al. Evaluation of MRCP compared to ERCP in the diagnosis of biliary and pancreatic duct. *Nippon Rinsho.* 1998;56:2874.
19. Varghese JC, Farrell MA, Courtney G, et al. Role of MR cholangiopancreatography in patients with failes or inadequate ERCP. *AJR.* 1999;73:1527.
20. Varghese JC, Liddell RP, Farrell MA, et al. The diagnostic accuracy of magnetic resonance cholangiopancreatography and ultrasound compared with direct cholangiography in the detection of choledocholithiasis. *Clin Radiol.* 1999;54:604.
21. Lam WW, Lam TP, Sing H, et al. MR cholangigraphy and CT cholangiography of pediatric patients with choledochal cyst. *AJR.* 1999; 173:401.
22. Magnuson TH, Bender JS, Duncan MD, et al. Utility of magnetic resonance cholangiography in the evaluation of biliary obstruction. *J Am Coll Surg.* 1999;189:63;discussion,71.
23. Laghi A, Pavone P, Catalano C, et al. MR cholangiography of the late biliary complications after liver transplantation. *AJR.* 1999;172:1541.
24. Norton KI, Glass RB, Kogan D, et al. MR cholangiography in children and young adults with biliary disease. *AJR.* 1999;172:1239.
25. Little AF, Smith PJ, Hennessy OF, et al. Magnetic resonance cholangiopancreatography: Non-invasive imaging for the biliary tree and pancreatic duct. *Med J Aust.* 1998;169:266.
26. Laghi A, Pavone P, Panebianco V, et al. Biliary complications of liver transplant. Role of cholangiography with MR. *Radiol Med* (Torino). 1998;95:66.
27. Ichikawa T, Haradome H, Hanoka H, et al. Improvement of MR cholangiopancreatography at .5 T: Three-dimensional half-averaged single-shot fast spin echo with multi breath hold technique. *J MRI.* 1998;8:459.
28. Merker EM, Nussle K, Glasbrenner B, et al. MRCP (magnetic resonance cholangiopancreatography): An assessment of current status. *Z Gastroenterol.* 1998;36:215.
29. Demartines N, Eisner L, Schnabel K, et al. Evaluation of magnetic resonance cholangiography in the management of bile duct stones. *Arch Sug.* 2000;135:148.
30. Harbin WP, Mueller PR, Ferrucci JT Jr. THC: Complications and use patterns of the fine-needle technique. *Radiology.* 1980;135:15.
31. Young AT, Cardella JF, Castañeda-Zúñiga WR, et al. The anterior approach to left biliary catheterization. *Semin Intervent Radiol.* 1985;2:31.
32. Saiki S, Chijiwa K, Komura M, et al. Preoperative internal biliary drainage is superior to external biliary drainage in liver regeneration and function after hepatectomy in obstructive jaundice rats. *Ann Surg.* 1999;230:655.
33. Braasch JW, Gray BN. Considerations that lower pancreatoduodenectomy mortality. *Am J Surg.* 1977;133:480.
34. Brooks JR, Culebras JM. Cancer of the pancreas: Palliative operation. Whipple procedure or total pancreatectomy? *Am J Surg.* 1976;131:516.
35. Feduska NJ, Dent TL, Lindenauer SM. Results of palliative operations for carcinoma of the pancreas. *Arch Surg.* 1971;103:330.
36. Maki T, Sata T, Kakisaki G, et al. Pancreaticoduodenectomy for periampullary carcinomas: Appraisal of two-stage procedures. *Arch Surg.* 1966;92:825.
37. Tsai CC, Mo LR, Lin RC, et al. Self-expandable metallic stents in the management of malignant biliary obstruction. *J Formosan Med Assoc.* 1996;95:298.
38. Rossi P, Bezzi M, Rossi M, et al. Metallic stents in malignant biliary obstruction: Results of a multicenter european study in 240 patients. *JVIR.* 1994;5:279.
39. Amigdalos MA, Haskal ZJ, Cope C, et al. Transjugular insertion of biliary stents (TIBS) in patients with malignant ascites and coagulopathy. *Cardiovasc Intervent Radiol.* 1996;19:107.
40. Pitt HA, Miyamoto T, Parapatis SK, et al. Factors influencing the outcome in patients with post-operative biliary strictures. *Am J Surg.* 1982;144:14.
41. Morrison MC, Lee MJ, Saini S, et al. Percutaneous balloon dilatation of benign biliary strictures. *Radiol Clin North Am.* 1990;28:1191.
42. Burhenne HJ. Garland lecture: Percutaneous extraction of retained biliary tract stones: 661 patients. *AJR.* 1980;134:889.
43. Kusano T, Masato F, Isa T, et al. Percutaneous transhepatic cholangioscopic lithotripsy and change of biliary manometry patterns. *Hepatogastroenterology.* 1999;46:2153.
44. Wittich GR, vanSonnenberg E, Goodacre BW. Radiologic management of hepatolitiasis. *Gastroenterologist.* 1998;6:21.

45. Bakke K, Navjord D, Nilsen BH. Percutaneous drainage of the gallblader in acute cholecystitis. *Tidsskr Nor Laegeforen.* 1999;119:3260.

46. Patel M, Miedema BW, James MA, et al. Percutaneous cholecystostomy is an effective treatment for high-risk patients with acute cholecystitis. *Am Surg.* 2000;66:33.

47. Sugiyama M, Tokuhara M, Atomi Y. Is percutaneous cholecistostomy the optimal treatment for acute cholecystitis in the very elderly? *World J Surg.* 1998;22:459.

48. Lee KT, Wong SR, Cheng JS, et al. Ultrasound-guided percutaneous cholecystostomy as an initial treatment for acute cholecystitis in elderly patients. *Dig Surg.* 1998;15:328.

49. Boggi U, Di Candio G, Campatelli A, et al. Percutaneous cholecystostomy for acute cholecystitis in critically ill patients. *Hepatogastroenterology.* 1999;46:121.

50. Joly JP, Duchmann JC, el Yamani A, et al. Percutaneous cholecystostomy: A study of 30 patients. *Gastroenterol Clin Biol.* 1998;22:127.

51. Daves CA, Landercasper J, Gundersen LH, et al. Effective use of percutaneous cholecystostomy in high-risk surgical patients: Techniques, tube management and results. *Arch Surg.* 1999;134:727;discussion, 731.

52. Kiviniemi H, Makela JT, Autio R, et al. Percutaneous cholecystostomy in acute cholecystitis in high-risk patients: An analysis of 69 patients. *Int Surg.* 1998;83:299.

53. Wong SK, Yu SC, Lam YH, et al. Percutaneous cholecystostojmy and endoscopic cholecystolithotripsy in the management of acute cholecystitis. *Surg Endosc.* 1999;13:48.

54. Probst P, Castañeda-Zúñiga WR, Amplatz K. Percutaneous transhepatic drainage catheter: A valuable therapeutic aid in obstructive jaundice. *Rofo.* 1978;128:443.

55. Mueller PR, vanSonnenberg E, Ferrucci JT Jr. Percutaneous biliary drainage: technical and catheter related problems-experience with 200 cases. *AJR.* 1982;138:17.

56. Carrasco C, Zornoza J, Bechtel W. Malignant biliary obstruction: Complications of biliary drainage. *Radiology.* 1984;152:343.

*I*ntestinal Surgery

Chapter Thirty-Nine (Part One) · · · · · ·

A ppendectomy

JORGE CUETO-GARCÍA and JOSÉ ANTONIO VÁZQUEZ-FRIAS

INTRODUCTION

Appendectomy is the most common emergency operation performed all over the world.[1] The fact that it is very common and considered a simple procedure has generated an unfounded trust in both the medical community and the general population, for the complications of the disease continue to produce protracted morbidity, considerable suffering and expense, and rarely the death of the patient. The most important aspect in the treatment of appendicitis is an early diagnosis so surgical treatment can be done as soon as possible. Laparoscopic surgery offers an excellent method for an early diagnosis and safe and efficient treatment in patients with clinical suspicion of acute appendicitis.[2–10]

HISTORICAL BACKGROUND

Since the classic papers of Morton,[11] McBurney,[12] Murphy,[13] and others were published, the surgical treatment of appendicitis had changed very little until the introduction of laparoscopic appendectomy, first performed in 1983 by Semm,[14] although Schreiber[15] was the first one to carry out laparoscopic appendectomy in cases of acute appendicitis, and Götz et al[8] was the first group to report large series of patients treated successfully by this method. Laparoscopic appendectomy (LA) has become more popular recently and there are several clinical studies that support its systematic use in the treatment of acute appendicitis and its complications.[5,8–10,14–42]

NATURAL HISTORY OF THE DISEASE AND COMPLICATIONS

Acute inflammation of the appendix with or without the presence of obvious obstruction usually results from a fecalith that progresses to acute suppuration, gangrene, perforation, and peritonitis.

The morbidity of acute appendicitis in general is approximately 3.1%, but it can increase in cases of perforation up to 47.2%.[3,4] Perforation of the appendix is the most feared complication of the disease and is present in up to 20 to 30% of patients. The average symptom duration in patients without perforation is approximately 22.4 hours and for those with perforation symptoms more than 56 hours.[25,27,28] The overall mortality is less than 1%, but if all cases with perforation and peritonitis are considered, mortality can be considerably higher;[3,4] this is why the most important aspect of the treatment of the disease is to establish an early diagnosis and perform surgery to avoid gangrene, perforation, diffuse peritonitis, abscess formation, and fistulas—complications that even now are associated with considerable morbidity and increased hospital costs, not to mention patient suffering and mortality.[43–45]

CLINICAL DIAGNOSIS

The clinical diagnosis of appendicitis can be found in many excellent textbooks, one of the best being the classic textbook by Dr. Cope.[46] The typical clinical picture is that of insidious epigastric and/or mesogastric pain or discomfort accompanied by nausea and, rarely, vomiting. The patient later develops intense lower right quadrant pain, when general symptoms such as low-grade fever and tachycardia usually appear, followed by ileus. If perforation ensues, the patient experiences generalized excruciating abdominal pain and the typical signs and symptoms of purulent peritonitis, such as high fever, rigid abdomen, rebound tenderness, and painful rectal examination may be present. A rectal examination is an important—and often neglected—part of the clinical examination.

It is also important to remember that in both extremes of age there may be an almost total absence of these symptoms. A common clinical presentation in older patients—particularly those with cardiovascular and/or pulmonary pathology—is that of ileus of several days' duration, nausea, vomiting, electrolyte imbalance, and evidence of systemic toxicity. The same can apply to patients receiving high doses of steroids and/or immunosuppressive agents.

It is inadequate to establish the diagnosis and decide to operate based primarily on the white blood cell count (WBC) because although most patients with acute appendicitis have leukocytosis, usually above 12,000 mm^3 (and perforation must be suspected when the WBC is above 16,000 mm^3), there are many patients with pathologically proven appendicitis with a normal WBC.

Chest and abdominal films should be taken, and in recent years the use of ultrasound (US) has become very popular, since it is a noninvasive method that can provide the clinician with valuable information, such as the presence of fluid in the abdomen and/or in the pelvis, and the data needed to rule out ovarian and/or tubal pathology or cholecystitis. In some instances, depending on the skill of the diagnostician, a distended appendix with or without an abscess can be diagnosed preoperatively. The test can also be repeated if the equipment is readily available. Computed tomography has also been used to diagnose appendicitis.

DIFFERENTIAL DIAGNOSIS

It is during the work-up to make the differential diagnosis where this mini-invasive method offers many advantages to the patient, the hospital, and the medical group. It has been well documented that up to 30% of female patients of reproductive age can have acute pelvic inflammatory disease and/or adnexal pathology which is clinically indistinguishable from appendicitis, and in some instances US will not aid in making the differential diagnosis. In this situation it is generally wise to operate rather than risk the consequences of perforation and peritonitis. If the patient presents with symptoms typical of an upper respiratory infection and/or diarrhea, this does not necessarily exclude the diagnosis of appendicitis. Occasionally one may also see a patient with so-called left-sided appendicitis.

One of the advantages of laparoscopy is that a complete inspection of the abdomen can be done easily, and a more thorough exam may be done than the exam that even an experienced surgeon can do through a 3- to 5-cm right lower quadrant incision. In older patients or in those in whom the diagnosis is not clear or may be obscured by the use of antibiotics or potent analgesics, the diagnosis is invariably established by laparoscopy.[47] The use of laparoscopy avoids the need for long and costly periods of observation, as well as the expense of repeated laboratory and imaging tests.[7,15,19–21]

SURGICAL TECHNIQUE

With the patient under general endotracheal anesthesia and having received 1 g of a second-generation cephalosporin intravenously, the umbilicus is infiltrated with 5 mL of 2% lidocaine with epinephrine and the pneumoperitoneum is established with a Veress needle. Usually a 10-mm 0° laparoscope is inserted to carry out the diagnostic laparoscopy. It is important to mention that there are many scopes available with smaller diameters such as 5, 3, and even 2 mm that can be helpful in these circumstances. If there is obvious abdominal distention an open technique can be used to establish the pneumoperitoneum.[47,48] Once the diagnosis of appendicitis is confirmed, a second 5-mm trocar is inserted, taking care not to injure the epigastric vessels by using transillumination and by direct inspection with the laparoscope. The surgeon will ma-

nipulate instruments through this trocar with the right hand. A third trocar is usually placed in the right side of the pubic area for a 3 to 5-mm reusable instrument that will be manipulated by the surgeon's left hand (Fig. 39–1). With the patient placed in a steep Trendelenburg position, sometimes with a left lateral inclination, the surgeon stands on the left side of the table at the level of the patient's thigh and the monitor is placed opposite from the surgeon (to the right of the table) (Fig. 39–1). The surgeon grasps the appendix with the 3-mm grasper (a very large, edematous appendix may require a 5-mm instrument) and with the right hand proceeds to carry out the dissection of the appendix, determining the location of its base and the condition of the mesoappendix. The authors use the technique initially described by Professor Götz in Germany,[8] in which the mesoappendix is desiccated (Fig. 39–2) with the aid of bipolar electrocautery (usually a 5-mm reusable instrument) which provides excellent hemostasis and when used carefully does not have the disadvantages of monopolar electrocautery (e.g., inadvertent damage to a neighboring structures, even those far from the site of cautery). This instrument can be used even if staples are present. The use of 5-mm harmonic scissors, particularly in complicated cases, has obvious advantages, such as excellent hemostasis and separation of the tissues without damage to surrounding organs, and the fact that it also saves operating time. Once the mesoappendix has been divided, a preformed loop of absorbable suture is introduced through the 5-mm left pubic trocar and tied at the base of the appendix (Fig. 39–3), with two such loops tied at the base of the appendix and one distally. In patients whose appendix is not distended, a 5- or 10-mm staple can be applied distally instead of the loop of suture. In cases where the base of the appendix is very wide or friable, a "figure of X" stitch is applied with 3-0 polyglactin.

Once the appendix has been divided and before extracting it, we move the patient out of the Trendelenburg position and carry out a thorough irrigation and cleansing of the lower abdomen and pelvic area and the pouch of Douglas. This is one of the most important advantages of using a laparoscopic approach.

The most expeditious way of dividing the mesoappendix and the appendix itself is using an endo-stapler, which saves 10 to 15 minutes operating time but adds considerable expense and

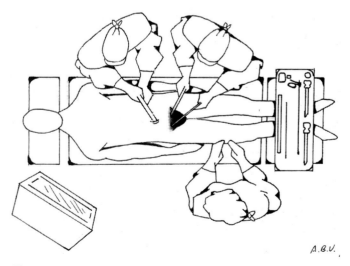

Figure 39–1. Position of the surgical team. The surgeon is using a 5-mm instrument with his right hand and using a 3-mm instrument with his left hand.

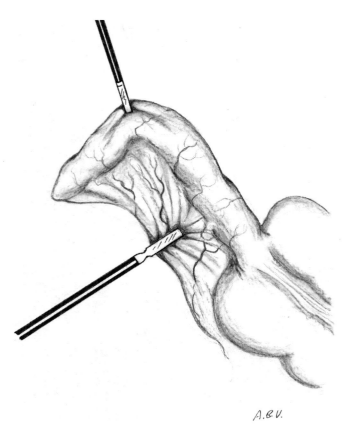

A.B.V.

Figure 39–2. Desiccation of the mesoappendix with the aid of a grasper and bipolar electrocautery.

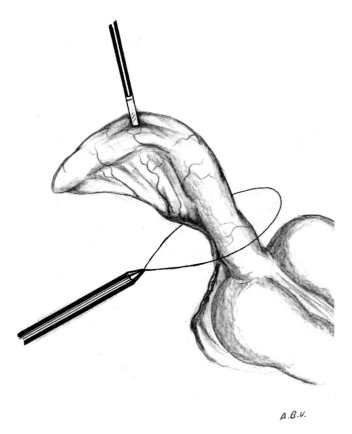

A.B.V.

Figure 39–3. Placement of the preformed loop of absorbable suture around the base of the appendix.

necessitates a 12 or 15-mm incision. Cost-benefit considerations and surgeon preference should play an important role in the selection of the instruments used, as in any other laparoscopic procedure.

In cases of retrocecal, ascending, or perforated appendicitis, this procedure is most useful and instead of making a larger incision (which may be difficult cosmetically for young female patients) that may become infected in the postoperative period, additional trocar(s), usually 3 or 5 mm in size, can be placed in the lower or upper right quadrant to accommodate a grasper, an irrigating cannula, or bipolar electrocautery. In patients with an abscess, careful irrigation and debridement is done under direct vision with increased pressure in the pneumoperitoneum, and a closed, semirigid drainage tube is placed and exteriorized through one of the pubic ports. No drainage is used for patients with diffuse peritonitis, because they require extensive irrigation and appropriate parenteral antibiotic therapy.

For the extraction of the specimen, the endoscope is exchanged for a 5-mm scope that is introduced in the left pubic port and an extraction forceps is introduced through the 10-mm port in the umbilicus. In cases of a very congested, dilated, gangrenous, or fragmented appendix or another type of infected specimen, a sterile plastic bag is introduced through the same port to avoid spillage and contamination of the abdominal cavity[49] (Fig. 39–4).

The umbilical wound is closed using a special reusable instrument[50] with 0 polydioxanone, and the 3- and 5-mm wounds are closed with subcutaneous 4-0 polyglactin. In patients with obvious contamination, the trocar wounds are scrubbed with povidone iodine foam mixed with hydrogen peroxide and then washed with isotonic solution.

It is noteworthy to mention that even in very complicated septic cases, we have not seen wound infections in the mini-incisions. In our clinical experience, of 36 perforated appendices—4 of which also had a pelvic abscess—there have been no residual abscesses.

Recently a new modification of this procedure has been introduced which may be used in patients who are not overweight, and who have uncomplicated appendicitis.[51] In this technique, the umbilical trocar is placed as described above, but the pubic trocars (a 3-mm and a 5-mm trocar) are placed in the unshaved but thoroughly scrubbed pubic area, careful cleansing being necessary to prevent infection. It has been shown that with even smaller mini-incisions, there is less postoperative pain, surgical trauma, and immunologic depression, and the cosmetic results are improved as well.[52,53]

DISCUSSION

A well-controlled prospective randomized trial is considered to be the gold standard for evaluating the benefits and disadvantages of a new procedure.[54] To date, about 20 prospective randomized trials (PRTs)[10,25,31–39,55–64] comparing laparoscopic and open appendectomy (OA) have been published in some prestigious journals. Most studies have found significant advantages of LA over OA, while some have not (Table 39–1). There have

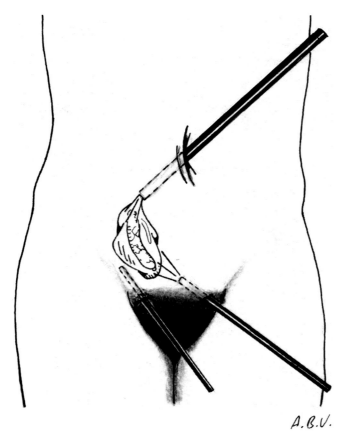

A.B.V.

Figure 39–4. Extraction of the specimen with the aid of a sterile plastic bag.

also been at least 6 meta-analyses[65–70] and 5 reviews[41,54,71–73] (Table 39–2) that in some cases found flaws (i.e., intention-to-treat analysis, small sample sizes, and a lack of blind selection, among others) in the methodology of the original studies, that may have yielded misleading results. Despite this, most of the PRTs,[10,25,31,32,35,37–39,55,56,61–64] the 6 meta-analyses, and 4 of the reviews[41,54,71,72] agree that LA yields superior results, especially in terms of more accurate diagnosis, less pain, reduction in wound infection, and quicker return to daily activities. On the other hand, two major disadvantages of LA are frequently mentioned: longer operative time and higher costs. In a few reports there was also a trend toward increasing numbers of postoperative abscesses.[67]

As the Society of the American Gastrointestinal Endoscopic Surgeons (SAGES) stated in 1992:[74] "The safety and effectiveness of LA have been demonstrated; it is neither experimental nor investigational." The European Association for Endoscopic Surgery (EAES) also reported in their Consensus Development Conference on LA in 1995,[20] that "LA is an efficacious new technology. Its safety and feasibility have been shown in the published literature, mainly from centers with a special interest in endoscopic surgery."

We strongly believe, as do other surgical groups, that the advantages of LA over OA outweigh any increased risks of LA.[40,75–78] Regarding the finding that LA takes longer to perform and costs more, we would only comment that as surgeons obtain more experience and become more skillful at performing LA, operative time decreases (LA takes only 12 to 17 minutes longer than OA when done by an experienced surgeon), as do conversion rates and complications. This has also been the experience worldwide with other types of laparoscopic procedures. Further decreases in costs may be had by using less disposable equipment.[79] A recent prospective randomized study examining the cost effectiveness of

TABLE 39–1. PROSPECTIVE RANDOMIZED STUDIES COMPARING OPEN WITH LAPAROSCOPIC APPENDECTOMY (LA)

Author	Year	Sample Size	Conclusions
Atwood[10]	1992	62	LA: Earlier discharge, quicker recovery, less complications.
Tate[34]	1993	140	No significant differences.
Kum[32]	1993	137	LA: Fewer wound infections, earlier return to normal activities.
Frazee[31]	1994	75	LA: Shorter duration of analgesics, quicker return to normal activities.
Hebebrand[55]	1994	57	LA: Less analgesia and time until resumption of regular diet, shorter hospital stay.
Ortega[25]	1995	253	LA: Less pain, more rapid return to full activities, shorter hospital stay.
Martin[33]	1995	169	No significant differences.
Henle[57]	1996	170	No significant differences.
Hansen[35]	1996	151	LA: Longer surgical time, fewer wound infections, less requirement of narcotic analgesia, earlier return to normal activity.
Mutter[58]	1996	100	No significant differences.
Hart[38]	1996	81	LA: Quicker return to normal activity, fewer intra-abdominal abscesses, fewer narcotic injections.
Cox[39]	1996	64	LA: Shorter hospital stay, quicker return to daily activities.
Lejus[59]	1996	63	No significant differences.
Williams[60]	1996	57	No significant differences.
Macarulla[61]	1997	210	LA: Shorter hospital stay, earlier resumption of diet, higher operative but lower total cost, less postoperative analgesia.
Kazemier[56]	1997	201	LA: Less pain and fewer wound infections, longer surgical time.
Reiertsen[37]	1997	108	LA: Reduced risk of unnecessary appendectomy, shorter postoperative convalescence, longer surgical time.
Laine[62]	1997	50	LA: Lower rate of negative appendectomies, better diagnostic accuracy.
Minne[36]	1997	57	LA: Longer operative time, higher direct charges.
Hellberg[63]	1999	500	LA: Less pain, quicker recovery, longer operative time.
Ozmen[64]	1999	70	LA: Shorter hospital stay, fewer postoperative complications, better diagnostic accuracy.

TABLE 39–2. CONCLUSIONS OF SEVERAL META-ANALYSES AND REVIEWS

Author	Year	Conclusions
1. Kazemier[65] (MA)	1997	LA results in longer operative time, faster postoperative recovery, fewer postoperative complications and shorter hospital stay.
2. Sauerland[66] (MA)	1998	LA results in fewer wound infections and eases postoperative recovery.
3. Golub[67] (MA)	1998	LA reduces the incidence of wound infections and shortens recovery times, but a trend toward increased intra-abdominal abscess is worrisome.
4. Temple[68] (MA)	1999	Operating time is significantly longer but return to normal activities is significantly earlier with LA.
5. Chung[69] (MA)	1999	LA offers reduced postoperative pain and wound infection rate and a faster convalescence, but a longer procedure which translates into higher cost.
6. Garbutt[70] (MA)	1999	LA offers reduced postoperative pain and wound infection rates and a more rapid return to normal functioning, but an increased operating time.
7. McCall[41] (R)	1997	LA is associated with longer operating time, minimal reduction in hospital stay, and reduced wound infections with no increase in other complications, and probably also results in an earlier return to normal activity.
8. Moberg[71] (R)	1997	LA causes less trauma and has better diagnostic accuracy and cosmetic results, at the price of a longer operating time.
9. Slim[54] (R)	1998	No significant differences. Perhaps increased direct cost of LA.
10. Fingerhut[72] (R)	1999	LA has consistently longer operating times, minimal reduction in hospital stay, and perhaps an earlier return to normal activity.

LA, laparoscopic appendectomy; MA, meta-analysis; R, review.

OA vs. LA concluded that although hospital expenses are higher for LA, it offers significant cost savings due to increased productivity resulting from shorter convalescence.[80]

The issue of residual intra-abdominal abscesses deserves special attention. Some authors found them more frequently after LA,[67,81,82] while others did not.[77,83–85] Our group has not seen an increase in this complication to date.[36] We believe that a careful dissection and extensive lavage are key factors in avoiding postoperative intra-abdominal abscesses. As mentioned before, no wound infections were seen in our group of patients, even in the most complicated cases, a finding that has also been reported by other surgeons.[25,41,62,86]

A perforated appendix, far from being a contraindication for LA,[85] could in fact be one of the main indications to use this approach. It is our impression as well as that of other groups, that patients that benefit the most from LA are those with a difficult diagnosis or complicated appendicitis, obese patients, and those for whom cosmesis is of utmost importance. Cosmetic results are clearly enhanced by using a laparoscopic approach; furthermore, when the modified technique described above is used, the scars are not visible just 3 months after surgery. Postoperative incisional hernias have also been reported to occur less frequently compared with open appendectomies.[25–28]

As with other laparoscopic procedures, the need for conversion to larger instruments and/or to laparotomy may arise once the diagnosis is established or during the procedure, but this should not result in any increase in morbidity due to the operation. Also, in female patients with pelvic inflammatory disease, endometriosis, or other pelvic pathology, our group advocates an incidental appendectomy, because there should be no increased morbidity associated with the procedure compared to diagnostic laparoscopy,[87] and it could affect the patient's future differential diagnosis of abdominal pain.

Finally, as Kazemier[65] and his group also pointed out, the fact that LA has some advantages over OA does not necessarily mean that conventional appendectomies should not be done for the safety and well being of patients. As in many other areas of medical and surgical treatment, sound clinical judgment must be used and criteria must be followed, and the patient and his or her family needs to be given objective facts, and the decision of how to treat should not be based on any bias on the part of the surgeon.

The postoperative management it is no different from that for a conventional procedure, and patients with uncomplicated disease that are operated early in the morning can usually be discharged the same day with oral pain medication. For patients with purulent peritonitis, abscesses, fistulas, or other serious complications, the treatment should focus on the local and systemic complications.

ADDENDUM: CONSENSUS OF THE EUROPEAN ASSOCIATION OF ENDOSCOPIC SURGERY IN REFERENCE TO LAPAROSCOPIC APPENDECTOMY[20]

I. Safety and Efficacy

a) Laparoscopic appendectomy (LA) has the same indications as traditional appendectomy.

b) There is no evidence that LA is less efficient than conventional appendectomy.

c) Operative time is directly related to the amount of experience the surgeon has in performing it, thus it can be shorter or longer than conventional appendectomy.

d) There is no evidence that postoperative complications are more frequent in LA than in traditional appendectomy.

e) There are no contraindications for LA, even in the presence of abscess and/or diffuse peritonitis.

II. Benefits for the Patient

a) A quicker and more precise diagnosis is provided for patients with pain in the right lower quadrant, primarily in children and women.

b) It is associated with less pain and postoperative discomfort.

c) Hospitalization time is the same or shorter than in uncomplicated conventional appendectomy.

d) There are fewer postoperative adhesions.

e) There is less risk of wound infection.

f) LA yields better cosmetic results.

g) It is concluded that LA has advantages over conventional appendectomy.

III. Technical Aspects

a) Conversion to laparotomy is needed when the appendix cannot be found by laparoscopy.

b) If the diagnostic laparoscopy is negative, it is not mandatory to perform an appendectomy.

c) Bipolar coagulation must be the method of choice for desiccation of the mesoappendix. Monopolar electrocautery can be used **with proper precautions.** The use of staples can be combined with electrocoagulation.

d) When the base of the appendix is not inflamed, simple ligature is recommended; if it is edematous or very enlarged, two ligatures are recommended. Staples alone are not recommended; automatic staplers are very expensive and are not required in the vast majority of cases.

e) The appendix must be sectioned 5 mm above the ligature and it is unnecessary to carry out invagination.[63]

f) It is recommended that the appendix be extracted in a bag to avoid infection of the wounds.

g) It is recommended that peritoneal irrigation be used in cases of intra-abdominal contamination.

h) Antibiotics must be used exactly as in conventional appendectomy.

IV. Recomendations for Training for Laparoscopic Appendectomy

Laparoscopic appendectomy must be part of the training program of all surgical residents. Residents must perform at least 20 laparoscopic appendectomies during the training program.

CONCLUSION

Laparoscopic appendectomy has become more popular everywhere, but it does require a surgical group with experience in advanced laparoscopic surgery and a well-equipped surgical unit. LA is extremely useful and can provide an accurate diagnosis with the concomitant well-known advantages of mini-invasive surgery.

REFERENCES

1. Cooperman M. Appendicectomy complications. *Surg Clin North Am.* 1983;6:1229.
2. Hauswald KR, Bivins BA, Meeker WR, et al. Analysis of the causes of mortality from appendicitis. *Am Surg.* 1976;42:761.
3. Lewis FR, Holcroft JW, Boey L, et al. Appendicitis: A critical review of diagnosis and treatment in 1000 cases. *Arch Surg.* 1975;110:667.
4. Cueto JG, Ribe J, Giorgana L, et al. Morbilidad y mortalidad de la apendicitis. *Rev Gastroent Mex.* 1977;42:126.
5. Easter D, Cuschieri A. The utility of diagnostic laparoscopy for abdominal disorders. *Arch Surg.* 1992;127:379.
6. Berci G. Elective and emergency laparoscopy. *World J Surg.* 1993; 17:8.
7. Llanio R. *Laparoscopia de Urgencia.* Científico-Técnica:1977.
8. Götz P, Pier A, Götz F, Bacher C. Laparoscopic appendectomy in 625 cases: From innovation to routine. *Surg Laparosc Endosc.* 1991;1:8.
9. Nowzaradan Y, Barnes JP, Westmoreland J, et al. Laparoscopic appendectomy: Treatment of choice for suspected appendicitis. *Surg Laparosc Endosc.* 1993;3:411.
10. Atwood SE, Hill AD, Murphy PG, et al. A prospective randomized trial of laparoscopic versus open appendectomy. *Surgery* 1992;112:497.
11. Morton TG. The diagnosis of pericaecal abscess and its radical treatment by removal of the vermiform appendix. *JAMA.* 1888;10:733.
12. McBurney C. Experience with early operative interference in cases of disease of the vermiform appendix. *NY State Med J.* 1889;50:676.
13. Murphy JB. Two-thousand operations for appendicitis and deductions from his personal experience. *Am J Med Sci.* 1904;125. Cited in Ref. 4.
14. Semm K. Endoscopic appendectomy. *Endoscopy* 1983;15:59.
15. Schreiber JH. Early experience with laparoscopic appendectomy in women. *Surg Endosc.* 1987;1:211.
16. Reddick EJ, Saye WB. Laparoscopic appendicectomy. In: Zucker KA, Baley RW, Reddick EJ, eds. *Surgical Laparoscopy.* Quality Medical Publishing:1991;227.
17. Schultz LS, Piettrafita JJ, Graber JN, et al. Retrograde laparoscopic appendicectomy: Report of a case. *J Laparoendosc Surg.* 1991;1:111.
18. Leahy PF. Technique of laparoscopic appendicectomies. *Br J Surg.* 1989;76:616.
19. Nowzaradan Y, Barnes JP, Westmoreland J, et al. Laparoscopy appendectomy: Treatment of choice for suspected appendicitis. *J Laparoendosc Surg.* 1991;1:247.
20. The European Association for Endoscopic Surgery (EAES) Consensus development conferences on laparoscopic cholecystectomy, appendectomy and hernia repair. *Surg Endosc.* 1995;9:550.
21. Jain A, Marcado PD, Grafton KP, et al. Out-patient appendectomy. *Surg Endosc.* 1995;9:424.
22. DesGroseillieres S, Fortin M, Lokanathan R, et al. Laparoscopic appendectomy versus open appendectomy: Retrospective assessment of 200 patients. *Can J Surg.* 1995;38:2:178.
23. Constantini M, Pianalto S, Baldan N, et al. Laparoscopic versus conventional surgery for suspected appendicitis in women. *Surg Endosc & Percutan Tech.* 2000;10:211.
24. Connor TJ, Garcha IS, Ramshau BJ, et al. Diagnostic laparoscopy for suspected appendicitis. *Am Surg.* 1995:61:2:187.
25. Ortega AE, Hunter JG, Peers GH, et al. Prospective, randomized, comparison of laparoscopic appendectomy with open appendectomy: Laparoscopic appendectomy study group. *Am J Surg.* 1995;169:2:208.
26. Pruett B, Pruett G. Laparoscopic appendectomy: Have we found a better way? *J Miss State Med Assoc.* 1994;35:12:647.
27. Vargas HI, Aberbook A, Staimos NG. Appendiceal mass: Conservative therapy followed by interval laparoscopic appendectomy. *Am Surg.* 1994;60:10:753.
28. Neal GE, McClintic EC, Williams JS. Experience with laparoscopic and open appendectomies in a surgical residents program. *Surg Laparosc Endosc.* 1994;4:4:272.
29. Pearl RH, Hale DA, Molloy M, et al. Pediatric appendectomy. *J Pediatr Surg.* 1995;30:2:173.
30. Richards KF, Fisher KS, Flores JH, et al. Laparoscopic appendectomy: Comparison with open appendectomy in 720 patients. *Surg Laparosc Endosc.* 1996;6:205.
31. Frazee RC, Roberts JW, Symmonds RE, et al. A prospective randomized trial comparing open versus laparoscopic appendectomy. *Ann Surg.* 1994;219:725.
32. Kum CK, Ngoi SS, Goh PM, et al. Randomized controlled trial comparing laparoscopic and open appendectomy. *Br J Surg.* 1993;80:1599.
33. Martin LC, Puente I, Sosa JL, et al. Open versus laparoscopic appendectomy. A prospective randomized comparison. *Ann Surg.* 1995; 222:256.

34. Tate JJ, Dawson JW, Chung SC, et al. Laparoscopic versus open appendicectomy: Prospective randomized trial (see comments). *Lancet* 1996;342:633.

35. Hansen JB, Smithers BM, Schache D, et al. Laparoscopic versus open appendectomy. Prospective randomized trial. *World J Surg.* 1996;20:17.

36. Minne L, Varner D, Burnell A, et al. Laparoscopic vs. open appendectomy. *Arch Surg.* 1997;132:708.

37. Reiertsen O, Larsen S, Trondsen E, et al. Randomized controlled trial with sequential design of laparoscopic versus conventional appendicectomy. *Br J Surg.* 1997;84:842.

38. Hart R, Rajgopal C, Plewes A, et al. Laparoscopic versus open appendectomy: a prospective randomized trial of 81 patients. *Can J Surg.* 1996;39:457.

39. Cox MR, McCall JL, Toouli J, et al. Prospective randomized comparison of open versus laparoscopic appendicectomy in men. *World J Surg.* 1996;20:263.

40. Johnson AB, Peetz ME. Laparoscopic appendectomy is an acceptable alternative for the treatment of perforated appendicitis. *Surg Endosc.* 1998;12:940.

41. McCall JL, Sharples K, Jadallah F. Systematic review of randomized controlled trials comparing laparoscopic with open appendectomy. *Br J Surg.* 1997;84:1045.

42. Chae FH, Stiegmann GV. Current laparoscopic gastrointestinal surgery. *Gastrointest Endosc* 1998;47:500.

43. Koespell TD, Inui TS, Farewell VT. Factors affecting perforation appendicitis. *Surg Gynecol Obstet.* 1981;153:508.

44. Bradley EL, Isaacs J. Appendiceal abscess revisited. *Arch Surg.* 1978;113:130.

45. Scher KS, Coil JA. The continuing challenge of perforation appendicitis. *Surg Gynecol Obstet.* 1980;150:535.

46. Cope Z. *The Early Diagnosis of the Acute Abdomen*, 14th ed. Oxford Medical:1972.

47. Cueto J, Rojas O, Garteiz D, et al. The efficacy of laparoscopic surgery in the diagnosis and treatment of peritonitis: Experience with 107 cases in Mexico City. *Surg Endosc.* 1997;11:366.

48. Weber A, Cueto J. Neumoperitoneo y sugerencias para facilitar las técnicas de cirugía miniinvasiva. In: *Cirugía Laparoscópica*, 2nd ed. McGraw Hill Interamericana:1994:40.

49. Weber SA, Vázquez JA, Valencia MS, et al. Retrieval of specimens in laparoscopy using disposable zipper-type plastic bags. A simple, cheap and useful method. *Surg Laparosc Endosc.* 1998;8:457.

50. Cueto J, Garteiz D, Melgoza C, et al. A simple and safe technique for closure of trocar wounds using a new instrument. *Surg Laparosc Endosc.* 1996;6:392.

51. Cueto GJ, Valencia-Reyes MS, Vázquez-Frias JA, et al. Technical modifications for laparoscopic appendectomy and other pelvic procedures using microinstruments. *Surg Laparosc Endosc Percutan Tech.* 2000;10(4):211–214.

52. Allendorf JDF, Bessler M, Whelan RL, et al. Postoperative immune function varies inversely with the degree of surgical trauma in a murine model. *Surg Endosc.* 1997;11:427.

53. Vittimberga FJ, Foley DP, Meyers WC, et al. Laparoscopic surgery and the systemic immune response. *Ann Surg.* 1998;227:326.

54. Slim K, Pezet D, Chipponi J. Laparoscopic or open appendectomy: critical review of randomized, controlled trials. *Dis Colon Rectum.* 1998;4:398.

55. Hebebrand D, Troidl H, Spangenberger W, et al. Laparoskopische oder klassische appendektomie? Eine prospektiv random-isierte studie. *Chirurg.* 1994;65:112.

56. Kazemier G, de Zeeuw GR, Lange JF, et al. Laparoscopic vs. open appendectomy. A randomized clinical trial. *Surg Endosc.* 1997;11:336.

57. Henle KP, Beller S, Rechner J, et al. Laparoskopische vs. konventionelle appendektomie: eine prospektiv, randomiserte studie. Chirurg 1996;67:526–530.

58. Mutter D, Vix M Bui A, et al. Laparoscopy not recommended for routine appendectomy in men: results of a prospective randomized study. *Surgery* 1996;120:71.

59. Lejus C, Delile L, Plattner V, et al. Randomized, single-blinded trial of laparoscopic vs. open appendectomy in children: effects on postoperative analgesia. *Anesthesiology* 1996;84:801.

60. Williams MD, Collins JN, Wright TF, et al. Laparoscopic vs. open appendectomy. *South Med J.* 1996;89:668.

61. Macarulla E, Vallet J, Abad JM, et al. Laparoscopic versus open appendectomy: a prospective randomized trial. *Surg Laparosc Endosc.* 1997;4:335.

62. Laine S, Rantala A, Gullichsen R, et al. Laparoscopic appendectomy—is it worthwhile? *Surg Endosc.* 1997;11:95.

63. Hellberg A, Rudberg C, Kullman E. Prospective randomized multicentre study of laparoscopic versus open appendicectomy. *Br J Surg.* 1999;86:48.

64. Ozmen MM, Zulfikaroglu B, Tanik A, et al. Laparoscopic versus open appendectomy: prospective randomized trial. *Surg Laparosc Endosc Percutan Tech.* 1999;9:187.

65. Kazemier G, Steyerberg EW, Bonjer HJ. Meta-analysis of randomized clinical trials comparing open and laparoscopic appendectomy. Scientific Session. The Society of Gastrointestinal Endoscopic Surgeons (SAGES) Meeting of the Americas. San Diego, California, March 19–22,1997.

66. Sauerland S, Lefering R, Holthausen U, et al. Laparoscopic vs conventional appendectomy—a meta-analysis of randomised controlled trials. *Lagenbecks Arch Surg.* 1998;383:289.

67. Golub R, Siddiqui F, Pohl D. Laparoscopic versus open appendectomy: a meta analysis. *J Am Coll Surg.* 1998;186:545.

68. Temple LK, Litwin DE, McLeod RS. A meta-analysis of laparoscopic versus open appendectomy in patients suspected of having acute appendicitis. *Can J Surg.* 1999;42:377.

69. Chung RS, Rowland DY, Li P, et al. A meta-analysis of randomized controlled trials of laparoscopic versus conventional appendectomy. *Am J Surg.* 1999;177:250.

70. Garbutt JM, Soper NJ, Shannon WD, et al. Meta-analysis of randomized controlled trials comparing laparoscopic and open appendectomy. *Surg Laparosc Endosc.* 1999;1:17.

71. Moberg AC, Montgomery A. Appendicitis: laparoscopic versus conventional operation: a study and review of the literature. *Surg Laparosc Endosc.* 1997;7:459.

72. Fingerhut A, Millat B, Borrie F. Laparoscopic versus open appendectomy: time to decide. *World J Surg.* 1999;23:835.

73. Slim K, Bousquet J, Kwiatkowski F. Analysis of random-ized controlled trials in laparoscopic surgery. *Br J Surg.* 1997;84:610.

74. The Society of Gastrointestinal Endoscopic Surgeons (SAGES) Statement on Policy. Laparoscopic Appendectomy. SAGES Standards of Practice Committee. Approved by the Board of Governors of SAGES, October 1992.

75. Prado E, Garcia-Alcala H, Dominguez-Cocco A. Estudio comparativo de apendicectomia laparoscopica vs apendicectomia abierta. *Rev Gastroenterol Mex.* 1997;62:254.

76. Anderson DG, Edelman DS. Laparoscopic appendectomy versus open appendectomy: a single institution study. *J Soc Laparoendosc Surg.* 1997;1:323.

77. Paya K, Rauhofeer U, Rebhandl W, et al. Perforating appendicitis. An indication for laparoscopy? *Surg Endosc.* 2000;14:182.

78. Alvarez C, Voitk AJ. The road to ambulatory laparoscopic management of perforated appendicitis. *Am J Surg.* 2000;179:63.

79. Weber A, Valencia S, Rodríguez M, et al. Análisis del costo entre apendicectomía abierta versus laparoscópica. *Anales Médicos del Hospital ABC.* Abril–Junio 1997;42:59.

80. Heikkinen TJ, Haukipuro K, Hulkko A. Cost-effective appendectomy. Open or laparoscopic? A prospective randomized study. *Surg Endosc.* 1998;12:1204.

81. Tang E, Ortega AE, Anthone GJ, et al. Intraabdominal abscesses following laparoscopic and open appendectomies. *Surg Endosc.* 1996;10:327.

82. Paik PS, Towson JA, Anthone GJ, et al. Intraabdominal abscesses following laparoscopic and open appendectomies *J Gastrointest Surg.* 1997;1:188.

83. Klingler A, Henle KP, Beller S, et al. Laparoscopic appendectomy does not change the incidence of postoperative infectious complications. *Am J Surg.* 1998;175:232.

84. Reid IR, Dobbs BR, Frizelle FA. Risk factors for post-appendectomy intra-abdominal abscess. *Aust NZ J Surg.* 1999;69:373.

85. Khaili TM, Hiatt JR, Savar A, et al. Perforated appendicitis is not a contraindication to laparoscopy. *Am Surg.* 1999;65:965.

86. Meynaud-Kraemer L, Colin C, Vergnon P, et al. Wound in-fection in open versus laparoscopic appendectomy. A meta-analysis. *Int J Technol Assess Health Care.* 1999;15:380.

87. Greason KL, Rappold JF, Liberman MA. Incidental laparoscopic appendectomy for acute lower quadrant abdominal pain. Its time has come. *Surg Endosc.* 1998;12:223.

Chapter Thirty-Nine (Part Two) ● ● ● ● ● ●

*M*eta-Analysis of Trials Comparing Laparoscopic and Open Appendectomy

GEERT KAZEMIER, EWOUT W. STEYERBERG, and HENDRIK J. BONJER

INTRODUCTION

Laparoscopic techniques have revolutionized general surgery in many fields. Particularly, laparoscopic cholecystectomy has gained widespread popularity. Laparoscopic removal of the gallbladder is now considered by many to be the gold standard in the treatment of symptomatic gallbladder stones.[1,2] Laparoscopic appendectomy is also being performed on a regular basis in many hospitals, but has not yet become the treatment of choice in every patient with acute appendicitis. Reports on patients who had laparoscopic removal of the appendix were published prior to the first experiences with laparoscopic cholecystectomy.[3,4] In those first reports, possible advantages were described of minimally invasive appendectomy.[3] A number of randomized trials comparing laparoscopic (LA) and open appendectomy (OA) have been reported in the past years. Most of these trials showed considerable advantages of the laparoscopic technique.[5–19]

In spite of these results and although appendectomy accounts for over 6% of all surgical procedures in daily practice and over 700,000 appendectomies are performed yearly in the European Union, widespread employment of LA did not follow.[20] Reluctance to create a pneumoperitoneum in patients with peritonitis, the use of small incisions for OA, frequent performance of appendectomy at night, or presumed higher costs associated with laparoscopic appendectomy might have prevented many surgeons from converting from the open to the laparoscopic technique. One other factor that might possibly contribute to the hesitation to embrace this new technique is the seemingly inconsistent outcome or statistically insignificant results of some randomized trials. In order to provide a more definitive answer to the question of how LA differs from OA, we combined data of all published, randomized clinical trials comparing LA and OA for acute appendicitis in a meta-analysis.

MATERIALS AND METHODS

A MEDLINE (Silver Platter MEDLINE version 3.11) search was performed covering the period from January 1, 1966 to January 1, 1998 using the key words **appendectomy, laparoscopy,** and **randomized.** Using these items, randomized, clinical trials comparing LA and OA for acute appendicitis in adults were selected by two independent reviewers (G.K. and H.J.B.).

Published data from these papers were used to perform a meta-analysis. Trials focusing only on the diagnostic value of laparoscopy or on specific subgroups of patients were excluded, as were experimental or nonrandomized studies and editorials and abstracts. Each included study was reviewed independently by two investigators (G.K. and H.J.B.). They were blinded to the name of the journal, authors, and date of publication. Consensus was reached by both investigators afterwards on conflicting scores by reviewing these data together. Data on operative time, postoperative pain, restoration of diet, hospital stay, postoperative complications, and return to normal activities were extracted from each study. Results of this analysis were based solely on trials that provided data on that specific aspect. Only data on items scored in three or more studies were analyzed.

Postoperative pain was scored differently in several studies. To overcome some of these problems, visual analogue scale (VAS) scores for postoperative pain on day 1 and day 2 were all recalculated to percentages of the maximum score. Total dosages of parenteral and oral pain medication were scored as stated in the studies.

Outcomes were distinguished as continuous or dichotomous. We pooled differences between LA and OA as calculated within each study, using standard meta-analytic techniques, assuming homogeneity between studies.[21]

Continuous Outcomes

Operative time, VAS scores for pain on postoperative day 1 and day 2, total number of dosages of parenteral and oral pain medication, number of days until tolerance of liquid and solid diets, number of postoperative days spent in the hospital, and number of postoperative days until restoration of normal activities were analyzed as continuous outcomes. For these continuous outcomes, variances (var) of differences were determined. Not all studies provided variances for all items. A mean variance was calculated using variances from the other studies. For every study and item a standard error (SE) was determined as $SE = \sqrt{var} \cdot \sqrt{(1/N_{LA} + N_{OA})}$. The weight (w) of each study was calculated as $w = 1/SE^2$. For each continuous outcome the precision-weighted pooled difference (i.e., pooled mean difference [PMD]) was calculated as the weighted sum of the results per study: $PMD = \Sigma wb / \Sigma w$, where b is the difference between OA and LA in each study. The standard error of the PMD was calculated as $SE_{PMD} = 1/\sqrt{\Sigma w}$. Ninety-five percent confidence intervals (95% CI) were calculated as $95\% \; CI = PMD \pm 1.96 \cdot SE_{PMD}$. To test for statistical significance, a Z-test was performed: $Z = PMD/SE_{PMD}$. The corresponding p value indicates the likelihood that the observed difference between the laparoscopic and the open group did exist while the difference was in fact zero.

A chi-square test was used to test for heterogeneity between studies: $X^2 = \Sigma w(b - PMD)^2$. Calculations were performed using a spreadsheet program.

Dichotomous Outcomes

Complications were classified into four groups: total, wound infection, early bowel obstruction, or intra-abdominal abscess, and analyzed as dichotomous outcomes. Odds ratios were calculated per item per study and were pooled using the Mantel-Haenszel method.[22] Calculations, including tests on heterogeneity, were performed using exact variance formulas as implemented in StatXact software (StatXact Version 2, Cytel Software Corporation, Cambridge, MA).

We also calculated the means (averages, weighted by number) and percentages (events divided by total N) in the laparoscopic and open group separately for illustrative purposes. The differences between these averages are not necessarily equal to the PMD for continuous outcomes. Similarly, pooled odds ratios can differ from those calculated with average percentages for dichotomous outcomes.

P values of less than 5% (two-sided) were considered statistically significant.

RESULTS

The MEDLINE search identified 44 studies. Fifteen studies were selected that described the results of a randomized, clinical trial comparing LA and OA.[5–19] In Table 39–3 the studies are shown with the number of patients randomized, number of patients analyzed, and reason for exclusion of analysis of patients. Differences between open and laparoscopic groups with respect to demographic and preoperative clinical data and data on number of inflamed and perforated appendices were small; they are not shown because all studies were randomized. In the study by Lujan Mompean et al,[11] it is stated that formal randomization was precluded by instrument availability. How the actual allocation to either LA or OA was done in this study is unclear. A total number of 1907 patients was enrolled in these trials. Eighty-two randomized patients were not analyzed for various reasons (Table 39–3). Operative techniques for LA and OA were comparable in each study, with the exception of the study by Ortega et al.[12] In this study, 253 patients were randomized to either OA (86 patients) or LA using an endoscopic linear stapler (78 patients) or LA using catgut ligature (89 patients). In the meta-analysis, all patients operated upon laparoscopically (167 patients) were pooled as LA and analyzed as one group.

Table 39–4 shows differences between LA and OA for continuous and dichotomous outcomes of different trials. Negative values indicate lower levels or rates in the LA group.

TABLE 39–3. TRIALS INCLUDED IN THE META-ANALYSIS

First Author	Year of Publication	Journal	Number of Patients Randomized	Number of Patients Analyzed	Number of Patients Excluded from Analysis after Randomization
Attwood	1992	*Surgery*	62	62	—
Kum	1993	*Br J Surg*	137	109	28, normal or perforated appendix
Tate	1993	*Lancet*	140	140	—
Frazee	1994	*Ann Surg*	75	75	—
Hebebrand	1994	*Chirur*	57	48	9, conversion from LA to OA
Lujan Mompean	1994	*Br J Surg*	200	200	—
Martin	1995	*Ann Surg*	169	169	—
Ortega	1995	*Am J Surg*	253	253	—
Hansen	1996	*World J Surg*	158	151	7, normal appendix or conversion from OA to midline laparotomy
Williams	1996	*South Med J*	39	37	2, conversion from LA to OA
Henle	1996	*Chirurg*	170	169	1, conversion from OA to LA
Hart	1996	*Chirurg*	170	169	1, conversion from LA to OA
Kazemier	1997	*Surg Endosc*	201	201	—
Reiertsen	1997	*Br J Surg*	108	84	24, normal appendix, other pathology or conversion from LA to midline laparotomy
Mimé	1997	*Arch Surg*	57	50	7, use of ketorolac or tromethamine
		Total	1907	1825	82

TABLE 39–4. DIFFERENCES OF OUTCOMES BETWEEN LA AND OA IN DIFFERENT TRIALS

Outcomes	Attwood	Tate	Kum	Heberbrand	Lujan Mompean	Frazee	Ortega	Martin	Hansen	Williams	Henle	Hart	Kazemier	Reiertsen	Mimé
No. of patients analyzed	62	140	109	48	200	75	253	169	151	37	169	77	201	84	50
Operative time (min)	10	24	3		5	22	10	20	23	6	4	29	19	26	15
VAS pain day 1 (0–100)		−6.0		−14.5			−14.6						−23.4	−4	−3
VAS pain day 2 (0–100)				−12.6			−6.7						−15.3		
Total parenteral pain medication (dosages)		0.0	−0.3	−0.5					−2.0			−1.5	−0.9	−1.1	
Total oral pain medication (dosages)			−2.2	−0.2					1.0				−0.8	0.1	
Days to liquid diet		−0.1	−0.3										−0.1		
Days to solid diet		−0.1	0.0			−0.8			−0.5	−0.7			−0.1		
Days in hospital		−0.1	−1.0	−2.3	−1.2	−0.8	−0.2	−2.1	0.0	−0.4	−1.0	0.2	−0.7	0.3	−0.1
Days until normal activity	−1.3		−13			−11.0	−5.0	−0.6	−7.0		−7.0	−7.2		−4.7	0.0
Complications (%)		−2.9	−8.8	4.7	−4.0	2.5		1.0	−7.9	4.4	2.7		−3.3	14.3	10.5
Total	−12.5	−2.9	−8.8	−4.3	−6.0	−0.1	−10.4	−3.1	−8.6	−0.3	−2.9	−0.6	−5.8		
Wound infection	−3.1	1.4	0.0	0.0	−1.0	0.0	4.4	3.8	1.1	−0.3	3.4		2.3		
Early bowel obstruction	−3.1	1.4	0.0	0.0	2.0	2.6	3.6	0.3	0.0	0.0	−1.3	3.1	−1.0	−2.4	3.1
Intra-abdominal abscess	0.0														

VAS, visual analogue scale.

Values in table represent outcomes in LA minus outcomes in OA group.

TABLE 39–5. RESULTS OF META-ANALYSIS OF CONTINUOUS OUTCOMES AND HETEROGENEITY OF OUTCOMES

Outcomes	LA[1]	OA[1]	Pooled Mean Difference (95% CI)		Effect p Value	Homogeneity p Value
Operative time (min)	63	50	−15	(−12 to −18)	$<10^{-5}$	$<10^{-3}$
VAS pain score day 1 (0–100)	35	51	13	(10 to 17)	$<10^{-5}$	0.005
VAS pain score day 2 (0–100)	11	25	11	(7 to 15)	$<10^{-5}$	0.111
Parenteral pain medication[2]	1.8	2.7	0.92	(0.69 to 1.16)	$<10^{-5}$	$<10^{-4}$
Oral pain medication[2]	2.4	3.5	0.42	(−0.08 to 0.92)	0.26	0.003
Days to liquid diet	1.2	1.4	0.15	(−0.02 to 0.31)	0.22	0.59
Days to solid diet	1.9	2.1	0.27	(0.12 to 0.42)	0.006	0.03
Days in hospital	3.2	3.9	0.69	(0.41 to 0.98)	$<10^{-5}$	0.01
Days until normal activity	14.7	19.3	4.8	(3.7 to 5.9)	$<10^{-5}$	$<10^{-5}$

[1]Mean values of outcomes in laparoscopic (LA) and open appendectomy (OA) group.
[2]Total number of doses.
VAS, visual analogue scale.

Table 39–5 shows the results of the meta-analysis of continuous outcomes. The combined evidence from the trials indicated a statistically significantly longer operative time, less postoperative pain and less use of parenteral pain medication, faster restoration of solid diet, shorter hospital stay, and faster restoration of normal activity for LA as compared to OA. Studies were heterogeneous for the exact results of several continuous outcomes (operative time, VAS day 1, total doses of parenteral and oral pain medication, days to solid diet, hospital stay, and days to normal activity).

Table 39–6 shows results of the meta-analysis of dichotomous data (i.e., complications). We observed a statistically significant reduction in postoperative wound infections and no statistical differences in total number of complications, intra-abdominal abscesses, and early bowel obstruction following LA as compared to OA. Insignificant trends were noticed towards increased percentages of early postoperative bowel obstruction and intra-abdominal abscesses following LA as compared to OA. All studies were rather homogenous for these outcomes.

DISCUSSION

Laparoscopic removal of inflamed appendices has been performed for more than a decade.[3] However, the majority of general surgeons have not adopted this technique. Laparoscopic appendectomy has been considered cumbersome and time-consuming, with few clinical advantages. The advent of laparoscopic cholecystectomy has incited renewed interest in the laparoscopic approach to acute appendicitis, but this has not yet resulted in its widespread application. Surprisingly, laparoscopic removal of the gallbladder

became the gold standard treatment for symptomatic gallbladder stones even before solid evidence of its superiority over open cholecystectomy was evident.[23] Laparoscopic appendectomy has by now been evaluated in 15 randomized clinical trials. Although the numbers of patients were small in some of these studies, advantages of the laparoscopic approach to appendicitis were shown in almost all studies. Due to the small numbers of patients included in individual studies, trends rather than significant differences were shown for some outcomes. Conflicting results also became apparent while reviewing these trials. In order to allow proper evaluation of the merits of laparoscopic appendectomy, a meta-analysis was done. This analysis graded the impact of the studies, depending on the number of patients included in each study. A qualitative weighting factor was not introduced, because qualitative scoring adds the analyst's subjective bias to the results and is therefore generally not advocated.[24] Some studies showed major flaws in the statistical analysis. One of the shortcomings was a lack of intention-to-treat analysis. Another flaw was found in 8 studies that only documented ranges of outcomes, without standard deviation, standard error, or 95% confidence interval. In the study by Lujan Mompean et al,[10] formal randomization was precluded by instrument availability. Because consecutive patients were studied and because instrument availability might only be a minor influence on outcomes, this study was nevertheless included in this meta-analysis. With exception of the trial by Lujan Mompean, however, no substantial differences with the initial meta-analysis were noticed. Blinding of the patients and postoperative observers to the surgical approach was only partially performed in one study.[12]

In this analysis, outcomes of trials were largely heterogeneous for 7 out of 9 continuous outcomes. This means that outcomes of different trials were poorly comparable with respect to the actual

TABLE 39–6. RESULTS OF META-ANALYSIS OF DICHOTOMOUS OUTCOMES AND HETEROGENEITY OF OUTCOMES

Complications	LA[1]	OA[1]	Pooled Mean Difference (95% CI)	Effect p Value	Homogeneity p Value
Total	12.6%	13.8%	0.89 (0.66–1.21)	0.48	0.18
Wound infection	3.3%	7.7%	0.37 (0.23–0.57)	$<10^{-5}$	0.29
Early bowel obstruction	4.7%	2.2%	1.68 (0.96–3.01)	0.076	0.69
Intra-abdominal abscess	2.2%	1.1%	1.78 (0.83–4.03)	0.19	0.28

[1]Mean percentage of outcomes in laparoscopic (LA) and open appendectomy (OA) group.

numeric value of the outcome. However, in all cases a negative or positive effect of laparoscopy was consistently reported by the majority of trials. For instance, every trial reported longer operative time for LA, but differences between LA and OA for operative time ranged from 3 to 29 minutes among the trials. This large range resulted in clear statistical heterogeneity between trials for operative time, although all trials were highly homogeneous on the question of whether LA took longer than OA.

Operative times were on average 15 minutes longer for LA compared to OA. Part of this increased operative time for LA could perhaps be attributed to the fact that most surgeons have less experience with the laparoscopic approach than the open. The impact of a learning curve could not be assessed, because the experience of the operative teams was not reported consistently in the reviewed studies. In our experience, LA remains technically more demanding even with growing experience, particularly in those patients with extensive inflammatory adhesions between the appendix and surrounding structures. When dissecting these adhesions, the surgeon relies more on tactile sensations, which are diminished in laparoscopic surgery. Operative time has become increasingly important in this era of increased financial scrutiny of surgical practice, and the longer operative time for LA appears to be a financial disadvantage. However, LA was associated with significantly shorter hospital stay and earlier return to normal activities. These variables are all of paramount importance when considering direct and indirect costs, but other factors such as instrument costs, cost of medication, and costs related to possible (late) readmissions should be taken into account as well in a proper cost-effectiveness assessment.

Assessing acute postoperative pain is difficult, and comparing different scoring systems might be even more difficult. However, less pain was shown following LA by objective standards such as visual analogue scale scores on postoperative days 1 and 2. Diminished postoperative pain was also shown by less use of parenteral analgesia after LA, but use of oral pain medication was not clearly different, indicating an advantage of LA for pain immediately after the procedure, when most parenteral pain medication is used. Although postoperative pain and postoperative recovery are very important factors in the postoperative course, safety of the procedure must never be jeopardized for these reasons.

In this analysis, the published percentages of complications in the trials were pooled. The percentage of early small bowel obstructions was not clearly different between LA and OA, although a trend towards increased incidence was seen following LA. Surprisingly, general restoration of solid diet was significantly faster following LA, although the clinical significance of a difference of 0.27 days may be quite small. The general belief that laparoscopic surgery is associated with faster recovery of normal bowel function was not supported by the studies included in this analysis.

LA resulted in fewer wound infections. However, intra-abdominal abscesses were seen more frequently in the LA group, although the overall incidence was low in both groups and not significantly different. This finding is in accordance with the findings of earlier studies.[25,26] The reason for this seemingly increased number of intra-abdominal abscesses could be the fact that the entire laparoscopic operation is performed intra-abdominally, while the open operation is performed mainly extra-abdominally, causing more wound infections. On the other hand, larger uncontrolled series of laparoscopic appendectomies have shown considerably lower incidences (0.2 to 0.3%) of intra-abdominal abscesses.[27,28]

Thus insufficient laparoscopic irrigation of the abdominal cavity during early experience or other factors related to the learning curve effect could explain the insignificantly higher number of intra-abdominal abscesses in the LA group. The consequences of a learning curve were assessed in one study, which showed 60% of complications occurred in the first 20% of patients operated laparoscopically.[15]

Late complications were not reported in any of these trials as follow-up was either not stated or very short. The majority of these late complications following appendectomy were bowel obstructions due to adhesions, which were reported in previous studies to occur in 5 to 10% of patients who underwent OA.[28,29] De Wilde[31] showed that at second-look laparoscopy, performed 3 months after appendectomy, 80% of patients developed adhesions following OA compared to 10% following LA.[31] Although not yet firmly proven, late bowel obstruction could be less common following LA.

Reduction in the number of unnecessary appendectomies might be another possible advantage of LA not assessed in this analysis. Due to the highly variable clinical picture of acute appendicitis, especially in women of child-bearing age, the rate of removal of normal appendices can be as high as 20 to 35%.[20,32] When a grid-iron incision is made for suspected acute appendicitis, it is common practice to remove the appendix even if it is normal. Laparoscopy has been shown to improve diagnostic accuracy for acute appendicitis with a reported sensitivity and specificity of over 95%.[33] With the introduction of laparoscopic inspection of the abdominal cavity instead of laparotomy and standard removal of the appendix, reduction of redundant appendectomies has been shown to be possible in 30 to 35% of patients presenting with acute right lower abdominal pain.[18,34,35]

In this analysis LA was shown to result in less postoperative pain, faster restoration of solid diet, fewer wound infections, shorter hospital stay, and faster recovery to normal activities. On the other hand, operative time was shown to be longer compared to OA. It is true that laparoscopic appendectomy can be performed safely, with certain benefits for the patient, but only a long-term cost-effectiveness analysis can show whether laparoscopic appendectomy is the optimal approach to treat every patient with acute appendicitis in every hospital by every surgeon.

REFERENCES

1. The Southern Surgeons Club. A prospective analysis of 1518 laparoscopic cholecystectomies. *N Engl J Med.* 1991;213:2.
2. Neugebauer E, Troidl H, Spangenberger W, et al. Conventional versus laparoscopic cholecystectomy and the randomized controlled trial. *Br J Surg.* 1991;78:150.
3. Semm K. Endoscopic appendectomy. *Endoscopy* 1983;15:59.
4. Dubois F, Icard P, Berthelot G, et al. Coelioscopic cholecystectomy. Preliminary report of 36 cases. *Ann Surg.* 1990;211:60.
5. Attwood SEA, Hill ADK, Murphy PG, et al. A prospective randomized trial of laparoscopic versus open appendectomy. *Surgery* 1992;112:497.
6. Kum CK, Ngoi SS, Goh PMY, et al. Randomized controlled trial comparing laparoscopic and open appendicectomy. *Br J Surg.* 1993;80:1599.
7. Tate JJT, Dawson JW, Chung SCS, et al. Laparoscopic versus open appendectomy: prospective randomized trial. *Lancet* 1993;342:633.
8. Frazee RC, Roberts JW, Symmonds RE, et al. A prospective randomized trial comparing laparoscopic versus open appendectomy. *Ann Surg.* 1994;219:725.

9. Hebebrand D, Toidl H, Spangenberger W, et al. Laparoskopische oder klassische Appendektomie? *Chirurg* 1994;65:112.

10. Lujan Mompean JA, Robles Campos R, et al. Laparoscopic versus open appendicectomy: a prospective assessment. *Br J Surg.* 1994;81:133.

11. Martin LC, Puente I, Sosa JL, et al. Open versus laparoscopic appendectomy; a prospective randomized comparison. *Ann Surg.* 1995; 222:256.

12. Ortega AE, Hunter JG, Peters JH, et al. A prospective randomized comparison of laparoscopic appendectomy with open appendectomy. *Am J Surg.* 1995;169:208.

13. Hansen JB, Smithers BM, Schache D, et al. Laparoscopic versus open appendectomy: prospective randomized trial. *World J Surg.* 1996;20:17.

14. Williams MD, Colloins JN, Wright TF, et al. Laparoscopic versus open appendectomy. *South Med J.* 1996;89:668.

15. Henle KP, Beller S, Rechner J, et al. Laparoskopische versus konventionelle Appendektomie: eine prospektive, randomisierte Studie. *Chirurg* 1996;67:526.

16. Hart R, Rajgopal C, Plewes A, et al. Laparoscopic versus open appendectomy: a prospective randomized trial of 81 patients. *Can J Surg.* 1996;39:457.

17. Kazemier G, de Zeeuw GR, Lange JF, et al. Laparoscopic versus open appendectomy: a randomized clinical trial. *Surg Endosc.* 1997;11:336.

18. Reiertsen O, Larsen S, Trondsen E, et al. Randomized controlled trial with sequential design of laparoscopic versus conventional appendectomy. *Br J Surg.* 1997;84:842.

19. Minné L, Varner D, Burnell A, et al. Laparoscopic vs open appendectomy. *Arch Surg.* 1997;132:708.

20. De Dombal FT, Clamp SE, Wardle KS. Measuring surgical performance in acute abdominal pain: Some reflections from international studies. *Eur J Surg.* 1997;163:323.

21. Greenland S. Quantitative methods in the review of epidemiologic literature. *Epidemiol Rev.* 1987;9:1.

22. Robins JM, Greenland S, Breslow NE. A general estimator for the variance of the Mantel-Haenszel odds ratio. *Am J Epidemiol.* 1986; 124:719.

23. Majeed AW, Troy G, Nicholl JP, et al. Randomized, prospective, single-blind comparison of laparoscopic versus small-incision cholecystectomy. *Lancet* 1996;347:989.

24. Greenland S. Invited commentary: a critical look at some popular meta-analytic methods. *Am J Epidemiol.* 1994;140:290.

25. Frizelle FA, Hanna GB. Pelvic abscess following laparoscopic appendectomy (letter). *Surg Endosc.* 1996;10:947.

26. Tang E, Ortega AE, Anthone GJ, et al. Intraabdominal abscesses following laparoscopic and open appendectomies. *Surg Endosc.* 1996;10:327.

27. Pier A, Gotz F, Bacher C, et al. Laparoscopic appendectomy. *World J Surg.* 1993;17:29.

28. EI Ghoneimi A, Valla JS, Limonne B, et al. Laparoscopic appendectomy in children; report of 1379 cases. *J Pediatr Surg.* 1994;29:786.

29. Metger U, Schwartz H. Bridenileus oder Perforationsperitonitis. *Helv Chir Acta.* 1975;42:571.

30. Zbar IR, Crede WB, McKahnn CF, et al. The postoperative incidence of small bowel obstruction following standard open appendectomy and cholecystectomy: a six-year retrospective cohort study at Yale-New Haven Hospital. *Conn Med.* 1993;57:123.

31. De Wilde RL. Goodbye to late bowel obstruction after appendicectomy (letter). *Lancet* 1991;338:1012.

32. Berry J, Malt R. Appendicitis near its centenary. *Ann Surg.* 1984; 200:567.

33. Wagner M, Aronsky D, Tschudi J, et al. Laparoscopic stapler appendectomy. A prospective study of 267 consecutive cases. *Surg Endosc.* 1996;10:895.

34. Olsen JB, Myren CJ, Haahr PE. Randomized study of the value of laparoscopy before appendicectomy. *Br J Surg.* 1993;80:922.

35. Jadallah FA, Abdul-Ghani AA, Tibblin S. Diagnostic laparoscopy reduces unnecessary appendectomy in fertile women. *Eur J Surg.* 1994; 60:41.

Chapter Forty ......

Small Bowel Obstruction and Adhesiolysis

BERNARD DALLEMAGNE

The treatment of postoperative abdominal adhesions was one of the first applications of laparoscopic surgery. Initially, patients with chronic abdominal pain syndromes were explored, and the adhesions thought likely to be causing the pain were divided, but only a few experienced surgeons have attempted to treat acute obstructions.[1-3]

With the development of instrumentation and the growing experience with laparoscopic surgical technique, acute bowel obstructions are increasingly being treated with this modality. Acute intestinal obstructions constitute a chronic surgical challenge, owing to their frequency, their predominantly postoperative origin, and the frequent complications that arise after laparotomy. Laparoscopy has a reputation for producing fewer postoperative adhesions, among other advantages, and this has caused many surgeons to consider its use in emergency situations.

INDICATIONS

There are many causes of intestinal obstruction (Table 40–1).

The diagnosis of small bowel obstruction is based initially on the patient's history, and results of contrast radiologic imaging (enemas, enteroclysis, and computed tomography scan). The diagnostic can be made with water-soluble enemas, which allow imaging up to the jejunum if Bauhin's valve is closed. This often shows the exact site of the obstruction, can detect multiple obstructions, and allows visualization of the intestinal loops. In the case of an isolated obstruction, a mark placed over the patient's abdomen near the site of the obstruction allows the surgeon to orient the placement of the trocars. The selection of patients who might benefit from a laparoscopic approach to acute small bowel obstruction is difficult, because there is no way for the surgeon to know before surgery exactly how significant the obstructions are and their exact nature. However, one element that we believe to be predictive is a history of repeated laparotomies to treat adhesions; in this case, use of lap-

aroscopy may not be indicated. In most other cases, however, we believe that an initial laparoscopic approach can be attempted.

TECHNIQUE

The procedure is performed under general anesthesia, with the patient lying supine, with the arms next to the body. The patient's shoulders, torso, and legs are secured to the operating table. This position allows the surgeon to move freely around the patient, and change the working position as dictated by the surgical findings. It also allows the table to be moved and the patient repositioned (e.g., Trendelenburg or lateral inclination) to provide surgical exposure and use gravity to help move intestinal loops out of the way.

The initial abdominal approach is in the left hypochondrium. If intestinal distention is not severe, a Veress needle is inserted and the pneumoperitoneum is created. The Veress needle can be carefully used to palpate the hypochondrium and evaluate it. If it is found to be free, then the first trocar is inserted over the needle. However, in most cases an "open" laparoscopy technique is required: a 10-mm incision is made in the left hypochondrium, then dissection is performed until the peritoneum can be incised under direct visual control. Once this is accomplished, the first trocar can be inserted and the abdomen can be insufflated, permitting visualization of the peritoneal cavity to help ensure the proper placement of the other trocars. Their exact placement will depend on the adhesions that are found, as well as the patient's history and preoperative examination. Generally, three trocars are sufficient; one for the camera, and two for the surgeon's hands. A 30° or 45° lens is recommended because the view of deep structures is difficult due to the distended small bowel.

The choice of instruments is important because the wall of the distended small bowel is fragile. The instruments must be absolutely atraumatic and we recommend the use of scissors for the section of adhesions.

TABLE 40–1. CAUSES OF BOWEL OBSTRUCTION

	Occurrence (%)
Single adhesion	49
Multiple adhesions	22
Fibrous bowel stenosis	2
Strangulated hernia (internal recurrence)	2
Appendix or sigmoid abscess	4
Crohn's disease	3
Bowel tumor	2
Biliary ileus	1
Unknown	1

Electrocoagulation should not be used except for vascularized bands, and even here the use of the hook is dangerous. If a tumor is found, the lesion is exteriorized by a short central incision and resection is performed. An intestinal resection can also be performed under laparoscopic guidance, but extraction of the specimen will require a shorter incision. In the case of a strangulated hernia, the reduction may require incision (with scissors) of the herniated ring. A careful evaluation of the herniated loop's vascular status allows judgment of its viability. Correction of the hernia is then performed. We recommended a complete examination of the entire intestine, from the jejunum to the distal ileus, so that no other sites of obstruction are overlooked.

COMPLICATIONS

The most common and feared complication is intestinal perforation, which can occur under two circumstances: when the Veress needle is inserted, or when intestinal loops are manipulated, either after simple mobilization or after liberating the loop responsible for the obstruction.

The first instance may be avoided by using care in placing the Veress needle, and use of a systematic open approach. The second and more problematic situation depends in part on the state of the small bowel wall, and injury can be avoided by the use of atraumatic instruments. If perforation does occur, an intestinal clamp is placed over the affected loop and a primary suture is performed under laparoscopy. The perforation can also be managed by clamping it under laparoscopic control, then through a short incision the intestinal segment can be exteriorized and a conventional sutured repair performed. In both cases, extensive peritoneal lavage must be performed. In cases of massive abdominal contamination or extensive bowel injury, a laparotomy is recommended.

In some cases the small bowel distention is so prominent that it makes the creation of the pneumoperitoneum difficult. Under such circumstances movement of the instruments is difficult and dangerous, risking organ perforation. In these cases an early laparotomy is preferable.

RESULTS

Between 1991 and 1998, 86 patients with acute small bowel obstruction were treated via an initial laparoscopic approach; 45 patients had a history of pelvic, gynecologic, or appendicular surgery, and 41 patients had had other surgical procedures. The causes of bowel obstruction are listed in Table 40–1.

A conversion to laparotomy was required in 23 patients (26.7%): 11 patients had multiple adhesions, small bowel perforations occurred in 4, and in 8 patients the manipulation of the small bowel and the accessibility to the adhesion was impossible and/or dangerous.

The most frequent cause of obstruction was adhesions, either single or multiple, and these were found in 71 patients. The overall success rate of the laparoscopic approach was 68% in this group of patients. If the patient had previous gynecologic, pelvic, or appendiceal surgery (n = 45), the success rate was 83%, compared to 43% for patients with other types of previous surgical procedures (n = 41).

The postoperative hospital stay averaged 4.3 days for the laparoscopy group, and 9.6 days for the converted group. Three patients died in the postoperative course (mortality, 3.4%). Causes were cardiac decompensation in a 93-year-old patient (on the 15th day) after a laparoscopic procedure, and pulmonary failure in one 83-year-old and another 85-year-old patient after laparotomy.

DISCUSSION

The treatment of small bowel obstruction is difficult; the diagnosis and choice of treatment, whether surgical or conservative, and the timing of the surgery, as well as the operative morbidity and mortality, are some of the factors to consider.

Hernias, adhesions, and tumors cause approximately 80% of intestinal obstructions.[4] Parietal hernias are generally recognizable and easily treatable; however, the therapeutic decision in patients with internal hernias and adhesions is still troublesome due to the difficulty in predicting success. A prolonged conservative treatment regimen can be painful for the patient, and may produce an ischemic perforation.[5,6] Survival rates are then much lower and operative mortality can reach 15 to 20%.[7,8]

Conventional surgery has a morbidity of about 24 to 27%, mainly due to pulmonary and parietal complications. The advantages of laparoscopic surgery have been proven for gallbladder and gastroesophageal reflux surgery, among many other procedures. Success has also been reported by gynecologists, who after years of performing exploratory laparoscopies for female infertility observed that the occurrence of postoperative adhesions is reduced by using a laparoscopic approach. These two factors have caused experienced surgeons to adopt this approach for the exploration of abdominal pain due to adhesions, as well as for the diagnosis and treatment of intestinal obstructions.

The results that have been published indicate that a laparoscopic approach is better. The morbidity and mortality rates are lower than those seen with conventional surgery; however, larger long-term studies are needed to confirm these impressions. If they are confirmed, then the operative decision could become easier, and the risk of visceral complications due to conservative treatment will also be reduced. However, a laparoscopic approach to treat intestinal occlusion is still technically difficult.

For novice surgeons, this approach should be reserved for ideal patients. Patients with a history of appendicular or genital surgery will derive the greatest benefit from this approach. But for patients who have had many abdominal procedures, the decision to take a laparoscopic approach should be considered carefully, and many of these patients will need quick conversion to laparotomy.

ADDITIONAL READING

1. Adams S, Wilson T, Brown AR. Laparoscopic management of acute small bowel obstruction. *Aust NZ J Surg*. 1993;63:39.
2. Franklin ME Jr., Dorman J, Pharand D. Laparoscopic surgery in acute small bowel. *Surg Laparosc Endosc*. 1994;4:289.
3. Cueto J, Diaz O, Gartiez D, et al. The efficacy of laparoscopic surgery in the diagnosis and treatment of peritonitis. *Surg Endosc*. 1997;11:366.
4. Oscher R, Frank R, Baumann A, et al. Results of surgical treatment of mechanical ileus of the small intestine. *Chirurg* 1991;62:614.
5. Cheadle WG, Garr EE, Richardson JD. The importance of early diagnosis of small bowel obstruction. *Am Surg*. 1988;54:565.
6. Pain JA, Colier DS, Ilanka R. Small bowel obstruction: computer-assisted prediction of strangulation at presentation. *Br J Surg*. 1987; 74:981.
7. Otamiri T, Sjodahl R, Ihse I. Intestinal obstruction with strangulation of the small bowel. *Acta Chirurgica Scandinavica* 1987;153:307.
8. Zadeh BJ, Davis JM, Canizaro PC. Small bowel obstruction in the elderly. *Am Surg*. 1985;51:470.

*L*arge Bowel Surgery

Chapter Forty-One • • • • • • •

*L*aparoscopic Colectomy

GUSTAVO PLASENCIA, MANUEL VIAMONTE, III, and MOISÉS JACOBS

Since its inception, laparoscopic colectomy has been controversial, especially as regards cancer. Several questions need to be answered: Is laparoscopic colectomy safe? Is it practical? Is it feasible? During the course of this chapter, these questions will be answered.

INDICATIONS

Although controversies exist regarding laparoscopic colectomy for cancer, very little doubt exists regarding laparoscopic colectomy for benign disease. As such, colectomies are done for diverticulitis, inflammatory bowel disease, functional disorders, polyps not amenable to colonoscopic removal, and iatrogenic trauma. Recent studies have also shown that laparoscopic colectomies for cancer show similar recurrence and survival rates to open colectomy, and are not considered a contraindication.[1,2]

BENEFITS

The benefits of laparoscopic colectomy are similar to those of laparoscopy in general. There is faster recovery, more rapid return to everyday activities. There is less pain, less ileus. The question persists, if laparoscopic colectomy offers these benefits, why the slow adoption?

First, this is difficult surgery, with learning curves that may extend to 50 cases. Second, laparoscopic colectomy involves surgery in all four quadrants and involves several different operations (right, left, transverse, sigmoid colectomies, low anterior and abdominoperineal resections). Finally, advanced laparoscopic surgery including colectomies is not being taught consistently in residency programs; as recently as 1999, only about 7% of residency programs taught advanced laparoscopic surgeries consistently.

LIMITING FACTORS

Surgeon inexperience and limited skills are probably the best reasons not to perform laparoscopic colectomy. But this is probably true of any procedure, open or laparoscopic.

As for as the anatomic limiting factors of laparoscopic colectomy, inability to safely handle the bowel and inability to dissect tissue planes are the most important reasons for conversion to open laparotomy. From very early on in our experience with laparoscopic colectomies, because at that time we were using primitive instrumentation, we have never grasped the bowel; rather, we grab the mesentery, the fat, the appendix epiploica to manipulate the bowel. We believe that grasping the bowel with laparoscopic instrumentation, without tactile sensation, may lead to bowel injuries and microperforations (which also may lead to trocar site recurrences). Therefore, when it is difficult to manipulate the bowel, as in very distended bowel, we consider this an indication for conversion.

When inflammatory or malignant reactions are such that tissue planes cannot safely be identified or separated, we also consider this an indication for conversion; this happens most often in diverticulitis or in extraserosal cancers.

FIVE STEPS OF LAPAROSCOPIC COLECTOMY

Identification

Without tactile sensation, small polyps or cancers that don't affect the serosa may be missed. Therefore, it is imperative in these cases to have preoperative identification of the site of these lesions (Fig. 41–1). Radiologic studies, such as barium enema or computed tomography, may be very helpful. Also, an x-ray showing the colonoscope at the site of the lesion is useful (Fig. 41–2). Another useful preoperative technique is to tattoo the site of the lesion by injecting dye, such as India ink. These dyes may last up to weeks and are helpful when identifying a site of

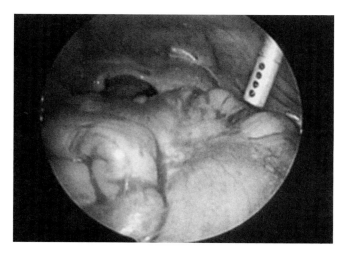

Figure 41–1. Colon cancer. See Color Section.

previous colonoscopic polyp removal that requires a colectomy at a later time.

Of course, when faced with a situation where a lesion cannot be identified intraoperatively, intraoperative colonoscopy may be indicated, especialy for left-sided lesions. When intraoperative colonoscopy is performed, care must be taken not to distend the

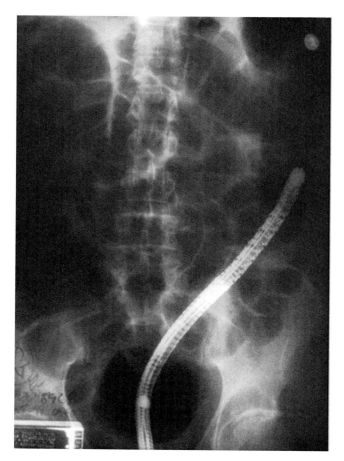

Figure 41–2. Colonoscope.

bowel. Therefore, proximal control with bowel clamps must be exerted so as to not distend the proximal bowel. Once the site has been localized, colonoscopic decompression of the distended bowel should be done.

Obviously, if the lesion cannot be identified, the operation should be converted to open laparotomy.

Mobilization

As we practice laparoscopic colectomy, it is a laparoscopic-assisted procedure where the bowel is exteriorized through a small incision. Thus the object of the mobilization of the colon is to let it reach, without tension, the anterior abdominal wall where the extraction site is to be placed.

Devascularization

Once the bowel has been mobilized, devascularization must be performed. This can be done extracorporeally or intracorporeally. When dealing with malignancy, it must be done intracorporeally, as in this method, the base of the mesentery can be reached and an oncologic resection performed.

In laparoscopy, efficiency is of the utmost concern. If one thinks of the anatomy of the colon as a tree trunk, and one divides the right and left side of the colon into two trees and the inferior mesenteric artery (IMA) becomes the tree trunk for the left side of the colon, it becomes more efficient and becomes an oncologic resection if the IMA is transected at its base, rather than staying close to the bowel walls and transecting, ligating individual tributaries.

In this fashion, by ligating and transecting the IMA at the base of the mesentery and by ligating and dividing the right ileocolic, the right colic, and the right branch of the middle colic at their bases, one can perform an efficient and oncologic resection of the left and right colon.

Resection

In laparoscopic-assisted colectomy, the bowel is brought out extracorporeally and resected. The bowel can either be brought out as a loop or as a tube. In cases of cancer, the extraction site is a muscle-transecting incision and must be large enough so as not to squeeze the colon. In addition, the extraction site must be protected with a plastic sleeve, so as to not allow direct contact between a tumor and the abdominal wall.

Anastomosis

The anastomosis, in the case of a right colectomy, transverse colectomy, or true left colectomy, is done extracorporeally. In the case of a sigmoid colectomy or low anterior resection, the anastomosis is done intracorporeally.

TECHNICAL TIPS

1. Tuck both arms by the patient's side. This gives the surgeons full 360-degree access to the patient without having to worry about the arm boards.
2. Work in the direction of the scope. This makes the hand-eye coordination much easier.
3. Do not grasp the bowel—use atraumatic instruments. It is thought that one of the modes of trocar and extraction site

implantations is tumor cells transported through instrumentation. By not grasping the bowel, but rather by pushing, pulling, or grasping the mesentery or fat about the bowel, one minimizes the risk of tumor transplantation and bowel injuries.

4. Use gravity as a second assistant to minimize the use of trocars. Let gravity push the small bowel away from the colon.

5. Patient positioning: Allow the use of gravity to bring the portion of the colon being manipulated to the forefront. For example, right side up brings the right colon to the front.

6. Use angled scopes. These give a perspective more similar to open surgery, "looking down at the bowel." This is especially useful when looking at the rectosigmoid region and into the pelvis for a low anterior resection or abdominoperoneal resection, or when looking down at the mesentery.

7. Use both hands, as in open surgery; therefore two surgeons and four trocars are required. The surgeon should stand opposite the side of the pathology. The trocars should be placed in a way to avoid "sword-fighting."

8. By placing tension on the mesentery, blood vessels become taut and bow out like violin strings, making the named blood vessels easy to identify even in obese patients.

9. Minimize irrigation when there is blood in the field. Aspirate instead of irrigating the blood all over the abdominal cavity.

10. Use an ultrasonic scalpel. This is more efficient and decreases the length of surgery, because one instrument dissects, coagulates, and transects, instead of requiring other equipment.

LAPAROSCOPIC RIGHT COLECTOMY

Preoperative Setup and Trocar Placement

The operating room setup and trocar placement for laparoscopic right hemicolectomy are shown in Figure 41–3. The operating room setup consists of two television monitors positioned to the patient's right—one at the patient's head and the other at the foot of the table. The surgeon and assistant stand on the left side of the patient.

Four trocars are required. The first trocar is inserted into the umbilicus. The location of the secondary trocars is as follows: suprapubic (midway between the pubis and umbilicus); subxyphoid (two fingerbreadths below the costal margin and to the left of the midline); and left lateral to the left of the midclavicular line, midway between the umbilical and subxyphoid trocars. The patient is placed in a Trendelenburg position with a left lateral oblique rotation.

Mobilization and Devascularization

The peritoneal attachments to the right colon are sharply incised by using ultrasonic scissors. Mobilization of the peritoneal attachments continues from the terminal ileum to the hepatic flexure. Takedown of the hepatic flexure is facilitated by the 30-degree angled laparoscope. The patient is repositioned in a reverse Trendelenburg position.

Dissection of the peritoneal attachments of the right colon progresses toward the transverse colon. The duodenum must be identified at this point (Fig. 41–4). Next the hepatocolic ligament is transected (Fig. 41–5). Dissection progresses to the midtransverse colon. The terminal ileum, cecum, ascending colon, and proximal transverse colon are completely mobilized, and the right colon should reach the anterior abdominal wall without tension.

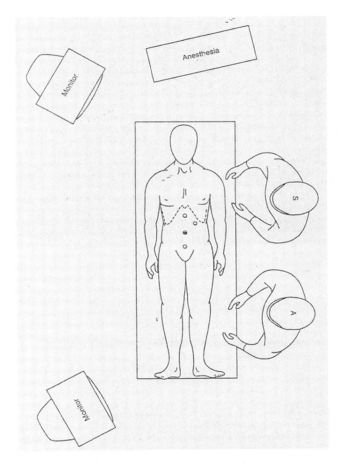

Figure 41–3. Operating room setup, right colon.

The surgeon and assistant place upward traction on the mesentery, causing the ileocolic, right colic, and right branch of the middle colic arteries to become pronounced and taut (Fig. 41–6). The vessels are controlled using vascular endostaples or sutures.

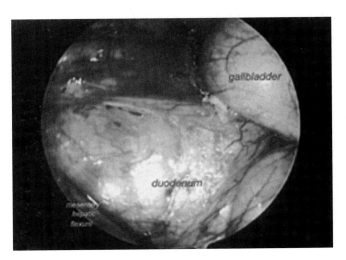

Figure 41–4. Exposure of duodenum. See Color Section.

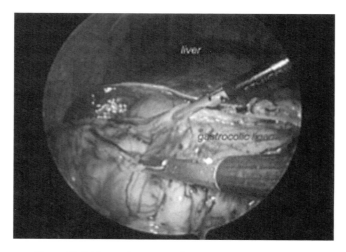

Figure 41–5. Transecting gastrocolic ligament. See Color Section.

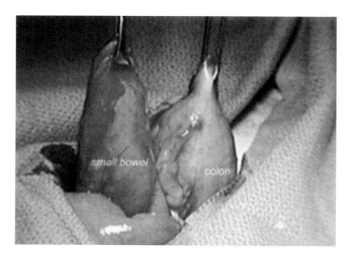

Figure 41–7. Exteriorization, right colon. See Color Section.

Resection and Anastomosis

After mobilization and devascularization are accomplished, the bowel should reach the anterior abdominal wall without tension. If sufficient mobilization and devascularization have been accomplished, a 4 to 6-cm muscle-splitting incision in the right lower quadrant is created. If the operation is performed for suspected malignancy, a plastic sleeve is used to protect the incision. The colon is now delivered extracorporeally through this protected incision (Figs. 41–7 to 41–9).

The exteriorized colon is resected and an extracorporeal anastomosis is performed.

Clinical Caveats

• When performing laparoscopic colorectal surgery for malignancy, avoid bulky lesions.
• When dissecting the peritoneal attachments of the right colon, avoid wide dissection. The common error is to dissect far more laterally than usual; this may lead to additional hemorrhage and possible ureteric injury.

• The duodenum and its developmental adhesions must be dissected before any vascular ligation is carried out.
• The patient must be secured to the operating room table because patient slippages have occurred.
• Before making an incision, place the colon at the point of exteriorization and make the incision there. Proper location of the incision will facilitate the procedure. It is important to have the colon reach the anterior abdominal wall without tension.
• Always reintroduce the pneumoperitoneum and observe trocar sites and anastomosis before the conclusion of the procedure.

LAPAROSCOPIC SIGMOID COLECTOMY/ LOW ANTERIOR RESECTION

Preoperative Setup and Trocar Placement

The preoperative setup of the operating room and the trocar placement for either laparoscopic sigmoid resection or low anterior resection is the same (Fig. 41–10). Two television

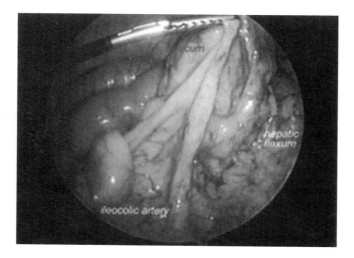

Figure 41–6. Ileocolic artery. See Color Section.

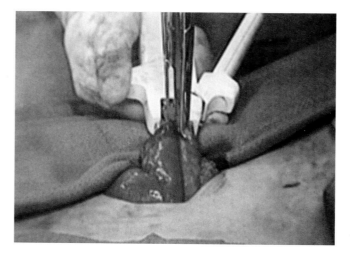

Figure 41–8. Ileocolic anastamosis. See Color Section.

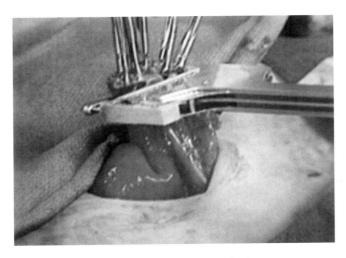

Figure 41–9. Closure. See Color Section.

monitors are positioned at either side of the patient's feet. The surgeon stands to the right of the patient while the camera operator/assistant is to the left of the patient. The patient is placed in a modified lithotomy position. The first trocar is inserted through the umbilicus. A diagnostic laparoscopy is performed before the secondary trocars are placed. The second trocar is inserted in the left midclavicular line, approximately two fingerbreadths below the left costal margin. The video camera is subsequently reinserted into this trocar before additional trocars are placed. The third trocar is placed laterally in the anterior axillary line (left flank) at the level of the umbilicus. The fourth trocar is inserted into the suprapubic area.

Mobilization and Devascularization

The peritoneal attachments of the sigmoid colon are sharply incised and the sigmoid is resected superiorly and medially. The pulsation of the iliac artery is visualized and serves as an anatomic landmark for identifying the ureter (Fig. 41–11).

The inferior mesenteric artery and vein are identified, and can be identified anteriorly when appropriate traction is placed on the mesentery. The proper traction bows the mesentery and vessels like violin strings.

The surgeon develops the avascular plane proximal to the inferior mesenteric artery (IMA). Inspection through this window allows visualization of the ureter to minimize potential iatrogenic injury to the ureter before IMA ligation. A vascular stapling device (Fig. 41–12) is used to secure the vessel. If there is any doubt before vascular ligation that the ureter is not clearly identified, this may be an indication for conversion.

Resection and Anastomosis

For a sigmoid colectomy, the distal margin of resection is at the level of the rectosigmoid junction; for a low anterior resection, the distal margin will be at the appropriate level determined by the anatomic location of the lesion. The devascularization of the mesentery is completed so that the bowel is cleared of mesentery at the distal point of resection. The endolinear stapling device is applied to the bowel at the distal resection margin and the bowel is transected (Fig. 41–13).

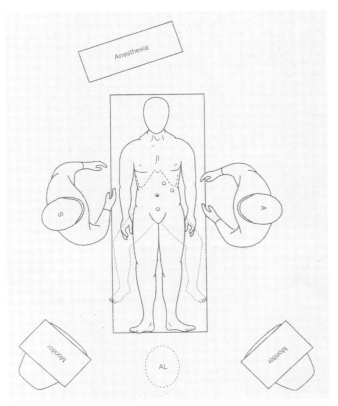

A

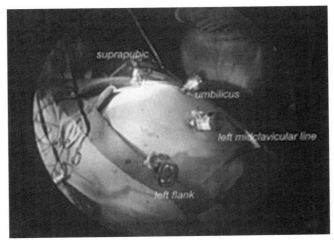

B

Figure 41–10. A. Operating room setup, sigmoid colon. **B.** Sigmoid trocars.

An incision is made incorporating the previously made suprapubic trocar site and the proximal bowel is delivered through this incision. We routinely use a plastic sleeve to protect the incision from potential contamination. The proximal margin of resection is selected (Fig. 41–14). A purse-string suture is applied to the proximal margin of resection. The bowel is then resected extracorporeally. After selecting the appropriate circular stapler size, the surgeon places the anvil and head of the circular stapler in the proximal colon and the purse-string is securely tied (Fig. 41–15). The proximal bowel is

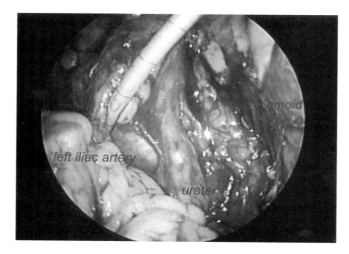

Figure 41–11. Left ureter, iliac artery. See Color Section.

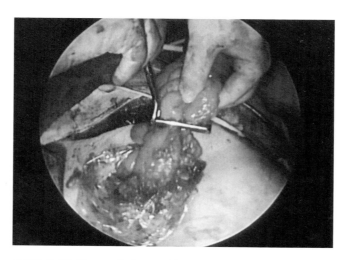

Figure 41–14. Placement of purse-string sutures, proximal margins; bowel exteriorized through plastic sleeve. See Color Section.

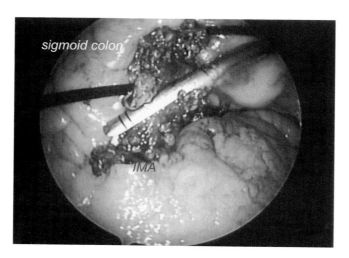

Figure 41–12. Stapler transecting IMA. See Color Section.

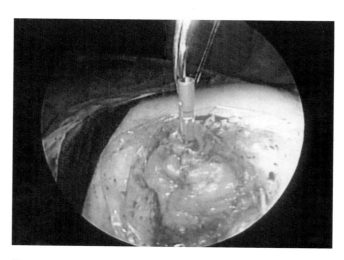

Figure 41–15. Proximal bowel with head of circular stapler. See Color Section.

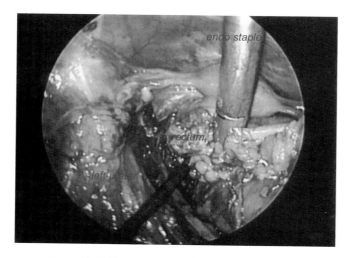

Figure 41–13. Rectosigmoid transection. See Color Section.

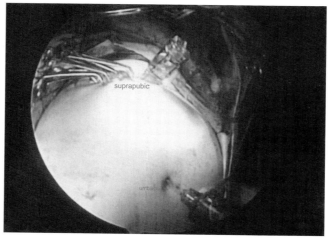

Figure 41–16. Extraction site with towel clips. See Color Section.

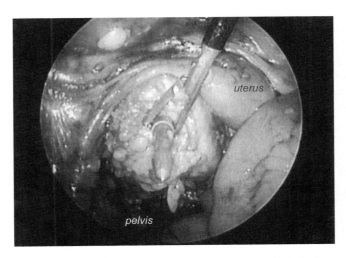

Figure 41–17. Circular stapler penetrating rectal stump. See Color Section.

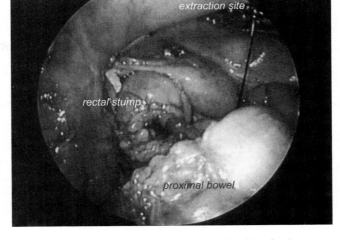

Figure 41–18. Marriage of circular stapler. See Color Section.

returned to the abdominal cavity. The incision is closed with towel clips and a pneumoperitoneum is reestablished (Fig. 41–16).

Intracorporeal Anastomosis

The shaft of the circular stapling device is passed transanally and the spearhead is extruded through the rectal stump's staple line (Fig. 41–17). The surgeon and assistant marry the head and anvil with the shaft. When union between the anvil and shaft has been accomplished, the circular stapler is closed (Fig. 41–18).

The "doughnuts" are visually inspected and the integrity of the anastomosis is tested by insufflating air through a sigmoidoscope passed transanally while the anastomosis is submerged in saline.

If anastomotic leak is demonstrated, the surgeon has several options: direct intracorporeal suture repair of a small anterior defect, extending the suprapubic incision in a transverse fashion for a directed open repair, proximal diverting ostomy, and conversion to an open procedure.

Clinical Caveats

- During the mobilization and devascularization phase of laparoscopic sigmoid resection and low anterior resection, the pulsation of the iliac artery serves as an anatomic landmark for the identification of the ureter.
- An avascular plane developed proximally to the inferior mesenteric artery allows visualization of the ureter before vascular ligation. This serves as an important safeguard to minimize iatrogenic injury to the ureter.

Postoperative Course

GI Function. Most laparoscopic colectomy patients have bowel sounds within 24 to 48 hours and can therefore be given liquids during this time. The diet is gradually advanced over the third or fourth postoperative day and a passage of flatus or bowel movement usually occurs within this time. The incidence of an ileus is between 10 and 20%.

Narcotics. Pain is very subjective. Therefore, the use of narcotics/analgesics depends on the individual patient. However, studies by Wexner, Nelson, and others have shown significant decrease in the time that patients require analgesia, and in the amount of narcotics required. This is probably due to the smaller incisions and less manipulation done in laparoscopic colectomies. By inference, as has been shown by Milson, there is faster recovery of pulmonary function and therefore fewer pulmonary complications.

Disability. Again, as has been shown by multiple authors, including Wexner and Nelson, postoperative recuperation is significantly faster for laparoscopic patients versus those undergoing conventional open colectomies. It can be said that return to normal activities after laparoscopic colectomies is twice as fast as after open colectomy.

REFERENCES

1. Lujan G, Pasencia M, Jacobs M, et al. Long term survival after laparoscopic colon resection for cancer: complete five year follow up. *Dis Colon Rectum* 2002;45:491.
2. Lacy AM, Garcia-Valdecasas JC, Delgado S, et al. Laparoscopy-assisted colectomy versus open colectomy for treatment of non-metastatic colon cancer: a randomised trial. *Lancet* 2002;359:2224.

Chapter Forty-Two ● ● ● ● ● ●

Colonic Resection in the Treatment of Colorectal Carcinoma: Multicentric Study with Prospective Comparison of Traditional and Laparoscopic Methods

MORRIS E. FRANKLIN, JR., JORGE E. BALLI, and J. ARTURO ALMEIDA

Early in 1990, as the value of minimally invasive surgery particularly for laparoscopic cholecystectomy, appendectomy, and diagnostic purposes became apparent, we became extremely interested in application of this method to patients with colonic-related diseases and in particular carcinoma. We took the initiative of going to the laboratory to perform a series of experiments on animals, including laparoscopic resection, maintenance of sterility, minimization of contamination, and maintenance of oncologic principles. After 6 months in the laboratory and the successful completion of a number of totally intracorporeal laparoscopic colectomies in animals, in which we demonstrated short- and long-term results and equivalency of operations, we felt that a human trial was in order. We took the information gleaned, as well as our experience in laparoscopic surgery for benign disease in our patient population (including the treatment of appendectomies, perforated ulcers, hernia, cholecystectomy with common bile duct exploration, and intestinal obstruction), to the attention of the surgery department of our hospital and the Institutional Review Board and obtained approval to initiate a human trial.[1-4]

MATERIALS AND METHODS

The ensuing human trial is the basis of this discussion as well as subsequent long-term follow-up. We felt that a comparison between open and laparoscopic surgery was indeed indicated, but because of logistics in private practice, we were unable to establish a randomized prospective study of laparoscopic versus open surgery. Therefore, we embarked upon a prospective comparison of open and laparoscopic colon surgery between our group of laparoscopic surgeons and a group of well-known open colorectal surgeons in San Antonio, Texas. The study proposal was to compare the outcome in a prospective manner in a group of patients undergoing either open or laparoscopic colon resection for carcinoma.[5]

The initial study started in June 1990 and extended through April 1996,[6] but long-term follow-up continued through the year 2000. The purpose of the study was to demonstrate the effects of laparoscopic colon surgery for cancer, compare long-term survival and recurrence data, and to have this in the form of a prospective study. The study was designated to evaluate sequential patients with no patients being excluded. The same pathologists were used in each limb of the study. The follow-up was to be at designated intervals in an organized manner, and the data gathering was to be performed by third parties other than the surgeons. The parameters to be considered were the stage of the disease at the time of surgery, type of resection performed, length of hospitalization, complications, recurrence of carcinoma, and deaths. Also evaluated in the study were pathologic evaluations such as number of lymph nodes retrieved and margins of resection. Return to full function was also evaluated.

There were 266 patients in the laparoscopic group and 224 patients in the open group. The male-female ratio in each of the groups was comparable. The mean age was 64 years in the open group and 67 years in the laparoscopic group (Table 42–1). There was a concern about the unequal number of patients who underwent one type of procedure compared to another in either group. Thus, a careful analysis of the types of resections was carried out, and it was found that, within a few percentage points, both the laparoscopic and the open group had comparable numbers (Figs. 42–1 and 42–2). It was interesting that there was a tremendous amount of criticism of initial laparoscopic surgery with the performance of an inordinate number of abdominoperineal resections (APR), but

TABLE 42–1. DEMOGRAPHICS

	LCR	OCR
Total number	266	224
Male	119	123
Female	147	101
Average age	67 years	64 years

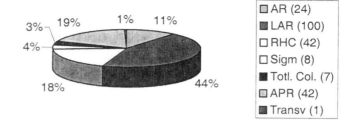

Figure 42–2. Open colon resection (OCR), by type of procedure. (AR, anterior resection; LAR, low anterior resection; RHC, right hemicolectomy; Sigm, sigmoidectomy; Totl. Col., total colectomy; APR, abdominoperineal resection; Transv, transverse colectomy.)

when this study was evaluated carefully, it was found that the open group had almost 19% APRs compared to 14% for the laparoscopic group. The remainder of the types of resections were essentially the same.

The intraoperative, perioperative, and postoperative complications were also compared (Tables 42–2 and 42–3). The primary intraoperative complication for open colon resection was bleeding. There was one visceral perforation and one ureteral injury in the open group. In the laparoscopic group, the primary complication again was either bleeding or visceral perforation. The laparoscopic visceral perforations occurred in both sigmoid and low anterior resection cases of the laparoscopic group. These were recognized at the time of surgery, and were repaired without difficulty. The majority of these perforations were in response to taking down severe adhesions from prior surgery. There were no instances of missed visceral perforations in the laparoscopic group. There were several patients with stage IV cancer who had massive bleeding and were converted to open surgery.

The conversions of laparoscopic surgery were evaluated by stage and by type of surgery (Table 42–4). There was no pattern established in the type of surgical procedure that resulted in laparoscopic conversion, however; the conversions appeared to be primarily related to the disease process. There were 11 conversions (3%) to open in the laparoscopic group, one of which was for concurrent stomach cancer. The blood loss was compared between the laparoscopic and open groups, and it was found that the laparoscopic group in all categories and stages of cancer, had less blood loss compared to the open group. The only deviance was that of a total colectomy, where the estimated blood loss for the laparoscopic group was 250 mL and the open group was 220 mL.

The staging of the cancer was felt to be very important, and a comparison was made between the numbers of patients in the open group versus the laparoscopic group by stage. It was found

that the groups were comparable, and there was not an overly heavy weighting of laparoscopic surgery for early-stage cancer. As a matter of fact, the greatest number of cancers was in stage II in each of the groups, with 113 patients in the open group and 108 in the laparoscopic group. This is represented in Figure 42–3.

The most difficult part of any long-term ongoing study is that of follow-up. A significant number of patients, particularly in the open group, were lost to follow-up. In the laparoscopic group in this study, however, there were no patients lost to follow-up. The laparoscopic group had an overall follow-up of 37 months in stage I and the open group had and overall follow-up of 25 months. This held true dynamically for the years of this study. Stage II and stage III patients had similar follow-up data. The overall hospital stays of these patients were also compared. The average hospital stay for the laparoscopic group was 5.2 days and for the open group was 9.35 days depending on the concurrent problems with the patient. It must be mentioned that a significant number, almost 10% of the patients in the laparoscopic group, were patients who had been turned down for open surgery as being too sick to survive an open procedure.

In the later stages of the study, we began to look at survival, recurrence, and death rates by stage, comparing the laparoscopic group with the open group. We found in all groups that the laparoscopic patients fared as well or perhaps better than the open group. This was most noticeable in the stage II and stage III patients, as outlined in Tables 42–5 to 42–8. In the cumulative data, it is to be noted that there was a 12.4% death and recurrence rate at 6 years into the study with the laparoscopic group compared to a 19.1% cumulative death and recurrence rate in the open group (Table 42–9).

DISCUSSION

While no definite conclusions can be drawn from this study because of the lack of randomization, nevertheless it appears that laparoscopic surgery at least has long-term results similar to those obtained with open surgery. The results of this study were compiled for a report in 1996.[6] Since that time, we have continued to follow our patients in great detail, with 357 in the laparoscopic group (Table 42–10), but have been unable to obtain adequate data on the patients who had undergone open colon resection. Now 10 years into our study with an overall follow-up of greater than 80 months, but with more than half of our patients having more than

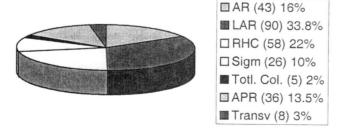

Figure 42–1. Laparoscopic colon resection (LCR), by type of procedure. (AR, anterior resection; LAR, low anterior resection; RHC, right hemicolectomy; Sigm, sigmoidectomy; Totl. Col., total colectomy; APR, abdominoperineal resection; Transv, transverse colectomy.)

TABLE 42–2. COMPLICATIONS OF LCR

Early (<30 Days)		Late (>30 Days)	
Urinary tract Infection	11	Pulmonary	2
Pulmonary	17	Anastomotic stenosis	3
Ileus	8	Intra-abdominal abscess	1
Bleeding	7	Fistula	1
Pelvic hematoma	1	Urinary tract infection	2
Wound infection	1	Intestinal obstruction	3
Intra-abdominal abscess	1	Diarrhea	1
Deep vein thrombosis	1	Rectal bleeding	1
Anastomotic stenosis	3		
Acute acalculous cholecistitis	1		
TOTAL	51 (19%)		14 (5.2%)

TABLE 42–3. COMPLICATIONS OF OCR

Early (<30 Days)		Late (>30 Days)	
Urinary tract infection	5	Post incisional hernia	2
Pulmonary	6	Anastomotic recurrence	4
Ileus	11	Intra-abdominal abscess	1
Bleeding	1	Fistula	1
Intestinal obstruction	1	Urinary tract infection	2
Wound infection	14	Intestinal obstruction	6
Intra-abdominal abscess	1	Wound infection	3
Deep vein thrombosis	1	Parastomal hernia	1
Anastomotic dehiscence	4		
Peritonitis	1		
Pulmonary embolus	1		
TOTAL	51 (23.8%)		20 (8.9%)

TABLE 42–4. CONVERSIONS FROM LCR TO OCR

Stage	Type of Procedure	Reason for Conversion
I	AR	Concurrent gastric carcinoma
I	RHC	Bleeding
II	LAR	Bleeding
III	LAR	Big tumor and visceral perforation
III	LAR	Obstructed sigmoid colon
III	RHC	Bleeding
III	AR	Visceral perforation
IV	RHC (2 cases)	Massive tumor in right upper quadrant
IV	APR	Massive bleeding
IV	RHC	Tumoral invasion in sup. mesenteric vein, bleeding
IV	APR	Massive tumor

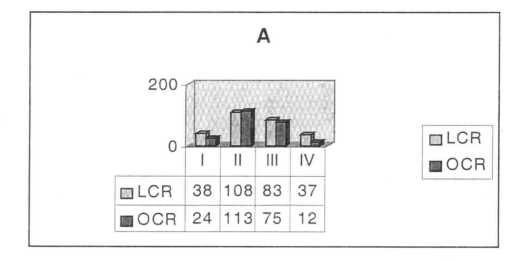

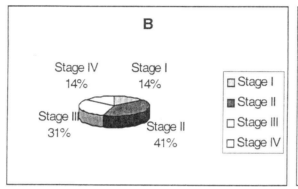

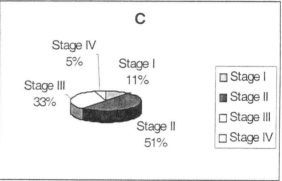

Figure 42–3. A. Number of cases by stage in the laparoscopic colon resection group (LCR) and the open colon resection group (OCR). B. Percent of cases by stage in the LCR group. C. Percent of cases by stage in the OCR group.

5 years since the time of the surgery, our death and recurrence rate remains essentially the same. As a matter of fact, when comparing our results with those of a recently published study by Bokey et al,[7] laparoscopic surgery seems to have better results, as our overall death and recurrence rate is less than 25% at 5 years for all patients compared to 49% for Bokey et al.

In summary, when we look at the 5-year study described earlier, we have demonstrated no deleterious effects of laparoscopy. When oncologic principles are observed and care is taken to prevent trocar site implants, these patients do not have an increased risk for this problem, and in this particular group of patients there were no implantations found. We have found that the resections are comparable, and similar complications occur. There is a definite shorter hospitalization with the laparoscopic group. There is equal survival, but obviously more studies and longer follow-up are needed.

One of the most important aspects of laparoscopic surgery is a virtual lack of wound problems. The impact of wound-related complications from open surgery has never been studied in detail. However, in this study we found that the incidence of open wound complications approached 14% when wound infections and hernias in the wound sites were included. However, in the laparoscopic group this remains less than 1%. We feel that this is

TABLE 42–5. SURVIVAL, RECURRENCE, AND MORTALITY, STAGE I TUMORS

	LCR		OCR	
	#	%	#	%
Alive with no evidence of disease	36	95	23	96
Alive with evidence of disease	1	2.6	1	4
Mortality	1	2.6	0	0
TOTAL	38		24	

TABLE 42–6. SURVIVAL, RECURRENCE, AND MORTALITY, STAGE II TUMORS

	LCR		OCR	
	#	%	#	%
Alive with no evidence of disease	90	83.3	96	85
Alive with evidence of disease	8	7.4	10	9
Mortality	10	9.2	7	6
TOTAL	108		113	

TABLE 42–7. SURVIVAL, RECURRENCE, AND MORTALITY, STAGE III TUMORS

	LCR		OCR	
	#	%	#	%
Alive with no evidence of disease	62	74.6	50	66.6
Alive with evidence of disease	9	11	16	21
Mortality	12	14.4	9	12
TOTAL	83		75	

TABLE 42–8. SURVIVAL, RECURRENCE, AND MORTALITY, STAGE IV TUMORS

	LCR		OCR	
	#	%	#	%
Alive with no evidence of disease	0	0	0	0
Alive with evidence of disease	23	62	9	75
Mortality	14	38	3	25
TOTAL	37		12	

TABLE 42–9. RECURRENCE RATE AND MORTALITY (CUMULATIVE DATA 6 YEARS INTO THE STUDY).

	LCR		OCR	
	#	%	#	%
Stage I	2		1	
Stage II	18		17	
Stage III	21		25	
TOTAL	41[1]	15	43	19

[1]8 patients died for different causes without evidence of cancer. Corrected rate (12%).

TABLE 42–10. UP-TO-DATE[1] SERIES OF LAPAROSCOPIC COLON RESECTIONS FOR CANCER.[2]

Total	357	laparoscopic colon resections for cancer
Male	187	(52.3%)
Female	170	(47.6%)
LAR	123	
Sig	35	
AR	54	
RHC	80	
Transv	11	
APR	47	
Total colectomy	7	
Conversion to open procedure	20 cases (5.6%)	

[1]As of January 2001.

[2]0% trocar site implants.

extremely significant and stands alone as a fairly good reason to pursue performance of laparoscopic surgery for a variety of conditions, perhaps even cancer if long-term survival data remains constant.

TROCAR SITE IMPLANTATIONS

There is no doubt that trocar site implantations with recurrent cancer have occurred. There was an alarming jump in this entity in the early to mid 1990s, and it continues to be a problem.[8–11] When one looks very carefully at the basic science data and at the patients who had trocar site implants, several problems become apparent. The first is that the majority of the trocar site implants reported in the literature have been at extraction sites where cancer-laden tissue was pulled through a tight wound without adequate protection. The second is that trocar site implantations occur in advanced disease processes such as stage III and stage IV carcinoma. Third, most trocar site implants have occurred in the hands of surgeons who are not experienced in laparoscopic colon resection and, as a matter of fact, initiated laparoscopic colon surgery for cancer prior to perfecting techniques with benign disease.

We have identified, and have practiced from day one, based on our laboratory work and common sense, several precautions that we think can aid in prevention of trocar site implants. These are given in Table 42–11.[12]

TABLE 42–11. AIDS AND TECHNIQUES IN PREVENTION OF TROCAR SITE IMPLANTS

Preresection

- Minimize tissue trauma by proper placement of trocars, perpendicular to peritoneum
- Trocar fixation
- Prevent CO_2 leakage
- Minimize handling of tumor
- Colonoscopy and intraluminal irrigation with Betadine
- Clean instruments with Betadine after each use

Resection

- Do not cut through or handle the tumor
- High vascular ligature
- Control colon lumen specifically of resected specimen

Postresection

- Irrigation of trocars with 3.5% Betadine prior to removal
- Bagging the specimen
- Protect extraction site
- Drain peritoneal cavity prior to deflating, to prevent the "slosh" phenomenon
- Trocar site closure
- Deflate the abdomen with trocars in place
- Avoid liquid spillage when closing the trocar site
- Closed suction drain use
- Irrigation of trocar and extraction site with Betadine and water

Other Aids

- Adequate training
- Adequate technique
- Proper patient selection
- Surgical team training
- Adequate laparoscopic equipment for colon resection

The first issue is that of adequate training. We feel that no surgeon should embark upon laparoscopic colon resection for cancer without first having adequate training by spending time with someone who is well-versed in laparoscopic colon resection. Initial experiences with colon resections should be for benign disease, not cancer, except perhaps stage IV cancers. We feel that when adequate experience has been obtained in benign disease, one can progress to cancer resection with better results.

The second issue in the prevention of trocar site implantation is to meticulously avoid handling the tumor. Chipping, manipulating, or perforating a colon cancer all lead to problems, whether the procedure is done laparoscopically or is open.[13,14] Third, the trocars must be securely attached to the abdominal wall. Loss of a trocar with subsequent loss of pneumoperitoneum, bathing of the site with intraperitoneal fluid, and contamination of the wound with tumor cell-laden instruments, is believed to be a primary cause of remote trocar site implantations.[15,16] Therefore, meticulous attention should be paid in placing trocars, and they should be securely attached with sutures to the skin of the abdomen so that they are not inadvertently removed during the procedure. Oncologic principles must be observed in laparoscopic colon surgery. This includes controlling the ends of the colon initially as well as high ligation of vessels and isolation of the specimen as soon as possible.

The fourth issue is that of bagging the specimens, and we recommend bagging all colon specimens resected for cancer prior to removal.[17] We have on occasion used wound protectors, but do not feel this is the best method available. Fifth, we perform intraoperative colonscopy with Betadine lavage of the colon in 100% of our patients. We feel that this helps in preventing exfoliation and, to this date, have had absolutely no implantations or recurrent cancer at the line of resection.[18]

Sixth, all trocars must be thoroughly washed with a tumoricidal solution prior to removal.[19,20] We have preferred 3.5% Betadine, as this appears to be the most effective and economical solution to irrigate trocars. We also irrigate the trocar site very thoroughly with Betadine after removal. Closure of the trocar site with intraoperatively placed sutures seems to be very important, and there are several basic science studies that have demonstrated the need to close trocar sites to prevent cancer implantations.[15,21,22]

CONCLUSIONS

We feel that there has been a tremendous amount of adverse publicity in regard to laparoscopic colon resection for cancer as well as laparoscopic oncologic treatment of cancer in general. Some of this criticism has been well founded, and is the fault of laparoscopic surgeons for not having more thorough basic science evidence for their observations. This basic science material is now available and demonstrates that, for the most part, laparoscopic surgery is as safe as open surgery for a variety of oncologic maneuvers. In laparoscopic colon surgery, a tremendous learning curve is present. However, in the hands of skilled surgeons who practice colorectal surgery and laparoscopic colon resection for cancer and who observe oncologic principles, this is a feasible, safe, and effective procedure with equal or better long-term results compared with those reported in the literature for open surgery.

REFERENCES

1. Phillips EH, Franklin ME, Carroll BJ, et al. Laparoscopic colectomy. *Ann Surg.* 1992;216:703.
2. Franklin ME, Ramos R, Rosenthal D, et al. Laparoscopic colonic procedures. *World J Surg.* 1993;17:51.
3. Jacobs M, Verdeja JC, Goldstein HS. Minimally invasive colon resection. *Surg Endosc.* 1991;1:144.
4. Franklin ME, Dorman JP. Laparoscopic surgery in acute small bowel obstruction. *Surg Endosc.* 1994;4:1289.
5. Franklin ME, Rosenthal D, Norem RF. Prospective evaluation of laparoscopic colon resection versus open colon resection for adenocarcinoma: A multicenter study. *Surg Endosc.* 1995;9:811.
6. Franklin ME, Rosenthal D, Abrego-Medina D, et al. Prospective comparison of open vs. laparoscopic colon surgery for carcinoma. *Dis Colon Rectum.* 1996;39:S53.
7. Bokey EL, Chapuis PH, Fung C, et al. Postoperative morbidity and mortality following resection of the colon and rectum for cancer. *Dis Colon Rectum.* 1995;38:480.
8. Alexander RJ, Jaques BC, Mitchell KG. Laparoscopically assisted colectomy and wound recurrence. *Lancet.* 1993;341:249.
9. Fusco MA, Paluzzi MW. Abdominal wall recurrence after laparoscopic-assisted colectomy for adenocarcinoma of the colon: A report of a case. *Dis Colon Rectum.* 1993;36:858.
10. Vukasin P, Ortega AE, Greene FL, et al. Wound recurrence following laparoscopic colon cancer resection: Results of the American Society of Colon and Rectal Surgeons laparoscopic registry. *Dis Colon Rectum.* 1996;39:S20.
11. Wexner SD, Cohen SM. Port site metastases after laparoscopic colorectal surgery for cure of malignancy. *Br J Surg.* 1995;82:295.
12. Balli JE, Franklin ME, Almeida JA, et al. How to prevent port site metastasis in laparoscopic colorectal surgery. *Surg Endosc.* 2000; 14:1034.
13. Reilly WT, Nelson H, Schroeder G, et al. Wound recurrence following conventional treatment of colorectal cancer: A rare but perhaps underestimated problem. *Dis Colon Rectum.* 1996;39:200.
14. Martínez J, Targarona EM, Balgue C, et al. Port site metastasis. An unresolved problem in laparoscopic surgery: A review. *Int Surg.* 1995;80:315.
15. Schneider C, Jung A, Reymond MA, et al. Efficacy of surgical measures in the prevention of port-site recurrences in a porcine model. *Surg Endosc.* 2001;15:121.
16. Kim SH, Milson JW, Gramlich TL, et al. Does laparoscopic vs. conventional surgery increase exfoliated cancer cells in the peritoneal cavity during resection of colon cancer? *Dis Colon Rectum.* 1998;41:971.
17. Franklin ME, Diaz JA, Balli JE. Mechanical means for prevention of trocar site cancer implantation. In: Reymond MA, Bonjer HJ, Kockerling F. eds. *Port-Site Wound Recurrences in Cancer Surgery.* Springer; 998:91.
18. Franklin ME, Balli JE. Intracorporeal anastomosis. In: Wexner SD, ed. *Protocols in General Surgery and Laparoscopic Colorectal Surgery.* Wiley;1998.
19. Neuhaus SJ, Watson DI, Ellis T, et al. Efficacy of cytotoxic agents for the prevention of laparoscopic port-site metastases. *Arch Surg.* 1998;133:762.
20. Docherty JG, McGregor JR. Purdie CA, et al. Efficacy of tumoricidal agents in vitro and in vivo. *Br J Surg.* 1995;82:1050.
21. Reymond MA, Schneider C, Kastl S, et al. Pathogenesis of port-site recurrences. *J Gastrointest Surg.* 1998;2:406.
22. Lacy AM, Delgado S, García-Valdecasas JC, et al. Port site metastases and recurrence after laparoscopic colectomy. A randomized trial. *Surg Endosc.* 1998;12:1039.

Chapter Forty-Three • • • • • •

Colonic Carcinoma Implants at Port Sites

**ANTONIO MA DE LACY, S. DELGADO, C. BALAGUÉ, A. CASTELLS,
J.C. GARCÍA-VALDECASAS, and J.M. PIQUÉ**

INTRODUCTION

The advantages offered by laparoscopy in general surgery has made its use almost routine for certain procedures. However, one of the more controversial topics involving laparoscopic surgery remains laparoscopic resection of malignancy. Colon cancer is the malignancy which is treated laparoscopically most often, and there are a number of reports of patients with colon cancer.

Although laparoscopic colorectal resection yields more patient comfort than open surgery, there are two points to be addressed before laparoscopy is widely accepted for this indication: (1) what the oncologic criteria are that would make its use feasible; and (2) whether its use induces increases in recurrence and changes dissemination patterns.

Several series have shown that laparoscopy is technically feasible, and tumors can be resected to the same extent and lymph nodes harvested similarly to open laparotomy (Table 43–1). But several reports of early tumor recurrence at port sites after laparoscopic resection, including Dukes A lesions (Table 43–2), have led some to believe that the pattern of disease recurrence may be altered by the laparoscopic approach. That is likely the main reason laparoscopic resection of colorectal cancer has not been widely accepted.[1]

The question is whether the incidence of wound implants is increased by laparoscopy. There is a low incidence of wound implants (less than 1%) in large series of colorectal cancer cases treated with open surgery (Table 43–3). The logical explanation for these implants is that they are due to manipulation of the tumor and resulting direct implantation of viable exfoliated tumor cells. Surgeons have tried different lavage fluids to reduce the number of free tumor cells in the abdominal cavity, and consequently the risk of implants. But this is not a new problem that came with increased use of laparoscopy, though the incidence of implants appears to be higher with the use laparoscopy than in laparotomy.[2]

In the search for answers to this phenomenon, a great number of experimental studies have been developed and some parameters have been proposed to evaluate the possible influence of the differential factors of laparoscopy.

IMMUNE RESPONSE

When surgery is performed to resect the tumor, the surgery also has a negative impact on host immune defenses due to temporary suppression of immune function that may encourage tumor growth. Before the introduction of laparoscopy, several experimental studies demonstrated this negative influence of surgery. Laparotomy is associated with accelerated tumor growth and an increased rate of metastatic tumor formation in the early postoperative period, as compared with results of use of anesthesia alone.[3,4]

With regard to the pneumoperitoneum, during in vitro incubation of colonic cancer cells, the elevated pressure caused suppression of tumor cell growth. However, the same increased intraperitoneal pressure is associated with promotion of subcutaneous and intraperitoneal tumor growth in a rat model.[5] These contradictory results could be explained by immunosuppression caused by higher intraperitoneal pressures. When laparotomy and CO_2 laparoscopy have been compared with regard to tumor growth in either a subcutaneous location or in the lungs, some studies have demonstrated an increase in tumor size or in the incidence of metastases, with the rate being lowest in the anesthesia control group, followed in ascending order by the CO_2 pneumoperitoneum group and the sham laparotomy group. The results in the CO_2 pneumoperitoneum group, although worse than those of the anesthesia control group, are significantly better (smaller or fewer tumors) than the results in the laparotomy group.[6–8] Some experimental studies[9–11] have been done using gasless laparoscopy in hopes of improving the results, and there was significantly less tumor growth

TABLE 43–1. OPEN LAPAROTOMY VERSUS LAPAROSCOPY

Author	Year	No. of Pts.	Margins	n Lymph Nodes
Hoffman	1994	63	ns	ns
Musser	1994	41	—	ns
Saba	1995	45	—	ns
Franklin	1996	406	ns	ns
Gellman	1996	75	—	ns
Lord	1996	81	ns	ns
Stage	1997	29	ns	ns
Lacy	1997	122	ns	ns
Schwenk	1997	60	ns	ns
Milsom	1998	109	ns	ns

ns = nonsignificant.

after gasless than after CO_2 laparoscopy. However, the use of abdominal lifting systems is still problematic due to pressure and tissue trauma in the abdominal wall, and significant technical difficulties remain.

Major open surgery results in a period of relative immunosuppression, with alterations in serum cytokine levels, macrophage and neutrophil function, lymphocyte proliferation rates, delayed-type hypersensitivity (DTH) response, and differential expression of lymphocyte and mononuclear cell surface antigens.[12–16] When the immune response of laparotomy and CO_2 pneumoperitoneum were compared, some studies found that laparoscopic procedures were associated with significantly less immunosuppression than open procedures.[17–19]

The group led by Lee[20] found that cancer cells incubated in vitro with plasma from mice that had undergone sham laparotomy proliferated significantly faster than cells incubated with plasma from animals that had undergone CO_2 insufflation or anesthesia alone. The authors believe that these results suggest the existence of a laparotomy-related plasma-soluble factor that is responsible, at least in part, for the increase in tumor growth seen after laparotomy, and that this substance could be platelet-derived growth factor (PDGF).

There is definitely an early postoperative period of immunosuppression, but it appears to be less severe with laparoscopy than laparotomy. This improved immune response after laparoscopy

TABLE 43–2. PORT-SITE METASTASES

Without Tumor Manipulation		
Author/Year	Procedure	Tumor
Siriwardena/93	Conventional and laparoscopic	ADK pancreas
Watson/95	Gastroenterostomy	ADK pancreas
Jorgensen/95	Laparoscopic diagnosis	ADK pancreas
Nieveen/96	Laparoscopic diagnosis	ADK pancreas
Nieveen/96	Laparoscopic diagnosis	ADK stomach
Early Tumors		
Author/Year	Tumor	Stage
Nduka/94	Gallbladder carcinoma	No invasion
Prasad/94	Colon ADK	Dukes A
Lauroy/94	Colon ADK	Dukes A
Fingerhut/95	Colon ADK	Dukes A

ADK = adenosine kinase.

TABLE 43–3. LAPAROTOMY: INCIDENCE OF WOUND RECURRENCE

Author/Year	No. of Patients	Incidence
Hughes/1983	1603 patients	1%
Reilly/1996	1711 patients	0.6%

could result in better clinical results in a long-term follow-up, but this requires further study. On the other hand, if laparoscopy is associated with a lower rate of tumor growth that may be caused by a more intact immune response, how do we explain the appearance of port-site metastases? It is clear that other factors are at work here.

Port-site metastases can be thought of as local recurrences. It is possible that local factors might influence the incidence of port-site metastases. These factors may well be related to the differences of the laparoscopic vs. the open approach: elevated intra-abdominal pressure and CO_2 insufflation.

LOCAL FACTORS

Pneumoperitoneum creates a closed environment with elevated pressure. It has been theorized that the presence of a pneumoperitoneum creates a pressure gradient with a subsequent outflow of gas and aerosolized tumor cells through the port wounds, called the chimney effect (Fig. 43–1).[2] These cells may become trapped in the trocars via a mechanism described by Murthy et al.[21] With the removal of the trocars, these cells could become implanted in the abdominal wall, a process facilitated by the ischemia and local necrosis. But the chimney effect requires the aerosolization of the cells, a factor not yet clearly demonstrated. Furthermore, even if this factor exists, some believe that it is irrelevant.[22,23] Other investigations have shown that tumor cell movement within the abdominal cavity seems to be more influenced by instrumental contamination than by the aerosolization of tumor cells by the insufflated gas.[24,25]

Study by electronic microscopy has been carried out on the effects of high pressure on mesothelial cells, and alterations are seen in cell shape, the number of microvilli, and the intercellular junctions.[26] Disruption of the peritoneal surface seems to increase tumor cell adherence.[27,28]

It has also been observed that tumor cells grow more rapidly in a CO_2 environment compared with helium or room air. Additionally, CO_2 has been shown to cause intracellular acidosis and increased intracellular calcium levels (Fig. 43–1).[29]

Another local factor to consider is wound conditions. Local factors such as ischemia and necrosis probably influence local tumor adherence, but this has not been definitively proven. Using rat laparoscopic models, Jacobi et al[30] and Bouvy et al[31] observed that local ischemia or necrosis could help explain the significant increase in metastases at trocar sites where ischemia was induced by crushing or electrocautery.

MANIPULATION AS A FACTOR

Though the factors listed above may have some influence on port-site metastases, it appears that manipulation of the tumor plays an important role in the induction of port-site metastases.[32] The

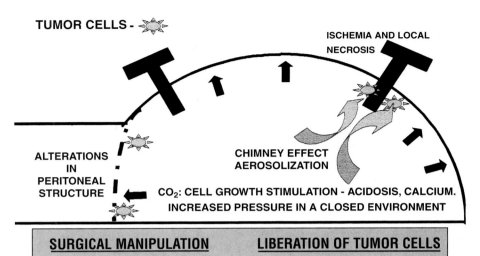

Figure 43–1. Local factors influencing port-site metastases.

surgical technique used and experience of the surgeon have been shown to play a major role in tumor metastasis in both laparoscopic and conventional cancer surgery.[33,34] Since the introduction of laparoscopy, there has been a decreased incidence of port-site metastases secondary to improved technique and more careful tumor manipulation in patients with malignancy. The wide variation in the incidence of port-site metastases reported after colorectal surgery might also be explained by the differences in level of experience of surgical teams and differences in intraoperative manipulation of the tumors.

It is impossible to evaluate metastasis using tumor cells in suspension because they do not effectively simulate the human milieu. These models indicate that tumor cells are liberated, but do not permit the study of how the cells become separated from the primary tumor, which is the most important event in the entire process, and has obvious relevance to analyzing the effects of surgical manipulation.

Although it is not known how many cells are liberated during cancer resection, when we see the high incidence of trocar and intra-abdominal implants occurring in many of the animal studies, we can postulate that the concentration of cells in the inoculum is

quite high. Wu et al[35] determined the port-wound tumor incidence after laparotomy and laparoscopy using two different tumor inoculum concentrations. Significantly more animals developed wound tumors after CO_2 pneumoperitoneum with the high-dose tumor inoculum, while little difference was seen in the open surgery group with low-dose inoculum (Fig. 43–2).

Lee et al,[36] carried out experiments using a murine solid tumor model in spleen. In four studies, they observed a reduction in the rate of laparoscopic port-site implants from the first to the second study, with the rate declining to a level similar to that for open splenectomy (Fig. 43–3). The results of the third and fourth studies confirmed the results of the first two. The port-site tumor rate was directly related to the laparoscopic experience level of the surgeon. This influence of tumor manipulation seems agree with the recent clinical results. Initially the incidence that authors reported was more than 1%. Wexner and Cohen[37] reviewed several series and found an incidence of around 4%. But when we examine more recent larger series, we see that currently the incidence is no more than 1% (Table 43–4). The most recent data from two large laparoscopic colectomy series with mean follow-up of >2 years indicate an incidence of 0 to 1.2%.[38,39]

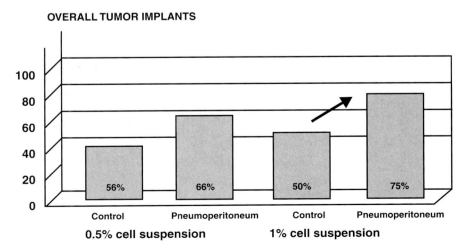

Figure 43–2. Influence of tumor inoculum concentration on tumor implantation. *(Reproduced from Wu et al.[35])*

PORT-SITE METASTASES (%)

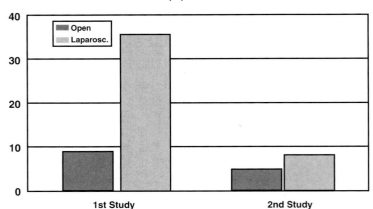

Figure 43–3. Influence of the learning curve on port-site metastases. *(Reproduced from Lee et al.[36])*

This suggests that the learning curve could have a strong influence, and that perhaps port-site metastases are not an inevitable result of tumor manipulation during laparoscopic surgery. However, manipulation is just one factor to consider, and perhaps it's possible that the degree of manipulation coupled with a higher or lower rate of liberated tumor cells may determine the level of influence of the other local factors.

Although several recent investigators have described favorable experiences with laparoscopic cancer surgery, an issue of such magnitude demands prospective randomized trials that can provide the statistical power to definitively resolve the issue. Only such large trials can definitively determine if port-site metastases are the inevitable result of the technical approach, or if their development is more closely related to the learning curve.

TABLE 43–4. LAPAROSCOPIC COLON SURGERY FOR CARCINOMA—INCIDENCE OF PORT-SITE METASTASES

Author	Patients (n)	Incidence (%)
Laparoscopic Surgery		
Berends (1994)	14	21
Drouard (1995)	507	2.4
Fingerhut (1995)	92	3.2
Boulez (1996)	117	2.5
Gellman (1996)	58	1.7
Hoffman (1996)	130	0.8
Franklin (1996)	192	0
Kohler (1997)	47	0
Fielding (1997)	149	0
Lacy (1998)	130	0.7
Milsom (1998)	55	0
Balli (1999)	320	0
Köckerling (1999)	>500	0.4
Hatley (2000)	57	0
Conventional Surgery		
Hughes (1983)	1.603	1
Reilly (1996)	1.711	0.6

RESULTS OF A CONTROLLED TRIAL OF LAPAROSCOPICALLY-ASSISTED COLECTOMY VERSUS OPEN COLECTOMY FOR THE TREATMENT OF ADENOCARCIONOMA OF THE COLON

There remains significant controversy surrounding the use of laparoscopic techniques in curative colorectal cancer surgery. We believe significant benefits to patients may be derived from laparoscopic surgery in cancer. Also, we do not believe there are increased risks of early recurrences in these patients if they are operated on by surgical teams experienced in laparoscopic colorectal cancer surgery. At present, laparoscopy represents the standard surgical procedure for many abdominal disorders. However, there is still some reluctance to accept this approach for oncologic therapy, because it has been suggested that it may favor tumor dissemination. In order to clarify this concern, we developed a protocol in the Hospital Clínic of Barcelona to establish the efficacy of laparoscopically-assisted colectomy (LAC) in the treatment of colon cancer, regarding short-term outcome, tumor relapse, and survival, by means of a randomized clinical trial in which this approach was compared with conventional open colectomy (OC). In previous reports, our group and others have demonstrated that pathological staging of the specimen is not influenced by the surgical procedure, and also that laparoscopic technique is associated with a lower degree of immunosuppression. In addition, short-term outcome clearly favors minimally invasive surgery, and no differences in the probability of recurrence and survival have been found in preliminary analysis from ongoing clinical trials. Nevertheless, to definitively rule out any meaningful negative influence of laparoscopy on patient prognosis, results regarding both tumor recurrence and survival from a large series of patients that were carefully selected and followed for a long period of time were needed.

We included patients from September 1993 to July 1998. All patients with nonmetastatic colon cancer admitted in the Institute of Digestive Diseases of the University of Barcelona were evaluated for entry into the study. Patients were stratified by tumor location and subsequently allocated to LAC or OC in a random fashion. The inclusion criterion was diagnosis of adenocarcinoma of the colon above 15 cm from the anal verge. Exclusion criteria were: colon cancer located at the transverse colon, presence of distant metastases or adjacent organ invasion, intestinal obstruction, past surgical history of previous colon operation, and refusal to participate in the study. Adjuvant therapy and postoperative follow-up were identical in both treatment groups. Postoperative surveillance consisted of medical history, physical examination, and laboratory studies including serum carcinoembryonic antigen (CEA) levels 1 month after surgery and every 3 months thereafter. At each visit, the patient's symptoms were recorded and wound scars were examined for subcutaneous metastases. Abdominal ultrasonography/computed tomography and chest radiographs were performed every 6 months, and total colonoscopy once a year. When colonoscopy was incomplete, a combination of sigmoidoscopy and barium enema was undertaken.

Results

Of the 208 patients included in the study, 106 patients were allocated to LAC and 102 patients to OC. Both groups were identical regarding baseline characteristics, except for age (LAC, 68 ± 12 years vs. OC, 71 ± 11 years; $p = 0.03$) and serum CEA level (LAC, 16 ± 40 ng/mL vs. OC, 6 ± 11 ng/mL; $p = 0.02$). LAC was converted to laparotomy in 12 (11%) patients because of tumor invasion of adjacent organs. One patient from each group was lost to follow-up. Patients of the LAC group recovered faster than those of the OC group in regard to passing flatus (36 ± 31 hours vs. 53 ± 32 hours; $p < 0.001$), oral intake (54 ± 42 hours vs. 81 ± 45 hours; $p < 0.001$), and postoperative stay (5.3 ± 2.1 days vs. 7.1 ± 3.3 days; $p < 0.001$). Associated morbidity was also significantly lower in the LAC group (RR: 0.50; 95% CI: 0.29 to 0.84), although it did not influence perioperative mortality (RR: 0.65; 95% CI: 0.36 to 1.16). After a median follow-up of 39 months (range: 22 to 80 months), the probability of cancer-related survival was higher in the LAC group ($p < 0.02$). The Cox model identified LAC as independently associated with a reduction in the risk of tumor relapse (RR, 0.39; 95% CI, 0.19 to 0.82), death from any cause (RR, 0.48; 95% CI, 0.23 to 1.01), and cancer-related death (RR, 0.38; 95% CI, 0.16 to 0.91) relative to OC.

The results of ongoing large multicenter trials will definitively prove or disprove a higher survival rate in patients with colon cancer treated laparoscopically. The results of the current study definitively rule out any negative impact of the laparoscopic approach in colon cancer related either to port-site metastases or to inappropriate oncologic resections. This result seems to prove the benefits of laparoscopy for short-term outcome, and the technique appears to be the preferable approach for colon cancer resection, as it is for other surgical indications. Confirmation of these data may have some meaningful implications. Since results obtained in patients with stage III tumors from the LAC group were similar to those seen in patients with stage II lesions from the OC group, the role of adjuvant therapy should be re-evaluated both in terms of eligibility criteria and actual benefit.

Conclusion

LAC is more effective than OC for the treatment of colon cancer in terms of morbidity, tumor recurrence, and survival.

REFERENCES

1. Whelan RL. Laparotomy, laparoscopy, cancer, and beyond. *Surg Endosc.* 2001;3:??.
2. Hubens G, Pauwels M, Hubens A, et al. The influence of a pneumoperitoneum on the peritoneal implantation of free intraperitoneal colon cancer cells. *Surg Endosc.* 1996;10:809.
3. Eggermont AM, Steller EP, Marquet RL, et al. Local regional promotion of tumor growth after abdominal surgery is dominant over immunotherapy with interleukin-2 and lymphokine-activated killer cells. *Cancer Detect Prev.* 1988;12:421.
4. Goshima H, Saji S, Furata T, et al. Experimental study on preventive effects of lung metastases using LAK cells induced from various lymphocytes: special references to enhancement of lung metastases after laparotomy stress. *J Jpn Surg Soc.* 1989;90:1245.
5. Lee SW, Whelan RL, Southall JC, et al. Abdominal wound tumor recurrence after open and laparoscopic-assisted splenectomy in a murine model. *Dis Colon Rectum.* 1998;41:824.
6. Allendorf JD, Bessler M, Kayton M, et al. Tumor growth after laparoscopy and laparotomy in a murine model. *Arch Surg.* 1995;130:649.
7. DaCosta ML, Redmond HP, Finnegan N, et al. Laparotomy and laparoscopy differentially accelerate experimental flank tumor growth. *Br J Surg.* 1998;85:1439.
8. DaCosta ML, Redmond P, Boucher-Hayes DJ. The effect of laparotomy and laparoscopy on the establishment of spontaneous tumor metastases. *Surgery* 1998;124:516.
9. Jones DB, Guo LW, Reinhard MK, et al. Impact of pneumoperitoneum on trocar site implantation of colon cancer in hamster model. *Dis Colon Rectum.* 1995;38:1182.
10. Jacobi CA, Sabat R, Ordemann J, et al. Peritoneal instillation of taurolidine and heparin for preventing intraperitoneal tumor growth and trocar metastases in laparoscopic operations in the rat model. *Langenbecks Arch Chir.* 1997;382:31.
11. Bouvy ND, Marquet RL, Jeekel H, et al. Impact of gas(less) laparoscopy and laparotomy on peritoneal tumor growth and abdominal wall metastases. *Ann Surg.* 1996;224:694.
12. Eilber FR, Morton DL. Impaired immunologic reactivity and recurrence following cancer surgery. *Cancer* 1970;25:362.
13. Heys SD, Deehan DJ, Eremin O. Interleukin-2 treatment in colorectal cancer current results and future prospects. *Eur J Surg Oncol.* 1994;20:622.
14. Lee SW, Gleason NR, Ssenymanturno K, et al. Colon cancer tumor proliferative index is higher and tumor cell death rate is lower in mice undergoing laparotomy vs insufflation. *Surg Endosc.* 1998;12:514.
15. Nakashima M, Sonoda K, Watanabe T. Inhibition of cell growth and induction of apoptotic cell death by the human tumor-associated antigen RCAS1. *Nat Med.* 1999;5:938.
16. Hansbrough JF, Bender EM, Zapata-Sirvent R, et al. Altered helper and suppressor lymphocyte populations in surgical populations in surgical patients: a measure of postoperative immunosuppression. *Am J Surg.* 1984;148:303.
17. Allendorf JDF, Bessler M, Whelan RL, et al. Postoperative immune function varies inversely with the degree of surgical trauma in a murine model. *Surg Endosc.* 1997;11:427.
18. Allendorf JDF, Bessler M, Whelan RL, et al. Better preservation of immune function after laparoscopic-assisted vs open bowel resection in a murine model. *Dis Colon Rectum.* 1996;10:s67.
19. Griffith JP, Everitt NJ, Lancaster F, et al. Influence of laparoscopic and conventional cholecystectomy upon cell-mediated immunity. *Br J Surg.* 1995;82:677.
20. Lee SW, Gleason N, Zhai C, et al. Increased platelet-derived growth factor (PDGF) release after laparotomy stimulates systemic tumor growth in mice. *Surg Endosc.* 2000;14(Suppl. 1):S155.
21. Murthy S, Summaria L, Miller R, et al. Inhibition of tumor implantation at sites of trauma by plasminogen activators. *Cancer* 1991;68:1724.

22. Prasad A. Avery C. Abdominal wall metastases following laparoscopy. *Br J Surg.* 1994;81:1693.
23. Lacy AM, Delgado S, Garcia-Valdecasas JC, et al. Port site metastases and recurrence after laparoscopic colectomy. A randomized trial. *Surg Endosc.* 1998;12:828.
24. Hewett PJ, Thomas WM, King G, et al. Intraabdominal cell movement during abdominal carbon dioxide insufflation and laparoscopy. *Dis Colon Rectum.* 1996;39(Suppl):7.
25. Thomas WM, Eaton MC, Hewett PJ. A proposed model for the movements of cells within the abdominal cavity during CO_2 insufflation and laparoscopy. *Aust NZ J Surg.* 1996;66:105.
26. Schaeff B, Paolucci V, Henze A. Electron microscopic study on mesothelial cells after laparoscopic operations. Data presented at the Second Workshop of Experimental Laparoscopic Surgery, 1998, Rotterdam, The Netherlands.
27. Goldstein DS, Lu ML, Hattori T. Inhibition of peritoneal tumor cell implantation: model for laparoscopic cancer surgery. *J Endourol.* 1993;7:237.
28. Farrell TM, Johnson AB, Metreveli RE, et al. Fascial closure limits metastases after pneumoperitoneum. *Surg Endosc.* 1999;13(Suppl):33.
29. Wildbrett P, Jacobi CA. Influence of carbon dioxide and helium on intracellular calcium and pH levels in tumor cells and peritoneal macrophages. Data presented at the Second Workshop of Experimental Laparoscopic Surgery, 1998, Rotterdam, The Netherlands.
30. Jacobi CA, Ordemann J, Bohm B, et al. Inhibition of peritoneal tumor cell growth and implantation in laparoscopic surgery in a rat model. *Am J Surg.* 1997;174:359.
31. Bouvy ND, Giuffrida MC, Tseng LN, et al. Effects of carbon dioxide pneumoperitoneum, air pneumoperitoneum, and gasless laparoscopy on body weight and tumor growth. *Arch Surg.* 1998;133:652.
32. Lee SW, Southall J, Allendorf J, et al. Traumatic handling of the tumor independent of pneumoperitoneum increases port site implantation rate of colon cancer in a murine model. *Surg Endosc.* 1998; 12:828.
33. Leather AJM, Kockan G, Savage F, et al. Detection of free malignant cells in the peritoneal cavity before and after resection of colorectal cancer. *Dis Colon Rectum.* 1994;37:814.
34. Balli H. How to prevent port-site metastases in laparoscopic colorectal surgery. *Surg Endosc.* 1999;13(Suppl 1):4.
35. Wu JS, Jones DB, Guo LW, et al. Effects of pneumoperitoneum on tumor implantation with decreasing tumor inoculum. *Dis Colon Rectum.* 1998;41:141.
36. Lee SW, Bessler M, Whelan RL. Port-site tumor recurrence rates in a murine laparoscopic splenectomy model decreased with increased experience. *Surg Endosc.* 1998;12:514 (Abstract).
37. Wexner SD, Cohen SM. Port site metastases after laparoscopic colorectal surgery for cure of malignancy. *Br J Surg.* 1995;82:295.
38. Franklin ME, Rosenthal D, Abrego-Medina D, et al. Prospective comparison of open versus laparoscopic colon surgery for carcinoma: five year results. *Dis Colon Rectum.* 1996;39:S35.
39. Fleshman JW, Nelson H, Peteers WR, et al. Early results of laparoscopic surgery for colorectal cancer: retrospective analysis of 372 patients treated by Clinical Outcomes of Surgical Therapy (COST) study group. *Dis Col Rectum.* 1996;39:S53.

Appendix: Conclusions of the Consensus of the E.A.E.S., Published with the Authorization of the Secretary of the Association, Dr. Jack Jackimowicz

EAES Experts' Opinion Conference on Colonic Cancer by Elective Laparoscopy, European Association for Endoscopic Surgery, Eighth International Congress

TECHNICAL PROCEDURES: TIPS AND TRICKS

LAPAROSCOPIC RESULTS VERSUS EVIDENCE-BASED SURGERY

Edited by the EAES
J. Mouiel and A. Montori
J. Mouiel, University of Nice Sophia-Antipolis, Dept. of Digestive Surgery, Video-Surgery and Liver Transplantation Hopital L'Archet 2, BP 3079, 06202 Nice Cedex 3
A. Montori, Dept. of Surgery University of Rome, La Sapienza, 00 199 Roma, Italy
Thursday, June 29, 2000
Nice, France

Does laparoscopic surgery involve specific risks in oncology? That is the question facing surgeons following several reports of neoplastic contamination of port sites after laparoscopic colectomies for cancer.

Indeed an alarming rate of port-site metastases was published in the first reports, even in patients with Dukes A and Dukes B tu-

mors, so it was recommended to avoid colectomy for colonic cancer, except in controlled trials and several randomized studies that were organized by national societies.

Criteria for Evaluating the New Technologies. The criteria for evaluating the new technologies are based on the recommendations of B. Jennett and served as a basis for the consensus conferences of the European Association for Endoscopic Surgery (EAES).

The 5 states of technological evaluation

1. FEASIBILITY: Technical performance, applicability, safety, complications, morbidity, mortality.
2. EFFICACY: Benefit for the patient demonstrated in the centers of excellence.
3. EFFICIENCY: Benefit for the patient under normal conditions, in other words, reproducible results with broad application.
4. COST: Benefit in terms of cost-efficiency.
5. GOLD STANDARD: This methodology is essential if we wish to avoid making the same mistakes as have been made in the past with surgical procedures that were widely used and then abandoned, such as surgery for prolapsed organs, internal ligature of the mammary in myocardial infarction, treatment of hypertension with sympathectomy, hypothermia for gastric bleeding, internal carotid/external carotid anastomoses for stroke, and the use of the laser in angioplasty.

The evidentiary value depends on the scientific value of the studies.

The scientific value of the studies includes 4 levels: controlled randomized study, 3; controlled prospective study (parallel or historical controls), 2; study with review of the literature, database analysis, expert reports, 1; and noncontrolled study, anecdotal report, 0.

The strongest scientific proof is provided by prospective studies with randomized control, which avoids bias due to contingency of recruitment, technique, and follow-up.

This acknowledgment applies to the evaluation of all of the new technologies, since before proceeding with a controlled prospective study, the feasibility of the procedure must be first determined in order to make it easily reproducible without complication. As an example, we cite renal dialysis, where half of the first 30 patients did not benefit from the method in any way; and heart valve surgery, where somewhat fewer than half of the patients died.

Current Level of Evaluation of Colectomy for Cancer.
Feasibility has been determined as we did a comparison of the technical performance, applicability, safety, complications, morbidity, and mortality with the recommended conventional surgical procedures, based on the many publications accumulated to date.

Efficacy has been established, in other words, the benefit for the patients has been demonstrated in centers of excellence which accumulated several hundred patients each. The preliminary results of the EAES experts suggest that the rate of the port-site metastasis is actually very low in comparison with the previous reports. It has been suggested that this may be due to the learning curve of laparoscopic colectomy for cancer. Indeed, skilled surgeons apply oncologic rules without manipulation of the tumor and use preventive measures to avoid dissemination.

Efficiency of the procedure, demonstrating the benefit to the patient under normal conditions, in other words, adequate reproducible results with broad application, is **not yet established.** The penetration rate of laparoscopic colectomy for cancer is very low, either by lack of experience or by fear of dissemination.

The direct as well as the indirect costs have not been fully evaluated with respect either to the surgical procedures themselves or with respect to surgical treatment versus medical treatment. Thus at the present time the procedure cannot be considered the gold standard in the treatment of this disease.

Recommendations of the EAES. Laparoscopic colectomy for cancer is probably **highly surgeon-dependent** as are all other surgical procedures. This is why the EAES recommendations specify to:

- Perform laparoscopic colectomy for cancer only after a personal experience of 20 colectomies for benign disease;
- Select the patients and choose the cases. It is recommended to begin with technically simpler cases such as right colectomy, and to perform more complex cases after acquisition of skills. The best method is to be assisted by an experienced surgeon.
- Respect oncologic principles and avoid manipulation of the tumor; first approach the vascular pedicles, perform an adequate resection with large margins and complete lymphadenectomy; Use preventive measures. Avoid multiple passages of instruments through the trocars that are secured to the abdominal wall; use a wound protector and port-site irrigation with tumoricidal agents such as povidone iodine; carefully close all peritoneal wounds; perform aspiration of the pneumoperitoneum instead of exsufflation; and above all, until the results of the large randomized studies are in, perform no laparoscopic colectomy for cancer outside a prospectively randomized trial.

Indeed it is mandatory to be sure that patients are not penalized by use of a minimal procedure which, under the pretext of less invasive surgery and reduced pain, shorter hospitalization, and easier rehabilitation, actually ends up having the maximal negative influence on long-term results.

References

Presentations Made During the Expert's Opinion Conference on Colonic Cancer by Elective Laparoscopy During the Eighth International Congress of Endoscopic Surgery of the E.A.E.S. in Nice, France, June 28 to July 1, 2000

H.J. Bonjer, Ph. Wittich, G. Kazemier: Port-Site Recurrences in Laparoscopic Surgery.

M.E. Franklin Jr., J.A. Almeida, A.A. Santos, J.L. Glass, D. Abrego: Laparoscopic Colectomy for Cancer: 8-Year Experience and Follow-Up.

E. Lezoche, F. Feliciotti, A.M. Paganini, M. Guerrieri, R. Campagnacci, A. De Sanctis: Colonic Cancer by Elective Laparoscopy versus Open Procedures. Quality Control of Laparoscopic Curative Resections for Colorectal Cancer.

F. Kockerling, M.A. Reymond, and the Laparoscopic Colorectal Surgery Study Group: Laparoscopic Colectomy vs. Conventional Surgery in the Treatment of Colon Carcinoma. A Randomized Study.

A.M. Lacy, S. Delgado, J.C. Garcia Valdecasas, M. Pera: Lap Results vs. Evidence-Based Surgery. Results of Randomized Studies and National Trials.

Chapter Forty-Four • • • • • •

*L*aparoscopic Colectomy for Benign Disease

THOMAS BIRDAS, PAVLOS PAPASAVAS, DANIEL GAGNÉ,
and PHILIP CAUSHAJ

The surgical world has witnessed a true revolution during the last decade of the 20th century and the beginning of the 21st with the advent of laparoscopic surgery. The first hesitant steps with laparoscopic cholecystectomy have led to an explosion, a result of which is that no intra-abdominal organ or disease process is considered beyond laparoscopic reach. Jacobs, Verdeja, and Goldstein[1] published the first report of laparoscopic-assisted colectomy in 1991. Since then an increasing number of applications in the field of colorectal surgery have been developed, although significant controversy still exists for some diseases, particularly colorectal malignancies.

INDICATIONS IN BENIGN DISEASE

Essentially the entire spectrum of colorectal disorders can be and has been approached laparoscopically. A substantial body of literature exists on the laparoscopic management of diverticular disease as well as inflammatory bowel disease. These entities are covered elsewhere in this text and will not be reviewed again here. The main focus of this chapter will be on the management of colonic polyps and rectal prolapse.

Polyps

Little controversy exists on the optimal management of colonic polyps. Endoscopic removal is the rule. This is particularly true of pedunculated polyps. Size is an important determinant of endoscopic resectability, with variation depending on the expertise and comfort level of the endoscopist. For large sessile polyps (Figure 44–1), the threshold for surgical referral is lower. Malignant polyps can be treated adequately with polypectomy alone if there is no vascular or lymphatic invasion of the stalk, if they are not poorly differentiated, and if the resection margin is negative for cancer by at least 2 mm. Although open segmental colon resection is still the gold standard

for those polyps that cannot be removed endoscopically, a laparoscopic approach is intuitively logical (Figure 44–2). In these cases, communication between the endoscopist and the surgeon is of crucial importance, since elimination of tactile stimuli during laparoscopic surgery severely impairs the surgeon's ability to localize the polyp, an often painstaking task even in open colectomies. If the gastroenterologist has not tattooed the polyp, it is imperative that intraoperative colonoscopy be performed. An interesting concept suggested by Prohm et al[2] is for the colonoscopic resection of a polyp under laparoscopic guidance and assistance in particular for polyps located in unfavorable sites or large polyps associated with an increased risk for perforation or incomplete removal. Laparoscopic resection (total colectomy) has also been advocated in the management of patients with familial adenomatous polyposis (FAP).

Rectal Proplapse

Rectal prolapse is one of the most controversial conditions when it comes to its operative management. Over 200 different operations have been described in the surgical literature. Hippocrates was perhaps the first to suggest a "minimally invasive" approach: "The patient, hanging by his heels, be shaken, for so the gut, by this shaking, will return to its place." A variety of transabdominal and perineal procedures have recently become popular. Of these, transabdominal rectopexy with or without resection of the redundant sigmoid can be performed laparoscopically. The final word on the role of laparoscopy in the management of rectal prolapse has not been written.

Other Indications

Laparoscopically assisted colectomy has also been described in the management of other, less common conditions, such as sigmoid volvulus, arteriovenous malformations, and colonic inertia. The literature is limited to isolated case reports and anecdotal studies.

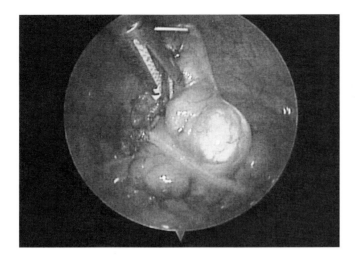

Figure 44–1. Colon polypectomy. See Color Section.

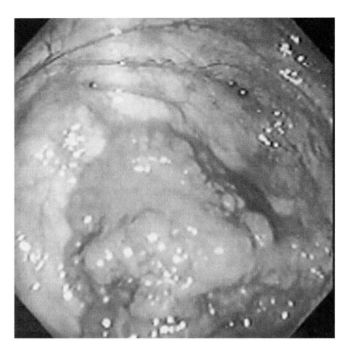

Figure 44–2. Cecal polyps as seen with the colonoscope. See Color Section.

OPERATIVE TECHNIQUES

Segmental colonic resections for polyps are performed in the standard fashion, as described elsewhere in the text. The obvious difference is that the resection margins do not need to be as wide as for malignant processes. Once again, the importance of preoperative localization of the polyp cannot be overemphasized. We will review the technique for transverse colectomy for benign polyps, as there are some special technical considerations.

The operating room setup is similar to that for other laparoscopic colon surgery. The positions of the surgeon and the assistant change during the operation, as the surgeon mobilizes the flexures unless the surgeon is positioned between the lower extremities. Four trocars are usually inserted: umbilicus, at each midclavicular line just superior to the umbilicus, and at the left anterior axillary line. Mobilization begins at the splenic flexure and proceeds toward the hepatic flexure, which is also taken down. The lateral peritoneal attachments are divided with electrocautery or preferably the harmonic scalpel. Countertraction is provided by the assistant through the ipsilateral midclavicular trocar. Once the transverse colon is mobilized, the greater omentum is either separated from or included in the specimen. The mesentery is then retracted anteriorly to allow visualization of the middle colic vessels. This is a critical part of the operation, and transillumination or ultrasonic guidance may be applied for the surgeon's assistance. Care must be exerted to identify mid-colic and insure that the superior merenteric artery is not divided. Once identified, the vessels are divided with a vascular stapler. Subsequently, a small incision is made and the fully mobilized transverse colon is delivered through it, resected and reanastomosed with staplers or by a hand-sewn technique. The mesenteric defect is not routinely closed.

Of considerable interest is the combination of laparoscopy and colonoscopy for removal of "difficult" polyps. As described by Franklin et al,[1] after laparoscopic mobilization of the involved segment of the colon, the proximal bowel is cross-clamped and the colonoscope passed to the involved portion of the colon. The polyp is then presented to the colonoscopist by appropriate laparoscopic manipulation to facilitate removal. The serosal surface is monitored for any indications of full-thickness injury, and if so, the area is repaired primarily. With this approach up to 50% of polyps that would otherwise require a segmental resection can be removed safely and with minimal morbidity.[2]

For performance of a laparoscopic rectopexy, the operating room setup is similar to sigmoid resection. Two monitors are at the foot of the table. The surgeon stands to the right of the patient and the assistant to the left. Four trocars are used: umbilical, left upper quadrant, left flank, and suprapubic. The camera is inserted through the left upper quadrant trocar.

The operation begins with the mobilization of the sigmoid colon. The assistant and surgeon apply traction and countertraction through the left flank and umbilical trocars, respectively. The lateral peritoneal reflection is then divided sharply, exposing the retroperitoneum. Using the iliac artery pulsations as a landmark, the ureter is identified and preserved.

By placing traction on the mesentery, the inferior mesenteric vessels become taut and easily identified. This bowing technique has been previously described by the author's reference. The peritoneum is incised distal to the inferior mesenteric vessels and the retrorectal space is entered. Anterior traction is then applied through the left flank and suprapubic trocars. A cautery spatula or a harmonic scalpel is then inserted through the umbilical port and used to separate the rectum from the presacral fascia, down to the levator ani muscles.

The sacral promontory is then exposed using blunt and sharp dissection. The promontory is located by direct palpation using the instruments. Dissection in this area should be gentle to avoid bleeding from the presacral vessels. Once the middle of the promontory is cleared to the bone, dissection is continued several centimeters into the sacral hollow. At this point, a 6 by 4 cm piece of prolene mesh is inserted through the suprapubic trocar and deployed. A stapler is then used to secure the mesh onto the sacrum, by firing two parallel rows of staples in the midline of the mesh. Before the two lateral wings of the mesh are secured to the rectum, reduction of the prolapse must be verified, with a rectal exam by a third person, and reduction maintained by continued traction to the rectum in an anterior and superior direction. The wings of the mesh can be either stapled or, preferably, sutured to the lateral walls of the rectum, leaving the anterior wall uncovered. If staples are used, they should not be applied full thickness, but rather to the fat of the rectum and mesentery. This technique probably makes this less secure fixation than by suture.

At the completion of the procedure, the rectum is once again examined to ensure that the prolapse is reduced. A rigid proctoscopy is also performed to verify that the staples have not penetrated the rectal mucosa.

RESULTS

Polyps

Young-Fadok et al[3] reported on 38 patients undergoing laparoscopic right hemicolectomy for polyps. These patients were matched with similar patients undergoing an open resection. The operative time was longer in the laparoscopy group, but the length of postop ileus, need for narcotics, and length of stay were all significantly shorter. The conversion rate was 18.7% in the early patients and 10% later in the studies.

Joo et al[4] noted similar results. In their series of 45 patients, half of whom were treated laparoscopically, length of stay, duration of ileus, postop pain, and return to work were better in the laparoscopy group. Of interest, no significant difference in cost was seen, although the study was of rather limited size.

Eijsbouts et al[5] reported their experience with 20 patients with polyps that could not be removed endoscopically. Six of twenty patients had a colotomy and closure, while the rest had a segmental or anatomic resection. No comparative data to open removal were given.

Familial Adenomatous Polyposis (FAP)

Milsom et al[6] presented preliminary data on the feasibility of laparoscopic total abdominal colectomy with ileorectal anastomosis. Comparative studies between open and laparoscopic approaches in FAP, however, are lacking. In one study, Marcello et al[7] noted earlier return of bowel function and shorter hospital stay in the laparoscopy group.

Rectal Prolapse

A number of reports in the literature have documented the efficacy of laparoscopic repair of rectal prolapse.[8–10] Overall, good functional results are obtained that are not different from open repairs. The hospital stay seems shorter, as is the return to normal activities. It should be noted, however, that particularly in the case of rectal prolapse, other, even less invasive procedures are available. We have shown that perineal rectosigmoidectomy has results similar to laparoscopic repairs and is tolerated very well, if not better, by the patients.

CONCLUSIONS

Benign conditions of the colon represent an ideal field for the application of laparoscopic surgery. The common concerns about laparoscopy and malignant disease (adequacy of resection, port site recurrences) obviously do not apply. Apart from improved cosmesis, laparoscopic colectomy for benign disease is associated with faster and less morbid recovery, although it requires special skills on the surgeon's part.

REFERENCES

1. Franklin ME Jr, Diaz-EJA, Abrego D, et al. Laparoscopic-assisted colonoscopic polypectomy: The Texas Endosurgery Institute experience. *Dis Colon Rectum.* 2000;43:1246.
2. Prohm P, Weber J, Bonner C. Laparoscopic-assisted coloscopic polypectomy. *Dis Colon Rectum.* 2001;44:746.
3. Young-Fadok TM, Radice E, Nelson H, Harmsen WS. Benefits of laparoscopic-assisted colectomy for colon polyps: A matched series. *Mayo Clin Proc.* 2000;75:344.
4. Joo JS, Amarnath L, Wexner SD. Is laparoscopic resection of colorectal polyps beneficial? *Surg Endosc.* 1998;12:1341.
5. Eijsbouts QA, Heuff G, Sietses C, et al. Laparoscopic surgery in the treatment of colonic polyps. *Br J Surg.* 1999;86:505.
6. Milsom JW, Ludwig KA, Church JM, Garcia-Ruiz A. Laparoscopic total abdominal colectomy with ileorectal anastomosis for familial adenomatous polyposis. *Dis Colon Rectum.* 1997;40:675.
7. Marcello PW, Milsom JW, Wong SK, et al. Laparoscopic restorative proctocolectomy: case-matched comparative study with open restorative proctocolectomy. *Dis Colon Rectum.* 2000;43:604.
8. Zittel TT, Manncke K, Haug S, et al. Functional results after laparoscopic rectopexy for rectal prolapse. *J Gastrointest Surg.* 2000;4:632.
9. Heah SM, Hartley JE, Hurley J, et al. Laparoscopic suture rectopexy without resection is effective treatment for full-thickness rectal prolapse. *Dis Colon Rectum.* 2000;43:638.
10. Kellokumpu IH, Kairaluoma M. Laparoscopic repair of rectal prolapse: A prospective study evaluating surgical outcome and changes in symptoms and bowel function. *Surg Endosc.* 2000;14:634.

Chapter Forty-Five • • • • • •

*L*aparoscopic Surgery for Diverticular Disease

RENE F. HARTMANN, SERGIO MARTINEZ, and CARLOS A. BAPTISTA

Diverticular disease of the colon and its clinical consequences have become increasingly prevalent in the United States and other economically developed countries with each passing decade. Now, while the proportion of the aged in our population rapidly rises, their probable risk of developing diverticula is estimated at nearly 50% at age 60.

The prevalence of colonic diverticulosis in western societies is often contrasted to the rarity with which it is observed in tropical countries and in Japan. Such prevalence has been reported as follows: 10 to 20% for patients more than 40 years of age, 30% by the age of 60 years, and 60% for people older than 80 years. The frequency of diverticular disease of the colon is strikingly correlated with advancing age.

The impressive geographic and ethnic distribution may be due in some measure to genetic influences and environmental causes. Patients with diverticular disease have a significant increase in frequency of gallbladder stones, ischemic heart disease, varicose veins, hiatal hernia, and hemorrhoids.

In industrialized countries the most frequent site of colonic diverticular disease is the sigmoid colon, involved alone in 65% and in combination with other areas in 95% of cases. It has been estimated that 10 to 25% of patients with known diverticulosis will develop one or more episodes of diverticulitis; successful response to medical management drops from 70% after the first attack to 6% after the third attack. Thus, sigmoid resection is usually indicated after the second attack.

Laparoscopic colon surgery is performed as an alternative to the open approach. In 1990, Jacobs et al performed the first laparoscopically assisted colectomy. By 1991 there were at least half dozen reports of laparoscopic colon resections published in the English-language literature.[1]

Laparoscopic surgery for colon and rectal disease has increased in importance. Currently, both malignant and benign disease are being treated with minimally invasive surgery because of the touted advantages regarding cosmesis, as well as similar safety and feasibility when compared to open surgery. However, drawbacks of laparoscopic colorectal surgery, such as increased costs due to longer operative time and expensive laparoscopic equipment, have been criticized. A growing number of experiences regarding laparoscopic surgery for colorectal disease are being reported.

PREOPERATIVE CONSIDERATIONS

Laparoscopic procedures performed for the colon and rectum are far more complex than those for the gallbladder. There are multiple and variable trocar sites, the bowel must be placed on traction to be mobilized, and the techniques for gaining and applying traction vary. The operative field is dynamic and must change as certain objectives have been achieved during the course of the operation.

Essential to the performance of these more advanced procedures is a grasp of the fundamentals of laparoscopic surgery. Before initiating a laparoscopic colorectal surgery protocol, it is important to develop a laparoscopic team familiar with the necessary instrumentation and equipment. The ability to position Babcock clamps and bowel clamps automatically and insure traction can prevent complications. There must be interactive coordination between the surgeon and the first assistant. Countertraction is necessary to minimize iatrogenic injury to the bowel and mesentery. The camera operator and surgeon must coordinate their efforts. For example, when bleeding occurs, the operative field must not change, because it may prove difficult to find the same exposure, which can force conversion of a salvageable laparoscopic procedure to an open one. We believe strongly that a decision to convert a laparoscopic procedure to an open approach is not a complication but the exercise of good surgical judgment.

INDICATIONS

The indications for laparoscopic colorectal surgery and conventional open surgery are identical. Among the surgical indications for elective diverticular disease are the following.

1. Resection following recurrent attacks of diverticulitis (after two attacks or after a single attack in either young patients or patients requiring chronic immunossupresive therapy).
2. Diverticulitis associated with fistulas to the bladder or vagina.
3. Elective resection following previously percutaneously drained pericolic abscesses (Hinchey stages I and II).

The Hinchey grading system is as follows.

I. Pericolic abscess.
IIA. Distant abscess amenable to percutaneous drainage.
IIB. Complex abscess associated with fistula.
III. Generalized purulent peritonitis.
IV. Fecal peritonitis.

CONTRADICTIONS

Patient selection is as important in laparoscopic surgery as it is in open surgery. A patient who is not a good candidate for an open procedure is not an appropriate candidate for laparoscopic intervention. The indication for conventional surgery must be identical for laparoscopic surgery. Laparoscopy is a tool in the armamentarium of the surgeon, but its use does not supplant the necessity for standard surgical indications to be present.

There are contraindications to the use of the laparoscopic technique. Portal hypertension remains the Achilles heel of surgeons; when present, as in open surgery, any laparoscopic procedure becomes more difficult. Bowel obstruction is a difficult problem to handle laparoscopically; intestinal distention makes handling of the bowel treacherous and increases the risk of perforation and fecal contamination. Patients who have undergone previous surgical operations and who have significant adhesions may not be appropriate candidates, although previous surgery is not a contraindication because the surgeon can remove the adhesion lapaproscopically.

There are relative contraindications that are partially predicated on the surgeon's experience. Although originally considered an absolute contraindication, a palpable mass associated with benign disease may be approached laparoscopically. An inflammatory mass is usually secondary to adhesions of the omentum and small bowel. We consider a palpable mass in the presence of malignancy a relative contraindication to use of the laparoscopic technique. The presence of a colovaginal or colovesicular fistula secondary to diverticular disease does not mandate open surgery; however, these are technically challenging even for experienced surgeons.

A patient with compromised hemodynamic stability secondary to sepsis or with cardiogenic or hypovolemic circulatory instability may benefit more from open surgery expeditiously performed by an experienced surgeon. However, as the surgeon gains experience with laparoscopic techniques, it may be advantageous to use laparoscopy for selected, appropriately resuscitated patients. Several contraindications must be absolutely maintained by the surgeon early in his or her laparoscopic learning curve. Patients with coagulopathy, inability to tolerate general anesthesia, extensive intraperitoneal adhesion, and hemodynamic instability should be managed with conventional open techniques.

SIGMOID DIVERTICULAR DISEASE—SURGICAL TECHNIQUE

Positioning of the patient for laparoscopic surgery is crucial, as attention to arrangement details will facilitate the procedure. First, the patient should be placed in the Lloyd Davies position, which allows the performing of the subsequent anastomosis or eventually an intraoperative endoscopy. Second, the thighs should be placed almost parallel to the pelvis, so movement of the external shaft of the laparoscopic instruments can be done without interference. Third, the upper extremities should be tucked toward the body to allow the surgeons to change position during the operation. Finally, frequent tilting of the table will be used during the procedure, so the patient must be firmly secured to the operating table.

The surgeon stands on the right side of the patient. The assistant/camera operator is on the left. Two monitors are used to allow simultaneous visualization of the operative field by the surgical team. The monitor at the left is temporally moved toward the patient's head when the proximal descending colon or splenic flexure needs mobilization. If this is required, the assistant/camera operator also stands at the right side during this step.

After general anesthesia is induced, both nasogastric and vesical catheters are inserted. Pneumatic sequential compression stockings are used to prevent deep vein thrombosis. The patient is positioned as described above, and the abdomen and pelvis are prepared and draped exposing the area by the pubis, the xiphoid, and both anterior superior iliac spine. In positioning of the trocar, caution should be taken to avoid the epigastric vessels, which run parallel to the edge of the rectus muscles. All trocars should be 10 to 12 mm, so that repositioning of the instruments can be easily done.

The pneumoperitoneum is achieved either by closed or open technique based on the existence of previous abdominal operations. Moreover, a semiclosed technique (incision of the subcutaneous fat and insertion of a Veress needle in the anterior fascia under direct vision) may facilitate the creation of pneumoperitoneum in the obese patient. The zero-degree laparoscope is introduced, and the abdomen is explored. The operative table is placed in the Trendelenburg position, and tilted to the right to move bowel loops away from the surgical field. It is essential that the surgeon should use the two-handed technique, so traction and countertraction are provided in a coordinated fashion. The port sites located in the left upper quadrant and in the left flank are used for introducing laparoscpic graspers (Babcock type). Such instruments are used to pull the sigmoid colon away from the lateral abdominal wall and expose the white line of Toldt. The sigmoid colon is mobilized with a combination of sharp and blunt dissection with the use of a laparoscopic scissors introduced through the suprapubic trocar. Lately, the use of the ultrasonic dissector/coagulator (Harmonic Scalpel, Ethicon Endosurgery, Cincinnati) has increased. The touted advantages are less chance of thermal injury to adjacent organs, better visibility due to less smoke production, and transection of some vascularized areas (such as the mesorectum) without the need of clips or stapler. In cases with severe inflammation and scarring, we recommend starting the dissection away from the affected area, and subsequently proceeding to the "difficult" area. It is important to carry the dissection up to the splenic flexure, which would be taken down to create a tension-free anastomosis in many cases. The crucial steps while doing the dissection are as follows. Remain above the Gerota's fascia, to avoid creation of "windows" in the mesocolon, and most importantly to achieve clear identification of the left ureter and gonadal vessels. It cannot be overemphasized that failure to identify the left ureter is an indication to convert the procedure. Finally, the colonic mobilization should be accomplished in the first hour of surgery.

Once the dissection is achieved, the next step is the vascular transection. To do this, the respective region of mesentery is pulled up with the use of the laparoscopic Babcock grasper. The pulsating area corresponding to the inferior mesenteric vessels is carefully scored. The vessels are identified and dissected with a laparoscopic right-angle dissector. Afterward, the vessels can be transected either with the use of laparoscopic clips (two or three clips are placed in the mesentery and one clip is placed on the bowel side) or with an endoscopic stapler. Occasionally, the inferior mesenteric vein will run separately from the artery.[1] In this scenario, the vein is ligated separately, which frequently eases bringing down the descending colon, thus decreasing the tension in the anastomosis. Then attention is turned to the transection of the mesorectum. Such a maneuver can be accomplished by either the use of an endovascular stapler or with an ultrasonic dissector/coagulator as stated before. Next, the colon is transected at the rectosigmoid junction with a 60-mm endoscopic stapler. Usually two cartridges are required to complete the transection. It is important to transect the colon below the rectosigmoid junction, so that recurrence of the diverticular disease is avoided. Benn et al[2] showed that diverticulitis recurred in 12.5% of patients with anastomosis to the distal sigmoid colon compared to only 6.7% of patients undergoing a complete sigmoid colectomy. The following landmarks are used to identify the rectosigmoid junction: the area where spreading of the taenia coli occurs with absence of epiploic appendages and haustrae, the colonic region next to promotorium of the sacrum, and the point corresponding to the upper limit of the mesorectum.

The resection of the distal colon is extracorporeally performed. The suprapubic trocar site is extended for 3 to 4 cm. A muscle-splitting incision is performed, and the proximal colon is extracted through this site. A supple colonic area with no thickening of the wall is chosen. A purse-string suture is placed in the colonic edge and the anvil of the widest circular stapler is used (28 to 31 mm in diameter). The purse-string suture is tied and the colon is reintroduced into the abdomen. The fascia of the corresponding trocar site is closed with an absorbable suture, and the pneumoperitoneum is reestablished. The circular stapler is introduced through the anus and the spike is advanced through the rectal wall close to the suture line. Placement of a small loop of silk in the tip of the spike of the Auto Suture stapler (if that is the instrument used) will expedite the retrieval of the spike. After the anvil and the shaft are joined, the stapler is fired to perform the anastomosis. The integrity of the "doughnuts" is checked. A laparoscopic Babcock grasper is applied to the area proximal to the suture line, and the pelvis is filled with saline solution for air testing of the anastomosis under water. The use of a rigid proctoscope for rectal insufflation also allows the inspection of the anastomosis to assure hemostasis. Alternatively, for complex cases a Pfannenstiel incision can be made after the laparoscopic dissection of the colon.[3,4] Then vessel transection, sigmoid colon resection, and performing the anastomosis

can be completed through such an incision following standard surgical techniques. Finally, the fascia of the trocar incisions is closed with absorbable suture and the skin closed with staples. At the conclusion of the procedure, the nasogastric tube is removed. The patient can start a liquid diet on the first postoperative day. Early ambulation is also encouraged. Oral intake is advanced by the third or fourth day to a regular diet. At that time, the patient is usually having bowel movements, and is discharged.

Recently, Franklin et al published experiences with the use of laparoscopic surgery for complicated colonic diverticular disease.[5] We found that complications of diverticular disease may be managed by minimally invasive surgery. However, the following technical details should be noted. First, profuse irrigation of the abdomen and any abscess cavity is highly endorsed. Placement of subsequent drains[6] can be done through the trocars. Second, the use of atraumatic laparoscopic bowel graspers is recommended to avoid enterotomies while handling the edematous bowel. Third, the inflammatory process makes vascular dissection difficult, so it should be performed close to the colon. In addition to the specified reasons, it is especially important to identify and transect the sigmoid below the rectosigmoid junction, so that the subsequent Hartman procedure takedown may be done with no need of a distal repeated resection.

The treatment of internal sigmoid fistula secondary to diverticulitis has also been reported.[7–9] The technique involves dissection of the sigmoid colon from the abdominal wall, and subsequent transection of vessels laparoscopically. Afterward, the fistula between the involved organs can be dissected with laparoscopic instruments. Alternatively, a Pfannenstiel incision is performed and the fistulous tract can be pinched off between the fingers of the surgeons to free the sigmoid from the compromised organ. The conversion rate for these cases ranged from zero[8] to 25%. The feasibility of laparoscopic surgery for this condition may be certain, even though its complexity demands considerable experience in laparoscopic colorectal surgery.

Sigmoid diverticulitis is associated with severe scarring and tissue inflammation, so its management through laparoscopic surgery is challenging. Therefore, the conversion rate is higher than observed for other colonic conditions (such as colon cancer treated by laparoscopic surgery).[10,11] The main reason for conversion during laparoscopic sigmoid colectomy for diverticulitis is severe adhesions, which preclude safe dissection. In this setting, the injury of structures is certain. As stated earlier, inability to identify the left ureter during laparoscopic sigmoid colectomy is a powerful indication for converting the laparoscopic surgery. In addition, other reasons, including stapler perforation of the rectum, perforation of the transverse colon during mobilization of the splenic flexure, and simply failure to progress,[3,12] have been reported as grounds for conversion to open surgery.

REFERENCES

1. Jacobs M, Verdeja JC, Goldstein HS. Minimally invasive colon resection (laparoscopic colectomy). *Surg Laparosc Endosc.* 1991;1:144.
2. Benn PL, Wolff BG, Illstrup DM. Level of anastomosis and recurrent colonic diverticulitis. *Am J Surg.* 1986;151:269.
3. Eijsbouts QA, Cuesta MA, de Brauw LM, et al. Elective laparoscopic-assisted sigmoid resection for diverticular disease. *Surg Endosc.* 1997;11:750.
4. Martinez SA, Cheanvechai V, Alasfar FS, et al. Staged laparoscopic

resection for complicated sigmoid diverticulitis. *Surg Laparosc Endosc Percutan Tech.* 1999;9(2):99–105.

5. Franklin ME Jr, Dorman JP, Jacobs M, et al. Is laparoscopic surgery applicable to complicated colonic diverticular disease? *Surg Endosc.* 1997;11:1021.

6. Verdeja JC, Jacobs M, Goldstein HS. Placement of drains in laparoscopic procedures. *J Laparoendosc Surg.* 1992;2:193.

7. Hewett PJ, Stitz R. The treatment of internal fistulae that complicate diverticular disease of the sigmoid colon by laparoscopically assisted colectomy. *Surg Endosc.* 1995;9:411.

8. Puente I, Sosa JL, Desai U, et al. Laparoscopic treatment of colovesical fistulas: Technique and report of two cases. *Surg Laparosc Endosc.* 1994;4:157.

9. Joo JS, Agachan F, Wexner SD. Laparoscopic surgery for lower gastrointestinal fistulas. *Surg Endosc.* 1997;11:116.

10. Hoffman GC, Baker JW, Fitchett CW, et al. Laparoscopic-assisted colectomy. Initial experience. *Ann Surg.* 1994;219:732; discussion, 740.

11. Falk PM, Beart RW Jr, Wexner SD, et al. Laparoscopic colectomy: A critical appraisal. *Dis Colon Rectum.* 1993;36:28.

12. Stevenson AR, Stitz RW, Lumley JW, et al. Laparoscopically assisted anterior resection for diverticular disease: Follow-up of 100 consecutive patients. *Ann Surg.* 1998;227:335.

Chapter Forty-Six . . . .

*L*aparoscopy for Inflammatory Bowel Disease

HENRY J. LUJAN, GUSTAVO PLASENCIA, and MOISÉS JACOBS

Since the first series of successful laparoscopic colon resections described in 1991 by Jacobs et al,[1] laparoscopic techniques have seen widespread application for colorectal procedures. A natural progression to the spectrum of colectomies for both benign and malignant disease has evolved. The indications for the use of laparoscopic surgery continue to expand, and there are very few procedures that have not been performed laparoscopically. But laparoscopic techniques may not be appropriate for all types of surgery. Prospective, randomized, controlled studies are still needed to fully evaluate and determine the safety, cost-effectiveness, and efficacy of laparoscopic techniques as compared to conventional surgery.

Laparoscopy has been used extensively in the treatment and management of inflammatory bowel disease. However, for the most part, these technically demanding and specialized procedures, as they are applied to Crohn's disease and ulcerative colitis, are limited to a number of major laparoscopic centers (UCLA Medical Center; Mount Sinai Medical Center, NY; Cleveland Clinic Foundation, OH; Cleveland Clinic Florida; Leiden University Medical Center, Netherlands; Free University Hospital, Amsterdam; University Hospital Saarland, Homburg; Laparoscopic Center of South Florida). It is at these centers that advancements in technology and expertise are defining the applications of and limitations to laparoscopic surgery for inflammatory bowel disease at this time.

Inflammatory bowel disease encompasses Crohn's disease and ulcerative colitis. There is little controversy in regard to long-term outcome and survival when performing laparoscopy for benign colorectal disorders. The feasibility and safety have been confirmed by numerous studies.[2-5] But many questions and concerns remain unresolved. In experienced hands, laparoscopic procedures can be performed for inflammatory bowel disease. However, the long operative times and limited long-term benefits (or at least difficult to prove long-term benefits), combined with a steep learning curve and technically demanding procedures, make the use of laparoscopy less widespread and less appealing to the average surgeon and thus limited to specialized centers. Nevertheless, the po-tential advantages of less postoperative pain, less ileus, shorter hospital stay, and better cosmesis have attracted laparoscopic and colorectal surgeons to the young group of patients who often require numerous operations throughout their lifetime. Table 46–1 lists the generally recognized advantages and disadvantages of laparoscopic surgery for inflammatory bowel disease. Many of these benefits and disadvantages apply to laparoscopic surgery for other general and colorectal disease processes. Whether these advantages and disadvantages apply universally to all laparoscopic procedures for inflammatory bowel disease remains unclear. For example, many of the theoretical advantages associated with other laparoscopic procedures—including shorter duration of ileus, shorter hospital stay, and fewer complications—have not been seen with laparoscopic-assisted restorative proctocolectomy.[6] Yet some would argue that subjectively these patients do better and that patient satisfaction is higher.

There are a number of procedures that need to be specifically addressed and compared to conventional open surgery. These procedures include laparoscopic ileostomy and colostomy, laparoscopic ileocolectomy for Crohn's disease, laparoscopic total abdominal colectomy with or without ileostomy for Crohn's disease or ulcerative colitis, laparoscopic repair of enteric and colonic fistula in Crohn's disease, laparoscopic total proctocolectomy with ileostomy, and ulcerative colitis with ileal J-pouch anal anastomosis (restorative proctocolectomy).

CROHN'S DISEASE

Crohn's disease can involve any part of the gastrointestinal tract and anorectal region. The true etiology of Crohn's disease has yet to be determined. The objective of surgery is to relieve symptoms, correct complications, restore health and function when medical management fails, withdraw or minimize medications, and restore normal quality of life.[7-9]

TABLE 46–1. ADVANTAGES AND DISADVANTAGES OF LAPAROSCOPIC SURGERY FOR INFLAMMATORY BOWEL DISEASE

Advantages	Disadvantages
Less postoperative pain	Loss of tactile sensation
Less ileus	Longer operative times
Shorter hospital stay	Steep learning curve
Improved cosmesis	Technically demanding
Less adhesion formation	Difficult logistics (setup, video, equipment)
Less morbidity	Cost
Fewer wound complications	
Earlier return to work	
Psychological (improved body image, self image)	
Cost	
Less immunologic/inflammatory response	
Less physiologic trauma	

Many of the unique features of Crohn's disease—such as the skip areas of intestinal involvement, incidence of enteric fistulae, presence of inflammatory masses or phlegmons, need for bowel-sparing approaches, and difficulties with anastomotic leaks and subsequent fistula formation—have significantly limited the opportunities to even consider a laparoscopic approach.[10] However, the literature supports the claim that laparoscopic techniques can be safely and effectively applied to the treatment of patients with various manifestations of Crohn's disease. Ileocolectomy, total colectomy, diverting loop ileostomy, and a number of other procedures have been performed laparoscopically in the treatment of Crohn's disease. For the most part, laparoscopic approaches to Crohn's disease have been predominantly applied to ileocecal resections in selected patients. Laparoscopic total colectomy with or without proctectomy is a more significant undertaking, and some argue that long operative times and possibly increased incidence of complications and few benefits compared to open total colectomy make it a relative contraindication.[11]

A number of articles have been written on experience with laparoscopy and Crohn's disease. Issues specific to Crohn's have defined the advantages and disadvantages. Advantages include earlier return of intestinal function, earlier tolerance of diet, reduced postoperative pain, minimizing adhesions, better wound healing and cosmesis, reduced hospital stay, and less ileus. Disadvantages include fragile intestinal tissue, thickened mesentery, malnutrition, immunosuppression, adhesions, prolonged operative time, expense, and difficult learning curve.[3,4,12]

Indications for Surgery in Crohn's Disease

When to operate on a patient with Crohn's disease has been a subject of controversy and beyond the scope of this chapter. In general, the most common indications for surgery are intractability to medical treatment, bowel obstruction, fistula, fulminant colitis, toxic megacolon, perforation, hemorrhage, and severe growth retardation.[7,8] The decision and timing of surgery requires careful evaluation, clinical experience, and sound judgment. The decision to proceed laparoscopically depends on a number of factors as well. Level of expertise, time constraints, multiple previous laparotomies, and available experienced assistance all influence decision making. Having said that, relatively few absolute contraindications exist. However, certain conditions arise that make laparoscopic management less likely to be efficient or successful, and a number of authors have documented common reasons for conversion to an open procedure in their experience; these include palpable mass, complicated fistulas, presence of dilated bowel, and obesity.[12–15] The most common scenarios for laparoscopic surgical techniques to be applied to Crohn's disease are briefly reviewed below.

Ileocolic Crohn's Disease

The most common application for laparoscopic techniques in patients with inflammatory bowel disease is ileocolic resection for Crohn's disease (Table 46–2). Most authors[3,15–24] advocate a similar laparoscopic-assisted approach to ileocolectomy in this clinical scenario. Full mobilization of the right colon and terminal ileum is performed laparoscopically, and then the cecum is delivered through an umbilical or right lower quadrant transverse incision that is kept to 4 to 6 cm. Extracorporeal vascular division of the thick, often friable mesentery usually encountered in Crohn's disease is most common, and bowel division and anastomosis are

TABLE 46–2. LAPAROSCOPIC ILEOCOLECTOMY FOR CROHN'S DISEASE

Author	Center	Study Period	No. Patients	Conversions to Open (Patients)	Mean Operative Time and Range (min)	Mean Length of Stay and Range (days)	Morbidity (%)
Milsom et al[18]	Cleveland Clinic Foundation	1991–1992	9	3	170[1] (150–210)	7[1] (5–12)	0
Ludwig et al[14]	Cleveland Clinic Foundation	1992–1994	23	3	NR	3–7	3
Reissman et al[2]	Cleveland Clinic Florida	1992–1995	32	7	144 (36–270)	5.1 (3–18)	14
Alabaz et al[28]	Cleveland Clinic Florida	1991–1996	26	3	150 (NR)	7 (NR)	15
Bemelman et al[26]	Leiden University Medical Center	1995–1998	30	2	138 (NR)	5.7 (NR)	10
Hildebrandt et al[32]	University of Saarlandes	1993–1997	45	NR	NR (90–280)	11 (NR)	12.3
Canin-Endres et al[15]	Mt. Sinai Medical Center	1993–1998	70	0	183 (96–400)	4.2 (3–11)	14
Wu et al[24]	Washington University	1992–1996	46	5	143 (75–300)	4.5 (NR)	7
Meijerink et al[4]	Leiden University	1995–1997	26	2	138 (NR)	5.6 (NR)	8

[1]Median.

NR, not reported.

performed using standard techniques. A two-handed technique for running the bowel in retrograde fashion from the terminal ileum to the duodenojejunal junction is recommended in all cases to rule out previously unidentified fistula, which is said to occur in 6% of patients.[25] If encountered, these fistulas can be addressed through the small incision used for the ileocolic resection. Care is taken to avoid enterotomy or mesentery tears, which can result in bleeding. Enlargement of the planned incision is usually considered a conversion to an open procedure.

Milsom et al[18] reported on 9 patients at the Cleveland Clinic Foundation who underwent laparoscopically assisted ileocolectomy for patients with Crohn's disease of the terminal ileum. They encountered no complications and concluded that the procedure was safe and feasible for selected patients. Ludwig et al[14] later reported on a group of 23 carefully selected patients, with similar excellent results. Encountering complete or near-complete obstruction with dilated bowel, intra-abdominal abscess, intra-abdominal sepsis, and intra-abdominal fistulas were considered relatively strong contraindications for the laparoscopic approach.

Reissman et al[2,16] reported their overall experience with 51 patients with Crohn's disease, 30 of whom had ileocolic resections. Bleeding in 2 patients and a large inflammatory mass in 5 patients resulted in conversion to an open procedure (14%). Mean operative time was 144 minutes and the mean length of hospital stay was 5.1 days. The authors concluded that laparoscopy could be safely offered to most patients who require elective surgery for localized Crohn's disease.

A number of comparative studies have also been reported. Bemelman et al[26] compared 30 consecutive patients with Crohn's disease who underwent laparoscopic ileocolectomy at the Leiden University Medical Center, to 48 patients who underwent open ileocolic resection at the Academic Medical Center in Amsterdam during the same time period. They found slightly longer operative times for the laparoscopic group (138 ± 36 versus 104 ± 34 minutes), but laparoscopic patients were discharged earlier (an average of 5.7 versus 10.2 days) after the operation and postoperative morbidity did not differ significantly. Furthermore, improved cosmesis was felt to be a significant advantage for the laparoscopic group. This advantage was thought to be particularly significant for a group of patients whose peak incidence of disease is 20 to 30 years of age and who will likely require operation again in their lifetime. They cited other investigators who have shown better cosmetic and body image scores in Crohn's patients undergoing laparoscopic rather than open ileocolectomy.[27] They also included that laparoscopic-assisted ileocolectomy is as safe as open surgery. Alabaz et al[28] reported on 74 patients who had ileocolic resection and anastomosis for Crohn's disease, 48 in the open group and 26 in the laparoscopic group. Operating time was significantly shorter in the open group, with a mean of 90.5 minutes compared to 150 minutes in the laparoscopy group. However, the open group patients stayed in the hospital significantly longer than the laparoscopic patients (9.6 compared with 7 days). Interestingly, after a mean follow-up of 30 months, significantly more patients in the conventional group developed symptomatic bowel obstruction. No differences in early complication rate or cost of admission could be demonstrated. The authors concluded that the laparoscopic approach was not only safe but had less morbidity than conventional laparotomy. Talamini et al[20] reported similar results and conclusions. They were able to achieve laparoscopic advantages without increasing operative times.

Singh et al,[29] from Bedford Hospital in the United Kingdom, reported experience with 38 patients in whom laparoscopy was used as a diagnostic tool or aid. Twenty-three patients were suspected of having Crohn's disease. Out of this group, 11 were found not to have Crohn's disease and were spared a laparotomy. The other 12 were confirmed to have Crohn's disease and underwent appropriate therapy. The authors also found the laparoscopic approach especially useful in the treatment of small-bowel fistulas. Three patients had bowel fistulas (ileo-ileal, ileo-transverse, and transverse-cutaneous) and were successfully treated by dissecting out the fistula and simply transecting the fistula with a GIA linear endoscopic stapler. Traditionally, enteric fistulas in Crohn's disease mandate a resection of the primary site of the fistula and simple closure of the secondary site. At 2-year follow-up in the 3 patients treated with simple laparoscopic transection of the fistula and without bowel resection, no evidence of recurrence was found. The authors proposed that perhaps Crohn's disease fistulas could be handled with minimally invasive surgery with good results as in their 3 patients.

A number of series of laparoscopic ileocolic resections for patients with Crohn's disease have shown that this technique is feasible, safe, and offers "good results."[14,16,18,20,27,29,30] The contraindications to the laparoscopic approach for ileocolic disease have yet to be clearly defined. Some authors have expressed concerns that local complications of terminal ileitis in patients with Crohn's disease, such as abscess, phlegmon, or recurrent disease around a previous anastomosis, might be contraindications to a laparoscopic resection. Others have noted a higher rate of conversion to laparotomy in cases with the associated findings mentioned. Wu et al[24] attempted to address this issue and reported their experience with laparoscopy and Crohn's disease. In their study, patients were divided into four groups: abscess or phlegmon treated with bowel rest before surgery, recurrent Crohn's disease at the previous ileocolic anastomosis, no associated abscess or phlegmon, and open ileocolic resection. Blood loss, morbidity, and length of hospital stay were all higher for the open ileocolectomy group. The authors concluded that abscesses, phlegmons, or recurrent disease did not constitute contraindications to a laparoscopic approach in patients with Crohn's disease. They also suggested that concurrent enteric fistulas could be managed with minimally invasive techniques, and laparoscopic ileocolectomy compared favorably with the conventional approach.

Canin-Endres et al[15] reported the Mount Sinai Medical Center New York experience with laparoscopic management of Crohn's disease. Between 1993 and 1998, 70 of the 88 patients they reported on underwent ileocolic resection. Acute obstruction, generalized peritonitis, and toxic colitis were felt to be absolute contraindications. The combination of a mass and fistula often indicated a difficult dissection. Early postoperative obstruction was the most common complication encountered. Morbidity was reported in 10 patients (14%). Unlike many previous reports, the presence of an abscess, fistula, or inflammatory mass did not alter plans for a laparoscopic approach. Fistulas were usually transected with a laparoscopic stapling device or transected sharply with repair of the normal viscus using intracorporeal suturing techniques. The presence of these conditions was not considered contraindicated in experienced hands, but the authors did believe that these exclusion criteria were appropriate in a surgeon's early experience because of the steep learning curve. The only absolute contraindications to a laparoscopic approach were acute obstruction, generalized peritonitis, and toxic colitis. They found advantages similar to other studies, which included less pain, less ileus, decreased length of hospitals stay, and better cosmetic results.[17,22–24]

Table 46–2 summarizes the major published experience with laparoscopic ileocolic resection for Crohn's disease. Nearly all of the studies seem to support similar conclusions, namely the safety and feasibility of the procedure. Most agree that benefits include decreased pain, shorter duration of ileus, shorter hospital stay, earlier return to usual activities, and improved cosmesis. Furthermore, potential benefits include less morbidity possibly due to less adhesion formation,[28,29] less physiologic stress,[30] and less immunosuppression.[31] For the experienced laparoscopist, inflammatory mass, abscess, and fistula are not necessarily contraindications to the laparoscopic approach.

Our own experience is reinforced by these authors' conclusions. We offer laparoscopic ileocolectomy with well-informed consent in the elective setting. Extensive experience with both surgical management in Crohn's disease and advanced laparoscopic skills allows for a high rate of success in performing ileocolic resection for Crohn's disease. Finally, the management of fistulas appears to be amenable to minimally invasive techniques.[24,29]

Colonic Crohn's Disease

Laparoscopic total abdominal colectomy with ileorectal anastomosis or total proctocolectomy with ileostomy can be offered to patients with colonic Crohn's disease. A number of authors have reported cosmetic advantages, but the similar long operative times, no difference in length of hospital stay, increased cost, and possibly increased morbidity, when compared to conventional surgery, have made it difficult to justify the laparoscopic approach in these patients. As experience and expertise increases and instrumentation and technique continue to evolve, more patient benefit may be demonstrated in the future.[4,6,9,11,12,23,32–35] However, at this time there is little support for the laparoscopic approach in the published literature.

Wexner et al[11] reported a prospective study comparing laparoscopic total abdominal colectomy (5 patients) to conventional total abdominal colectomy (5 patients). However, patients had ulcerative colitis (n = 2), familial adenomatous polyposis (n = 6), or colonic inertia (n = 2). The time required for the laparoscopic procedures was 35% longer than for the open colectomies. The authors agreed there was some cosmetic advantage; however, the procedure was lengthy, and associated with a longer hospitalization and increased morbidity, when compared to open surgery.

Reissman et al[2] described a series of 72 patients also at the Cleveland Clinic Florida with inflammatory bowel disease who underwent laparoscopic operation. Eleven patients had Crohn's colitis. Patients undergoing total colectomy had a worse outcome in terms of operating room time, average length of stay, and overall morbidity. The authors concluded that based on their experience with laparoscopic colectomy for Crohn's disease, they could not recommend laparoscopic total abdominal colectomy.[2]

There are a number of other reports on laparoscopic total abdominal colectomy, but only a few scattered reports of patients with Crohn's disease undergoing laparoscopic total abdominal colectomy.[4,15,19,33] The combined experience found in the published literature with laparoscopic total abdominal colectomies for Crohn's colitis is not extensive. We have drawn similar conclusions from our own experience; however, we have encountered a

number of patients whose personal beliefs and body image makes cosmesis their main priority. For these, often younger, patients, smaller incisions outweigh other factors in their choice of approach. Unanswered questions remain regarding the theoretical benefits of less physiologic trauma, less immunologic response, and possibly less adhesion formation; and other long-term advantages will need to be followed. Crohn's disease patients in particular are quite demanding in regard to management of their disease. Dunker et al set out to compare body image, cosmesis, and quality of life in patients with Crohn's disease who underwent either open or laparoscopic ileocolic resection. Higher satisfaction with cosmesis was seen in patients who had laparoscopic resection. Furthermore, body image correlated strongly with cosmesis and with quality of life. The hospital experience was similar in both groups. However, as experience, instrumentation, and techniques continue to advance and operative times decrease, we are likely to see this procedure done more commonly by elite laparoscopic centers if patient benefit can be more clearly demonstrated.

Anorectal Crohn's Disease

A subgroup of patients will require temporary or permanent fecal diversion. Laparoscopic loop ileostomy can be performed safely. Usually only two 5-mm and one 10/12-mm trocars at the site of the stoma are needed. A description of the procedure can be found elsewhere.[36] Intraoperative assessment can easily be achieved at the same time to determine the presence of small bowel involvement. A number of authors have reported their experience with laparoscopic colostomy and ileostomy for various indications.[37–39] Success rate, operative times, and hospital stay compare favorably when the stoma is constructed laparoscopically.[2,19,39] Complications are relatively few and the procedure is usually easily accomplished. This procedure can generally be performed with two 5-mm trocars and one 12-mm trocar at the site of the previously marked stoma location.

Summary

High patient expectations, patient acceptance, excellent success rates, relatively low complication rates, and outcomes consistent with the current economic pressure of limiting medical costs suggest that laparoscopy will likely become part of the standard surgical therapeutic regimens for many surgeons treating patients with Crohn's disease.[10] In carefully selected patients with Crohn's disease, laparoscopic ileocolectomy, colostomy, and ileostomy can all be performed safely and with advantages. Laparoscopic total colectomy can also be performed safely, but advantages are difficult to prove and, in fact, some significant disadvantages exist.

ULCERATIVE COLITIS

Ulcerative colitis is a chronic inflammatory condition confined to the large bowel mucosa. The etiology and pathogenesis are not completely understood. Thorough preoperative evaluation is mandatory in this population of patients.[7] The majority of patients with inflammatory bowel disease who present for surgery have been on high-dose corticosteroids and immunosuppressive agents. These patients also have varying degrees of malnutrition based on the severity and length of illness. These factors obviously affect healing and postoperative recovery. A thorough physical exam along with endoscopy, small bowel series, and CT scan of the abdomen and pelvis are useful in ruling out evidence of Crohn's disease.

Indications for Surgery in Ulcerative Colitis

The indications for surgery in the elective setting are failed medical treatment, growth retardation in a child, and the development of dysplasia or invasive cancer. The indications for emergency surgery include acute severe colitis unresponsive to medical management, toxic megacolon, perforation, and massive hemorrhage.[8] The surgical options available in the treatment of ulcerative colitis are the following:

- Total proctocolectomy and end ileostomy.
- Total abdominal colectomy with ileorectal anastomosis.
- Total proctocolectomy with continent ileostomy (Koch's pouch).
- Restorative proctocolectomy with ileal pouch anal anastomosis with or without loop ileostomy.

Total abdominal colectomy with ileorectal anastomosis or end ileostomy and total proctocolectomy with end ileostomy have been performed laparoscopically in the management of ulcerative colitis. Laparoscopic total proctocolectomy with continent ileostomy to our knowledge has not been reported in the literature. Although feasible, the construction of a continent ileostomy is technically difficult and has a high incidence of complications associated with both pouch construction and function. This, combined with the growing popularity of restorative proctocolectomy, which most consider a better alternative, has made the continent ileostomy procedure more of historical interest; it is not widely applied in the surgical management of ulcerative colitis.

Laparoscopic total colectomy and total proctocolectomy, however, has been evaluated for its feasibility, safety, and practicality. The procedure is described elsewhere. Recommendations on trocar placement, order of dissection, management of flexures, and technical hints have been provided by numerous authors.[36,41] A significant amount of improvisation and tailoring to patient body habitus and anatomy are required of the surgeon. Operating times are still relatively long, on the order of 4 to 6 hours, and the benefits are not easily demonstrated. But most authors agree that cosmesis is superior to conventional surgery.[12,27]

In 1992, Peters[34] reported 2 cases of laparoscopic total proctocolectomy with ileostomy for ulcerative colitis. Neither patient required a blood transfusion and blood loss was reported to be less than 500 mL for each case. Although operative times were not reported, the author felt that this was an appropriate treatment option due to the perceived benefits of less pain, fewer wound complications, and earlier advancement of diet.

Thibault and Poulin[33] reported 4 cases of laparoscopic proctoclectomy and ileostomy, for 3 Crohn's disease patients and one ulcerative colitis patient, as mentioned earlier. Average operating time was 438 minutes. Average blood loss was 493 mL. Complications were limited to urinary retention and nausea. The authors suggested waiting for further studies before formulating opinions on the advantages of the procedure.

Meijerink et al[4] reported their experience with laparoscopic proctococolectomy in 13 patients with inflammatory bowel disease (3 patients with Crohn's disease and 10 with ulcerative colitis). Seven of the 10 colectomies in the patients with ulcerative colitis were for toxic megacolon and performed in the acute setting. In these 7 patients, no procedure-related complications were encountered. Operative time averaged 300 minutes (range, 225 to 360 minutes) and there were no conversions to an open procedure. Perioperative blood loss was low, ranging from 100 to 500 mL. Complications included urinary tract infection, wound infection, candidaiasis sepsis, and a subphrienic abscess. Length of stay ranged from 7 to 36 days, which was similar to that for conventional surgery. The limited Pfannenstiel incision and its location away from stoma formation were viewed as potential benefits. They also concluded that the procedure could be completed safely and with minimal blood loss.

A prospective trial was undertaken at the Cleveland Clinic Florida to assess the impact of laparoscopy on the outcome of total abdominal colectomy.[11] Laparoscopic total abdominal colectomy with ileorectal anastomosis or ileal pouch anal anastomosis was compared to open surgery for the same procedures. Patients in both groups had ulcerative colitis, familial adenomatous polyposis, or colonic inertia. This preliminary prospective study indicated that laparoscopically assisted total abdominal colectomy resulted in slightly longer lengths of ileus and hospitalization, but the differences were not statistically significant. Moreover, the length of time required for the laparoscopic procedures was 35% longer than for the open procedures. Thus, this study failed to demonstrate any differences in rates of postoperative recovery. Although technically feasible, laparoscopic total abdominal colectomy did not offer any immediately recognizable advantages to the patients when compared with open surgery. An update on the series of 74 laparoscopic and laparoscopically assisted colon and rectal procedures was also reported.[2] A variety of procedures were included in the study, but for those 20 patients who underwent total abdominal colectomy, the mean duration of the procedure was 234 minutes (range, 150 to 390 minutes), the median length of ileus was 3.5 (range, 2 to 7) days, and the median length of hospitalization was 7 (range, 4 to 20) days. There was no specific analysis for patients with ulcerative colitis but intra-operative complications occurred in 14% and postoperative complications in 20% of patients. Again, laparoscopic colectomy for ulcerative colitis was demonstrated as feasible, but offered no clear advantage over open surgery.[11,16]

Laparoscopic Restorative Proctocolectomy With Ileal Pouch Anal Anastomosis With or Without Loop Ileostomy

The results of laparoscopic restorative proctocolectomy in the literature are summarized in Table 46–2. Most groups used similar techniques although trocar placement varied somewhat; most felt some individualization is necessary depending on flexure locations. The laparoscopic total colectomy was performed intracorporeally, as was the division of the mesentery and devascularization. Some performed rectal dissection and proctectomy by laparoscopic techniques, arguing that they provide better visualization and ease of identifying planes. Others took advantage of the Pfannenstiel incision to complete this portion of the procedure, and sometimes a combined approach was used. The construction of the ileal J-pouch, ileoanal anastomosis, and ileostomy were performed in a conventional open fashion using the suprapubic incision universally.

Liu et al[3] reported on a series of patients with inflammatory bowel disease that included 5 laparoscopic restorative proctocolectomies. The only complication was a delayed peri-ileostomy fistula. They had a mean follow-up time of 15 months with no anastomotic complications, and all patients uniformly rated cosmetic results as excellent. Operative times were long, at slightly over 8 hours (range, 380 to 710 minutes). One was converted to an open procedure due to technical reasons. The hospital stay was a median of 7 (range, 6 to 13) days. Morbidity was 20% for the group overall.

In a recent study from the Cleveland Clinic Foundation, Cleveland, Ohio, Marcello et al[42] reported on 20 consecutive laparoscopic restorative proctocolectomies (13 mucosal ulcerative colitis, 7 familial adenomatous polyposis), which were compared to 20 matched open cases. No laparoscopic cases were converted to open. The authors reported quicker return of bowel function and shorter hospital stay for the laparoscopic cases. The median operative time was approximately 100 minutes longer in the laparoscopic group when compared to the open group [330 (range, 180 to 480) versus 225 (range, 180 to 300) minutes, $P < .001$]. Postoperative morbidity was comparable between groups and there was no significant difference in operative blood loss. Complications encountered included 3 patients who developed an ileus or partial small bowel obstruction and one patient who had a pelvic abscess. The authors concluded that there were several advantages but no apparent disadvantages or increase in complication rates in the laparoscopic group compared to the open group.

Potenti and Wexner[9] reported on 28 laparoscopic restorative proctocolectomies with ileal J pouch performed at the Cleveland Clinic Florida. Twenty-three were for mucosal ulcerative colitis and 6 for familial adenomatous polyposis. There were no differences in length of hospital stay when compared to a matched group of patients who underwent conventional restorative proctocolectomies. The mean length of surgery was 240 (range, 120 to 330) minutes in the laparoscopic group and 140 (range 120 to 300) minutes in the open surgery group. Sixteen patients required transfusion in the laparoscopic assisted group and only 7 in the open group ($P < .05$). Morbidity was also significantly higher for laparoscopic restorative proctocolectomy patients compared to open restorative proctocolectomy (43 vs. 30%, $P < .05$). Because of these findings, laparoscopic restorative proctocolectomy and laparoscopic total proctocolectomy could not be routinely justified for the treatment of ulcerative colitis, according to the authors.[6,9,12,42]

Santoro et al[43] reported the experience at the Regina Elena Cancer Institute in Rome. They performed 5 laparoscopic restorative proctocolectomies (3 for ulcerative colitis and 2 for familial adenomatous polyposis). No patients were converted and the only complication was bleeding from a drain site that resolved spontaneously. Long-term and functional results were excellent. The authors concluded that this procedure is safe, feasible, and effective. Furthermore, advantages included less intraoperative fluid loss, less ileus, less pain, and less psychological discomfort.

As with laparoscopic total abdominal colectomy, it has been difficult to demonstrate any short-term advantages to laparoscopic restorative proctocolectomy such as shorter hospital stay, earlier return to work, or less pain (Table 46–3). But other advantages such as less morbidity and fewer wound complications—as well as theoretical benefits of less adhesion formation, less physiologic trauma, and less immunologic response—may prove to be important, although they have not been proven at this time. Little argument about improved cosmesis exists, but certainly this is more important to some patients than others. No prospective randomized studies have been performed to date comparing these approaches.

Our own center's early experience with 3 laparoscopic restorative proctocolectomies resulted in longer operative times, minimal subjective advantage, and limited enthusiasm to pursue this approach (Plasencia G et al, personal communication, 2000). However, this area is being revisited at our institution because laparoscopic total abdominal colectomies are being performed with shorter, more acceptable operative times. It is possible that as skill, technique, and instrumentation continue to improve, operative times will decrease sufficiently to make this procedure practical for some centers with adequate volume and experience. Many questions remain unanswered and theoretical issues unresolved.

Other Considerations

Contraindications. Very few absolute contraindications exist. However, based on their experience, a number of authors have proposed relative contraindications to laparoscopic management of inflammatory bowel disease (Table 46–4). The importance of taking these relative contraindications into consideration to ensure proper patient selection cannot be overemphasized. Some of the contraindications are more specific to Crohn's disease and many apply to laparoscopic colorectal surgery in general. The patient's safety and best interest are weighed most heavily in making the decision to proceed with a laparoscopic approach. Obviously, the surgeon's experience and laparoscopic expertise factor heavily into the equation.

Immunology and Surgical Stress. Postsurgical immune suppression occurs as a consequence of a complex sequence of events which currently is not well understood. Major surgery is known to

TABLE 46–3. LAPAROSCOPIC RESTORATIVE PROCTOCOLECTOMY

Author	Center	Study Period	No. Patients	Conversions to Open	Mean Operative Time and Range (min)	Mean Length of Stay and Range (days)	Morbidity (%)
Liu et al[3]	UCLA	1993–1994	5	0	175 (120–235)	7 (6–13)	20
Marcello et al[42]	Cleveland Clinic Foundation	1993–1999	13	0	330* (180–480)	7* (4–14)	20
Schmitt et al[6]	Cleveland Clinic Florida	1991–1993	22	NR	240 (120–330)	8.7 (7–13)	55
Santoro et al[43]	Regina Elena Cancer Institute	1993–1996	5	0	364 (290–480)	12 (10–18)	0
Hildebrandt et al[32]	University of Saarlands	1994–1996	5	0	NR (305–420)	NR (13–16)	0
Jacobs et al[36]	Laparoscopic Center South Florida	1994–1995	3	0	253 (180–343)	7.3 (6–9)	0

NR, not reported.

TABLE 46–4. RELATIVE CONTRAINDICATIONS TO LAPAROSCOPIC MANAGEMENT OF INFLAMMATORY BOWEL DISEASE

Carcinoma

Peritonitis

Obesity

Perforation

Comorbidities (cardiopulmonary risk)

Toxic megacolon

Multiple prior operations

Coagulopathy

Recurrent Crohn's disease at previous ileocolic anastomosis

Fistula

Bowel obstruction or marked bowel dilatation

Abscess or phlegmon

---

result in impairment of immunologic function. In particular, cell-mediated immune function is known to be inhibited by surgical stress. The extent of suppression roughly correlates with the degree of trauma caused by surgery. Evidence exists that suggests laparoscopic techniques better preserve immune function when compared to equivalent open surgical procedures. Several recent studies have reported that laparoscopic surgery results in better preservation of lymphocyte and macrophage function and lower serum levels of potentially harmful cytokines such as tumor necrosis factor and interleukin-1.[31] The implications of such differences may be far reaching. Improved postoperative immune function may translate into lower rates of sepsis and infectious complications. This may be especially important in patients with inflammatory bowel disease, the etiology and pathogenesis of which are thought to be intimately related to immune system processes. That particular group of patients may benefit most by less alteration in immune function, allowing for more rapid healing and quicker recovery. Whether endoscopic and surgical recurrence rate are altered by laparoscopic or minimally invasive approaches will have to be addressed by comparative studies with long-term follow-up after laparoscopic resection in Crohn's disease.[21,23]

These theoretical advantages may be especially important in the patient with inflammatory bowel disease who is already under significant physiologic stress and immunologic suppression. Laparoscopy may offer advantages regarding surgical stress and recovery in patients with Crohn's disease. The severity of surgical trauma associated with laparoscopic procedures may be less than that for similar open procedures.[30,47]

Cost. Whether the laparoscopic approach in general makes sense from a cost-effective standpoint is not yet resolved. With an increase in technology, there has been increased emphasis on proving cost-effectiveness in a variety of medical therapies, especially laparoscopic surgery. The new therapy must either be vastly superior if it is more expensive, or at least equal in efficacy if it is less expensive, to gain widespread usage.[44] A number of variables need to be evaluated, including the use of reusable instruments versus disposables, reasonable lengths of operative time, low conversion rates, shorter hospital stays, and complication rates equal to or less than the open alternative. These are the main issues evaluated by most of the studies presented in this chapter; specifically for the type of procedures described, the justification for increased cost becomes more difficult. But the verdict is still out. These pro-

cedures are technically complex and have steep learning curves. Much will depend on improved instrumentation and trained laparoscopic surgeons. Anticipated increasing future demands for laparoscopic colorectal procedures mandates continued educational expansion and improvement.

Learning Curve. There is a learning curve associated with becoming proficient with laparoscopic surgery, and much has been written on the subject.[45–49] Laparoscopic colorectal procedures tend to have a longer learning curve than less complex procedures. To offer laparoscopic surgery to inflammatory bowel disease patients, the surgeon must not only be experienced with open colorectal procedures but with laparoscopic colorectal procedures as well. There appears to be yet another step or plateau when learning to do laparoscopic surgery for inflammatory bowel disease. Many cases are necessary to learn and to gain proficiency in laparoscopic techniques in the management of inflammatory bowel disease. Only those centers with a large volume and extensive experience with inflammatory bowel disease are in a position to advance significantly in this specialized area.

LAPAROSCOPIC PROCEDURES

Complete technical details on the different laparoscopic procedures as they are applied to colorectal disease and specifically to inflammatory bowel disease can be found elsewhere.[36,41] A brief description of laparoscopic ileocolectomy for Crohn's disease and laparoscopic total abdominal (procto) colectomy for inflammatory bowel disease will follow. General recommendations and clinical caveats are included as well.

Laparoscopic Ileocolectomy

The operating room setup and trocar placement for laparoscopic ileocolectomy are identical to those for laparoscopic right hemicolectomy. The operating room setup consists of two television monitors positioned to the patient's right—one at the patient's head and the other at the foot of the operating table. The surgeon and assistant stand on the left side of the patient. Two 5-mm and one 12-mm trocars are required. An optional 5-mm trocar can be added in the left upper quadrant so the assistant can help with counter traction. The first trocar is inserted into the umbilicus, and a diagnostic laparoscopy is performed with a 5-mm, 30-degree laparoscope. The entire small bowel is inspected to exclude synchronous proximal radiographically unidentified strictures using a "hand-over-hand" technique.

The peritoneal attachments to the right colon are sharply incised by the surgeon using cautery scissors or "harmonic" scalpel (Ethicon Endo-surgery) through the umbilical trocar, while the assistant places anteromedial traction using a laparoscopic Babcock clamp or grasper through the left upper quadrant trocar. Mobilization of the peritoneal attachments continues from the terminal ileum to the hepatic flexure. The patient is repositioned in a reverse Trendelenburg position. The hepatic flexure is mobilized by applying inferior traction to the colon via Babcock clamps directed by the surgeon and first assistant, through suprapubic and left upper quadrant trocars, respectively.

Devascularization is often accomplished extracorporeally in Crohn's disease because of the thick, inflamed mesentery usually encountered. However, if tenting of the mesentery is possible to allow clear isolation of the ileocolic and right colic vessels, this portion of the surgery may be completed intracorporeally in the usual fashion. We favor the 45-mm vascular (2.5) linear cutter (Ethicon Endosurgery) for the vessels and the ultrasonic scalpel for the mesentery.

After mobilization and devascularization are accomplished, the bowel should reach the anterior abdominal wall without tension. If sufficient mobilization and devascularization have been accomplished, a 4 to 6-cm muscle-splitting incision in the right lower quadrant, or alternatively, an incision through the umbilical trocar site, is created. The colon is now delivered extracorporeally through the incision. The exteriorized colon is resected and an extracorporeal anastomosis is performed in the standard manner. The mesenteric defect may be closed, if this can be easily accomplished. If the mesenteric defect cannot be easily closed, we leave it open. The incision is then closed, pneumoperitoneum is reestablished, and completion laparoscopy is performed. Completion laparoscopy allows examination of the anastomosis for torsion, enables withdrawal of secondary trocars under direct vision, and facilitates inspection of the abdominal cavity for hemostasis. The pneumoperitoneum is then slowly released under direct vision, and trocar sites and skin incisions are closed.

Clinical Caveats

- Careful patient selection is critical (Table 46–4).
- Perform a full preoperative and medical evaluation along with appropriate contrast studies and CT scans to avoid intraoperative surprises.
- Preserve potential stoma sites by keeping extraction incisions away from the right and left lower quadrants.
- The extraction site must be large enough to allow safe delivery of the thick, friable mesentery.
- The importance of an experienced assistant cannot be overemphasized.
- When dissecting the peritoneal attachments of the right colon, avoid wide dissection. The common error is to dissect far more laterally than necessary; this may lead to additional bleeding and possible ureteric injury.
- Dissect the duodenum and its developmental adhesions before any vascular ligation is carried out.
- The patient must be secured to the operating table with arms tucked to allow maximum unrestricted room, and so that steep positioning can be safely used to assist with gravity traction.
- Before making the incision, place the colon at the point of exteriorization to identify the proper site for the incision. The subsequent steps of devascularization and anastomosis will be facilitated by this maneuver. It is important to have the colon reach the anterior abdominal wall without tension.
- Always reintroduce the pneumoperitoneum and slowly release the pneumoperitoneum under direct vision and observe trocar sites and anastomosis for bleeding before the conclusion of the procedure.

Laparoscopic Total Abdominal and Total Proctocolectomy

Total abdominal colectomy and total proctocolectomy are probably the most challenging procedures performed laparoscopically. After induction of general endotracheal anesthesia, an orogastric tube and Foley catheter are inserted. Patients are placed in the supine, perineal lithotomy position using Allen stirrups (Allen Medical, Bedford Heights, OH). This allows the surgeon access between the patient's legs for mobilization of flexures, intraoperative colonoscopy, and circular stapler devices. The legs should be carefully positioned with the hips and knees gently flexed. The hip flexure needs to be kept to a minimum to allow greater range of mobility with the laparoscopic instruments. In other words, the thighs should be parallel to the floor. The surgeon will require use of the suprapubic trocar. This will insure less collision between the surgeon's forearm or instrument shaft and the patient's thigh, especially during mobilization of a high splenic flexure or when operating in the upper abdomen. We do not routinely use ureteral stents; indications for their use should be the same as for conventional surgery.

Port site placement for total abdominal colectomy and total proctocolectomy can be variable and need to be tailored to the patient's body habitus and anatomy. In general, port site placement is similar to that for left or sigmoid colectomies: umbilical, suprapubic, left upper quadrant, and left lateral. Usually the procedure can be accomplished using only these four ports. Sometimes a fifth port can be placed in the right lower quadrant to assist with retraction in particular stages of the operation. If placed strategically, this port site can also be used for the ileostomy site. Often other port sites can be used for drain placement. Trocar placements are simply recommendations, and there is much room for improvisation, surgeon ingenuity, and adjusting according to the clinical situation.

For the novice, the 30-degree, 10-mm camera is recommended, as this gives optimal visualization. We mainly use 5-mm trocars and add 10/12-mm trocars if technical difficulties arise. The peritoneal attachment of the sigmoid and descending colon is sharply incised using the ultrasonic scalpel (Ethicon Endosurgery). Once the left colon mobilization and identification of the left ureter are complete, the splenic flexure is mobilized. Dissection continues in the avascular plane between the greater omentum and transverse colon if it is not to be removed. Intracorporeal devascularization of the inferior mesenteric vessels is performed using 45-mm (2.5) vascular laparoscopic linear staplers (Ethicon Endosurgery), and the remainder of the mesentery is divided with the harmonic scalpel down to the sacral promontory. Right colon mobilization and devascularization is conducted as for a standard laparoscopic right colectomy. Once the ileocolic vessels have been divided, a mesenteric window becomes evident. The right and middle colic vessels are then sequentially clipped and ligated or transected using the 45-mm linear stapler with vascular reloads. Finally, the terminal ileum is transected intracorporeally with the endolinear stapling device and the specimen is delivered through a small suprapubic or Pfannenstiel incision. For restorative proctocolectomy, the rectal dissection is carried out laparoscopically down to the level of the levator ani before transection. Alternatively this can be accomplished in an open fashion or using a combined approach. We recommend placing an endoloop around the terminal ileum to allow for easy retrieval at this point. Then, depending on the operation, intracorporeal anastomosis is accomplished or an ileoanal reservoir constructed and anal anastomosis completed. The options are ileorectal anastomosis, an ileal pouch anal anastomosis, or creation of a Hartmann's pouch with end ileostomy. Minor variations and more detailed accounts of each sequential step in mobilization can be found in the references.[6,9,18,33,34,36,41,43]

Clinical Caveats

- Left colon mobilization and takedown of the splenic flexure should be performed first, because this is the most technically challenging portion of the procedure.
- Monitors are required on both sides of the patient and need to be easily relocated from patient's feet to shoulders on either side, as described.
- When ligating the middle colic vessels, anatomic certainty is crucial to avoid ligation of celiac vessels or superior mesenteric vessels.
- Use of the ultrasonic "harmonic" scalpel minimizes the smoke that interferes with visualization.
- Before devascularization, the ureter should be visualized through the mesenteric windows to safeguard against iatrogenic injury.

REFERENCES

1. Jacobs M, Verdeja JC, Goldstein HS. Minimally invasive colon resection (laparoscopic colectomy). *Surg Laparosc Endosc.* 1991;1:144.
2. Reissman P, Salky BA, Pfeifer J, et al. Laparoscopic surgery in the management of inflammatory bowel disease. *Am J Surg.* 1996;171:47.
3. Liu CD, Rolandelli R, Ashley SW. Laparoscopic surgery for inflammatory bowel disease. *Am Surg.* 1995;61:1054.
4. Meijerink WJ, Eijsbouts QA, Cuesta MA, et al. Laparoscopically assisted bowel surgery for inflammatory bowel disease. *Surg Endosc.* 1999;13:882.
5. Breen EM, Ashley SW. Laparoscopic surgery for Crohn's disease? A conditional Yes. *Inflamm Bowel Dis.* 2000;6:43.
6. Schmitt SL, Cohen SM, Wexner SD. Does laparoscopic-assisted ileal pouch anal anastomosis reduce the length of hospitalization? *Int J Colorectal Dis.* 1994;9:134.
7. Gordon PH, Nivatvongs S, eds. *Principles and Practice of Surgery for the Colon, Rectum, and Anus.* St. Louis: Quality Medical Publishing, 1999.
8. Wexner SD, Vernava AM III, eds. *Clinical Decision Making in Colorectal Surgery.* New York: Igaku-Shoin Medical Publishers, 1995.
9. Potenti FM, Wexner SD. Laparoscopy for benign colonic disease. In: Zuker KA, ed. *Surgical Laparoscopy,* 2nd ed. Lippincott Williams & Wilkins: 2001.
10. Hurst RD, Cohen RD. The role of laparoscopy and strictureplasty in the management of inflammatory bowel disease. *Semin Gastrointest Dis.* 2000;11:10.
11. Wexner SD, Johansen OB, Nogueras JJ, et al. Laparoscopic total abdominal colectomy. A prospective trial. *Dis Colon Rectum.* 1992;35:651.
12. Sardinha TC, Wexner SD. Laparoscopy for inflammatory bowel disease: Pros and cons. *World J Surg.* 1998;22:370.
13. Salky B. Is Laparoscopic surgery for most, a few, or no patients with Crohn's disease? 2000;6:40.
14. Ludwig KA, Milsom JW, Church JM, et al. Preliminary experience with laparoscopic intestinal surgery for Crohn's disease. *Am J Surg.* 1996;171:52.
15. Canin-Endres J, Salky B, Gattorno F. Laparoscopically assisted intestinal resection in 88 patients with Crohn's disease. *Surg Endosc.* 1999;13:595.
16. Reissman P, Salky BA, Edye M, et al. Laparoscopic surgery in Crohn's disease. *Surg Endosc.* 1996;10:1201.
17. Bauer JJ, Harris MT, Grumbach NM, Gorfine SR. Laparoscopic-assisted intestinal resection for Crohn's disease. *Dis Colon Rectum.* 1995;38:712.
18. Milsom JW, Lavery IC, Bohm B, et al. Laparoscopically assisted ileocolectomy in Crohn's disease. *Surg Laparoscop Endosc.* 1993;3:77.
19. Ludwig KA, Jerby BL. Laparoscopic procedures in patients with Crohn's disease. *Semin Colon Rectal Surg.* 1999;10:85.
20. Talamini MA, Moesinger RC, Kaufman H. Laparoscopically assisted bowel resection for Crohn's disease: The best of both worlds. Presented at Digestive Disease Week, Washington, DC, May 1997.
21. Hildebrandt U, Schiedeck T, Kreissler-Haag D, et al. Laparoscopically assisted surgery in Crohn's disease. *Zentralbla Chir.* 1995;123:357.
22. Jess P, Moller EH, Ladefoged K, et al. Laparoscopic assisted ileocecal resection for Crohn's disease. *Scand J Gastroenterol.* 1996;31:302.
23. Bemelman WA, van Hogenzand RA, Meijerink WJHJ, et al. Laparoscopic-assisted bowel resection in inflammatory bowel disease: State of the art. *Neth J Med.* 1998;53:39.
24. Wu JS, Birnbaum EH, Kodner IJ, et al. Laparoscopic-assisted ileocolic resections in patients with Crohn's disease: Are abscesses, phlegmons or recurrent disease contraindications? *Surgery.* 1997;122:682.
25. Wexner SD. General principles of surgery in ulcerative colitis and Crohn's disease. *Semin Gastroenterol.* 1991;2:90.
26. Bemelman WA, Slors JF, Dunker MS, et al. Laparoscopic-assisted vs. open ileocolic resection for Crohn's disease. *Surg Endosc.* 2000;14:721.
27. Dunker MS, Stiggelbout AM, vanHogezand RA, et al. Cosmesis and body image after laparoscopic-assisted and open ileocolic resection for Crohn's disease. *Surg Endosc.* 1998;12:1334.
28. Alabaz O, Augustine JNI, Nessim A, et al. Comparison of laparoscopically assisted and conventional ileocolic resection for Crohn's disease. *Eur J Surg.* 2000;166:213.
29. Singh K, Prasad A, Saunders JH, et al. Laparoscopy in the diagnosis and management of Crohn's disease. *J Laparoendosc Adv Surg Tech A.* 1998;8:39.
30. Kishi D, Nezu R, Ito T, et al. Laparoscopic-assisted surgery for Crohn's disease: Reduced surgical stress following ileocolectomy. *Surg Today.* 2000;30:219.
31. Lee SW, Whelan RL. The immunologic effects of laparoscopic colectomy. *Semin Colon Rectal Surg.* 1999;10:74.
32. Hildebrandt U, Lindemann W, Kreissler-Haag, et al. Laparoscopically-assisted proctocolectomy with ileoanal pouch in ulcerative colitis. *Zentralbla Chir.* 1998;123:403.
33. Thibault C, Poulin EC. Total laparoscopic proctocolectomy and laparoscopy-assisted proctocolectomy for inflammatory bowel disease: Operative technique and preliminary report. *Surg Laparosc Endosc.* 1995;5:472.
34. Peters WR. Laparoscopic total proctocolectomy with creation of an ileostomy for ulcerative colitis: Report of two cases. *J Laparoendosc Surg.* 1992;2:175.
35. Hildebrandt U, Pistorius G, Lindemann W, et al. Laparoscopic resection in Crohn's disease. *Chirurgie.* 1995;66:807.
36. Jacobs M, Plasencia G, Caushaj P, eds. *Atlas of Laparoscopic Surgery.* Williams & Wilkins: 1996.
37. Oliveira L, Reissman P, Nogueras J, et al. Laparoscopic creation of stomas. *Surg Endosc.* 1997;11:19.
38. Schmidt WU, Muller FP, Hesterberg R, et al. Laparoscopic ileostomy and colostomy in Crohn's disease patients. *Chirurgie.* 1996;67:1261.
39. Romero CA, James KM, Cooperstone LM, et al. Laparoscopic sigmoid colostomy for perianal Crohn's disease. *Surg Laparosc Endosc.* 1992;2:148.
40. Watanabe M, Ohgami M, Teramoto T, et al. Laparoscopically-assisted surgery for Crohn's disease. *Nippon Geka Zasshi. J Jpn Surg Soc.* 1997;98:418.
41. Milsom JW, Boohm B. *Laparoscopic Colorectal Surgery.* Springer-Verlag: 1996.
42. Marcello PW, Milsom JW, Wong SK. Laparoscopic restorative proctocolectomy: Case-matched comparative study with open restorative proctocolectomy. *Dis Colon Rectum.* 2000;43:604.
43. Santoro E, Carlini M, Carboni F, et al. Laparoscopic total proctocolectomy with ileal J pouch-anal anastomosis. *Hepatogastroenterology.* 1999;46:894.

44. Senagore AJ, Luchtefeld MA. The economics of laparoscopic surgery. *Semin Colon Rectal Surg.* 1999;10:69.

45. Larach SW, Gallagher J, Ferrara A. Lessons learned from laparoscopic colectomy. *Semin Colon Rectal Surg.* 1999;10:59.

46. Beck DE. Education and training for laparoscopic colon and rectal surgery. *Semin Colon Rectal Surg.* 1999;10:64.

47. Hildebrandt U, Kessler K, Pistorius G, et al. Granulocyte elastase and systemic cytokine response after laparoscopic-assisted and open resections in Crohn's disease. *Dis Colon Rectum.* 1999;42:1480.

48. Wishner JD, Baker JW Jr, Hoffman GC, et al. Laparoscopic assisted colectomy: The learning curve. *Surg Endosc.* 1995;9:1179.

49. Simons AJ, Anthone GJ, Ortega AE, et al. Laparoscopic assisted colectomy learning curve. *Dis Colon Rectum.* 1995;38:600.

Chapter Forty-Seven • • • • • •

*L*aparoscopic Management of Colonic Emergencies

EDDIE GOMEZ, MOISÉS JACOBS, and SASHIDHAR GANTA

The first laparoscopic colon resection was reported by Jacobs et al in 1991.[1] Though several surgeons adopted this technique, the majority of colon resections are still being performed by the open technique. Critics of the laparoscopic approach for colon resections state that it has not been proven in a randomized prospective trial. There are few standard surgical procedures ever supported by randomized prospective trials; rather, most are established with the test of time and large retrospective analyses. The authors believe that laparoscopic colon resection is a procedure here to stay, and as long as the time-tested, basic general surgical and oncologic principles are adhered to, the patient outcome will be better. It is our opinion that laparoscopic colon resection can be safely performed by most community general surgeons who have advanced laparoscopic skills and the ability to apply the principles of surgery to the laparoscopic setting. The management of laparoscopic colonic emergencies adds an extra level of expertise to colonic surgeries because of the patient's general status and because of operative field conditions.

Not surprisingly, only a small fraction of emergency colon surgeries are attempted laparoscopically. Apart from the fact that it is a difficult technical procedure, other factors such as availability of expert assistance and capable OR staff, immediate availability of reliable equipment including a colonoscope, and the next day's schedule play a significant role in the surgeon's decision.

This chapter discusses the role of laparoscopy in emergency colon surgery. The authors categorize the various emergencies and includes the technical details of the procedures not featured elsewhere in this book.

GENERAL PRINCIPLES OF LAPAROSCOPIC COLON SURGERY

The same principles that are essential in the open operation are applied in the laparoscopic approach. Both the surgeon and the assistant need advanced laparoscopic skills for safe and successful outcome. The surgeon embarking on this procedure should have his or her team well trained and organized so that cases can be successfully completed, benefiting the patient. Be aware that change in the position of the patient, monitor, and personnel is frequently required, and the procedure algorithm should be well thought out prior to the incision so that each step can proceed in a deliberate fashion.

Emergency Surgery and Special Precautions

Most emergencies operations on the colon are performed using the open technique. Several additional factors should be considered before deciding to approach the problem laparoscopically. Availability of good assistance and OR staff capable of handling the situation is mandatory. Perhaps the most important decision is whether a laparoscopic approach is beneficial to the patient. Can the procedure be performed with the same safety as an open operation without increase in morbidity? Most often common sense gives the answer. It is important to consider the adequacy of bowel preparation, if any; antibiotic coverage; and overall condition of the patient.

Preoperative Preparation of the Patient

Mechanical and antibiotic bowel preparation is not possible in most emergency situations. Prophylaxis for thromboembolism and perioperative antibiotics are routine practice. All the options should be discussed in detail with the patient and family. A list of possible complications and outcomes should also be part of the discussion and informed consent.

The surgeon should check that all the required apparatus and instruments are available in the operating room. Careful thought given to the details of the planned procedure and availability of any additional equipment (such as for intraoperative colonoscopy) saves time. If one expects to have to perform an intraoperative colonoscopy, the patient should be placed in low lithotomy position for easy access to the perineum.

Room Setup and Port Placement

1. When positioning the patient it is very important to place both arms along the side of the trunk and secure the pressure points with cushions. This gives unrestricted access to both sides of the patient.

2. Care should be taken to pad all potential pressure areas of the patient when positioning. An extreme Trendelenburg position is used at times and the patient should be adequately secured to the table.

3. Positioning of the monitor depends on the operation, but the principles should be adhered to. When the surgeon, laparoscope, site of operation, and monitor are in one straight line, optical correctness is achieved.

4. Trocar placement and OR setup depend on the nature of the procedure being performed. Many times, a surgeon won't know the etiology of the emergency until after a diagnostic laparoscopy has been performed; therefore the surgeon and OR personnel must be flexible enough to accommodate the diagnosis and placement of monitors and trocars. Usually a preoperative work-up including CT scans is performed to give the surgeon as much information as possible. Sometimes colonoscopy performed preoperatively reveals the diagnosis, as in an obstructing or bleeding lesion. If the diagnosis is known preoperatively, then the trocar and monitor setup should be done as in an elective operation (as described elsewhere in this book).

Patient Selection

Which patients to operate upon laparoscopically during an emergency depends on many factors. These include the surgeon's experience, skill, and comfort with laparoscopy; patient stability; and the patient's ability to tolerate pneumoperitoneum. If any of these criteria are negative, the operation should be done conventionally; or if the patient deteriorates while a laparoscopic procedure is being performed, the surgeon should convert to laparotomy.

COMMON COLONIC EMERGENCIES

Table 47–1 lists common colonic emergencies that may be suitable for laparoscopic management when the clinical condition of the patient permits. These are discussed in the following sections.

Iatrogenic Perforation of Colon

Colorectal perforations secondary to colonoscopy form the majority of the iatrogenic perforation group (Fig. 47–1). Therapeutic colonoscopy has a higher incidence of this complication. One large study from the Mayo clinic reviewed over 57,000 procedures and noted one perforation per 1333 procedures, a rate of 0.075%.[2] The incidence of perforation during diagnostic procedures was 0.1 to 0.8% and for therapeutic procedures was 0.5 to 3%.[3] Reported mortality from this complication was highly variable (0.14 to 17%), but there was consensus that with delay in treatment, mortality rose steeply, to as high as 50% in 24 hours. It is therefore important to

TABLE 47–1. COLON EMERGENCIES AMENDABLE TO LAPAROSCOPY

- Iatrogenic perforation of colon
- Acute diverticulitis and perforation
- Colonic obstruction
- Volvulus
- Ogilvie's syndrome
- Localized bleeding from colon

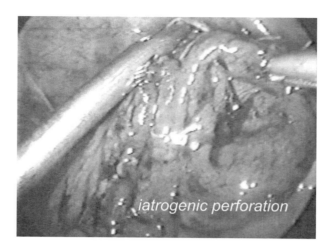

iatrogenic perforation

Figure 47–1. Iatrogenic perforation.

recognize the complication and institute therapy at the earliest possible time.[4] Most patients underwent exploratory laparotomy and a few were managed nonoperatively.

Etiology and Mechanism. Colonoscopy was the most common cause of iatrogenic perforation. Other causes included air insufflation during barium enema and trauma. The majority of perforations occured in the sigmoid colon (52 to 65%).

Several mechanisms have been proposed to explain this complication.[3] The most common cause in diagnostic colonoscopy is forceful insertion of the scope. Multiple serosal lacerations due to excessive stretching are usually associated. It is not uncommon for the endoscopist not to recognize this complication immediately. Most of these patients require surgical intervention. Forceful passage of the tip through the wall is another mechanism. This is more common in the diseased segment of the colon or due to failure to recognize a large diverticulum. Stretching may also cause laceration of segments of colon fixed by previous adhesions. Mechanisms of perforation in therapeutic colonoscopy are different; most common is excessive heat during the use of electrocautery, which results in a small perforation. Perforation with biopsy forceps is rare.

Diagnosis. The clinical presentation depends on the site, size of the perforation, amount of soiling, and condition of the patient.[5] A high index of suspicion is needed to diagnose this catastrophe early. Signs of generalized or local peritonitis may be elicited on physical examination. Once suspected, the diagnosis may be confirmed by plain films (free air, extracolonic air), water-soluble rectal contrast studies, or CT scan. Sometimes after extensive imaging, the diagnosis is not established and the surgeon is forced to manage the patient on an empiric basis or to consider diagnostic laparoscopy.

Surgical Options. Management of colonoscopic perforations is based on several factors, including the mechanism of perforation, adequacy of bowel preparation, time from incident to diagnosis, physical signs, and general condition of the patient.[6] Most patients with perforations after diagnostic colonoscopy require surgery, and most patients after therapeutic colonoscopy can be managed nonoperatively.[3,7] A subset of patients exists in whom imaging fails to confirm the suspicion, and diagnostic laparoscopy should be considered rather than empiric management.

The surgical options depend on the intraoperative findings and preexisting disease of the colon. Even though the perforation is suitable for primary closure, if the original disease of the colon requires other definitive surgery, then the definitive surgery should be performed if the patient's clinical condition permits.

Procedure. Port placement and room setup are as described earlier in this chapter. Initially, a diagnostic laparoscopy is performed to evaluate the location and extent of injury and local tissue conditions. After this step, a decision may be reached as to the exact procedure.

If the contamination is limited, as is usually the case in colonoscopically prepped bowel, and if the diagnosis is made early enough, two options exist for primary closure. The edges of the perforation are trimmed to healthy tissue. The defect is closed transversely either with interrupted sutures (Fig. 47–2) or Endo stapler. If there is a long linear tear, it is better to perform a resection and anastomosis than closure of the perforation. If the perforation occurs in the left colon, as is usually the case, colonoscopy should be performed to check the patency of the lumen and to assure an airtight seal.

Acute Diverticulitis

Acute diverticulitis is the most common indication for an emergency Hartman's procedure in the Western world. Clinical conditions permitting, some surgeons opt to perform a resection and primary anastomosis with or without lavage/diverting stoma. The majority of these operations are performed by the open technique. A proportion of the procedures might benefit from a laparoscopic approach. Though technically possible to perform these procedures laparoscopically, wisdom is needed to exercise proper judgment as to the risk versus benefit to the individual patient. Careful consideration should be given to factors such as previous abdominal operations, sepsis and shock, respiratory status, and anticipated time in the operating room. An expeditious open operation may be far less traumatic than a prolonged laparoscopic procedure. In patients in whom surgery is required where there is no fecal contamination, but rather a purulent peritonitis/or abscess, laparoscopy has a place.

The authors have reported a series[8] in which patients who did not have fecal peritonitis, and in whom the perforation had sealed (proven by intraoperative sigmoidoscopy), peritoneal lavage was done, IV antibiotics administered for 1 to 2 weeks postoperatively, and subsequently the patient was brought for an elective colectomy at an appropriate time. This approach usually is in patients who do not respond to IV antibiotics or in whom an abscess (Fig. 47–3) is not amenable to percutaneous drainage. Alternatively, a resection may also be done laparoscopically (Fig. 47–4). In these cases, the mesentery is friable and cheesy, and staying closer to the bowel may be easier than trying to access the base of the mesentery. Usually the mesenteric fat breaks and disintegrates, leaving only blood vessels that can easily be controlled using regular endoclips or an ultrasonic scalpel. Because usually in these cases the mesentery also becomes foreshortened, proximal colonic mobilization also has to be performed, and a primary anastomosis may not be able to be done laparoscopically, necessitating a Hartman's procedure.

The laparoscopic approach should be converted in patients in whom there is fecal contamination, or in patients with inflammation so severe that tissue planes cannot be identified or separated. Also, when the left ureter cannot be identified, laparoscopic resection should be abandoned.

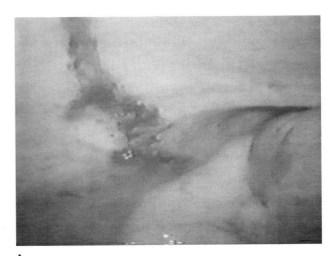

A

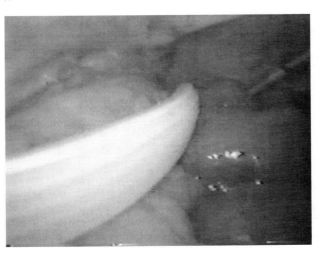

B

Figure 47–3. A. Collection of pus in pelvis. B. Diverticular abscess.

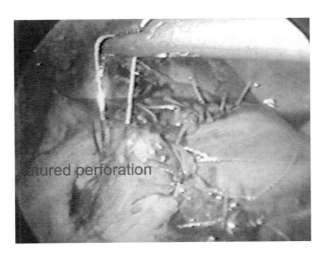

Figure 47–2. Sutured perforation.

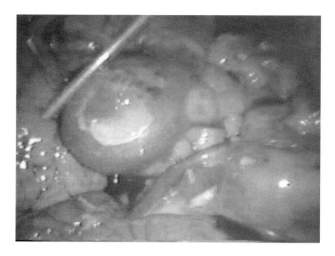

Figure 47–4. Necrotic diverticulum. See Color Section.

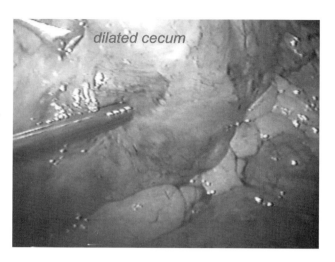

Figure 47–5. Ogilvie's syndrome. See Color Section.

Colonic Obstruction

Several options exist for management of colonic obstruction. A right hemicolectomy or extended right hemicolectomy with anastomosis is the choice for right or transverse colon obstruction. With a left-sided obstruction the decision is more difficult. Traditional two or three-stage procedures are being replaced by the single-stage procedure consisting of resection and primary anastomosis.[8] More recently, experience is accumulating in the use of self-expandable metal stents to relieve the left colon obstruction.[9] These patients can then undergo a bowel preparation prior to the definitive surgical procedure. This is a very promising new approach, and has the potential to make the staged procedures obsolete. A large proportion of patients successfully treated with stents would be able to undergo laparoscopic resection. In a proportion of all of the situations described, a laparoscopic approach is possible. The surgeon should decide which patient is appropriate to undergo a laparoscopic resection based on the factors discussed earlier. In patients in whom obstruction is caused by cancer, if the base of the mesentery cannot be reached because of the bulkiness of the tumor, or in patients in whom the mesentery is so fixed that it cannot be lifted, conversion to an open procedure should be considered. In patients in whom the colonic or enteric distension is such that exposure is precluded or the bowel can't be handled safely without the risk of perforation, conversion should be considered.

However, a proximal diverting colostomy/ileostomy may be able to be done in these patients, creating a two-stage procedure. This is done by localizing the segment that needs to be exteriorized, creating a window in the mesentery, and then under direct vision making a counter-incision in the abdominal wall and delivering the bowel for diversion.

Colonic Volvulus

Volvulus requires a similar technique, and has similar contraindications, as for obstruction. However, sometimes in these very mobile colons, once the diagnosis is made, a small counter-incision can be made and the bowel exteriorized through this small incision, without the requirement of a major laparotomy.

Ogilvie's Syndrome

Ogilvie's syndrome (pseudocolonic obstruction; Fig. 47–5) can be treated with laparoscopic decompression using "gastrostomy" kits through the cecum (Fig. 47–6). Once the colon is decompressed, a decision can be made as to whether a resection or repair of tears and microperforations is required; and these can be done laparoscopically.

Localized Bleeding

If bleeding is uncontrolled or a subtotal colectomy is required in septic patients (toxic megacolon), laparoscopy should only be done for diagnostic purposes. If bleeding is localized to a segment of the colon and if it is not massive, laparoscopically assisted resection could be undertaken.

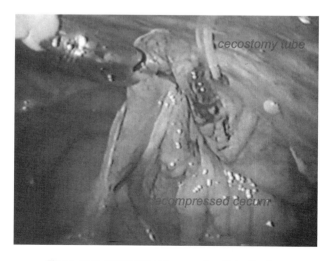

Figure 47–6. Decompressed cecum. See Color Section.

FUTURE DIRECTIONS

A decade after the first laparoscopic colon resection, only a minority of colon emergencies are handled by this approach. Lack of experience in elective resections and the advanced skills required are among the causes. Advances in teaching methods and technology will continue to instill confidence in the surgeon. The use of self-expandable metal stents to temporarily relieve left colon obstruction is a promising approach, because this would be amenable to, and benefit from, laparoscopic resection.

REFERENCES

1. Jacobs M, Verdeja JC, Goldstein HS. Minimally invasive colon resection (laparoscopic colectomy). *Surg Laparosc Endosc.* 1991;1:144.
2. Farley DR, Bannon MP, Zietlow SP, et al. *Mayo Clin Proc.* 1997;72:729.
3. Hymie Kavin, Sinicrope F, Esker AH. Management of perforation of the colon at colonoscopy. *Am J Gastroenterol.* 1992;87:161.
4. Kockerling F. Repair of perforations of the colon and rectum. In: Kremer K, Platzer W, Schreiber HW, et al, eds. *Minimally Invasive Abdominal Surgery.* Thieme: 2001:364.
5. Gedebou TM, Wong RA, Rappaport WD, et al. Clinical presentation and management of iatrogenic colon perforations. *Am J Surg.* 1996; 172:454.
6. Adair HM, Hishon S. The management of colonoscopic and sigmoidoscopic perforations of the large bowel. *Br J Surg.* 1981;68:415.
7. Berry MA, Rangraj M. Conservative treatment of recognized laparoscopic colonic injury. *J Soc Laparoendosc Surg.* 1998;2:195.
8. Franklin MC, Jr, Dorman JP, Jacobs M, et al. Is laparoscopic surgery applicable to complicated colonic diverticular disease? *Surg Endosc.* 1997;11:1021.
9. Deen KI, Madoff RD, Goldberg SM, et al. Surgical management of left colon obstruction: The university of Minnesota experience. *J Am Coll Surg.* 1998;187:573.
10. Tamin WZ, Ghellai A, Counihan TC, et al. Experience with endoluminal colonic wall stents for the management of large bowel obstruction for benign and malignant disease. *Arch Surg.* 2000; 135:434.

Chapter Forty-Eight · · · · · · ·

*L*aparoscopic Rectopexy for Complete Rectal Prolapse

MIGUEL A. CUESTA and RICHELLE J.F. FEET-BERSMA

Complete rectal prolapse is defined as the protrusion of all layers of the rectal wall through the anal sphincter complex. If the rectal wall is prolapsed but does not protrude through the anal sphincter, it is called an occult rectal prolapse or a rectal intussusception. About 75% of patients with rectal prolapse suffer from anal incontinence.[1,2] The standard treatment for complete rectal prolapse consists of either transabdominal or perineal surgery; more than 50 different operative procedures have been described. Until recently, abdominal rectopexy has been advocated as the treatment of choice for complete rectal prolapse. Recurrence rates are low (0 to 8%)[2,3] and continence improves in the majority of patients (50 to 88%).[1,4,5] As most patients are elderly and not always fit enough to undergo an abdominal procedure, various perineal approaches, such as the Delorme procedure or proctosigmoidectomy, are preferred. They have recurrence rates varying from 5 to 21%, depending on the type and the extent of the operation.[6–9] A possible alternative is laparoscopic rectopexy, which has been performed in our department since 1991.[10] This method, being the laparoscopic counterpart of the abdominal Ripstein procedure, aims to combine the good functional outcome of abdominal procedures with the low postoperative morbidity of minimally invasive surgery. Laparoscopic rectopexy has been proven technically feasible.[10–16] However, postoperative results including manometric and/or endosonographic findings have not been published until now.

The purpose of this study was to evaluate the clinical outcome of laparoscopic rectopexy and to determine whether clinical improvements are associated with changes in manometric and endosonography findings.

MATERIALS AND METHODS

Between June 1991 and September 1997, 28 consecutive patients (25 women and 3 men) referred to our clinic with complete rectal prolapse were treated by laparoscopic rectopexy according to a modified sling repair procedure. The median age of the patients was 73 years (range, 57 to 86 years). A detailed history, physical examination (inspection, digital examination, and proctoscopy), manometry, and endosonography were performed preoperatively and 3 months postoperatively. Seventeen patients had normal bowel habits and 11 had constipation. Twenty-one had different grades of fecal incontinence.

One patient had undergone two operations for fistula in ano and 14 patients an abdominal hysterectomy because of leiomyomas and prolapse. Continence was scored according to Parks,[17] with grade 1 meaning full continence, grade 2 difficult control of flatus and diarrhea, grade 3 no control of liquid stools, and grade 4 no control of solid stools.

Anal Manometry, Rectal Sensitivity, and Anal Endosonography

Anorectal function tests were performed according to the technique published by our group elsewhere.[18]

Operative Procedure

All patients received low-dosage subcutaneous heparin and had a preoperative mechanical cleansing of the bowel. After introducing an indwelling catheter, patients are placed supine with the legs in leg rests to allow for inspection and digital examination during the operation. The video monitor is placed between the legs. The surgeon and the second assistant (camera) stand on the right side of the patient, and the operating nurse on the surgeon's right side and the first assistant in front of the surgeon. Pneumoperitoneum was established using a Veress needle introduced via a subumbilical wound. The needle was then replaced with a 10-mm trocar in order to introduce the laparoscope. Three auxilliary trocars were placed under direct vision: two in the right iliac fossa and another in the left iliac fossa.[10] The patients were placed in a moderately steep Trendelenburg tilt.

If present, the uterus was fixed to the ventral abdominal wall using a temporary suture. The sigmoid and rectum were subsequently mobilized, with care taken to identify the ureters. Anteriorly, the rectum was mobilized up to the high limit of the vagina; posteriorly, the presacral space was entered and dissected to the level of the coccyx. The lateral ligaments and the nervi erigentes were left intact. The limit of the posterior dissection was determined by rectal examination. Following this, a 4×8 cm polypropylene mesh, tightly rolled like a cigarette, was introduced into the abdomen and attached to the promontorium and presacral fascia using an endoscopic "hernia" stapler device (Ethicon, Cincinnati, OH). After determining that the mesh was firmly attached to the sacrum, the rectum was held under tension and the mesh was fixed to the anterolateral wall of the rectum using three nonabsorbable seromuscular sutures on each side, so that one third of the circumference of the bowel was left free.

RESULTS

There were no major preoperative complications. One patient had a transient brachial plexus apraxia due to hyperextension of the upper arm during the operation. The median duration of the procedure was 2 hours and 45 minutes (range, 2 hours and 10 minutes to 4 hours and 30 minutes). There were no conversions during surgery. Blood losses were less than 100 mL in each case. Commencement of bowel movements appeared at 24 hours postoperatively, with passage of stools on the fourth postoperative day (range, 2 to 7 days). No wound complications occurred, and the median hospital stay was 10 days (range, 6 to 11 days) and postoperative stay was 7 days (range, 5 to 10 days).

No recurrences took place during a median follow-up of 18 months (range, 4 to 24 months). Three patients needed additional rubber band ligation of persisting and mucosal prolapse (2 patients at 2 months, one patient at 1 year after surgery). Seven out of 28 patients were continent before surgery and remained so afterwards. There was a marked increase in continence in 16 of 21 patients who suffered from either grade 4 or grade 3 incontinence before operation. One patient showed only a mild improvement and 4 patients did not improve, remaining incontinent for liquid stools. Eleven out of 28 patients were constipated before the rectopexy and remained so after the surgical procedure. Three patients suffered from postoperative constipation. In all of these patients, constipation was treated successfully with a fiber-enriched diet and/or bulk-forming agents.

Anal Manometry

Postoperatively, the basal pressure increased significantly from 20 to 25 mm Hg ($P < .01$), whereas the squeeze pressure did not change after operation.

Rectal Sensitivity

Rectal sensitivity did not change significantly after laparoscopic rectopexy.

Anal Endosonography

Preoperative endosonography showed asymmetry of the internal anal sphincter in the majority of patients. Also, thickening of the internal anal sphincter was found (IST, 3.0 mm). After surgery, IST decreased significantly ($P = .02$) compared to preoperative

values, but the asymmetrical aspect of the internal anal sphincter persisted. The external anal sphincter was normal before and after surgery.

DISCUSSION

Recurrence rates of the different abdominal rectopexy procedures are low (up to 8%), and incontinence improves in the majority of patients (50 to 88%).[1–5] Even if all rectopexy procedures are considered to increase constipation (up to 50%), the combination of resection with any form of rectopexy could improve this symptom in almost three fourths of patients.[5] The perineal procedures have recurrence rates varying from 5 to 21% depending on the type of operation, and the persistent incontinence is higher in comparison to abdominal operations.[6–9] Along with this, the constipation rates remain unchanged. A possible alternative to both approaches is laparoscopic rectopexy. This method aims to combine the good functional outcome of abdominal procedures with the low postoperative morbidity of minimally invasive surgery.

Laparoscopic rectopexy is a feasible and effective treatment for complete rectal prolapse. In the group of patients, here presented, the procedure was associated with only one minor complication. The postoperative recovery of these patients was rapid, with resumption of bowel function and normal activities within a few days after surgery. The median hospital stay was 10 days. This is shorter than the 16 days recorded approximately 20 years ago in our department[19] and less than the 13 to 15 days reported by McKee et al[20] for different open procedures. However, the median hospital stay of 10 days certainly did not reflect the full advantages of laparoscopic surgery regarding postoperative recovery. These elderly patients (median 73 years) were often single and admission was frequently prolonged on a social indication to allow for arranging of additional help at home after their hospital stay. Blaker et al[21] have compared laparoscopic assisted and open resection rectopexy. Hospital stay was significantly shorter for the laparoscopic assisted group (4 versus 8 days).

One difference with the open procedure is the fixation of the mesh, which is performed using "hernia" staplers in the laparoscopic version of rectopexy. So far, this modification of the technique has not been associated with increased recurrence rates compared to the 0 to 8% described for the open procedures.[2,3] Continence improved in 16 of 21 preoperatively incontinent patients, and this is comparable to the open technique. Both manometric basal pressure representing internal anal sphincter function, and squeeze pressure representing external anal sphincter function, are strongly associated with fecal incontinence.[22] An increase in squeeze pressure after abdominal rectopexy has been described by Delemarre et al.[23] In our patients, improved continence was associated with a small but significant increase in basal pressure, suggesting a restoration of the internal anal sphincter. An increase in this basal pressure has been previously described after open procedures.[1,24–27] It is believed that this improvement after surgery might be due to relief of rectoanal inhibition, which is induced by the prolapsed bowel distending into the lower rectum.[5,26,27] Also of importance might be the simple anatomic restoration of the prolapsed bowel, which prevents further dilatation of the anal sphincters.[1]

A major drawback of abdominal rectopexy is constipation. Previous studies have reported an increased incidence of postoperative constipation (up to 50%), probably related to the division of the lateral ligaments.[28,29] Three of our patients developed mild constipation postoperatively, which was treated successfully with a fiber-enriched diet and intermittent use of bulk-forming agents. These satisfactory results regarding postoperative constipation can be explained by the fact that we did not dissect the lateral ligaments and the nervi erigentes. This is sustained by our finding that rectal sensitivity, which has been proven to be impaired after lateral ligament division,[29] was not changed significantly in our patients after the operation. Although the St.-Mark's group found a higher recurrence rate after not dividing these ligaments,[23] we found no complete recurrences. These results were confirmed by Scaglia et al.[29]

Different laparoscopic rectopexy techniques have been described, from laparoscopic suture rectopexy to the most elaborate resection rectopexy. Most of the series include patients with a full-thickness rectal prolapse, and some include patients with intussusception. Our results, concerning feasibility, recurrence rate, control of incontinence, and appearance of constipation, are concordant with the results obtained by Heath et al[13] with the suture rectopexy technique, Himpens et al[16] with the rectopexy according to Wells, and Boccasanta et al.[15] In the series of Kellokumpu et al,[14] in which an analysis was made of the results (not randomized) of suture and resection rectopexy (two groups of 17 patients each), a longer operative time was found in the resection than in the suture group (255 versus 150 minutes), with the same outcomes concerning operative stay, median time off work, improvement of incontinence, constipation, and recurrence.

There are no reports of anal endosonography in rectal prolapse. This technique has been proven of value in the assessment of anal sphincter defects and is capable of giving excellent images of the internal as well as the external anal sphincter.[30–32] The asymmetry and the thickening of the internal anal sphincter, with the underlying thickened submucosa, supplies a rather striking image. Thickening of the internal anal sphincter could be expected in these elderly patients, since evidence exists that it is a physiologic process of aging.[33,34] However, the decrease of internal sphincter (IST) after surgery suggests a partially reversible process, such as edema, that might occur as a result of irritation of the rectum protruding into the anal canal. Decrease of IST after surgery gives us further evidence toward restoration of internal anal sphincter function. These results confirm those previously obtained in our department with a reduced number of patients.[35]

In conclusion, laparoscopic rectopexy is a technically feasible method that resulted in improved continence in the majority of our patients. This was associated with a significant increase in continence grade in our patients without important worsening of the constipation rate. Anorectal function study demonstrated a (partial) recovery of the internal anal sphincter. Moreover, laparoscopic rectopexy combines the low morbidity of minimally invasive surgery with the good clinical outcome of abdominal rectopexy.

REFERENCES

1. Madden MV, Kamm MA, Nicholls RJ, et al. Abdominal rectopexy for complete prolapse: Prospective study evaluating changes in symptoms and anorectal function. *Dis Colon Rectum.* 1992;35:48.

2. Keighley MRB, Fielding JWL, Alexander-Williams J. Results of Marlex mesh abdominal rectopexy for rectal prolapse in 100 consecutive patients. *Br J Surg.* 1983;70:229.

3. Tjandra JJ, Fazio VW, Church JM, et al. Ripstein procedure is an effective treatment for rectal prolapse without constipation. *Dis Colon Rectum.* 1993;36:501.

4. McCue JL, Thomson JPS. Clinical and functional results of abdominal rectopexy for complete rectal prolapse. *Br J Surg.* 1991;78:921.

5. Duthie GS, Bartolo DCC. Abdominal rectopexy for rectal prolapse: A comparison of techniques. *Br J Surg.* 1992;79:107.

6. Ramanujam PS, Venkatesh KS, Fietz MJ. Perineal excision of rectal procidentia in elderly high risk patients. A ten-year experience. *Dis Colon Rectum.* 1994;37:1027.

7. Lechaux JP, Lechaux D, Perez M. Results of Delorme's procedure for rectal prolapse. Advantage of a modified technique. *Dis Colon Rectum.* 1995;38:301.

8. Johansen OB, Wexner SD, Daniel N, et al. Perineal rectosigmoidectomy in the elderly. *Dis Colon rectum.* 1993;36:767.

9. Graf W, Ejerblad S, Krog M, et al. Delorme's operation for rectal prolapse in elderly or unfit patients. *Eur J Surg.* 1992;158:555.

10. Cuesta MA, Borgstein PJ, De Jong D, et al. Laparoscopic rectopexy. *Surg Laparosc Endosc.* 1993;3:456.

11. Berman IR. Sutureless laparoscopic rectopexy for procidentia: Technique and implications. *Dis Colon Rectum.* 1992;35:689.

12. Cuschieri A, Shimi SM, Vander VG, et al. Laparoscopic prosthesis fixation rectopexy for complete rectal prolapse. *Br J Surg.* 1994;81:138.

13. Heath SM, Hartley JE, Hurley J, et al. Laparoscopic suture rectopexy without resection is effective treatment for full-thickness rectal prolapse. *Dis Colon Rectum.* 2000;43:638.

14. Kellokumpu IH, Vironen J, Scheinin T. Laparoscopic repair of rectal prolapse. A prospective study evaluating surgical outcome and changes in symptoms and bowel function. *Surg Endosc.* 2000;14:634.

15. Boccasanta P, Venturi M, Reitano MC, et al. Laparotomic vs laparoscopic rectopexy in complete rectal prolapse. *Dig Surg.* 1999;16:415.

16. Himpens J, Cadiere GB, Bruyns J, et al. Laparoscopic rectopexy according to Wells. *Surg Endosc.* 1999;13:139.

17. Parks AG. Anorectal incontinence. *Proc R Soc Med.* 1975;68:681.

18. Felt-Bersma RJF, Klinkenberg-Knol EC, Meuwissen SGM. Investigation of anorectal function. *Br J Surg.* 1988;75:53.

19. Hoitsma HFW, Meijer S, Klinkenberg-Knol EC, et al. The treatment of complete rectal prolapse by transabdominal posterior rectopexy. *Neth J Surg.* 1984;36:73.

20. McKee RF, Lauder JC, Poon FW, et al. A prospective randomized study of abdominal rectopexy with and without sigmoidectomy in rectal prolapse. *Surg Gynecol Obstet.* 1992;174:145.

21. Blaker R, Senagore AJ, Luchtefeld MA. Laparoscopic assisted vs. open resection. Rectopexy offers excellent results. *Dis Colon Rectum.* 1995;38:199.

22. Felt-Bersma RJF, Klinkenberg-Knol EC, Meuwissen SGM. Anorectal function investigations in incontinent and continent patients. Differences and discriminatory value. *Dis Colon Rectum.* 1990;33:479.

23. Delemarre JBVM, Gooszen HG, Kruyt RH, et al. The effect of posterior rectopexy on fecal continence. A prospective study. *Dis Colon Rectum.* 1991;34:311.

24. Broden G, Dolk A, Holmstrom B. Recovery of the internal and sphincter following rectopexy: A possible explanation for continence improvement. *Int J Colorectal Dis.* 1988;3:23.

25. Williams JG, Wong WD, Jensen L, et al. Incontinence and rectal prolapse: A prospective manometric study. *Dis Colon Rectum.* 1991;34:209.

26. Farouk R, Duthie GS, Bartolo DCC, et al. Restoration of continence following rectopexy for rectal prolapse and recovery of the internal and sphincter electromyogram. *Br J Surg.* 1992;79:439.

27. Farouk R, Duthie GS, MacGregor SAB, et al. Rectoanal inhibition and incontinence in patients with rectal prolapse. *Br J Surg.* 1994; 81:743.

28. Speakman CT, Madden MV, Nicholls RJ, et al. Lateral ligament

division during rectopexy causes constipation but prevents recurrence: Results of a prospective randomized study. *Br J Surg.* 1991; 78:1431.

29. Scaglia M, Fasth S, Hallgren T, et al. Abdominal rectopexy for rectal prolapse: Influence of surgical technique on functional outcome. *Dis Colon Rectum.* 1994;37:185.

30. Bartram CI. Anal endosonography. *Ann Gastroenterol Hepatol.* 1992;28:185.

31. Cuesta MA, Meijer S, Derksen EJ, et al. Anal sphincter imaging in fecal incontinence using endosonography. *Dis Colon Rectum.* 1992; 35:59.

32. Felt-Bersma RJF, Van Baren R, Koorevaar M, et al. Unsuspected sphincter defects shown by anal endosonography after anorectal surgery: A prospective study. *Dis Colon Rectum.* 1995;38:249.

33. Nielsen MB, Hauge C, Rasmussen OO, et al. Anal sphincter size measured by endosonography in healthy volunteers. Effect of age, sex and parity. *Acta Radiol.* 1992;33:453.

34. Burnett S, Bartram CI. Endosonographic variations in the normal internal anal sphincter. *Int J Colorectal Dis.* 1991;6:2.

35. Poen AC, de Brauw LM, Felt-Bersma RJF, et al. Laparoscopic rectopexy for complete rectal prolapse. Results regarding clinical outcome and anorectal function tests. *Surg Endosc.* 1996;10:904.

*S*plenic, Adrenal, and Pancreatic Surgery

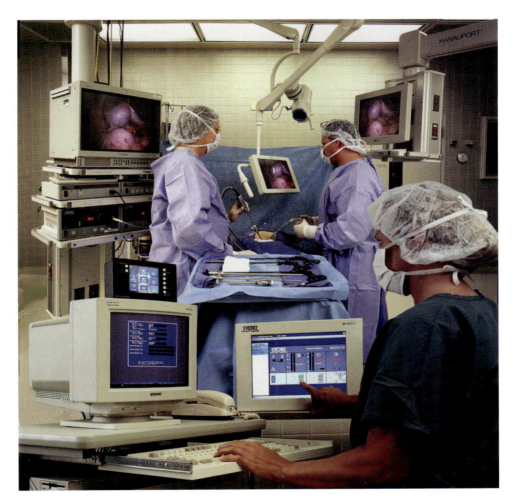

Courtesy of K. Storz, Germany.

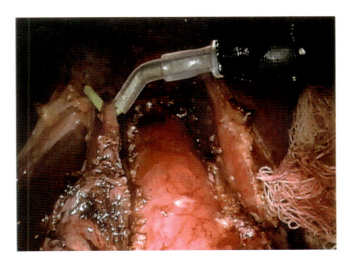

Figure 17–6. Esophageal myotomy with the Da Vinci Robotic System (Intuitive Surgical, Mountview, CA).

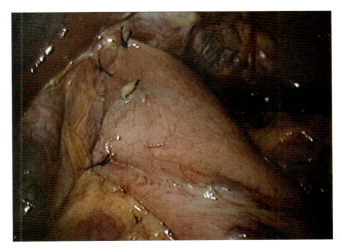

Figure 17–7. Dor anterior fundoplication.

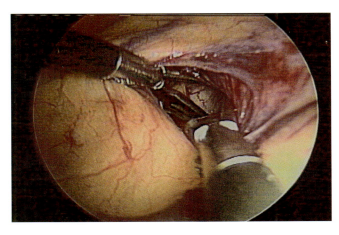

Figure 26–4. Dissection between the gastric branches of the anterior vagus nerve and gastric wall.

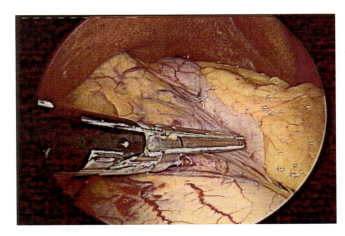

Figure 26–5A. Stapling of the stomach to create the gastric pouch.

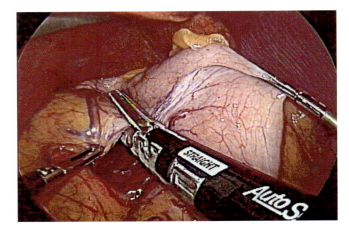

Figure 26–5B. Further stapling of the stomach to create the gastric pouch.

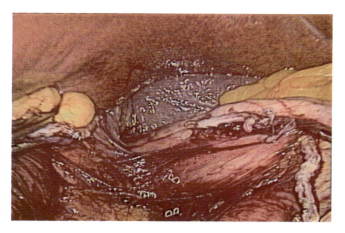

Figure 26–6. Completed separation of the proximal gastric pouch from the distal portion.

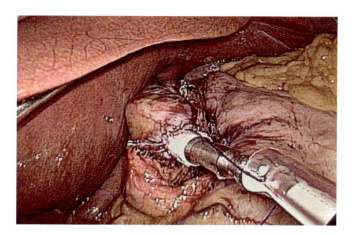

Figure 26–10. The nasogastric tube is pulled until the anvil appears through the staple line.

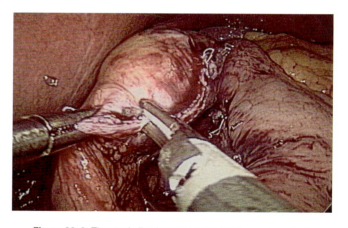

Figure 26–8. The staple line is opened with the harmonic scalpel.

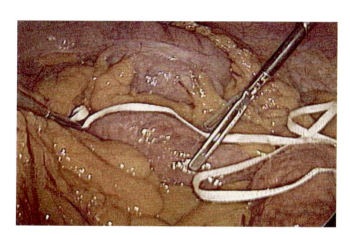

Figure 26–11. Roux limbs are measured with a precut umbilical tape.

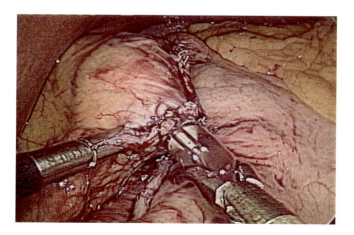

Figure 26–9. The nasogastric tube is grasped and pulled into the abdominal cavity.

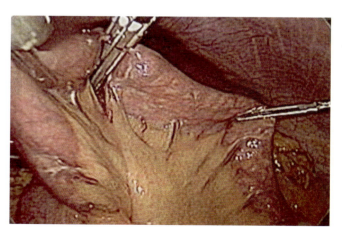

Figure 26–12. The bowel is transected with a stapler.

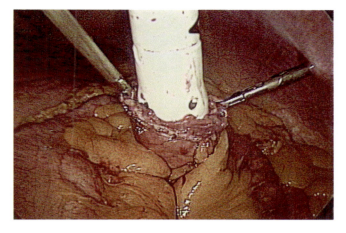

Figure 26–14. The circular stapler is introduced into the jejunal loop.

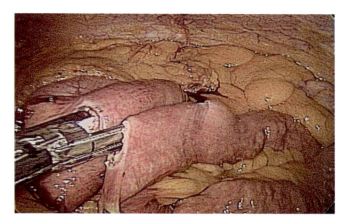

Figure 26–17. A side-to-side jejunojejunostomy is performed with a stapler.

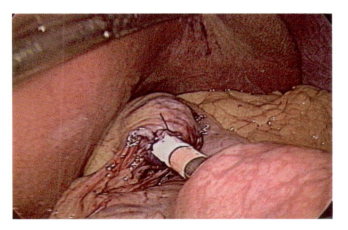

Figure 26–15. The stapler is brought up to the staple line to perform the gastrojejunostomy.

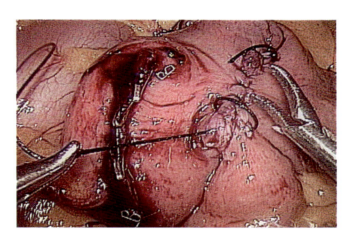

Figure 26–18. The enterotomies are closed with a running suture.

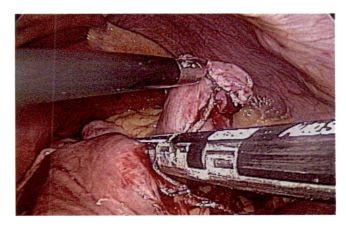

Figure 26–16. The remaining jejunal loop is transected with a stapler.

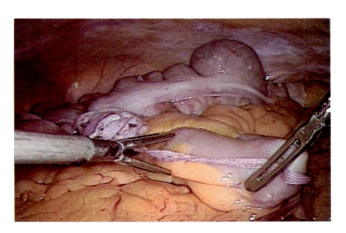

Figure 27–4. Measurement of small bowel.

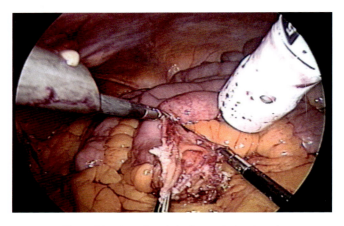

Figure 27–6. Insertion of circular stapler into bowel.

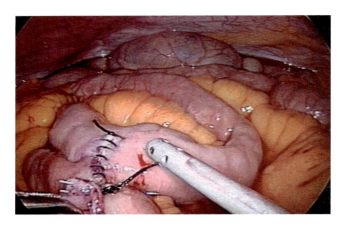

Figure 27–9. Intracorporeal side-to-side anastomosis of small bowel.

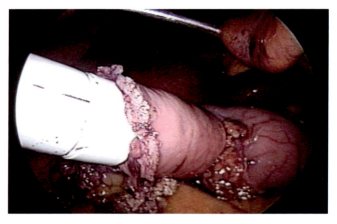

Figure 27–7. Insertion of circular stapler into bowel.

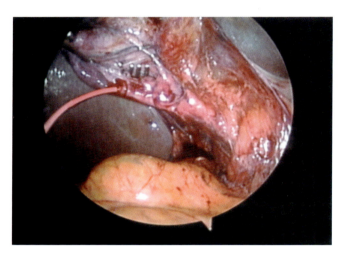

Figure 30–3. Transcystic duct passage of a no. 4 Fogarty embolectomy catheter.

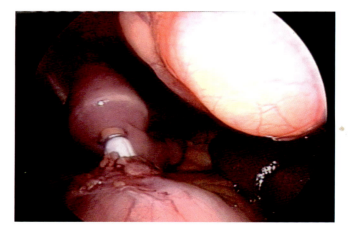

Figure 27–8. Joining the two ends of the stapler.

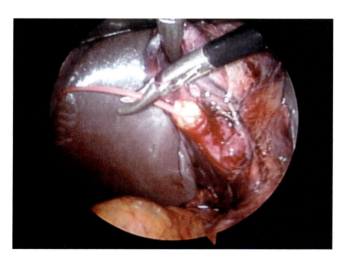

Figure 30–5. Transcystic stone extraction using a Fogarty embolectomy catheter.

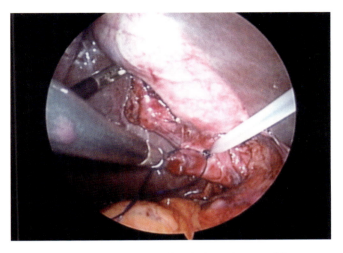

Figure 30–6. Closure of dilated cystic duct using an endoloop.

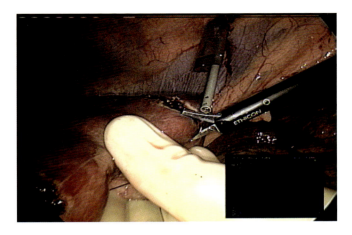

Figure 34–10. Liver resection using an ultrasonic dissector.

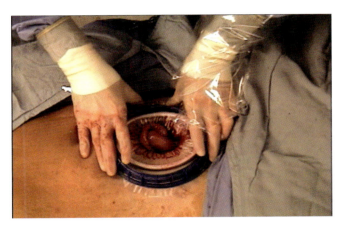

Figure 34–7. Hand-assisting device.

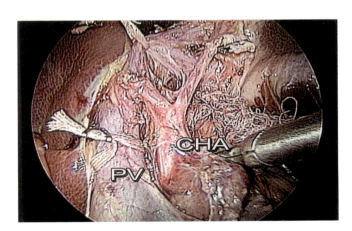

Figure 36–1. Dissection of the portal vein (PV), common hepatic artery (CHA), and common bile duct at the hepatic hilum.

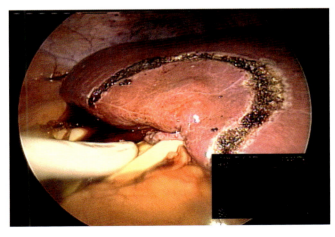

Figure 34–9. Tumor margins are marked with electrocautery.

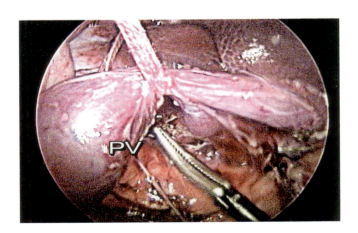

Figure 36–2. The portal vein is encircled with an umbilical tape.

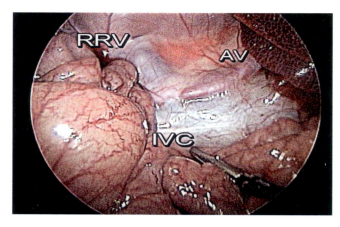

Figure 36–3. After retracting the bowel, the inferior vena cava (IVC), right renal vein (RRV), and right adrenal vein (AV) are identified.

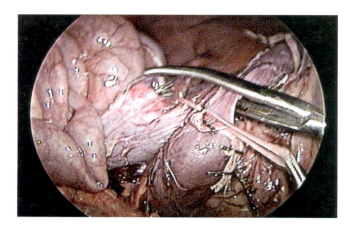

Figure 36–6. Cross-clamping of the portal vein (PV) and inferior vena cava (IVC).

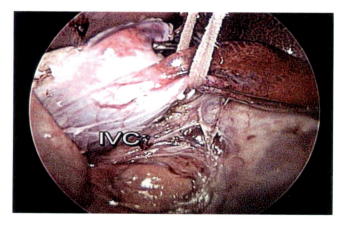

Figure 36–4. The inferior vena cava (IVC) is encircled with an umbilical tape.

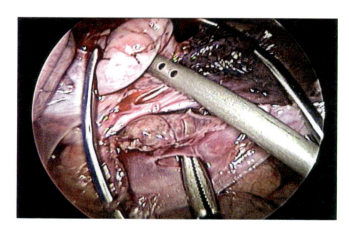

Figure 36–7. The phlebotomies are performed.

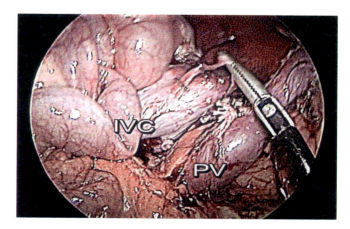

Figure 36–5. The portal vein (PV) and inferior vena cava (IVC) are approximated before clamping.

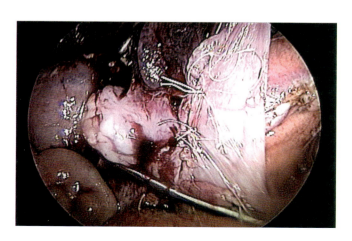

Figure 36–8. Final side-to-side portocaval shunt.

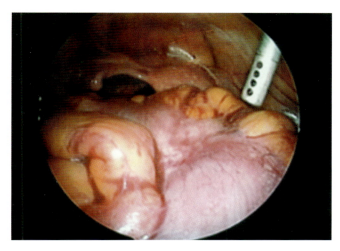

Figure 41–1. Colon cancer.

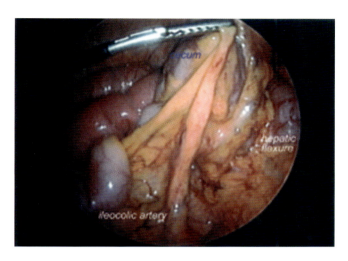

Figure 41–6. Ileocolic artery.

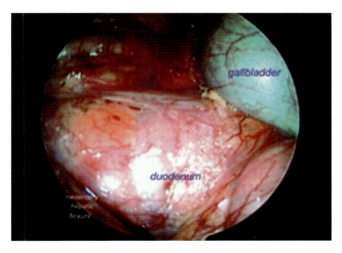

Figure 41–4. Exposure of duodenum.

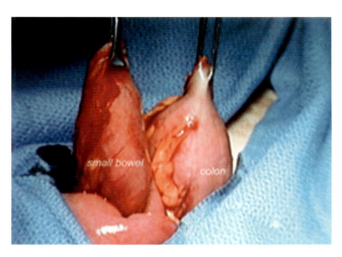

Figure 41–7. Exteriorization, right colon.

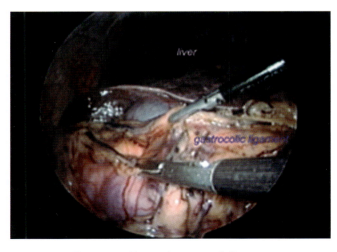

Figure 41–5. Transecting gastrocolic ligament.

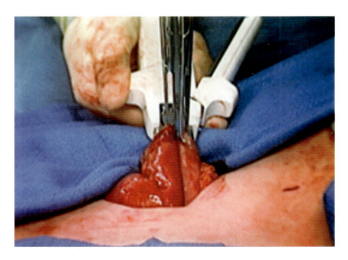

Figure 41–8. Ileocolic anastamosis.

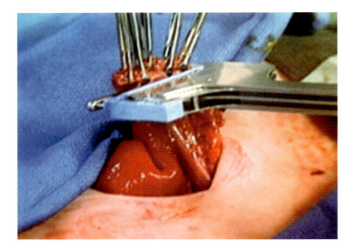

Figure 41–9. Closure.

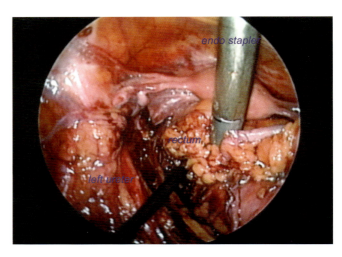

Figure 41–13. Rectosigmoid transection.

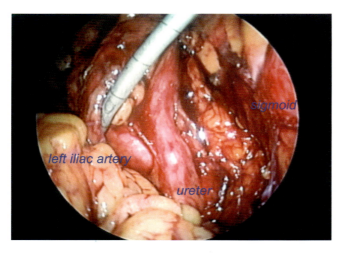

Figure 41–11. Left ureter, iliac artery.

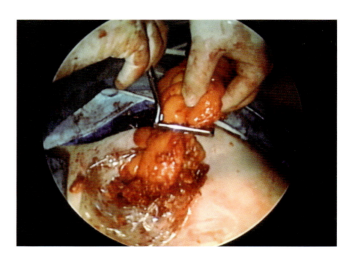

Figure 41–14. Placement of purse-string sutures, proximal margins; bowel exteriorized through plastic sleeve.

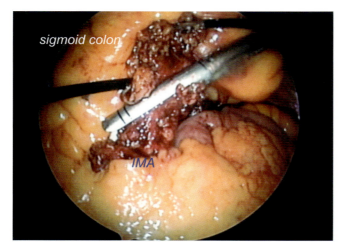

Figure 41–12. Stapler transecting IMA.

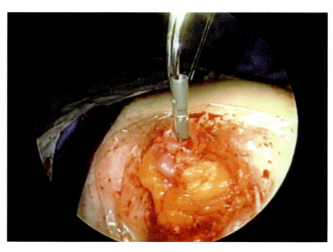

Figure 41–15. Proximal bowel with head of circular stapler.

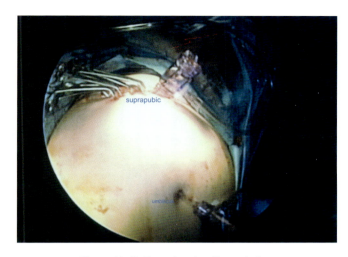

Figure 41–16. Extraction site with towel clips.

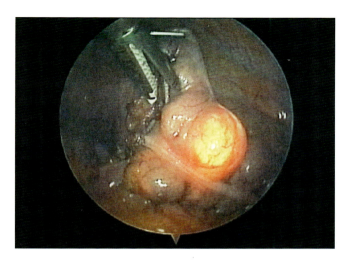

Figure 44–1. Colon polypectomy.

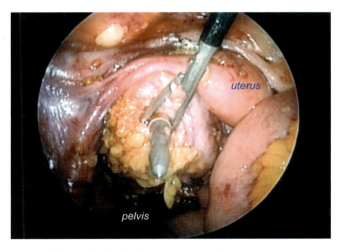

Figure 41–17. Circular stapler penetrating rectal stump.

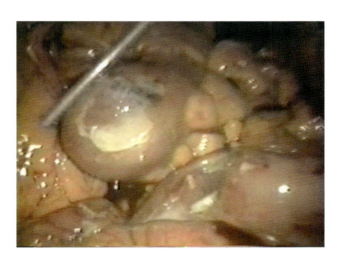

Figure 47–4. Necrotic diverticulum.

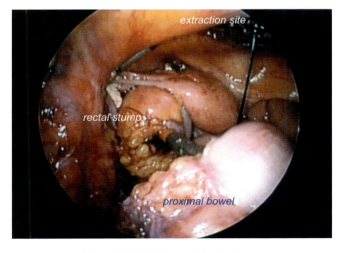

Figure 41–18. Marriage of circular stapler.

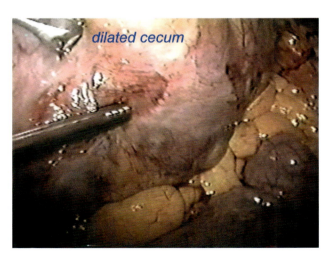

Figure 47–5. Ogilvie's syndrome.

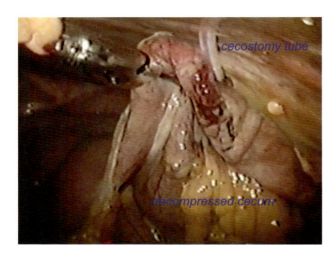

Figure 47–6. Decompressed cecum.

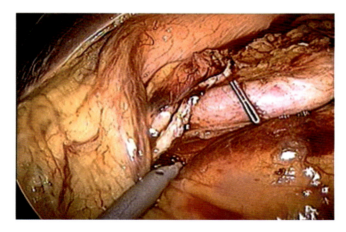

Figure 54–14. Completed laparoscopic distal pancreatectomy with splenic preservation.

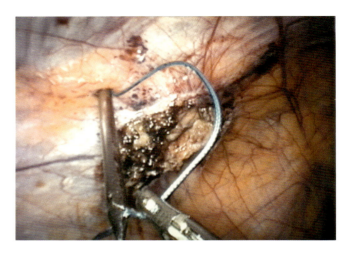

Figure 63–2. Carter-Thomason needlepoint suture passer introducing the suture.

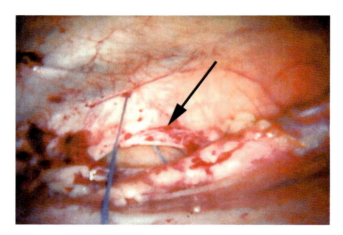

Figure 63–3. Suture being retrieved through the other side of defect.

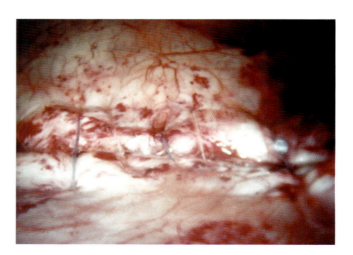

Figure 63–4. Defect closed.

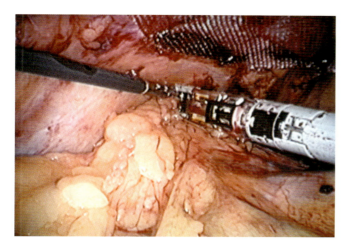

Figure 63–12. Omentum fixed with staples in pelvis, separating bowel from mesh.

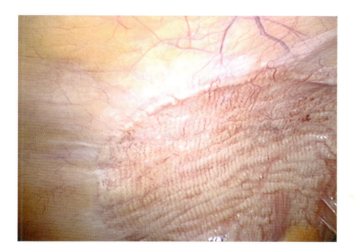

Figure 63–13. Intraperitoneal mesh seen 8 months postoperation. No adhesions noted.

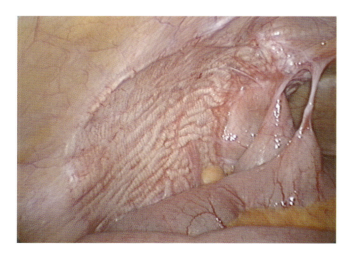

Figure 63–14. Intraperitoneal mesh seen 13 months postoperation. Mild adhesions that were easily taken down.

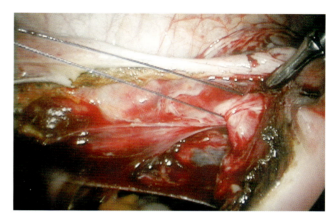

Figure 68–2. After dissection of the left uterine artery, 0 Vicryl on a CTB-1 needle is placed around the left uterine artery.

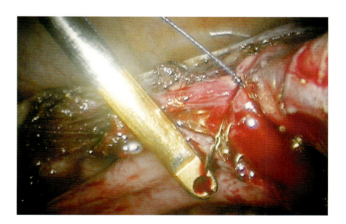

Figure 68–3. The suture around the left uterine artery is tied extracorporeally using a Clarke-Reich knot pusher.

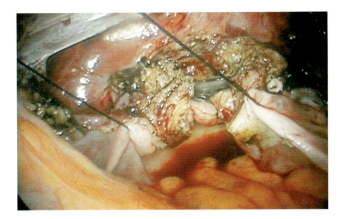

Figure 68–4. A single 0 Vicryl suture includes the uterosacral and cardinal ligaments along with the posterior vaginal wall.

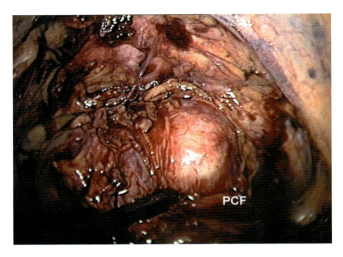

Figure 72–2. Elevation of the right pubocervical fascia with the vaginal hand.

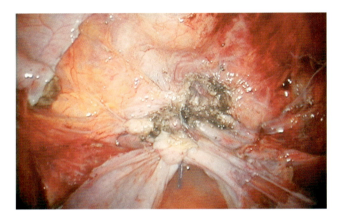

Figure 68–5. The vaginal closure is completed with a second interrupted midline suture.

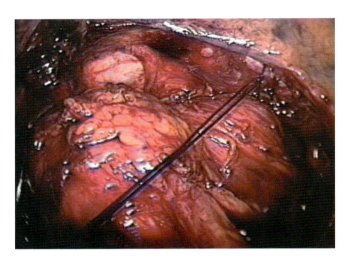

Figure 72–3. Suture placed through the right Cooper's ligament.

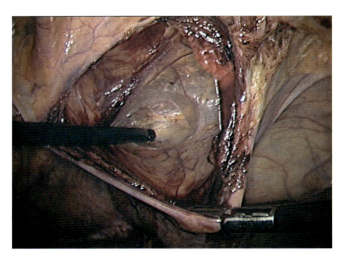

Figure 72–1. Opening the space of Retzius. Note the filmy areolar tissue.

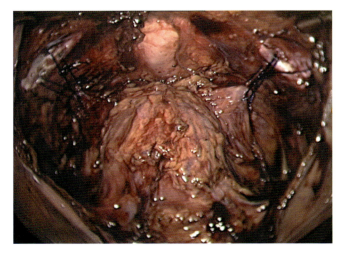

Figure 72–4. Completed Burch procedure. Note the "dog ears" formed as the pubocervical fascia is used to form a hammock under the bladder neck and urethra.

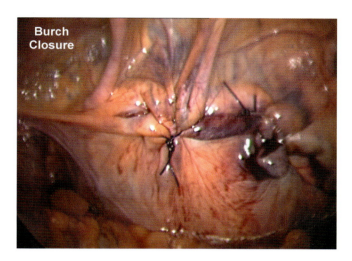

Figure 72–6. Closure of the space of Retzius.

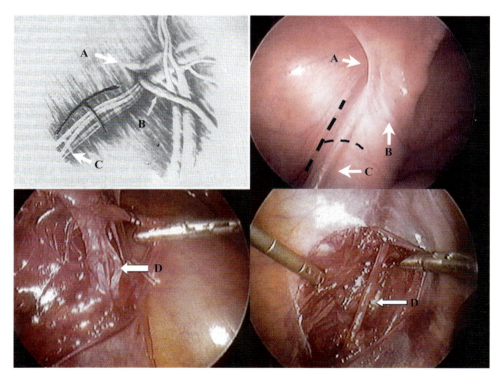

Figure 75–2. A "T" incision (A, B, C) is made in the peritoneum. Identification of the spermatic arteries (D) and clippage of the spermatic veins.

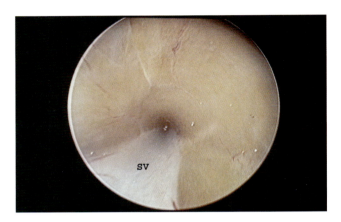

Figure 83–2. The saphenous vein is identified with a 5-mm endoscope through the Vasoview, and the balloon is inflated every 2 cm over it to create the tunnel.

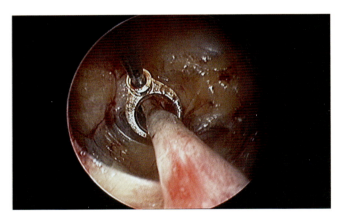

Figure 83–4. The saphenous vein is completely detached from its tributaries with the orbital dissector.

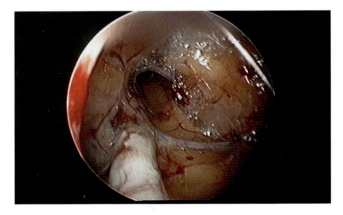

Figure 83–3. Once the CO_2 is insufflated, the tunnel distends and the saphenous vein is seen suspended from fibrous elements and tributaries.

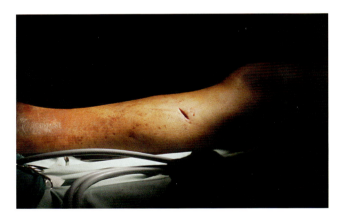

Figure 84–3. Final appearance of the leg after endoscopic interruption of perforating veins.

Chapter Forty-Nine ▪ ▪ ▪ ▪ ▪ ▪

*L*aparoscopic Staging in Pancreatic Cancer

CARLOS FERNÁNDEZ DEL CASTILLO

Two basic approaches prevail in the management of the patient with recently diagnosed pancreatic cancer. In one, all patients are surgically explored soon after the clinical diagnosis has been established. In the other, a series of tests are carried out in an attempt to preoperatively stage the cancer, and tailored treatment is instituted based on these findings. The advantages of preoperative staging in pancreatic cancer are the following: (1) further surgery and potential iatrogenic injury are avoided in patients with advanced disease; (2) patients with resectable tumors are identified and transferred to specialized centers where pancreatic resection can be carried out safely; (3) new treatment protocols complementing or extending surgery can be implemented (in order to improve the poor long-term results following resection); (4) radiation therapy is limited to patients without metastatic disease; and (5) minimally invasive treatments can be planned.

If precise preoperative staging is desired, laparoscopy needs to be part of the protocol. Peritoneal and superficial liver metastases are the second most common sites of extranodal metastases in pancreatic cancer (following the liver), and will be present in over 50% of patients at autopsy.[9] Because these implants very commonly measure only a few millimeters, being beyond the resolution power of CT or ultrasound, they can only be detected by direct visualization at the time of laparotomy or laparoscopy. They are frequently multiple and can be located on the peritoneal surfaces of the liver, abdominal and pelvic wall, stomach, intestines, and omentum.

TECHNIQUE FOR LAPAROSCOPIC EXAMINATION IN PANCREATIC CANCER

The procedure is typically performed in an outpatient setting. Our preference is to perform the procedure under general anesthesia, although local anesthesia and intravenous sedation can also be used. After adequate pneumoperitoneum is obtained, a large trocar and camera are inserted, usually through an infraumbilical incision.

Visual examination of the lower abdomen and pelvis is completed first. Peritoneal and omental metastases may be found in this location even in the absence of implants elsewhere. Free fluid is aspirated for cytologic evaluation. The laparoscope is then rotated to inspect the upper abdomen. Examination of the surface of the liver is particularly relevant, and to inspect the undersurface adequately it is necessary to insert a rod through a second, smaller trocar (5 mm) in the right upper quadrant of the abdomen.

Biopsies of peritoneal or omental nodules can be taken with forceps inserted through the second trocar. Implants in the liver are most easily sampled with a Tru-Cut® needle inserted directly through the abdominal wall. Nodules smaller than 1 mm can be accurately sampled under direct vision. For samples on the pelvic peritoneum it is sometimes necessary to insert another trocar in the lower midline or the biopsy forceps, although the cutting needle inserted percutaneously can also be used. Enlarged lymph nodes can be successfully sampled with the cutting needle or by fine-needle aspiration.

Laparoscopy also permits visualization of the body and tail of the pancreas by using either a supragastric approach (through the lesser omentum) or entering below the stomach (through the gastrocolic omentum or the mesocolon). This procedure, which has also been called pancreatoscopy, was first proposed by Meyer-Burg[18] and was further developed by Ishida[11] and Cuschieri et al.[6] Others have proposed a more extensive laparoscopic evaluation for staging pancreatic cancer, including examination of the hilum of the liver and mesenteric and celiac vessels,[4] or use of laparoscopic ultrasound for detection of intraparenchymal liver metastases, vascular invasion, or lymphadenopathy.[1,13]

Cholangiography can also be performed at the time of laparoscopy, with injection of contrast transhepatically either to the gallbladder or to a dilated bile duct.[6] Laparoscopic cholecystojejunostomy has recently been described in patients with pancreatic cancer who at the time of laparoscopic staging are found to be unresectable,[19] and gastrojejunostomy is feasible as well.

It has been our practice to use laparoscopy to help stage pancreatic cancer because of its unique capacity to detect small peritoneal metastatic disease. We do not think that direct visualization of the pancreatic tumor or involvement of the major vessels is necessary since a CT scan has already been obtained in the great majority of cases. Furthermore, the tumor can be biopsied percutaneously in most cases and perhaps should not be attempted in patients with potentially resectable tumors, as will be discussed later on. Diagnostic cholangiography is rarely needed by the time the patient is being staged; if there was any question about the diagnosis of pancreatic cancer, or if relief of jaundice was required prior to surgery, endoscopic retrograde cholangiopancreatography (ERCP) and stenting are done prior to staging. Furthermore, one of the attractive features of laparoscopy should be its simplicity, making it a feasible study in any hospital and thereby allowing for triage of potentially resectable patients to specialized centers.

RESULTS FROM CLINICAL STUDIES

The use of laparoscopy for staging in pancreatic cancer predates by many years the current surge of laparoscopic surgical procedures. As early as 1911, Bernheim from Johns Hopkins reported on a patient with pancreatic cancer who was evaluated with "cystoscopy of the abdominal cavity," and proposed that this technique could be useful to identify patients who would not benefit from further surgery.[2] Before the widespread availability of computerized tomography, laparoscopy was used extensively in Europe for the diagnosis and staging of various gastrointestinal cancers, including those of the pancreas.[3,7,14,23] Results of several published series describing the use of diagnostic laparoscopy in pancreatic cancer[1,5,6,8,11,12,21,22] include a more recent series of 114 patients staged by us over a 5-year period (April 1989 through April 1994).

The series published by Ivanov and Keranov,[12] and the second series from Cuschieri,[5] both show prevalences of peritoneal and liver metastases identified by laparoscopy of 70% or more. This is much higher than the range of 35 to 43% previously described by us and also reported by Ishida.[11] This discrepancy is explained by our exclusion of patients with liver or other distant metastases already identified by CT or ultrasound. These patients clearly derive no further benefit from laparoscopy, since they are not candidates for resection or radiation and tissue for diagnosis can be obtained percutaneously with little morbidity. The series by Conlon et al[4] involved a variety of peripancreatic malignancies. In that study, the use of "extended" laparoscopic assessment allowed for identification of unresectability in 41 of 108 patients, in some cases because of liver or peritoneal metastases, and in others because of vascular invasion or nodal metastases.[4]

Our experience from 1989 to 1994 shows that the prevalence of liver and peritoneal involvement identified by laparoscopy was 27 of 114 patients (23.6%). Eleven of these patients had metastases to the liver surface, 3 to the peritoneum, 2 to omentum, and 11 to more than one site. Metastases were 2.4 times more common in tumors of the body and tail of the pancreas (11 of 25 patients, 44%) than in pancreatic head cancers (16 of 89 patients, 17.9%) ($P < .05$). This is probably due to a relative delay in diagnosis of tumors of the distal pancreas, which remain "silent" in the absence of jaundice.

The current trend for more aggressive multimodality treatments in which radiation and chemotherapy precede resection underscores even more the necessity to exclude metastatic disease, since the morbidity, costs, and time commitment required by this approach are not negligible. Other institutions share this belief and include laparoscopy in their protocols before including patients for neoadjuvant therapy.[10,25]

In our current staging scheme for patients with presumptive pancreatic cancer we use spiral CT as the initial test. If this shows absence of metastases, we proceed with laparoscopy in all patients with tumors of the pancreatic body and tail and in those with pancreatic head tumors larger than 2 cm, since in smaller lesions the likelihood of metastases is very low. The information obtained by spiral CT and its curvilinear and three-dimensional reconstructions makes the use of angiography obsolete in most cases.

PERITONEAL CYTOLOGY

Pancreatic cancer implants on the serosal surfaces are presumably the result of transperitoneal seeding from the primary tumor. To investigate the prevalence of malignant cells within the peritoneal cavity in patients with small, apparently contained tumors, we performed peritoneal washings in 40 patients with "early" pancreatic cancer (localized by CT and angiography).[20] Washings were performed during laparoscopy or laparotomy by instilling 100 mL of normal saline into the subhepatic space, allowing it to disperse in the peritoneal cavity by tilting the operating table and agitating the abdominal wall, and then aspirating under direct vision. Cytologic smears and cell blocks prepared from centrifuged specimens were examined for the presence of malignant cells using strict criteria for malignancy in order to avoid potential confusion with reactive mesothelial or inflammatory cells.

Malignant cells were found in 12 of those first 40 patients (30%). A disturbing finding of the study was that positive cytologic results were significantly increased in patients who had undergone percutaneous needle biopsy earlier compared to those who had not (75 versus 19%). This is consistent with observations made by other investigators of rapid intra-abdominal spread and implantation after tumor manipulation and biopsy,[17,24] and cautions against the use of preoperative biopsy in potentially resectable patients. The likelihood of resectability was higher in patients with negative cytological findings (13 of 25) as compared to those with positive malignant cells (1 of 10), a fact which was also reflected in a significantly better survival rate. In another report of a small series of patients, peritoneal cytology was positive preoperatively in 2 of 7 patients who had undergone a previous percutaneous biopsy with fine-needle aspiration, and negative in all 8 patients without prior biopsy.[26] Although our more recent experience[8] and that of others[15,16] has failed to confirm a statistically significant increased risk of peritoneal dissemination with needle biopsy, the phenomenon does exist. We therefore continue to recommend that whenever histologic diagnosis is mandatory (for example, if the patient is to enter a protocol of intensive preoperative radiation and chemotherapy), the biopsy be done transduodenally guided by endoscopic ultrasound.

In our experience of 1989 to 1994, peritoneal cytology was positive in only 16 of 94 patients (17%).[8] A positive peritoneal cytology had a very close correlation with the presence of liver or peritoneal implants (10 of 22 patients with metastases versus 6 of 72 without, $P < .001$). Although the majority of the cytologies are seen in conjunction with visible metastases, 38% of positive cases occur without other evidence of spread, and this still amounts to 8% of all resection candidates.

REFERENCES

1. Bemelman WA, de Wit LTh, Van Delden OM, et al. Diagnostic laparoscopy combined with laparoscopic ultrasonography in staging of cancer of the pancreatic head region. *Br J Surg.* 1995;82:820.

2. Bernheim BM. Organoscopy. Cystoscopy of the abdominal cavity. *Ann Surg.* 1911;53:764.

3. Chissov VI, Maksimov IA, Vinogradov AL. Laparoscopy in the diagnosis of gastric carcinoma spread. *Khirurgiia (Mosk).* 1981;11:13.

4. Conlon KC, Dougherty E, Klimstra DS, et al. The value of minimal access surgery in the staging of patients with potentially resectable peripancreatic malignancy. *Ann Surg.* 1996;223:134.

5. Cuschieri A. Laparoscopy for pancreatic cancer: Does it benefit the patient? *Eur J Surg Oncol.* 1988;14:41.

6. Cuschieri A, Hall AW, Clark J. Value of laparoscopy in the diagnosis and management of pancreatic carcinoma. *Gut.* 1978;19:672.

7. Dagnini G, Caldironi MW, Marin G, et al. Laparoscopy in abdominal staging of esophageal carcinoma. Report of 369 cases. *Gastrointest Endosc.* 1986;32:400.

8. Fernández-del Castillo C, Rattner DW, Warshaw AL. Further experience with laparoscopy and peritoneal cytology in staging for pancreatic cancer. *Br J Surg.* 1995;82:1127.

9. Fernández-del Castillo C, Warshaw AL. Peritoneal metastases in pancreatic carcinoma. *Hepato-gastroenterology.* 1993;40:430.

10. Fuhrman GM, Charnsangavej C, Abbruzzese JL, et al. Thin-section contrast-enhanced computed tomography accurately predicts the resectability of malignant pancreatic neoplasms. *Am J Surg.* 1994;167:104.

11. Ishida H. Peritoneoscopy and pancreas biopsy in the diagnosis of pancreatic diseases. *Gastrointest Endosc.* 1983;29:211.

12. Ivanov S, Keranov S. Laparoscopic assessment of the operability of pancreatic cancer. *Khirurgiia (Sofiia).* 1989;42:12.

13. John TG, Greig JD, Carter DC, et al. Carcinoma of the pancreatic head and periampullary region. Tumor staging with laparoscopy and laparoscopic ultrasonography. *Ann Surg.* 1995;221:156.

14. Kriplani AK, Kapur BM. Laparoscopy for preoperative staging and assessment of operability in gastric carcinoma. *Gastrointest Endosc.* 1991;37:441.

15. Leach SD, Rose JA, Lowy AM, et al. Significance of peritoneal cytology in patients with potentially resectable adenocarcinoma of the pancreatic head. *Surgery.* 1995;118:472.

16. Lei S, Kini J, Kim K, et al. Pancreatic cancer: Cytologic study of peritoneal washings. *Arch Surg.* 1994;129:639.

17. Martin JK Jr, Goellner JR. Abdominal fluid cytology in patients with gastrointestinal malignancies. *Mayo Clin Proc.* 1986;61:467.

18. Meyer-Burg J. The inspection, palpation and biopsy for the pancreas. *Endoscopy.* 1972;4:99.

19. Shimi S, Banting S, Cuschieri A. Laparoscopy in the management of pancreatic cancer: Endoscopic cholecystojejunostomy for advanced disease. *Br J Surg.* 1992;79:317.

20. Warshaw AL. Implications of peritoneal cytology for staging of early pancreatic cancer. *Am J Surg.* 1991;161:26.

21. Warshaw AL, Gu Z-y, Wittenberg J, Waltman AC. Preoperative staging and assessment of resectability of pancreatic cancer. *Arch Surg.* 1990;125:230.

22. Warshaw AL, Tepper JE, Shipley WU. Laparoscopy in the staging and planning of therapy for pancreatic cancer. *Am J Surg.* 1986; 151:76.

23. Watt I, Stewart I, Anderson D, et al. Laparoscopy, ultrasound and computed tomography in cancer of the oesophagus and gastric cardia: A prospective comparison for detecting intra-abdominal metastases. *Br J Surg.* 1989;76:1036.

24. Weiss SM, Skibber JM, Mohiuddin M, et al. Rapid intra-abdominal spread of pancreatic cancer. *Arch Surg.* 1985;120:415.

25. Yeung RS, Weese JL, Hoffman JP, et al. Neoadjuvant chemoradiation in pancreatic and duodenal carcinoma. A phase II study. *Cancer.* 1993;72:2124.

26. Zerbi A, Balzano G, Bottura R, et al. Reliability of pancreatic cancer staging classifications. *Int J Pancreatol.* 1994;15:13.

Chapter Fifty · · · · · · ·

*L*aparoscopic Splenectomy

ALFONS POMP and MICHEL GAGNER

Following early reports of laparoscopic splenectomy by Delaitre and Maignien in 1991[3] and Carroll and Poulin's groups in 1992[2,14] this technique has become increasingly popular. In 1992 our group first introduced the posterolateral approach for adrenalectomy[6] and this was subsequently adapted for splenectomy.[12] Most authors who have embraced this operation as the gold standard have described excellent clinical results, primarily with patients with idiopathic thrombocytopenic purpura (ITP).[4,9,12] Laparoscopic splenectomy can be a challenging procedure given the fragile, well-vascularized nature of the spleen and its proximity to the pancreas, stomach, and colon. Perioperative morbidity may also be influenced by specific features associated with hematologic disease, including thrombocytopenia and the immunocompromised state of patients with leukemia or lymphoma.

SURGICAL TECHNIQUE

Our surgical technique has been described previously.[12] Following induction of general anesthesia, the patient is placed in the right lateral decubitus position (Fig. 50–1). The left arm is supported, the right brachial plexus is protected with a pillow roll, and pneumatic compression stockings are applied. Pneumoperitoneum is established using an open (Hasson) technique by making a 10-mm incision in the left subcostal area, on the midaxillary line. A 10-mm trocar is introduced, followed by a 30° laparoscope. Under direct vision the second and third trocars (5- or 10-mm) are introduced following an imaginary line approximately 6 cm below the left costal margin, and one trocar is placed 10 cm medial and the other 10 cm lateral of this line. The surgeon and assistant stand on the patient's right side (Fig. 50–2). We sequentially dissect the splenic flexure of the colon, the lateral peritoneal attachments of the spleen, and the splenorenal and splenophrenic ligaments. We attempt to leave a 1-cm cuff of peritoneum along the lateral aspect of the spleen to act as a handle to manipulate the organ. The splenic hilum is approached from the lower pole and dissection is continued cephalad. Regardless of whether the splenic artery is of a magistral or distributed configuration, a lower pole vessel is usually present; this is either divided by

clips or taken with an ultrasonic dissector. The splenic artery and vein are divided using a linear cutter following or prior to division of the short gastric vessels.

Placing the completely detached spleen into a durable extraction bag is the final and often challenging step. The spleen is morcellated within the bag and extracted piecemeal using sponge forceps. Occasionally a muscle splitting or infraumbilical incision is used to remove large spleens. All incisions are closed and drains are usually not necessary.

RESULTS AND DISCUSSION

We recently described our experience of 138 patients who underwent splenectomy. The procedure was completed laparoscopically in 129 patients and converted to an open procedure in 9 patients (6%). Bleeding from hilar vessels, portal hypertension, splenic laceration, and a generalized coagulopathy were the primary reasons for conversion. Only two patients were unable to be completed laparoscopically because of the technical difficulty of dissecting large spleens. Patient demographics are listed in Table 50–1 and the indications for splenectomy are listed in Table 50–2.

Accessory spleens were identified in 21 patients (15%). Mean operative time was 170 minutes (range, 52 to 560). Estimated blood loss was less than 250 mL in 99 patients, between 250 and 500 mL in 21 patients, and greater than 500 mL in 18 patients. Fourteen patients (10%) required transfusions in the perioperative period. The median postoperative stay was 3 days (mean, 5.5 days; range 1 to 81 days), including patients converted to open procedures.

Concomitant surgical procedures were performed in 25% of patients and included hepatic biopsy (12), distal pancreatectomy (11), cholecystectomy (5), and others (7).

Significant perioperative complications occurred in only 17 patients (12%) including 5 complications in the 12 patients operated for thrombotic thrombocytopenic purpura (TTP). Complications included infections in 4 patients and a left subphrenic collection (hematoma/abscess) in 4 patients, one of whom also developed a deep vein

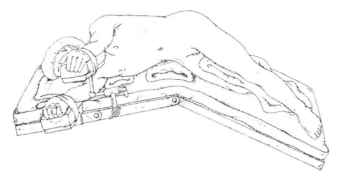

Figure 50–1. Patient in right lateral decubitus position in preparation for laparoscopic splenectomy.

thrombosis (DVT). Two patients developed pneumonia and 2 patients had mild pancreatitis that was treated medically. One patient had a sigmoid volvulus that was decompressed by colonoscopy in the immediate postoperative period. Another patient with a concomitant cholecystectomy had a bile leak from the cystic duct remnant that required drainage. One patient developed an ileus that required rehospitalization for intravenous hydration following discharge after the laparoscopic splenectomy. To our knowledge only 1 patient has developed a postoperative incisional hernia. This patient with severe splenomegaly (due to lymphoma) had a lower midline incision to remove the spleen and developed a ventral hernia that required laparoscopic repair.

There were two postoperative deaths: multiple organ system failure in an AIDS patient and severe perioperative anemia in a patient refusing blood transfusion on religious grounds.

Open splenectomy is not considered a technically difficult operation. Nonetheless, the organ's fragile, well-vascularized anatomy and its intimate proximity to other intra-abdominal organs combined

with the traction and surgical maneuvers necessary for exposure often results in technical complications. Reported complications include bleeding, subphrenic collection, pulmonary problems, and pancreatic tail injury. Splenectomy for malignant disease is associated with morbidity that ranges from 40 to 60%.[8] Continued advances in technology coupled with the progressive mastery of laparoscopic skills by surgeons have naturally evolved to the laparoscopic removal of solid organs. In theory this type of excisional surgery should share the physiologic advantages of laparoscopic cholecystectomy, with decreased surgical pain and improved postoperative pulmonary function expediting recovery, reducing hospital stay, and decreasing the period of disability.[11] Laparoscopic splenectomy also has the potential advantage of decreasing complications related to open surgery because of the great visual magnification obtained for dissection and avoidance of manipulation of the left side of the diaphragm. Although these affirmations seem logical, various factors, but primarily patient demand for a minimally invasive approach, have limited the institution of controlled randomized trials.[1,5,13]

The major difference in surgical morbidity following laparoscopic splenectomy when compared with historical controls is in the severity of the complications. In large series of open splenectomies, subphrenic abscesses (requiring a second procedure), bleeding requiring re-exploration, and pulmonary complications are noted in about 5% of patients.[10] In our series the total complication rate is 13%; however, only 4 patients (3%) developed a subphrenic collection and only 2 (1.5%) developed pneumonia. This experience is mirrored in other published series. Although

TABLE 50–1. PATIENT DEMOGRAPHICS

Number: 138
Sex: male, 54 (39%), female, 84 (61%)
Age (y): mean, 45; range, 2–83
Weight (kg): mean, 68; range, 12–135
Previous abdominal surgery: 43 (32%)

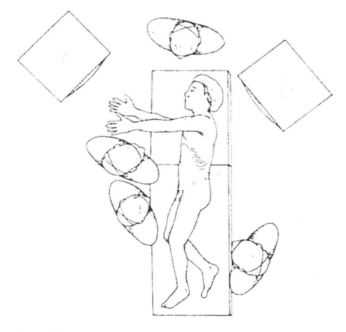

Figure 50–2. Surgeon and assistant positions for laparoscopic splenectomy.

TABLE 50–2. INDICATIONS FOR LAPAROSCOPIC SPLENECTOMY

Autoimmune thrombocytopenia: 67
  Idiopathic thrombocytopenic purpura: 63
  Evans syndrome: 2
  Lupus: 2
Malignant neoplasms: 23
  Non-Hodgkin's lymphoma: 15
  Chronic myeloid leukemia: 3
  Chronic lymphocytic leukemia: 1
  Hairy cell leukemia: 1
  Others: 3
Thrombotic thrombocytopenic purpura: 12
Autoimmune hemolytic anemia: 10
Distal pancreatic lesions: 7
Spherocytosis: 5
Sickle cell anemia: 3
Others: 11
  HIV: 4
  Hypersplenism: 3
  Lymphangioma: 1
  Abscess: 1
  Splenic infarct: 1
  Felty syndrome: 1

there are potential complications specifically related to laparoscopy, including those secondary to the type of access (trocar insertion), we did not observe these complications. Deep vein thrombosis prophylaxis is indicated for all advanced laparoscopic procedures, and our results and those of others[7] have underscored the need for at least sequential compression stockings, especially in cases of malignant hematologic disease.

Age, increased spleen weight, and particularly malignant hematologic disease have been associated with surgical morbidity;[8] however, the only significant increase in the complication rate we saw was in our group of TTP patients who, although representing only 9% of the cohort, suffered 28% of the complications. Theoretically, TTP patients have small spleens that would be ideally amenable to laparoscopic splenectomy. However, this is a difficult group with an unpredictable response to splenectomy that is not well documented in the literature.[9] The multisystemic nature of the disease and the variable response of the coagulopathy and immune response following plasmapheresis may contribute to the increased complication rate seen in this patient group.

Conversion to an open procedure, while often a manifestation of good surgical judgment, is definitely the least cost-effective alternative for splenectomy. The high cost of instrumentation is now combined with the increased hospital stay of the open procedure. Conversion rates in published series vary from 3 to 8%.[5,9,13] There is no apparent correlation to the patient having had previous surgery and also no temporal relationship to the surgeon's learning curve. In our series conversion occurred because of bleeding in most patients, and the mean blood loss for these patients was 2250 mL. We no longer advocate laparoscopic splenectomy for patients who have clinical or imaging evidence of portal hypertension.

Splenic artery embolization has been described to improve patient morbidity by decreasing the incidence and severity of intraoperative bleeding and possibly decrease surgical time;[5,15] however, this has not been advocated by others.[9,13] We believe that the increased presurgical pain, often requiring narcotics, and the possible complications of angiography including infection, pancreatitis, and migration of coils outweigh the possible benefits of embolization.

In order to be cost effective, operative time has to be minimized; our mean time of 170 minutes compares with published data.[1,5,9,13,14] We believe this surgical time may possibly be slightly improved. However, in our institutions, these procedures are in large part performed by senior residents and fellows who turnover yearly and need this operative experience to acquire advanced laparoscopic skills. It is more difficult to analyze why our length of stay is 1 to 2 days greater than other comparable series.[1,5,7,9,13,14] Our length of stay reflects that our institution is a tertiary center with a relatively dispersed geographical patient referral base. The relatively high incidence of patients with malignancy (17%) and thus significant comorbidities, and patients with TTP (9%) often requiring postoperative plasmapheresis also contribute to these results.

It is particularly troubling in the analysis of laparoscopic literature that the incidence of the recovery of accessory spleens may be lower than that found in open surgery. Gigot et al[7] noted residual splenic tissue in 50% of their patients after laparoscopic splenectomies, although in this series there were a significant number of perioperative splenic tears. We believe the published incidence of accessory spleens compares favorably to that of the open literature[1,5,9,13,14] as well as autopsy studies.[16] We agree with Katkhouda et al[9] that meticulous surgical technique to prevent splenosis secondary to splenic trauma during dissection is as important as a thorough search for accessory spleens. If ITP is refractory to laparoscopic splenectomy, every effort should be made to rule out the presence of an accessory spleen. Unfortunately, preoperative imaging with computed tomography (CT) or nuclear studies generally have an unsatisfactory yield for the identification of accessory spleens because the vast majority are so near the hilum.

Mention should be made of the hand port or hand-assisted laparoscopic surgical (HALS) technique for splenectomy. There is general consensus that this technique is not required for routine laparoscopic splenectomy. However, it has been suggested that this may serve as a learning bridge for those surgeons who are still perfecting their laparoscopic skills. Hand-assisted technique may also be helpful for splenectomy for trauma or for less common indications such as partial splenectomy.

SUMMARY

Laparoscopic splenectomy is a safe procedure for a variety of splenic pathologies. It also permits an appropriate abdominal exploration, particularly for accessory spleens, and is associated with a low incidence of major complications. Surgeons require advanced laparoscopic abilities to deal with the challenge of splenectomy given the spleen's fragile anatomy and its relationship to other abdominal viscera, especially the pancreas. Trauma to the spleen during laparoscopic dissection may result in splenosis. Prudence is indicated in patients with portal hypertension and TTP because they have a higher incidence of intraoperative bleeding and postoperative complications. In order to justify the increased cost of laparoscopic equipment, hospital length of stay should be minimized; this may be difficult to achieve in patients operated for TTP or hematologic malignancy. Concomitant surgery including liver biopsy, cholecystectomy, and distal pancreatectomy may be performed with acceptable morbidity. The laparoscopic technique is the procedure of choice for most indications for splenectomy.

REFERENCES

1. Brunt LM, Langer JC, Quasebarth MA, et al. Comparative analysis of laparoscopic versus open splenectomy. *Am J Surg*. 1996;172:596.
2. Carroll BJ, Phillips EH, Semel CJ, et al. Laparoscopic splenectomy. *Surg Endosc*. 1992;6:183.
3. Delaitre B, Maignien B. Splenectomie par voie laparoscopique, 1 observation (letter). *Presse Med*. 1991;20:2263.
4. Friedman RL, Faallas MJ, Carroll BJ, et al. Laparoscopic splenectomy for ITP, the gold standard. *Surg Endosc*. 1996;10:991.
5. Friedman RL, Hiatt JR, Korman JL, et al. Laparoscopic or open splenectomy for hematologic disease: which approach is superior? *J Am Coll Surg*. 1997;185:49.
6. Gagner M, Lacroix A, Prinz RA, et al. Early experience with laparoscopic approach for adrenalectomy. *Surgery* 1993;114:1120.
7. Gigot JF, Jamar F, Ferrant A, et al. Inadequate detection of accessory spleens and splenosis with laparoscopic splenectomy: a shortcoming of the laparoscopic approach in hematological diseases. *Surg Endosc*. 1998;12:101.

8. Horowitz J. Smith JL, Weber TK, et al. Postoperative complications after splenectomy for hematological malignancy. *Ann Surg.* 1996; 223:290.

9. Katkhouda N, Hurwitz MB, Rivera RT, et al. Laparoscopic splenectomy: outcome and efficiency in 103 consecutive cases. *Ann Surg.* 1998;228:568.

10. Musser G, Lazar G, Hocking W, et al. Splenectomy for hematological disease: the UCLA experience with 306 patients. *Ann Surg.* 1984;200:40.

11. National Institutes of Health. Consensus conference statement on gallstones and laparoscopic cholecystectomy. *JAMA.* 1993;269:1018.

12. Park A, Gagner M, Pomp A. The lateral approach to laparoscopic surgery. *Am J Surg.* 1997;173:126.

13. Park A, Marrcaccio M, Sternbach M, et al. Laparoscopic versus open splenectomy. *Arch Surg.* 1999;134:1263.

14. Poulin EC, Mamazza J. Laparoscopic splenectomy: lessons from the learning curve. *Can J Surg.* 1998;41:28.

15. Thibault C, Mamazza J, Letourneau R, et al. Laparoscopic splenectomy: operative technique and preliminary report. *Surg Endosc.* 1992;2:248.

16. Wadham BM, Adams PB, Johson MA. Incidence and localization of accessory spleens (letter). *N Engl J Med.* 1981;304:1111.

Chapter Fifty-One ·······

*L*aparoscopic Adrenalectomy

THERESA M. QUINN and MICHEL GAGNER

BACKGROUND

Since the first laparoscopic adrenalectomy was performed in 1992, the minimally invasive approach to the adrenal gland has become the preferred operation.[1–18] The features of adrenalectomy that make the operation amenable to a minimally invasive approach include the small size of the glands, their superior retroperitoneal location, the benign nature of most adrenal tumors, and the morbidity of an open incision. Laparoscopic adrenalectomy is superior to the conventional open operation with significantly decreased operative blood loss, reduced narcotic requirements, and shorter hospital stay/recovery time demonstrated in several series. As with the open method, anterior, lateral, and posterior approaches can be used to remove the adrenal gland laparoscopically.

Laparoscopic adrenalectomy was initially performed through an anterior transperitoneal approach; however, with the patient supine, gravity effects on the surrounding organs limited the operative window and made exposure of the gland difficult. To facilitate the exposure of the adrenal glands, most surgeons now use a lateral transperitoneal approach. With the patient in the lateral decubitus position, gravity retracts structures and simplifies the exposure of the adrenal gland. As with any operative procedure, the keys to successful adrenal surgery remain careful preoperative evaluation and deliberate intraoperative conduct. The preoperative evaluation should include a comprehensive endocrine evaluation and thorough radiographic localization utilizing diagnostic imaging and functional studies as needed. Even more imperative than for the open operation, laparoscopic adrenalectomy requires knowledge of the three-dimensional anatomy, meticulous hemostasis, and delicate tissue handling.

PREOPERATIVE EVALUATION

Clinical Examination

The clinical examination is targeted to detect the signs and symptoms of aldosterone, catecholamine, or cortisol excess. A history of hypertension is present in nearly all patients with hyperaldosteronism and in 60% of patients with pheochromocytoma.[19] In addition, nearly 90% of patients with pheochromocytoma experience nonspecific symptoms that include headache, diaphoresis, palpitations, abdominal pain, nervousness, nausea, vomiting, chest pain, and weakness. A history of multiple endocrine neoplasia (MEN) type 2A or 2B can also be helpful in diagnosing pheochromocytoma because 40% of this group of MEN patients will ultimately develop this endocrine tumor.

A glucocorticoid-producing adenoma is extremely rare in the absence of signs of hypercortisolism—easy bruising, striae, and myopathy. Functioning adrenocortical carcinoma is suspected by the abrupt onset of Cushing's syndrome, virilization, pyrexia, and abdominal pain. Only 10% of adrenocortical carcinomas are small and present asymptomatically as an incidentaloma on a radiographic study. Most adrenocortical carcinomas are symptomatic and large at presentation, with a mean diameter of 12.4 cm.[20]

Biochemical Evaluation

Adrenal lesions are detected on 0.3 to 5.0% of all CT scans of the abdomen performed for other reasons.[21] However, serum and urine testing need to be performed to detect functional masses that will require excision. For the patient with no evidence of a functioning adrenal tumor after the biochemical evaluation, a repeat CT scan should be done within 6 months to monitor evolution. Tumors that are larger than 4 cm or growing at the follow-up study should be resected owing to the concern for adrenocortical carcinoma. The general biochemical evaluation for a patient with an adrenal mass should begin with a serum potassium level and a 24-hour urine collection for metanephrines, vanillylmandelic acid, 17-hydroxycorticosteroids, and free cortisol. Hypokalemia in a hypertensive patient suggests an adrenal hyperaldosteronoma. The patients have an elevated plasma aldosterone level with decreased plasma renin activity.

Pheochromocytoma patients may be normotensive or have episodic hypertension or chronic hypertension. Urinary measurement of metanephrines, vanillylmandelic acid, and plasma catecholamines allow biochemical confirmation of the diagnosis. CT or magnetic resonance imaging is used to localize the tumor. Further radiographic evaluation with scintigraphy using 131-metaiodobenzylguanidine can exclude multiple or bilateral tumors or the presence of metastases.[22]

Cushing's syndrome is caused by excess glucocorticoid secretion. For the patient with an adrenal etiology for Cushing's syndrome—glucocorticoid-producing adenoma, adrenal carcinoma, or macronodular adrenal hyperplasia—adrenalectomy is indicated. However, a patient with a pituitary adenoma or ectopic ACTH production may benefit from bilateral adrenalectomy for control of symptoms if pituitary surgery or a primary tumor resection has failed to control cortisol hypersecretion. Differentiation of the cause of the hypercortisolism is based upon biochemical and radiographic evaluation. Free cortisol and 17-hydroxycorticosteroid levels are elevated in patients with Cushing's disease and syndrome. A normal or slightly elevated ACTH level suggests pituitary disease, whereas a markedly elevated level is usually of ectopic origin. Suppressed levels of ACTH suggest adrenal production of glucocorticosteroids. A CT scan can differentiate adrenal tumors from macronodular adrenal hyperplasia. While adrenocortical carcinoma is a rare condition, it should be suspected in a patient with elevated 17-ketosteroid level, a large adrenal mass (more than 6 cm), and evidence of local invasion or of distant metastases.

Twenty-four-hour urine collection for 17-ketosteroids, plasma testosterone, and dehydroepiandrosterone levels must be determined in case of virilizing syndromes to confirm the presence of an androgen-producing adrenal tumor.

Radiographic Evaluation

Patients with adrenal masses first diagnosed by ultrasound or CT scan should undergo further evaluation with either helical CT scanning or MRI. In most cases, a thin-cut (3-mm) helical CT scan is adequate to determine the adrenal origin of the tumor, its size, and its relationship to contiguous structures. MR imaging adds the advantage of T2-weighted ratios between the adrenaloma and the liver. Pheochromo-cytomas have a characteristic increased signal using the T2-weighted ratio.

In selected cases of suspected aldosterone-producing tumors, adrenal venous sampling can be used to differentiate an incidentaloma from a cortical adenoma that produces aldosterone.

The role of fine-needle aspiration (FNA) cytology is limited owing to the inability of this test to distinguish an adenoma from a well-differentiated carcinoma on cytology. In addition, a needle biopsy in a patient with a pheochromocytoma can lead to a fatal hypertensive crisis. FNA is not generally recommended.[23]

ADRENAL GLAND ANATOMY

The adrenal glands are located in the lateral retroperitoneal area and surrounded by perirenal fascia. Each adrenal gland is placed like a cap on the superomedial pole of each kidney. The glands weigh approximately 6 g each, measure $5.0 \times 3.0 \times 0.6$ cm, and are located in front of the 12th rib on the right and in front of the 11th and 12th ribs on the left. The dorsal and lateral anatomic relationships of the right and left adrenal glands are similar, while their ventral and medial relationships are different. Differences in the blood supply also have important implications for surgical technique.

Both of the adrenal glands have dorsal and lateral relationships that are almost identical. Through the pararenal fat and the perirenal fascia, the posterolateral aspect of the adrenal gland is in contact with the superior part of the posterior abdominal wall. Each gland lies in close proximity to the diaphragmatic crus and to the lateral arcuate ligament. The crus and arcuate ligament separate the adrenals from the reflection of the pleura, the 11th and 12th ribs, and the subcostal, sacrospinalis, and latissimus dorsi muscles.

The ventrolateral relationships of the right adrenal gland are to the peritoneum between the liver and kidney. Exposure of the gland is achieved by opening the peritoneum after mobilizing the right lobe of the liver cephalad and medially. The ventromedial relation of the right adrenal gland is to the inferior vena cava. The right adrenal vein emerges from this aspect of the gland before emptying directly into the inferior vena cava.

The ventrolateral relationships of the left adrenal gland are the attachments of the kidney and occasionally the splenic flexure of the colon. Mobilization of the splenic flexure of the colon and incision of the peritoneal layer overlying Gerota's fascia expose the lateral aspect of the left adrenal gland. The ventromedial relations of the left adrenal gland are the spleen, pancreas, and fundus of the stomach. There are three major approaches to the left adrenal. The splenorenal ligament can be divided along the lateral aspect of the spleen to allow medial displacement of the spleen, the tail of the pancreas, and the fundus of the stomach. The splenic vein can be seen coursing along the posterior margin of the pancreas and the splenic artery along the superior border. The body of the pancreas separates the adrenal gland from the lesser sac and from the stomach. A second approach to the left adrenal gland is direct access through the lesser sac after division of the gastrocolic ligament. The adrenal gland can be exposed by a peritoneal incision along the inferior or superior border of the pancreatic body. Finally, a third approach entails dissection of the transverse mesocolon to give direct access to the posterior side of the pancreas and the adrenal gland.

Vascular Anatomy

The adrenal glands receive their arterial blood from three sources: a superior adrenal artery arising from the inferior phrenic artery, a middle adrenal artery from the abdominal aorta, and an inferior adrenal artery derived from the renal artery.

The arrangement of the adrenal veins is more straightforward than that of the arteries. There is one dominant vein and smaller accessory veins that follow the arteries. During adrenalectomy for the treatment of tumor with excess hormonal production, and especially in cases of pheochromocytoma, the flow of the main adrenal vein is controlled at the beginning of the adrenal dissection. On the left side, vascular control of the adrenal vein is relatively straightforward because the adrenal vein is long (up to 30 mm) and empties into either the left inferior phrenic vein or the left renal vein. However, it takes more time and a longer dissection to expose the left adrenal vein compared to the right. After identifying the inferior pole of the left adrenal, dissection for 1 to 2 cm along the medial margin of the adrenal gland will reveal the left adrenal vein.

On the right side, vascular control of the adrenal vein is more precarious because the adrenal vein is significantly shorter (less than 6 mm) and empties directly into the posterior wall of the inferior vena cava. This anatomic arrangement increases the risk of major venous injury with disastrous hemorrhage. For both adrenal glands, numerous accessory adrenal veins follow the arteries and empty into the inferior phrenic vein, renal vein, or branches that enter the azygos and posterior gastric veins. The collateral vessels may significantly enlarge in cases of large tumors.

OPERATIVE INDICATIONS

Since the introduction of laparoscopic adrenalectomy in 1992, the minimally invasive approach has become the gold standard for adrenalectomy for selected patients with a variety of conditions (Table 51–1). Successful laparoscopic adrenalectomy requires advanced laparoscopic skills, knowledge of the three-dimensional anatomy, meticulous hemostasis, and delicate tissue handling. As with any adrenal operation, there should be a thorough preoperative evaluation and localization of the adrenal pathology by radiographic and biochemical means.

There are several distinct contraindications to laparoscopic adrenalectomy (Table 51–2). As with any laparoscopic operation, the main contraindication is surgeon inexperience with the technique. In addition, patients with suspected adrenal carcinoma based on radiographic evaluation or a lesion greater than 10 cm in size should undergo an open operative approach to assure complete excision of the lesion along with an en bloc resection of surrounding organs as necessary. Additional contraindications include coagulopathy and portal hypertension, conditions that limit the exactitude of the laparoscopic procedure and increase the risk of perioperative bleeding.

PREOPERATIVE PREPARATION

Routine bowel preparation and antibiotics are unnecessary. Intermittent pneumatic compression stockings or subcutaneous heparin should be used to prevent thromboembolism.

In patients with pheochromocytoma, severe hypertension can occur with mild tumor manipulation intraoperatively, and hypotension can occur after tumor removal owing to inadequate preoperative volume resuscitation. Preoperative preparation with alpha- and beta-blockage is recommended.[19] Several options are available; however, we prefer the use of phenoxybenzamine for at least 1 week preoperatively. A reasonable alternative oral medication is the selective alpha-antagonist Prazosin. Success has also been reported with the regimen of intravenous phentolamine and esmolol, or calcium channel blockers starting the day before surgery. Beta-blockers can be given to control intraoperative arrhythmias but must be initiated after alpha-blockade is achieved. Patients with aldosteronomas should have potassium deficits corrected before operation. The preoperative administration of spironolactone can counteract the activity of tumor production of aldosterone.

While two approaches, transperitoneal and retroperitoneal, to laparoscopic adrenalectomy have been described in the literature, we advocate the transperitoneal approach because the anatomy is more familiar to most surgeons, the approach is better for enlarged glands, and the liver can be assessed for metastases. The retroperitoneal approach involves creation of a retroperitoneal space similar to the open posterior approach and has been recommended for a patient with adhesions due to previous abdominal surgery.[24–26] However, over half of our transperitoneal operations have been performed in patients with previous abdominal surgery without difficulty. We advocate the lateral transperitoneal approach for most cases of adrenal pathology. The following description will delineate the steps for the lateral transperitoneal approach to laparoscopic adrenalectomy. The retroperitoneal technique will be described later.

PATIENT POSITIONING

After placement of intermittent compression stockings and a Foley catheter, the patient is placed in the lateral decubitus position on a beanbag with the side of the adrenal pathology facing up. An axillary roll is placed to protect the brachial plexus and a rolled blanket under the flank enhances the opposite flank exposure. The flank must be positioned over the table break to allow table flexion at this joint to maximize the distance between the costal margin and the iliac crest. The arms are extended over boards and secured in a neutral position with padding of pressure points. The surgeon and assistant stand on the abdominal side of the patient. The area from the umbilicus to the vertebral column and from the nipple to the mid-iliac crest is prepared and draped. Video monitors are placed on either side of the head of the table.

INSTRUMENTATION

A 30-degree laparoscope is recommended for adequate vision of the operative field. A fan-type liver retractor is useful for liver retraction in the laparoscopic right adrenalectomy.

Laparoscopic adrenalectomy can be performed using a bowel grasper in the surgeon's nondominant hand. The flat surface of the atraumatic grasper is used to grasp and retract the tissue adjacent to the adrenal. In the surgeon's dominant hand, either scissors with cautery, a hook cautery, or an ultrasonic scalpel is used. All of these devices can generate thermal energy, and caution must be

TABLE 51–1. OPERATIVE INDICATIONS

Functional Masses
Cortisol-secreting adenoma (Cushing's)
Aldosterone-secreting adenoma (Conn's)
Adrenocortical hyperplasia (Cushing's) or other hypercortisolism
Syndromes
Pheochromocytoma
Virilizing/feminizing syndromes
Nonfunctional Tumors
Incidentaloma (>3 cm or growing)
Isolated adrenal metastases
Symptomatic angiomyolipoma
Symptomatic adrenal cyst

TABLE 51–2. OPERATIVE CONTRAINDICATIONS

- Surgeon inexperience
- Adrenal carcinoma
- Adrenal mass > 10 cm
- Coagulopathy (uncorrected)
- Portal hypertension

undertaken not to rest the scissors, hook, or active-blade of the ultrasonic scalpel against tissue that is not intended for division. A 5-mm curved ultrasonic endoshear is particularly valuable for dissection around the adrenal. The adrenal vein can be dissected with a right-angle dissector and clipped with either medium or large titanium clips. Arteries can be ligated with clips and divided with endoshears or divided with the ultrasonic scalpel directly. Laparoscopic ultrasound (5 to 7-MHz probe) can be useful for localizing the left adrenal when extensive perirenal and retroperitoneal fat is present.[27] Intraoperative ultrasound is particularly useful in cases of small tumors when the tumor is not directly visible, the adrenal appears normal, and a paraganglioma is present, and in evaluating venous anatomy, invasion, or metastases.[28] Laparoscopic biopsy forceps should be available for biopsy of the adrenal gland. An impermeable nylon laparoscopic bag is necessary for gland retrieval to prevent seeding of the abdomen or trocar sites.

OPERATIVE TECHNIQUE: LEFT ADRENALECTOMY

Lateral Transperitoneal Approach

Either three or four trocars can be used for this operation. The typical approach uses four 10-mm trocars along the left subcostal margin. The optional fourth port is the most posterior at the costovertebral angle. The fourth port is used for retraction of the spleen, but the need for this additional port can be prevented by adequate mobilization of the spleen and patient positioning in reverse Trendelenburg position and rotation toward the surgeon to allow the spleen to fall away from the operative field.

Using an open technique of abdominal access, the first port is placed medial to the anterior axillary line, 2 cm below and parallel to the costal margin. The abdomen is insufflated to 15 mm Hg and a 10-mm trocar is placed. The abdomen is visually explored. Under laparoscopic vision, two additional trocars are placed, one inferiorly and slightly medial to the tip of the 11th rib, and the next more anterior and medial to the initial trocar (staying lateral to the rectus sheath, approximated by a handbreadth from the midline, to avoid the epigastric vessels). The most anterior trocar is used for the camera, and the surgeon uses the lateral two ports. Trocars must be placed a minimum of 5 cm or, more optimally, 10 cm apart to allow adequate mobility of the instruments.

Using a laparoscopic bowel clamp (left hand) and harmonic endoshears (right hand), the splenic flexure is mobilized inferiorly and medially to reveal the inferior pole of the splenorenal ligament. Next the splenorenal ligament is divided along the lateral border of the spleen, from the inferior to the superior pole of the spleen, all the way to the diaphragmatic attachments. When the short gastric vessels and the fundus of the stomach are seen, the dissection is complete. Once the spleen is fully mobilized, it will fall medially, and the retroperitoneum will be in full view. The lateral and anterior portions of the adrenal gland will become visible in the perinephric fat, superior and medial to the kidney.

Next the adrenal gland is mobilized by grasping the perinephric fat and dividing lateral and anterior or medial and inferior attachments using the hook electrocautery or ultrasonic scalpel. The superior and posterior attachments act as an anatomic retractor of the gland: leaving these attachments for last facilitates the dissection of the adrenal vein. Grasping the periadrenal tissue

prevents tearing of the fragile adrenal capsule. Seeding of adrenal cells into the bed can occur with fracture of the capsule similar to that seen with spleen or parathyroid dissection. The initial goal of the dissection is to identify and clip the adrenal vein (two or three clips proximally and two distally). The inferior phrenic vein joins with the adrenal vein prior to the adrenal vein junction with the renal vein. The adrenal vein can be clipped above the junction with the inferior phrenic vein. Any branches from the inferior phrenic vein to the adrenal gland can be clipped as dissection continues along the medial/superior border of the adrenal. The final dissection of the adrenal gland is performed in the superior and posterior planes. The shaft of a closed instrument can be used to retract the adrenal or elevate it gently during the dissection. The adrenal is placed in an impermeable nylon bag and removed through the original trocar site by gentle spreading of the abdominal musculature using a clamp.

OPERATIVE TECHNIQUE: RIGHT ADRENALECTOMY

Lateral Transperitoneal Approach

Four trocars are used for the right adrenalectomy. The typical approach uses four 10-mm trocars spread evenly along the right subcostal line. The abdomen is accessed as described above and insufflated to 15 mm Hg. The most medial trocar is placed lateral to the ipsilateral rectus muscle, approximately a handbreadth from the midline, to avoid the epigastric vessels. The most anterior trocar is used for the liver retraction, the second for the camera, and the surgeon works in the two lateral ports.

A fan-type liver retractor is inserted through the most anterior port and the right hepatic lobe is gently reflected medially. The 30-degree angled laparoscope is inserted into the second trocar and liver mobilization is begun. Using a laparoscopic curved dissector (left hand) and harmonic endoshears (right hand), the right lateral hepatic attachments and the triangular ligament are divided along the diaphragm. Patient positioning is key to the exposure of the adrenal gland. The table is tilted to a reverse Trendelenburg position, permitting displacement of the surrounding organs and collection of irrigation or oozing away from the field of dissection. Airplaning of the patient toward the surgeon will also aid the liver in retraction. The peritoneum between the liver and the vena cava along the upper border of the renal vein to the triangular ligament is divided. The dissection permits more effective medial retraction of the liver. The adrenal gland, perinephric fat, and vena cava are generally seen at this point.

Dissection of the adrenal gland is undertaken along the lateral/inferior margin of the gland to identify the adrenal vein. The dissection continues medially and superiorly until the main adrenal vein coming directly off the vena cava is identified. The adrenal vein is defined with a right-angle clamp and clipped with medium or large titanium clips (three on cava side, two on adrenal side). A vascular TA or GIA stapler may be used if the vein is large. As the dissection progresses superiorly, small veins draining the adrenal gland directly into the inferior phrenic vein or vena cava can be encountered and will need to be clipped. The final dissection of the adrenal gland is performed in the superior and posterior planes. The adrenal is placed in an impermeable nylon bag and removed through the original trocar site by gentle spreading of the abdominal musculature using a clamp. The incision may have to be enlarged to remove the specimen.

Larger adrenal masses (>5 cm) may prevent visualization of the adrenal vein and preclude initial dissection and division of the adrenal vein. When a large right adrenal mass is encountered, we prefer to dissect laterally and superiorly first, and then continue caudally along the vena cava to reach the adrenal vein, being careful not to injure the superior pole renal arteries.

OPERATIVE TECHNIQUE: LAPAROSCOPIC BILATERAL ADRENALECTOMY

When a bilateral laparoscopic adrenalectomy is needed, the patient is placed in the lateral decubitus position. Either the left or right side may be performed first. After all wounds have been closed on the first side, the patient is repositioned and redraped to expose the other side. Repositioning may not be necessary, however, if one performs a posterior technique with the patient in the prone position. We prefer to do the left side in lateral decubitus position first and then the right side. Most cases of bilateral laparoscopic adrenalectomy are performed for Cushing's disease or for bilateral pheochromocytoma—either benign or malignant. Rarely, bilateral adrenalectomy is performed for neoplastic hypercortisolism that cannot be controlled medically or for bilateral macronodular hyperplasia associated with Cushing's syndrome.

OPERATIVE TECHNIQUE: RETROPERITONEAL ADRENALECTOMY

The laparoscopic retroperitoneal approach to the adrenal gland was first described by Mercan et al in 1995.[29–33] The patient is placed in the prone position, enabling bilateral adrenalectomy without repositioning the patient. A retroperitoneal space is created using a balloon dissector. Although a retroperitoneal approach reduces the risk of injury to intra-abdominal organs, there are fewer classic anatomic landmarks and it can be more challenging to identify the adrenal glands. Owing to the smaller operative field, this approach allows management only of smaller adrenal lesions. The accidental opening of the posterior peritoneal sheath allows gas to escape into the abdomen, a complication that can further reduce the retroperitoneal space and make dissection more difficult. Bonjer et al[5] reported their series of 111 consecutive endoscopic retroperitoneal adrenalectomies. The authors recommend the retroperitoneal approach only for tumors smaller than 6 cm in diameter.

POSTOPERATIVE CARE

Oral fluids are started on the day of surgery. Nasogastric tubes are unnecessary. Most patients need only oral pain medication. The postoperative course is similar to that for laparoscopic cholecystectomy, with the exception that some endocrine diseases require hormonal support (e.g., stress-dose steroids for glucocorticoid-producing tumors). Patients walk on the day of the operation and are generally discharged on the first postoperative day. Discharge may be delayed for patients who require perioperative stress-dose steroids or adjustment of blood pressure medications.

COMPLICATIONS

Bleeding

Operative bleeding can be prevented by meticulous attention to hemostasis. The retroperitoneal fat can be particularly difficult to dissect in the male patient. The fat is extensive and will bleed with even gentle manipulation. The ultrasonic scalpel is useful for this type of dissection.

Particular points about adrenal vein handling can reduce the incidence of perioperative bleeding: laparoscopic dissectors, when the jaws are opened, can create significant force that cannot be appreciated by the laparoscopic surgeon. Gentle spreading of the right angle without opening the jaws to their full extent can reduce the chance of tearing the vessel one is attempting to define. The laparoscopic suction tip can also be used for gentle, effective dissection around vessels. When using clips, they should be applied at right angles to the tissue. A twisting motion or application of the clip applier at any other angle can result in scissoring of the clip and division of the vessel. Double or triple clip application to the distal segment of the adrenal vein can reduce the chance of clip dislodgment. Suction devices should be used only under direct vision in the adrenal bed to prevent clip removal by the suction.

Clips should not be used indiscriminately or blindly if bleeding occurs. The renal vein, vena cava, and other retroperitoneal structures are at risk if blind clips are placed. The best approach to bleeding during any laparoscopic case is gentle pressure with an instrument or placement of an additional trocar to assist in pressure or exposure. The assistant holding the camera needs to stay calm and keep the field in view, but avoid blood on the lens.

Damage to Adjacent Organs

Damage to the pancreas and spleen (left adrenalectomy) or liver and vena cava (right), as well as to the renal arteries for either approach, should be carefully avoided by knowledge of the anatomy and close adherence to the technical details discussed earlier. In particular, the adrenal vein/left renal vein junction does not need to be identified. It is appropriate to trace the left adrenal vein back to the adrenal gland to confirm its identity and prevent injury to the left renal vein.

Damage to the spleen or pancreas can be prevented by adequate mobilization of the spleen by precluding the need for additional retraction of the spleen or pancreas.

Damage to the pancreas can present early as pancreatitis or late as a pancreatic pseudocyst. In addition to avoiding retraction injuries, keeping the dissection close to the adrenal gland and top of the kidney after dividing the splenorenal ligament reduces the chance of pancreatic damage.

A liver laceration can be controlled with gentle pressure, and a bowel laceration should be closed with an intracorporeal suture repair.

Deep Venous Thrombosis (DVT)

Deep venous thrombosis (DVT) was noted in 3% of patients from our series of 100 patients. We routinely use intermittent compression boots placed at the beginning of the operation to prevent this complication.

CLINICAL OUTCOME

Since the first report of laparoscopic adrenalectomy in 1992, over 1000 cases of laparoscopic adrenalectomy have been reported in the literature. While there are no prospective, randomized trials of this new technique, there is considerable evidence in the literature substantiating the effectiveness and safety of the procedure. A recent review of the English-language literature from 1995 to 1999 of studies consisting of more than 20 cases found 1052 patients for a total of 1082 adrenalectomies.[18] There were 30 bilateral resections. The patient age ranged from 17 to 84, with equal numbers of males and females. The lesions ranged in size from 0.5 to 14 cm. The lateral transperitoneal approach was used in the majority (88%) of patients, with the posterior retroperitoneal approach used in the remainder (12%).

In these series, the conversion rate to an open approach ranged from 0 to 18%. The most common indications for adrenalectomy were aldosteronoma (42.7%), followed by Cushing's syndrome (18.6%), incidentaloma (16.9%), and pheochromocytoma in 14.7%. Other less common indications included angiomyolipoma, metastases, small carcinoma, virilizing adenoma, and macronodular hyperplasia.

The studies comparing laparoscopic adrenalectomy to an open approach are retrospective in nature, revealing a shorter operating time for the open operations overall (149 versus 195 minutes). Recently authors have reported operating times for laparoscopic adrenalectomy as low as 109 minutes. The senior author's experience now encompasses over 200 cases of laparoscopic adrenalectomy.[18] In the first 100 cases, the mean operative time was 123 minutes, mean blood loss was 70 mL, and the average length of stay was 2.4 days.[2] More recently, adrenalectomy is performed in less than 60 minutes for a benign unilateral lesion and the median length of stay is one day.

Laparoscopic adrenalectomy has less blood loss compared to the open approach (153 versus 355 mL) and the length of stay is shorter (2.6 versus 6.5 days).[18] The complication rate is lower in the laparoscopic group (7%) compared to the open group (24%), with postoperative hematoma or need for transfusion approximately 3%, and wound complications, pulmonary complications, and DVT all less than 1%. The open adrenalectomy is complicated by respiratory problems such as pneumonia or atelectasis 6% of the time, wound infections (3%), and transfusion requirement (3%). The open approach is also complicated by splenic injury/splenectomy in 1.5% of cases. Late complications for the open approach (54%) are the most notable: chronic pain (14%), flank numbness (10%), and muscle laxity (30%). When performed by an experienced laparoscopic surgeon, laparoscopic adrenalectomy can be completed with no mortality, minimal morbidity, and no recurrences of hormonal excess. In the senior author's experience, conversions have been performed only for invasive or giant (>15 cm) tumors. There have been no conversions for bleeding.

Retrospective studies comparing the laparoscopic transperitoneal and retroperitoneal approaches show a slight decrease in the operating time and blood loss but no difference in the length of stay.[18] Although the retroperitoneal approach avoids intraperitoneal adhesions in a previously operated abdomen and saves repositioning time for a bilateral adrenalectomy, the adrenal anatomy is more difficult to discern and the working space is smaller. The liver and peritoneum cannot be surveyed for metastases from the retroperitoneal approach. In general, the laparoscopic retroperitoneal approach is ideal for a surgeon experienced with this approach and for benign adrenal tumors less than 6 cm in size.

Laparoscopic adrenalectomy has become the standard of care for most adrenal neoplasms. Although the open anterior approach still has a role for large tumors and obvious malignancy, the open posterior approach has been replaced by laparoscopic techniques. The choice of laparoscopic lateral transperitoneal versus retroperitoneal adrenalectomy is determined primarily by surgeon preference except with larger tumors, where the lateral transperitoneal approach is clearly superior.

CONCLUSIONS

Since the introduction of laparoscopic adrenalectomy in 1992, the minimally invasive approach has become the gold standard for adrenalectomy for a wide range of diseases, including Cushing's adenoma, hyperaldosteronism, pheochromocytoma, and nonfunctioning adrenal lesions. As for any adrenal operation, there should be a thorough preoperative evaluation and localization of the adrenal pathology by radiographic and biochemical means. Laparoscopic adrenalectomy in particular requires advanced laparoscopic skills, thorough knowledge of the three-dimensional anatomy to overcome the two-dimensional limitations in vision, meticulous hemostasis, and delicate tissue handling. Laparoscopic adrenalectomy causes less pain, fewer wound and respiratory complications, and allows a shorter hospital stay compared to open surgery. The choice of a laparoscopic transperitoneal versus retroperitoneal approach is determined primarily by surgeon preference, except in patients with larger tumors or possible intra-abdominal metastases, in whom the transperitoneal approach is clearly superior.

REFERENCES

1. Gagner M, Lacroix A, Bolte E. Laparoscopic adrenalectomy in Cushing's syndrome and pheochromocytoma. *N Engl J Med.* 1992;327:1033. Letter.
2. Gagner M, Pomp A, Heniford B, et al. Laparoscopic adrenalectomy: Lessons learned from 100 consecutive procedures. *Ann Surg.* 1997;226:238.
3. Gagner M, Breton G, Pharand D, et al. Is laparoscopic adrenalectomy indicated for pheochromocytoma? *Surgery.* 1996;120:1076.
4. Duh QY, Siperstein AE, Clark OH, et al. Laparoscopic adrenalectomy: Comparison of the lateral and posterior approaches. *Arch Surg.* 1996;131:870.
5. Bonjer HJ, Lange JF, Kazemeir G. Comparison of three techniques for adrenalectomy. *Br J Surg.* 1997;84:679.
6. Baba S, Miyajima A, Uchida A, et al. A posterior lumbar approach for retroperitoneoscopic adrenalectomy: Assessment of surgical efficacy. *Urology.* 1997;50:19.
7. Gagner M, Lacroix A, Prinz RA, et al. Early experience with laparoscopic approach for adrenalectomy. *Surgery.* 1993;114:1120.
8. Chapuis Y, Maignien B, Abboud B. Adrenalectomy under celioscopy: Experience of 25 operations. *Presse Med.* 1995;24:845.
9. Brunt LM, Doherty GM, Norton JA, et al. Laparoscopic adrenalectomy compared to open adrenalectomy for benign adrenal neoplasms. *J Am Coll Surg.* 1996;183:1.
10. Fernandez-Cruz L, Saenz A, Benarroch G, et al. Laparoscopic unilateral and bilateral adrenalectomy for Cushing's syndrome: Transperitoneal and retroperitoneal approaches. *Ann Surg.* 1996;224:727.
11. de Canniere L, Michel L, Hamoir E, et al. Multicentric experience of

the Belgian group for endoscopic surgery (BGES) with endoscopic adrenalectomy. *Surg Endosc.* 1997;11:1065.

12. Jacobs JK, Goldstein RE, Geer RJ, et al. Laparoscopic adrenalectomy: A new standard of care. *Ann Surg.* 1997;225:495.

13. Filipponi S, Guerrieri M, Arnoldi G, et al. Laparoscopic adrenalectomy: A report on 50 operations. *Eur J Endocrinol.* 1998;138:548.

14. Guazzoni G, Montorsi F, Bocciardi A, et al. Transperitoneal laparoscopic versus open adrenalectomy for benign hyperfunctioning adrenal tumors: A comparative study. *J Urol.* 1995;153:1597. See comments.

15. Janetschek G, Finkenstedt G, Gasser R, et al. Laparoscopic surgery for pheochromocytoma: Adrenalectomy, partial resection, excision of paragangliomas. *J Urol.* 1998;160:330.

16. Winfield HN, Hamilton BD, Bravo EL, et al. Laparoscopic adrenalectomy: The preferred choice? A comparison to open adrenalectomy. *J Urol.* 1998;160:325.

17. Janetschek G, Altarac S, Finkenstedt G, et al. Technique and results of laparoscopic adrenalectomy. *Eur Urol.* 1996;30:475.

18. Jossart G, Burpee SE, Gagner M. Endocrine incidentalomas. *Endocrinol Metab Clin.* 2000;29:57.

19. Grant C. Pheochromocytoma. In: Clark OH, Duh Q, eds. *Textbook of Endocrine Surgery.* Saunders:1997;513.

20. Icard P, Louvel A, Chapuis Y. Survival rates and prognostic factors in adrenocortical carcinoma. *World J Surg.* 1992;16:453.

21. Herrera MF, Grant CS, van Heerden JA, et al. Incidentally discovered adrenal tumors: An institutional perspective. *Surgery.* 1991;110:1014.

22. Gross MD, McLeod MK, Sanfield JA, et al. Scintigraphic evaluation of clinically silent adrenal masses. *J Nucl Med.* 1994;35:1145.

23. Silverman SG, Mueller PR, Pinkey LP, et al. Predictive value of image-guided adrenal biopsy: Analysis of results of 101 biopsies. *Radiology.* 1993;187:715.

24. Gasman D, Droupy S, Koutani A, et al. Laparoscopic adrenalectomy: The retroperitoneal approach. *J Urol.* 1998;159:1816.

25. Heintz A, Walgenbach S, Junginger T. Results of endoscopic retroperitoneal adrenalectomy. *Surg Endosc.* 1996;10:633.

26. Linos D, et al. Anterior, posterior, or laparoscopic approach for the management of adrenal diseases? *Am J Surg.* 1997;173:120.

27. Miyake O, Yoshimura K, Yoshioka T, et al. Laparoscopic adrenalectomy: Comparison of the transperitoneal and retroperitoneal approach. *Eur Urol.* 1998;33:303.

28. Heniford BT, Iannitti DA, Hale J, et al. The role of intraoperative ultrasonography during laparoscopic adrenalectomy. *Surgery.* 1997;122:1068.

29. Mercan S, Seven R, Ozarmagan S, et al. Endoscopic retroperitoneal adrenalectomy. *Surgery.* 1995;118:1071.

30. Takeda M, Go H, Watanabe R, et al. Retroperitoneal laparoscopic adrenalectomy for functioning adrenal tumors: Comparison with conventional transperitoneal laparoscopic adrenalectomy. *J Urol.* 1997;157:19. See comments.

31. Terachi T, Matsuda T, Terai A. Transperitoneal laparoscopic adrenalectomy: Experience in 100 patients. *J Endourol.* 1997;11:361.

32. Thompson GB, Grant CS, van Heerden JA, et al. Laparoscopic versus open posterior adrenalectomy: A case-control study of 100 patients. *Surgery.* 1997;122:1132.

33. Walz MK, Peitgen K, Saller B, et al. Subtotal adrenalectomy by the posterior retroperitoneoscopic approach. *World J Surg.* 1998;22:621.

Chapter Fifty-Two ■ ■ ■ ■ ■ ■

Laparoscopic Necrosectomy for Acute Necrotizing Pancreatitis

ANNE WAAGE and MICHEL GAGNER

The clinical presentation of acute pancreatitis varies from a mild, spontaneously resolving inflammation to a rapidly fatal disease in patients with local and systemic complications.[1-3] About 25% of patients develop a severe clinical course with mortality rates exceeding 30%.[2-5]

There is a strong morphologic correlation between clinical severity and extent of intrapancreatic and extrapancreatic necrosis.[1] Infected necrosis due to migration and colonization of bacteria develops in 30 to 70% of patients with acute necrotizing pancreatitis, and more than 80% of deaths among patients with acute pancreatitis are caused by septic complications as a consequence of bacterial infection of the pancreatic necrosis.[2-4]

The outcome in patients developing infected necrosis is fatal without intervention.[5] That is why this condition is regarded as an absolute indication for surgical treatment even if the timing and type of surgery remain controversial.[4,6-8]

DIAGNOSIS

Contrast-enhanced CT scan remains the gold standard for diagnosing necrotizing pancreatitis, with an accuracy of more than 90% if there is more than 30% glandular necrosis.[9] On the basis of CT observations, a significant direct correlation exists between mortality and the amount of pancreatic parenchymal necrosis.[10] For recognition of clinically severe acute pancreatitis patients, severity-of-illness classifications are used, both including clinical signs with prognostic importance (Ranson Score) and the Acute Physiology and Chronic Health Evaluation (APACHE II) based on physiologic variables. The number of Ranson signs within the first 48 hours of admission correlates with the incidence of systemic complications and the presence of pancreatic necrosis, while the APACHE II score allows classification of illness severity on admission and may be recalculated daily.[11]

TIMING OF SURGERY

The treatment of necrotizing pancreatitis requires a multimodal approach including the combination of intensive medical care and specific surgical debridement. The initial management of severe acute pancreatitis should be conservative.[2] Early deaths (within 1 to 2 weeks after onset of symptoms) are considered due to multisystem organ failure (MOF) and systemic inflammatory response system (SIRS) caused by the release of inflammatory mediators and cytokines, for which the best management consists of intensive medical care and prevention of infection.[2,4,28] In addition, the necrotic tissues are not well demarcated from the viable tissues in this phase, making it difficult to perform blunt radical necrosectomy. This may force the surgeon to perform formal resection or leave nonviable tissues behind.[12]

Surgical management in patients with sterile necrosis is controversial, as operative intervention has not been shown to lower the 10 percent mortality in this group.[5] Conversely, nonoperative therapy for infected necrosis is not recommended, and few question the necessity for surgical debridement in this situation, considering a 100% mortality rate without intervention.[4,6-8]

SURGICAL DEBRIDEMENT

Surgical methods for treating necrosis vary from conventional drainages to closed procedures.[3,13] High mortality rates and frequent reinterventions because of abdominal sepsis have been major drawbacks of the closed drainage procedures. This is why most surgeons prefer the open technique, although repeated debridement and manipulation of the abdominal viscera by laparotomy results in postoperative morbidity such as pancreatic fistulas, small and large bowel lesions, and bleeding from the pancreatic bed in 15 to 56% of patients.[8,14,16] Pancreatic or gastrointestinal fistulas occur in up to 41% of patients, and these complications often require additional surgery for closure.[15]

Avoiding hemorrhage is a major challenge in the management of necrotizing pancreatitis. Bleeding requiring transfusion may occur both intra- and postoperative in 20 to 26% of the cases. Complications from the abdominal wound, both as local infection and later hernia development, are also common.[17]

A prolonged hospital stay after surgery and a long convalescence are characteristic of the disease in which surgery has been performed, contributing to a huge amount of costs.[16]

THE ROLE OF LAPAROSCOPY IN NECROTIZING PANCREATITIS

The laparoscopic era brings new alternatives in the surgical management of pancreatic disease, but still the experience with laparoscopic debridement in this critically ill group of patients is limited.[19,22,24,27] Advances in laparoscopic technology and instrumentation allow a minimally invasive technique and lessen the stress of surgery in the already compromised pancreatic patient. The potential advantages of using this technique include a decrease in postoperative complications and shortness of hospital stay.

Learning laparoscopic techniques for performing laparoscopic staging in pancreatic malignancies enables the surgeon to perform more advanced and complex minimally invasive procedures on the pancreas and the peripancreatic region including the debridement of necrotic tissues. These include the laparoscopic Kocher maneuver, exploration of the lesser sack, and biopsies of pancreatic tissue and lymph nodes.[18–20,23]

ANATOMY AND EXPOSURE

The pancreas is a soft gland that lies in the peritoneum. It measures 15 cm in length and extends from the duodenum to the splenic hilum. The uncinate process, which lies in front of the aorta, surrounds the mesenteric vessels. The first portion of the duodenum delineates the upper border of the head of the pancreas, and the third and fourth portions of the duodenum are located inferiorly and to the right of the mesenteric vessels. The portal vein, common bile duct (CBD), and vena cava are all located posterior to the pancreas. A groove between the neck and the body of the pancreas cradles the gastroduodenal artery. The splenic vessels are found posterior to the pancreas and course along its body to enter the hilum of the spleen.

LAPAROSCOPIC TECHNIQUES

All patients receive a nasogastric tube for decompression of the stomach and a Foley catheter for decompression of the bladder. For the intraperitoneal approach, the patient is placed in a supine position. For the retroperitoneal approach, a left or right semilateral position is preferred.

The entire abdomen is prepped, from the nipple to midthigh. For the intraperitoneal approach, the placement of trochars largely depend of the localization of the necrotic tissues as assessed by preoperative CT scanning. For the direct retroperitoneal approach, the troacars are placed along the costal margins (Fig. 52–1).

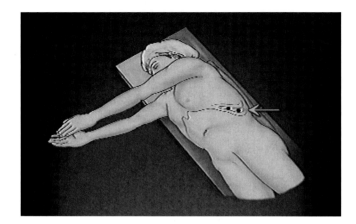

Figure 52–1. Patient position and trocar placement in the retroperitoneal approach.

A preoperative radiologic examination by intravenous loaded CT scan delineates where the maximum amount of the disease is located, and dictates whether the retroperitoneum is to be approached via the right or via the left side (Fig. 52–2). The necrotic tissues of the patient with infected necrotizing pancreatitis should be treated as abscess cavities, and careful removal of all nonviable tissues should be performed. Gentle debridement of pancreatic tissue is mandatory, avoiding major bleeding. Hydrodissection is very useful in this setting, and the suction–irrigation probe is used to gently aspirate and break the peripancreatic debris.

The initial aspirate should be sent for histologic and microbiologic examination to identify any offending organism in the pus. Debridement is performed by a spoon forceps, and the debris are placed in an endobag for retrieval (Fig. 52–3). At the end of the procedure, large sump drains are left in place through the trocar sites (Figs. 52–4 and 52–5).

The routine use of intraoperative ultrasound is recommended, being beneficial for evaluating the extent of pancreatic injury, for evaluating biliary or pancreatic stones, and for verifying whether pseudocysts are present.

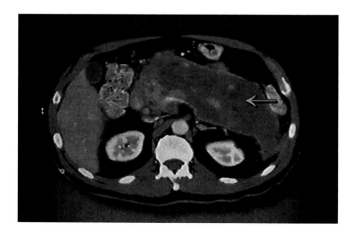

Figure 52–2. CT scan in a patient with necrotizing pancreatitis. Arrow indicates the approach is from the left.

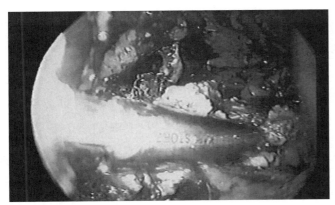

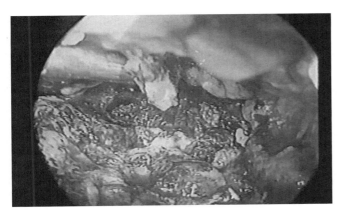

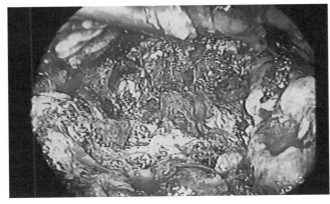

Figure 52–3. Laparoscopic removal (A through C) of peripancreatic necrotic tissue.

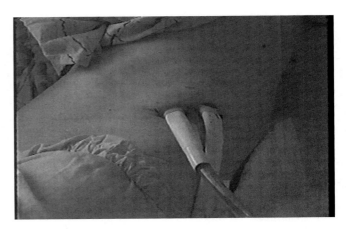

Figure 52–4. Postoperative drainage after performing debridement by retroperitoneal approach.

Intraperitoneal Approach

If necrosectomy is indicated early in the disease process, there is minimal fibrotic tissue, scarring, or thick inflammatory response, making the retroperitoneum easily accessible via the intaperitoneal approach. Whether to enter the abdominal cavity from the left or right side depends on the site of maximal damage to the pancreas and the localization of the peripancreatic necrosis.

Pneumoperitoneum is established via the open technique with CO_2 gas at a maximum level of 15 mm Hg. A 30-degree angled scope is inserted through the umbilicus, and an exploratory laparoscopy is performed. Two paramedian trocars are inserted under direct visualization.

Depending on the site of the necrosis the retroperitoneum can be entered via the following routes:

1. Opening of the gastrocolic ligament. Ultracision is recommended for opening the gastrocolic ligament to allow careful inspection and debridement of the entire body and tail of the pancreas and the peripancreatic and retrogastric area.
2. Opening of the gastrohepatic ligament. The lesser sac may be entered to get access to the retrogastric or perihepatic area, with great care being taken to avoid injury to the left gastric artery.

LAPAROSCOPIC APPROACHES

The different laparoscopic approaches for exposing the pancreatic or retroperitoneal necroses depend on the localization of the pathology, the alternatives being the intraperitoneal approach, direct entry of the retroperitoneal space, or an intraperitoneal transgastric approach.

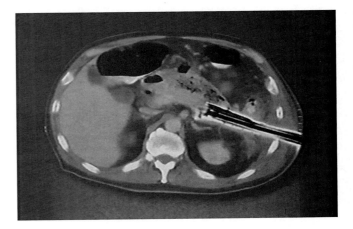

Figure 52–5. CT scan showing the position of postoperative drainage.

3. Mobilization of the right colon. By opening the lateral peritoneal attachments, the right colon is mobilized, exposing the retrocolic space extending from the right flexure and eventually down into the pelvis. Care is taken at this point to avoid injury of the right ureter. Assisted by a bowel forceps from the epigastic port, a Kocher maneuver may be performed to assess the pancreatic head.
4. Mobilization of the splenic flexure. Cutting the lateral peritoneal attachments of the left colon and dividing the splenic flexure opens the left retrocolic space. If the necrosis extends to the retrocolic pelvic space, it may be necessary to open the peritoneal lateral attachments all the way down to the rectum.
5. Through the transverse mesocolon. Care must be taken to avoid injury to the middle colic vessels and their tributaries when this route is taken.

In some cases, the hand-assisted technique may be useful to facilitate the intra-abdominal procedures.

Retroperitoneal Debridement

The retroperitoneal approach to the pancreas is almost solely used for maturing peripancreatic necrosis or infections. The patient is placed in the lateral decubitus position (see Fig. 52–1) and the retroperitoneum is entered from the right or left side, depending on the location of the maximal damage. A 0-degree scope is placed through a trocar in the flank between the iliac crest and twelfth rib posteriorly. The retro-peritoneum is insufflated to 15 mm Hg with CO_2 gas. The right and left kidneys are used for landmarks to progress toward the head or tail of the pancreas. The procedure for debridement and drainage is the same as described previously.

Laparoscopic Transgastric Pancreatic Necrosectomy

The laparoscopic transgastric pancreatic approach is recommended in a patient who presents with late onset of infected pancreatic necrosis, pancreatic abscess, or infected pseudocysts. The abdomen is entered after the establishment of pneumoperitoneum. Intraoperative gastroscopy is performed to visualize the posterior wall of the stomach for any bulging and for insufflation of the stomach throughout the procedure. The anterior wall of the stomach is punctured with a troacar having a balloon in the tip, which anchors it

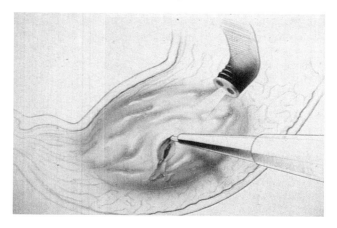

Figure 52–6. Transgastric approach.

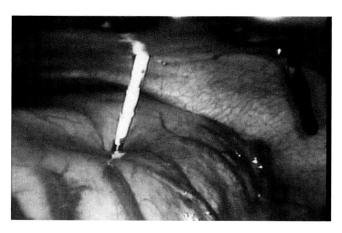

Figure 52–7. Transgastric incision for debridement/drainage.

during the intragastric portion of the procedure. An additional two or three trocars are placed through the anterior gastric wall. Laparoscopic ultrasound is mandatory to assess the anatomy and localize the pathology. Excising the bulging portion of the posterior gastric wall using ultracision performs a fenestration, making a cystogastrostomy (Figs. 52–6 and 52–7). Debridement is best performed using a 5-mm biopsy trocar. The necrotic tissue can be left in the stomach once adequate tissues are taken for sampling. No drains are left in the gastrostomy after the procedure. The anterior gastric wall incisions are closed using 2-0 laparoscopic suturing. If necessary, the debridement can be repeated using gastroscopy-assisted irrigation through the gastrocystostomy.

CONCLUSION

Necrosis is present in approximately 20 to 30% of the 185,000 new cases of acute pancreatitis per year in the United States, consuming huge amounts of economical resources. Despite advances in intensive care medicine, the morbidity and mortality rates of patients with acute necrotizing pancreatitis remain high, reflected by the postoperative short- and long-term complications in patients where open debridement has been performed.

The rationale for laparoscopic intracavitary debridement is to achieve adequate evacuation of the infection and necrotic pancreatic tissue while preserving the body's natural attempt to contain the process. The potential benefits of applying the minimally invasive technique are yet to be proven due to few reports in the literature on using laparoscopic therapy in this group of severely ill patients.

REFERENCES

1. Alexandre JH, Guerrieri MT. Role of total pancreatectomy in the treatment of acute pancreatitis. *World J Surg.* 1981;5:369.
2. Beger HG, Rau B, Mayer J, et al. Natural course of acute pancreatitis. *World J Surg.* 1997;21:130.
3. Rau B, Uhl W, Buchler MW, et al. Surgical treatment of infected pancreatic necrosis. *World J Surg.* 1997;21:155.
4. Baron TH, Morgan D. Acute necrotizing pancreatitis. *N Engl J Med.* 1999; 340:1412.

5. Banks PA. Infected necrosis: Morbidity and therapeutic consequences. *Hepatogastroenterology.* 1991;38:116.

6. Berger HG, Bittner R, Bucheler, et al. Necrosectomy and postoperative local lavage in necrotizing acute pancreatitis. *Br J Surg.* 1998;75:207.

7. Bradley EL, Allen K. A prospective longitudinal study of observation versus surgical intervention in the management of necrotizing pancreatitis. *Am J Surg.* 1991;161:19.

8. Beger HG, Isenman R. Surgical management of necotizing acute pancreatitis. *Surg Clin North Am.* 1999;79;783.

9. Balthazar EJ, Freeny PC, van Sonnenberg E. Imaging and intervention of acute pancreatitis. *Radiology.* 1994;193:297.

10. Isemann R, Buceler MW. Infection and acute pancreatitis. *Br J Surg.* 1994;81:1707.

11. Banks PA. Practice guidelines in acute pancreatitis. *Am J Gastroenterol.* 1997;92:377.

12. Mier J, Luque-de Leon EC, Castillo A, et al. Early versus late necrosectomy in severe necrotizing pancreatitis. *Am J Surg.* 1997;173:71.

13. Freeny PC, Lewis GP, Traverso LW, et al. Infected pancreatic fluid collection: Percutaneous catheter drainage. *Radiology.* 1998;167:435.

14. Rattner DW, Legermate DA, Lee MJ, et al. Early surgical debridement of symptomatic pancreatic necrosis is beneficial irrespective of infection. *Am J Surg.* 1992;163:105.

15. Tsiotos GG, Smith CD, Sarr MG. Incidence and management of severe pancreatic and enteric fistual after surgical management of severe necrotizing pancreatitis. *Arch Surg.* 1995;130:48.

16. Castillo CF, Rattner DW, Warshaw AL, et al. Debridement and closed packing for the treatment of necrotizing pancreatitis. *Ann Surg.* 1998;228:676.

17. Dogiletto GB, Gui D, Pacelli F, et al. Open vs closed treatment of secondary pancreatic infections: A review of 42 cases. *Arch Surg.* 1994;129:689.

18. Pietrabissa A, Di Candio G, Guilianotti PC, et al. Laparoscopic exposure of the pancreas and staging of pancreatic cancer. *Semin Laparosc Surg.* 1996;3:3.

19. Cuscheri A. Laparoscopic surgery of the pancreas. *J R Coll Surg Edinb.* 1994;76:539.

20. Gagner M, Pomp A, Herrera MF. Early experience with laparoscopic resection of islet cell tumors. *Surgery.* 1996;120:1051.

21. Gagner M, Pomp A, Herrara MF. Laparoscopic pylorus-preserving pancreaticoduodenectomy. *Surg Endosc.* 1994;8:408.

22. Gagner M. Laparoscopic treatment of acute necrotizing pancreatitis. *Semin Laparosc Surg.* 1996;3:10.

23. Minnard EA, Conlon KC, Hoos A, et al. Laparoscopic ultrasound enhances standard laparoscopy in the staging of pancreatic cancer. *Ann Surg.* 1998;228:182.

24. Gagner M. Laparoscopic pancreatic surgery. In: Eubanks WS, Swanström LL, Soper NJ, eds. *Mastery of Endoscopic and Laparoscopic Surgery.* Lippincott Williams & Wilkins:2000;291.

25. Uhl W, Buchler MW. Approach to the management of necrotizing pancreatitis, *Probl Gen Surg.* 1997;13:67.

26. Buchler MW, Malfertheiner P, Block S, et al. Morphologic and functional changes in the pancreas following acute necrotizing pancreatitis. *Gastroenterology.* 1985;23:79.

27. Alverdy J, Vargish T, Desai T, et al. Laparoscopic intracavitary debridement of peripancreatic necrosis: Preliminary report and description of the technique. *Surgery.* 2000;127:112.

28. Buchler M, Gloor B, Muller CA, et al. Acute necrotizing pancreatitis: Treatment strategy according to the status of infection *Ann Surg.* 2000;232:619.

Chapter Fifty-Three ∙ ∙ ∙ ∙ ∙ ∙

Laparoscopic Treatment of Acute Biliary Pancreatitis

VALERIE J. HALPIN and NATHANIEL J. SOPER

PATHOPHYSIOLOGY AND PRESENTATION

Biliary pancreatitis is a result of transient or persistent ampullary obstruction by a gallstone migrating from the gallbladder.[1] Patients typically present with abdominal pain in the upper abdomen radiating to the back with associated abdominal tenderness, nausea, and/or vomiting. The damage to the pancreas is usually reversible if the obstruction is relieved within 48 hours. Beyond this time period irreversible damage such as necrosis and autolysis of the gland may occur. Symptoms usually subside within a few days; however, in more severe cases the patient can develop sepsis and shock.

DIAGNOSIS

Diagnosis is based on history and physical examination in conjunction with laboratory and radiologic testing. Elevated serum amylase and lipase are diagnostic laboratory markers. The level of the serum amylase does not predict the etiology, prognosis, or severity of disease. Serum lipase is a more specific but less sensitive marker for pancreatic inflammation. Liver function test results are frequently elevated in patients with acute gallstone pancreatitis because of the presence of transient or ongoing biliary obstruction by a stone.

Radiologic imaging techniques include transabdominal ultrasonography (US), computed tomography (CT), and magnetic resonance cholangiopancreatography (MRCP). Abdominal ultrasound is generally the first imaging study performed in patients with symptoms or signs of biliary disease. Ultrasound is very sensitive for detecting gallstones in the gallbladder, but frequently misses common bile duct (CBD) stones. Ultrasound imaging of the pancreas may be limited due to overlying intestinal segments filled with gas. CT scanning provides more information regarding pancreatic inflammation and associated peripancreatic fluid collections, but is less accurate in detecting gallstones. CT scanning

should be reserved for patients with severe or complicated pancreatitis or for individuals who fail to improve with conservative therapy. MRCP is an emerging technique for biliary imaging that is noninvasive and does not require intravenous contrast material. The role of MRCP in the management of biliary pancreatitis is currently undefined.

TREATMENT

The initial treatment of patients with gallstone pancreatitis consists of bowel rest and resuscitation with IV fluids. The role of antibiotics in the management of acute pancreatitis is controversial and no definitive trials have answered this issue. However, there are several reasons to consider routine antibiotic prophylaxis in acute pancreatitis due to gallstones, including the possibility of associated cholangitis, the role of infected bile in influencing the severity of the pancreatitis, and the higher mortality of infected pancreatic necrosis compared to sterile necrosis. Antibiotics such as imipenem, which have excellent pancreatic penetration, should provide adequate coverage.

ROLE OF ENDOSCOPIC RETROGRADE CHOLANGIOPANCREATOGRAPHY

The role of endoscopic retrograde cholangiopancreatography (ERCP) in the therapeutic management of gallstone pancreatitis has been evolving since the development of laparoscopic cholecystectomy.[2] As laparoscopic techniques for CBD exploration have developed, there is decreasing need for preoperative ERCP (Table 53–1).[2,3] For mild pancreatitis, recent randomized studies have shown[2] that selective postoperative ERCP results in a shorter length of stay, decreased costs, performance of fewer procedures, and no increase in combined treatment failure rate compared to routine

TABLE 53–1. INDICATIONS FOR ERCP

Preoperative

Severe pancreatitis

Cholangitis

Jaundice

Poor surgical candidate

Lack of surgeons skilled in advanced laparoscopy

Postoperative

Persistent common bile duct stones and lack of advanced laparoscopic skills

preoperative ERCP.[4,5] Preoperative ERCP is indicated in those patients who have severe pancreatitis, cholangitis, or jaundice, are poor surgical candidates, or when no advanced laparoscopic skills are available.

SURGICAL MANAGEMENT

Cholecystectomy is indicated for all but the most debilitated patients with gallstone pancreatitis.[6] Over 90% of patients will be candidates for a laparoscopic approach. The patient should be taken to the operating room to undergo laparoscopic cholecystectomy with intraoperative imaging of the bile duct during the initial admission once the acute manifestations of pancreatitis have resolved. The exact timing of surgical intervention is debated, but we usually plan to operate the day prior to that of anticipated discharge. Intraoperative cholangiography (IOC) and laparoscopic intracorporeal ultrasound (LICU) are both acceptable techniques of intraoperative biliary imaging. IOC is the most widely used method of biliary imaging and is considered the gold standard. LICU is gaining popularity as it has been demonstrated to be more sensitive in detecting bile duct stones. If stones are detected on intraoperative imaging, laparoscopic stone removal should be attempted. Surgeons who are inexperienced in laparoscopic techniques can refer patients for postoperative ERCP for stone removal. Patients who develop severe pancreatitis with pancreatic necrosis will require pancreatic debridement. Overall, the results of laparoscopic treatment of acute biliary pancreatitis have been favorable (Table 53–2).

TECHNIQUES FOR BILE DUCT STONE MANAGEMENT

When CBD stones are detected during laparoscopic cholecystectomy, several treatment options are available to the surgeon (Table 53–3). The size and location of the CBD stones determine the best method for extraction. Small stones can usually be flushed into the duodenum after administering intravenous glucagon. CBD stones that are relatively few in number (<5), relatively small in size (<6 to 8 mm) and located in the distal CBD can usually be retrieved via the cystic duct. Multiple stones, stones located proximal to the CBD-cystic duct junction, and large stones (>6 to 8 mm) are likely to require laparoscopic choledochotomy as long as the CBD is greater than 8 mm in diameter. Both transcystic techniques and laparoscopic choledochotomy have demonstrated excellent results in the management of common bile duct stones.

TRANSCYSTIC EXPLORATION

Transcystic exploration and clearance of the common duct is highly effective. Using a transcystic technique, 80 to 90% of common duct stones can be cleared, precluding choledochotomy or ERCP. Initial port placement is the same as for standard laparoscopic cholecystectomy. Access to the cystic duct is usually aided by high placement of the midclavicular access port (<2 cm below the rib). After demonstrating choledocholithiasis by intraoperative imaging, the cystic duct is dissected further distally and is incised near its junction with the CBD. A hydrophilic guidewire is inserted through the cholangiogram catheter into the CBD. The catheter is then advanced over the guidewire. Normal saline is flushed through the cholangiocatheter in an attempt to wash small stones through the ampulla or out the ductotomy. Fluoroscopy allows the surgeon to observe whether the stones empty into the duodenum or remain in the CBD. Often, gently advancing the catheter pushes small stones through the ampulla. In addition, the resting tone of the ampullary sphincter may be decreased with 1 to 2 mg IV glucagon, nitroglycerin, or 1% lidocaine infused into the CBD.

Baskets may be passed over the guidewire into the common duct to extract stones under fluoroscopic guidance. Once a stone is captured, the stone and basket move together on fluoroscopy.

TABLE 53–2. RESULTS OF LAPAROSCOPIC CHOLECYSTECTOMY FOR BILIARY PANCREATITIS

Study	N	Converted		ERCP		Positive		IOC	Positive		Complications	
		n	(%)	n	(%)	n	(%)	n	n	(%)	n	(%)
Canal	29	0		4	17%	0		22	3	14%	1	3%
Soper	49	0		29	59%	9	31%	36	6	17%	2	4%
Tate	24	3	12.5%	23	96%	7	30%	1	0		2	8%
Delorio	59	7	12%	43	72%	19	44%	31	4	13%	4	7%
Tang	142	7	12%	31	23%	13	42%	104	9	9.6%	—	
Taylor	29	7	19%	1	3%	0		24	4	17%	5	16%
Ballestra	40	0		0		—		40	2	5%	8	20%
Cueto	32	2	6.2%	1	3.1%	0		30	12	37%	10	31%
Total	404	26	7.7%	132	35%	48	36%	288	40	14.1%	32	11.1%

IOC, intraoperative cholangiography, ERCP, endoscopic retrograde cholangiopancreatography.

From Cueto J, et al. Proceedings of the Seventh World Congress of Endoscopic Surgery. Monduzzi Editore, June 1–4, 2000.

TABLE 53–3. TECHNIQUES FOR MANAGEMENT OF COMMON BILE DUCT STONES

Transcystic exploration
  Flushing
  Baskets
  Balloon embolectomy catheters
Transcystic choledochoscopy
  Flushing
  Baskets
Laparoscopic choledochotomy
  Choledochoscopy
  Baskets
  Balloon catheters
Intracorporeal lithotripsy
Antegrade transcystic sphincterotomy
Transcystic balloon ampullary dilatation

Whenever fluoroscopic basket extraction is attempted, the surgeon must be careful not to open the basket in the CBD proximal to the stone and then advance the basket. This may push the basket with stone into the duodenum causing the basket to be trapped, and an open surgical procedure may be necessary to remove the stone from the basket. If the stone is impacted in the duct or the basket cannot open fully to trap the stone, a 4F embolectomy catheter may be advanced past the stone, the balloon inflated, and the stone gently pulled back into a more dilated portion of the proximal CBD.

TRANSCYSTIC DUCT CHOLEDOCHOSCOPY

Transcystic choledochoscopy directly visualizes the biliary tract and is used when fluoroscopic extraction techniques fail. Because choledocholithiasis usually results from stones migrating through the cystic duct into the CBD, the cystic duct is often of adequate diameter to accept a choledochoscope to extract stones. The diameter of the distal cystic duct and ductotomy must be as large as the largest CBD stone to successfully perform transcystic extraction. If necessary, the cystic duct may be balloon dilated to a maximum of 8 mm in diameter. A 3- to 5-cm long balloon is positioned with its proximal end protruding from the cystic duct and its distal end within the CBD. Contrast material is injected to confirm proper placement. The balloon is inflated to several atmospheres of pressure (pressure varies by balloon size) and held for 5 minutes under direct vision. The balloon is then deflated, removed, and the guidewire is left in place. A choledochoscope is passed over the guidewire into the CBD. Examination of the duct is optimal during withdrawal of the cholangioscope and is improved by continuous saline infusion. Because of the unusual angle of insertion of the cystic duct into the CBD, it is very difficult to perform transcystic choledochoscopy of the proximal biliary tree. Under visual guidance, a stone basket is introduced through the biopsy channel, then the tip is advanced beyond the stone and the basket opened. As the basket is pulled backward and rotated the stone is ensnared. The stone is removed under direct vision along with the scope through the ductotomy, and the stone is placed in a bag. Multiple passes are made with the endoscope until the duct is clear. A completion cholangiogram should be performed to conclusively demonstrate clearance of the duct. Because tissue edema develops secondary to ductal dilation and manipulation, the cystic duct stump is ligated (rather than clipped) for added security after choledochoscopy.

LAPAROSCOPIC CHOLEDOCHOTOMY

Laparoscopic choledochotomy is safe and effective in experienced hands, and has shorter hospitalization compared to open CBD exploration. The major disadvantage of laparoscopic CBD exploration is that it is technically difficult to close the ductotomy without narrowing the lumen. The diameter of the CBD must at least 6 to 8 mm in order to perform choledochotomy safely. A small (0.5- to 1.0-cm) longitudinal choledochotomy is made on the mid-anterior CBD distal to the cystic duct–CBD junction. Electrocautery should be avoided because of the potential for CBD stricture formation. A flexible choledochoscope is inserted through a 5-mm trocar. Sterile saline is infused through the working channel to dilate the duct and improve visualization, and balloons or baskets may be used to withdraw most stones. After stone removal a 12F to 14F T tube is placed in the duct, the choledochotomy is closed using intracorporeal suturing techniques with 4-0 absorbable monofilament suture, and the T-tube is brought out a lateral port site (Fig. 53–1). A completion cholangiogram should be performed to document clearance of the CBD and absence of leaks. The gallbladder is then removed and the cystic duct is loop ligated. The T-tube may be removed in 10 to 14 days, after a repeat T-tube cholangiogram to assure a stone-free duct. Complications of laparoscopic choledochotomy include laceration of the common duct, bile leakage, sewn-in T tubes, and postoperative strictures.

If the patient is stable with a retained stone on T-tube cholangiography, the T-tube should be left in place. The CBD is evaluated by T-tube cholangiography or percutaneous choledochoscopy at 4 to 6 weeks. Residual stones are safely and effectively removed through the tract using baskets, balloons, or a lithotripsy device. Complications include sinus tract perforation, cholangitis, pancreatitis, and vasovagal reactions.

OTHER TECHNIQUES

Intracorporeal lithotripsy can be used to fragment large or impacted stones. Stones may be fragmented using either pulsed-dye laser or electrohydraulic pulses. Laparoscopic antegrade transcystic sphincterotomy can be performed for patients with complex choledocholithiasis in whom transcystic CBD exploration and choledochotomy have failed. Another approach is laparoscopic transcystic ampullary balloon dilation with flushing of the CBD stones into the duodenum.

TECHNIQUES FOR DEBRIDEMENT IN PANCREATITIS

Reports of endoscopically-assisted debridement of infected pancreatic tissue are emerging as alternatives to the traditional open necrosectomy[7,8] The theoretical advantages include lower morbidity and decreased length of stay. Reported techniques include

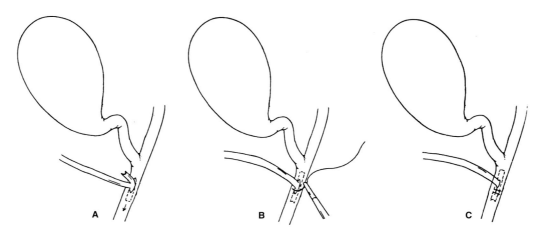

Figure 53–1. Laparoscopic T-tube placement following choledochotomy. A. A T-tube is inserted into the choledochotomy incision and brought out through a subcostal port. B. & C. The T-tube is sutured into place with 4-0 absorbable suture intracorporeally.

laparoscopically-assisted percutaneous drainage and intracavitary debridement and endoscopically-assisted retroperitoneal or "lumboscopic" drainage of abscess cavities and infected pancreatic necrosis. As further studies are performed, such approaches may succeed in further decreasing the morbidity associated with severe pancreatitis and infected pancreatic necrosis.

CONCLUSIONS

The management of acute biliary pancreatitis continues to evolve as new laparoscopic techniques for common bile duct evaluation and pancreatic debridement develop and surgeons become increasingly facile in laparoscopy. Given the success of laparoscopic common bile duct exploration and ERCP, it should be possible to manage the majority of patients with gallstone pancreatitis by minimally invasive techniques.

Acknowledgments. The authors gratefully acknowledge the Washington University Institute for Minimally Invasive Surgery as funded by an educational grant from U.S. Surgical Corporation.

REFERENCES

1. Acosta JM, Ledesma DL. Gallstone migration as a cause of acute pancreatitis. *N Engl J Med.* 1974;290:484.
2. Soper NJ, Brunt LM, Callery MP, et al. Role of laparoscopic cholecystectomy in the management of acute gallstone pancreatitis. *Am J Surg.* 1994;167:42.
3. Cueto J, Vazquez A, Weber A. Laparoscopic approach in patients with acute biliary pancreatitis. Sixth World Congress of Endoscopic Surgery, Rome, Italy, 1998; June 3–6, Rome, Monduzzi Eds, p. 737.
4. Chang L, Lo S, Stabile BE, et al. Preoperative versus postoperative endoscopic retrograde cholangiopancreatography in mild to moderate gallstone pancreatitis. *Ann Surg.* 2000;231:82.
5. Rhodes M, Sussman L, Cohen L, et al. Randomised trial of laparoscopic exploration of common bile duct versus postoperative endoscopic retrograde cholangiography for common bile duct stones. *Lancet* 1998;351:159.
6. McGrath MF, McGrath JC, Gabbay J, et al. Safe laparoendoscopic approach to biliary pancreatitis in older patients. *Arch Surg.* 1996;131:826.
7. Alverdy J, Vargish T, Desai T, et al. Laparoscopic intracavitary debridement of peripancreatic necrosis. Preliminary report and description of the technique. *Surgery* 2000;127:112.
8. Gambiez LP, Denimal FA, Porte HL, et al. Retroperitoneal approach and endoscopic management of peripancreatic necrosis collections. *Arch Surg.* 1998;133:66.

Chapter Fifty-Four ● ● ● ● ● ●

*L*aparoscopic Pancreatic Resection

PAOLO GENTILESCHI and MICHEL GAGNER

Laparoscopy is still evolving in its approach to pancreatic disease. Surgeons first started performing laparoscopy for the diagnosis and staging of pancreatic tumors.[1,2] Diagnostic laparoscopy has been shown to provide useful information in such patients.[1,2] The introduction and development of laparoscopic ultrasonography enhanced the ability of staging laparoscopy to determine resectability in pancreatic cancer.[3,4] In addition, surgical palliative procedures, such as laparoscopic biliary and intestinal bypass operations, have been developed and safely performed.[5,6] Recent technological improvements have made laparoscopic pancreatic resection possible.[7,8]

The types of reported laparoscopic pancreatic resections vary from enucleation of insulinomas to pancreaticoduodenectomy.[7–26] Current evidence shows that these procedures are not associated with an increase in morbidity and mortality compared with results in open pancreatic resections.[11,13,17,18,21,22,24,25] On the other hand, the advantages of performing pancreatic resections by laparoscopy are not still evident.[9] Obstacles to laparoscopic pancreatic surgery are related to long operative times; difficulty in retraction, particularly in obese patients; difficulty in safe parenchymal transection; and difficulty in assessing proper margins of resection due to the loss of tactile sensation. However, laparoscopic technology is in a rapid state of evolution and further advancements might play an important role for the future diffusion of laparoscopic pancreatectomy. These advancements include refinement in laparoscopic ultrasound, improvements in stapling instrumentation and techniques, availability of coagulating parenchymal transection tools such as the ultrasonic dissector (harmonic scalpel), and development of hand-assisted laparoscopic techniques.

The following is a review of our experience and of the world literature on laparoscopic pancreatic resection, including distal pancreatectomy, enucleation, and pancreaticoduodenal resection.

REPORTED EXPERIENCE

Laparoscopic Pancreaticoduodenectomy

Laparoscopic pancreaticoduodenectomy was first reported in 1992 in a patient with chronic pancreatitis.[7] An animal model for this procedure was described in 1994.[27] In a review article published in 1994, Cuschieri reported two patients treated by laparoscopic pancreaticoduodenectomy with no benefit to the postoperative period.[10] A case of a pancreaticoduodenectomy performed via a mini-laparotomy with the use of an abdominal wall-lift retractor and a laparoscope for better visualization of the operative site was reported in 1996.[28]

The first, and to the best of our knowledge the only, series of patients treated by laparoscopic pancreaticoduodenal resection was reported in 1997.[9] They were 6 women and 4 men with a mean age of 71 years (range, 33 to 82 years). Eight patients were affected by malignant periampullary tumors and 2 had chronic pancreatitis. The presenting symptoms were painless jaundice in 8 and chronic pain requiring constant narcotics in 2. The rate of conversion to an open procedure was 40%, and complications were seen in the nonconverted group. The average operative time required for a laparoscopic Whipple procedure was 8.5 hours (range, 5.5 to 12 hours) compared with 4.6 hours (range, 3.5 to 6.0 hours) for operations converted to open procedures. Average hospital stay was 22.3 days in the laparoscopic group (range, 7 to 62 days) and 20.1 days in the open group (range, 14 to 36 days). An average of 2.0 (range, 0 to 6) units of packed red blood cells was transfused perioperatively in the laparoscopic group and 1.5 (range, 0 to 4) units in the converted group.

Complications occurred in 3 patients who had a laparoscopic Whipple procedure while there were none in the converted group. The complications included delayed gastric emptying in one patient, splenic hemorrhage in one, and a pancreatic leak in one. Total parenteral nutrition was required for 2 weeks in the patient with delayed gastric emptying; splenectomy 24 hours after the initial operation was performed in the patient with splenic hemorrhage; the pancreatic leak, which was minor, was managed by total parenteral nutrition and drainage and eventually stopped by the second postoperative week. No difference was noted in the average number of nodes retrieved, which was 7 in the laparoscopic group (range, 3 to 14) and 8 in the open group (range, 6 to 11); nodes were positive in 3 patients of the laparoscopic group and in 2 patients of the converted group.

Although this series was small, no major benefit seemed to be derived from the use of a complete laparoscopic Whipple procedure. Although postoperative pain was more acceptable in the laparoscopic group, the postoperative period, recovery and convalescence were similar to those associated with open surgery.

Laparoscopic Distal Pancreatectomy and Enucleation

The world literature review that we have performed shows that 68 laparoscopic distal pancreatectomies and enucleations (42 distal pancreatectomies and 26 enucleations) have been attempted to date, with 13 conversions to open procedures (19.1%; Table 54–1).[8,9,11–26] The indications were islet cell tumors in 45 patients, chronic pancreatitis in 11 patients, cystadenomas in 10 patients, and infiltrative tumors in 2 patients.

In 37 of the 42 reported distal pancreatectomies, it was possible to know if a splenectomy was associated to the pancreatic resection. In 25 cases, the spleen was preserved; in 12 patients a splenectomy was also performed. This is related to the fact that most (11) of the pancreaticosplenectomies were reported by Cuschieri, who performed these procedures in patients with chronic pancreatitis, in which the fibrotic process renders the dissection of the pancreatic tail from the spleen often impossible.

There was no mortality after the 68 laparoscopic distal pancreatectomies and enucleations. The most common major postoperative complication was pancreatic leak, which occurred in a total of 5 patients (7.3%), in one case requiring reoperation. Based on the reports where mean hospital stay was mentioned, we calculated an average overall hospital stay of 9 days.

In our series, a total of 13 patients (8 women, 5 men; mean age, 41 years, with an age range from 29 to 74 years) have undergone laparoscopic distal pancreatectomy and enucleation. Twelve patients were affected by islet cell tumors (6 insulinomas, 4 of unknown origin, 2 gastrinomas) while one patient had chronic pancreatitis. The mean size of the lesions was 3 cm (range, 2 to 6 cm). There were four conversions to an open procedure. Two patients with gastrinomas were converted after diagnostic laparoscopy because of extensive intra-abdominal disease. They both underwent extensive debulking with distal pancreatectomy. A retroportal insulinoma was not localized by laparoscopy and laparoscopic ultrasonography and therefore the operation was converted to an open procedure. The tumor was finally localized with open ultrasound and enucleated. In the fourth case, a nonsecreting islet cell tumor was found to be too deep in the pancreatic parenchyma to be enucleated. The patient received an open pylorus-preserving pancreaticoduodenectomy, and histology showed a nesidioblastoma with positive antibodies to somatostatin and glucagons.

Mean operative time for the laparoscopic distal pancreatectomies was 6.3 hours, with an average hospital stay of 5 days. Mean operative time for enucleations was 3 hours, with a mean hospital stay of 4 days. Two complications were observed in the laparoscopic group: one case of significant intraoperative bleeding from the splenic vein, which was managed laparoscopically; and one pancreatic leak, which resolved in 3 months. Mean follow-up was 27 months (range, 15 to 40 months), in which no recurrences were observed.

PERSONAL SURGICAL TECHNIQUE

Laparoscopic Pancreaticoduodenectomy

In the first report of 1992, the procedure performed was a pylorus-preserving pancreaticoduodenectomy with a modification for the anastomosis between the pylorus and the jejunum, which was end-to-end. The original was a purely laparoscopic technique performed with the use of six trocars. Subsequently, the technique was modified with the introduction of a hand-assisted approach (Fig. 54–1).[29] Both techniques are feasible but the hand-assisted approach is associated with shorter operative times and tactile sensation, which can be very useful either in the staging of the tumor or during the procedure. The retraction, finger blunt dissection, and manual control of eventual bleeding afforded by the assisting hand are very useful tools for such a complex operation.

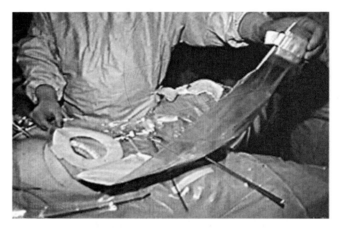

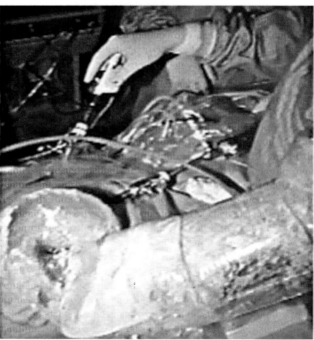

Figure 54–1. The Pneumosleeve.

Together with the insertion of 5 trocars, an 8-cm incision is made in the right subcostal area (Fig. 54–2) for the introduction of the nondominant (left) hand with a special plastic device (Dexterity Pneumosleeve; Fig. 54–1). During the whole procedure, while maintaining the left hand inside the abdomen and the pressure of the pneumoperitoneum, the dissection, transection, and reconstruction are carried out with laparoscopic instruments with the dominant (right) hand. The hand inside the area is useful for gentle retraction, performance of the Kocher maneuver, palpation of tumor extension, and evaluation of tumor resectability. In addition, bleeding can be controlled with finger compression, intracorporeal suturing is facilitated, and the incision is used for extraction of the specimen.

Intraoperative laparoscopic ultrasound examination is performed routinely for tumor staging, and to delineate the relationship between tumor, pancreas, and vessels. The procedure starts with the Kocher maneuver, achieved by the left hand dissecting the retroduodenal area as well as by endoscopic scissors taking down the adhesions. The maneuver is begun by opening the peritoneal reflection close to the lateral curve of the duodenum from the hepatoduodenal ligament above to the mesocolon below. After cauterizing the small vessels lying under this part of the peritoneum, blunt dissection between the pancreas in front, and the vena cava behind, is possible in an avascular plane. For complete mobilization, the right colonic flexure is freed and reflected downwards with the use of the left hand. The avascular peritoneal reflection covering the third portion of the duodenum is divided right up to the large vessels at the mesenteric root. In this way, the second, third, and fourth portions of the duodenum are dissected and mobilized and the vena cava is exposed. Also, the peritoneum covering the common bile duct is opened anteriorly and laterally. The peritoneal sheet of the hepatoduodenal ligament and lesser omentum is divided close to the hepatic hilum, thus exposing the structures within this ligament. A laparoscopic right-angled dissector is used to isolate the common bile duct, portal vein, and right hepatic artery. Cholecystectomy with cholangiogram is performed. The gastrocolic ligament is then opened with the harmonic scalpel, laterally to the gastroepiploic artery, which is preserved, and all the transverse branches are divided (Fig. 54–3). The dissection is continued towards the pylorus and the transection of the first portion

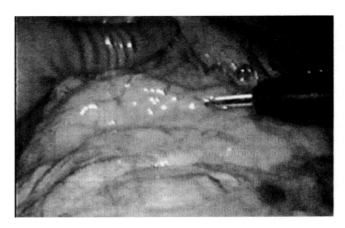

Figure 54–3. The gastrocolic ligament is opened with the harmonic scalpel.

of the duodenum is performed at 1 cm from the pylorus with an Endo-GIA stapler (US Surgical, Norwalk, CT) (Fig. 54–4). The bile duct is suspended with an umbilical tape and transected with a 30-mm Endo-GIA stapler approximately 3 cm above the superior border of the pancreas. The gastroduodenal artery is then exposed and transected with an endoscopic stapler. The superior mesenteric vein and portal vein are dissected from the head of the pancreas using a suction/irrigation probe in a blunt fashion. With this maneuver, the neck of the pancreas is carefully cleared from the portal vein by gentle blunt dissection and hand assistance.

The pancreas is then transected, starting inferiorly and moving toward the superior border anterior to the portal vein and the mesenteric vessels. The harmonic scalpel (Ethicon Endo-Surgery, Cincinnati) is extremely useful to achieve this goal with minimal blood loss (Fig. 54–5). The fourth portion of the duodenum, medial to the mesenteric vessels, is transected with the stapler (Fig. 54–6). Again, the harmonic scalpel is useful to clear the uncinate process from the mesenteric artery and vein. The specimen is placed in an impermeable nylon bag (Cook Surgical, Bloomington, IN) and pulled through the Pneumosleeve.

The three anastomoses are created by intracorporeal suturing techniques. The proximal jejunal loop is pulled behind the

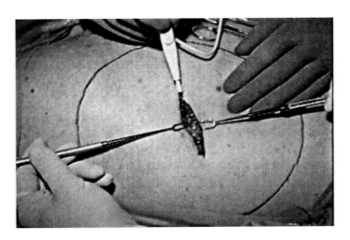

Figure 54–2. The incision in the right subcostal area for the left hand.

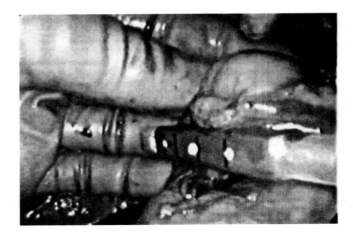

Figure 54–4. Transection of the first portion of the duodenum.

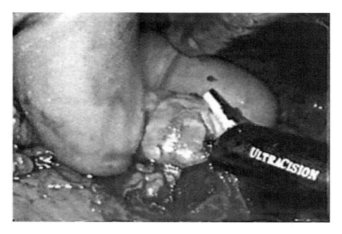

Figure 54–5. Transection of the pancreas with the harmonic scalpel.

mesenteric vessels and its antimesenteric side is approximated to the pancreatic duct in two layers. A 5-F pediatric tube is used as a stent and need only be 5 cm in length. One half of the stent is inserted into the pancreatic duct and sutured to the duct and jejunal opening with 4-0 monofilament absorbable sutures. A layer of 3-0 silk interrupted sutures is then applied between the anterior capsule of the pancreas and the serosal side of the jejunal loop (Fig. 54–7). The hepaticojejunostomy is then performed without tubes with a running posterior and running anterior 3-0 monofilament absorbable suture (Fig. 54–8). Finally, through the open incision with a wound protector, the third anastomosis is carried out with the same suture between the pylorus and the jejunum end-to-end. A feeding jejunostomy (T-tube, 14-French) is inserted through one of the trocar sites and two large Jackson-Pratt drains are left anterior and posterior to these anastomoses.

Laparoscopic Distal Pancreatectomy and Enucleation

The decision to perform either a distal pancreatectomy or enucleation is based on the pathology of the pancreatic lesion. Current indications for distal pancreatectomy and/or enucleation are benign

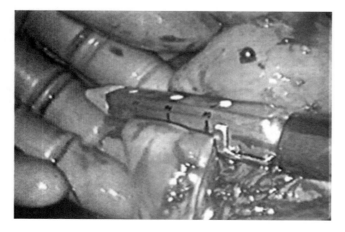

Figure 54–6. Transection of the fourth portion of the duodenum.

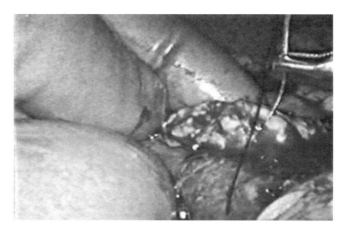

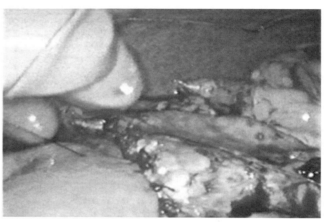

Figure 54–7. Pancreatico-jejunostomy.

neoplasms, islet cell tumors, exocrine tumors of the body and the tail, and chronic pancreatitis (Fig. 54–9).

On the operating table, the patient is rotated laterally 45 degrees so that the left side is up or in a full lateral and reverse Trendelenburg position (Fig. 54–10). The surgeon is positioned between the patient's legs, with the scrub nurse to the patient's left, and the first assistant on the patient's right. After placing an umbilical trocar, diagnostic laparoscopy is performed. Laparoscopic ultrasound is carried out, being useful to delineate the relationship between pancreas, tumor, and vessels. Biopsy of suspicious peritoneal nodules is usually performed and sent for frozen section.

The resection starts with the entry into the lesser sac and exposure of the pancreas. The gastrocolic ligament is opened with the harmonic scalpel, usually starting halfway along the greater curvature laterally to the gastroepiploic artery, thus exposing the anterior portion of the body and tail of the pancreas. For a better exposure of the tail of the pancreas, mobilization of the splenic flexure of the colon, and division of lower short gastric vessels are usually required. At this point of the procedure, ultrasonography is used to define the relationship between the lesion, the splenic vessels, and the pancreatic duct. Pancreatic resection includes splenectomy in cases of large tumors lying adjacent to the spleen or involving the vessels. Also when distal pancreatectomy is performed for chronic pancreatitis, preservation of the spleen is not always technically feasible, because inflammation and fibrosis of

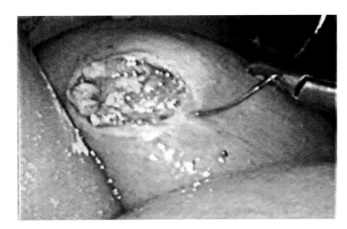

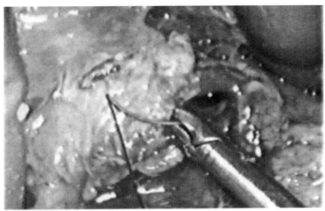

Figure 54–8. Hepaticojejunostomy is performed with a running posterior and running anterior 3-0 monofilament absorbable suture.

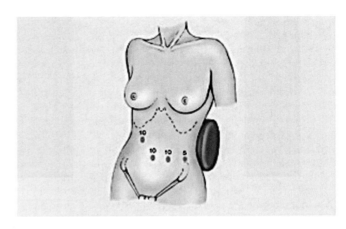

Figure 54–10. Patient position on the operating table, and trocar sites for laparoscopic distal pancreatectomy.

stapler. The pancreas is then mobilized, dissecting from the body to the tail. For resection of lesions located in the tail, an alternative approach can be used, in which the spleen and pancreas are mobilized prior to division of the splenic vessels and the pancreas. Ligamentous attachments of the spleen are divided, and the posterior spleen and tail of the gland are mobilized from the retroperitoneum, dissecting from lateral to medial. In all other cases, whenever possible, we prefer to preserve the spleen, splenic artery, and splenic vein. This is accomplished with gentle dissection and meticulous hemostasis when dissecting between the pancreas and vessels.

Once the plane of parenchymal transection is determined with the use of ultrasound, the pancreas can be mobilized. The mobilization starts with the dissection of the inferior border of the pancreas from the retroperitoneal fat, until the gland is mobile and the splenic vein is reached. This dissection is accomplished with the use of the harmonic scalpel. Gentle dissection to the right of the lesion is performed between the pancreas and the splenic vessels. A window is created with a right angle and then the pancreas is transected with a linear stapler (Fig. 54–11). Once the stapler is fired, bleeding from pancreatic vessels may require additional sutures. A U-stitch, using a fine nonabsorbable monofilament suture,

splenic vessels may make the dissection of the tail of the pancreas from the splenic hilum virtually impossible. If the decision to associate splenectomy with distal pancreatectomy is made, the splenic artery is divided at the planned line of pancreatic transection, using an endoscopic stapler reinforced with clips. The gland and the splenic vein are divided as a single unit with an endoscopic

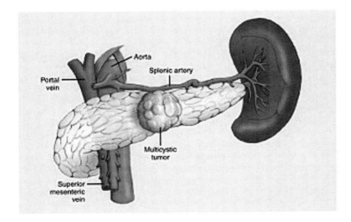

Figure 54–9. Example of a pancreatic multicystic tumor, suitable for laparoscopic distal pancreatectomy.

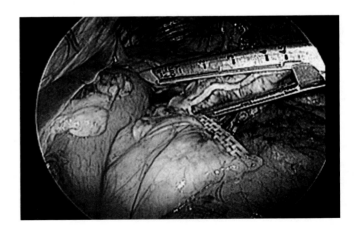

Figure 54–11. Transection of the pancreas with a linear stapler.

around the transected Wirsung duct, if it is well recognized, may be required.

Starting from the cut end of the pancreas, which is grasped and retracted anteriorly, the dissection is then continued towards the tail (Fig. 54–12). The transverse branches of the splenic artery and vein are well exposed, dissected with a right-angled instrument, and ligated (Fig. 54–13).

Continuing the lateral dissection, the tail of the pancreas is then completely mobilized. Additional attachments can be divided with the harmonic scalpel, and a careful control of hemostasis is carried out (Fig. 54–14). The specimen is extracted through the small incision by means of the left hand (Fig. 54–15). A Jackson-Pratt drain is placed near the pancreatic stump. At some point during the operation, the decision to convert the procedure to a hand-assisted approach can be made in difficult cases to render the dissection easier. This must be considered as an intermediary step before eventual conversion to open surgery, allowing the resection to be safer and faster but still minimally invasive.

When the decision to perform an enucleation of an islet cell tumor is made, the exposure is similar to the procedures described above. The islet cell tumor is usually localized with ultrasound, and the dissection is performed either with a hook or harmonic scalpel. The dissection plane is chosen between the tumor and parenchyma, ligating pancreatic vessels feeding the tumor with clips. Extraction of the specimen, placed in a plastic bag, is carried out through one of the operating ports, which is enlarged to the size of the tumor, and a Jackson-Pratt drain is positioned over the enucleation site.

DISCUSSION

Reports of laparoscopic pancreatic resections are still limited.[7–26] As a result, it is difficult to formulate any definite conclusions. However, some considerations can be made. Laparoscopic pancreatic surgery is rapidly evolving in relation to technological improvements and increasing experience among advanced laparoscopic surgeons. The literature review that we performed has shown that all kinds of pancreatic resection are feasible. Questions that remain to be answered regard safety,

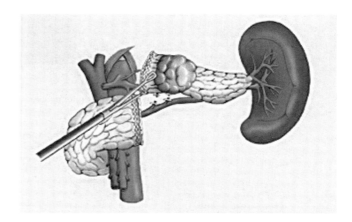

Figure 54–13. Gentle dissection between the pancreas and the splenic vessels during laparoscopic distal pancreatectomy with splenic preservation.

cost, and the potential benefits to the patients. As experience is gained, laparoscopic pancreatic resections might prove to be associated with real advantages during the postoperative period and convalescence. To date, a distinction must be made between pancreaticoduodenal resection and distal pancreatectomy and enucleation.

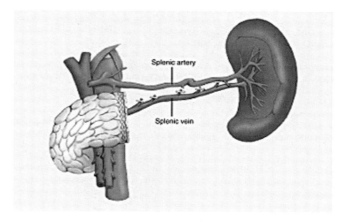

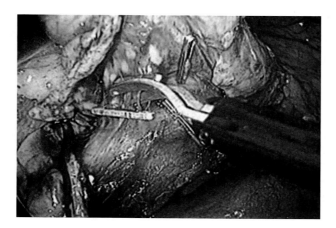

Figure 54–12. The dissection is continued towards the tail.

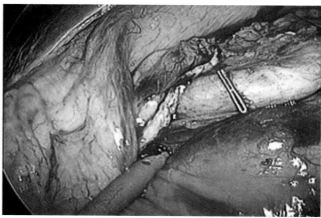

Figure 54–14. Completed laparoscopic distal pancreatectomy with splenic preservation. For bottom photo, see Color Section.

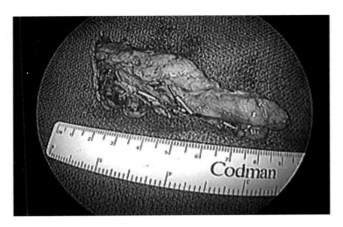

Figure 54–15. Specimen of distal pancreatectomy.

Laparoscopic Pancreaticoduodenectomy

Totally laparoscopic pancreaticoduodenectomy is technically challenging but feasible. However, in cases involving malignancy, lack of tactile sensation may lead to misdiagnosis, difficulty in localizing the lesion and inadequate assessment of tumor spread. This is one of the major reasons that laparoscopic surgery has not been widely used in the oncologic setting.[30] Obesity and previous abdominal surgery add an extra degree of difficulty in retracting organs or doing the dissection.

Our impression, based on initial experiences, is that the hand-assisted technique that we described should be able to make laparoscopic pancreaticoduodenectomy safer and easier. Since a limited laparotomy is required to remove the resected specimen, it seems logical to make the small incision at the beginning of the operation. This may address concerns regarding operating time, related costs, and oncologic safety of tumor removal through the abdominal wall. The hand-assisted technique can also be used as a replacement to conversion to open surgery, or as an intermediate step between laparoscopy and laparotomy. This could represent an attempt to preserve the advantages of minimally invasive surgery, with the improvements and safety afforded by the assisting hand.

Purely laparoscopic pancreaticoduodenectomy seems to offer no advantage in terms of patient outcome and may be associated with increased morbidity.[9] The reported experience with hand-assisted laparoscopic pancreaticoduodenectomy is too small to make any consideration about the incidence of overall morbidity and mortality and hand-technique-related morbidity. We believe that the hand-assisted technique should give substantial advantages to laparoscopic pancreaticoduodenectomy, improving the exploration of the abdominal cavity and exposure of major anatomic structures; determining a better organ retraction, especially in the obese; and permitting safer dissection and specimen removal.

Although the hand-assisted technique might improve the results of laparoscopic pancreaticoduodenectomy, many concerns are being raised with regard to attempting this operation. It has been suggested that patients might be put at risk during portions of this unconventional dissection. There is also concern that the patient undergoing either purely laparoscopic or hand-assisted laparoscopic pancreaticoduodenectomy receives a compromised cancer operation. In the report of 1997 about the 10 patients who received laparoscopic pancreaticoduodenectomy, we stated that the proce-

dure offered no advantages in terms of patient outcome and may be accompanied by increased morbidity. Cuschieri, in 1998,[17] concluded that pancreaticoduodenectomy should always be performed by the open approach, irrespective of whether the lesion in the proximal pancreas is benign or malignant. In pancreaticoduodenectomy, laparotomy forms only a small component of the total operative insult to the patient and, for this reason, avoidance of laparotomy does not influence recovery, convalescence, and postoperative disability. It is also obvious that further experience, especially with the hand-assisted approach, may be able to demonstrate potential advantages without putting the patient at risk of not having the required procedure.

Laparoscopic Distal Pancreatectomy and Enucleation

By contrast, distal pancreatic resection and enucleation are safe, associated with low morbidity, and seem to be accompanied by a postoperative recovery that compares favorably with the one after open pancreatic resection.

After open distal pancreatectomy and enucleation, morbidity follows in 10 to 30% of patients.[31,32] This morbidity is often secondary to a pancreatic leak and may result in pancreatitis, pancreatic fistulas, or subphrenic abscess formation. Mortality rates following open distal pancreatic resection range from zero to 6%.[31,33] In the present world literature review, there is no mortality and the morbidity rate seems acceptable. In particular, pancreatic leak occurred in 5 patients (7.3%), requiring reoperation in only one patient.

Two authors, Gagner and Cuschieri, have together reported a total of 28 distal pancreatic resections and enucleations. The remaining 40 pancreatic resections have been performed by a total of 13 centers, with 6 single case reports. The high number (approximate 20%) of cases that were converted to open surgery could be due to the high number of surgeons who have performed these new and complex procedures and therefore to their learning curve period. On the other hand, considering only the two largest experiences (Gagner and Cuschieri), the conversion rate is approximately the same (21.4%). Other possible reasons for this high conversion rate could be the complexity of pancreatic surgery and the difficulty in localizing small lesions in the pancreatic parenchyma by laparoscopic exploration and ultrasonography.

The average hospital stay of 9 days must be considered good, being influenced by some complications and by a prudent approach to discharge by most surgeons, dealing with a new and complex procedure.

Laparoscopic distal pancreatectomy and enucleation should be considered in patients with chronic pancreatitis, islet cell tumors, and benign cystadenomas. Preservation of the spleen is indicated for treatment of neuroendocrine pancreatic tumors, provided these are benign and well localized. Infiltrative lesions often require a pancreaticosplenectomy. Splenic preservation is feasible during laparoscopic distal pancreatectomy, as shown by the present literature review. Patients with chronic pancreatitis may have severe retroperitoneal fibrosis, which precludes safe splenic preservation.

Some concern arises for the laparoscopic treatment of cystic tumors of the pancreas, because some benign cystadenomas are found to be malignant on histologic examination of excised specimen. Because these tumors have a reasonably good long-term prognosis if radical resection is performed, suspicious cystadenocarcinomas during laparoscopy should still probably be treated by open pancreatectomy.

Case selection is, however, crucial, and should be based on pathology, clinical features, and past surgical history. Relative contraindications are obesity and previous upper abdominal surgery. Patients with operable pancreatic cancer should be approached by laparoscopy for staging and, provided the possibility of a curative resection is confirmed, should be converted to open surgery. Laparoscopic pancreatic surgery should be reserved for palliative procedures, benign tumors, benign islet cell tumors, and chronic pancreatitis. These operations should only be performed in centers with expertise in both pancreatic surgery and advanced laparoscopy.

REFERENCES

1. Warshaw AL, Gu ZY, Wittenberg J, et al. Preoperative staging and assessment of resectability of pancreatic cancer. *Arch Surg.* 1990;125:230.
2. Murugiah M, Paterson-Brown S, Windsor JA, et al. Early experience of laparoscopic ultrasonography in the management of pancreatic carcinoma. *Surg Endosc.* 1993;7:177.
3. Bemelman WA, de Wit LT, van Delden OM, et al. Diagnostic laparoscopy combined with laparoscopic ultrasonography in staging of cancer of the pancreatic head region. *Br J Surg.* 1995;82:820.
4. Minnard EA, Conlon KC, Hoos A, et al. Laparoscopic ultrasound enhances standard laparoscopy in the staging of pancreatic cancer. *Ann Surg.* 1998;228:182.
5. Hawsali A. Laparoscopic cholecysto-jejunostomy for obstructing pancreatic cancer. *J Laparoendosc Surg.* 1992;2:351.
6. Wilson RG, Varma JS. Laparoscopic gastroenterostomy for malignant duodenal obstruction. *Br J Surg.* 1992;79:1348.
7. Gagner M, Pomp A. Laparoscopic pylorus-preserving pancreatoduodenectomy. *Surg Endosc.* 1994;8:408.
8. Cuschieri A. Laparoscopic hand-assisted surgery for hepatic and pancreatic disease. *Surg Endosc.* 2000;14:991.
9. Gagner M, Pomp A. Laparoscopic pancreatic resection: Is it worthwhile? *J Gastroint Surg.* 1997;1:20.
10. Cuschieri A. Laparoscopic surgery of the pancreas. *J R Coll Surg Edinb.* 1994;39:178.
11. Gagner M, Pomp A, Herrera MF. Early experience with laparoscopic resections of islet cell tumors. *Surgery.* 1996;120:1051.
12. Sussman LA, Christie R, Whittle DE. Laparoscopic excision of distal pancreas including insulinoma. *Aust NZ J Surg.* 1996;66:414.
13. Cuschieri A, Jakimowicz JJ, Van Spreeuwel J. Laparoscopic distal 70%
14. Clark GJ, Onders RP, Knudson DJ. Laparoscopic distal pancreatectomy procedures in a rural hospital. *AORN J.* 1997;65:334.
15. Tihanyi TF, Morvay K. Laparoscopic distal resection of the pancreas with the preservation of the spleen. *Acta Chir Hung.* 1997;36:1.
16. Klingler PJ, Hinder RA, Menke DM, et al. Hand-assisted laparoscopic distal pancreatectomy for pancreatic cystadenoma. *Surg Laparosc Endosc.* 1998;8:180.
17. Cuschieri A, Jakimowicz JJ. Laparoscopic pancreatic resections. *Semin Laparosc Surg.* 1998;5:168.
18. Chapuis Y, Bigourdan JM, Massault PP, et al. Videolaparoscopic excision of insulinoma. A study of 5 cases. *Chirurgie.* 1998;123:461.
19. Ueno T, Oka M, Nishihara K, et al. Laparoscopic distal pancreatectomy with preservation of the spleen. *Surg Laparosc Endosc Percutan Tech.* 1999;9:290.
20. Matsumoto T, Kitano S, Yoshida T, et al. Laparoscopic resection of a pancreatic mucinous cystadenoma using laparosonic coagulating shears. *Surg Endosc.* 1999;13:172.
21. Vezakis A, Davides D, Larvin M, et al. Laparoscopic surgery combined with preservation of the spleen for distal pancreatic tumors. *Surg Endosc.* 1999;13:26.
22. Park A, Schwartz R, Tandan V, et al. Laparoscopic pancreatic surgery. *Am J Surg* 1999;177:158.
23. Collins R, Schlinkert RT, Roust L. Laparoscopic resection of an insulinoma. *J Laparoendosc Adv Surg Tech.* 1999;9:429.
24. Santoro E, Carlini M, Carboni F. Laparoscopic pancreatic surgery: Indications, techniques and preliminary results. *Hepatogastroenterology.* 1999;46:1174.
25. Berends FJ, Cuesta MA, Kazemier G, et al. Laparoscopic detection and resection of insulinomas. *Surgery.* 2000;128:386.
26. Spitz JD, Lilly MC, Tetik C, et al. Ultrasound-guided laparoscopic resection of pancreatic islet cell tumors. Surg *Laparosc Endosc Percutan Tech.* 2000;10:168.
27. Soper NJ, Brunt LM, Dunnegan DL. Laparoscopic distal pancreatectomy in the porcine model. *Surg Endosc.* 1994;8:57.
28. Uyama I, Ogiwara H, Iida S, et al. Laparoscopic minilaparotomy: Pancreaticoduodenectomy with lymphadenectomy using an abdominal wall-lift method. *Surg Laparosc Endosc.* 1996;6:405.
29. Southern surgeon's club study group. Handoscopic surgery: A prospective multicenter trial of a minimally invasive technique for complex abdominal surgery. *Arch Surg.* 1999;134:477.
30. Chi DS, Curtin JP. Gynecologic cancer and laparoscopy. *Obstet Gynecol Clin North Am.* 1999;26:201.
31. Lillemoe KD, Kaushal S, Cameron JL, et al. Distal pancreatectomy: Indications and outcomes in 235 patients. *Ann Surg.* 1999;229:693.
32. Trede M, Carter DC. *Surgery of the Pancreas*, 2nd ed. Churchill Livingstone:1997.
33. Proye C. Surgical strategy in insulinoma of adults: Clinical review. *Acta Chir Scand.* 1987;153:481.

pancreatectomy and splenectomy for chronic pancreatitis. *Ann Surg.* 1996;223:280.

*D*iagnostic Procedures

Chapter Fifty-Five ■ ■ ■ ■ ■ ■

*L*aparoscopic Surgery in the Diagnosis and Treatment of Peritonitis

JORGE CUETO-GARCÍA and JOSÉ ANTONIO VÁZQUEZ-FRÍAS

INTRODUCTION

Secondary peritonitis includes a spectrum of disease processes with different causes and clinical courses.[1] Even though major advances in medical technology, antibiotics, and surgical and intensive care have contributed to diminish the mortality and morbidity rates due to peritonitis, they still remain very high.[2–7]

The main goals of surgical treatment of peritonitis are: (1) early diagnosis, (2) elimination of the septic foci and repair of intraperitoneal visceral lesions, (3) reduction of the bacterial inoculum of the peritoneal cavity, and (4) prevention or treatment of persistent and/or recurrent infection.[3,4,8]

Jacobeus[9] is credited as the first physician to perform a direct visualization—after insufflation of air—of the peritoneal cavity and although the value of diagnostic laparoscopy has been recognized since the 1950s,[10–12] it was not used in the treatment of acute peritonitis until recently. The results obtained in laparoscopic cholecystectomy led surgeons to proceed with minimally invasive procedures in patients with acute cholecystitis, appendicitis (and its complications), pelvic surgical diseases, intestinal obstruction, perforated peptic ulcer, and colonic diverticulitis, among other procedures, with similar results.[13–16]

MATERIALS AND METHODS

Since October 1990 the authors have operated on 151 consecutive patients with acute abdominal syndrome (Table 55–1). Aggressive medical treatment was instituted preoperatively: hydration, widespectrum intravenous antibiotics, nasogastric suction, and urinary catheter and central venous lines were used as needed. All patients were hemodynamically stable and underwent general endotracheal anesthesia. Pneumoperitoneum was established at the umbilicus with a Veress needle except in patients with abdominal distention in whom the first trocar was placed with an open technique.[17,18]

The number and position of ports varied depending on the pathological disorder found after the diagnostic laparoscopy (Fig. 55–1).

RESULTS

Ninety-four patients were females and 57 were males, and average age was 50 years (range, 8 to 92). In 36 patients (23.8%) the diagnosis was questionable before laparoscopy. In all cases diagnostic laparoscopy established the diagnosis (Table 55–1) and in 138 of them (91.3%) the procedure was performed with this minimally invasive approach. Conversion to laparotomy due to technical problems was necessary in 13 patients (8.6%) without additional morbidity. Reoperation was required in 8 patients (5.2%), in three cases due to "residual" abscesses (in one patient with perforated colonic diverticula, one with perforated ulcer, and one with a severe intestinal obstruction due to adhesions), in three others because of persistent peritonitis, in one patient a pancreatic necrosectomy was done, and one laparotomy was negative. Six patients presented minor complications: three with postoperative ileus, one with a lesion of the epigastric vessels, and two with umbilical cellulitis. No complications related to the pneumoperitoneum occurred. Overall, five patients died (3.3%) (Table 55–2). A 91-year-old female operated on for an intestinal obstruction died from a myocardial infarction on the eleventh postoperative day, and an 87-year-old female had two laparotomies for recurrent sepsis and suffered respiratory failure due to chronic obstructive pulmonary disease. Two other deaths occurred due to multiple organ failure secondary to sepsis in elderly males 71 and 75 years old, both with chronic lung disease and one with acute liver failure due to obstructive jaundice of 3 weeks' duration and purulent cholangitis (treated elsewhere). The fifth death occurred in a 28-year-old female patient with postpartum endotoxic shock who was referred to us with acute cholecystitis from the ICU. She recovered from the laparoscopic

TABLE 55–1. ETIOLOGY OF ACUTE ABDOMEN

Causes	No. of Cases
Perforated appendicitis†	36
Perforated cholecystitis*	25
Pelvic disorders	23
(Ectopic pregnancy, 6; pelvic inflammatory disease, 4; adnexal torsion, 2; hemorrhagic ovarian cyst, 11)	
Bowel obstruction	21
Biliary pancreatitis	13
Blunt abdominal trauma	12
Perforated diverticulitis	7
Perforated peptic ulcer	4
Residual abscess	2
Penetrating abdominal trauma	2
Sigmoid volvulus	2
Small bowel volvulus	1
Epiploic appendagitis	1
Mesenteric ischemia	1
Mesenteric adenitis	1
Total	151

*Acute cholecistitis was excluded.

†Uncomplicated acute appendicitis was excluded.

cholecystectomy but went on to develop progressive irreversible multiple organ failure.

DISCUSSION

Acute abdominal syndrome remains one of the most common causes of admission to the emergency department and constitutes a continuing daily challenge even for experienced surgeons. It is important to establish an early and correct diagnosis and to administer rapid treatment to reduce morbidity, mortality, pain, and costs.[5] An incorrect preoperative diagnosis may lead to a delay in surgical treatment (with its obvious negative consequences), or an unnecessary laparotomy, which carries a morbidity rate of between 5 and 22%.[9,19,20]

Laparoscopy eliminates long, expensive periods of patient observation and monitoring (usually with a variety of tests) in cases of nonspecific acute abdominal pain. A recent randomized clinical trial[21] reported that early laparoscopy provides higher diagnostic accuracy than observation and improves quality of life postoperatively. Diagnostic accuracy of minimally invasive exploration in peritonitis has been reported to be between 81 and 100%.[13,14,22–26] Literature specifically dealing with peritonitis due to various conditions (i.e., laparoscopically diagnosed and treated) is scarce. Navez et al[27] reported diagnostic accuracy of 84.8%, Geis and Kim[28] reported accuracy of 99.3%, and as previously mentioned[29] our group found the correct diagnosis in 100% of cases. Following confirmation of the etiologic diagnosis, successful treatment by minimal invasive surgery by these groups was reported to be 70.1%, 96%, and 91.3%, respectively.

Several researchers report that the laparoscopic approach provides greater exposure of the abdominal and pelvic cavities in cases of acute abdomen.[12,15,30,31] A thorough and accurate exploration of intraperitoneal structures may be more easily done with lapa-

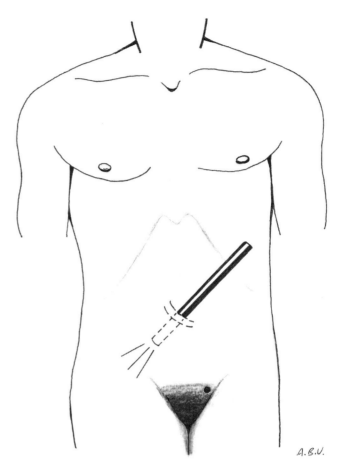

Figure 55–1. A zero degree laparoscope is inserted to perform diagnostic laparoscopy to establish the number and position of trocars needed for the procedure.

roscopy than with traditional open incisions, even if they are extended. Inspection of retroperitoneal organs can also be done, but requires more experience and different instrumentation.

In peritonitis, abdominal distention is common due to dilated bowel loops and inflammation. In these patients, pneumoperitoneum is often established with the open technique[17,18] which appears to be safer,[32–34] though not completely trouble-free, because some bowel and vascular lacerations have been reported using this technique.[35,36] In the group of patients reported above, there were no lesions in the establishment of pneumoperitoneum. Like other surgical groups,[27] our group stresses the use of the proper instruments, and that great care be used when working with inflamed,

TABLE 55–2. MORTALITY IN OUR SERIES OF ISI PATIENTS

Age	Sex	Initial Diagnosis	Cause of Death
91	Female	Bowel obstruction	Myocardial infarction
87	Female	Bowel obstruction	Respiratory failure
75	Male	Necrotic pancreatitis	Sepsis/MOF
71	Male	Purulent cholangitis	Sepsis/MOF
28	Female	Pelvic inflammatory disease	Sepsis/MOF

MOF, multiple organ failure.

dilated intestinal loops. The authors operated on two patients, both elderly females, in which an intestinal obstruction was resolved, but malaise, abdominal pain, and distention occurred 72 hours postoperatively, necessitating laparotomy. In both cases perforations were found at sites different from those of the original obstruction. After review of the surgical videos, no evidence of intraoperative lesions was seen, but the possibility exists that this complication could be related to bowel manipulation, perhaps of edematous, ischemic loops of small bowel.

The importance of meticulous lavage of the abdominal cavity with large amounts of isotonic solution in cases of generalized septic peritonitis or massive contamination is well known. Laparoscopic surgery facilitates this by allowing irrigation with pressure under direct vision with aspiration of pus, bile, blood, and fecal material, and by allowing drainage of abscesses in the subphrenic spaces, paracolic gutters, and the sac of Douglas. It also enables the surgeon to obtain culture samples and/or biopsies under direct vision, as well as removal of fibrinoid and purulent exudates from intra-abdominal structures.

A recent review of the literature evaluating the use of laparoscopic surgery in surgical infection[37] revealed that minimally invasive operations result in a lower incidence of infectious complications. This has been a controversial issue that has been argued mostly in papers dealing with complicated appendectomies (comparing laparoscopic vs. open surgery) and postoperative intra-abdominal abscesses. Some surgeons[38–40] have found more intra-abdominal abscesses after laparoscopic appendectomy, other authors[27,41–43] have concluded there is no difference at all, and there are groups[44–46] (like ours) that fortunately have not seen them yet, even in very complicated cases. Several meta-analyses[47–49] have proven that infectious morbidity of the mini-incisions is lower in comparison with the open surgery wound in the setting of appendicitis. A very important surgical aspect has to be stressed: following laparotomy in patients with peritonitis, most surgeons have seen and will continue to care for patients with large complicated incisional hernias that require long-term, multiple, expensive surgical procedures that often fail and produce severe physical limitations in patients. Furthermore, abdominal wound dehiscence (which is reported to be up to 3% and carry a mortality rate between 9 and 44%)[50] is virtually eliminated by minimally invasive surgery.[27]

Minimally invasive surgery is very useful in critical care patients in whom there is no time for a delayed diagnosis or a negative laparotomy, or in clinical situations in which the differential diagnosis is complicated due to the presence of other pathological entities or equivocal physical examination, laboratory, or imaging findings. Mention must be made of cases of mesenteric ischemia[51,52] in which a port may be left in situ, properly isolated (with topical antibiotics and a dressing) in order to have the ability to take a second look up to 24 hours later, as we have done in two patients in the ICU. In these patients diagnostic laparoscopy can be performed safely in the ICU under local anesthesia and sedation in selected cases[53–55] using small (2- to -3 mm) laparoscopes. This procedure (discussed elsewhere in this book) can be also performed in the emergency department or in an office setting with minimal morbidity.

In the last decade it has been demonstrated that minimally invasive surgery produces a significantly less severe inflammatory and metabolic response, as well as less immunosuppression, compared with laparotomy,[37,56–61] and this is thought to be due to the reduction in surgical trauma. All of this could mean fewer and less severe infections, and perhaps less local sepsis,[60,61] which if true, could be an important advantage in patients with abdominal sepsis and immunosuppression.

Use of CO_2 pneumoperitoneum was once considered to be contraindicated in the setting of peritonitis, due to the possibility of spread of the infection[62–63] and the potential for severe hypercapnia. In this regard, several studies comparing CO_2 pneumoperitoneum and laparotomy have found that both may increase the incidence of bacteremia,[64–68] and only one of them[64] favored the laparotomy group. On the other hand, a prospective study revealed that pneumoperitoneum itself is unlikely to disperse bacteria.[69]

The minimally invasive approach allows intestinal resection and anastomosis to be carried out completely within the abdominal cavity, as well as the construction of intestinal stomas simply by enlarging the port site incisions.[70–73] Gastrostomies or jejunostomies for enteral nutrition can also be performed with this approach.[74,75]

Laparoscopic surgery in patients with peritonitis usually requires varied and special skills and adequate equipment and instrumentation. If technical problems arise, it must be always kept in mind that the use of an extra trocar can make the difference between conversion to an open procedure or completion of the operation laparoscopically. In cases in which the procedure cannot be finished laparoscopically, conversion can be usually be performed through a smaller incision than is normally required without increasing morbidity or mortality.[29] At present, the hand-assisted procedures[76] that are becoming popular for some types of abdominal surgery (as discussed elsewhere in this book) are another option to consider before formal conversion to laparotomy is done. To avoid further contamination, in some instances the specimen can be retrieved from the abdomen while enclosed in a sterile plastic bag.[77]

Another worrisome aspect of peritonitis is that of adhesions. It is well known that minimally invasive surgery produces fewer postoperative adhesions because manipulation of the viscera is minimal and selective.[78–80] Ileus in peritonitis is not completely understood,[81] and although minimally invasive surgery is associated with less postoperative ileus, further studies are needed for clarification.[82,83]

Some reports have also documented a reduction in HIV and hepatitis transmission with the mini-invasive surgical method.[84–86]

Finally, it must be mentioned that the use of laparoscopic surgery in the diagnosis and treatment of peritonitis has many well known advantages, including less pain, shorter hospital stay, less pulmonary morbidity, fewer wound infections, and excellent cosmetic results.[5,48,49,57,87–89]

CONCLUSION

Laparoscopic surgery in the diagnosis and treatment of peritonitis is feasible and safe, though it requires special skills and an experienced and well-equipped surgical team. For establishing the diagnosis it may be considered the new gold standard, and its advantages for carrying out the procedure required to treat the disorder are many and frequently superior to the use of conventional surgery. Whatever the procedure being performed, it will always be the surgeon's expertise and judgement that determine whether laparoscopy should be continued or if conversion to laparotomy is necessary.

REFERENCES

1. Johnson CC, Baldessarre J, Levison ME. Peritonitis: update in pathophysiology, clinical manifestations, and management. *Clin Infect Dis.* 1997;24:1035.

2. Wittmann DH. World progress in surgery. Intraabdominal infections. *World J Surg.* 1990;14:145.

3. Bosscha K, van Vroonhoven ThJMV, van der Verken Ch. Surgical management of secondary peritonitis. *Br J Surg.* 1999;86:1371.

4. Wittman DH, Schein M, Condon RE. Management of secondary peritonitis. *Ann Surg.* 1996;224:10.

5. Easter D, Cuschieri A. The utility of diagnostic laparoscopy for abdominal disorders. *Arch Surg.* 1992;127:379.

6. Cueto GJ, Rojas DO, Weber SA. ?Es útil la laparoscopia en el diagnóstico y tratamiento del síndrome abdominal agudo? *Rev Gastroenterol Mex.* 1993;58:360.

7. Berci G. Elective and emergency laparoscopy. *World J Surg.* 1993;17:8.

8. Nathens AB, Rotstein OD, Marshall JC. Tertiary peritonitis: clinical features of a complex nosocomial infection. *World J Surg.* 1998;22:158.

9. Memon MA, Fitzgibbons RJ. The role of minimal access surgery in the acute abdomen. *Surg Clin North Am.* 1997;77:1333.

10. Llanio R, Sarle H. Interêt de la peritoneoscope chez politraumatismes. *Marseille Chirurcale* 1956;8:82.

11. Llanio R. *Laparoscopia de urgencia.* Ed. Científico-Técnica:1977.

12. Llanio R, Sotto A, Ferret O, et al. Diagnostique de l'abdomen aigu par laparoscopie: experience portant 6400 cas. 3rd European Congress of Gastrointestinal Endoscopy 1976. Abstract. Budapest, 1976.

13. Geis WP, Kim HC. Use of laparoscopy in the diagnosis of patients with surgical abdominal sepsis. *Surg Endosc.* 1995;9:178.

14. Navez B, D'Udekem Y, Cambier E, et al. Laparoscopy for the management of non-traumatic acute abdomen. *World J Surg.* 1995;193:382.

15. Connor TJ, Garcha IS, Ramshaw BJ, et al. Diagnostic laparoscopy for suspected appendicitis. *Am Surg.* 1995;61:187.

16. Cueto GJ, Weber SA, Serrano BF. Laparoscopic treatment of perforated ulcer. *Surg Laparosc Endosc.* 1993;3:216.

17. Hasson HM. Open laparoscopy: a report of 150 cases. *J Reprod Med.* 1974;12:234.

18. McKernan JB, Champion JK. Access techniques: Veress needle—initial blind trocar insertion versus open laparoscopy with the Hasson trocar. *Endosc Surg Allied Technol.* 1995;3:35.

19. Sugarbaker PH, Sanders JH, Bloom BS, et al. Preoperative laparoscopy in diagnosis of acute abdominal pain. *Lancet* 1995;1:442.

20. Petersen SR, Sheldon GF. Morbidity of a negative finding at laparotomy in abdominal trauma. *Surg Gynecol Obstet.* 1979;148:23.

21. Decadt B, Sussman L, Lewis MPN, et al. Randomized clinical trial of early laparoscopy in the management of acute non-specific abdominal pain. *Br J Surg.* 1999;86:1383.

22. Nagy AG, James D. Diagnostic laparoscopy. *Am J Surg.* 1989;157:490.

23. Vander Velpen GC, Shimi SM, Cuschieri A. Diagnostic yield and management benefit of laparoscopy: a prospective audit. *Gut* 1994;35:1617.

24. Salky BA, Edye MB. The role of laparoscopy in the diagnosis and treatment of abdominal pain syndromes. *Surg Endosc.* 1998;12:911.

25. Cuesta MA, Eijsbouts QAJ, Gordijin RV, et al. Diagnostic laparoscopy in patients with an acute abdomen of uncertain etiology. *Surg Endosc.* 1998;12:915.

26. Chung RS, Diaz JJ, Chari V. Efficacy of routine laparoscopy for the acute abdomen. *Surg Endosc.* 1998;12:219.

27. Navez B, Tassetti V, Scohy JJ, et al. Laparoscopic management of acute peritonitis. *Br J Surg.* 1998;85:32.

28. Geis WP, Kim HC. Use of laparoscopy in the diagnosis and treatment of patients with surgical abdominal sepsis. *Surg Endosc.* 1995;9:178.

29. Cueto J, Díaz O, Garteiz D, et al. The efficacy of laparoscopic surgery in the diagnosis and treatment of peritonitis. Experience with 107 cases in Mexico City. *Surg Endosc.* 1997;11:366.

30. Soper NJ, Brunt LM, Kerbl K. Laparoscopic general surgery. *N Engl J Med.* 1994;330:409.

31. Weber SA, Serrano BF, Cueto GJ. Puntos claves para facilitar la técnica, en cirugía laparoscópica. *Cir Gen.* 1994;17:88.

32. Byron JW, Markenson G, Miyazawa K. A randomized comparison of Veress needle and direct trocar insertion for laparoscopy. *Surg Gynecol Obstet.* 1993;177:259.

33. McKernan JB, Champion JK. Access techniques: Veress needle—initial blind trocar insertion versus open laparoscopy with the Hasson trocar. *Endosc Surg Allied Technol.* 1995;3:35.

34. Bonjer HJ, Hazabroek EJ, Kazemier G, et al. Open versus closed establishment of pneumoperitoneum in laparoscopic surgery. *Br J Surg.* 1997;84:599.

35. Penfield AJ. How to prevent complications of open laparoscopy. *J Reprod Med.* 1985;30:660.

36. Hanney RM, Carmalt HL, Merret N, et al. Use of the Hasson cannula producing major vascular injury at laparoscopy. *Surg Endosc.* 1999;13:1238.

37. Targarona EM, Balague C, Knook MM, et al. Laparoscopic surgery and surgical infections. *Br J Surg.* 2000;87:536.

38. Tang E, Ortega AE, Anthone GJ, et al. Intraabdominal abscesses following laparoscopic and open appendectomies. *Surg Endosc.* 1996;10:327.

39. Paik PS, Towson JA, Anthone GJ, et al. Intraabdominal abscesses following laparoscopic and open appendectomies. *J Gastrointest Surg.* 1997;1:188.

40. Frazee RC, Bohannon WT. Laparoscopic appendectomy for complicated appendicitis. *Arch Surg.* 1996;131:509.

41. Johnson AB, Peetz ME. Laparoscopic appendectomy is an acceptable alternative for the treatment of perforated appendicitis. *Surg Endosc.* 1998;12:940.

42. Klingler A, Henle KP, Beller S, et al. Laparoscopic appendectomy does not change the incidence of postoperative infectious complications. *Am J Surg.* 1998;175:232.

43. Khalili TM, Hiatt JR, Savar A, et al. Perforated appendicitis is not a contraindication to laparoscopy. *Am Surg.* 1999;65:965.

44. Paya K, Rauhofer U, Rebhandl W, et al. Perforating appendicitis. An indication for laparoscopy? *Surg Endosc.* 2000;14:182.

45. Alvarez C, Voitk AJ. The road to ambulatory laparoscopic management of perforated appendicitis. *Am J Surg.* 2000;179:63.

46. Reid RD, Dobbs BR, Frizelle FA. Risk factors for post-appendectomy intra-abdominal abscess. *Aust N Z J Surg.* 1999;69:373.

47. Meynaud-Kraemer L, Colin C, Vergnon P, et al. Wound infection in open versus laparoscopic appendectomy. A meta-analysis. *Int J Technol Assess Health Care.* 1999;15:380.

48. Garbutt JM, Soper NJ, Shannon WD, et al. Meta-analysis of randomized controlled trials comparing laparoscopic and open appendectomy. *Surg Laparosc Endosc.* 1999;1:17.

49. Chung RS, Rowland DY, Li P, et al. A meta-analysis of randomized controlled trials of laparoscopic versus conventional appendectomy. *Am J Surg.* 1999;177:250.

50. Ellis H. Management of the wound. In: Schwartz SI, Ellis H, eds. *Maingot's Abdominal Operations,* 9th ed. Appleton & Lange: 1990;195.

51. Navez B. Laparoscopy in the management of the nontraumatic acute abdomen. In: Felicien MS, Welter R, eds. *Minimally Invasive Surgery.* Quality Medical Publishing:1994;207.

52. Cuschieri A. Diagnostic laparoscopy and laparoscopic adhesiolysis. In: Cuschieri A, Buess G, Perissat J, eds. *Operative Manual of Endoscopic Surgery.* Springer-Verlag:1992;180.

53. Forde K, Treat M. The role of peritoneoscopy (laparoscopy) in the evaluation of the acute abdomen in critically ill patients. *Surg Endosc.* 1992;6:219.

54. Walsh RM, Popovich MJ, Hoadley J. Bedside diagnostic laparoscopy and peritoneal lavage in the intensive care unit. *Surg Endosc.* 1998;12:1405.

55. Rehm CG. Bedside laparoscopy. *Crit Care Clin.* 2000;16:101.

56. Lee SW, Southall JC, Gleason NR, et al. Time course of differences in lymphocyte proliferation rates after laparotomy vs CO_2 insufflation. *Surg Endosc.* 2000;14:145.

57. Kehlet H, Nielsen HJ. Impact of laparoscopic surgery on stress responses, immunofunction, and risk of infectious complications. *New Horiz.* 1998;6(2 Suppl):S80.

58. Vittimberga FJ, Foley DP, Meyers WC, et al. Laparoscopic surgery and the systemic immune response. *Ann Surg.* 1998;227:326.

59. Kuntz C, Wunsch A, Bay F, et al. Prospective randomized study of stress and immune response after laparoscopic vs conventional colonic resection. *Surg Endosc.* 1998;12:963.

60. Sietses C, Beelen RH, Meijer S, et al. Immunological consequences of laparoscopic surgery, speculations on the cause and clinical implications. *Langenbecks Arch Surg.* 1999;384:250.

61. Smit MJ, Beelen RH, Eijsbouts QA, et al. Immunological response in laparoscopic surgery. *Acta Gastroenterol Belg.* 1996;59:245.

62. Bloechle C, Emmermann A, Treu H, et al. Effect of a pneumoperitoneum on the extent and severity of peritonitis induced by gastric ulcer perforation in the rat. *Surg Endosc.* 1995;9:898.

63. Bloechle C, Emmermann A, Strate T, et al. Laparoscopic vs open repair of gastric perforation and abdominal lavage of associated peritonitis in pigs. *Surg Endosc.* 1998;12:212.

64. Ozmen MM, Col C, Aksoy AM, et al. Effect of CO_2 insufflation on bacteremia and bacterial translocation in an animal model of peritonitis. *Surg Endosc.* 1999;13:801.

65. Jacobi CA, Ordemann J, Bohm B, et al. Does laparoscopy increase bacteremia and endotoxemia in a peritonitis model? *Surg Endosc.* 1997;11:235.

66. Jacobi CA, Ordemann J, Zieren HU, et al. Increased systemic inflammation after laparotomy vs laparoscopy in an animal model of peritonitis. *Arch Surg.* 1998;133:258.

67. Gurtner GC, Robertson CS, Chung SCS, et al. Effect of carbon dioxide pneumoperitoneum on bacteraemia and endotoxaemia in an animal model of peritonitis. *Br J Surg.* 1995;82:844.

68. Ozguc H, Yizmazlar T, Zorlouglu A, et al. Effect of CO_2 pneumoperitoneum on bacteremia in experimental peritonitis. *Eur Surg Res.* 1996;28:124.

69. Taffinder NJ, Cruaud P, Catheline JM, et al. Bacterial contamination of pneumoperitoneum gas in peritonitis and controls: a prospective laparoscopic study. *Acta Chir Belg.* 1997;97:215.

70. Cueto J, Vázquez-Frias JA, Castañeda-Leeder P, et al. Laparoscopic assisted resection of a bleeding gastrointestinal stromal tumor. *JSLS.* 1999;3:225.

71. Milsom JW, Lavery IC, Church JM, et al. Use of laparoscopic techniques in colorectal surgery. Preliminary study. *Dis Colon Rectum.* 1994;37:215.

72. Roe AM, Barlow AP, Durdey P, et al. Indications for laparoscopic formation of intestinal stomas. *Surg Laparosc Endosc.* 1994;4:345.

73. Bohm B, Milsom JW, Stolfi VM, et al. Laparoscopic intraperitoneal anastomosis. *Surg Endosc.* 1993;7:194.

74. Rosser JC Jr., Rodas EB, Blancaflor J, et al. A simplified technique for laparoscopic jejunostomy and gastrostomy tube placement. *Am J Surg.* 1999;177:61.

75. Lo Gerfo P. Feeding gastrostomy. *Surg Endosc.* 1994;8:1049.

76. The HALS Study Group. Hand assisted laparoscopic surgery (HALS) with the hand port system. Initial experience with 68 patients. *Ann Surg.* 2000;231:715.

77. Weber SA, Vázquez JA, Valencia MS, et al. Retrieval of specimens in laparoscopy using reclosable zipper-type plastic bags: a simple, cheap and useful method. *Surg Laparosc Endosc.* 1998;6:457.

78. Garrard CL, Clements RH, Nanney N, et al. Adhesion formation is reduced after laparoscopic surgery. *Surg Endosc.* 1999;13:10.

79. Schippers E, Tittel A, Ottinger A, et al. Laparoscopic versus laparotomy: comparison of adhesion formation after bowel resection in a canine model. *Dig Surg.* 1998;15:145.

80. Shafer M, Krahenbul L, Buchler MW. Comparison of adhesion formation in open and laparoscopic surgery. *Dig Surg.* 1998;15:148.

81. Frantzides CT, Mathias C, Ludwig KA. Small bowel myoelectric activity in peritonitis. *Am J Surg.* 1993;165:681.

82. Ludwig KA, Frantzides CT, Carlson MA, et al. Myoelectric motility patterns following open versus laparoscopic cholecystectomy. *J Laparoendosc Surg.* 1994;3:461.

83. Bohm B, Milsom JW, Fazio VW. Postoperative intestinal motility following conventional and laparoscopic intestinal surgery. *Arch Surg.* 1995;130:415.

84. Eubanks S, Newman L, Lucas G. Reduction of HIV transmission during laparoscopic procedures. *Surg Laparosc Endosc.* 1993;3:2.

85. Buillot JL, Dehni N, Kazatchkine M, et al. Role of laparoscopic surgery in the management of acute abdomen in the HIV-positive patients. *J Laparoendosc Surg.* 1995;5:101.

86. Fry DE. Reduction of HIV transmission during laparoscopic procedures. *Surg Laparosc Endosc.* 1993;3:1.

87. Coskun I, Hatipoglu AR, Topaloglu A, et al. Laparoscopic versus open cholecystectomy: effect on pulmonary function tests. *Hepatogastroenterology* 2000;47:341.

88. Karayiannakis AJ, Makri GG, Mantzioka A, et al. Postoperative pulmonary function after laparoscopy and open cholecystectomy. *Br J Anaesth.* 1996;77:448.

89. Cueto GJ, Rojas DO, Weber SA. Laparoscopía como método diagnóstico y terapéutico de la peritonitis. In: Cueto J, Weber A, ed. *Cirugía Laparoscópica*, 2nd ed. McGraw-Hill Interamericana: 1994;181.

Chapter Fifty-Six • • • • • •

*L*aparoscopic Diagnostic Procedures in the ICU

**MORRIS E. FRANKLIN, JR., JORGE E. BALLI,
JOSÉ ANTONIO VÁZQUEZ-FRÍAS, and J. ARTURO ALMEIDA**

The diagnosis of acute abdominal processes in the intensive care unit is an ongoing problem in many institutions.[1,2] Frequently, the patient is subjected to specialized and expensive procedures such as computed tomography scans, magnetic resonance imaging, or even peritoneal lavage on the basis of a given clinical picture in the hope of aiming at a diagnosis.[3] This process often results in delay of diagnosis and frequently is not cost-effective, particularly in terminal patients or those requiring support who must be moved to specialized facilities and undergo further studies. Many studies are in fact performed in patients in whom, if the diagnosis was known earlier, were obviously not salvageable. This results in an unnecessary use of intensive care unit beds and a drain on vital resources. Laparoscopy offers an alternative to establish a diagnosis and, in selected patients, help in future therapy, also acting as a valuable tool in the decision-making process.[4,5]

INDICATIONS

Indications for laparoscopy in the intensive care unit (ICU) obviously include extremely ill patients with a suspected intraabdominal process. These patients are those in whom there is a tremendous risk for movement to the operating room or to a study at another location, and for whom there is a need to establish a diagnosis that may affect the course of the patient's treatment. An additional patient who would be a candidate for a diagnostic laparoscopic procedure would be one who has a low chance of survival but in whom a disease process may be present that surgical correction potentially could improve, but is too sick to undergo a series of stressful tests. Thus, laparoscopy can be used as a tool for the diagnosis of a given ailment prior to planning additional therapy. Generally speaking, patients who are intubated are those in whom this is easiest to do; however, a patient who is not intubated may also be a candidate under specific circumstances. The patients should have stable vital signs, no head injury, and not have falling blood pressure. Recently, however, Kelly et al[6] reported a successful diagnostic laparoscopy series in 17 ICU patients with systemic inflammatory response syndrome (SIRS)/septic state of unknown origin, in which all patients were unstable and required significant respiratory and hemodynamic support. Extreme care must be taken to ensure that all nurses and all personnel understand exactly what is expected and what the potential risk and expected outcome may be. The equipment used in the procedure must be mobile and often must be brought from a separate location. It is advisable to have an anesthesiologist available to control the respiratory movement of the patient, paralyze the patient if indicated, or in the case of a nonintubated patient, intubate the patient at a moment's notice. The patient does not need to be transferred to an operating table in order to complete the examination, as the procedure is diagnostic and, generally speaking, no therapeutic procedure should be undertaken.

CONTRAINDICATIONS

Contraindications include a morbid patient in whom there is no chance for survival, a patient who has unstable or falling blood pressure, or any other patient in whom there is no need to establish a diagnosis. A lack of basic and advanced laparoscopic experience and inability to take care of the problem in an open manner are absolute contraindications to attempting this procedure. Other contraindications include uncorrectable bleeding dyscrasias, massive abdominal distention, multiple prior operative procedures, and increased intracranial pressure. Relative contraindications should include unhelpful nurses, poor equipment, and an unwilling anesthesiologist (Table 56–1).

TABLE 56–1. CONTRAINDICATIONS

Absolute

Morbid, no chance of survival

Unstable vital signs

No need to establish diagnosis

Bleeding dyscrasias

Massive abdominal distention

Multiple prior operations

Increased intracranial pressure

Lack of surgical skills

Relative

Unhelpful nurses

Poor equipment

Unwilling anesthesiologist

Lack of basic advanced laparoscopic experience in the surgeon

TECHNIQUE

The procedure should be performed with at least basic laparoscopic equipment. A high-definition camera and monitor, as well as a powerful light source, are mandatory. The patient should have a Foley catheter and nasogastric tube in place, and all attempts should be made to diminish abdominal distention. Ideally, a bed should have Trendelenburg capabilities. Local anesthesia is generally used and minimal insufflation is needed (pressure 8 to 10 mm Hg). If local anesthesia is to be used, care should be exercised to avoid undue distention of the abdomen, as the CO_2 absorption may became excessive and acidosis will occur. A pressure of 8 to 10 mm Hg is recommended in patients in whom the procedure is to be performed under local anesthesia. Microinstrumentation greatly facilitates the procedure; however, the major problem with small scopes (2 mm or less) is lack of a wide field of vision, often requiring additional time for orientation and visualization of the entire abdominal cavity. Thus, this procedure should be used only in patients in whom one is attempting to rule in or out perforations, peritonitis, or the presence of dead bowel. No attempt should be made to quantify the amount of dead bowel with a mini-laparoscope (2 mm), as this may give an erroneous impression. A 10-mm scope will give a better idea of the extent of a given problem once identified. If the patient is intubated, a slightly higher CO_2 pressure can be established as control of respiration is achieved, and the elevation of the CO_2 can be readily dispersed. As mentioned earlier, an anesthesiologist should be present and available for paralysis and/or IV sedation if needed. As previously mentioned, patients with head injuries or those with increased intracranial pressure should not undergo a laparoscopic procedure, as there is good laboratory evidence that this may result in irreversible elevation of intracranial pressure.[7,8]

Access to the abdominal cavity with insufflation can be achieved with the Verres needle or the open Hasson technique. A

TABLE 56–2. RESULTS OF ICU LAPAROSCOPIES, TEXAS ENDOSURGERY EXPERIENCE

Age	Sex	Presenting Symptoms	Laparoscopic Findings	Decision Made	Length of Procedure	Outcome
74	F	Obstruction, sepsis, hypotension	Entire bowel necrosis	No heroic maneuvers (NHM)	30 min	Died same day
81	M	KUB—free air, sepsis, renal failure	Perforated colon, massive fecal contamination	NHM	25 min	Died same day
80	M	Nausea vomiting, acute renal, respiratory failure	No apparent problems	Continue medical treatment	45 min	Died 30 days PO. Pathology findings: small bowel with perforation and ischemic changes
79	M	Obstruction, nausea, vomiting, fever	Necrotic colon	NHM	55 min	Died next day
81	F	Nausea, vomiting, sepsis, hypotension, acidosis	Necrotic small bowel	NHM	45 min	Died same day
86	F	Abdominal pain, severe arteriosclerosis, acute MI	Infracted and dead small bowel secondary to volvulous or hernia	NHM	25 min	Died same day
78	M	Abdominal pain, septic shock	Dead bowel (mesenteric thrombosis)	NHM	45 min	Died same day
56	F	Abdominal pain, fever pneumonia	Normal bowel and gallbladder	Treat pneumonia	30 min	Survived, pneumonia subsided
66	M	Postoperative exploratory laparotomy and bowel resection, trocar left for second look	No further dead bowel	Supportive measures	40 min	Survived, discharged 30 days PO
75	M	Postoperative exploratory laparotomy and bowel resection, trocar left for second look	Remainder of the bowel dead	NHM	45 min	Died next day

PO = postoperative; KUB, kidney and upper bladder; NHM, no heroic maneuvers.

four-quadrant search should be carried out immediately. Any fluid present should be cultured and the color of the fluid noted. A greenish color obviously implies a perforation such as an ulcer and/or perforated proximal bowel; gray or red imply dead bowel; and brown implies colonic perforation. The small bowel should be checked for viability as much as can be done with local anesthesia. The gallbladder should be checked for gangrene and/or perforation. A ruptured appendix and other common problems such as intestinal obstruction and unsuspected strangulated hernia should be ruled out in a very short period of time.

It is important to have the operating room standing by ready to receive the patient should a misadventure occur or should a finding be present that would mandate an immediate operation. Obviously a thorough discussion should be carried out with the family and the patient, if at all possible, in regard to what is trying to be accomplished with this procedure. The family should be well aware that this is a diagnostic procedure upon which additional decisions can be based. It is an attempt to save the patient from an unneeded laparotomy should an uncorrectable problem or nothing be found. It is strongly advised to have 30 and 45-degree scopes as well as suction available. At this point in time, we do not recommend attempting therapeutic procedures unless an extremely unusual situation exists. The technique is to be used for biopsy and culture and decision-making only; one should avoid the temptation of a therapeutic procedure, as this will often lead to a disaster where there is no help available, with conversion to laparotomy virtually impossible or at least dangerous.

RESULTS

We have successfully performed this procedure on a number of patients over the past 9 years and have been uniformly satisfied based on our findings to recommend further therapeutic procedures. Table 56–2 shows the results for patients who have undergone this procedure.

CONCLUSION

Laparoscopy can be a valuable diagnostic tool in the intensive care unit in properly selected patients with grave medical conditions suspected of harboring an intra-abdominal process. The procedure often can be performed in the intensive care unit under controlled conditions to establish a diagnosis and thus can be the basis of further therapeutic decisions. Adequate family counseling, nurse training, and forethought will result in acceptable outcomes in the majority of patients who would benefit from this procedure. Additionally, expensive therapeutic tests can be avoided and earlier decision-making processes can be instituted to determine the best course of action in a given patient. Eventually this approach may become the standard of care for these extremely ill patients, possibly with a laparoscopic cart in each ICU.

REFERENCES

1. Sackier JM, Nibhanupudy B. Adult diagnostic laparoscopy. In: Toouli J, Gossot D, Hunter J, eds. *Endosurgery*. Churchill–Livingstone:1996; 197.
2. Sackier JM. *Laparoscopy*. Philadelphia, Current Medicine:1994;17.1.
3. Berci G, Sackier JM. Emergency laparoscopy. *Am J Surg*. 1991;161:332.
4. Bender JS, Talamini MA. Diagnostic laparoscopy in critically ill intensive care unit patients. *Surg Endosc*. 1992;6:302.
5. Walsh RM, Popovich MJ, Hoadley J. Bedside diagnostic laparoscopy and peritoneal lavage in the intensive care unit. *Surg Endosc*. 1998;12:1405.
6. Kelly JJ, Puyana JC, Callery MP, et al. The feasibility and accuracy of dagnostic laparoscopy in the septic ICU patient. *Surg Endosc*. 2000; 14:617.
7. Halverson A, Buchanan R., Jacobs L, et al. Evaluation of mechanism of increased intracranial pressure with insufflation. *Surg Endosc*. 1998;12:266.
8. Halverson A, Barrett WL, Iglesias AR, et al. Decreased cerebrospinal fluid absorption during abdominal insufflation. *Surg Endosc*. 1999;13:797.

Chapter Fifty-Seven ▪ ▪ ▪ ▪ ▪ ▪

*L*aparoscopy and Thoracoscopy in Trauma

NATAN ZUNDEL MAJEROWICK and JUAN DAVID HERNANDEZ RESTREPO

Trauma of the torso, both blunt and penetrating, is an important cause of morbidity and mortality, and has been a major concern for surgeons through history. When the patient has clear symptoms like hemorrhage, hemodynamic instability, peritoneal signs, or respiratory difficulty, the need for surgery is clear. The challenge comes when the history and the physical examination give insufficient information because of different reasons: the patient is hemodynamically stable and asymptomatic, has a head injury with loss or alteration of consciousness, or is under the effects of alcohol or drugs.

This picture is frequently present in patients with blunt abdominal trauma, anterior and especially tangential gunshot wounds, and abdominal and thoracoabdominal stab wounds. The current approach in these cases, with a stable patient perhaps with signs of internal organ injury but without an indication for urgent laparotomy, is the use of the diagnostic methods available to confirm or rule out the need for abdominal surgery. Along with the physical examination, the surgeon should perform a local wound exploration, diagnostic peritoneal lavage (DPL), ultrasonography, and CT scanning.

Although their use in trauma has been proposed for about a century, laparoscopy and thoracoscopy were left aside for many years, and only recently has new interest been shown.

HISTORY OF MINIMALLY INVASIVE SURGERY IN TRAUMA

Philipp Bozzini, in the beginning of the 19th century, was the first to address the main problem of using open tubes to observe hollow structures by creating a light-guidance system. He built a case with a candle inside and in one side attached different open tubes to look into the mouth and the rectum.[1] In 1877, Max Nitze created the first cystoscope with a set of optical lenses first illuminated with a platinum wire and later with Edison's filament globe miniaturized to fit in the device.[1]

In 1902, George Kelling, from Dresden, Germany, who previously created a flexible gastroscope, used a cystoscope and pneumoperitoneum to explore the peritoneal cavity of dogs in a procedure that he called coelioscopy.[2] The first mention of laparoscopy in trauma to diagnose hemoperitoneum among other uses was in 1925.[3] In 1935, Ruddock reported his experience with "peritoneoscopy" in patients,[4] and Zoeckler in 1958 published an analysis of 1000 procedures.[1]

Laparoscopy was cast to oblivion, and in spite of articles published[1] in the 1960s by a South African surgeon about peritoneoscopy in diagnosis of abdominal trauma,[5] it did not become popular. In the 1970s, gynecologists started to use this procedure in the diagnosis and treatment of pelvic diseases.[1] In the same decade a number of articles appeared reporting experience in diagnosis of blunt and penetrating abdominal trauma.[6,7] Gazzaniga et al reported on 37 cases of blunt and penetrating trauma and described in detail the positions and techniques used to view all the peritoneal cavity.[6] In the 1980s more articles appeared,[8,9] but nothing seemed to convince the surgeons.

In 1986, Erich Mühe practiced the first laparoscopic cholecystectomy in Böblingen, Germany, using the galloscope, an optical system he designed.[10] This experience was repeated in France by Mouret, Dubois, and Perissat.[11] The greatest problem was that only the surgeon was able to see the surgery looking through the lens, making the procedure uncomfortable for the surgeon and difficult for the assistant to follow. These reports, in addition to the invention of a computer chip that made it possible to attach a video camera to the lens, and the design of specialized instruments, caused the revolution we are experiencing now. Surgeons became familiar with the use of laparoscopic instruments and began to practice other procedures, and simultaneously new interest in laparoscopy in trauma arose.

Based on the earlier developments and using Nitze's cystoscope, in 1910 Professor Hans Christian Jacobaeus from Stockholm University practiced thoracoscopy first in dogs and later in humans to study pleural effusions.[13] Jacobaeus was the first to employ thoracoscopy as a therapeutic tool in a treatment called pneumolisis, using cautery to cut the adhesions in the pleural space to collapse the lung.[13] In the following years some reports appeared of the application of thoracoscopy in different pathologies, particularly in Europe, but it did not become popular until the appearance of video-assisted thoracoscopy and instruments specially designed for laparoscopic procedures.

CURRENT CONCEPTS

Today the frequency of blunt and penetrating trauma has increased in civilian life as a consequence of faster transportation, an increase in interpersonal violence, and easier access to different weapons. In this setting, the diagnostic and therapeutic measures have to be faster and more accurate. Today thoracoscopy and laparoscopy have a place in the diagnosis and management of trauma, with the advantages of minimal invasiveness, direct visualization, and the therapeutic option. Nevertheless, there are still some matters to clarify when thoracoscopy and laparoscopy are compared with other options.

LAPAROSCOPY IN ABDOMINAL TRAUMA

Trauma surgeons recommend that patients who sustain penetrating or blunt trauma and have symptoms or signs of a life-threatening intra-abdominal injury should have an exploratory laparotomy immediately.[15] However, patients with minimal findings or who are asymptomatic need a different approach. Routine laparotomy in these cases will lead to a high rate of negative explorations, while excessive trust in noninvasive tests and observation may carry an increase in missed injuries and therefore in morbidity and mortality. Weigelt and Kingman reviewed the outcome of 248 patients with abdominal trauma who had a negative exploratory laparotomy.[16] When the patients had one or more associated injuries, the postoperative morbidity was 65%; and when there were no associated lesions, the morbidity reached 22%. Renz and Feliciano, in a prospective study,[17] found complications in 41% of 254 patients who underwent unnecessary (nontherapeutic) laparotomy and in 19.7% of 80 patients with a completely negative laparotomy (no peritoneal penetration). Late complications are incisional hernias and small bowel obstruction, two very good additional reasons to avoid unnecessary laparotomies.[16,17]

The studies mentioned, among others, clearly indicate that a more accurate screening is needed in patients with a dubious history or physical examination. Repeated observation, wound exploration, diagnostic peritoneal lavage (DPL), ultrasonography, and CT scan have been used to reduce the number of unnecessary laparotomies with different grades of success, depending on the mechanism of trauma and the location of the injury.

As surgeons gained experience and confidence with elective laparoscopic procedures, the idea of using laparoscopy in the evaluation and treatment of patients with abdominal trauma seemed possible. Sosa et al[18] compared negative laparotomy and negative laparoscopy in abdominal gunshot wounds, and they found a dramatic diminution in morbidity and hospital stay. Other studies in both blunt and penetrating abdominal trauma came to light, rediscovering a long-known diagnostic and therapeutic tool. All of the studies emphasize that minimal access surgery is employed only in stable patients.

Blunt Trauma

Blunt abdominal trauma is an important cause of preventable deaths, because its evaluation is difficult and demands a high suspicion index and careful analysis. The decision to take the patient to the operating room is a lot more difficult than in penetrating trauma because the symptoms and signs are less obvious and frequently obscured by head trauma, associated injuries, and intoxication with alcohol or other substances.[19] In a trauma program in Toronto, Boulanger and McLellan found that the abdominal physical examination alone was unreliable in 65% of blunt trauma victims for initial assessment.[20] Besides, clear peritoneal signs may not appear for hours or days in stable patients with intestinal lesions.[21]

There is a special group of patients, those who will not be available for repeated examination because they will be under sedation or will be taken to surgery for associated injuries. In these patients, an intra-abdominal lesion has to be expeditiously ruled out.

The use of DPL worldwide for 35 years and the great experience acquired allows us to make some statements about it with certainty. DPL is a sensitive test with a low specificity, leading to an elevated number of negative or nontherapeutic laparotomies. It is also an invasive study that makes posterior physical examination unreliable. When a ruptured hollow viscus exists, the white blood cell count will rise, but only hours after the trauma,[19] and on the other hand, an important number of patients with isolated high leukocyte counts will have nontherapeutic laparotomies.[20] DPL's low specificity makes it impossible to identify the type or degree of injury to a specific organ, and cannot diagnose retroperitoneal and diaphragmatic lesions.[22] Some authors think that currently DPL is indicated in hemodynamically unstable patients in whom the question of whether there is an intra-abdominal hemorrage that requires urgent exploration has to be answered immediately.[20]

CT scanning is excellent in the evaluation of solid organ and retroperitoneal injuries, and is extensively used for the nonoperative management of intra-abdominal trauma,[19,20] which are the main indications for it in stable patients. CT has the problem of transportation and the time required to complete it. Although in an interesting retrospective study Sherck et al[21] obtained good accuracy in the use of CT for diagnosis of bowel perforation in blunt trauma, their experience has not been reproduced, and the findings were not specific for intestinal injury. Besides, CT needs the evaluation of an experienced radiologist, who is not always available. So CT still fails in recognizing intestinal, pancreatic, and urinary bladder lesions.[20] In reference to diaphragmatic injuries, CT has a similar sensitivity to DPL,[23] and cannot be used in these lesions, which have a not-negligible rate of 5% in blunt trauma.[24]

Focused assessment with sonography for trauma (FAST) is a well-established procedure in the initial approach to trauma patients in the United States.[25] It is used in the emergency department and has been reported as a 3-minutes procedure, with patent advantages over DPL and CT. It is highly sensitive in the detection of hemoperitoneum or intraperitoneal fluid, with an accuracy of 96%,[20] and in detecting solid organ injuries, and it is used as a screening method; but it cannot assess the bowel or diaphragm accurately.

The use of laparoscopy has been discouraged in the diagnosis of blunt trauma because of the number of missed injuries that have been reported, particularly splenic, small bowel, mesentery, colon, and retroperitoneal lesions.[5,22,26,27] There are some problems associated with the use of pneumoperitoneum in blunt trauma that will be discussed later.

Laparoscopy has been used as a tool to confirm the nonoperative management of hepatic and splenic injuries, with the intention of ruling out other injuries that would make it necessary to suspend the observation and practice laparotomy.[20] Zantut et al used laparoscopy in 21 patients to rule out hollow viscus injuries and recover blood for autotransfusion from injured solid organs, avoiding the use of contaminated blood and obtaining a significant elevation in hematocrit values.[28] A similar use was described by Collin and Bianchi,[29] who also examined the spleen to establish the need for surgery,[29] and other studies have used thrombostatic agents to stop bleeding in the spleen to warrant nonoperative management.[27] Townsend et al found that laparoscopy served to prevent the selection of two patients for nonsurgical management by finding unsuspected hollow viscus injuries missed in CT.[27] Other authors have reported the placement of closed drains as an adjunct in the nonoperative management of blunt hepatic trauma.[30] Gazzaniga et al,[6] in a classic paper, found splenic injuries and also jejunal perforations. They described the technique and maneuvers to examine all of the peritoneal cavity before the appearance of the video computer chip, and demonstrated a reduction in unnecessary laparotomies and hospital stay.

The use of local anesthesia and intravenous sedation has been advocated to make laparoscopy faster and cheaper in the emergency department.[22,31]

In a review of articles on laparoscopy as a screening test (a tool that reliably indicates the need for laparotomy in the trauma patient) in blunt trauma, Villavicencio and Aucar reported a sensitivity of 90 to 100%, a specificity of 86 to 100%, and an accuracy between 88 and 100%.[5] When used as a diagnostic test, that is, to diagnose all the injuries present in a patient, laparoscopy was less reliable, since an important number of lesions were missed.

In a recent article, experienced surgeons expressed the opinion that the role of laparoscopy in blunt trauma is as an adjunct to CT scanning to evaluate the injury and rule out associated lesions in order to select patients for nonoperative management; the study was limited by the small number of patients.[32] Others think that the function of laparoscopy is the same as for CT, except in retroperitoneum.[33] In our opinion, allowing of course for an appropriate learning curve, the systematic examination of the abdominal cavity will be more accurate, the number of injuries missed will be minimized, and the therapeutic options will increase, as laparoscopy becomes an important tool in blunt trauma.

Penetrating Trauma

Excluding patients with gunshot or stab wounds needing immediate exploratory laparotomy, a large number of patients require a deeper analysis to decide if they have to be operated upon or if they can be observed. The former approach, of exploring all of these patients, was abandoned long ago. There are a variety of options to study them. Patients who cannot be reexamined on a regular basis should not be included in a nonoperative protocol, because of the high risk of missed injuries.[15] The diagnosis has to be made rapidly.

Wound exploration under local anesthesia is useful to establish the depth of penetration and to see if the peritoneum has been injured in stab wounds. If the patient remains stable and penetration of the peritoneum is demonstrated, or if the wound tract is not clear, further diagnostic studies are indicated.[34] This test is not reliable in the thoracoabdominal area, flanks, and back owing to the difficulty in exploring these zones. Nearly one third of patients with abdominal stab wounds have superficial compromise and can be discharged safely.[35]

DPL is considered a better study than laparoscopy for blunt trauma, and its use in penetrating trauma is controversial.[35,36] DPL has a false-negative and false-positive rate of up to 20%, leading to a significant number of negative laparotomies.[8,15,22,25] DPL is highly unspecific and the positive results can be attributed to the damage suffered by the abdominal wall or a minor injury to the spleen or liver. It has been used regularly only to diagnose diaphragmatic injuries, with a low sensitivity.[35]

The use of FAST in penetrating trauma is increasing and some centers in the United States have algorithms that include it. Even so, FAST is focused upon detection of fluid in determined spaces in the peritoneal and thoracic cavities, and is not useful for diagnostic of specific organ injuries.[25,35]

CT has been associated with a high rate of false-negative studies on penetrating abdominal trauma, and may miss lesions to the diaphragm, hollow viscus, and mesentery.[22,37] CT scanning with the triple-contrast technique is useful in penetrating wounds in the back and flanks.[35]

In 1976, Gazzaniga et al found that laparoscopy avoided nontherapeutic laparotomy in 14 patients without false-negative results, and helped to shorten the hospital stay and reduced the rate of complications of a negative laparotomy.[6] Carnevale et al practiced laparoscopy on 20 patients with blunt and penetrating trauma, and 60% of them did not require laparotomy.[7] For Berci et al,[8,31] laparoscopy proved to be safer, faster, and more accurate than lavage, and allowed them to avoid exploration in 6 of 9 patients. Livingston et al found laparoscopy accurate in penetrating injuries to the peritoneal cavity localized in flanks, back, and lower chest, with 24% of patients avoiding laparotomy.[26] Livingston et al also consider mobilization of the colon feasible in the study of trauma patients. In an article in which laparoscopy was compared to DPL in screening abdominal trauma (both blunt and penetrating), Salvino et al conclude that laparoscopy benefits patients with stab wounds indicating nonsurgical management based on laparoscopic findings.[22] Ivatury et al found no disruption of the peritoneum and precluded laparotomy in 33.8% of 65 patients with stab wounds and in 60% of 35 patients with gunshot wounds.[38] They compared the groups of negative laparoscopy and negative laparotomy (those with peritoneal penetration who underwent exploration because of the study design) and found a shorter hospital stay and smaller incidence of complications in the laparoscopy group. Ditmars and Bongard had similar findings, with 64% of patients not requiring laparotomy and a substantial reduction in hospital stay and in hospital charges in laparoscopy patients compared to patients with negative laparotomy.[39] When speaking about tangential gunshot wounds, Ivatury et al consider laparoscopy a better screening tool than DPL, because laparoscopy can detect bowel injuries by a blast effect.[38] Sosa et al,[18] in an interesting study of abdominal gunshot wounds, found that laparoscopy had a 0% false-negative rate with a correct identification of peritoneal penetration in all patients. They recommend exploration in all patients with peritoneal disruption since this finding is associated with significant intra-abdominal injuries in 89 to 96% of cases. However, they consider that experienced surgeons can avoid nontherapeutic exploration in these patients. In a cooperative study with the largest number of patients, Zantut et al examined laparoscopic exploration in 510 patients following penetrating trauma.[40] Of this large patient group, 54.3% did not have penetration and were discharged uneventfully with an average of 1.7 days of hospital stay and avoiding a negative laparotomy. Laparoscopy was almost always used as a screening test, and none of the patients were diagnosed late. Although some lesions were not seen at laparoscopy, none of these patients had any indication for laparotomy.

A very important concern expressed in many papers is the difficulty in achieving a complete and accurate observation of the bowel.[18,41] Ponsky and Marks describe a method of systematically assessing the peritoneal cavity, with special emphasis on the colon and small bowel, and they achieved a complete evaluation in 15 patients without complications.[37] Zantut et al also found that with practice, they could "run the bowel" easier and could rule out lesions to it.[40] Another option is to use gasless laparoscopy with an abdominal wall retractor or laparolift.

There have been occasional reports of therapeutic maneuvers in laparoscopy for both blunt and penetrating trauma. These include diaphragmatic repair,[32,37,40] employment of hemostatic agents in solid organ injuries,[27,40] cholecystectomy for an injured gallbladder,[40] and suturing of gastrointestinal perforations.[32,40]

Problems and Pitfalls of Laparoscopy in Trauma.
Minimally invasive surgery in trauma was not considered a useful tool by surgeons, and has achieved general interest only since the appearance of video laparoscopy and video thoracoscopy. In this setting, it could be considered a new technique. As with every new procedure in surgery, it has to be proved and validated in clinical practice. What follows is a compilation of most of the serious issues that have arisen concerning the risks of using these procedures.

An important concern is the probable complications related to the CO_2 pneumoperitoneum. Holthausen et al published a series of studies with pigs analyzing the factors that may influence the use of laparoscopy in traumatized patients, especially in blunt trauma.[42] They found that pneumoperitoneum raised the intracranial pressure in a head injury model, an effect that they attributed to elevated intra-abdominal pressure due to decreased venous return and delayed cerebrovascular outflow. Even though in earlier studies using pneumoperitoneum in these patients there were no descriptions of complications attributed to it, this problem can be prevented using abdominal wall retraction instead of pneumoperitoneum.[34] Holthausen et al also found that CO_2 pneumoperitoneum induced lower levels of intestinal metabolism than helium, and also an impairment in microcirculation.[42] This has minimum clinical relevance in a healthy patient undergoing planned surgery, but it might acquire importance in a traumatized and hypovolemic

patient, as was suggested by Ho et al in an animal model.[43] They found that in pigs with hypovolemia, CO_2 pneumoperitoneum caused a decreased stroke volume and mean arterial pressure, and that these effects were not reversed with restoration of baseline values. These changes are due to the CO_2, and not to the pneumoperitoneum itself. Josephs et al,[44] using a head injury model in pigs, showed that a standard pneumoperitoneum increases ICP, apparently in a way independent of arterial pH, mean arterial pressure, PaO_2, or $PaCO_2$, suggesting a direct mechanical effect. This mechanical effect seems to be the elevation of venous pressure in the inferior vena cava with the establishment of the pneumoperitoneum, with a consequent rise in the vascular compartment of the spinal canal, which causes a rise in the intraspinal and intracranial pressure. Although some studies included head trauma patients and there were no complications attributable to it,[40] these findings, until different evidence is obtained, contraindicate laparoscopy in patients with associated head trauma.

Doubts have been expressed about the difficulty in completely observing the spleen and ruling out lesions in it, due to its location and interference of the omentum.[6,20,26] Nevertheless, the authors think that trauma surgeons could do as well as laparoscopic surgeons with experience in laparoscopic splenectomy for hematologic diseases, who are able to handle the spleen, and establish accurately the possible injuries, and possibly in the future repair them by laparoscopy.

We already mentioned the problem of achieving a complete inspection of the bowel and the solution proposed by Ponsky. For Gazzaniga et al,[6] jejunal perforation was the second most common finding in traumatized patients, and Berci et al[8] diagnosed hollow viscus perforations by indirect signs or by watching the perforation directly. We believe that the small bowel and colon can be observed with accuracy using the atraumatic instruments used in laparoscopic colonic surgery, and if this is not possible, the problem of "running the bowel" can be solved by gasless laparoscopy, in which it is possible to examine the intestine outside the abdominal cavity.

Delay in definitive treatment is another argument against laparoscopic evaluation in abdominal trauma.[38] It is important to remember that patients to be enrolled in this kind of protocol must be hemodynamically stable and without indications for urgent laparotomy—that is, patients who otherwise would be studied with CT scan or observed.

There are a number of complications attributable directly to the laparoscopic procedure. Tension pneumothorax was developed during pneumoperitoneum in a patient with a thoracoabdominal stab wound.[38] There is a theoretical risk of gas embolism related to the presence of ruptured vessels,[20,27,38] but this has never been reported in trauma patients as far as we know. Lesions caused by introduction of the Verres needle or trocars, such as enterotomies or injuries to the omentum,[22,27,31] can be prevented using the Hasson technique, which we strongly recommend. It is important to note that most of the articles reviewed report no complications.

In conclusion, we think that laparoscopy does have an important role in diagnostic and therapeutic assessment of abdominal trauma, but we agree with Berci et al[8] and Ivatury et al[38,40] that it is necessary that these procedures be performed by an experienced surgeon, ideally one experienced both in laparoscopic surgery and in trauma. It is essential for the surgeon to be familiar with the small bowel and colon mobilization and manipulation and the exposure of the spleen to warrant a complete inspection.

The surgeon will be able not only to diagnose all the injuries but also to repair many of them laparoscopically. In their analysis, Villavicencio and Aucar[5] found that laparoscopy as a screening test in penetrating injuries had a sensitivity of 93 to 100%, specificity of 80 to 100%, and accuracy of 84 to 100%. As a diagnostic study, a sensitivity of 80 to 100%, specificity of 38 to 86%, and accuracy of 54 to 89% have been reported, and consequently it cannot be recommended yet for a complete assessment of abdominal trauma, and still has to be used only in protocols of investigation. A demonstrated advantage of laparoscopy in penetrating trauma is the shortening of hospital stay, lower hospital charges, and avoidance of unnecessary laparotomy when used as a screening method.[5,32,40] The rest remains to be proven.

THORACOSCOPY IN THORACIC TRAUMA

Thoracotomy and median sternotomy remain the standard of treatment in patients with severe thoracic trauma, because it has been proven that conditions like major hemorrhage with profound shock and pericardial tamponade cannot be reversed with external resuscitation, and situations such as uncontrolled high-volume air leakage require urgent intervention.[45] Nevertheless, about 80% of patients suffer less severe injuries and can be treated with tube thoracostomy and suction.[46,47] A smaller number of patients with no other problem than a wound in the thorax have been assessed with noninvasive methods and observation.

Hirshberg et al[48] showed how diagnostic mistakes based on chest x-rays and in situations like a misplaced subclavian venous catheter led to interpreting transfused blood as persistent bleeding. This resulted in unnecessary thoracotomies. A tube insertion is a potential danger, as in cases with herniated organs of a diaphragmatic hernia. Mediastinal vascular and cardiac injuries are easily missed if not suspected, especially when they give no signs. Besides, chest x-rays may underestimate the volume of thoracic fluid collection. All of these dubious situations have to be elucidated in order to prevent serious complications of a delayed diagnosis of thoracic lesions. Until the last decade, this was achieved by a thoracotomy, a major surgical procedure with important consequences. The major causes of morbidity of any thoracotomy are the large incision, the spreading of the ribs while widening the intercostal space, and postoperative pain.[49] These considerations may cause the surgeon to delay a surgical treatment in patients with unusual presentations or subacute complications.[45]

Video-assisted thoracoscopic surgery (VATS) is now a real alternative in hemodynamically stable patients for diagnosis of those lesions that are occult to other methods and would require a thoracotomy for diagnostic purposes, perhaps nontherapeutic, or when the injuries need treatment but thoracotomy seems to be a very aggressive technique. The rigid conformation of the thoracic wall, and the possibility of collapsing the lung with selective intubation and one-lung ventilation, allows the practice of thoracoscopy without the use of CO_2 insufflation or the use of ports,[50] and makes possible the use of conventional surgical instruments. This diagnostic and therapeutic tool now has proven indications and is continuously being tested for new applications.

In some studies,[47,51] in the presence of continued hemorrhage after tube thoracostomy placement, usually originating in the intercostal vessels and occasionally in the internal mammarian vessels, thoracoscopy made it possible to identify the site of bleeding

if it still existed. It also made it possible to treat it with diathermy, endoclips, or suture placing. When thoracoscopic management is not possible, knowing the location of the vessel permits control with a limited thoracotomy.

Clotted hemothorax, defined as a residual clot with volume greater than 500 mL, appeared in 2 to 30% of patients with hemothorax managed even with two thoracostomy tubes.[46,49,51] The persistence of a clotted hemothorax or a retained hemothorax gives a higher risk of empyema or fibrothorax formation in patients with thoracic trauma.[14,46,52] Formerly, the only alternative for treatment when the diagnosis had been established was thoracotomy. Now, most patients can be treated with thoracoscopic irrigation and drainage of clots and retained blood. The early evacuation of these collections makes the procedure easier and favors its success, and most authors agree that this means before the first 7 to 10 days. In this period, the rate of success is close to 90%.[50,52] The early evacuation of clotted hemothorax shortened the hospital stay, reduced postoperative pain, and hastened the return to normal activities.[53] Villegas and Morales analyzed the outcome of 61 patients with clotted hemothorax treated thoracoscopically and concluded that after 7 days following the trauma, the risk of conversion to an open procedure was higher due to pleural thickening.[54] Empyema is a complication present in 2 to 25% of thoracic trauma patients,[14,45,47] and has been attributed to clotted hemothorax.[55] VATS has good results achieving the goals of drainage and obliteration of the pleural space with less morbidity than a thoracotomy, as reported by O'Brien et al,[49] who succesfully treated 8 patients with thoracoscopy alone, without other measures. Although there were complications with management of the pleural space in 2 patients, these were treated with thoracoscopy as well. Liu et al[45] found it easy to practice enucleation of the empyema cavity and decortication using conventional instruments during thoracoscopy. Heniford et al[55] observed that empyema was present in 2 patients operated upon more than 7 days after admission and in none of those operated on within 7 days of admission.

Of patients who arrive at the hospital with penetrating thoracic trauma and cardiac wounds, 20% do not show signs or symptoms of cardiac tamponade or injury.[14,56,57] There are some reports of thoracoscopic pericardial windows with good results. Morales et al[57] reported 108 pericardial windows and 30% of them were positive, in completely asymptomatic patients. They reported a 100% sensitivity, 96% specificity, and 97% accuracy rates, higher than those found in echocardiography and a subxiphoid pericardial window. Although some authors disagree,[45,58] we agree with Morales et al that VATS is a very good alternative to a subxiphoid pericardial window. It has the advantage of minimum invasion, accurate diagnosis, and the possibility of examining the complete thoracic cavity. Thoracoscopy is also useful in diagnosis of mediastinal injuries compromising the aorta or the esophagus.[14]

Thoracoscopy has also been used successfully with other diagnostic and therapeutic indications. Lang-Lazdunski et al[59] practiced in 5 patients with persistent air leak and pneumothorax removal of a rib fragment, stapling of ruptured blebs, and a parenchymal laceration and pleurabrasion. Schermer et al demonstrated that VATS reduced hospital stay in patients with persistent air leak compared to nonoperative management.[60] Intrathoracic foreign bodies like wire, bullets, and grenade splinters have also been removed in 4 patients. There are other reports of the retrieval of foreign bodies such as fragments of glass and bullets.[53,61] Reardon et al reported the thoracoscopic repair of a traumatic lung hernia of the chest wall.[62] All of these patients avoided a thoracotomy.

Mineo et al, in a study of blunt chest trauma, reported a substantial reduction of the number of thoracotomies due to the more frequent use of thoracoscopy in the assessment of these patients.[63] They succesfully treated clotted hemothorax, empyema, prolonged bleeding, and prolonged air leak, and suggested that video thoracoscopy has restricted the indications for open thoracotomy. Many other articles confirm the current importance of video thoracoscopy in diagnosis and treatment of thoracic trauma both blunt and penetrating when the aforementioned injuries are present,[64–68] and all of these results suggest that thoracoscopy actually reduces costs in terms of a shorter hospital stay and a diminution in the number of unnecesary thoracotomies.

Villavicencio et al reviewed 28 articles published since 1910 in the trauma setting,[69] and found that thoracoscopic control of bleeding and avoidance of thoracotomy was successful in 82% of cases with no procedure-related complications in all of the patients. In the evacuation of posttraumatic empyemas, VATS was successful in 86% of cases, with 2 complications. When used to evacuate retained hemothoraces or clots, the rate of success was 90%, with 3 procedure-related intraoperative complications corrected with the resumption of one-lung ventilation. The authors could not find a single study analyzing costs. A very interesting issue is the number of thoracotomies or laparotomies prevented with the use of VATS, 323 of 514 patients, equivalent to 62% of cases. Villavicencio et al also note that when thoracotomy is required, thoracoscopy helps to establish the location and extent of the incision. The risks include a 2% procedure-related complication rate and 0.8% missed injuries (3 of them in 1910, without video assistance). Villavicencio et al conclude that nonvideo thoracoscopy and VATS can be applied safely and effectively in the care of the injured patient.

As stated by Villavicencio et al,[69] these procedures have to be practiced by surgeons experienced in thoracic trauma or in thoracoscopy, and ideally in both areas. The learning curve to identify structures, handle instruments, manipulate the lung, and decide on management is long and has to be accomplished with adequate guidance.

The surgical techniques have been adequately described elsewhere, but it is important to note some issues. Almost all authors agree on the use of general anesthesia with selective intubation and one-lung ventilation to ease the procedure and allow a better visualization with the collapse of the lung. This is important to reach an adequate diagnosis and facilitate a therapeutic intervention.[14,70] The patient must be placed in full lateral decubitus position, which gives the surgeon an optimal view and if needed, allows the conversion to an open thoracotomy. Nevertheless, the supine position can be used in bilateral injuries to practice bilateral thoracoscopy, as it is done in bilateral resection of pulmonary metastases.[14,70] Usually three incisions are enough to practice therapeutic interventions, and only one port is used for the lens (0 or 30 degrees), in order to avoid contact with blood. This port has to be far enough from the diaphragm in order to achieve a good view of all its dome-shaped surface. The gasless condition of VATS gives the opportunity of employing both conventional or specially designed instruments.

THORACOABDOMINAL TRAUMA

Injuries located in the so-called thoracic abdomen have always been a diagnostic and therapeutic challenge, since they are frequently silent in symptoms and compromise portions of intra-abdominal and intrathoracic organs and the diaphragm. The thoracoabdominal area is defined as the part of the body bounded by a line between the nipples anteriorly and the tips of the scapula posteriorly (corresponding to the fifth and seventh intercostal spaces aproximately) and the costal margins inferiorly.

The capability of wounds located in this area to injure the diaphragm and organs in both the thoracic and abdominal cavities is the main problem. Patients with hemodynamic instability, hemorrhage, and peritoneal signs have a well-defined treatment,[24] but when the abdominal examination is equivocal, the assessment of the possible injuries needs the highest index of suspicion and the help of a variety of diagnostic techniques. The diaphragm is wounded in 10 to 15% of all penetrating thoracic injuries, and in 30% if the lesion is located anteriorly and below the nipples.[71] Even though the diaphragmatic perforation is less frequent in posterior wounds, some series have reported an incidence of up to 27%. Victims of penetrating diaphragmatic wounds will have associated organ injuries in 85% of cases. The concern generated by lesions to the diaphragm is the risk of a traumatic diaphragmatic hernia followed by all the associated complications.[72–74] Madden et al[74] found a 20% strangulation rate with a 36% mortality rate in patients with undiagnosed diaphragmatic lacerations.

In many cases a patient with a thoracoabdominal wound will arrive asymptomatic or with an equivocal abdominal examination, and the possibility of an injury to the diaphragm and other organs has to be discarded. Moore et al found that in 32% of cases, the physical examination was negative, and in an additional 9% the intoxication of patients avoided a correct diagnosis.[24] The assessment of a thoracoabdominal injury is very difficult, since the diagnostic studies lack sensitivity. Chest x-rays are normal in 85% of patients, and when a radioopaque nasogastric tube or a barium meal study are added, the results are even more disappointing.[9,24,72] Peritoneal lavage has also been used to rule out diaphragmatic wounds, with an important discussion of the RBC count to be used, with 5000 to 10,000 the most accepted range, but with the risk of increasing the number of negative laparotomies.[72] Isolated diaphragmatic injuries are often missed with this method with RBC counts of less than 1000,[73,74] or on the contrary, with a high red blood cell count caused by minor lacerations to liver or spleen, leading to a nontherapeutic laparotomy.[75] CT is not a good test for the diaphragm, with results similar to DPL.[23,71,72]

Because of the continuous movement of the diaphragm, the constant negative pressure in the thorax with the positive intra-abdominal pressure, and the frequent interposition of the omentum in the defect, there is not a small enough diaphragmatic tear to be considered innocuous.[24,72,75,76] Additionally, small tears facilitate the strangulation of bowel in the thorax, as happens in any other hernia. That is why any diaphragmatic rent has to be repaired. Accordingly, in the 1970s many authors recommended laparotomy for every patient with penetrating lower chest wounds that might injure the diaphragm,[73–75] but this led to as many as 40% negative laparotomies (A. Valencia, personal communication).

There is a controversy concerning which way to diagnose a diaphragm injury in terms of minimally invasive surgery. Some authors advocate the laparoscopic approach, arguing that diagnosis of intra-abdominal injuries cannot be done by a thoracoscopy, and that when time has passed since the trauma, pleural adhesions make the thoracic procedure difficult.[9] Ivatury et al considered laparoscopy a superior method for the detection of isolated, occult injuries to the diaphragm, reducing the number of unnecessary laparotomies in 34%

of stab wounds and in 60% of gunshot wounds, and also warned about the risk of tension pneumothorax caused by the pneumoperitoneum.[14,75] Adamthwaite[9] diagnosed 8 diaphragmatic tears using a laparoscope, 6 of them with herniated organs. He found the posterior aspects of the diaphragm difficult to visualize, requiring traction on the stomach. Successful diagnosis and repair of diaphragmatic acute and chronic ruptures has been reported, with a reduction in herniated content and assessment of intra-abdominal organs.[77–81] Zantut et al pointed out the impossibility of adequately assessing the right hemidiaphragm.[80] Other authors argue in favor of thoracoscopy, and we agree that this approach has several advantages: The access port can be placed in the same incision as the tube thoracostomy, avoiding disruption of the peritoneal cavity; the assessment of the posterior diaphragm is more accurate, and any rent can be repaired even using conventional instruments; the mediastinum can be inspected; it is possible to practice a pericardial window when indicated; and the hemothorax and clots can be drained.[14,47,71,76,79,81] The technique of thoracoscopy has already been discussed, but it is important to mention that the camera port has to be far enough from the diaphragm in order to visualize all the dome-shaped structure. We consider it more appropriate to practice thoracoscopy in thoracoabdominal trauma, and when a diaphragmatic lesion is found, to repair it and then to perform a laparoscopy to rule out intra-abdominal organ injuries and again, if possible, to repair them. Additionally, thoracoscopy in head-injured patients can be used instead of laparoscopy. Villavicencio et al recommended thoracoscopy, especially when a diaphragmatic injury is suspected.[69]

With all the information given and the experience accumulated by different groups, we believe that laparoscopy and thoracoscopy are very important elements in the diagnosis and treatment of trauma of the torso in stable patients. The problems that still exist will disappear when these procedures are performed by laparoscopic surgeons with experience in trauma, or trauma surgeons with experience in laparoscopic surgery after a necessary learning curve.

REFERENCES

1. Berci G, Forde KA. History of endoscopy. What lessons have we learned from the past? *Surg Endosc.* 2000;14:5.
2. Kelling G. Ueber Oesophagoskopie, Gastroskopie und Kolioskopie. *Munch Med Wochenschr.* 1902;49:21.
3. Short AR. The uses of coelioscopy. *BMJ.* 1925;2:254.
4. Ruddock JC. Peritoneoscopy. *Surg Gynecol Obstet.* 1935;65:623.
5. Villavicencio RT, Aucar JA. Analysis of laparoscopy in trauma. *J Am Coll Surg.* 1999;189:11.
6. Gazzaniga AB, Stanton WW, Bartlett RH. Laparoscopy in the diagnosis of blunt and penetrating injuries to the abdomen. *Am J Surg.* 1976;131:315.
7. Carnevale N, Baron N, Delany HM. Peritoneoscopy as an aid in the diagnosis of abdominal trauma: A preliminary report. *J Trauma.* 1977;17:634.
8. Berci G, Dunkelman D, Michel SL, et al. Emergency minilaparoscopy in abdominal trauma: An update. *Am J Surg.* 1983;146:261.
9. Adamthwaite DN. Traumatic diaphragmatic hernia: A new indication for laparoscopy. *Br J Surg.* 1984;71:315.
10. Mühe E. Die erste Cholecystectomie durch das Laparoskop. *Langensbecks Arch Klin Chir.* 1986;369:804.
11. Dubois F, Historia de la colecistectomia laparoscopica. In: Cueto J Weber A (eds.). *Cirugía Laparoscopica.* Chap. 22. McGraw-Hill Interamericana: 1997:139.
12. Alvarez-Tostado Ra, Alvarez-Tostado Ro. *Cirugía Toracoscopica* videoasistida, Chap. 56. In: Cueto J, Weber A (eds.). Cirugía Laparoscopica. McGraw-Hill Interamericana: 1997:415.
13. Jacobaeus HC. The cauterization of adhesions in pneumothorax treatment of tuberculosis. *Surg Gynecol Obstet.* 1921;32:493.
14. Simon RJ, Ivatury R. Current concepts in the use of cavitary endoscopy in the evaluation and treatment of blunt and penetrating truncal injuries. *Surg Clin North Am.* 1995;75:157.
15. Conell DB, Trunkey DD. Nonoperative management of abdominal trauma. *Surg Clin North Am.* 1990;70:677.
16. Weigelt JA, Kingman RG. Complications of negative laparotomy for trauma. *Am J Surg.* 1988;156:544.
17. Renz BM, Feliciano DV. Unnecessary laparotomies for trauma: A prospective study of morbidity. *J Trauma.* 1995;38:350.
18. Sosa JL, Baker M, Puente I et al. Negative laparotomy in abdominal gunshot wounds: Potential impact of laparoscopy. *J Trauma.* 1995;38:194.
19. McAnena OJ, Moore EE, Marx JA. Initial evaluation of the patient with blunt abdominal trauma. *Surg Clin North Am.* 1990;70:495.
20. Boulanger BR, McLellan BA. Blunt abdominal trauma. *Emerg Med Clin North Am.* 1996;14:151.
21. Sherck J, Shatney C, Sensaki K, et al. The accuracy of computed tomography in the diagnosis of blunt small bowel perforation. *Am J Surg.* 1994;168:670.
22. Salvino CK, Esposito TJ, Marshall WJ, et al. The role of diagnostic laparoscopy in the management of trauma patients: A preliminary assessment. *J Trauma.* 1993;34:506.
23. Hernandez JD, Castaneda JC. Heridas del diafragma en trauma toracoabdominal penetrante: Lavado peritoneal diagnostico vs Laparoscopia. Hospital de la Samaritana (unpublished data).
24. Moore JB, Moore EE, Thompson JS. Abdominal injuries associated with penetrating trauma in the lower chest. *Am J Surg.* 1980;140:724.
25. Boulanger BR, Rozycki GS, Rodriguez A. Sonographic assessment of traumatic injury: Future developments. *Surg Clin North Am.* 1999;79:1297.
26. Livingston DH, Tortella BJ, Blackwood J, et al. The role of laparoscopy in abdominal trauma. *J Trauma.* 1992;33:471.
27. Townsend MC, Flancbaum L, Choban PS, et al. Diagnostic laparoscopy as an adjunct to selective conservative management of solid organ injuries after blunt abdominal trauma. *J Trauma.* 1993;35:647.
28. Zantut LF, Machado MA, Volpe P, et al. Autotransfusion with laparoscopically salvaged blood in trauma: Report of 21 cases. *Surg Laparosc Endosc.* 1996;6:46.
29. Collin GR, Bianchi JD. Laparoscopic examination of the traumatized spleen with blood salvage for autotransfusion. *Am Surg.* 1997;63:478.
30. Zantut LF, Machado MA, Volpe P, et al. The role of laparoscopy in the nonoperative management of major blunt liver trauma. *Panam J Trauma.* 1995;5:63.
31. Berci G, Sackier JM, Paz-Partlow M. Emergency laparoscopy. *Am J Surg.* 1991;61:332.
32. Ivatury RR, Zantut LF, Yelon JA. Laparoscopy in the new millenium. *Surg Clin North Am.* 1999;79:1291.
33. Poole GV, Thomae KR, Hauser JH. Laparoscopy in trauma. *Surg Clin North Am.* 1996;76:539. Spanish edition.
34. Marx JA. Abdominal trauma. In: Rosen L, ed. *Emergency Medicine: Concepts and Clinical Practice,* 4th ed. Mosby Yearbook:1998.
35. Ferrada R, Birolini D. New concepts in the management of patients with penetrating abdominal wounds. *Surg Clin North Am.* 1999;79:1331.
36. Espinoza R, Rodriguez A. Traumatic and nontraumatic hollow viscera. *Surg Clin North Am.* 1997;77:1291.
37. Ponsky JL, Marks JM. Laparoscopic examination of the bowel in trauma patients. *Gastrointest Endosc.* 1996;43:146.
38. Ivatury RR, Simon RJ, Stahl WM. A critical evaluation of laparoscopy in penetrating abdominal trauma. *J Trauma.* 1993;34:822.
39. Ditmars ML, Bongard F. Laparoscopy for triage of penetrating trauma: The decision to explore. *J Laparoendosc Surg.* 1996;6:285.

40. Zantut LF, Ivatury RR, Smith RS, et al. Diagnostic and therapeutic laparoscopy for penetrant abdominal trauma: A multicenter experience. *J Trauma.* 1997;42:825.

41. Elliott DC, Rodriguez A, Moncure M, et al. The accuracy of diagnostic laparoscopy in trauma patients: A prospective, controlled study. *Int Surg* 1998;83:294.

42. Holthausen UH, Nagelschmidt M, Troidl H. CO_2 pneumoperitoneum: What we know and what we need to know. *World J Surg.* 1999;23:794.

43. Ho HS, Saunders CJ, Corso FA. The effects of pneumoperitoneum on hemodynamics in hemorraged animals. *Surgery.* 1993;114:381.

44. Josephs LG, Este-McDonal JR, Birkett DH, et al. Diagnostic laparoscopy increases intracranial pressure. *J Trauma.* 1994;36:815.

45. Liu DW, Liu HP, Lin PJ, et al. Video-assisted thoracic surgery in treatment of chest trauma. *J Trauma.* 1997;42:670.

46. Mancini M, Smith L, Nein A, et al. Early evacuation of clotted blood in hemothorax using thoracoscopy: Case reports. *J Trauma.* 1993;34:144.

47. Carrillo EH, Heniford T, Etoch SW, et al. Video assisted thoracic surgery in trauma patients. *J Am Coll Surg.* 1997;184:316.

48. Hirshberg A, Thompson SR, Bade PG. Pitfalls in the management of penetrating chest trauma. *Am J Surg.* 1989;157:372.

49. O'Brien JO, Cohen M, Solit R, et al. Thoracoscopic drainage and decortication as definitive treatment for empyema thoracis following penetrating chest injury. *J Trauma.* 1994;36:536.

50. Ramirez JC, Camacho F, Guzman F, et al. Videotoracoscopia: Indicaciones potenciales y experiencia inicial. *Rev Col Cirugia.* 1993;8:172.

51. Smith RS, Fry WR, Tsoi EKM, et al. Preliminary report on videothoracoscopy in the evaluation and treatment of thoracic injury. *Am J Surg.* 1993;166:690.

52. Osorio C, Salinas CM, Botero AC, et al. La toracoscopia. Evaluacion como metodo diagnostico y terapeutico. *Rev Col Cirugia.* 1994;9:62.

53. Salinas CM. La toracoscopia en el trauma. *Rev Col Cirugia.* 1994;9:11–14.

54. Villegas MI, Morales CH. Drenaje del hemotorax coagulado mediante toracoscopia: Factores predictivos de éxito. *Rev Col Cirugia.* 2000;15:29.

55. Heniford BT, Carrillo EH, Spain DA, et al. The role of thoracoscopy in the management of retained thoracic collections after trauma. *Ann Thorac Surg.* 1997;63:940.

56. Brewster SA, Thirlby RC, Snyder WH. Subxiphoid pericardial window and penetrating cardiac trauma. *Arch Surg.* 1988;123:937.

57. Morales CH, Salinas CM, Henao CA, et al. Thoracoscopic pericardial window and penetrating cardiac trauma. *J Trauma.* 1997;42:273.

58. Hoff WS, McMahon DJ, Schwab CW, et al. Thoracoscopic pericardial window. *J Trauma.* 1997;43:561. Letter.

59. Lang-Lazdunski L, Mouroux J, Pons F, et al. Role of videothoracoscopy in chest trauma. *Ann Thorac Surg.* 1997;63:327.

60. Schermer CR, Matteson BD, Demarest GB, et al. A prospective evaluation of video-assisted thoracic surgery for persistent air leak due to trauma. *Am J Surg.* 1999;177:480.

61. Bartek JP, Grasch A, Hazelrigg SR. Thoracoscopic retrieval of foreign bodies after penetrating chest trauma. *Ann Thorac Surg.* 1997;63:1783.

62. Reardon Mj, Fabre J, Reardon PR, et al. Video-assisted repair of a traumatic intercostal pulmonary hernia. *Ann Thorac Surg.* 1998; 65:1155.

63. Mineo TC, Ambrogi V, Cristino B, et al. Changing indications for thoracotomy in blunt chest trauma after the advent of videothoracoscopy. *J Trauma.* 1999;47:1088.

64. Sosa JL, Pombo H, Puente I, et al. Thoracoscopy in the evaluation and management of thoracic trauma. *Int Surg.* 1998;83:187.

65. Feliciano DV, Rozycki GS. Advances in the diagnosis and treatment of thoracic trauma. *Surg Clin North Am.* 1999;79:1417.

66. Velmahos GC, Demetriades D. Early thoracoscopy for the evacuation of undrained haemothorax. *Eur J Surg.* 1999;165:924.

67. Wong MS, Tsoi EK, Henderson VJ, et al. Videothoracoscopy: An effective method for evaluating and managing thoracic trauma patients. *Surg Endosc.* 1996;10:118.

68. Von Oppell UO, Bautz P, De Groot M. Penetrating thoracic injuries: What we have learnt. *Thorac Cardiovasc Surg.* 2000;48:55.

69. Villavicencio RT, Aucar JA, Wall MJ. Analysis of thoracoscopy in trauma. *Surg Endosc.* 1999;13:3.

70. Colt HG. Therapeutic thoracotomy. *Clin Chest Med.* 1998:19:383.

71. Feliciano DV, Cruse PA, Mattox KL, et al. Delayed diagnosis of injuries to the diaphragm after penetrating wounds. *J Trauma.* 1988;28:1135.

72. Kern JA, Tribble CG, Spotnitz WD, et al. Thoracoscopy in the subacute management of the patients with thoracoabdominal trauma. *Chest.* 1993;104:942.

73. Kessler E, Stein A. Diaphragmatic hernia as a long term complication of stab wounds of the chest. *Am J Surg.* 1976;132:34.

74. Madden MR, Paull DE, Finkelstein JL, et al. Occult diaphragmatic injury from stab wounds to the lower chest and abdomen. J Trauma. 1989;29:292.

75. Ivatury RR, Simon RJ, Weksler B, et al. Laparoscopy in the evaluation of the intrathoracic abdomen after penetrating injury. *J Trauma.* 1992;33:101.

76. Uribe RA, Pachon CE, Frame SB, et al. A prospective evaluation of thoracoscopy for the diagnosis of penetrating thoracoabdominal trauma. *J Trauma.* 1994;37:650.

77. Smith CH, Novick TL, Jacobs DG, et al. Laparoscopic repair of a ruptured diaphragm secondary to blunt trauma. *Surg Endosc.* Online publication, 24 March 2000.

78. Matz A, Alis M, Charuzi I, et al. The role of laparoscopy in the diagnosis and treatment of missed diaphragmatic rupture. *Surg Endosc.* Online publication, 8 May 2000.

79. Marks JM, Ramey RL, Baringer DC, et al. Laparoscopic repair of a diphragmatic laceration. *Surg Laparosc Endosc.* 1995;5:415.

80. Zantut LF, Autran M, Machado C, et al. Diaphragmatic injuries. Laparoscopic diagnosis and management. Report on two cases. *Panam J Trauma.* 1995;5:60.

81. Ochsner MG, Rozycki GS, Lucente F, et al. Prospective evaluation of thoracoscopy for diagnosing diaphragmatic injury in thoracoabdominal trauma: A preliminary report. *J Trauma.* 1993;34:704, 709.

Chapter Fifty-Eight • • • • • •

*L*aparoscopy in the Patient with Fever of Unknown Origin

RAIMUNDO LLANIO-NAVARRO and ROBERTO MILLÁN-SANDOVAL

INTRODUCTION

Fever is a subjective and objective symptom that is generally indicative of disease and is an important sign of imbalance between sickness and health. When present, whether associated or not with other symptoms known as the febrile syndrome, fever requires a careful examination of the patient to search for the cause.

When it is prolonged without an identifiable source it is known as fever of unknown origin (FUO), and it can adopt a classic fever pattern that indicates a certain disease state, or it can be prolonged, shedding no light on its origin. The classic definition of FUO was established in 1961 by Petersdorf and Benson,[1] and is based on the following criteria:

- Fever lasting over 3 weeks.
- Documented presence of fever over 38.3°C on two or more occasions.
- The patient is exhaustively investigated for over a week without establishing the diagnosis.

This concept can be modified, but it is obvious that FUO is a diagnostic challenge. It can be due to a benign condition, and in many cases it is the only persistent indicator of a disease that may be curable or not. It may carry prognostic importance, and requires a well-directed investigation to avoid useless, cumbersome, and expensive tests.[2]

INDICATIONS AND CONTRAINDICATIONS

The authors have employed laparoscopy for years in cases of FUO, and it has proven valuable for peritoneal lesions as well as for lesions in other organs visible under laparoscopy. It also provides better views of areas that are difficult to explore via laparotomy and provides an excellent means for obtaining cytological samples and directed biopsies, as well as for extracting peritoneal fluid. When the surgeon is experienced, there are very few contraindications to performing laparoscopy, and these are addressed elsewhere.[3,4]

The authors have performed 119,700 laparoscopies, and only 2.5% were unsuccessful, and 2% were explored but incomplete due to unsatisfactory views of the abdomen due to adhesions. This series includes planned as well as emergency laparoscopies, particularly for acute abdomen.

RESULTS

At the Instituto de Gastroenterología in Havana, Cuba, there have been 119,700 laparoscopies since 1970, of which 60,300 were urgent due to spontaneous or traumatic acute abdomen. Out of the remaining 59,400 laparoscopies, 2% (1,188) were indicated to aid in the diagnosis of FUO.

The disease states most frequently found were infectious diseases, neoplasms, granulomatous lesions, parasitic diseases, collagen vascular diseases, primary biliary cirrhosis, and chronic active hepatitis.[5,6,7]

Laparoscopy demonstrated lesions that were either macroscopically characteristic or required aspiration cytology, biopsy, or culture to determine the diagnosis in 85% of the cases; in the remaining 15% there was no finding that justified an examination of a certain area, in which case a blind cytology study or biopsy was performed. In 8% of cases the diagnosis was established with these complementary methods or through cultures that showed a disorder in some other site, such as salmonellosis, bacterial endocarditis, connective tissue disease, pyelonephritis, or factitious fever. In some cases the febrile syndrome disappeared before the cause was established. The final result could not be established in the remaining 7% of patients because of incomplete follow-up.[5]

DESCRIPTION OF THE LAPAROSCOPIC CHARACTERISTICS OF SOME COMMON LESIONS

Hodgkin's Disease (Lymphadenoma)

Laparoscopy is very useful for diagnosing Hodgkin's disease in contrast to other diffuse reticular diseases. On many occasions, the diagnosis is made during a laparoscopy for FUO. The different presenting forms of Hodgkin's disease can be divided into four groups:[7]

- *Type I:* Miliary form—This can be distinguished from other miliary forms through biopsy. The endoscopic appearance is of small white, round, pleomorphic lesions that protrude only slightly.
- *Type II:* Conglomerated form—Miliary lesions are grouped together forming characteristic conglomerations.
- *Type III:* Nodular or tumoral form—Prominent whitish-yellow tumors found over liver surfaces, commonly at the borders of the lobules, that can be differentiated from other types of nodules or tumors by the fact that they are perfectly round. This diagnosis must be confirmed by directed biopsy.
- *Type IV:* Diffuse form—The liver is diffusely affected in the form of whitish macules that are not prominent, having an appearance similar to that of hepatic sarcoidosis.

All cases require definitive confirmation via biopsy, which when directed has an almost 100% efficacy. This classification refers to endoscopic changes and is not related to the clinical staging of Hodgkin's disease.

Systemic Hematological Diseases

The systemic hematologic diseases and myeloproliferative syndromes that most frequently cause FUO are large cell lymphoma, hepatic lymphosarcoma, plasmacytoma, and some forms of leukemia. The lesions that these diseases produce in the liver are atypical, and are generally seen as multiple yellowish micronodules (large cell lymphoma), more confluent less isolated micronodules (cellular lymphoid reticulosis), or small prominent nodules that give a granular aspect to the hepatic and splenic surfaces.[7]

Infectious Diseases and Granulomas

Different processes that form granulomas can be found in the liver, spleen, or peritoneum, they can be distributed diffusely throughout the liver, and can sometimes be confirmed by blind biopsy, although false negatives may occur if the granuloma is not included in the sample. However, some granulomas like the ones formed in tuberculosis, sarcoidosis, Wegener's granulomatosis, polyarteritis nodosa, and syphilis among others, tend to develop thicker, more focal changes that are not detectable by simple biopsy, and justify the use of laparoscopy and directed biopsy not only in cases of FUO, but also in cases in which the diagnosis is thought to be known.

It should be noted here that there is a group of granulomatous lesions whose cause cannot be proven in spite of histologic confirmation, known as granulomatous hepatitis, which almost always responds to steroid treatment.[7,8]

In general, granulomatosis presenting with alterations in Glisson's capsule adopts one of these patterns: macular, exudative, isolated nodules, granular, or an elongated form. Some patterns are more common in certain granulomatous diseases, which aids in the endo-scopic diagnosis, but endoscopy should always be accompanied by a directed biopsy.

Tuberculosis

FUO may be caused by asymptomatic tuberculosis, or less frequently by early splenohepatic tuberculosis.[9] In typical cases multiple miliary white nodules of a uniform size are observed in the liver or in rare cases in the spleen or peritoneum, sometimes accompanied by fibrinous exudates or adhesions between the liver surface and the diaphragm or between intestinal loops. On occasion serofibrinous ascites can be found that is clinically undetectable.[7,10]

Sarcoidosis

Sarcoidosis affects the liver in stages II and III of this disease, but it can also appear earlier in an isolated form in this organ. The surface presents a complex picture: some cases present with isolated spots, and in others the entire liver is filled with miliary nodules (similarly to other granulomatous processes, and even in massive steatosis); on rare occasions it adopts a rounded nodular form that is endoscopically indistinguishable from neoplasia.[7]

Wegener's Granulomatosis

This presents with lesions similar to the ones found in the nodular form of sarcoidosis, with nodules of varying size distributed irregularly throughout the liver.[7]

Polyarteritis Nodosa

The liver has an enlarged aspect but the surface is slick, and there are signs of arteritis in Glisson's capsule such as narrowing of the arterioles and formation of a whitish layer around them that correspond histologically with the infiltrative-granulomatous lesions as described by Solis-Herruzo et al.[11]

PARASITOSIS AND INFECTIONS

Some parasitic infections in the larval phase pass through the liver towards the lung to infect the digestive tract, and there are some parasites that remain in the liver throughout their larval phase and produce not only FUO, but entire syndromes characterized by anorexia, asthenia, and weight loss, which can simulate tuberculous lesions, lymphomas, or other neoplasias. The characteristic lesions produced by the so-called visceral larva migrans have been described, allowing diagnosis based on laparoscopy alone. The lesions produced by *Toxocara cati* and *Toxocara canis*, as well as *Fasciola hepatica*, *Clonorchis sinensis*, *Capillaria hepatica*, *Angiostrongylus costaricensis* and others can also be distinguished.

Whitish-yellow linear lesions, sometimes convoluted and twisting in nature, are prominent on the surface and may sometimes correspond histologically with granulomas. A directed biopsy can sometimes reveal special histologic characteristics that are produced by the larva, generally at the end of the lesion, making it necessary to take samples from this portion to obtain portions of the larva. If special dyes are employed (e.g., Mason's trichromic) granulomas can be seen with periodic acid–Schiff (PAS)-positive fragments that correspond to larval portions.[12–14]

Amebic Hepatic Abscess

Most cases can be diagnosed with ultrasonography, but on occasion a small abscess or one in a previously damaged liver can be difficult to visualize, making laparoscopy a valuable tool. Two fundamental lesions can be observed: a large elevated lesion that is white or pink color, or a thickening of Glisson's capsule with an increase in vascularity, sometimes having adhesions that attach to the lateral wall of the abdomen or diaphragm. In either case the lesion should be pierced and aspirated to evacuate it and to introduce medication, and to test for the presence of amebic infection. Healing is much faster when pus is evacuated and an antiparasitic agent is left in the cavity.[10]

Hepatocholangitis

When bacterial cholangitis is present, the hepatic surface has patchy lesions ranging from delicate opacities to dense perihepatic deposits that simulate frost, forming adhesions to the abdominal wall or diaphragm or both. The lesions are macular and have a red-gray color, and in cases of recurrent cholangitis whitish-gray areas can be seen which are remnants of previous abscesses.[7]

HEPATIC NEOPLASIA

Hepatocarcinoma

There are three anatomical presentations, each of which has its own laparoscopic image. The most frequent are the single nodule form, characterized by a large nodule (sometimes up to 10 cm) that is yellow color with many dilated and irregular vessels on the surface; and the multiple nodule form with prominent, rounded white lesions that range from 1 to 4 cm in size. These can easily be confused with hepatic metastasis from different carcinomas, although these generally have an umbilicated center as a result of tumor necrosis. Either lesion is an important finding in a patient with FUO. A directed biopsy in the peripheral region of the nodules allows histologic assessment. Hepatic cirrhosis is frequently concurrently found. The diffuse form, which is the rarest, can be difficult to distinguish laparoscopically from fibrosis or hepatic cirrhosis, and it is only via biopsy that the diagnosis can be established.[7,15]

Peritoneal Carcinomatosis

This entity can cause FUO, and laparoscopy allows visualization of small white-yellow nodules that tend to coalesce and are easily viewed on the epiploon, over intestinal loops, or below the diaphragm (generally on the right side). This entity can be distinguished from peritoneal tuberculosis because the nodules in the latter are much smaller and more disseminated.[7,10]

Other Neoplasms

Some other neoplasms (e.g., of the gallbladder, pancreas, or colon) can cause FUO and can be demonstrated by laparoscopy.

HEPATIC DISEASES

Chronic Active Hepatitis

The liver has an enlarged aspect, with a surface that tends to undulate or show a granular aspect, with thickening of the capsule and an increase in vascularity and a pale red color.[7,10]

Primary Biliary Cirrhosis

Also called primary chronic destructive or nonsuppurative cholangitis, this disease has differing appearances according to its stage; in the most typical form, a large liver spotted with small greenish nodules and white scars with depressions in between is seen.

OTHER DISEASES

Crohn's Disease

FUO has been seen as the presenting symptom of Crohn's disease in some patients, in whom laparoscopy reveals thickened, reddish intestinal loops (particularly at the terminal ileum), with increased vascularity, absence of peristalsis, and immobility, with slight dilation of the anterior loops and a noted thickening of the mesentery in the affected areas.[10,16]

Giant Cell Arteritis and Systemic Lupus Erythematosus

These diseases frequently present with FUO. In some cases laparoscopy can reveal slight changes in the hepatic or splenic capsules. A biopsy should always be done when the liver or spleen are explored, which can provide valuable results when the clinical diagnosis is obscure.[7,10]

CONCLUSIONS

Many authors advocate the use of an exploratory laparotomy to determine the diagnosis in cases of FUO,[19,20] and we believe that laparoscopy should be performed before laparotomy, augmented by aspiration or biopsy, because in experienced hands it can be of great help in determining or confirming the exact diagnosis. The procedure is simple, minimally invasive, and can be performed under light sedation if necessary.

REFERENCES

1. Petersdorf RG, Benson PE. Fever of unexplained origin: Report of 100 cases. *Medicine* 1961;40:1.
2. Pérez Caballero MD, Rodríguez Silva H. Fiebre de origen desconocido. *Rev Cubana Med.* 1992;31:120.
3. Llanio R, Sotto A, et al. *Laparoscopia en Urgencias.* Científico-Técnica:1977.
4. Solis-Herruzo JA, et al. *Atlas de Diagnostico Diferencial Laparoscópico.* Paz Montalvo:1975.
5. Llanio R. Archivos del Departamento de Endoscopia. Instituto de Gastroenterología. Havana, Cuba, 1994.
6. Solis-Herrzo JA, Muñoz Yagu T, Colina RD. Laparoscopy in fever of unknown origin. *Endoscopy* 1981;13:207.
7. Beck K, Llanio R. *Atlas en Colores de Laparoscopia*, 3rd ed. Editorial Ciencias Médicas:1991.
8. Moreto M, Testillano M, Zaballa M, et al. Diagnostic yield and endoscopic patterns of laparoscopy in the diagnosis of granulomatous hepatitis. *Endoscopy* 1988;20:294.
9. Llanio R. Tuberculosis esplénica primitiva: Diagnostico de un síndrome hepatosplénico. *Revista Kuba* 1956;12:38.
10. Llanio R. Personal experience. Instituto de Gastroenterología. Havana, Cuba.

11. Solis-Herruzo JA, Muñoz-Yagu? T, Colins RD. Laparoscopic findings in polyarteritis nodosa. *Endoscopy* 1981;13:9.

12. Llanio R, Sotto A. Laparoscopic diagnosis of the visceral larva migrans. Endoscopy of the Digestive System Proceedings of the First European Congress of Digestive Endoscopy. Praga, 1968. Karger-Basel:1969.

13. Llanio R, Sotto A. Diagnosis of the visceral larva migrans. Fourth World Congress of Gastroentererology. Copenhagen, Denmark, July 1970.

14. Llanio R, Sotto A. Larva migrans visceralis: Diagnostique par laparoscopie. *Semaine Hopitaux* 1972;48:1223.

15. Vázquez-Puello R, Bel CC, et al. Hepatocarcinoma como causa de fiebre de origen desconocido. Cartas al Editor. *An Med Intern.* 1993;10:566.

16. Domínguez A, Peña JM, Barbado FG, et al. Fiebre de larga evolución como forma de presentación de la enfermedad de Crohn. *An Med Intern.* 1990;7:39.

17. Boyce HW, Palmer ED. *Techniques of Clinical Gastroenterology.* Charles Thomas:1975.

18. Kortsik C, Winckelmann G, Beck K, et al. Was leistet die Laparaskopie bei der K1 rung von Fieber unbekannter Ursache? *Dtsch Med Wschr.* 1987;112:1657.

19. Geraci JE, Weed LA, Nichols DR. Fever of obscure origin: The value of abdominal exploration in diagnosis. *JAMA.* 1959;169:1306.

20. Keller JW, William RD. Laparotomy for unexplained fever. *Arch Surg.* 1965;90:494.

Chapter Fifty-Nine • • • • • •

Laparoscopic Ultrasonography

FREDERICK GREENE

The laparoscope has proved to be a valuable tool not only for diagnosis but now for therapeutic intervention within the abdomen, chest, and retroperitoneum. The use of conventional radiologic imaging has proved beneficial in that CT scans, magnetic resonance imaging, and percutaneous ultrasonography have played a role in identifying disease processes amenable to laparoscopic diagnosis and resection. More recently, introduction of intraoperative ultrasound using hand-held probes has supported resectional techniques done by open approaches to the abdomen.[1,2] It was only logical that these same principles should now be applied through laparoscopic ports, and that the use of laparoscopic ultrasound, while not standard, will become more prevalent and useful.

Laparoscopic diagnosis is limited by the ability to see only surface lesions, which may be enhanced slightly by paplation techniques using solid rods or other accessories. Using laparoscopic ultrasound probes passed through 10-mm trocar sites, the surgeon is now able to appreciate lesions within the hepatic parenchyma, pancreas, retroperitoneum, and other solid areas within the abdomen (Fig. 59–1). This technology has also facilitated direct needle biopsy and therapeutic intervention such as cryotherapy, which may be directed by ultrasound findings.[3] It has been estimated that the combination of laparoscopy and ultrasound-guided biopsy is 98% sensitive and accurate.[4]

The technique of laparoscopic ultrasound can be performed either as an inpatient or outpatient procedure, and may be used under both general and local anesthesia techniques. We prefer general anesthesia because of the ability to distend the abdominal wall using pneumoperitoneum without associated discomfort to the patient. In addition, general anesthesia allows the luxury of a detailed, unhurried exam.

It is obvious that there is a learning curve in the interpretation of ultrasound findings, and it is strongly recommended that the surgeon work with his or her radiologic colleague in the early cases in order to understand the variety of images that can be developed by ultrasound. The use of split-screen video monitoring also enables the ultrasound image to be directly placed on the monitor as the intra-abdominal image is also displayed. Early work with laparoscopic ultrasonography dealt with hepatic lesions, and simple differentiation between benign and malignant masses showed that diagnostic accuracy could exceed 90% when using laparoscopic ultrasonography.[5]

The importance of laparoscopic ultrasound investigation is to avoid unnecessary resections or open abdominal exploration in patients with pancreatic or esophageal lesions who may benefit from other therapeutic modalities. This is less clear in patients with colorectal cancer with hepatic metastases, since resection of the colon may still be standard even in the face of metastases. The real advantage in patients with metastatic colorectal disease to the liver is to identify lesions that may either be resected or treated with other modalities such as cryotherapy. Because conventional imaging techniques may underestimate involvement in the liver, laparoscopic ultrasound can prove quite beneficial in identifying small lesions under the size of 2 cm in diameter. Similar application is seen in the evaluation of patients with primary hepatic tumors such as hepatocellular carcinoma and cholangiocarcinoma of the bile ducts or liver.[6,28] Multiple lesions may occur in hepatocellular cancer and may not be appropriately treated by resection techniques. An additional use of laparoscopic ultrasound is to evaluate the retroperitoneum looking for abnormal lymph nodes, which may be biopsied especially during staging procedures for Hodgkin's disease.[7,23]

TECHNICAL ISSUES

Laparoscopic ultrasonography has been made possible because of continued development of ultrasound technology during the last decade.[5] Small scanning probes as well as flexible tips on the laparoscopic instruments allow more accurate placement on the surfaces of the liver, pancreas, and retroperitoneum. Laparoscopic intraoperative ultrasonography was first described in 1958 by Yamakawa et al,[8] but limitations of ultrasound technology and a lack of laparoscopic therapeutic application inhibited further development. In 1989, Ido et al[9] reported the use of laparoscopic intraoperative ultrasonography to guide ethanol injections into the liver for treatment of small hepatocellular carcinomas.[28]

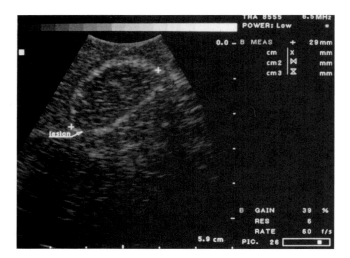

Figure 59–1. B-mode laparoscopic ultrasound image showing benign liver lesion which is isoechoic with a hyperechoic "halo."

Jakimowicz et al[10] and Yamashita et al[11] reported the use of laparoscopic intraoperative ultrasonography as a screening procedure during laparoscopic cholecystectomy.[23]

The ultrasound equipment consists of two main components, a dedicated digital electronic system (scanner) and the transducer probe. The scanner provides the electrical signal, which is used to stimulate the crystal in the transducer probe. The crystal images a series of ultrasonic pulses, part of which are reflected from the structure being scanned and are detected by the transducer crystal and converted into electrical signals. These electrical signals are transmitted to the scanner, amplified, and finally displayed in two-dimensional real-time image on the video screen. A variety of ultrasound transducers are available; sector scanners, convex (radial) array, and linear array. For laparoscopic intraoperative ultrasonography, linear and convex array and sector transducers are used. The higher-frequency transducers provide greater axial resolution, but the depth of ultrasound visualization is decreased and inversely proportional due to frequency of the sound waves used. Intraoperative examination involves contact screening of the organ, which allows the use of a high-frequency transducer probe that has a limited depth of field but high resolution.

The laparoscopic ultrasound probe is generally placed through a 10-mm port site. The distance from the access port to the examined area may be very long and thus the length of the transducer probe may need to be 35 to 40 cm in length to provide contact screening. The transducer probe should provide high-quality images with lateral resolution of less than 1 mm, thus necessitating the use of high-frequency transducers (6.5 to 10 MHz). The depth of view in laparoscopic intraoperative ultrasonography may be limited to 5 to 10 cm because the transducer is placed directly on the area of interest.

The examination technique depends on the target area and the ultrasound transducer used. The rigid transducer probe is passed through one of the access trocars and placed under visual control on the organ to be examined. The ability to have "picture in picture" is useful in order to show both the ultrasound and the laparoscopic image at the same time. The common bile duct may be examined by placing the transducer on the anterior or anterolateral aspect of the common bile duct. The best images are achieved by

slow withdrawal of the transducer toward the examiner through the access port.[12] It is essential to keep the common bile duct continuously in the field of view, and to try and examine as long a segment of the common bile duct as possible (Fig. 59–2). The common bile duct may be traced from the proximal area to the region of the pancreas. Landmarks such as the portal vein, behind the common bile duct, and the right hepatic artery, located between the proximal part of the duct and the portal vein, may be visualized. The distal part of the bile duct is surrounded by pancreatic tissue and the inferior vena cava lies posterior to the distal duct. This area may be screened through the duodenum using compression by the transducer. Saline infusion around the hepatoduodenal ligament may allow better acoustic contact between the screening surface and the ultrasound probe. Better acoustic contact and a more convenient angle for examination can be achieved by partial reduction of the pneumoperitoneum.

It is important to examine the liver carefully especially because of the involvement of small metastases (Fig. 59–3). Examination is begun with evaluation of the right lobe of the liver. The transducer is placed in approximation to the diaphragm and screening is performed in several directions starting from lateral to medial and then from medial to lateral. Since the penetration of high-frequency transducers is limited, screening the liver from both the anterior and superior aspects must be considered. The left lobe of the liver is usually smaller and can be more easily examined either from the anterior or posterior aspects.

The ultrasound probe may also be used for examining specific lymph node areas. Good approximation and contact between tissue and the transducer probe is mandatory. This may also be heightened by instillation of saline solution.

CLINICAL RESULTS

Jakimowicz[13] reported 176 patients who had laparoscopic intraoperative ultrasonography using a rigid transducer probe. The majority of these patients had the technique used for screening of the biliary tract during laparoscopic cholecystectomy or prior to common bile duct exploration. Approximately 30 patients out of this

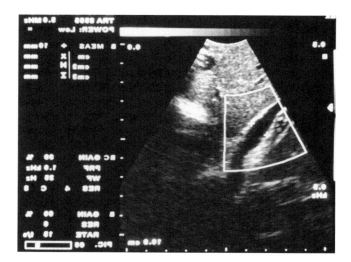

Figure 59–2. Dilated common bile duct with thickened wall.

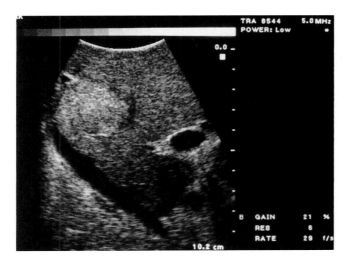

Figure 59–3. Metastatic liver lesion adjacent to hepatic vein.

group had laparoscopic ultrasound studies during staging procedures for cancer.[23,24,26,29] The ability to visualize the common bile duct and to assess for both anatomy and intraductal stones is available using intraoperative ultrasound techniques. Once the initial learning curve is passed, accurate studies may be achieved. The time needed for screening in this situation is approximately 5 to 10 minutes and therefore does not add a significant amount of time to routine laparoscopic cholecystectomy. During staging procedures, however, careful attention to ultrasound examination of the liver, pancreatic area, and nodal regions may add 25 to 30 minutes to the diagnostic laparoscopy time-frame.[23,24,26,29] While assessment of the common bile duct for stone disease and anatomy can be achieved and is comparable to intraoperative cholangiography,[12] we still believe that intraoperative cholangiography is the standard and should be routinely done in these procedures.

In addition to routine ultrasound examination, use of color Doppler for laparoscopic intraoperative ultrasonography is available. Using this equipment, easier identification of anatomic structures and better identification of vascular patterns of tumors have been noted.[14,25] Color Doppler imaging relates to the application of real-time pulse Doppler measurements of the entire ultrasound image with the resulting areas of flow superimposed on the gray-scale picture. The system produces an anatomic image, using a different color for each flow direction (toward and away from the transducer) with the brightness of color representing flow velocity. The majority of current commercially available ultrasound scanners provide conventional B-mode imaging, pulse Doppler, and color Doppler imaging options. The Doppler capability provides information about the speed and flow pattern of blood within the vessel being examined. When an ultrasound signal is reflected by flowing blood, a spectrum of frequencies is received correlating with distribution of flow-velocity vectors in the volume sampled by the transducer. The first Doppler systems provided only audio output when the operator's ear was in essence the frequency analyzer. This subjective approach is now supplemented by real-time digital frequency analysis. To identify flow direction toward or away from the transducer, the positive and negative Doppler frequencies are assigned to the colors on opposite sides of the color bar—red and blue. Differentiation of arteries from veins is rapid

and easy by color Doppler imaging. Information provided through these techniques enhances ultrasound examination and reduces the time needed to complete the patient evaluation. Using these techniques, encouraging results have been published on the identification of benign lesions such as hepatic focal nodular hyperplasia[15] and malignant tumors such as hepatocellular carcinoma.[16,28] Focal nodular hyperplasia (FNH) is a rare benign hypervascular liver lesion that shows a specific vascular pattern consisting of a feeding artery entering the central zone, branching at the periphery, and supplying the lesion centrifugally.[15] Color Doppler enables the identification of this vascular pattern with greater accuracy than angiography, particularly in lesions smaller than 3 cm in diameter. The identification of tumor thrombus in patients with renal carcinoma and hepatocellular carcinoma has also been documented using color Doppler imaging.[17,25,28]

During diagnostic ultrasonography, color Doppler imaging enables differentiation between pseudocysts, malignant tumors, and fluid collections.[23,25] The main criterion for differentiation is the presence of internal vascularization in malignant tumors in contrast to cysts or fluid collections.[23] Machi et al[18] identified five advantages of operative color Doppler imaging over operative conventional B-mode ultrasound imaging:

1. Detection and localization of relatively small blood vessels that are impossible or difficult to find by B-mode imaging or surgical exploration alone.
2. Rapid and definitive differentiation of blood vessels from other hypoechogenic areas, such as tissue spaces, ducts, and cystic lesions.
3. More precise assessment of the relation of tumors and other lesions to vascular structures including vascular invasion by cancer.
4. Confirmation of adequate blood flow to critical organs after completion of major surgical procedures.
5. Easier and more precise targeted needle biopsy or guidance of needle placement for other purposes.[25]

Combinations of intraoperative laparoscopic ultrasonography as well as color Doppler imaging may be beneficial both in routine screening of the biliary tract during laparoscopic cholecystectomy and in the evaluation of intra-abdominal malignancy.[26] It has been stated that color Doppler imaging during laparoscopic intraoperative ultrasound examination not only enhances the screening procedure but curtails the learning curve for operators with limited experience in ultrasound techniques. During hepatic scanning, primary liver tumors and metastatic deposits are clearly depicted by virtue of their vascularity using color Doppler imaging. These techniques are especially important when cryotherapy of metastatic liver tumors is used, because proximity to vessels may be a contraindication to freezing of metastatic implants.[19] Determining the relation of tumors to major vessels and documentation of vascular invasion are possible with laparoscopic color Doppler imaging, which should be routinely used when cryotherapy is performed (Fig. 59–4). In addition, evaluation of pancreatic cancer may be enhanced in that vascular invasion by pancreatic tumors may be more easily recognized and therefore open operative extirpation of pancreatic lesions avoided.[20] Similarly, evaluation of abnormal lymph nodes and biopsy of these areas may be more safely carried out using color Doppler imaging and ultrasound guidance when these nodes are in the vicinity of major vessels. This will ultimately enhance the TNM staging of pancreatic cancer.

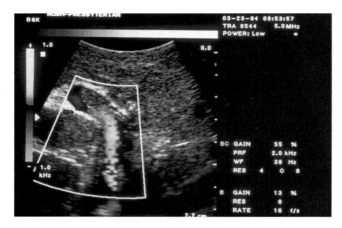

Figure 59–4. Color Doppler study showing arterial and venous flow around metastatic liver lesion.

The assessment of blood supply is an important indicator of organ function and is also used for the enhancement and thus the identification of tumors. Newer techniques may use ultrasound contrast agents in the form of microbubbles small enough to cross capillaries.[14] These gas-filled bubbles provide enhanced reflection during ultrasound examination and give improved accuracy of Doppler recording. Use of these contrast agents may enhance the diagnosis of hepatic tumors, particularly hepatocellular carcinoma.[28] In addition, laparoscopic cryosurgery may be better monitored using ultrasound contrast agents. More accurate monitoring of the size and volume of the cryo-lesion with respect to the tumor being ablated may be a by-product of this technology. This will obviously lead to greater total tumor kill by freezing techniques.

Conventional ultrasound techniques facilitated by laparoscopic placement in addition to newer concepts of color Doppler imaging with or without contrast agents will surely be the "stethoscope" for the modern surgeon performing laparoscopic surgery. It is imperative that current diagnostic evaluation of intraoperative cancer be performed with ultrasound techniques as an adjunct. The team approach with radiologist and surgeon is strongly recommended in order to allow both disciplines to bring their experience to the management of the patient undergoing minimal-access surgical techniques. Through this approach, the surgeon and radiologist will learn together and create an environment where healthy collaboration will benefit all parties. An approach such as this should enhance the selection of patients for laparoscopic resection of tumors of the liver[21] and other solid organs, the dissection and harvest of lymph nodes, and the monitoring of the parenchymal effects during laparoscopic hepatic cryotherapy or radiofrequency ablation.[22]

REFERENCES

1. Machi J, Isomoto H, Yamashita Y, et al. Intraoperative ultrasonography in screening for liver metastases from colorectal cancer: Comparative accuracy with traditional procedures. *Surgery.* 1987;101:678.
2. Luck AJ, Maddern GJ. Intraoperative abdominal ultrasonography. *Br J Surg.* 1999;86:5.
3. Crews KA, Kuhn J, McCarty T, et al. Cryosurgical ablation of hepatic tumors. *Am J Surg.* 1997;174:614.
4. Cooperman AM, Hurt K. Laparoscopy and liver cancer. *Surg Oncol Clin North Am.* 1994;3:653.
5. Jakimowicz J. Laparoscopic intraoperative ultrasonography: Equipment and technique. *Semin Laparosc Surg.* 1994;1:51.
6. John TG, Greig JD, Crosbie J, et al. Superior staging of liver tumors with laparoscopy and laparoscopic ultrasound. *Ann Surg.* 1994;220:711.
7. Greene FL, Cooler AW. Laparoscopic evaluation of lymphomas. *Semin Laparosc Surg.* 1994;1:13.
8. Yamakawa K, Naito S, Azuma K, et al. Laparoscopic diagnosis of the intra-abdominal organs. *Jpn J Gastroenterol.* 1958;55:741.
9. Ido K, Kawamoto C, Ohtani M, et al. Intratumoral injection of absolute ethanol under peritoneoscopic ultrasound imaging for treatment of small hepatocellular carcinoma. *Endoscopia Digestiva (Jpn).* 1989;9:1255.
10. Jakimowicz JJ, Ruers TJM. Ultrasound-assisted laparoscopic cholecystectomy: Preliminary experience. *Dig Surg.* 1991;8:114.
11. Yamashita Y, Jurohiji T, Kimitsuki H, et al. A clinical experience of intraoperative ultrasound at laparoscopic cholecystectomy. *Rinshoto Kenkyo (Jpn).* 1991;68:3497.
12. Birth M, Ehlers KU, Delinikolas K, Weiser HF. Prospective randomized comparison of laparoscopic ultrasonography using a flexible-tip ultrasound probe and intraoperative dynamic cholangiography during laparoscopic cholecystectomy. *Surg Endosc.* 1998;1:30.
13. Jakimowicz JJ. Intraoperative ultrasonography during minimal access surgery. *J R Coll Surg Edinb.* 1993;38:231.
14. Jakimowicz JJ, Stultiëns G. Laparoscopic intraoperative ultrasonography, color Doppler and power flow application. *Semin Laparosc Surg.* 1997;4:110.
15. Kudo M, Tomila S, Minowa K. Color Doppler flow imaging of hepatic focal nodular hyperplasia. *J Ultrasound Med.* 1992;11:553.
16. Tanaka S, Kitamara T, Fujita M, et al. Small hepatocellular carcinoma: Differentiation from adenomatous hyperplastic nodule with color Doppler flow imaging. *Radiology.* 1992;182:161.
17. Hübsch P, Schurawitzki H, Susani M. Color Doppler imaging of inferior vena cava: identification of tumor thrombus. *J Ultrasound Med.* 1992;11:639.
18. Machi J, Sigel B, Kurohiji, et al. Operative color Doppler imaging for general surgery. *J Ultrasound Med.* 1993;12:455.
19. Onik G, Rubinsky B, Zemel R, et al. Ultrasound-guided hepatic cryosurgery in the treatment of metastatic colon carcinoma. *Cancer.* 1991;67:901.
20. John TG, Wright A, Allan PL, et al. Laparoscopy with laparoscopic ultrasonography in the TNM staging of pancreatic carcinoma. *World J Surg.* 1999;23:870.
21. Rahusen FD, Cuesta MA, Borgstein PJ, et al. Selection of patients for resection of colorectal metastases to the liver using diagnostic laparoscopy and laparoscopic ultrasonography. *Ann Surg.* 1999;230:31.
22. Curley SA, Izzo F, Delrio P, et al. Radiofrequency ablation of unresectable primary and metastatic hepatic malignancies: Results in 123 patients. *Ann Surg.* 1999;230:1.
23. Hurst BS, Tucker KE, Awoniyi CA, et al. Endoscopic ultrasound. *J Reprod Med.* 1996;41:67.
24. Van Dickum EJ, de Wit LT, van Delden OM, et al. Staging laparoscopy and laparoscopic ultrasonography in more than 400 patients with upper gastrointestinal carcinoma. *J Am Coll Surg.* 1999;189:459.
25. Liu JB, Feld IR, Goldberg BB, et al. laparoscopic gray-scale and color Doppler ultrasonography. *Radiology.* 1995;184:851.
26. Misawa T, Koike M, Suzuki K, et al. Ultrasonographic assesement of the risk of injury to branches of the middle hepatic vein uring laparoscopic cholecystectomy. *Am J Surg.* 1999;178:418.
27. Den Boer KT, de Wit LT, Dankelman J, et al. Preoperative time-motion analysis of diagnostic laparoscopy with laparoscopic ultrasonography. *Br J Surg.* 1999;86:951.
28. Lo CM, Lai EC, Lui CL, et al. Laparoscopy and laparoscopic ultrasonography avoid exploratory laparotomy in patients with hepatocellular carcinoma. *Ann Surg.* 1998;227:527.
29. Romijn MG; van Overhagen H, Spillernaar Bilgen EJ, et al. Laparoscopy and laparoscopic ultrasonography in staging of oesophageal and cardial carcinoma. *Br J Surg.* 1998;85:1012.

Chapter Sixty • • • • • •

*L*aparoscopy and Oncology: Diagnostic and Therapeutic Staging in Digestive Oncology

MIGUEL A. CUESTA and S. MEIJER

The growing development of minimally invasive surgery (MIS) in its diagnostic and therapeutic aspects assigns an increasing role to this approach in the diagnosis and treatment of tumors of the digestive tract.[1,2] The surgeon, who usually works in oncological surgery and at the same time has experience with laparoscopic surgery, will try to take advantages of what this laparoscopic surgery may offer for the solution of diagnostic and staging problems caused by gastrointestinal tumors, as well as for their radical or palliative treatment.

The goal of this chapter is to describe the laparoscopic staging of different gastrointestinal tumors; if only palliative treatment is indicated, a description is given of how to perform it laparoscopically.

LAPAROSCOPIC STAGING OF TUMORS

Laparoscopy has been widely used for many years by gastroenterologists as an important diagnostic tool in undiagnosed ascites, liver and spleen diseases, and abdominal masses.[3] In the last 20 years, its use has been replaced by the development of modern imaging techniques and guided fine-needle biopsies. However, with the expansion of minimally invasive surgery, laparoscopic techniques are also playing an increasingly valuable role in the preoperative staging of tumors.

Imaging of abdominal organs, especially the liver and pancreas, has greatly improved with the introduction of ultrasound (US), enhanced computed tomography (CT), and magnetic resonance imaging (MRI).[4,5] Despite these techniques, the surgeon dealing with patients having malignancies in these organs is often faced with a wide discrepancy between pre- and perioperative staging, mainly due to the presence of liver and lymph nodes and peritoneal metastases.

More accurate staging before the operation is desirable, especially for cancer of the esophagus, stomach, liver, bile ducts, and pancreas. In these cases, the presence of metastases means that surgery is neither the only nor always the best palliative treatment.[1,6,7] In the case of hepatic tumors, moreover, determining their exact diagnosis, and their number (in the case of metastases) and localization in the liver segments, is imperative when considering liver resection or adjuvant therapy.

Laparoscopy performed prior to a planned laparotomy will, upon inspection of the liver, abdominal cavity, and lesser sac, visualize these metastases, allow for biopsies, and therefore prevent an unnecessary laparotomy. Laparoscopy is still limited in the assessment of less obvious hepatic and retroperitoneal tumors, but it is here where ultrasound performed during laparotomy has proven its value.[8,9] Nowadays, it is possible to perform laparoscopic ultrasound by introducing an ultrasound transducer via the cannula,[10] combining visualization of the abdominal cavity and ultrasound of the liver, biliary tract, pancreas, and retroperitoneal lymph nodes.

Another sign in which diagnostic laparoscopy can demonstrate its value can be in the presence of ascites and/or abdominal masses remaining undiagnosed or unclearly staged in a specific patient after several advanced imaging investigations. Diagnostic laparoscopy will, by visualization of the abdominal cavity and the masses and with the possibility of taking biopsies, establish the diagnosis and stage the tumor.[3]

We will explain first the possibilities, instruments, and technique of diagnostic laparoscopy (DL) alone or in combination with ultrasound (laparoscopic ultrasound, LUS); and second, the use of imaging modalities (US, CT, and MRI) for staging of these tumors.[4,5,11,12] However, there are substantial differences in resolution, costs, and availability of the various techniques, leading to conflicting statistics when comparing alternative modalities.

ULTRASOUND

Transabdominal US still plays a crucial role in detecting, diagnosing, and evaluating liver and bile duct malignancies, but less in the case of pancreatic and retroperitoneal lymph nodes and peritoneal metastases. It provides multiplanar imaging with excellent spatial resolution. Hepatic vascular (portal and hepatic venous) anatomy and patency are accurately displayed using color Doppler flow techniques. US is, however, highly operator dependent and easily restricted by patient habitus or interference by bowel gas and the rib cage. Although sensitivity as high as 94% has been reported for detection of small hepatomas, results are generally much more variable, with sensitivities ranging from 20 to 76% in the detection of colorectal liver metastases. And it is here where an exact diagnosis, and knowledge of the number of the metastases and their localization in the liver segments, are mandatory before the laparotomy.

US is especially suited to screening liver metastases during follow-up of colorectal cancer, and in following the development of hepatocellular carcinoma in patients with liver cirrhosis.

COMPUTED TOMOGRAPHY

The principal imaging methods used in the preoperative assessment of intra-abdominal tumors are based on CT scanning. Various enhancement techniques exist, including helicoid CT scan, dynamic contrast bolus, delayed scanning, and arterial portography (CTAP). Conventional CT will detect hepatic involvement in 90% of cases, but only 70% of actual lesions are reliably documented. Thirty to 50% of individual lesions remain undetected. Conventional CT is unable to visualize hepatic (and peritoneal) nodules under 1 cm in size due to the partial volume effect. The detection rate of helicoid CT is better. In the case of pancreatic tumors, CT is a good diagnostic method for determining the size of the tumor, but is not reliable for detection of small peritoneal or liver metastases. Because of its ability to provide general information regarding tumor growth and spreading, CT remains the primary imaging modality for the staging of patients with intra-abdominal malignancies.

INDICATIONS FOR DIAGNOSTIC LAPAROSCOPY

1. Staging of upper gastrointestinal cancers
   - Hepatic tumors (primary and metastases)
   - Bile duct cancer (Klatskin tumors)
   - Esophageal and gastric cardia cancer
   - Gastric cancer
   - Head of the pancreas and ampulla cancer
   - Pancreatic cancer
   - Colorectal cancer
2. Diagnosing and staging abdominal masses (and/or ascites)

SURGICAL TECHNIQUE

General Aspects

Diagnostic laparoscopy (DL) (with laparoscopic ultrasound, LUS) is usually planned as a separate procedure, as this allows the most efficient planning of operating room time and may have psycho-logical advantages in discussing therapeutic options. Alternatively, it may be done directly before the planned laparotomy.

The operation is performed under general anesthesia as this allows the greatest freedom for complete and precise information. The entire procedure takes approximately 40 minutes. Patients may be discharged after several hours, making it possible to use outpatient facilities if available.

Performing the LUS examination in collaboration with a radiologist is certainly advisable during the learning phase. It also provides an independent observer for interpreting the US images, one who is less likely to be biased by a motivation for resection.

Positioning (Patient and Trocars)

The patient is placed in the supine position and supported to allow tilting of the operating table as necessary. The surgeon and radiologist stand on the left side with the assistant opposite. Video monitor and ultrasound screen are on the upper right side. After inducing pneumoperitoneum, the laparoscope (10 mm, 0 degrees) is introduced through the lower aspect of the umbilicus and connected to the video camera. The placement of trocars obviously depends on the existing abdominal scars (especially during the assessment of patients with colorectal metastases). The safest technique in these cases is through open placement of a Hasson trocar in the right upper abdomen (after left colon surgery) or left subcostal region (after right-sided colon resections). Once the laparoscope has been introduced, secondary trocars are placed under visual control, which may require taking down adhesions. Generally DL and LUS examination requires access from the right subcostal region, preferably introduced between the midclavicular and anterior axillary lines. A second port is needed for full examination and may be introduced left subcostal. These auxiliary trocars are preferably 10/11 mm disposable ones if laparoscopic ultrasonography is also planned, to avoid damaging the LUS transducer surface with the metallic valves. When only diagnostic laparoscopy is planned, 5-mm trocars are sufficient. An ultrasonographic transducer (linear or sector, generally 7.5 MHz) is introduced through these 10-mm cannulas in order to perform the LUS of different organs.

For direct contact ultrasonography of the liver, our group uses a rigid probe with a 7.5-mHz 10-mm linear array transducer, coupled to a mobile US unit (SSD 650, Aloka Co., Tokyo). To allow better contact between the convex liver surface and the rigid probe, about 1000 mL of normal saline solution is routinely instilled in the upper abdomen to provide an acoustic window. The abdomen is mostly desufflated to further improve contact with the liver. Maintaining visual guidance of the probe's position on the liver with the laparoscope aids in orientation. Essential in examination of the liver is to be acquainted with its segmental anatomy (according to Couineaud). The exact location of the tumor/metastases relative to the central vascular structures is assessed.

The following types of information can be obtained by diagnostic laparoscopy:

1. Visualization of abdominal organs
   - Primary tumor
   - Surface of liver and spleen
   - Ascites and peritoneal metastases
   - Hepatoduodenal ligament
   - Inspection of the pancreas through the gastrohepatic ligament (Meyer-Burg's approach) and the gastrocolic ligament (Strauch's approach)

- Intestines, internal genitals, and Douglas space
- Mesenteric axis
2. Taking of biopsies and cytology
   - Peritoneal lavage
   - Biopsy forceps
   - Tru-cut needle
   - Chiba needle
3. Laparoscopic ultrasound for assessment of
   - Solid organs
   - Retroperitoneum
   - Lymph nodes (e.g., coeliac axis)

LIVER AND BILIARY TRACT TUMORS

Selection Criteria for Laparoscopic Ultrasound

The inclusion criteria for undergoing DL and LUS in patients with hepatic lesions were (1) the presence of hepatic lesions with no certainty regarding the diagnosis (e.g., lesions other than cysts and hemangiomas found during workup of abdominal pain); (2) hepatic lesions found during staging of tumors other than gastrointestinal cancer (e.g., breast cancer) and where the correct diagnosis is essential for outlining further treatment; (3) ascertaining resectability of hepatic metastases (from colorectal cancer) when during the preoperative studies doubt still existed about the number or localization in the liver segments; (4) follow-up of patients with colorectal cancer in whom an increase in carcinoembriogenic antigen (CEA) is found without liver metastasis or local recurrence; (5) evaluation of extension and/or multicentricity of hepatocellular carcinoma in patients with and without liver cirrhosis with determination of its resectability; (6) follow-up of other cancers such as ovarian, melanoma, sarcoma, and gastric cancer in order to ascertain the resectability of metastases; (7) liver adenomas found on ultrasonography during evaluation for symptomatic gallstones and considered suitable for laparoscopic resection; and (8) preoperative assessment of the operability of Klatskin tumors, gallbladder cancer, and common bile duct cancer.[13]

Diagnostic Laparoscopy

All peritoneal deposits are best considered suspect and require biopsy to exclude malignancy. Occasionally, benign mesothelial proliferations may appear as multiple peritoneal metastases and small hamartomas in the liver surface will also appear as multiple metastases (von Meyenburg complex). The visual aspect of lesions seen on the liver surface is often diagnostic. Cysts are greenish-blue in appearance when visible at the surface. Small metastases are usually easily identified, and larger ones have a typical umbilicated/crater appearance. The recognition of satellite lesions is difficult when there are regeneration nodules in a cirrhotic liver.

Laparoscopic Ultrasound

Most intrahepatic lesions can be characterized by their ultrasound appearance. Cysts show an empty cavity with acoustic shadowing. Hemangiomas are hyperechoic, homogeneous, and compressible. Hepatocellular carcinoma and metastases have poor echoic deposits that are alternatively hyperechoic or have a bulls-eye appearance. In all cases where LUS indicated inoperability, biopsies were taken of the peritoneum, liver metastases, and/or lymph nodes to confirm this finding from frozen section diagnosis.

Criteria for Resectability on Laparoscopic Ultrasound

The criterion for resectability of patients with liver metastases from colorectal cancer is the presence of fewer than four metastases in the entire liver parenchyma.[13]

For hepatocellular carcinoma, the only criterion was the possibility of performing radical resection, up to extended right or left hemihepatectomy or even liver transplantation. Extension of the cancer to outside the liver indicated unsuitability for resection.

For gallbladder carcinoma, the spread of the tumor outside the gallbladder and its hepatic bed, such as metastases in the liver, obstruction of the confluence of the hepatic duct, and peritoneal metastases, means unresectability.

For Klatskin tumors and common bile duct carcinoma, criteria for unresectability were the presence of liver or peritoneal metastases or lymph node metastases outside the hepatoduodenal ligament, visualization of the tumor in the hepatoduodenal ligament, the presence of portal hypertension, and encasement or thrombosis of the portal vein.

Confirmation of the Diagnosis by Laparoscopic Ultrasound

It is important to realize that the indiscriminate biopsy of lesions may result in needle-tract or port-site metastases, and should not be performed when there is a possibility of performing curative surgery. The lesions can be identified by their visual and ultrasonographic aspect.

Discussion

Yamakawa and Wagai introduced laparoscopic ultrasonography in the evaluation of gallbladder cancer in 1963.[14] Since then, other authors have described similar examinations for the diagnosis of hepatic and pancreatic lesions using linear array and sector scanners.[15–23] Using a laparoscopic linear array scanner, we obtained additional information leading to a change in surgical approach in 28 of 45 patients (62%) with different liver lesions. In 13 patients this information was provided solely by visualizing the abdominal cavity using laparoscopy, and in another 9 patients by a combination of data obtained through laparoscopy and ultrasound; in another 6 patients with less visible tumors, this information was obtained primarily by ultrasonography.[18]

John et al[20] assessed by laparoscopic ultrasonography a cohort group of 50 consecutive patients diagnosed as having potentially resectable liver tumors (9 primary tumors, 37 secondary, and 6 nonmalignant). The presence of adhesions precluded laparoscopic assessment in 4% of the patients. Six patients had liver cirrhosis. Laparoscopic exploration precluded curative resection in 23 (46%) patients. Factors such as extrahepatic tumor spread, bilobar dissemination of disease, and unexpected extrahepatic tumor sites were described by laparoscopy and ultrasonography.

Our group has studied the value of DL and LUS in the staging and selection of patients with colorectal liver metastases.[24] Fifty consecutive patients were considered to be candidates for resection on the basis of preoperative imaging studies (ultrasonography and CT). Diagnostic laparoscopy could not be performed in 3 out of 50 patients because of adhesions. On the basis of DL and LUS, 18 (38%) patients were found not to be candidates for resection. Reasons included the presence of extrahepatic metastases, more metastases in the liver, or no metastases at all. In these patients an explorative laparotomy could be avoided. Of the 29 patients who subsequently underwent laparotomy and ultrasonography, another 6 (13%) were deemed unresectable.

Laparoscopic ultrasonography, at the present time in its development, is a reliable technique that will contribute to a more accurate preoperative staging of liver and biliary tract malignancies. According to the previous studies, approximately 50% of the patients considered resectable preoperatively by external ultrasonography and CT were finally selected for resection on the basis of DL and LUS. The technique should be compared with other proven methods such as open ultrasonography, and in selected groups of patients will replace other preoperative imaging techniques. With the development of small transducers, this procedure will be performed on an outpatient basis in the near future.

ESOPHAGUS AND GASTRIC CARDIA CANCER

Preoperative staging of esophageal and gastric cardia cancers includes the assessment for metastases by US of the neck and CT scan of the abdomen (with special attention to the liver and lymph nodes of the coleiac axis) and local staging by endoscopic US and in the case of proximal esophageal tumors by tracheobronchoscopy. Metastases are confirmed by biopsy guided by US or CT.

Diagnostic Laparoscopy

The main goal of diagnostic laparoscopy in preoperative staging of carcinoma of the esophagus or gastric cardia is to avoid an unnecessary explorative laparotomy in patients with incurable disease. Special technical pitfalls during the DL are the inspection of the hiatus and the coeliac axis. The left lobe of the liver will be elevated by a probe, followed by opening the gastrohepatic ligament in order to visualize the hiatus and the coeliac axis. Extraesophageal extension of the tumor or carcinomatosis or extensive mass in the coeliac axis will indicate biopsy.

Watt et al[6] have demonstrated the value of diagnostic laparoscopy for the preoperative evaluation of intra-abdominal metastases in patients with cancer of the esophagus and gastric cardia, comparing it with preoperative US and CT. They demonstrated, in a prospective study, that laparoscopy was significantly more sensitive than US or CT for the demonstration of hepatic metastases. Furthermore, laparoscopy was much more reliable for the identification of secondary lymph node involvement even if it was statistically significant only when compared to US. As for demonstration of peritoneal metastases, laparoscopy was able to detect them in 8 of 9 cases, contrary to US and CT, which had not shown any. The authors conclude that laparoscopy is a safe and reliable method for the preoperative evaluation of cancer of the esophagus and gastric cardia and may avoid, in view of alternative palliative therapies, an unnecessary laparotomy.

Dagnini,[25] with a series of 280 patients with esophageal and 89 with gastric cardia cancer assessed by laparoscopy, found metastases or extension of the tumor beyond resection in 14% of the patients and liver cirrhosis in another 14% of the patients that excluded them from resection.

Laparoscopic Ultrasound

Bemelman et al[26] studied a group of 56 patients who were selected for curative resection of carcinoma of the esophagus (n = 38) or gastric cardia with involvement of the distal esophagus (n = 18) after a routine preoperative workup. During laparoscopic ultrasound, the abdominal cavity was assessed for metastatic spread and ultrasonography was performed of the liver and coeliac axis. In all patients without histologically proven metastases, laparotomy was then performed.

Laparotomy was avoided in 2 (11%) patients and the preoperative stage changed in 7 patients (41%), all of whom had cancer of the distal esophagus and gastric cardia. This was also the case in one (3%) and 2 (6%) patients with middle and distal carcinoma of the esophagus, respectively. The authors concluded that preoperative staging by DL and LUS is of little value in patients with carcinoma of the middle and lower esophagus. The probable role of LUS in staging patients with cancer of the gastric cardia remains to be confirmed in a larger series. Staging laparoscopy might be indicated when a transthoracic approach of the tumor is chosen as the first step of surgery. Future protocols with neoadjuvant multichemotherapy, more effective than single-modality chemotherapy, will need a pretreatment correct staging of the cardia cancer by laparoscopy in order to evaluate results.

Criteria of incurability for cancer of the esophagus and gastric cardia assessed by preoperative and diagnostic laparoscopy are as follows:

- Incurable. Due to local factors: ingrowth in bronchotracheal tree, aorta, or pancreas. Distal metastases: hematogenic metastases, peritoneal metastases, lymph nodes, neck, or coeliac axis.
- Potentially curable. Due to local factors: limited ingrowth in diaphragm. Distal metastases: lymph node metastases in the chest or along the (root of) left gastric artery.

GASTRIC CANCER

Patients with symptomatic gastric cancer, such as obstruction or bleeding, do not need to be assessed by laparoscopy because the surgeon may be committed to resection even if only palliation may be achieved.[27] But in the case of an asymptomatic patient with gastric cancer, if laparoscopy demonstrates peritoneal or liver metastases, it is a matter of judgment whether or not to perform a palliative resection to improve the quality of life.

Another indication for DL will be in cases with local advanced gastric cancer, T3 and T4 by endoscopic ultrasound, in which laparoscopy can determine the T and M stage with greater precision than established imaging methods can provide in order to start some multimodality neoadjuvant chemotherapy before surgical exploration.

Diagnostic Laparoscopy and Laparoscopic Ultrasound

Kriplani and Kapur,[28] in a series of 40 patients with gastric cancer potentially resectable by preoperative study, found metastases in 12.5% and locally advanced unresectable tumors in another 11 patients (27%). Because there were no signs of obstruction or hemorrhage in 40% of patients, an explorative laparotomy could be avoided. These results were confirmed by Possik et al,[29] who in a series of 360 patients with gastric cancer found peritoneal and liver metastases by laparoscopy in 37% and 18%, respectively. Laparoscopy detected these metastases with an accuracy of 89% and 96%, respectively. Similar results were found by Burke et al,[30] with a 37% prevalence of metastases in 110 patients with gastric cancer judged to be free of intra-abdominal metastases on preoperative CT. In their series, in 24% of patients an unnecessary laparotomy could be avoided.

Ungeheuer et al[31] investigated 170 patients with gastric cancer (T3 or T4) by DL and LUS. A significant part of the study was the complete assessment of the stomach by laparoscopy, including the anterior and posterior wall of the stomach (by opening the gastrocolic ligament with inspection of the pancreas and coeliac axis) and the gastroesophageal junction (opening the gastrohepatic ligament). LUS included not only the liver but also the stomach wall by introducing 300 mL saline into the stomach.

In 50% of patients the staging was confirmed by DL and LUS and in another 50% the staging was changed by laparoscopy—that means a change in the initially planned treatment in 41% of patients. LUS findings accounted for 7% of the changes.

The preoperative staging needed to be upgraded in 24% of patients (peritoneal carcinomatosis and tumor invasion of pancreas and liver), whereas a downgrading was achieved in 16%.

Conclusion

DL and LUS in patients with gastric cancer are mandatory if suspicion exists of unconfirmed peritoneal or liver metastasis in patients with asymptomatic gastric cancer (nonobstructed, nonbleeding patients). Also, diagnostic laparoscopy is considered a prerequisite for the determination of adequate therapy in a multimodal approach to locally advanced (T3 or T4) gastric cancer.

TUMORS OF THE PANCREATIC HEAD REGION

Pancreatic cancer has the worst prognosis of all gastrointestinal malignancies. According to the National Cancer Institute, only 3% of patients will be alive 5 years after diagnosis. A good preoperative staging is therefore mandatory in order to select patients for effective intent to cure. According to the staging, patients who cannot be cured will be selected for palliative therapy.

Cuschieri[32] has indicated that DL is a good method for the diagnosis and staging in patients with cancer of the pancreas, visualizing the abdominal cavity and the lesser omental sac and being able at the same time to obtain biopsies and cytology of the primary tumor and possible metastases.

Warshaw et al[7] and Fernanadez del Castillo et al[33] furthermore showed us that even if the CT scan may supply useful information about the size of the primary tumor, it is not meaningful for the discovery of the small hepatic and peritoneal metastases typical of pancreatic cancer.

Radiologic assessment by CT scan focuses on the following:

- Tumor size and location.
- Presence or absence of hepatic or peritoneal metastases or ascites.
- Presence of extrahepatic tumor extension.
- Presence or absence of lymph nodes, particularly coeliac, peripancreatic, or periportal.
- Vascular encasement.

Radiologic criteria for unresectability were hepatic or peritoneal metastases, definitive vascular encasement, or obstruction. The presence of lymph nodes, minimal ascites, or the appearance

of vascular encroachment were considered relative criteria for unresectability. Patients with relative criteria or a normal CT scan are considered candidates for DL.

Criteria for Resectability on Laparoscopy and Ultrasonography

For the preoperative assessment of resectability of tumors of the pancreatic head, diagnostic laparoscopy plays a very important role because of its ability to visualize small distant metastases and tumor deposits in the lymph nodes, both of which are difficult to assess by the preoperative studies. Other criteria for unresectability are visualization of the tumor in the hepatoduodenal ligament or outside of the duodenum, and the presence of portal hypertension.[7,13,33–35,52]

Diagnostic laparoscopy can be used in three ways. These are, in order of increasing difficulty, (1) diagnostic laparoscopy "scan," (2) extensive diagnostic laparoscopy, and (3) diagnostic laparoscopy with laparoscopic ultrasonography.

Diagnostic Laparoscopy "Scan"

The so-called diagnostic laparoscopy scan is a diagnostic procedure in which the surgeon, in a sitting previously to the planned duodenopancreatomy, performs a simple inspection of the peritoneum, surface of the liver, hepatoduodenal ligament, duodenum, mesocolon, and coeliac axis. If metastases are present, these are biopsied. No other investigation is conducted (such as an extensive inspection of the inframesocolic areas or washing cytology). This exploration is performed with three trocars, an infraumbilical trocar for the laparoscope and two others of 5 mm placed under the subcostal margins. It is a reliable method, simple to perform and to interpret, and takes only about 15 minutes.

In our experience with this method, performed in 32 patients with a "curable" tumor in the pancreatic head, 12 patients had small liver metastases and 2 had an extension of the tumor through the duodenal wall. Therefore, in 43% of the patients an explorative laparotomy could be avoided. The rest of the patients were operated on; 6 of them (18%) were found unresectable because of invasion of the tumor into the portal vein (5) or the caval vein (1). Finally, in the remaining 12 patients (40%), a duodenopancreatectomy could be performed.

Extensive Diagnostic Laparoscopy

Warshaw and others,[7,33,35,36] in a series of 114 patients (89 with pancreatic cancer in the head of the pancreas and 25 in the body or tail) potentially resectable according to the preoperative CT scan, performed a diagnostic laparoscopy for preoperative assessment. Patients with cystoadenocarcinoma and ampullomas were not included in the series.

Simple laparoscopic inspection of the whole abdominal cavity (peritoneum, liver, lesser sac, coeliac axis, porta hepatis, duodenum, and transverse mesocolon) was performed along with peritoneal lavage and a biopsy of suspected metastases. Metastases were found in 27 patients (24%). Intra-abdominal spread was more common in tumors of the body or tail of the pancreas (44%) and less in the head (18%). None of the patients with proved metastases underwent further surgery. Jaundice was palliated with endoscopic or percutaneous stents or both.

Of the 87 patients without intra-abdominal spread, 42 were found to have vascular invasion by angiography and were offered radiation therapy. Finally, 40 patients were explored with intent to resection, and this was accomplished in 30 (75% of surgically explored patients and 26% of those who underwent laparoscopy). Resectability was 26% in previous series. Sensitivity of the procedure was 93%.

This study demonstrated that unsuspected intra-abdominal metastases were identified by diagnostic laparoscopy in 24% of patients previously screened by CT. This prevalence is lower than that reported by the same authors in the period between 1982 and 1989, when it was 41%. Other authors have reported figures of 39%, 44%, and 73%.[33,35,36] Reasons for this decrease could be due to tumors being diagnosed earlier, the improved capacity of the CT scanner to diagnose small metastases (seems unlikely given the typical size of these metastases, 1 to 2 mm), and perhaps the favorable change in the benignity of the tumor.

Diagnostic Laparoscopy With Laparoscopic Ultrasonography

What can laparoscopic ultrasound add to these figures? Bemelman et al[34] described the value of diagnostic and laparoscopic ultrasonography in a group of 73 patients (stage I according to the American Committee for staging of cancer) suitable for curative resection (after US and Doppler examination).

Laparoscopic ultrasonography will add important information for finding (1) metastases in the rest of the hepatic parenchyma, (2) invasion of vascular structures (portal vein and superior mesenteric vein), and (3) involved N3 lymph nodes in the hepatoduodenal ligament or coeliac axis. Proven involvement will mean inoperability. Biopsies were taken under direct laparoscopic or ultrasonographic guidance using biopsy forceps or Tru-cut needles and Rotex biopsy needles. Biopsies from the lymph nodes were taken if the examination fullfilled these criteria: larger than 1 cm, hypoechoic appearance, and disappearance of the hyperechoic hilum. Patients with a negative laparoscopy underwent a laparotomy for resection.

Sixteen of the 21 patients with distant metastases were diagnosed by DL (10 patients) and LUS. Forty-nine patients had surgical exploration and trial dissection to assess local resectability. Twenty-nine patients (41%) had resectable cancers. Positive predictive value of local invasion by LUS was 93%. Laparotomy was avoided in 19% of patients, and the preoperative stage was changed in 41%.

An interesting point is the predictive value of LUS in the assessment of local invasion into large vessels: 22 patients were considered resectable (no tumor contact with large vessels) by LUS, whereas 21 patients were resectable during the operation. Thirteen patients were considered probably resectable (tumor contact with large vessels), but only 7 could definitely not be resected. And finally, of 14 patients considered unresectable (tumor infiltration of large vessels and loss of white plane) by LUS, only 2 could be radically resected. The authors concluded that visualization of local tumor extension in major vessels by LUS is technically demanding and ultrasonographically guided biopsies are difficult to take. An important shortcoming for this technique is that LUS probes are not equipped for this. Surgical exploration must always be carried out if histologic proof of metastastic disease is not obtained.

Comparable results to those reported by Bemelman et al were obtained by our group and by John et al.[37] In a series of 40 pa-

tients they found unsuspected peritoneal and/or liver metastases in 14 patients (35%). LUS was responsible for upstaging the disease to unresectable status in 10 patients (25%) following negative laparoscopy.

Conclusions

Diagnostic laparoscopy is a mandatory exploration for patients who are candidates for resection due to pancreatic head tumors (Table 60–1). In spite of several publications favoring this technique, until now it has not been taken up by the general surgeon, whose current extensive experience with laparoscopic techniques and equipment is facilitating the introduction of DL for the preoperative assessment of pancreatic head cancer.

The three methods described here represent an increasing difficulty grade. The scan method of DL is within the reach of every general surgeon coping with pancreatic cancer surgery. The more extensive diagnostic laparoscopy, and especially the addition of laparoscopic ultrasonography to DL, will increase the difficulty grade of interpretation. Decisions concerning whether or not to perform an explorative laparotomy on ultrasonographic imaging of invasion of the tumor into the portal vein or the presence of lymph nodes with malignant characteristics without pathologic confirmation are not ethically responsible. Nowadays, these LUS studies belong to the chapter of fundamental clinical investigations and in the future will have important consequences for surgical decision-making.

Trial dissection should be performed to confirm the findings of LUS on local unresectability until sufficient experience has been obtained with this new diagnostic modality. Development of better ultrasonographically guided biopsy devices will help to solve these problems. On the other hand, noninvasive procedures such as MERCP (magnetic resonance cholangiopancreatography) and positron emission tomography (PET) can mean a better staging procedure without the necessity for the more invasive diagnostic laparoscopy. Studies and trials will be performed to find the most reliable and noninvasive method for the patient.

For patients with unresectable pancreatic head cancer following diagnostic laparoscopy, a palliative biliodigestive anastomosis can be performed laparoscopically. Also, trials will be performed here to establish which of the present methods of palliation—placement of stents, or open or laparoscopic surgery—will provide better results and quality of life to these disabled patients. This laparoscopic staging is only of value in the case that patients can be palliated endoscopically. If conventional palliation by laparotomy is needed, in order to perform a gastro- and choledocho-jejunostomy, all of the potential advantages of endoscopic staging will disappear.

TABLE 60–1. ALGORITHM FOR STUDY AND TREATMENT OF CARCINOMA OF PANCREATIC HEAD AND PERIAMPULLARY REGION

1. Preoperatory assessment: conventional ultrasound and CT
2. ERCP and introduction of biliary stent. If unresectable, the patient is already palliated
3. Diagnostic laparoscopy (and ultrasonography). If peritoneal or liver metastases, the patient is already palliated with the biliary stent
4. Laparotomy
   If metastases or vascular infiltration, palliation (stent)
   Otherwise, duodeno-pancreatectomy

PANCREATIC CANCER

Warshaw et al[7] found intra-abdominal metastases in 11 of a series of 25 patients with body and tail pancreatic cancer (44%). This figure was 62% (18 of 29 patients) in his 1982 to 1989 series. Diagnostic laparoscopy will therefore be routinely employed as a preoperative assessment tool in all patients with this type of pancreatic cancer.

COLON CANCER

Diagnostic laparoscopy and ultrasound should be performed in every laparoscopic intervention for colorectal cancer. Staging of this colorectal cancer is an essential part of the operation. The lack of manual palpation of the liver will necessitate the use of DL and LUS in order to stage this cancer correctly. Hartley et al found a superior detection of hepatic lesions with laparoscopic ultrasound compared to preoperative ultrasound and similar to MRI.[38] Abdominal lavage for cytology, liver inspection and ultrasonography, and inspection of the peritoneum and mesentery of the small bowel and colon are mandatory diagnostic steps before resection.

ABDOMINAL MASSES AND/OR ASCITES

In most patients the cause of the ascites can be determined by clinical and laboratory assessment including cytology of the ascitic fluid. But inability to determine the cause of ascites is a clear indication for diagnostic laparoscopy.[39] Macroscopically, the ascitic fluid observed at laparoscopy may indicate the nature of the underlying disease and can be classified as serious (yellow/green), chylous, myxomatous (colloidal), or blood-stained.

Sometimes, despite radiologic studies (ultrasonography and CT scan), the presence of a palpable abdominal mass(es) with or without ascites remains undiagnosed. In order to establish a diagnosis and a therapeutic program, a diagnostic laparoscopy should be performed. This permits a definitive diagnosis, staging, and therapeutic planning through inspection of the tumor, the relation of the tumor with the rest of the organs, the presence of liver and peritoneal spreading, and the possibility for taking cytology and biopsies. This exploration will be performed at a point that can by its effectiveness reduce unnecessary cost to patients (in both time and expense).

Retroperitoneal nodal enlargement without the existence of enlarged lymph nodes in other more accessible areas (neck and groin) will mean the necessity of taking biopsies to confirm or exclude the existence of a lymphoma. A percutaneous biopsy cannot always be taken, and therefore laparoscopy will by inspection and exposure of the retroperitoneum permit these biopsies by means of forceps, Tru-cut needles, and so forth.

PALLIATIVE TECHNIQUES FOLLOWING DIAGNOSIS AND STAGING

For the surgical treatment of cancer of the head of pancreas, there is the growing trend to preoperatively evaluate its resectability using diagnostic laparoscopy. Traditionally, if the cancer is not resectable with radical criteria, because of the presence of distant or local metastases or by invasion into the portal vein, the surgeon will perform a digestive bypass and occasionally prophylactically a gastrojejunal anastomosis to bypass the partially obstructed duodenum.

Following recent publications with report of an 18% mortality in doing this palliative surgery,[40] there is a growing interest in noninvasive palliative treatment of obstructive jaundice, placing a biliary endoprosthesis by the transpapillary route (via ERCP).[41] Recent evaluation of stent palliation versus conventional surgical palliation (gastrojejunostomy and choledochojejunostomy) show that the last procedure has better outcome then the stent in terms of septic complications, obstruction, and hospital stay, with no mortality at all (D. Gouma, personal communication).

Laparoscopic biliodigestive anastomosis is technically possible. But at the same time it is well known that a gastrojejunostomy will be necessary at least in one third of patients. Therefore a good alternative to the conventional double bypass will be the laparoscopic double anastomosis. Rothlin et al performed a case-controlled study and found that laparoscopic palliation (gastro- and hepaticojejunostomy) can reduce the three drawbacks of the open bypass surgery— high morbidity and mortality and long hospital stay.[42]

The published technique, technically easier, entails the anastomosis between the gallbladder and the jejunum in the form of a cholecystojejunostomy or hepaticojejunostomy, which may be performed manually or with the use of an endostapler.[42–44]

After the introduction of trocars, the technique essentially consists of the insertion of a needle in the gallbladder, to perform an intraoperative cholangiogram, to verify if the cystic duct is patent and if it is in direct communication with the common hepatic duct. The content of the gallbladder has been suctioned to make the procedure easier. The first jejunal loop is grasped and moved towards the gallbladder. A needle introduced through the right subcostal trocar is used to suture the gallbladder to the jejunal loop. With the help of the hook or the scissors, a small incision is made on either one of the structures, and through this a 3-cm endostapler is introduced to perform a side-to-side anastomosis. The opening is then closed with an endostapler or through a manual running suture in two layers, at the end of which it is important to check that the loop has not been obstructed at the level of the anastomosis.

Protocols will demonstrate the place of these interventions in comparison with palliative methods such as stents introduced percutaneously or through ERCP and endoscopic papillotomy.

Similarly to cancer of the head of the pancreas, as a matter of principle a gastrojejunostomy is indicated in cases of inoperable tumors of the duodenum or the first jejunal loop, or in the case of distal cancer of the stomach in patients in whom the resection is not possible. This procedure can be performed by the laparoscopic route, both manually and with the endostapler.[45–47] The technique is the same already described for the cholecystojejunostomy. After having performed the pneumoperitoneum and after having placed the trocars, with the help of sutures the anterior gastric wall on the greater curvature and the chosen jejunal loop are connected; a small incision is made on both organs, and twice the 3-cm endostapler is introduced and fired to perform a 6-cm anastomosis. The opening is then closed, either manually in two layers or with the use of the endostapler. Abdominal pain can be treated by bilateral thoracoscopic splanchnicectomy with encouraging results of pain relief.[48]

Other applications of endoscopic surgery in cancer palliation include the introduction of feeding gastrostomy and jejunostomy in patients with unresectable oropharyngeal and esophageal cancer,[49] percutaneous or laparoscopic treatment of liver tumors by cryosurgery or radiofrequency after exact localization by ultrasound,[50] palliative colonic resection in patients with metastatic disease,[51] creation of stomas in unresectable colorectal cancer, placement of port-a-cath systems in the hepatic artery for local chemotherapy for treatment of liver metastasis, placement of a peritoneo-jugular shunt for treatment of ascites, and the intra-abdominal placement of radiotherapy devices.

REFERENCES

1. Cuschieri A. Diagnosis and staging of tumours by laparoscopy. *Semin Laparosc Surg.* 1994;1:3.
2. Cuesta MA, Meijer S, Borgstein PJ. Laparoscopy and assessment of digestive cancer. *Br J Surg.* 1992;79:486.
3. Kalk H, Bruhl W. *Manual de Laparoscopia y Gastroscopia.* Madrid, Editorial Alhambra, 1957.
4. Sitzmann JV, Coleman J, Pitt HA, et al. Preoperative assessment of malignant hepatic tumors. *Am J Surg.* 1990;159:137.
5. Goulet RJ, Seekri I, Inman M, et al. The diagnosis and definition of hepatic malignancies by use of arterial enhanced computerized tomographic scanning. *Surgery.* 1990;108:694.
6. Watt I, Stewart I, Anderson D, et al. Laparoscopy, ultrasound and computed tomography in cancer of the oesophagus and gastric cardia: A prospective comparison for detecting intra-abdominal metastases. *Br J Surg.* 1989;76:1036.
7. Warshaw AL, Zhuo-yun-Gu, Wittenberg J, et al. Preoperative staging and assessment of resectability of pancreatic cancer. *Arch Surg.* 1990; 125:233.
8. Rifkin MD, Rosato FE, Branch HM, et al. Intraoperative ultrasound of the liver. An important adjunctive tool for decision-making in the operative room. *Ann Surg.* 1987;205:466.
9. Paul MA, Sibinga Mulder L, Cuesta MA, et al. Impact of intraoperative ultrasonography on treatment strategy for colorectal cancer. *Br J Surg.* 1994;81:1660.
10. Okita K, Kodama T, Oda M, et al. Laparoscopic ultrasonography. Diagnosis of liver and pancreatic cancer. *Scand J Gastroenterol.* 1984; 19(suppl 94):91.
11. Zerhouni EA, Rutter C, Hamilton SR, et al. CT and MR imaging in the staging of colorectal carcinoma: Report of the radiology diagnostic group II. *Radiology.* 1996;200:443.
12. Balfe DM. Hepatic metastases from colorectal cancer: Radiological strategies for improved selection. *Radiology.* 1992;185:18.
13. Cuesta MA, Meijer S, Borgstein PJ, et al. Laparoscopic ultrasonography for hepatobiliary and pancreatic malignancy. *Br J Surg.* 1993;80: 1571.
14. Yamakawa K, Wagai T. Diagnosis of intra-abdominal lesions by laparoscope. Ultrasonography through laparoscope. *Jpn J Gastroenterol.* 1963;55:741.
15. Bonhof JA, Frank K, Loch EG, et al. Laparoscopic sonography. *Ann Radiol.* 1985;28:16.
16. Frank K, Bliesze JA, Bonhof JA, et al. Laparoscopic ultrasonography: A new approach to intraabdominal disease. *J Clin Ultrasound.* 1985; 13:60.
17. Fornari F, Civardi G, Cavanna L, et al. Laparoscopic ultrasonography in the study of liver diseases. Preliminary results. *Surg Endosc.* 1989;3: 33.
18. Cuesta MA, Meijer S, Sibinga Mulder L. Laparoscopic ultrasonography for assessment of hepatic tumors. In: Cuesta MA, Nagy AG, eds. *Minimally Invasive Surgery in Gastrointestinal Cancer.* London, Churchill Livingstone, 1993;73.
19. John TG, Garden OJ. Laparoscopic ultrasonography: Extending the scope of diagnostic laparoscopy. *Br J Surg.* 1994;81:5.
20. John TG, Greig JD, Crosbi JL, et al. Superior staging of liver tumors with laparoscopy and laparoscopic ultrasound. *Ann Surg.* 1994;220: 711.
21. Miles WFA, Paterson-Brown S, Garden OJ. Laparoscopic contact hepatic ultrasonography. *Br J Surg.* 1992;79:419.
22. Jakimowicz JJ. Technical and clinical aspects of intraoperative ultrasound applicable to laparoscopic ultrasound. *Endosc Surg.* 1994;2:119.
23. Barbot DJ, Marks JH, Feld RI, et al. Improved staging of liver tumors using laparoscopic intraoperative ultrasound. *J Surg Oncol.* 1997;64:63.
24. Rahusen FD, Cuesta MA, Borgstein PJ, et al. Selection of patients for resection of colorectal metastases to the liver using diagnostic laparoscopy and laparoscopic ultrasonography. *Ann Surg.* 1999;230:31.
25. Dagnini G. Esophageal carcinoma. *Laparoscopy and Imaging Techniques.* Berlin, Springer Verlag, 1989;173.
26. Bemelman WA, van Delden OM, van Lanschot JJB, et al. Laparoscopy and laparoscopic ultrasonography in staging of carcinoma of the esophagus and gastric cardia. *J Am Coll Surg.* 1995;181:421.
27. Meijer S, de Bakker OJGB, Hoitsma HFW. Palliative resection in gastric cancer. *J Surg Oncol.* 1983;23:77.
28. Kriplani AK, Kapur BML. Laparoscopy for preoperative staging and assessment of operability in gastric carcinoma. *Gastrointest Endosc.* 1991;37:441.
29. Possik RA, Franco EL, Pires DR, et al. Sensitivity, specificity and predictive value of laparoscopy for the staging of gastric cancer and for detection of liver metastases. *Cancer.* 1986;58:1.
30. Burke EC, Karpeh MS, Conlon KC, et al. Laparoscopy in the management of gastric carcinoma. *Ann Surg.* 1997;225:262.
31. Ungeheuer A, Kraemer SJM, Feussner H, et al. Staging laparoscopy for gastric cancer. In: Phillips EH, Rosenthal RJ, eds. *Operative Strategies in Laparoscopic Surgery.* Berlin, Springer Verlag, 1995;159.
32. Cuschieri A. Laparoscopy for pancreatic cancer: Does it benefit the patient? *Eur J Surg Oncol.* 1988;14:41.
33. Fernandez del Castillo C, Rattner DW, Warshaw AL. Further experience with laparoscopy and peritoneal cytology in the staging of pancreatic cancer. *Br J Surg.* 1995;82:1127.
34. Bemelman WA, de Wit LTh, van Deelden OM, et al. Diagnostic laparoscopy combined with laparoscopic ultrasonography in staging of cancer of the pancreatic region. *Br J Surg.* 1995;82:820.
35. Conlon KC, Dougherty E, Kimstra DS, et al. The value of minimal access surgery in the staging of patients with potentially resectable peripancreatic malignancy. *Ann Surg.* 1996;223:134.
36. Ishida H. Peritoneoscopy and pancreas biopsy in the diagnosis of pancreatic diseases. *Gastrointest Endosc.* 1983;29:211.
37. John TG, Greig JD, Carter DC, et al. Carcinoma of the pancreatic head and periampullary region: Tumor staging with laparoscopy and laparoscopic ultrasonography. *Ann Surg.* 1995;221:156.
38. Hartley JE, Kumar H, Drew PJ, et al. Laparoscopic ultrasound for the detection of hepatic metastasis during laparoscopic colorectal surgery. *Dis Colon Rectum.* 2000;43:320.
39. Dagnini G. In: *Laparoscopy and Imaging Techniques.* Berlin, Springer Verlag, 1990;77.
40. Pretre R, Huber O, Robert J, et al. Results of surgical palliation for cancer of the head of the pancreas and periampullary region. *Br J Surg.* 1992;79:795.
41. Huibregtse K, Katon RM, Coene PP, et al. Endoscopic palliative treatment in pancreatic cancer. *Gastrointest Endosc.* 1986;32:334.
42. Rothlin MA, Schob O, Weber M. Laparoscopic gastro- and hepaticojejunostomy for palliation of pancreatic cancer: A case controlled study. *Surg Endosc.* 1999;13:1065.
43. Fletcher DR. Palliative surgery in pancreatic cancer. In: Cuesta MA, Nagy AG, eds. *Minimally Invasive Surgery in Gastrointestinal Cancer.* New York, Churchill Livingstone, 1993;112.
44. Cuschieri A. Laparoscopic surgery of the pancreas. *J R Coll Surg Edinb.* 1994;39:178.
45. Nagy AG, Brosseuk D, Hemming A, et al. Laparoscopic gastroenterostomy for duodenal obstruction. *Am J Surg.* 1995;169:539.

46. Fowler DL. Palliative surgery in upper digestive cancer. Laparoscopic gastroenterostomy. In: Cuesta MA, Nagy AG, eds. *Minimally Invasive Surgery in Gastrointestinal Cancer.* New York, Churchill Livingstone, 1993;123.

47. Bergamaschi R, Marvik R, Thoresen JE, et al. Open versus laparoscopic gastrojejunostomy for palliation in advanced cancer. *Surg Laparosc Endosc.* 1998;8:92.

48. Buscher HC, Jansen JJ, van Goor H. Bilateral thoracoscopic splanchnicectomy in patients with chronic pancreatitis. *Scand J Gastroenterol.* 1999;230(Suppl):29.

49. Weaver DW, Bouwman DL. Gastrostomy and jejunostomy by laparoscopic placement. In: Cuesta MA, Nagy AG, eds. *Minimally Invasive Surgery in Gastrointestinal Cancer.* London, Churchill Livingstone, 1993.

50. Cuschieri A, Bracken J, Boni L. Initial experience with laparoscopic ultrasound-guided radiofrequency thermal ablation of hepatic tumors. *Endoscopy.* 1999;31:318.

51. Molenaar CB, Bijnen AB, de Ruyter P. Indications for laparoscopic colorectal surgery. Results from the Medical Centre Alkmaar, the Netherlands. *Surg Endosc.* 1998;12:42.

52. Jimenez RE, Warshaw AL, Rattner DW, et al. Impact of laparoscopic staging in the treatment of pancreatic cancer. *Arch Surg.* 2000;135:409.

Chapter Sixty-One ·······

*I*mmunologic Consequences of Laparoscopic Surgery

COLIN SIETSES and MIGUEL A. CUESTA

INTRODUCTION

Today, the laparoscopic approach has become the operation of choice for a variety of procedures, including treatment of symptomatic gallstones, gastroesophageal reflux, and benign colonic diseases. Moreover, reports have shown that laparoscopic colon surgery is technically feasible and capable of fulfilling oncologic criteria for cancer surgery.[1–5] In general, laparoscopic techniques are thought to provide enormous benefits to patients, including faster recovery, shorter hospital stay, reduced postoperative morbidity, prompt return to normal activities, and superior cosmetic results.

One of the most important putative advantages of laparoscopic surgery is thought to be the reduction of the extent of surgical trauma.[6] Postoperative changes in the systemic immune response are proportional to the degree of surgical trauma, and subsequent immune suppression may be implicated in the development of septic complications and tumor metastasis.[7–9] In this review, an overview is given of the available literature, including our own data concerning laparoscopic surgery and postoperative immune function.

SYSTEMIC IMMUNE RESPONSE

The immunologic response to surgery has been increasingly studied since the introduction of minimally invasive techniques. Laparoscopic surgery reduces the magnitude of operative trauma. If alterations in the systemic immune response are proportional to the extent of injury, the response to minimally invasive technique will be reduced compared to that of conventional surgery. Comparative studies between the two techniques of a given surgical procedure offers the biological foundation of the advantages of laparoscopic surgery. In recent years a number of studies have been performed concerning the systemic immune response to laparoscopic surgery, both in animal models and in the clinical setting.

Cytokines and the Acute Phase Response

Cytokines and the acute phase response (APR) are vital to the immune function of the host, but overproduction or production at noninflammatory sites in some cases may lead to deleterious effects on the surrounding tissue.[10–11] Reduced production of cytokines and thereby a reduction in the inflammatory response is therefore thought to be beneficial for the patient's postoperative course.

Many of the nonhepatic manifestations of the APR such as fever, leukocytosis, and tachycardia, have been attributed to tumor necrosis factor-α (TNF-α) and interleukin-1 (IL-1),[12] whereas changes in hepatic protein synthesis are mainly caused by interleukin-6 (IL-6).[13] TNF-α and IL-1 are important cytokines in the activation of the systemic immune response and play a central role in initiating the cascade of inflammatory mediators and the subsequent activation of leukocytes that make up the immune response. Elevated plasma levels are usually not seen after conventional or laparoscopic surgery; however, significantly higher levels of IL-1, during and 6 hours after conventional cholecystectomy when compared to the laparoscopic approach have been described.[14]

Both IL-I and TNF-α mediate their actions through receptors on the surface membrane that, apparently in response to the same stimuli known to induce their production, are shed into the circulation (IL-1ra and sTNFr-P55 and P75). These soluble receptors are thought to antagonize and regulate the activity of both cytokines.[15] Unpublished data from our laboratory show that both types of sTNFr can be demonstrated after laparoscopic and conventional surgery, but no significant difference between the two procedures was observed. IL-Ira has also been demonstrated after both laparoscopic and conventional surgery. In contrast to the sTNFr levels, plasma levels of IL-Ira were significantly lower after the laparoscopic procedure, indicating less inflammation.[16]

IL-6 is a multifunctional cytokine that is involved in the modulation of host defense mechanisms such as local inflammation, and coordinates the systemic reaction known as the acute phase response (APR).[13] Plasma IL-6 levels are known to be proportional to the magnitude of the surgical procedure, and are predictive of postoperative complications.[17] Roumen et al[18] describe significant differences in postoperative IL-6 levels after laparoscopic chole-cystectomy, an observation that has frequently been confirmed by others (Fig. 61–1).[14,16,19–27]

However, the results concerning other surgical procedures show conflicting data. Hill et al[28] reported that the response of inflammatory mediators to hernia repair is not modified by undertaking the procedure laparoscopically. Perhaps the magnitude of the surgical injury from an open hernia repair is not large enough to demonstrate any significant reduction in the cytokine response after a minimally invasive laparoscopic repair. However, reports on more advanced laparoscopic procedures are also inconclusive. Harmon et al[29] described a significant blunting of the IL-6 response with the use of laparoscopic techniques for colectomy compared with standard laparotomy, but these data were not confirmed by others. Postoperative IL-6 levels have even been found to be higher after a laparoscopic approach by some researchers. Johnson et al[30] studied IL-6 levels after conventional and laparoscopically-assisted colectomy in dogs, and found significantly higher IL-6 levels after the laparoscopic approach. Stage et al[31] confirmed these results in a clinical study comparing laparoscopic versus open colonic resection for adenocarcinoma.

One possible explanation for the observed differences in postoperative IL-6 responses after colonic resection may be found in the techniques that were used (laparoscopically-assisted or the more invasive facilitated approach) or in the diversity of the patients included. Also, both benign and malignant diseases were studied. More studies are necessary to elucidate whether the observed advantages of the reduced inflammatory response seen after laparoscopic cholecystectomy also hold for other laparoscopic procedures.

The most frequently studied acute phase protein after laparoscopic surgical trauma is C-reactive protein (CRP). Postoperative CRP levels have been found to be significantly lower after the laparoscopic approach the first 2 days after surgery.[14,18–19,22,25–27,32–33] Measurement of other acute phase proteins does not show similar results. Vander Velpen et al[34] measured postoperative fibrinogen levels and found a significant increase after both procedures, but no difference between the procedures. These results were confirmed by Pike et al.[35] McMahon et al[36] measured various other acute phase proteins, such as albumin and transferrin, but found no differences between the laparoscopic and mini-laparotomy cholecystectomy. However, in contrast to various other studies, they also reported similar CRP levels after both approaches.

Interestingly, the reduced inflammatory response is not only seen after abdominal surgery. In a prospective randomized study of the inflammatory response after minimally invasive surgery of pneumothorax compared to standard thoracotomy, Gebhard et al[37] demonstrated that the release of inflammatory and vasoactive mediators was significantly lower after the laparoscopic procedure.

In summary, the data in the available literature on the postoperative inflammatory response to laparoscopic surgery were mostly obtained in patients undergoing cholecystectomy, and suggest reduced activation (IL-1ra, IL-6, and CRP) when compared with the conventional approach. However, less frequently studied cytokines (sTNFr and IL-8), acute phase proteins (fibrinogen, albumin, and transferrin), and other surgical procedures show a less clear picture.

Nonspecific Immune Response

Neutrophils play a central role in host defense, and dysfunction is clearly associated with an increased risk of infection. It is well recognized that the ability of neutrophils to phagocytose bacteria is reduced following trauma.[38] The impaired capacity of neutrophil phagocytosis is thought to be due to serum factors rather than intrinsic cellular defects.[39] There are several reports of decreased chemotaxis after surgery.[22,40] Furthermore, studies on intrinsic metabolic functions have showed increased leukotriene production and a increase in the production of superoxide anions.[22,41]

Comparative studies between laparoscopic and conventional cholecystectomy showed a transient increase in the total number of granulocytes after open surgery, but not after laparoscopic surgery.[21] After Nissen fundoplication, both techniques resulted in a significant increase in the number of granulocytes, and no differences in the number of white blood cells between the two approaches were observed; however, there are differences in postoperative granulocyte function between the two approaches.[42] Phagocytosis by polymorphonuclear leukocytes was significantly lower after a conventional Nissen fundoplication. No decrease in phagocytosis was observed after the laparoscopic Nissen fundoplication. This difference with the conventional procedure could be explained by a difference in the ability of the patients' plasma to

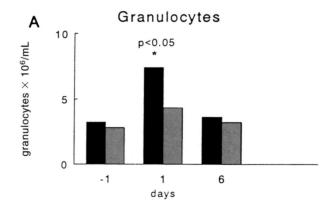

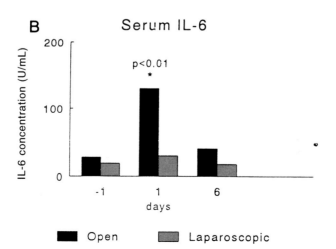

Figure 61–1. Median values of blood granulocytes (**A**) and serum IL-6 levels (**B**) in patients before and after open and laparoscopic cholecystectomy. *(Reproduced, with permission, from Kloosterman et al.20)*

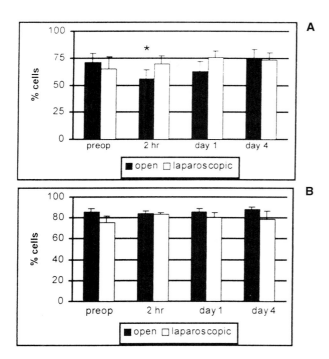

Figure 61–2. Phagocytic capacity of polymorphonuclear leukocytes (PMN). Preoperative and postoperative phagocytic capacity of PMN after open and laparoscopic Nissen fundoplication. *(Reproduced, with permission, from Sietses et al.[42])*

support opsonization of bacteria for phagocytosis (Fig. 61–2). Complement, antibodies, and fibronectin all contribute to the opsonic capacity of serum, which has repeatedly been found to be reduced after conventional surgery.[40] These effects are thought to be secondary to increased consumption during the postoperative inflammatory response.

This study also showed a significant difference in stimulated oxygen radical production between the conventional and the laparoscopic approach, suggesting a higher state of activation after conventional surgery. This difference in polymorphonuclear leukocyte (PMN) activation was further substantiated by the significant difference in CD11b expression between the laparoscopic and conventional technique. The CD11b receptor, a β_2-integrin, plays an important role in the emigration of PMN to sites of infection and inflammation. Cellular activation has also been studied by measuring postoperative hypochlorous acid generation, a potent neutrophil antimicrobial oxidant. In contrast to laparoscopic surgery, 1 day after conventional surgery hypochlorous acid production fell significantly compared with preoperative values.[43] It should be noted that a diverse group of patients was studied, including those with laparoscopic and laparoscopically assisted procedures. In a randomized prospective study, Redmond et al[22] reported significantly increased monocyte and neutrophil superoxide anion production and increased chemotaxis in open vs. laparoscopic cholecystectomy and correlated these differences with a significantly higher number of septic complications in the open group.

Interleukin-8 (IL-8) is one of the most important chemotactic cytokines (chemokine) for neutrophils. Decker et al[16] reported significantly higher plasma levels after conventional surgery when compared with a laparoscopic approach. Glaser et al[14] also studied postoperative IL-8 levels, but could not confirm the significant

difference between the two procedures. Another soluble factor which represents neutrophil activation is elastase. Postoperative levels have been found to be increased after both open and laparoscopic cholecystectomy; however, neutrophil elastase levels had returned to preoperative levels within 3 days after laparoscopic surgery, but remained elevated after the conventional approach.[44]

In the last few years it has become clear that the monocyte/macrophage has strong inflammatory, phagocytic, and tumoricidal functions and plays a central role in immune activation. The monocyte/macrophage is essential for recognition and processing of foreign antigens and it is responsible for antigen presentation to the lymphocytes, thus initiating the specific immune response. The major histocompatibility complex class II surface antigen, human leukocyte antigen-DR (HLA-DR), that is expressed on the surface of monocytes/macrophages is critical in this interaction.[45]

Kloosterman et al[20] studied monocyte HLA-DR expression as a parameter for trauma-induced immune suppression. They reported a significant reduction of HLA-DR expression 1 day after conventional surgery, but not after laparoscopic surgery (Fig. 61–3). These data were later confirmed by others.[46,47] Expression of the HLA-DR antigen on monocytes is a prerequisite for effective antigen presentation and processing and plays a central role in the generation of the immune response to infection.

Brune et al[47] demonstrated that the proliferative response of T cells stimulated by SEA, SEB, and TSST-1 was not impaired after either laparoscopic or conventional surgery. They therefore concluded that the loss of HLA-DR, in spite of being significant, does not affect the antigen-presenting capacity of monocytes. However, clinically it has clearly been demonstrated that reduced HLA-DR expression on monocytes and slow restoration to preoperative values after surgical intervention is associated with an increased incidence of infection.[7,8] Data concerning HLA-DR expression after conventional and laparoscopic Nissen fundoplication show that both procedures result in a reduction of expression as compared to preoperative values within 2 hours after surgery. However, after the laparoscopic approach, HLA-DR expression returned to preoperative values within 1 day after surgery, this in contrast to the conventional technique, after which the expression was still significantly reduced 1 day after surgery.[48] These results confirm the

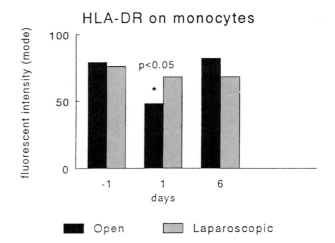

Figure 61–3. Median values of HLA-DR expression on monocytes after open and laparoscopic cholecystectomy. *(Reproduced, with permission, from Kloosterman et al.[20])*

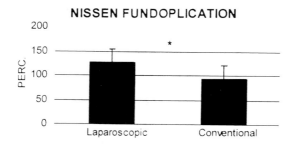

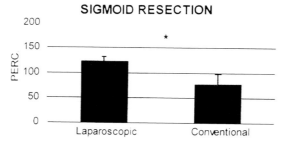

Figure 61–4. Differences in percentages of monocyte-mediated cytotoxicity 1 day after surgery. Laparoscopic versus open Nissen fundoplication and sigmoid resection. *(Reproduced, with permission, from Sietses et al.[49])*

study of Brune et al,[47] who reported reduced HLA-DR expression after both laparoscopic and conventional cholecystectomy and significantly faster recovery to normal values after laparoscopy.

Monocyte function has also been studied by measuring the cytotoxicity capacity against SW 948 adenocarcinoma cells. In vitro, monocyte-mediated cytotoxicity is known to correlate very closely with Kupffer (liver macrophage) cell-mediated cytotoxicity. Kupffer cells and monocytes play a crucial role in controlling tumor growth in the liver. Monocyte-mediated cytotoxicity was found to be suppressed after conventional surgery and preserved or slightly increased after laparoscopic procedures (Fig. 61–4).[49]

Based on these data, the nonspecific immune response appears to be better preserved after laparoscopic surgery. Most authors postulate that these preserved functions may prevent the development of septic complications.

Specific Immune Response: Humoral Immunity

There is an apparently normal number of circulating B cells after conventional surgery, although their capacity to mature into functional, intact, antibody-secreting plasma cells is significantly impaired. Furthermore, analysis of the B cells' capacity to secrete the different subclasses of immunoglobulin (IgA, IgG, and IgM) following trauma showed an abnormal antibody responsiveness.[50]

Cristaldi et al[51] studied the absolute number of lymphocytes expressing CD19 and found no postoperative reduction after either the laparoscopic or the conventional approach, indicating no significant difference in the total number of B cells between the two procedures.

Specific Immune Response: Cell-Mediated Immunity

Cellular immunity has traditionally been studied using delayed hypersensitivity skin testing, using either the mitogen phytohemag-

glutinin (PHA) or the keyhole limpet hemocyanin (KLH) skin tests. Anergy has clearly been shown to correlate to poor outcome after surgery, with patients having an increased risk of infectious complications and higher mortality. The duration of anergy relates to the severity of injury or infection.[52,53]

Various authors have studied the influence of laparoscopic surgery on postoperative immune functions in animal models. Horgan et al[54] were among the first to show that laparoscopic surgery is less immunotraumatic than laparotomy. They described significantly suppressed spontaneous lymphocyte proliferation and response to mitogen PHA after laparotomy, but not after laparoscopy. Trokel et al[55] tested both the KLH and the PHA skin tests in a rat model of laparoscopy. They found significantly reduced areas of induration after laparotomy as compared to control animals or the insufflation group, using both the KLH and PHA responses. Allendorf et al[56] later confirmed these data, describing better preserved cell-mediated immunity after laparoscopic-assisted as compared with open bowel resection. Because both the KLH and PHA responses were suppressed, they suggested that postoperative immune dysfunction occurs in activation of the effector phases of the responses and not in the cognitive phase of antigen presentation.

Clinically, Kloosterman et al[20] compared PHA skin tests after laparoscopic and conventional cholecystectomy and reported that PHA responsiveness could hardly be detected 1 day after conventional surgery, this in contrast to the laparoscopic approach, which did not influence the patient's responsiveness. PHA skin tests provide a sensitive indicator of T-cell function, regardless of antigen specificity. Griffith et al[57] studied T-cell proliferation in response to different mitogens in vitro, and found significant depression of T-lymphocyte proliferation to PHA, SEB and TSST.

A study examining the effects of surgery on the various T-cell subpopulations revealed defects in both the immunoregulatory T lymphocytes and NK cells. Following minor surgery, a fall in circulating T-helper cells occurs, thus altering the balance of the immunoregulatory helper:suppressor ratio in favor of suppressor lymphocytes. After major surgery, both the helper and the suppressor arms of the balance are affected, and the numbers of NK cells are suppressed.[58]

Cristaldi et al[51] studied lymphocyte subpopulations after open and laparoscopic cholecystectomy. They found a trend toward lower levels of the total lymphocyte count after the open procedure when compared with the laparoscopic technique during a 7-day observation period. They also reported differences in CD4 (T helper) and CD8 (T suppressor) expression on postoperative day one, favoring the laparoscopic approach. The number of CD4+ cells remained decreased 15 days after conventional surgery. Vallina et al[59] compared lymphocyte subpopulations after laparoscopic surgery with a historical group of Hansbrough. They reported that even though the laparoscopic approach did influence the ratio of T helper:T suppressor towards the suppressor side, the overall effect was significantly less than after conventional surgery.

Decker et al[46] reported marked differences in the Th1/Th2 balance between laparoscopic and conventional surgery. Surgical trauma causes a shift in the balance towards Th2, suggesting that cell-mediated immunity is downregulated and antibody-mediated immunity is upregulated after surgery. Downregulation of cell-mediated immunity makes patients more susceptible to infections with viruses and intracellular bacteria. Changes that reflect an increase in Th2-type immune activity were more pronounced in conventional cholecystectomy when compared with the laparoscopic technique; furthermore, they also reported reduced Th1-type activity after the conventional approach.

Little is known about NK cells after laparoscopic surgery. Cristaldi et al[51] reported a reduced number of NK cells after both laparoscopic and conventional surgery, which persisted until 30 days after surgery. A significant difference between the two procedures was observed 1 day after surgery, in favor of the laparoscopic approach. The authors suggested that depression of this cellular subset after conventional surgery may reduce resistance against viable tumor cells. In an animal model, Sandoval et al[60] studied natural antitumoral immunity in a small animal model. They reported decreased natural killer cell cytotoxicity after both laparoscopic and conventional surgery.

The above mentioned literature suggests a preservation of the specific immune response after laparoscopic surgery. However, more advanced laparoscopic procedures again fail to show the same results. Even though until now only one study has examined changes in lymphocyte subpopulations after laparoscopic-assisted versus open bowel resection, the current results show no significant differences between the groups.[61]

SPECULATIONS ON THE CAUSES

Why does surgical trauma appear to cause immune suppression just when there is increased demand on the body's defense mechanisms? The answer may lie in the wound itself.[62,63] A wound contains devitalized tissue and exposed self-antigens which must be cleared to allow healing to take place. It is a site of intense immunologic activity, with both neutrophils and macrophages, and at a later stage lymphocytes, playing an active role in regulating the inflammatory and healing processes. There are potent immunosuppressive factors present, which prevent local autoimmune destruction. Immunosuppression therefore makes sense. This supports the view that the degree of posttraumatic immunosuppression correlates with the extent of injury. This theory is further supported by a study by Allendorf et al,[64] who investigated the effects of incision length and exposure method for bowel resection with respect to postoperative immune function in a murine model and concluded that cell-mediated immune function varies inversely with the degree of surgical trauma.

The most logical explanation for the relatively preserved immunologic defenses after laparoscopic surgery would therefore be the reduction of the size of the wound. However, comparative studies between laparoscopic and conventional surgery have revealed that some aspects required to accomplish laparoscopy, such as the exclusion of air or CO_2 insufflation, could also be of importance. Little et al[65] studied the effects of surgical trauma on the cellular immune response in procedures that did or did not involve opening the peritoneum. Laparotomy was compared with a near-laparotomy in a murine model. The near-laparotomy consisted of a similar midline incision without involving the peritoneum. A significant impairment in cellular immune function was associated with opening of the peritoneum. Watson et al[66] subjected mice to laparoscopy with CO_2 or air and compared these results with a standard laparotomy. A significant increase in peritoneal macrophage release of TNF-α and the production of oxygen radicals was observed after laparoscopy with air and after laparotomy in comparison with laparoscopy with CO_2 insufflation. However, the ingestion of *Candida albicans* by peritoneal macrophages was significantly decreased after air insufflation and after laparotomy when compared with CO_2 insufflation. They also reported significant translocation of FITC-labeled lipopolysaccharide (LPS) into the peritoneal cavity and the systemic circulation after air laparoscopy and laparotomy only. They concluded that factors in circulating air can induce LPS translocation and subsequent stimulation of postoperative immune responses. The beneficial effects of laparoscopic surgery may therefore be partly explained by the minimal air contamination of the peritoneal cavity.

Recently West et al[67] reported an alternative hypothesis. West's group investigated the effect of CO_2 insufflation on peritoneal macrophages both in vivo and in vitro and compared these results with air and helium insufflation. Macrophages incubated in CO_2 produced significantly less TNF-α and IL-I in response to LPS compared to incubation in air and helium. Exposure to CO_2, but not to air or helium, caused a marked cytosolic acidification. The effects of CO_2 could be reproduced after pharmacologically-induced intracellular acidification.[67] It should be noted that the in vitro experiments were performed with insufflation pressures of 12 to 15 mm Hg, which is three times higher than the insufflation pressures normally used in rats.[68] The authors proposed that cellular acidification induced by peritoneal insufflation contributes to the blunting of the local inflammatory response during laparoscopic surgery. In another study they further investigated the effect of CO_2 on inhibition of LPS-stimulated cytokine release by examining the duration of CO_2 exposure needed to observe this inhibition, the duration of the inhibited response, and comparing inhibition of TNF-α and IL-I gene transcription to gain some insights into the mechanisms involved. They reported that inhibition of IL-1 occurred 15 minutes after CO_2 exposure, it was associated with decreased IL-1 mRNA, and it was rapidly lost following incubation in the control atmosphere. In contrast, TNF-α inhibition was seen despite normal levels of mRNA, it required more than 30 minutes of CO_2 exposure, and it persisted after CO_2 removal. These data suggest that different mechanisms exist for CO_2-induced inhibition of IL-1 and TNF-α, but that the inhibitory effects are transient. The authors postulated that these results may partly explain the lack of systemic symptoms after laparoscopic surgery.[69]

Currently, both theories are under investigation in a clinical study comparing CO_2 and helium for peritoneal insufflation with exposure to circulating air (using the abdominal wall lifting technique) on various immunologic parameters in patients undergoing laparoscopic cholecystectomy.

CLINICAL IMPLICATIONS

Immune suppression has been implicated in the development of postoperative infectious complications. Defects in PMN function after conventional surgery have been shown to correlate with subsequent development of postoperative complications. Wakefield et al[70] described that both CD11b expression and hydrogen peroxide production were significantly higher in surgical patients who were destined to develop postsurgical sepsis. Polk et al[38] reported that a reduced ability of a patient's serum to support phagocytosis is predictive of fatal outcome in severely injured patients. The tempered activation and the preserved opsonic capacity after laparoscopic surgery may therefore indicate a lower risk of postoperative complications.

Patients undergoing surgery for diseases complicated by inflammatory processes and peritonitis are at risk for postoperative infectious complications and could theoretically benefit the most from the preserved immunologic defenses associated with minimally invasive techniques. However, there is some theoretical concern that the elevated intra-abdominal pressure may increase the incidence of bacteremia and thereby the systemic inflammatory response after laparoscopic surgery.[71] It is speculated that the elevated intra-abdominal pressure, which is responsible for increased lymphatic absorption through which bacteria are removed from the peritoneal cavity, is responsible for the bacteremia. Both Collet et al[72] and Jacobi et al[73] studied the functional consequences of the preserved postoperative immune function in an animal model of peritonitis. They reported that laparotomy and laparoscopy both increased the release of inflammatory mediators; however, the inflammatory response was significantly higher in the laparotomy group. Furthermore, Jacobi's group found a significantly higher number of abscesses after laparotomy as compared to the laparoscopy group. Collet et al reported a significantly increased bacterial count in the peritoneal exudate after laparotomy when compared to laparoscopy. Both studies indicate that tempered inflammatory responses of peritoneal macrophages result in more effective bacterial clearance, but a more critical appraisal is warranted. To study the effects on severe peritonitis, Bloechle et al[74] reported on a pig model of laparoscopic versus open repair of gastric perforation. They found that for long-standing peritonitis (duration >12 h), use of the laparoscopic approach resulted in significantly higher mortality compared to the conventional approach (22 versus 78%); the increased risk was not observed if the peritonitis was less severe (duration <12 h).[74,75]

Though there are few clinical studies that directly address the issue of postoperative complications and laparoscopic surgery, most available reports indicate a lower incidence of postoperative infective complications.[76–79] A recently published meta-analysis of randomized controlled trials of laparoscopic versus conventional appendectomy showed that the overall complication rate was comparable between the two methods. However, the percentage of wound infections was significantly lower after the laparoscopic technique (–4.2%).[80]

Immune suppression may also be implicated in postoperative tumor metastasis. Especially important in this respect is the protection of the patient's immunity during the first days after surgery. The rate and incidence of tumor growth is known to be higher in immunocompromised patients. Hansen et al[81] demonstrated circulating tumor cells in 36% of patients who underwent surgery for colorectal cancer. We can speculate that these circulating cells can metastasize and grow more readily if the patient's immune status is compromised as a consequence of operative trauma. Several authors have demonstrated that conventional surgery is related to increased tumor growth in animal models. Eggermont et al[9] demonstrated increased tumor growth after intraperitoneal injection of tumor cells in rats that underwent laparotomy as compared to control animals. Oka et al[82] demonstrated that tumor cells injected into the portal vein grow more aggressively after small bowel resection as compared to laparotomy without resection, correlating the subsequent tumor growth rate with the amount of surgical trauma. Laparoscopic surgery is known to be less traumatic than conventional surgery and is thought to have less influence on postoperative immune function. There are now various animal studies which have shown that cancer cells grow more aggressively and metastasize more easily after laparotomy than after peritoneal insufflation with CO_2. Allendorf et al[83] found that tumor cells implanted intradermally in mice grew significantly faster after laparotomy than those in the control and CO_2 insufflation groups. Bouvy et al[84] reported that laparoscopic surgery was associated with decreased tumor spread when compared to laparotomy. Experimental studies have also shown that tumor growth that was stimulated by laparotomy can be reduced by immunomodulation.[9] We can speculate that the observed difference in tumor growth rate between laparoscopy and laparotomy could be explained by the postoperative preservation of immunologic functions after laparoscopic surgery. The described differences in NK cells and monocyte-mediated cytotoxicity after the laparoscopic approach suggest that the preservation of postoperative immunologic defenses is at least partly responsible for the observed reduction in postoperative tumor growth. Allendorf et al[85] demonstrated the correlation between reduced tumor growth after laparoscopic surgery and preserved immune function. They reported that the difference in tumor growth after open versus laparoscopic surgery was lost in an athymic model, implicating T-cell function as a causal factor. There are, however, alternative hypotheses that should be considered. There are various experimental studies which suggest that the CO_2 used for abdominal insufflation stimulates tumor growth. Jacobi et al[86] measured the growth of colon adenocarcinoma in vitro after incubation with either helium or CO_2, and found that tumor growth was significantly less after exposure to helium. As for the possible immunologic advantages, this point deserves further investigation to help identify any possible consequences for clinical practice.

With regard to the issue of port-site metastasis, current data suggest that the origin of these metastases is unrelated to immunologic factors, but is facilitated by implantation of malignant cells, either from contaminated instruments, or indirectly due to the mechanical effects of the insufflating gas. Literature concerning port-site metastases has been reviewed thoroughly elsewhere.[87]

CONCLUSION

Surgery (conventional or laparoscopic) involves controlled trauma and thus influences the systemic immune response. The extent and duration of postoperative immunosuppression will depend on the magnitude and type of the initial injury. The current review shows that the influence of laparoscopic surgery on the postoperative systemic immune response is significantly less after laparoscopic cholecystectomy when compared with the conventional approach. Unfortunately, few of these studies were randomized. Furthermore, to date few immunologic data are available concerning more advanced laparoscopic procedures; moreover, those that exist show conflicting data. Various animal model studies on postoperative septic complications and tumor growth show that the postoperative preservation of the systemic immune response after laparoscopic surgery can have enormous clinical advantages. In the future this may mean a lower rate of infection, less local recurrence, and even lower rates of distant metastasis. Prospective randomized studies are needed to discover whether these suspected advantages can be demonstrated in clinical practice. The concept that laparoscopic surgery causes fewer immunologic alterations may well prove to be the most important aspect favoring the minimally invasive approach.

REFERENCES

1. Reddick EJ, Olsen DO. Outpatient laparoscopic laser cholecystectomy. *Am J Surg.* 1990;160:485.

2. Johnson A. Laparoscopic surgery. *Lancet* 1997;349:631.

3. Dallemagne B, Weerts JM, Jehaes C, et al. Techniques and results of endoscopic fundoplication. *Endosc Surg Allied Tech.* 1993;1:72.

4. Eijsbouts QAJ, Cuesta MA, Brauw de LM, et al. Elective laparoscopic-assisted sigmoid resection for diverticular disease. *Surg Endosc.* 1997;11:750.

5. Falk PM, Beart RW, Wexner SD. Laparoscopic colectomy: critical appraisal. *Dis Colon Rectum.* 1993;36:28.

6. Vittimberga FJ, Foley DP, Meyers WC, et al. Laparoscopic surgery and the systemic immune response. *Ann Surg.* 1998;227:326.

7. Wakefield CH, Carey PD, Foulds S, et al. Changes in major histocompatibility complex class II expression in monocytes and T cells of patients developing infection after surgery. *Br J Surg.* 1993;80:205.

8. Cheadle WG, Hershman MJ, Wellhausen SR, et al. HLA-DR antigen expression on peripheral blood monocytes correlates with surgical infection. *Am J Surg.* 1991;161:639.

9. Eggermont ANM, Steller EP, Sugerbacker PH. Laparotomy enhances intraperitoneal tumour growth and abrogates the antitumor effects of interleukin-2 and lymphokine-activated killer cells. *Surgery* 1987;102:71.

10. Bone RC. Sir Isaac Newton, sepsis SIRS and CARS. *Crit Care Med.* 1996;24:1125.

11. Strieter RM, Standiford TJ, Huffnagle GB, et al. "The good, the bad, and the ugly." The role of chemokines in models of human disease. *J Immunol.* 1996;156:2095.

12. Dinarello CA. Interleukin-1. *Rev Infect Dis.* 1984;6:51.

13. Biffle WL, Moore EE, Moore FA, et al. Interleukin-6 in the injured patient. Marker of injury or mediator of inflammation. *Ann Surg.* 1996;224:647.

14. Glaser F, Sannwald GA, Buhr HJ, et al. General stress response to conventional and laparoscopic cholecystectomy. *Ann Surg.* 1995;221:372.

15. Zee van KJ, Kohno T, Fischer E, et al. Tumor necrosis factor soluble receptors circulate during experimental and clinical inflammation and can protect against excessive tumor necrosis factors in vitro and in vivo. *Proc Natl Acad Sci USA.* 1992;89:4845.

16. Decker D, Lindemann C, Low A, et al. Verdänderung der zytokinkonzentration (IL-6, IL-8, IL-1 RA) und der zellulär expression von membranmolekülen (CD25, CD 30, HLA-DR) nach operativem trauma. *Zentralbl Chir.* 1997;122:157.

17. Sakamoto K, Arakawa H, Mita S, et al. Elevation of circulating interleukin 6 after surgery: factors influencing the serum levels. *Cytokine* 1994;6:181.

18. Roumen RME, van Meurs PA, Kuypers HHC, et al. Serum interleukin-6 and C-reactive protein in patients after laparoscopic or conventional surgery. *Eur J Surg.* 1992;158:541.

19. Karayiannakis AJ, Makri GG, Mantzioka A, et al. Systemic stress response after laparoscopic or open cholecystectomy: a randomised trial. *Br J Surg.* 1997;84:467.

20. Kloosterman T, von Blomberg ME, Borgstein P, et al. Unimpaired immune function after laparoscopic cholecystectomy. *Surgery* 1994;115:424.

21. Maruszynski M, Pojda Z. Interleukin-6 levels in the monitoring of surgical trauma, a comparison of serum IL-6 concentrations in patients treated by cholecystectomy via laparotomy or laparoscopy. *Surg Endosc.* 1995;9:882.

22. Redmond BP, Watson RWG, Houghton T, et al. Immune function in patients undergoing open vs laparoscopic cholecystectomy. *Arch Surg.* 1994;129:1240.

23. Ueo H, Honda M, Adachi M, et al. Minimal increase in serum interleukin-6 levels during laparoscopic cholecystectomy. *Am J Surg.* 1994;168:358.

24. Cho JM, La Porta AJ, Clark JR, et al. Response of serum cytokines in patients undergoing laparoscopic cholecystectomy. *Surg Endosc.* 1994;8:1380.

25. Jakeways MSR, Mitchell V, Hashim IA, et al. Metabolic and inflammatory responses after open or laparoscopic cholecystectomy. *Br J Surg.* 1994;81:127.

26. Joris J, Cigarini I, Legrand M, et al. Metabolic and respiratory changes after cholecystectomy performed via laparotomy or laparoscopy. *Br J Anaesth.* 1992;69:341.

27. Mealy K, Gallangher H, Barry M, et al. Physiological and metabolic responses to open and laparoscopic cholecystectomy. *Br J Surg.* 1992;79:1061.

28. Hill ADK, Banwell PE, Darzi A, et al. Inflammatory markers following laparoscopic and open hernia repair. *Surg Endosc.* 1995;9:695.

29. Harmon GD, Senagore AJ, Kilbride MJ, et al. Interleukin-6 response to laparoscopic and open colectomy. *Dis Colon Rectum.* 1994;37:754.

30. Johnson DRE, Spencer UT, Cerra FB, et al. Laparoscopic versus open colectomy: a comparative study of the systemic stress response. *Surg Endosc.* 1994;8:447(abstract).

31. Stage JG, Schulze S, Moller P, et al. Prospective randomised study of laparoscopic versus open colonic resection for adenocarcinoma. *Br J Surg.* 1997;83:391.

32. Halevy A, Lin G, Gold-Deutch R, et al. Comparison of serum C-reactive protein concentrations for laparoscopic versus open cholecystectomy. *Surg Endosc.* 1997;9:280.

33. Squirrell DM, Majeed AW, Troy G, et al. A randomised, prospective, blinded comparison of postoperative pain, metabolic response, and perceived health after laparoscopic versus small incision cholecystectomy. *Surgery* 1998;123:485.

34. Vander Velpen G, Pennickx F, Kerremans R, et al. Interleukin-6 and coagulation-fibrinolysis after laparoscopic and conventional cholecystectomy. *Surg Endosc.* 1994;8:1216.

35. Pike GK, Bessell JR, Mathew G, et al. Changes in fibrinogen levels in patients undergoing open and laparoscopic Nissen fundoplication. *Aust NZ J Surg.* 1996;66:94.

36. McMahon AJ, O'Dwyer PJ, Cruikshank AM, et al. Comparison of metabolic responses to laparoscopic and minilaparotomy cholecystectomy. *Br J Surg.* 1993;80:1255.

37. Gebhard FT, Becker BP, Gemgross H, et al. Reduced inflammatory responses in minimal invasive surgery of pneumothorax. *Arch Surg.* 1996;131:1079.

38. Polk HC, George CD, Hershman MJ, et al. The capacity of serum to support neutrophil phagocytosis is a vital host defence mechanism in severely injured patients. *Ann Surg.* 1988;207:686.

39. Cohen IR, Sciutto MS, Brown GL, et al. Failure of opsonization as a sign of lethal sepsis. *J Infect Dis.* 1984;149:651.

40. Dijk v WC, Verburgh HA, Rijswijk v REN, et al. Neutrophil function, serum opsonic activity and delayed hypersensitivity in surgical patients. *Surgery* 1982;92:21.

41. Utoh J, Yamamoto T, Utsunomiya T, et al. Effects of surgery on neutrophil functions; superoxide and leukotriene production. *Br J Surg.* 1983;75:682.

42. Sietses C, Wiezer MJ, Eijsbouts QAJ, et al. The influence of laparoscopic surgery on postoperative polymorphonuclear leukocyte function. *Surg Endosc.* 2000;14:812.

43. Carey PD, Wakefield CH, Thayeb A, et al. Effects of minimal invasive surgery on hypochlorous acid production by neutrophils. *Br J Surg.* 1994;81:557.

44. Gal I, Lantos L, Roth E. Changes of PMN-elastase and C-reactive protein following traditional and laparoscopic cholecystectomy. *Surg Endosc.* 1996;10:552(abstract).

45. Johnston RB. Current concepts: monocytes and macrophages. *N Engl J Med.* 1988;318:747.

46. Decker D, Schondorf M, Bidlinger F, et al. Surgical stress induces a shift in the type 1/type 2 cell balance, suggesting down-regulation of

cell-mediated and upregulation of antibody-mediated immunity commensurate to the trauma. *Surgery* 1996;119:316.

47. Brune IB, Wilke W, Hensler T, et al. Normal T lymphocyte and monocyte function after minimally invasive surgery. *Surg Endosc.* 1998;12:1020.

48. Sietses C, Wiezer MJ, Eijsbouts QAJ, et al. A prospective randomized study of the systemic immune response after laparoscopic and conventional Nissen fundoplication. *Surgery* 1999;126:5.

49. Sietses C, Havenith CEG, Eijsbouts QAJ, et al. Laparoscopic surgery preserves monocyte-mediated tumor cell killing in contrast to the conventional approach. *Surg Endosc.* 2000;14:456.

50. Ertel W, Faist E. The influence of mechanical trauma on the B-cell system. In: Faist, Ninnemans, Greenberg, eds. *Immune Consequences of Trauma, Shock and Sepsis.* Springer-Verlag:1989;143.

51. Cristaldi M, Rovatti M, Elli M, et al. Lymphocyte subpopulation changes after open and laparoscopic cholecystectomy: a prospective and comparative study on 38 patients. *Surg Laparosc Endosc.* 1997;7:255.

52. Christou NV, Meakins JL, Gordon J, et al. The delayed type hypersensitivity response and host resistance in surgical patients, 20 years later. *Ann Surg.* 1995;222:534.

53. Christou NV, Meakins JL, MacLean LD. The predictive value of delayed type hypersensitivity in preoperative patients. *Surg Gynecol Obstet.* 1981;152:297.

54. Horgan PG, Fitzpatrick M, Couse NF, et al. Laparoscopy is less immunotraumatic than laparotomy. *Minimally Invasive Therapy* 1992;1:241.

55. Trokel MJ, Bessler M, Treat MR, et al. Preservation of immune response after laparoscopy. *Surg Endosc.* 1994;8:1385.

56. Allendorf JDF, Bessler M, Whelan RL, et al. Better preservation of immune function after laparoscopic assisted vs. open bowel resection in a murine model. *Dis Colon Rectum.* 1996;39:S67.

57. Griffith JP, Everitt NJ, Lancaster F, et al. Influence of laparoscopic and conventional cholecystectomy upon cell-mediated immunity. *Br J Surg.* 1995;82:677.

58. Lennard TWJ, Shenton BK, Borzotta A, et al. The influence of surgical operations on components of the human immune system. *Br J Surg.* 1985;72:771.

59. Vallina VL, Velasco VM. The influence of laparoscopy on lymphocyte subpopulations in the surgical patient. *Surg Endosc.* 1996;10:481.

60. Sandoval BA, Robinson AV, Sulaiman TT, et al. Open versus laparoscopic surgery: a comparison of natural antitumoral immunity in a small animal model. *Am Surg.* 1996;62:625.

61. Hewitt PM, Ip SM, Kwok SPY, et al. Laparoscopic-assisted vs open surgery for colorectal cancer, comparative study of immune effects. *Dis Colon Rectum.* 1998;41:901.

62. Regan MC, Barbul A. The role of the wound in posttraumatic immune dysfunction. In: Faist, Meakins, Schildberg, eds. *Host Defence Dysfunction in Trauma, Shock and Sepsis.* Springer-Verlag:1992;1043.

63. Barbul A, Regan MC. The regulatory role of T lymphocytes in wound healing. *J Trauma.* 1990;30:S97.

64. Allendorf JDF, Bessler M, Whelan RL, et al. Postoperative immune function varies inversely with the degree of surgical trauma in a murine model. *Surg Endosc.* 1997;11:427.

65. Little D, Regan M, Keana RM, et al. Perioperative immune modulation. *Surgery* 1993;114:87.

66. Watson RWG, Redmond HP, McCarthy J, et al. Exposure of the peritoneal cavity to air regulates early inflammatory responses to surgery in a murine model. *Br J Surg.* 1995;82:1060.

67. West MA, Hackam DJ, Baker J, et al. Mechanism of decreased in vitro macrophage cytokine release after exposure to carbon dioxide, relevance to laparoscopic surgery. *Ann Surg.* 1997;226:179.

68. Gutt CN, Riemer V, Brier C, et al. Standardized technique of laparoscopic surgery in the rat. *Digest Surg.* 1998;15:135.

69. West MA, Baker J, Bellingham J. Kinetics of decreased LPS-stimulated cytokine release by macrophages exposed to CO_2. *J Surg Res.* 1996;63:269.

70. Wakefield CH, Carey PD, Foulds S, et al. Polymorphonuclear leukocyte activation, an early marker of the postsurgical sepsis response. *Arch Surg.* 1993;128:390.

71. Tsilibary EC, Wissing SL. Lymphatic absorption from the peritoneal cavity: regulation of patency of mesothelial stomata. *Microvasc Res.* 1983;25:22.

72. Collet D, Vitale GC, Reynolds M, et al. Peritoneal host defenses are less impaired by laparoscopy than by open operation. *Surg Endosc.* 1995;9:1059.

73. Jacobi CA, Ordemann J, Zieren HU, et al. Increased systemic inflammation after laparotomy vs laparoscopy in an animal model of peritonitis. *Arch Surg.* 1998;133:258.

74. Bloechle C, Emmermann A, Strate T, et al. Laparoscopic vs open repair of gastric perforation and abdominal lavage of associated peritonitis in pigs. *Surg Endosc.* 1998;12:212.

75. Bloechle C, Emmermann A, True H, et al. Effect of pneumoperitoneum on the extent and severity of peritonitis induced by gastric ulcer perforation in the rat. *Surg Endosc.* 1995;9:898.

76. Chiarugi M, Buccianti P, Celona G, et al. Laparoscopic compared with open appendicectomy for acute appendicitis; a prospective study. *Eur J Surg.* 1996;162:385.

77. Frazee RC, Bohannon NW. Laparoscopic appendectomy for complicated appendicitis. *Arch Surg.* 1996;131:509.

78. Tate JJT. Laparoscopic appendectomy. *Br J Surg.* 1996;83:1169.

79. Viljakka MT, Luostarinen NM, Isolauri JO. Complications of open and laparoscopic antireflux surgery: 32-years audit at teaching hospital. *J Am Coll Surg.* 1997;185:446.

80. Sauerland S, Lefering R, Holthausen U, et al. Laparoscopic vs conventional appendectomy—a meta-analysis of randomised controlled trials. *Langenbecks Arch Surg.* 1998;383:289.

81. Hansen E, Wolff N, Knuchel IR, et al. Tumour cells in blood shed from the surgical field. *Arch Surg.* 1995;130:387.

82. Oka M, Hazama S, Suzuki M, et al. Depression of cytotoxicity of nonparenchymal cells in the liver after surgery. *Surgery* 1994;116:877.

83. Allendorf JDF, Bessler M, Kayton NM, et al. Increased tumour establishment and growth after laparotomy vs laparoscopy in a murine model. *Arch Surg.* 1995;130:649.

84. Bouvy ND, Marquet RL, Hamming JF, et al. Laparoscopic surgery in the rat: beneficial effect on body weight and tumour take. *Surg Endosc.* 1996;10:490.

85. Allendorf JDF, Bessler M, Whelan RL, et al. Differences in tumor growth after open versus laparoscopic surgery are lost in an athymic model and are associated with differences in tumor proliferative index. *Surg Form.* 1996;47:150.

86. Jacobi CA, Sabat R, Böhm B, et al. Pneumoperitoneum with carbon dioxide stimulates growth of malignant colonic cells. *Surgery* 1997;121:72.

87. Neuhaus SJ, Texler M, Hewett PJ, et al. Review: Port site metastases following laparoscopic surgery. *Br J Surg.* 1998;85:735.

*H*ernia Surgery

Chapter Sixty-Two ● ● ● ● ● ● ●

Laparoscopic Inguinal Hernioplasty

EDWARD FELIX

INTRODUCTION

When we began our study of laparoscopic hernia repair in 1991, we were using a tension-free anterior mesh repair modeled after the Lichtenstein repair,[1] but did not appreciate the rapid recovery and minimal morbidity described by its originators. We felt that a laparoscopic approach offered an advantage over open repairs, because the repair utilized laparoscopic techniques that had previously decreased recovery time in comparison to other open procedures.[2] Because the repair was based on an open posterior mesh buttressed approach that had a low recurrence rate,[3] we felt that laparoscopic hernioplasty would reduce recovery time, but still have low recurrence rates.

Our first laparoscopic approach was patterned after the posterior repair of Nyhus,[4] but we gained access to the extraperitoneal space via a transabdominal laparoscopic route.[5] From the beginning, our dissection was extremely aggressive and the size of our patch was large.[6] Other investigators were initially critical of our exuberance, because they felt the complication rate from such extensive laparoscopic dissection would be too great. The opposite proved to be true, and it has since become the standard procedure for most surgeons. The key to success for laparoscopic hernioplasty is a wide dissection of the entire inguinal floor and repair of all three potential hernias with a large sheet of polypropylene mesh.[7] Over the last 10 years, as we gained experience, our approach has been modified and refined to further improve results and reduce the incidence of complications. Although the majority of repairs performed by our center each year are now done using a totally extraperitoneal approach (TEP), we feel that the transabdominal preperitoneal approach (TAPP) is equally effective and has an important place in the laparoscopic surgeon's armamentarium.

Although laparoscopic hernioplasty remains controversial in the minds of some surgeons, there is now no doubt that in the hands of experienced laparoscopic surgeons, the approach does what it was designed to do. Recurrence rates of less than 1% are possible[7-10] and complication rates comparable to those of open repairs are achievable.[11-13] There are, however, reviews in which results have not been as good.[14-16] The reasons for this difference may

be that laparoscopic hernioplasty is an extremely difficult operation to master and it has a long learning curve.[17] To achieve the desired results, the surgeon must be an experienced laparoscopist, have a comprehensive knowledge of anatomy, and perform enough procedures under the guidance of a skilled laparoscopic hernia surgeon to overcome the learning curve.

Choosing when to use a laparoscopic approach may be as important as how to perform it. Complications can be reduced or eliminated by choosing the right procedure for each patient. Early in our experience we accepted virtually all patients with groin hernias who were good candidates for general anesthesia.[5] With experience, we learned that patients who potentially have an obliterated extraperitoneal space due to previous pelvic surgery should undergo an anterior tension-free repair rather than a laparoscopic repair. Also patients that have had extensive intra-abdominal pelvic infections may have bowel tissue adherent to the posterior wall, making any attempt to gain access to the extraperitoneal space too risky.[11] The choice of the type of laparoscopic repair (TAPP or TEP) also influences the outcome. Some hernias are better repaired via an extraperitoneal route, while others are better suited for the transabdominal approach.

Recently there has been a trend away from the transabdominal preperitoneal (TAPP) approach and toward totally extraperitoneal (TEP) repairs. It is essential that surgeons understand both techniques, however, since some TEP repairs need to be converted to TAPP repairs to be completed successfully, and others are best begun with a TAPP approach. No matter which approach is used, there are some basic principles that must be followed. In our multicenter study that compiled data from 7 centers' experience with laparoscopic hernioplasty, four basic principles were found to be common to all successful laparoscopic hernioplasties: (1) The entire posterior floor must be dissected; (2) the mesh must cover the entire posterior floor; (3) the mesh must be completely covered by peritoneum; and (4) the mesh must be adequately anchored to the floor. This last principle has recently come into question, and a definitive answer remains to be established. In addition, there are specific techniques that we have found helpful during the last 10 years in performing over 5000 laparoscopic repairs and that have contributed to our group's consistently good results.

TOTALLY EXTRAPERITONEAL APPROACH (TEP)

We begin the TEP hernioplasty with the surgeon standing on the side of the patient opposite the dominant hernia. A small transverse incision is made just below the umbilicus off the midline on the side of the hernia. Using "S" refractors, the anterior fascia is identified and incised with a no. 11 blade. The rectus muscle is retracted laterally, exposing the posterior rectus sheath. A balloon dissector is slid along the posterior sheath until the pubis is palpated. The procedure should be converted to a TAPP procedure if the resistance met is such that the peritoneum may be torn by the dissector. An alternative technique is to use the scope to bluntly dissect the extraperitoneal space, but this is more difficult. After the central extraperitoneal space is created, a blunt trocar is placed and CO_2 is insufflated to a pressure of 10 to 12 mm Hg. Two 5-mm trocars are placed in the midline under direct vision. The first is placed as close to the video trocar as possible, and the second is placed three fingerbreadths (5 to 7 cm) below the first. If the lower trocar is placed too close to the pubis, it will interfere with mesh placement.

Dissection begins with identification of Cooper's ligament and the inferior epigastric vessels, landmarks essential to continuing safe dissection of the direct, indirect, and femoral spaces. If a direct hernia is present, it is reduced by gentle traction on the sac. Care is taken not to injure the bladder if it is incarcerated in the hernia. After the direct hernia is reduced or the direct floor is adequately cleaned of fat to determine that there is no direct hernia, the space of Bogros is opened by sweeping the dissector downward just lateral to the inferior epigastric vessels. The peritoneal sac or edge is identified at this point. The lipoma, the most lateral component of the cord, must be reduced to prevent recurrence. It should be stripped off the cord structures and placed in the retroperitoneum above the dissection. The sac is then completely dissected off the vas deferens and testicular vessels as originally described by Stoppa et al.[3] If a hole is made in the sac it is ligated with an endo-loop. The surgeon must identify the iliopubic tract at this point. If it is still covered with fat, a lipoma remains in the canal and needs to be reduced.

After the entire posterior floor has been dissected, including the femoral space, the mesh is cut to fit the floor. The mesh is trimmed from a flat 6 × 6-inch piece of polypropylene mesh. It usually measures approximately 5 × 4½ inches, but may be as large as 6 × 6 inches, and is always wider on its medial half. The mesh overlaps the pubis, crosses the midline, and extends far lateral to the internal ring. It is anchored to Cooper's ligament, the transversalis fascia above the direct space, and lateral to the inferior epigastric vessels above the iliopubic tract. One hand is placed on the abdominal wall to palpate the stapler as it is pressed against the wall. This maneuver prevents misfiring anchors below the iliopubic tract into the area of the lateral cutaneous femoral branch of the genitofemoral or femoral nerves. Care should be taken not to push the stapler too firmly into the wall. In a thin patient, staples placed too deeply can catch the ilioinguinal and iliohypogastric nerves, causing severe localized abdominal wall and groin pain. We have recently begun using a contoured mesh that requires no fixation. Although we have not seen any early recurrences from this mesh, it is too soon to comment on its long-term use.

When the surgeon is satisfied that the mesh is in place without folds or wrinkles, the CO_2 is evacuated. The most common cause of failure of a laparoscopic hernioplasty is lateral lifting of the mesh by the peritoneum.[7] Therefore, the gas should be evacuated slowly while the inferior lateral corner of the mesh is held down. The peritoneum thus expands slowly over the mesh, holding it in place rather than elevating it. The 10-mm fascial incision is closed and local anesthetic injected around the incisions if this was not done at the beginning of the procedure. If CO_2 has inflated the scrotum, it is evacuated with a needle. In addition, any CO_2 trapped in the peritoneal cavity is evacuated with a Veress needle before closing the fascia.

TRANSABDOMINAL PREPERITONEAL APPROACH (TAPP)

Because the working space is larger, the anatomy more easily recognized, and the laparoscopic technique more familiar to most laparoscopic surgeons, the TAPP repair is technically easier to perform than the TEP repair. However, injuries to the viscera or vessels are potential risks when a trocar or Veress needle is inserted into the peritoneal cavity. If the TAPP approach is employed, care must to be taken to avoid potential trocar complications. Once the 10-mm umbilical trocar and two lateral 5-mm trocars at the level of the umbilicus are in place, the hernia is reduced by gentle traction on the omentum or bowel. An incision in the peritoneum is made from lateral to medial and above the internal ring. The lower peritoneal flap is dissected off the wall and the peritoneal sac reduced. If the indirect sac is extremely adherent to the cord structures or is difficult to reduce, the sac is transected. The sac is opened on its superior lateral edge in order to avoid injury to the cord structures, and then dissected free of the cord. After the sac is completely dissected off the cord, it is ligated. Just as in open repairs, the distal sac along the cord can be left open without increased risk of forming a hydrocele.

The floor dissection and repair are continued as described for the TEP. If necessary a double buttressed repair can be employed as we described in our first published reports of laparoscopic hernioplasty,[5,6] using a piece of mesh with a slit for the cord covered by a second piece of mesh. This technique is now reserved for extremely large or difficult hernias, or when the cord structures tent the mesh upwards, potentially leading to recurrence. We feel a slit in the mesh may cause increased fibrosis along the cord, leading to an increased incidence of testicular pain and hydrocele formation, and we therefore now limit use of the slit. Once the floor is repaired, the peritoneum is completely closed with a running suture to prevent entrapment of bowel or exposure of bowel to mesh.

RESULTS

There has been a gradual evolution in the laparoscopic approach to hernia repair over the last 10 years. It has gone from an experimental repair[2] to a reliable hernioplasty with an extremely low recurrence rate and low morbidity.[7–10] Many experienced laparoscopic surgeons have demonstrated that laparoscopic hernia repair is safe and offers the appropriate patient a viable alternative to open surgery. My own results have mirrored those of other experienced laparoscopic surgeons. In over 2100 repairs performed under general anesthesia, there have been no anesthetic complications. The recurrence rate has been less than 1% (9/2104 procedures) with a median follow-up of more than 4 years. The incidence of serious complications has improved with experience,[11] and in the last 2 years there have been no intraoperative complications. The overall incidence of complications is similar to that of comparable reviews of open hernioplasties.

Whether the TAPP or TEP repair is better is no longer a valid question. There is now sizeable experience with both approaches in the U.S. and around the world. Using a variety of approaches based on the principles outlined in this chapter, different centers have consistently reproduced the same excellent results. The choice of a TAPP or a TEP approach should be based on surgeon expertise and preference, as well as the patient's clinical presentation. The incidence of complications and failures for the two approaches is equal in the hands of experienced laparoscopic surgeons.

Although some of the most ardent opponents to laparoscopic hernia repair now admit that the approach is useful,[18] it is doubtful that laparoscopic hernia repair will ever become as popular as simpler, open, tension-free repairs. Laparoscopic repairs must be reserved for those surgeons willing to undergo the extensive training period required to perfect the approach and overcome the learning curve.

There are sure to be future refinements of the laparoscopic approach. The most recent, laparoscopic hernioplasty without fixation,[9] may increase the technique's popularity. This approach reduces the cost slightly and also reduces the potential for nerve injury. In my opinion, as well as that of others,[18,19] further studies are required to prove that recurrence rates will not increase when the mesh is not fixed to the abdominal wall. To continue to improve our results we must continue to examine this and other new techniques, and make changes in the procedure as deemed appropriate.

REFERENCES

1. Lichtenstein IL, Shulman AL, Amid PK, et al. The tension-free hernioplasty. *Am J Surg.* 1989;157:188.
2. Schultz L, Graber J, Pietrafitta J, et al. Laser laparoscopic herniorrhaphy: a clinical trial—preliminary results. *J Laparoendosc Surg.* 1990;1:98.
3. Stoppa R, Rives JL, Walamount C, et al. The use of Dacron in the repair of hernias of the groin. *Surg Clin North Am.* 1984;64:269.
4. Nyhus L. Recurrent groin hernia. *World J Surg.* 1989;13:541.
5. Felix EL, Michas C. Double-buttress laparoscopic herniorrhaphy. *J Laparoendosc Surg.* 1993;3:1.
6. Felix EL, Michas C, McKnight RL. Laparoscopic herniorrhaphy-transabdominal preperitoneal repair. *J Surg Endosc.* 1994;8:100.
7. Felix E, Scott S, Crafton B, et al. Causes of recurrence after laparoscopic hernioplasty—A multicenter study. *Surg Endosc.* 1998;12:226.
8. Leibl B, Schmidt J, Daubler P, et al. A single institution's experience with transperitoneal laparoscopic hernia repair. *Am J Surg.* 1998;1715:446.
9. Ferzli G, Sayad P, Huie F, et al. Endoscopic extraperitoneal herniorrhaphy. A 5 year experience. *Surg Endosc.* 1998;12):1311.
10. Ramshaw B, Frankum C, Young D, et al. 1000 total extraperitoneal herniorrhaphies: After the learning curve. *Surg Endosc.* (in press).
11. Felix E, Habertson N, Varteian S. Laparoscopic hernioplasty: Significant complications. *Surg Endosc.* 1999;13:328.
12. Payne JH Complications of laparoscopic herniorrhaphy. *Semin Lap Surg.* 1997;4:166.
13. Leim M, Van der Graff Y, Van Steensel C, et al. Comparison of conventional anterior surgery and laparoscopic surgery for inguinal hernia repair. *N Engl J Med.* 1997;23:1541.
14. Cooper S, McAlhany J. Laparoscopic inguinal hernia repair: is the enthusiasm justified? *Am J Surg.* 1997;63:103.
15. Beets GI, Dirksen CD, Go P, et al. Open or laparoscopic preperitoneal mesh repair for recurrent inguinal hernia repair? A randomized controlled trial. *Surg Endosc.* 1999;13:323.
16. Go P. Overview of randomized trials in laparoscopic inguinal hernia repair. *Semin Laparosc Surg.* 1998;5:238.
17. Wright D. The learning curve for laparoscopic hernia repair. *Semin Laparosc Surg.* 1998;5:227.
18. Brooks D. Laparoscopic herniorrhaphy. Where are we now? *Surg Endosc.* 1999;13:321.
19. Macintyre I. Does the mesh require fixation. *Semin Laparosc Surg.* 1998;5:224.

Chapter Sixty-Three •••••••

*I*ncisional Hernia

JORGE E. BALLI, MORRIS E. FRANKLIN, JR., and J. ARTURO ALMEIDA

Laparoscopic repair of ventral and incisional hernia has steadily gained recognition as an alternative to open procedures over the past decade. Reports of the use of polytetrafluoroethylene (PFTE), Marlex, and other polypropylene mesh prosthetic materials have shown this to be a viable option for therapy,[1-4] using laparoscopy as the means to dissect the hernia sac, remove the bowel and omental tissue, and then apply a prosthesis, usually with a stapling technique. Ventral incisional herniorrhaphy has not enjoyed great success in the history of surgical attempts to obtain a reliable and durable repair. High recurrence rates have been reported in the literature not only with the first repair but also subsequent reattempts at repair followed by increasingly higher recurrence rates.[5,6] It is for this reason that we have sought an alternative to conventional open surgical treatment of ventral and incisional hernia. The technique reported in this chapter makes use of three phases of the laparoscopic procedure, which we feel help to insure the security of the repair and may ultimately decrease the recurrence rate.[7] Laparoscopic dissection of abdominal wall adhesions is followed by placement of fascia-approximating nonabsorbable suture, fixation of the polypropylene mesh with staples, and finally, use of percutaneous sutures to further fixate the mesh.[8] We report on 275 patients to serve as a basis for this technique, while experience and follow-up continue.

MATERIALS AND METHODS

From February 1991 through September 2000, a total of 275 patients were treated in two different hospital institutions by laparoscopic technique for primary umbilical hernias, recurrent umbilical or ventral incisional hernias, and Spigelian hernias. For purposes of this discussion, the recurrent umbilical hernias were all appropriately grouped with the ventral incisional hernias. The distribution of patients in this study is outlined in Table 63–1. During the above time frame, 97% of the hernia repairs were accomplished laparoscopically. The reasons for conversion were bowel distention not allowing proper visualization and mobilization, massive adhesions, and enterotomies encountered during the

procedure. The types of hernias are outlined in Tables 63–2 to 63–4. About 10% of the hernia repairs were performed at the same time of a concomitant operation, usually laparoscopic cholecystectomy, but also with appendectomies (where no mesh was used) and laparoscopic inguinal herniorrhaphy (Table 63–5). All patients had a routine preoperative evaluation consisting of CBC, blood chemistries, chest x-ray, and EKG. Patients were prepared for surgery with a mild bowel catharsis or a formal bowel preparation with laxatives and oral antibiotics if colon involvement in the hernia was suspected.

TECHNIQUE

The technique demands general anesthesia as well as placement of a nasogastric tube and a Foley catheter. The patient must be firmly attached to the table to allow for alterations in position to Trendelenburg, reverse Trendelenburg, or extreme side-to-side "airplaning" to allow bowel displacement and adhesions to be dissected. We prefer to secure the patient to the table with tape at the shoulder level. Sequential compression devices are applied to the legs and the video monitors are positioned at the foot of the table, or at a place convenient for viewing by all involved. The authors prefer pneumoperitoneum access with a Verres needle at an alternate site away from the incision scar or hernia, usually in the upper quadrants lateral to the rectus muscle. Rarely, an open Hasson technique is chosen (3 of 275 patients), but we have for the most part abandoned this technique. The adhesions opposite to the initial ports are carefully taken down and additional ports are placed as adhesions are cleared. Each of these additional trocars should be considered as a port through which a stapler (or laparoscope) can be placed. Therefore, 10 to 12-mm trocars are desirable at all ports, although we have drifted to all 5-mm ports except for the ones used to introduce the mesh and staples (Fig. 63–1). Bleeding must be meticulously controlled and bowel injury avoided as the anterior abdominal wall is being cleared. All large defects should be closed with sutures, if at all possible, and can be placed either percutaneously or laparoscopically. In our practice this is usually

TABLE 63–1. DEMOGRAPHICS

February 1991–September 2000	275
Total patients	
Male	122
Female	153
Average age	58.2 years
Range	27–100 years
Average height	5.51 ft
Average weight	194.87 lb

TABLE 63–2. TYPES OF HERNIAS

Hernia Type	Number
Umbilical	81
Ventral/incisional	192
Spigelian	2

TABLE 63–3. UMBILICAL HERNIAS

Uncomplicated	27
Complicated	54
Incarcerated fat	28
Incarcerated bowel	10
Strangulated bowel	16
TOTAL	81

TABLE 63–4. VENTRAL/INCISIONAL HERNIAS

Uncomplicated	63
Complicated	129
Incarcerated omentum	92
Incarcerated bowel	24
Strangulated bowel	13
Recurrent	34
TOTAL	192

TABLE 63–5. CONCOMITANT PROCEDURES

Procedure	No. Patients
Ventral herniorrhaphy with laparoscopic cholecystectomy and intraoperative cholangiogram	6
Ventral herniorrhaphy with laparoscopic antireflux procedure	3
Ventral herniorrhaphy with laparoscopically monitorized colon polypectomy	1
Ventral herniorrhaphy with laparoscopic inguinal herniorrhaphy	1
Umbilical herniorrhaphy with laparoscopic cholecystectomy and intraoperative cholangiogram	10
Umbilical herniorrhaphy with laparoscopic inguinal herniorrhaphy	3
Umbilical herniorrhaphy with appendectomy (purulent appendicitis, no mesh placed)	3

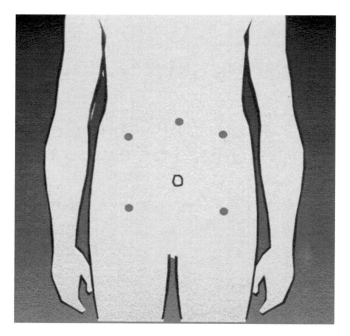

Figure 63–1. Trocar positions for a midline hernia repair.

accomplished percutaneously, using the Carter-Thomason needle point suture passer[9] (Inlet Medical, Eden Prairie, MN) with placement of #2 Tycron (Ethicon, Somerville, NJ) as individual sutures (Figs. 63–2 to 63–4).

Taking into consideration the thickness of the abdominal wall, polypropylene mesh (Surgipro, USSC, Norwalk, CT) is tailored to approximately 10% smaller than the area judged adequate for coverage of the defect, as estimated by laying the mesh out on the skin. As many defects as possible should be covered with each piece of mesh, while at the same time maintaining minimum margins of 3 to 5 cm circumferentially around each defect. Although one piece of mesh is ideal, it may not be possible in all instances, especially for those abdomens where extensive or multiple, widely

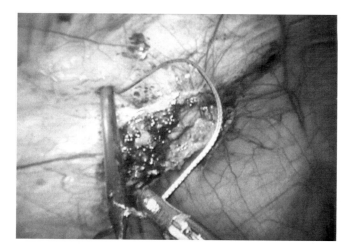

Figure 63–2. Carter-Thomason needlepoint suture passer introducing the suture. See Color Section.

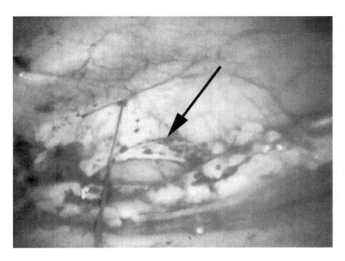

Figure 63–3. Suture being retrieved through the other side of defect. See Color Section.

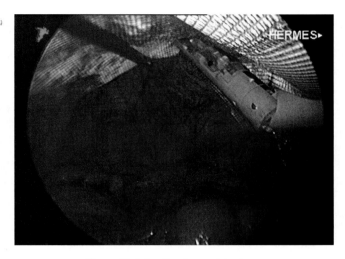

Figure 63–6. Stapling the mesh in place.

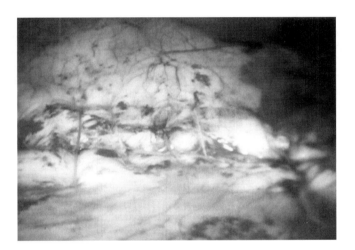

Figure 63–4. Defect closed. See Color Section.

spaced defects are present. The mesh must be placed over the defect and held in place with staples (Figs. 63–5 and 63–6) and, in most circumstances, transfascial sutures placed (Figs. 63–7 to 63–9). The presence of frank pus or necrotic bowel is consider a contraindication to mesh placement. If the peritoneal fluid is not cloudy on initial exam and strangulated bowel immediately has resumption of normal color, a mesh could be placed after a culture of the peritoneal fluid is obtained. There were no concomitant bowel resections in this group; however, since this study was concluded 2 patients were found to have necrotic bowel. One was resected laparoscopically and one extracorporeally; in the first patient a Vicryl mesh was placed and the later patient was repaired with sutures alone. Neither of these patients have had recurrence to this date. The trocar ports should all be carefully and completely closed (Figs. 63–10 and 63–11) (again, we prefer the Carter-Thomason needle point suture passer, Inlet Medical) and the abdomen desufflated after covering the repaired area with omentum (Fig. 63–12). The omentum is then spread over and tacked

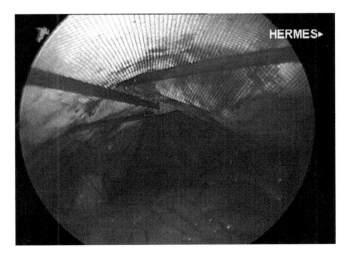

Figure 63–5. Holding and positioning the mesh in the abdominal cavity anterior wall covering defects >3 cm.

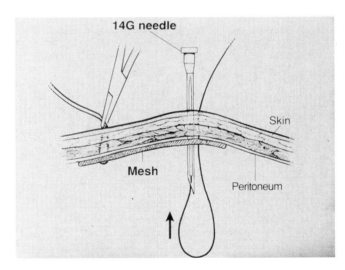

Figure 63–7. Mesh fixed to abdominal wall using transfascial Prolene sutures.

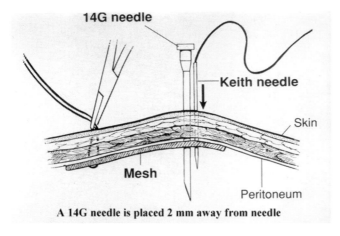

Figure 63–8. Technique of attachment of mesh with transfascial sutures.

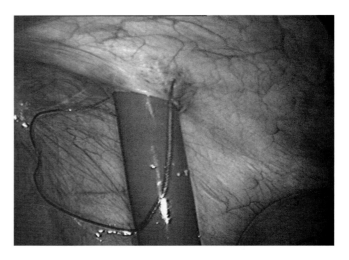

Figure 63–11. 12-mm trocar closure.

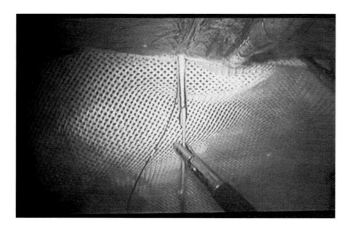

Figure 63–9. The straight needle returns through the 14 gauge-needle.

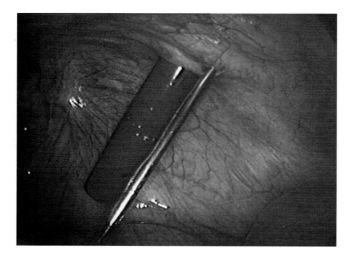

Figure 63–10. 12-mm trocar closure.

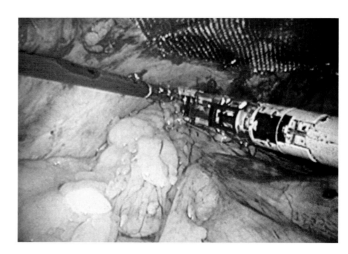

Figure 63–12. Omentum fixed with staples in pelvis, separating bowel from mesh. See Color Section.

(stapled) in place to serve as a barrier to separate the mesh from the bowel. Operation times vary with severity of adhesions, number of defects, bowel involvement, and need for concurrent procedures (Table 63–6).

The postoperative course is relatively benign, with the nasogastric tube and Foley catheter being removed in the recovery room in most instances. When excessive bowel manipulation is present due to adhesions or hernia involvement it is preferable to leave the nasogastric tube for 12 to 24 hours postoperatively. Hemoglobin, hematocrit, and electrolyte levels are checked the next day. We expect to occasionally see subcutaneous fluid in the hernia sites (serous), and explain this possibility to the patient preoperatively. This occurs at a much lower rate when the fascial defects are closed and "dead space" obliterated. The patient is given a diet when bowel sounds are present, which can vary from immediately to several days postoperative, depending on the amount of dissection,

TABLE 63–6. OPERATING TIMES

Hernia Type	Average (min)	Range (min)
Ventral hernia		
Uncomplicated	40	30–60
Complicated	105	72–165
Incisional hernia		
Uncomplicated	60	47–118
Complicated	120	70–210
Umbilical hernia		
With mesh	60	52–86
Without mesh	40	25–58

TABLE 63–7. COMPLICATIONS

Mortality	0
Morbidity	10.1%
Intraoperative complications	0
Early complications (<30 days)	(3.6%)
Trocar site infection	3
Urinary tract infection	2
Pulmonary	2
Prolonged ileus (>7 days)	2
Pseudo-obstruction	1
Late complications (>30 days)	(6.5%)
Mesh infection	1
Seroma/induration	10
Recurrent pain	5
Neuralgia at suture site	2
Recurrence	(0.72%)
Umbilical hernia	1
Ventral/incisional hernia	1
Spigelian hernia	0

handling of bowel, and bleeding. Patients are allowed to go home when they are afebrile, their wounds are clean, a regular diet is tolerated, and minimal pain is present.

EXPERIENCE

This procedure has been undergone by 275 patients during the past 9 years. Of the 275 patients, 172 had ventral incisional hernias (34 were recurrent), 20 with primary ventral hernia, 81 had primary umbilical hernias, and 2 had Spigelian hernias. Ninety-seven percent of the hernia repairs were completed laparoscopically. Follow-up has been for an average of 39.1 months (range, 1 to 116 months). Intraoperative complications have not been noted, but we have had 10 patients (3.6%) with early postoperative complications (<30 days) that included trocar site infection, prolonged ileus, urinary tract infection, pseudo-obstruction, and pulmonary problems. Late postoperative complications (>30 days) occurred in 18 patients (6.5%) and included seromas, recurrent pain, neuralgia, and mesh infection. Mesh infection occurred in only one patient, requiring its removal at 14 months postoperative. All patients had been instructed preoperatively that a "swelling" was anticipated at the site of the ventral hernia that could require several weeks to resolve. However, they were instructed to immediately report fever, increasing warmth at the site of the anticipated seroma, or an increase in local pain. Significant seromas were noted in only 2 patients, but the temptation to aspirate was overcome and the fluid collections finally resolved on their own (average time, 6 weeks).

The length of stay for these patients varied from 1 to 12 days, with the primary reason for prolonged stay related to combined cardiac and pulmonary problems in many of our patients, making any comparison of stay inaccurate.

Patients had been instructed to anticipate local discomfort associated with the repair. Recurrent pain in the ventral hernia area was noted in 2 patients without clinical evidence of recurrence. A prolonged period of "tightness" or "pulling" was reported by many in the subsequent weeks after surgery. Recurrence was noted in 2 patients (0.72%); one with a primary umbilical hernia at 4 months postoperatively that was not repaired with mesh, and one with a ventral incisional hernia repair at 14 months postoperative. There have been no mortalities in the series (Table 63–7).

DISCUSSION

Recurrence after open ventral herniorrhapy has been associated with multiple factors; infection at the time of the initial operation,[10] the size of the original hernia, tissue weakness, smoking, and poor blood supply of the scar tissue remain the most implicated.[5] Hesselink et al[5] noted a 60-month, 41% cumulative recurrence rate, with the second, third, and fourth incisional hernia repairs having 56, 48, and 47% recurrence rates, respectively. Unfortunately, the problem of the incisional hernia remains unresolved. Laparoscopic repair of ventral and incisional hernias has been studied as an innovative approach to this difficult problem. Polypropylene mesh has good tensile strength and has been shown to be a superior medium for tissue ingrowth, making it a suitable material to be used in laparoscopic repairs. Gore-Tex (polytetrafluoroethylene) prostheses have gained popularity in laparoscopic repair[1,11] because of apparent reduced

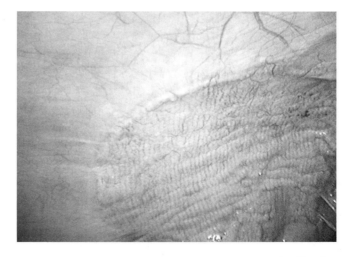

Figure 63–13. Intraperitoneal mesh seen 8 months postoperation. No adhesions noted. See Color Section.

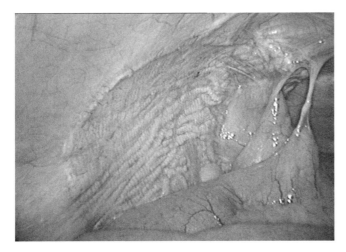

Figure 63–14. Intraperitoneal mesh seen 13 months postoperation. Mild adhesions that were easily taken down. See Color Section.

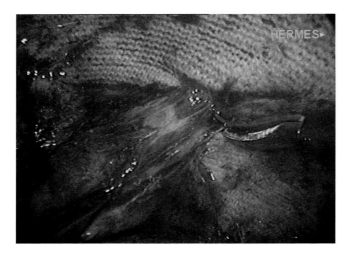

Figure 63–15. Intraperitoneal mesh seen 10 months postoperation. Severe adhesions present, partially liberated.

tissue reactivity (adhesion). It is therefore reliant on the inherent tensile strength of the material and on the continued integrity of the suture attachments of the prosthesis to the fascia. Newer dual prosthetic materials with polypropylene on one side and Gore-Tex (or some similar composite) on the opposite may be the ultimate answer.

In 192 patients with incisional hernias, we have noted only one recurrence (0.5%). The mean follow-up period for this subgroup is 4.1 years, with some patients now followed for up to 9 years. The complication rate has been quite acceptable in our opinion, with no intraoperative problems and a low overall complication rate of 10% in all categories of hernia repair (3.6% early, 6.5% late). In only one instance did infection lead to removal of the mesh. This occurred following a recurrent ventral herniorrhaphy with a staphylococcal mesh infection 14 months postoperatively. Two patients developed recurrent hernias; one umbilical repair without mesh failed at 4 months and was found to have the repairing sutures torn through the tissues. A laparoscopic repair with fascial sutures and mesh has now been in place for 45 months with no evidence of recurrence. The incisional recurrence followed infection of a graft as discussed earlier.

Although we have revisited laparoscopically only 4 patients in this series, including an umbilical recurrence and a patient with infected mesh, at times when an emergency surgery arose we have relaparoscoped 27 patients who had previously undergone inguinal intraperitoneal onlay mesh and ventral hernia repairs, and found that one third of the patients had no adhesions at all, one third had mild benign adhesions, but one third had severe adhesions (Figs. 63–13 to 63–15). All of this latter group had had prior surgery and needed adhesions taken down to complete the repair. There have been no instances of fistula formation of mesh migration into bowel to date. Thus this experience has let us to feel comfortable placing polypropylene mesh alone as a prosthetic material.

REFERENCES

1. Leblanc K, Booth WV. Laparoscopic repair of incisional abdominal hernias using expanded polytetrafluoroethylene, preliminary findings. *Surg Laparosc Endosc.* 1993;3: 39.
2. Sewell RW. Ventral hernia repair. In: MacFadyen BV, Ponsky JL, eds. *Operative Laparoscopy & Thoracoscopy.* Lippincott–Raven: 1996;807.
3. Gillion JF, Bégin GF, Marecos C, et al. Expanded polytetrafluoroethylene patches used in the intraperitoneal or extraperitoneal position for repair of incisional hernias of the anterolateral abdominal wall. *Am J Surg.* 1997;174:16.
4. Park A, Gagner M., Pomp A. Laparoscopic repair of large incisional hernias. *Surg Laparosc Endosc.* 1996;6:123.
5. Hesselink VJ, Luijendijk RW, de Wilt JWH, et al. An evaluation of risk factors in incisional hernia recurrence. Gynecol Obstet. 1993;176: 228.
6. George CD, Ellis H. The results of incisional hernia repair: A twelve year review. *Ann R Coll Surg Engl.* 1986;68:185.
7. Franklin ME. Laboratory rationale for intrapereitoneal placement of mesh in inguinal hernia repair. Abstract in: *Hernia 93: Advances or Controversies.* Indianapolis, 1993.
8. Rosenthal D, Franklin ME. Use of percutaneous stitches in laparoscopic mesh hernioplasty. *Surg Gynecol Obstet.* 1993;176:491.
9. Carter JE. A new technique of fascial closure for laparoscopic incisions. *J Laparoendosc Surg.* 1994;4:143.
10. Bucknall TE, Cox PJ, Ellis H. Burst abdomen & incisional hernia: A prospective study of 1129 major laparotomies. *Br Med J.* 1982;284: 931.
11. Toy FK, Smoot RT. Laparoscopic hernioplasty update. *J Laparoendosc Surg.* 1992;2:197.

Chapter Sixty-Four ● ● ● ● ● ●

*L*aparoscopic Incisional Preperitoneal Hernioplasty

SERGIO ROLL and WAGNER C. MARUJO

INCISIONAL HERNIAS

Incidence

Incisional hernias represent one of the more common complications of abdominal surgical procedures. The true incidence of incisional hernias has not been well defined, although a number of reports suggest that 3 to 13% of patients undergoing laparotomy will develop a fascial defect in their abdominal scar.[1] The majority of incisional hernias occur within the first postoperative year. However, the limited follow-up of most series may underestimate late hernia occurrence.

Diagnosis

Most patients with small and uncomplicated incisional hernias are asymptomatic or have only minor or intermittent complaints. However, these postoperative hernias may be a significant source of morbidity. Patients with incisional hernias alter their lifestyles so as not to exacerbate their abdominal wall hernia and often complain of their aesthetic appearance or suffer from discomfort, pain, or, occasionally, intestinal obstruction.

Predisposing Factors

Predisposing factors for the development of incisional hernias include patient characteristics such as advanced age and male gender; and systemic diseases such as obesity, cancer, chronic hepatic and cardiopulmonary failures, severe anemia, and malnutrition.[2,3] The underlying pathologic process, such as prostatism, radiotherapy, and steroid therapy, plus operative techniques, are also fundamental factors. Although the clinical experience seems to suggest that vertical celiotomy and the type of suture used (e.g., continuous suture and mass tissue closure) may increase the risk of incisional hernias, randomized studies have failed to show that any of these factors significantly alter the incidence of postoperative incisional hernia. Wound infection is associated with a fivefold increase in the risk of developing hernia.[1,4]

PRINCIPLES OF TREATMENT

The classical principles of ventral hernia repair are wound closure with no excessive tension, sutures placed in healthy tissue, and the use of strong material to support the wound through the critical period of healing. In many cases of incisional hernia with small-size defects, fascial closure can be achieved by apposing the fascial edges, closing the wound. When the fascial defect is large, a number of techniques have been proposed, including relaxing incisions, internal retention sutures, muscle or fascial flaps, fascial grafts, and the mesh repair.[5] However, the results have been often disappointing. Primary repair with suture only has been associated with 25 to 52% failure rates.[6] The use of a prosthetic material to cover the hernia defect has substantially reduced the incidence of recurrence. In a multicenter randomized trial enrolling 100 patients on each arm, Luijendijk et al compared the results of suture alone to mesh repair for incisional hernias.[7] After a follow-up of 36 months, the 3-year cumulative rates of recurrence among patients who had suture only and those who had mesh repair of a primary hernia were 43 and 24%, respectively. The recurrence rates were 58 and 20% for repair of the first recurrence. The risk factors for recurrence were suture repair, infection, prostatism, and previous surgery for abdominal aortic aneurysm. The size of the hernia did not affect the rate of recurrence. Most recurrences appear in the first 2 years after the repair. The same factors involved in the genesis of incisional hernias may contribute to these results.

Prosthetic Materials

The use of prosthetic materials to assist in incisional hernioplasty usually demands a more extensive dissection and may slightly increase the risk of wound healing complications.[5,8] The synthetic material should be physically unmodified by tissue fluid, chemically inert, and noncarcinogenic. It should also induce no inflammatory or foreign-body reaction, allergy, or hypersensitivity.[9,10] Finally, it should be able to resist mechanical stress, be tailored in the form required, and be easily and fully sterilized. The most popular prosthesis materials are made of polypropylene (PP), polyester (POL), and expanded polytetrafluorethylene (ePTFE). They are all nonabsorbable and there is no clear evidence from the literature that supports a preference for the clinical use of any one of the three main materials.[11] PP showed a relatively small inflammatory response with a far lesser degree of foreign-body reaction than the POL mesh. Expanded PTFE elicits less chronic inflammatory-cell reaction but greater foreign-body reaction. Mesh infection rates in selected laparoscopic series for repair of ventral and incisional hernias vary from 0.5 to 12%.[12] Despite different characteristics regarding fibroblastic reaction and time of incorporation, all of these prosthetic materials are associated with a high incidence of dense adhesions, and the reported low risk of adhesions and fistula formation by placing the mesh in contact with the peritoneum is not indisputable.[13] On the basis of current data, it seems that cost should be the deciding factor.

Repair Strategies

Although the modern era of hernia repair began more than a century ago, controversies continue about the optimal surgical technique to repair incisional hernias. Open techniques involve a large incision and extensive subcutaneous and intrabdominal dissection, and often necessitate the placement of drains. Complication rates range from 8 to 19% after open ventral repair.[14,15] Fistula rates after elective open hernia mesh repair vary from 2 to 5%.[6] Moreover, the infected prosthesis should be taken off, demanding a further more complicated repair. Transabdominal approaches carry the risk of injuring the viscera adherent to the undersurface of the scar. The basic strategy of the open repair is based on the Stoppa technique: The peritoneal cavity should not be entered and the mesh is secured to the fascial edges in the preperitoneal space.[16] However, the risk of reentering the site of a previous incision is an inadvertent enterotomy. The open repair allows the concomitant excision of a usually wide, irregular, and aesthetic scar. If this is the case, it is not unusual to enter the abdominal cavity.

Surgical laparoscopy has become an increasingly popular mode of treatment for many diseases because it potentially offers cost savings as a result of shorter hospital stays, less postoperative pain, and more rapid return to work.[17] Laparoscopic hernioplasty has been reported to be a safe and feasible technique with low morbidity and low rates of early recurrence. LeBlanc and Booth[18] first

reported the laparoscopic approach to repair incisional hernias in 1993, and several series have now demonstrated the efficacy of minimally invasive surgery in incisional hernia repair. The laparoscopic repair involves no long incision, no wide fascial dissection or flap creation, and usually no drains. It also minimizes the manipulation of a potentially contaminated site because the trocars are placed far distant from the original wound.[19] Moreover, the pneumoperitoneum facilitates the necessary adhesiolysis in order to identify the edges of the defect and the hernia sac. Enterotomy rates in selected laparoscopic series of ventral hernia repair, including incisional hernias and many with previous open mesh repair, vary from 0 to 14% (Table 64–1). Mesh infection rates vary from 0.5 to 12%.[12] One of the drawbacks of the laparoscopic approach is that it does not allow an aesthetic reconstruction of the abdominal wall, because the old scar that covers the hernia defect is left untouched. The need for an overall aesthetic result cannot be underestimated because this is frequently demanded by the patient.

INDICATIONS FOR LAPAROSCOPIC REPAIR

The size of the defect and the characteristics of a particular patient should dictate the best technical strategy. Patient selection for laparoscopic incisional hernioplasty is usually based on a demonstrable fascial defect over a previous abdominal incision or a highly suspected abdominal wall defect in a very obese patient such as seen in Spigelian hernia. The patient must be able to tolerate general anesthesia and abdominal insufflation.[20] Patient size is not a prohibiting factor, nor is the history of previous abdominal explorations or previous attempted repairs with or without placement of prosthetic material.

A massive incisional hernia with the protrusion of a substantial portion of the abdominal viscera might be a contraindication for a laparoscopic approach. A significant loss of the abdomen domain by the intestine might preclude the placement of the functional trocars because of insufficient lateral space. A densely scarred abdomen, inability to safely establish a pneumoperitoneum, and the presence of infected material in the abdomen may also contraindicate the laparoscopic approach.

It should be noted that intensity and extension of the adhesion formation is unpredictable. This way, multiple previous abdominal operations do not preclude laparoscopy, because an entry port for the first trocar can be obtained. The so-called "Swiss cheese" hernia is a good indication for the laparoscopic approach, because it allows a very clear delineation of the wall defects and

TABLE 64.1. RESULTS OF LAPAROSCOPIC VENTRAL/INCISIONAL HERNIOPLASTY

Author	Year	Reference	No. Patients	Complications		Hospital Stay (days)	Follow-up (months)	Recurrence
				Intraoperative	Postoperative			
Costanza et al	1998	14	31	0	2	2.0	18	1
Franklin et al	1998	34	176	0	9	2.2	30	2
Toy et al	1998	24	193	4	28	2.0	22	9
Sanders et al	1999	35	12	0	3	3.5	12	1
Scott-Roth et al	1999	20	73	2	14	2.9	17	7
Heniford et al	2000	6	415	5	48	1.8	23	14
Roll et al	2000	25	28	1	3	1.2	36	0

a more precise repair. Hernias very close to the costal margin may be difficult to treat through an open approach because they usually lack a good rim of strong tissue to secure the mesh. In this situation, the laparoscopic approach is more appropriate, considering that the mesh can be easily tacked to the internal face of the abdominal cavity. Moreover, full-thickness stitches around this area are usually followed by pain.

LAPAROSCOPIC TRANSABDOMINAL PREPERITONEAL (TAPP) REPAIR

Patient Preparation and Room Setup

A thorough preoperative evaluation is performed. The patient is fully informed about the risks of recurrence and the chances for conversion into an open procedure. Educational handouts are given in order to help convalescence, emphasizing pain control. Factors that might increase the recurrence rate are corrected if at all possible in the preoperative period. Special attention is given to respiratory care before admitting the patient to the hospital. In-hospital standard guidelines to prepare patients for abdominal surgery are followed. Mechanical bowel preparation is not usually necessary. The patient is asked to void just before leaving the ward.

The patient is placed on the operating table in a dorsal recumbent position with the arms padded along the body. It is important that the patient be securely belted to the operating table in order to permit the extremes of table positioning occasionally necessary for visceral retraction. General anesthesia is instituted and an orogastric tube is inserted for gastric decompression. Patients are given prophylactic antibiotic, usually a first-generation cephalosporin.

For most midline hernias, the surgeon stands on either the patient's left or right side. The video monitor is positioned on the opposite side, so the surgeon's view on the screen is parallel and in line with the laparoscopic repair of the hernia within the abdomen. The assistant stands opposite the surgeon, and a second monitor is placed in a suitable position.

Operative Technique

Good laparoscopic skills are mandatory, since each anatomic situation may be unique. The surgeon must always keep a low threshold for conversion to an open repair. Access to the abdominal cavity is obtained in an area away from the hernia using the Veress needle or, more frequently, by the open technique. Pneumoperitoneum is established by insufflating the abdomen to 12 mm Hg with carbon dioxide. A 30-degree laparoscope is introduced through the initial trocar, and the abdomen is explored. The hernia defect and any associated adhesions are identified. Usually two or three additional trocars are inserted under direct vision. The ultimate number and the exact site of the trocars depend on each individual case. For an optimal view and exposure, it is better to place the working ports as far away from the hernia defect as possible. Since the mesh will overlap the defect by about 3 cm, a very lateral or inferior position of the trocar sites maximizes the view and the efficiency of the instruments.

The repair technique is based on the Stoppa technique used in the open surgical procedure, in which the prosthetic material is placed posteriorly to the anterior fascia.[21] An adhesionlysis is performed to free the bowel from the abdominal wall and the margins

of the hernia defect are clearly defined. External manual pressure on the abdominal wall helps to delineate the edges of the hernia defect. It also changes the angles of vision and usually facilitates the dissection. Once the entire abdominal wall is cleared up and any incarcerated omentum or bowel reduced, the hernia defect is measured by introducing a sterile ruler into the peritoneal cavity. The surgeon must be very cautious when dissecting the bowel wall or omentum from the hernia sac, which typically encompasses attenuated fascia and peritoneum. The adhesionlysis is almost always the most challenging part of this procedure, especially if a previous mesh repair has already been attempted. Any energy source is capable of causing a full-thickness injury to the bowel wall. A harmonic scalpel may obviate the chances of an inadvertent injury. The standard approach in the advent of an enterotomy is the immediate simple suture. If this injury is complicated by a significant spillage of luminal fluids, an open primary repair might be performed or a staged laparoscopic mesh placement be devised.

The hernia sac contents are reduced and the peritoneal sac is now opened, followed by the precise delineation of the fascial defect, with at least 4 cm of healthy tissue surrounding it. Whenever possible, small-size fascial defects can be primarily closed by simply suturing the edges of the defect without tension. The suture is then covered by a mesh to reinforce the herniorrhaphy. This procedure may prevent the annoying sensation of the mesh just underlying the skin.

Dissecting within the preperitoneal plane in attempting to develop an intact layer to separate the mesh from the abdominal contents might be extremely difficult in some patients. If unsuccessful, this might result in a large peritoneal defect, leaving the mesh internally exposed. This is especially true in those patients with only a thin layer of subcutaneous fat and skin overlying the hernia. In this case, some authors recommend interfacing the omentum between the mesh and the bowel. However, we struggle to interface the sac layer between the mesh and the abdominal contents (Fig. 64–1). With some hernias it is easier to dissect out the healthy fascial edges within the preperitoneal space; these include incisional hernias secondary to extraperitoneal surgical incisions, such as lumbotomies or Pfannenstiel's, and defects away from the

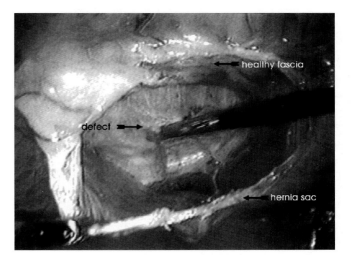

Figure 64–1. The hernia sac is opened and the healthy fascia along the defect rim is clearly defined.

midline. If the preperitoneal technique is deemed impossible, the hernia sac is not reduced, resected, or opened, and the mesh is positioned intraperitoneally according to the onlay technique.[22]

Prosthetic materials have been used with increasing confidence in direct contact with the abdominal contents. Complications have been few and may reflect selective reporting of good results. We always attempt to perform a transabdominal preperitoneal repair that uses mesh prosthesis to cover and close the hernia defect. The mesh, under some tension, should be secured to the abdominal wall using a hernia stapler or a tacking device, or sutured into position with full-thickness transabdominal stitches buried in the subcutaneous tissues. The stitches along the outer border of the mesh should leave a 3-cm margin lateral to the edges of the fascial defect (Fig. 64–2). Drains are not used. The trocar sites are then closed in the usual fashion.[23]

The most common early complications after the laparoscopic repair are suture site pain, when using the transabdominal stitches, and seroma. The former is probably related to some muscular ischemia and nerve entrapment. The development of seroma is secondary to the creation of a dead space and a secretory reaction to the prosthetic material. Only large and symptomatic collections should be aspirated.

Immediate Postoperative Care

Postoperatively, patients are given narcotics for appropriate analgesia. Liquid diet is started on the same day, and patients are

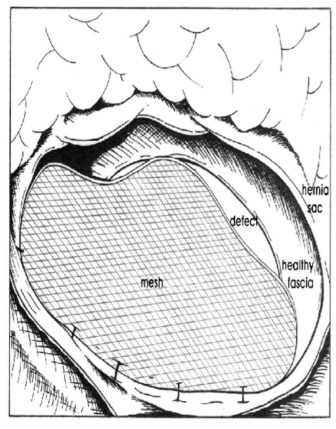

Figure 64–2. The mesh is positioned into the preperitoneal space and secured to the abdominal wall. The stitches along the outer border of the mesh must overlap the rim of the hernia defect by at least 3 cm.

encouraged to ambulate as soon as possible. Bowel function usually resumes very early on.[24] Selected patients may go home on the same day but most are discharged on the first postoperative day. Most patients develop an area of induration at the previous hernia site, but this resolves without complications or treatment within 4 to 6 weeks. In general, the patient is oriented to return to work at his or her convenience, and heavy physical activities are allowed 2 to 4 weeks later.

PERSONAL SERIES RESULTS

From January 1997 to October 2000, 28 patients underwent attempted laparoscopic incisional hernia repair.[25] We excluded from this series Spigelian hernias and incisional hernias that ended up requiring the intraperitoneal onlay technique. Total hernia repairs were 28 (one patient with two incisional hernias), one of which required conversion to an open repair because of dense adhesions and an inadvertent intestinal injury. Thirteen were females and 15 males. The defect size ranged from 64 to 225 cm². The original surgical procedures were hysterectomy (3), appendectomy (10), prostatectomy (4), gastrectomy (2), nephrectomy (3), laparotomy (2), epigastric herniorrhaphy (4), and umbilical herniorrhaphy (1). In all cases except one (the patient with two incisional hernias), the defect was covered with a single large piece of mesh. In all but 3 patients (POL mesh), we used a PP mesh for the repair. The average operating time was 60 minutes (range, 30 to 240 minutes), varying in relation to the degree of adhesionlysis required. All patients were discharged in the first 24 hours, with the exception of one patient who had an enterotomy recognized during the procedure. The mean length of hospital stay was 1.2 days (1 to 4 days). Patients required minimal amounts of postsurgical analgesia. Bowel function returned quickly in most patients.

There were no deaths. Four complications were recorded (14.8% of patients), most of them minor: two seromas, one hematoma, and one accidental small bowel enterotomy. Patients were closely followed postoperatively from 1 to 58 months (mean, 36 months), with no evidence of hernia recurrence. Most patients developed an area of induration at the hernia site, but this resolved without any treatment within 4 to 6 weeks. Apart from this transient induration, we have encountered no complications as a result of excising the hernia sac.

COMPARATIVE STUDIES OF OPEN VERSUS LAPAROSCOPIC REPAIR

Two retrospective studies and only one prospective study were designed to compare the results of open surgery techniques versus the laparoscopic approach for the repair of ventral hernias, which mostly included incisional defects (Table 64–2). In 1997, Holzman et al compared 21 patients with ventral/incisional hernias repaired laparoscopically with a group of 16 patients who had undergone the conventional open mesh repair. The mean follow-up was similar and two recurrences occurred in each group. The investigators concluded that the advantages of the laparoscopic approach seem to be a reduced rate of postoperative complications and wound healing problems, and more rapid recovery after surgery.[26] In 1998, Park et al compared 56 laparoscopic prosthetic repairs of large incisional hernias with 49 open surgical procedures.[27] The mean

TABLE 64–2. COMPARISON STUDIES OF LAPAROSCOPIC VERSUS OPEN REPAIR OF VENTRAL/INCISIONAL HERNIA

Study	Year	Cost (US$)	Repair Type	No. Patients	Size (cm²)	Time (min)	Complications Intraoperative	Complications Postoperative	Reop.	Hosp. Stay (days)	Follow-up (months)	Recurrence
Holzman et al[26]	1997	7299	Open	16	148	98	0	5	2	4.9	18	2
		4395	Lap	21	105	128	1	4	0	1.6	20	2
Park et al[27]	1998		Open	49	105	78	1	17	0	6.5	53	17
			Lap	56	99	95	0	10	2	3.4	24	6
Carbajo et al[28] (prospective study)	1999		Open	30	141	111	0	35	1	9	27	2
			Lap	30	139	87	0	5	1	2	27	0

follow-up was 24 months for the laparoscopic group and 53 months for the open procedure. The hernia recurred in 6 patients in the laparoscopic group (11%) and in 17 patients in the open repair group (34%), but the investigators could not make a meaningful comparison of the recurrence rates because of the large difference in the follow-up period. They found that the laparoscopic procedure took longer to perform but it was associated with fewer complications and shorter postoperative hospital stay. In the only prospective randomized study of laparoscopic repair versus open repair, Carbajo et al randomized 60 patients over a 3-year period into two homogeneous groups to be operated on for major ventral hernias using mesh.[28] Two recurrent hernias occurred in the open repair group and none in the laparoscopic group, with an average follow-up of 27 months. They concluded that laparoscopic repair reduces complications and the recurrence rate and offers several advantages over the classic surgical repair of abdominal wall defects.

ADVANTAGES AND DISADVANTAGES OF DIFFERENT LAPAROSCOPIC TECHNIQUES

The critical assessment of the reported results is difficult and potentially misleading due to the significant variations in terminology, patient selection, and operative techniques.[29] There are no available data to unequivocally support an overt advantage of any particular technique to repair incisional hernias. Clinical judgment, previous experience, and surgical team skills should guide the decision of which technique to apply to a particular patient. Despite the pitfalls of the available data, mainly from retrospective studies of selected patients, recurrence and complication rates do not seem to be much different regardless of the technique employed: open versus laparoscopic, and laparoscopic intraperitoneal versus preperitoneal.

The most popular laparoscopic technique of incisional hernia repair proposes a transperitoneal approach using a composite mesh prosthesis in intraperitonel location.[30,31] Biomaterials have become an important tool because they can permanently replace the defective transversalis fascia and permit the creation of a true tension-free hernioplasty. However, use of biomaterials is associated with four major concerns: rejection, infection, early adhesion and fixation, and host tissue incorporation. It is well known that a peritoneal defect or the presence of a foreign body in the abdominal cavity creates adhesions.[13] This in turn may result in major complications, including intestinal obstruction, migration of the foreign body and erosion into the bowel, fistula, and infection. In general, complications resulting from intraperitoneal adhesions account for a significant number of emergency surgical admissions and abdominal operations.[7] These concerns have prompted the development of a further refinement in the transabdominal laparoscopic approach: the preperitoneal laparoscopic mesh repair. Dissecting within the preperitoneal plane in order to create anatomic room for the mesh may sometimes be extremely difficult. On the other hand, our own experience shows that this approach is technically feasible in many circumstances, and indeed, this procedure is an extension of our current laparoscopic techniques for repairing inguinal hernias.[32] However, we should also underscore the fact that even the preperitoneal repair of inguinal hernias has not been free of adhesions and associated bowel complications. Only a longer follow-up will be able to determine if the theoretical advantages of positioning the mesh in the preperitoneal location will overcome the possible disadvantages of a more tedious procedure that usually demands a longer operative time.[33]

SUMMARY

The laparoscopic route has made possible the introduction of new surgical techniques for the repair of major abdominal wall defects. The laparoscopic surgeon is able to minimize the great degree of tissue traumatism involved in the classic surgery, typically associated with large fascial dissections, tense sutures, and postoperative drainages.

Laparoscopic repair of incisional hernias is a promising but still new technique that may be seen as a further refinement of the current surgical armamentarium to treat this common problem in general surgery. As with any new operation, we should initially be more careful about patient selection before embarking in a broader application of this technique. Adequate training and judicious indication can certainly ensure good surgical outcomes.

Up to now, patients in several series have tolerated the procedure well and had shorter postoperative hospitalizations in comparison to open procedures. Accordingly, given the potentially lower morbidity due to the smaller abdominal wall incisions, the overall hospital cost may be reduced, making this a more attractive approach to incisional hernias. Moreover, laparoscopy allows a comprehensive exploration of the abdominal cavity, an adequate assessment of the adherences in the hernia process, and a clear delineation of the topography. It may be the procedure of choice in patients who develop recurrence following a prior open hernia repair.

Laparoscopic incisional hernia repair can be safely performed with no increased morbidity or mortality, but the ultimate outcome in assessing the success of any hernia repair must be the rate of recurrence. The literature suggests that the laparoscopic approach, regardless of where the mesh is placed, has a midterm recurrence rate at least as good as that seen after the open operation. However, long-term assessment from large and well-controlled prospective studies is needed to confirm the expected advantages of the laparoscopic approach.

REFERENCES

1. Santora TA, Roslyn JJ. Incisional hernia. *Surg Clin North Am.* 1993; 73:557.
2. Makela JT, Kivinieme H, Juvonen T, et al. Factors influencing wound dehiscence after midline laparotomy. *Am J Surg.* 1995;170:387.
3. Niggebrugge AH, Hansen BE, Trimbos JB, et al. Mechanical factors influencing the incidence of burst abdomen. *Eur J Surg.* 1995;161:655.
4. Meissner K, Jirikowski B, Szecsi T. Repair of parietal hernia by overlapping onlay reinforcement or "gap-bridging" replacement polypropylene mesh: Preliminary results. *Hernia.* 2000;4:29.
5. Larson GM. Ventral hernia repair by the laparoscopic approach. *Surg Clin North Am.* 2000;80:1329.
6. Heniford BT, Park A, Ramshaw BJ, et al. Laparoscopic ventral and incisional repair in 407 patients. *J Am Coll Surg.* 2000;190:645.
7. Luijendijk RW, Hop WCJ, Tol P, et al. A comparison of suture repair with mesh repair for incisional hernia. *N Engl J Med.* 2000;343:392.
8. Leber GE, Garb JL, Alexander AI, et al. Long-term complications associated with prosthetic repair of incisional hernias. *Arch Surg.* 1998; 133:378.
9. Amid PK, Shulman G, Lichtenstein I, et al. Preliminary evaluation of composite materials for the repair of incisional hernias. *Ann Chir.* 1995;49:539.
10. Amid PK. Classification of biomaterials and their related complications in abdominal wall hernia surgery *Hernia.* 1997;1:15.
11. Morris-Stiff H. The outcomes of nonabsorbable mesh. *J Am Coll Surg.* 1998;186:352.
12. Koehler RH, Voeller G. Recurrences in laparoscopic incisional hernia repairs: A personal series and review of the literature. *JSLS.* 1999;3:293.
13. Marchal F, Brunaud L, Sebbag H, et al. Treatment of incisional hernias by placement of an intraperitoneal prosthesis: a series of 128 patients. *Hernia.* 2000;3:141.
14. Costanza MJ, Heniford BT, Arca MJ, et al. Laparoscopic repair of recurrent ventral hernias. *Am Surg.* 1998;64:1.
15. Luijendijk RW, Lemmen MHM, Hop WCJ, et al. Incisional hernia recurrence following "vest-over-pants" or vertical Mayo repair of primary hernias of the midline. *World J Surg.* 1997;21:62.
16. Stoppa R. The treatment of complicated groin and incisional hernias. *World J Surg.* 1989;13:545.
17. Park A, Gaguer M, Pomp A. Laparoscopic repair of large incisional hernias. *Surg Laparosc Endosc.* 1996;6:123.
18. Le Blanc KA, Booth WV. Laparoscopic repair of incisional abdominal hernias using expanded polytetrafluoroetilene: Preliminary findings. *Surg Laparosc Endosc.* 1993;3:39.
19. Hashizume M, Migo S, Tsugawa Y, et al. Laparoscopic repair of paraumbilical ventral hernia with increasing size in an obese patient. *Surg Endosc.* 1996;10:933.
20. Scott-Roth J, Park AE, Witzke D, et al. Laparoscopic incisional/ventral herniorrhaphy: A five-year experience. *Hernia.* 1999;4:209.
21. Wants GE. Incisional hernioplasty with Mersilene. *Surg Gynecol Obst.* 1991;172:129.
22. Barie PS, Mack CA, Thompson WA. A technique for laparoscopic repair of herniation of the anterior abdominal wall using a composite mesh prosthesis. *Am J Surg.* 1995;170:62.
23. Larson GM. Laparoscopic repair of ventral hernia. In: Scott-Conner CEH, ed. *The SAGES Manual.* Springer:1998;379.
24. Toy FK, Bailey RW, Carey S, et al. Prospective multicenter study of laparoscopic ventral hernioplasty. *Surg Endosc.* 1998;12:955.
25. Roll S, Benatti M, Roncada P, et al. Laparoscopic incisional preperitoneal hernioplasty. Seventh world congress of endoscopic surgery, Singapore, 2000.
26. Holzman MD, Purut CM, Reintgen K, et al. Laparoscopic ventral and incisional hernioplasty. *Surg Endosc.* 1997;11:32.
27. Park AE, Birch DW, Lovrics P. Laparoscopic and open incisional hernia repair: A comparison study. *Surgery.* 1998;124:816.
28. Carbajo MA, Martín del Olmo JC, Blanco JI, et al. Laparoscopic treatment vs open surgery in the solution of major incisional and abdominal wall hernias with mesh. *Surg Endosc.* 1999;113:250.
29. Chevrel JP, Rath AM. Classification of incisional hernias of the abdominal wall. *Hernia.* 2000;4:7.
30. Alexandre JH, Aouad K, Bethoux JP, et al. Recent advances in incisional hernia treatment. *Hernia.* 2000; 4:1.
31. Balique JC, Alexandre JH, Arnaud JP, et al. Intraperitoneal treatment of incisional and umbilical hernias: Intermediate results of a multicenter prospective clinical trial using an innovative composite mesh. *Hernia.* 2000;4:10.
32. Roll S, DePaula AL, Miguel P, et al. Laparoscopic transabdominal inguinal hernia repair with a preperitoneal mesh. *Surg Endosc.* 1994;8: 484.
33. Saiz AA, Willis IH, Paul DK, et al. Laparoscopic ventral hernia repair: A community hospital experience. *Am Surg.* 1996;62:336.
34. Franklin ME, Dorman JP, Glass JL, et al. Laparoscopic ventral and incisional hernia repair. *Surg Laparosc Endosc.* 1998;8:294.
35. Sanders LM, Flint LM. Initial experience with laparoscopic repair of incisional hernias. *Am J Surg.* 1999;177:227.

Gynecologic Surgery

Chapter Sixty-Five • • • • • • •

Laparoscopic Surgery of the Tubes and Ovaries

RAFAEL F. VALLE

INTRODUCTION

Laparoscopic surgery has been performed since the beginning of the century, but its impact on gynecology was not felt until the end of the 1960s, when a multitude of applications for it were found, particularly in therapeutic procedures. Among the factors that have contributed to the development of laparoscopic technique is the availability of better endoscopes and more appropriate instruments. The refinement of electrical instruments for use intra-abdominally, such as bipolar coagulation, endocoagulation, and lasers, has contributed greatly to the advancements in operative laparoscopy.[1–7]

The use of laparoscopic technique for reconstructive surgery of the oviduct and ovaries grew during the 1970s and the early 1980s, particularly with the increasing use of microsurgery. The results obtained with conventional surgery for the treatment of pathologic states that affect the fallopian tubes and ovaries were disheartening. Laparoscopy, however, with its increased magnification and meticulous technique used to preserve vascularization and restore anatomic structure, will undoubtedly improve results.[8,9] This chapter will review laparoscopic techniques employed for the treatment of benign conditions affecting the tubes and ovaries, particularly those that affect fertility.

ANATOMIC AND PHYSIOLOGIC CONSIDERATIONS

Despite their embryonic origins, the fallopian tubes and ovaries form an anatomically and physiologically related complex. During the fifth week of gestation, the gonadal bud develops in the dorsal wall of the celomic cavity, via proliferation of the celomic epithelium and condensation of the mesoderm. The mesonephros and the gonadal bud are formed from a common mesodermic mass, and develop along with the paramesonephric ducts as an extension with a central distal fusion, which develops into the uterus and the

upper third of the vagina. The distal and upper parts of the paramesonephric ducts become the fallopian tubes.

The uterine tubes, which are about 10 to 12 cm long, share their vasculature, innervation, and lymphatic drainage with the ovaries. Several segments can be distinguished:

- The intramural portion connects the tube to the uterine body and is about 1 to 2 cm long; its narrowest diameter is 0.2 to 0.5 mm.
- The isthmus is 2 to 3 cm long and has an internal diameter of 0.5 to 3 mm.
- The ampulla, where the tubes increase in diameter from 1 to 10 mm in the distal portion, measures about 5 to 8 cm.
- The infundibulum contains numerous finger-like extensions called fimbria, one of which, the ovarian fimbria, joins the distal portion to the ovary.

As a duct, the ovarian tube has a complex physiology, which allows transportation of the sperm, uptake of the ovum, and fertilization and transportation of the embryo. Many anatomic and hormonal interactions participate in these processes. Although no single portion of the tubes is essential for reproduction and fertility, damage to the ampulla and the fimbria can gravely affect reproductive function.

INDICATIONS FOR SURGERY OF THE UTERINE TUBES AND PREOPERATIVE EVALUATION

Most therapeutic procedures performed on the uterine tubes are directed at promoting or preserving fertility, which should be thoroughly evaluated before considering doing one of these procedures, which will be described. Laparoscopy and hysterosalpingography are valuable elements in the evaluation of peritoneal and tubal factors for infertility. This is why laparoscopy should not be performed until all factors for infertility not requiring endoscopy have been evaluated. All cases should have a hysterosalpingography performed as part of an infertility evaluation, not only because it allows detection of intrauterine disease, but because it shows the anatomy clearly and demonstrates the permeability and architecture of the tubes. This method can evaluate the site of obstruction, the presence of diverticuli, the preservation of tubal folds, and the degree of obstruction (partial or total) in the tube, enabling preparation for definitive surgical treatment. The tube can be affected at different sites, owing to adhesions, and concomitant damage to the tubal epithelium, generally as sequelae of an infection. A pure segmental obstruction can be seen after elective tubal sterilization.

Of the many classifications proposed for tubal disease, the one adopted by the International Fertility Society is probably the most understandable and practical (Table 65–1). The classification of therapeutic procedures performed on the tubes includes adhesiolysis and plastic surgery of the tubes in their intramural portions and the middle and distal segments. While the obstruction of the cornual tube not treatable by catheterization requires a microsurgical laparoscopic approach, the distal segment can be treated by laparoscopy. Currently, obstructions in the middle segment are not routinely treated by laparoscopy, due to the difficulty in aligning

TABLE 65–1. CLASSIFICATION OF SURGERY USED TO TREAT TUBOPERITONEAL FACTORS AFFECTING INFERTILITY

A. Adhesiolysis: Surgery for lysis of adhesions
  1. Ovariolysis: removal of periovarian adhesions
    a) Minimal adhesions: 1 cm or less of ovary affected
    b) Moderate adhesions: ovary partially surrounded
    c) Serious adhesions: encapsulated periovarian adhesions
  2. Salpingolysis: removal of peritubarian adhesions
    a) Minimal adhesions: 1 cm affected
    b) Moderate adhesions: tube partially surrounded
    c) Serious adhesions: peritubarian adhesions
  3. Extra-adnexal lysis of adhesions
    a) Minimal adhesions
    b) Moderate adhesions
    c) Serious adhesions
B. Surgery of the fallopian tube
  1. Tubo-uterine implantation
    a) Isthmic
    b) Ampullar
    c) Combined
  2. Tubotubal anastomosis
    a) Interstitial cornual or intramural: isthmus
    b) Interstitial cornual or intramural: ampulla
    c) Isthmus-isthmus
    d) Isthmus-ampulla
    e) Ampulla-ampulla
    f) Combined
  3. Salpingoneostomies
    a) Terminal
    b) Ampullar
    c) Isthmic
    d) Combined
  4. Fimbrioplasties
    a) For liberation and dilatation
    b) With serosal incision (for completely occluded tubes)
    c) Combined
  5. Other reconstructive tubal operations (for specific indications)
  6. Combination of several types of operations
    a) Bipolar: occlusion of both ends of the tube, proximal and terminal
    b) Bilateral: several operations on the right and left sides

Revised from Cognat MA. Classification of the operations for tuboperitoneal infertility. *Acta Europ Fertil.* 1982;13:47.

the tubal segments after eliminating fibrosis, and the ability to perfectly align them microsurgically.[83,84]

Laparoscopy: Instrumentation and Energy Sources

Operative laparoscopy requires special preparation of the patient. The instrumentation needed is extensive, and the needed instruments must be available to ensure that the procedure is performed with ease and security. A variety of instruments may be needed: clamps, scissors, cannulas, hemostatic agents, staples, and sutures, among others.

Electrosurgical or laser units should also be available. The laparoscopes that are most useful in performing advanced laparoscopic surgery have a diameter of at least 10 mm, which allows adequate observation with a wide angle. The quality of the image is directly related to the type of telescope, the sensitivity of the videocamera, the integrity of the light cable, and the quality of the light source. A powerful xenon or halogen light source is best. Numerous trocars from 5 to 10 mm may be required, which makes it essential to have a high-flow insufflator available that can be controlled electronically to achieve quick filling of the abdomen, with a safety interlock to regulate pressure; this is particularly important when a CO_2 laser is used, because it requires continuous evacuation of the smoke produced. These units should be capable of providing 5 to 9 L of CO_2 a minute.

A number of clamps, scissors, and other instruments are required during operative laparoscopy, but two are indispensable for advanced laparoscopic surgery: an irrigation-aspiration system and bipolar Kleppinger-type clamps.

The irrigation-aspiration system is useful not only to keep the operative field free of blood clots and detritus, but also to allow clear dissection of the peritoneal surface under optimal vision and to allow retroperitoneal dissection. Kleppinger clamps are also useful, allowing coagulation of tissues using bipolar energy during dissection, and allowing dissections employing both bipolar and monopolar energy to avoid damaging adjacent tissues. Monopolar energy is best applied with needle electrodes, to dissect specific areas of adhesion, and to perform procedures on the tubes when they have been liberated from other tissues.

Laser energy is also useful, especially because of its precision and the reduction in tissue damage. The CO_2 laser is the most useful for this type of surgery due to its penetration, which can be controlled to within 0.2 mm, and to its scalpel-like precision, which is especially useful for adhesiolysis and accurate dissection of tissues. However, fiberoptic lasers can also be used for this, although the fibers should be kept a safe distance from the tissue, which can be done with the tips pointing outwards, allowing better focus of laser energy.

The Nd:YAG laser, originally used for endometrial ablation because of its deep penetration (4 to 5 mm) when applied with the fibers, can also be used without the fibers when shallower penetration is needed for cutting and coagulation.

LAPAROSCOPIC SURGERY OF THE FALLOPIAN TUBES

The original applications of operative laparoscopy were for tubal sterilization, extraction of foreign bodies, and taking tissue for biopsy. Although thin adhesions were sometimes lysed, extensive dissection was not attempted. Gomel[1,10] began doing operative laparoscopy of the uterine tubes and ovaries in the early 1970s, including salpingo-ovariolysis, fimbrioplasty, neosalpingostomy, salpingo-oophorectomy, and treatment of tubal pregnancy. In Europe, Semm had developed techniques to perform these and other procedures at the end of the 1960s.[2,4] However, advancements in technology in general, in videocameras, in light sources, and in instrumentation, only made these applications a practical reality for most gynecologists in the last decade.

ADHESIOLYSIS

Pelvic and abdominal adhesions are common sequelae of pelvic infection and major abdominal surgery, and can affect fertility when they afflict the tubes or ovaries (Fig. 65–1). Most adhesions are thin and avascular, but some are thick and richly vascularized, and still others involve adjacent organs such as intestine. The key to success and safety in these procedures is clearly recognizing the structures, and having enough space to allow a safe division. At least two trocars are needed for these procedures: one to insert the instrument (scissors, laser, etc.) and one for traction and irrigation. If the CO_2 laser is used to aid dissection, it can be introduced through the laparoscope. This gives the surgeon more flexibility, allowing use of the instrument as a scalpel to cut and dissect tissues, while the other trocars are used to manipulate the structures. Most thin vascular adhesions can be incised, but if they are thicker, it is easier to divide them in layers, applying traction to expose their origins and divide them safely. Continuous irrigation with Ringer's lactate is important when these procedures are performed.[10–18]

Gomel[19] published a series of 92 patients in whom salpingo-ovariolysis was performed laparoscopically after a period of involuntary infertility of over 20 months; the rate of viable pregnancies was 58.7% after the intervention (Table 65–2). The results of other groups using similar techniques are shown in Tables 65–3 and 65–4.

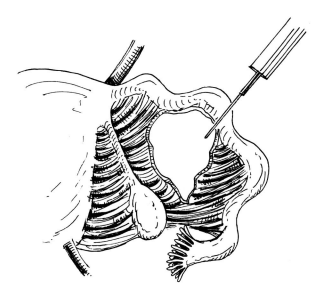

Figure 65–1. Lysis of adhesions (peritubarian and periovarian) with the use of a monopolar electrode tip or CO_2 laser.

TABLE 65–2. RESULTS OF LAPAROSCOPIC SALPINGO-OVARIOLYSIS IN 92 PATIENTS WITH INFERTILITY OF MORE THAN 20 MONTHS' DURATION

Results	Number of Patients
Viable births	54 (58.7%)
Voluntary termination	2
Spontaneous abortions	(4*) + 1
Ectopic pregnancy	(2*) + 3
Without pregnancy	32

*These patients also achieved term pregnancies.
From Gomel.[19]

FIMBRIOPLASTY AND NEOSALPINGOSTOMY

Distal obstruction as a consequence of pelvic inflammatory disease or previous surgery is the most common pathologic state found in the fallopian tube treated with surgery (Fig. 65–2). Unfortunately the results obtained with macroscopic and microscopic surgery have not been satisfactory, with a pregnancy rate ranging between 20 and 35%. Gomel[19] has treated this condition laparoscopically since 1970, but laparoscopic surgery was reserved for patients in whom microsurgical tubal reconstruction failed, which made comparison between the techniques difficult. In spite of this, the results of laparoscopic reconstruction of the occluded tubes seemed promising.

Tubal fibrosis or partial occlusion of the tubes can result in agglutination of the distal fimbria by the fibrous tissue covering the distal portion, or in stenosis of the distal ampulla, in which case the external appearance of the fimbria is relatively normal, but there is a ring constricting the infundibulum, which can be made apparent with chromoperturbation. Some excellent alternatives for performing these procedures are the CO_2 laser, fine-fiber fiberoptic lasers, monopolar needle electrodes, and microscissors; however, precise identification of the anatomic landmarks is required to avoid unnecessary damage to the tubes. Transcervical tubal chromoperturbation is very convenient for orientation and to confirm that the procedure has been completed successfully. Gomel[19] reported a successful pregnancy rate of 47.5% in 40 patients subjected to laparoscopic fimbrioplasty (Table 65–4 and Fig. 65–3). A study by Fayez[17] reported 5 pregnancies in 14 women subjected to laparoscopic fimbrioplasty.

Fimbrioscopy and salpingostomy, introduced by Nezhat, are also of use in the intraoperative evaluation of the fallopian tubes.[6] By suspending the fimbria in liquid and using a 3-mm salpingoscope to view the ostium tubarii with a videocamera (which

TABLE 65–3. RESULT OF LAPAROSCOPIC PROCEDURES PERFORMED TO PROMOTE FERTILITY

Procedure	Number of Patients	Total Pregnancies (%)
Ovariolysis	19	4 (21)
Salpingolysis	25	9 (36)
Fimbrioplasty	51	16 (31)
Salpingostomy	38	10 (26)

From Mettler et al.[18]

TABLE 65–4. RESULTS OF LAPAROSCOPIC FIMBRIOPLASTY IN 40 PATIENTS WITH INFERTILITY OF MORE THAN 22 MONTHS' DURATION

Result	Number of Patients
Viable births	9 (47.5%)
Spontaneous abortions	(1*) + 1
Ectopic pregnancy	2
Without pregnancy	18

*This patient also had a viable pregnancy.
From Gomel.[10]

enhances the image by magnifying the structures) any folds and adhesions requiring treatment can be detected.[20–22]

Dissection of the fimbria cannot be accomplished when the fallopian tube is affected by hydrosalpinx. In these cases a neosalpingostomy is performed; an incision in the form of a cross is made in the distal portion of the tube, and the intratubal mucosa is examined (Fig. 65–4).

The operation begins in the central part of the occluded distal portion, where a depression caused by scarring can be seen. Once the serosa has been incised, a cannula is inserted, and the incisions are performed from this site, if possible where the scar tissue is seen, generally where the tube is thinnest. This incision can be made with the CO_2 or fiberoptic laser and monopolar needle, and the distal portion of the tube is injected with indigo carmine to outline the salpinx during the procedure. Once the neosalpingostomy is completed, new leaflets are made out of the tube, they are everted using Bruhat's technique, and an unfocused CO_2 laser is used to coagulate the base of the new sheets. A bipolar coagulator at a low intensity or a regular endocoagulator can also be used.[20–22]

In 1977 Gomel[23] reported the results of laparoscopic salpingostomy performed on 9 women who had a previous laparotomy performed and had subsequently reoccluded; four of these patients had intrauterine pregnancies. Other studies reported success rates of 14 to 44% after laparoscopic salpingostomy. It is clear that the results obtained with microsurgery are the same as those obtained with laparoscopy, which has made laparoscopy the first line method for performing neosalpingostomy.

Canis et al[24] reported a series of 87 patients who were subjected to operative laparoscopy for distal tubal occlusion and followed for 4 years; 33.3% achieved pregnancy, and 6.9% presented with ectopic pregnancies. Many authors classify the damage to the distal tube in four stages, based on the hysterosalpingographic appearance of the damaged submucosa, the degree of obstruction, and the laparoscopic appearance of the tube. The patients in stages 3 and 4 had the worst prognosis, making in vitro fertilization (IVF) their best alternative, laparoscopy being performed only when this technique failed. The results obtained were similar to those obtained with microsurgery, with 86.7% of the pregnancies occurring during the first postoperative year, after which the fertility rate declined dramatically. IVF is recommended for any patients who have not achieved pregnancy 18 months after the procedure (Table 65–5).[25–27]

LAPAROSCOPIC TREATMENT OF ECTOPIC PREGNANCY

According to the Centers for Disease Control and Prevention (CDC) the incidence of ectopic pregnancy is increasing.[28] In the last 10 to 15 years the number of cases per 1000 pregnancies has almost doubled, from 9.4 in 1978 to 16.8 in 1987. The most important cause for this increase is the prevalence of pelvic inflammatory disease and surgery of the tubes; however, measurement of beta human chorionic gonadotrophin (β-hCG) and the use of

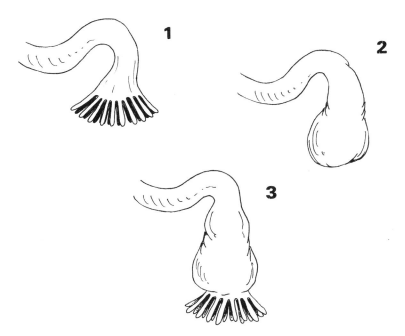

Figure 65–2. Normal and diseased fallopian tubes. **1.** Normal fallopian tube, with its fimbriae free of adhesions. **2.** Complete occlusion of the distal fallopian tube. **3.** Phimosis of the distal Fallopian tube.

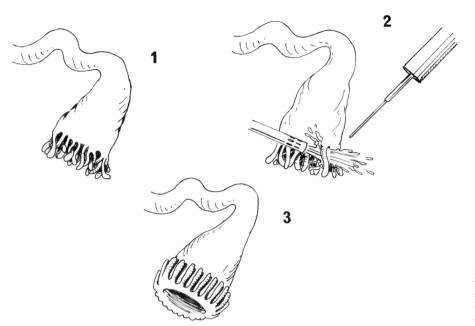

Figure 65–3. Laparoscopic fimbrioplasty. **1.** Agglutination of the distal fimbriae. **2.** Dissection and lysis of adhesions using a hydrodissector and a monopolar tip. **3.** Eversion of the fimbriae after laparoscopic treatment.

transvaginal ultrasonography have aided in the early detection of ectopic pregnancy.[29–31] At one time, the only treatment for ectopic pregnancy was total salpingectomy, but the use of linear microsurgical salpingostomy gained popularity during the 1970s because it improved the reproductive prognosis.[32–35] Later in that decade the condition began to be treated laparoscopically, and in 1980 this method was adopted with excellent results (Table 65–6).[36–40]

When selecting patients it is important to evaluate the hemodynamic state, which should be stable and without signs of hypovolemic shock. An intact gestational sac from an ectopic pregnancy is evaluated by laparoscopy, a small incision is made with laser,

electrosurgery, or microscissors, along the antimesenteric border of the tube adjacent to the sac (Fig. 65–5). The tubal pregnancy is extracted by hydroperturbation with an irrigation cannula through the salpingostomy incision. Dilute vasopressin can be injected at the base of the ectopic pregnancy to reduce bleeding. This method works best when the sac is in the ampullar portion, which is the most frequent site (78%), but in some instances it can be attempted in the isthmic portion, where the subsequent fibrosis may require a future segmental resection.

Vermesh and Presser[39] analyzed the prognosis for reproduction after a linear salpingostomy in a study with patients randomly

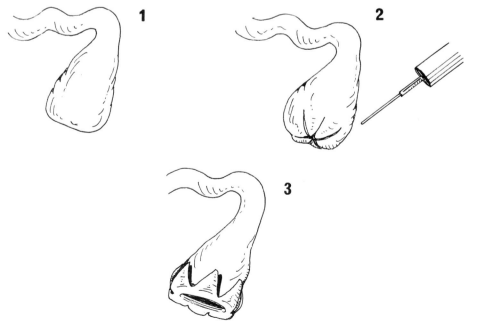

Figure 65–4. Laparoscopic neosaplingostomy. **1.** Total tubal occlusion. **2.** In neosalpingostomy, the incisions are made with a monopolar needle tip or with a CO_2 laser. **3.** Final result of the procedure.

TABLE 65–5. RESULTS OF LAPAROSCOPIC NEOSALPINGOSTOMY

Authors	Number of Patients	Number IUP* (%)	Number EP† (%)
Gomel[23]	9	4 (44)	—
Fayez[17]	19	0 (0.0)	2 (10.0)
Daniell and Herbert[1]	21	3 (14.0)	1 (5.0)
Reich[21]	7	2 (28.5)	0 (0.0)
Nezhat et al[8]	33	13 (36.0)	0 (0.0)
Bruhat et al (see table source note)	62	17 (34.0)	3 (5.0)
Canis et al[24]	87	29 (33.3)	6 (6.9)

*IUP, intrauterine pregnancy.

†EP, ectopic pregnancy.

From Bruhat MA, Mage G, Pouly JL, et al. *Coelioscopie Operatoire*. McGraw-Hill: 1989.

assigned to laparotomy or laparoscopy. While the total number of pregnancies did not differ, analysis proved that pregnancy occurred sooner in the laparoscopy group; 75% of all pregnancies after laparoscopy occurred within the first 16 months, whereas only 54% occurred after laparotomy. The total percentage of pregnancies after laparoscopy was from 44 to 63% after laparoscopy and from 36 to 52% after laparotomy. The reproductive potential after two consecutive ectopic pregnancies was very low, in this series only 20% (n = 10) of the patients who presented two consecutive ectopic pregnancies had term pregnancies, and four of them have presented with another ectopic pregnancy.[39] With the results obtained with IVF and embryo transfer, these methods should be suggested to these patients.

Pouly et al[40] reported a series of 223 patients treated for ectopic pregnancy by laparoscopy who wanted a future pregnancy. The incidence of intrauterine pregnancies was 67% (n = 149) and the incidence of recurrent ectopic pregnancies was 12% (n = 27). However, the condition of the tubes varies from patient to patient, so these authors proposed a scale to distinguish women who would benefit from conservative treatment from those who require a salpingectomy. While reproductive potential was independent of the characteristics of the ectopic pregnancy itself (size of the hematosalpinx, hemoperitoneum volume, and presence of tubal rupture), it was dramatically affected by the presence of ipsilateral periadnexal adhesions; 127 patients (67.5%) of the group in whom no adhesions were found (n = 188) achieved pregnancy, but only 16

TABLE 65–6. SUCCESS OF SUBSEQUENT PREGNANCY FOLLOWING LAPAROSCOPIC TREATMENT OF ECTOPIC PREGNANCY

Authors	Patients Desiring Pregnancy (n)	Intrauterine Pregnancies (%)	Repeated Ectopic Pregnancies (%)
Pouly et al[37]	118	74 (64)	26 (22)
DeCherney et al[42]	79	49 (62)	13 (16)
Reich et al (see table source note)	38	19 (50)	11 (28.9)
Total	235	142 (61.2)	50 (21.2)

From Reich H, Johns DA, De Caprio J, et al: Laparoscopic treatment of 109 ectopic serial pregnancies.

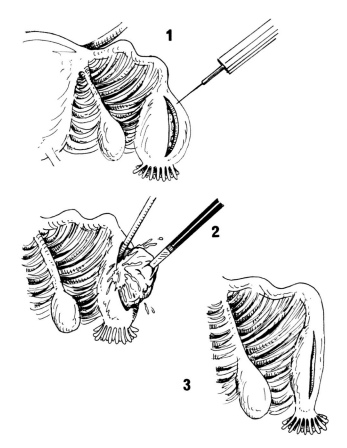

Figure 65–5. Conservative laparoscopic treatment of a tubal ectopic pregnancy. **1.** Ampullar neosalpingostomy performed with a monopolar needle tip. **2.** Extraction of the ectopic pregnancy; a grasper is used to provide traction while hydrodissection facilitates the procedure. **3.** Alignment of the salpingostomy edges after the removal of the ectopic pregnancy.

patients (45.7%) from the group in whom adhesions were found (n = 35) achieved pregnancy.

The state of the contralateral tube also played an important part in the prognosis for fertility. In 21.1% of the cases (n = 47), the contralateral tube was considered nonfunctional (absent or occluded). In these patients the rates of intrauterine pregnancy, recurrence, and infertility were 21.3% (n = 10), 21.3% (n = 10), and 57.4% (n = 27), respectively; the risk of a recurring ectopic pregnancy should be weighed against the possibility of having an intrauterine pregnancy.

A history of ectopic pregnancy, infertility, solitary tube, salpingitis, previous microsurgery, or laparoscopic adhesiolysis increases the risk of future ectopic pregnancies. Based on these factors, a grading system was developed to help decide between conservative treatment and salpingectomy for patients desiring future IVF or ET. Grades 0 to 3 are indications for conservative laparoscopic treatment, grade 4 indicates a radical laparoscopic treatment (salpingectomy), and grade 5 or higher indicates radical laparoscopic treatment (salpingectomy with contralateral sterilization). If there are no programs for IVF or ET, then a special effort should be made to attempt conservative treatment.[40]

Conservative laparoscopic treatment can conserve the remainder of trophoblast in the tube in 5% of patients, so follow-up measurement of β-hCG should be continued until serum levels are at zero. If the values are maintained or increase, additional treatment with oral or IM methotrexate (1 mg/kg) offers a 96% success rate and has minimal adverse effects. Another option is the IM administration of methotrexate (50 mg/m^2) without leucovorin, but if this fails to reduce β-hCG levels, then the patient should undergo a second laparoscopy with surgical excision of the tube.[41–44]

When applying conservative treatment, several issues should be taken into consideration: (1) complete extraction of the gestational tissue; (2) careful hemostasis; (3) preservation of as much healthy tube as possible; (4) use of an atraumatic technique (similar to microsurgery); (5) when the procedure is completed, all clots and blood should be aspirated and the pelvis should be irrigated with warm Ringer's lactate; and (6) weekly evaluation of β-hCG should be done to verify complete extraction of trophoblastic tissue. Depending on the size and condition of the gestation, conservative laparoscopic treatment can require coagulation, segmental resection, or linear salpingectomy. Subtotal or total salpingectomy is performed when conservative treatment fails, or when it is not possible or not indicated, whereas linear salpingostomy is mainly used for ampullar pregnancies, and segmental resection is employed for ectopic pregnancies located in the isthmus or the proximal portion.

SALPINGECTOMY

Partial salpingectomy as a method of tubal sterilization was performed in the late 1960s and early 1970s; however, total salpingectomy has not been used frequently until recent years, particularly in cases of ruptured ectopic pregnancies in which the tube is found to be damaged, or in cases of significant torsion. The procedure is performed with careful dissection and coagulation in the isthmic portion in a fashion similar to partial salpingectomy, but the incision is made close to the union with the uterus (Fig. 65–6).

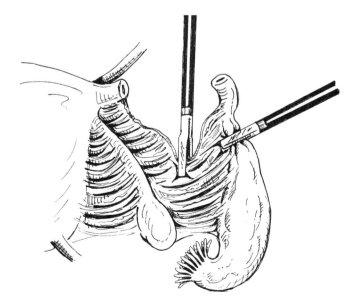

Figure 65–6. Laparoscopic salpingectomy for ectopic surgery. A bipolar grasper is used for hemostasis and the mesosalpinx is severed with a CO$_2$ laser or scissors.

This is followed by cutting and coagulation of the mesosalpinx at 1- to 2-cm intervals in the direction of the tubo-ovarian ligament. Finally the tubo-ovarian ligament is coagulated and divided. The divided tube is extracted from the abdominal cavity through a secondary port (5- or 10-mm, depending on the size of the specimen). Great care must be taken to preserve ovarian circulation. Cutting and coagulation of the mesosalpinx can be done with a CO$_2$ laser at 30 to 80W of power in superpulse mode, or it can be done with endoscissors once it has been coagulated with a Kleppinger bipolar clamp. Nezhat et al[45] reported a series of 100 salpingectomies performed by laparoscopy without complications or significant sequelae.

LAPAROSCOPIC SURGERY OF THE OVARIES

One of the sequelae of abdominal and pelvic surgery as well as pelvic infections is adhesions, which can interfere with fertility, produce pain, and on some occasions cause intestinal obstruction. The best treatment is prevention by meticulous surgical techniques; however, adhesions can develop in spite of proper technique. In such cases the treatment is surgical, and the laparoscopic method has proven to be the most effective, not only in avoiding recurrences of old adhesions, but in preventing the formation of new ones. Many variants of the technique can be used including scissors, bipolar coagulation, monopolar coagulation, and laser. Well-controlled studies on animals have not shown differences in the thermal lesion, the scarring pattern, and the postoperative formation of adhesions, between use of CO$_2$ laser or electromicrosurgery. These techniques present many options for the versatile surgeon who can combine them at will.[12–16]

The laparoscopic technique for lysis of periovarian adhesions is the same as for peritubal adhesions. However, the ovary must be freed of the adhesions, especially when they join it to the lateral pelvic wall. The dissection must be meticulous to avoid damaging other structures, particularly the ureter and important vascular structures. The ovary is lifted with a clamp and dissection to divide the adhesions begun, it is important to use atraumatic clamps to avoid damaging the ovarian cortex or the utero-ovarian ligament.

Ovarian Cystectomy

With the exception of small functional cysts, the extraction of ovarian cysts has traditionally been carried out via laparotomy until recently, when use of laparoscopic techniques have been expanded to allow more ample excisions; however, there is concern about discovering malignant ovarian neoplasms and locally disseminating the disease, or of being unable to perform the appropriate surgery during the laparoscopy. This is one of the main reasons for establishing criteria that allow adequate selection of patients, their evaluation, and the choice of appropriate techniques for treatment.

In premenopausal women most adnexal masses are benign, making minimally invasive surgery ideal for these patients. This is the case for patients with ovarian endometriomas, benign cysts, and some dermoid cysts. However, it is important to apply specific criteria for the selection of these patients, as well as using intraoperative evaluation and refined laparoscopic technique, in order to avoid operating by laparoscopy when laparotomy is indicated.[46–52]

Specific factors such as age, history of surgery for similar adnexal masses, pelvic examination and ultrasound suggestive of a benign mass, and some tumor markers like CA125, β-hCG levels, and alpha fetoprotein levels are involved in the selection of patients, especially in the very old or very young patient. Size, consistency, and bilaterality of the mass can be evaluated by transvaginal sonography, and in some cases with MRI. In general, pelvic masses that are cystic, uniloculated, and unilateral are benign; the presence of septated lesions, with papillae and solid components are ominous, because such masses can be malignant. By applying these strict evaluation criteria, a benign ovarian cyst is diagnosed in nearly 96% of cases. As experience with ultrasonographic evaluation of pelvic masses grows, specific signs give clues about their composition, allowing differentiation between endometriomas and simple cysts. Of course, the presence of ascites, bilateral masses, irregularity in the borders, size over 10 cm, adherence to the intestine, formation of papillas and solid components, and walls thicker than 2 mm strongly suggest that the lesion is malignant, and these patients should be treated by laparotomy.[49-54]

Due to their low specificity, tumor markers such as CA125 are most useful in postmenopausal women, but when they are found to be elevated they should alert one to the possibility of a malignant neoplasm. The combination of transvaginal ultrasonography and detection of CA125 increases the possibility of eliminating malignancy in nearly 96% of premenopausal women.

In spite of transvaginal sonography and tumor markers that help rule out malignancy, it is important to consider other factors intraoperatively; preoperative evaluation is not conclusive in all cases. The patient should be warned that a laparotomy may be required if a malignant tumor is found. Consultation with an oncologic gynecologist is desirable, particularly if the ovarian masses are over 8 cm and do not meet the preoperative criteria for being benign. A complete evaluation of the pelvic and abdominal cavities should be carried out before manipulation, and thorough lavage of the pelvis and superior abdomen should be performed before dissection. The mass should be carefully inspected, to look for any suspicious areas such as papillae or growths on the surface, and if these are found, samples should be taken. Percutaneous aspiration of the cyst using a small needle or through a secondary trocar is most useful, and endoscopic inspection of the cyst wall should be performed immediately and the liquid aspirated should be sent for cytologic evaluation. If any of these intraoperative samples show malignancy, then the procedure should be converted to laparotomy.[50-54]

Technique for Resection of Cysts

While the technique for cyst extraction varies according to size, the clinical impression, and surgeon preference, the main goals of the procedure are to remove all tissue for pathologic examination, obtain hemostasis, and preserve the ovarian cortex without unnecessary destruction. In some instances, oophorectomy must be performed instead of simply removing the cyst. Fortunately, in most cases of benign ovarian cysts, the resection can be performed via laparoscopy (Fig. 65–7). Draining the cyst generally aids in dissection, particularly for endometriomas and simple cysts; however, when a dermoid cyst is suspected, it should be aspirated with great care to avoid spillage, and it is advisable

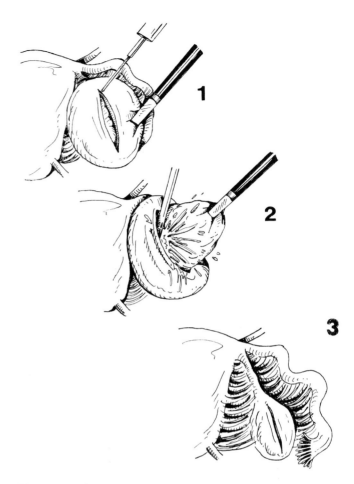

Figure 65–7. Ovarian laparoscopic cystectomy. **1.** The ovarian cortex is opened with a CO_2 laser to successfully dissect the ovarian cyst. **2.** Hydrodissection of the ovarian cyst is performed. **3.** After removal of the cyst, the edges of the cortex are approximated without sutures.

to remove it intact after drainage. In most cases the collapsed cyst can be removed through an auxiliary 10-mm trocar. Otherwise it is best to extract the cyst through a colpotomy having previously placed it in a plastic bag. The objective is to avoid spillage of the contents of a dermoid cyst onto the pelvic floor. In spite of the potential for profusely irrigating the zone, hydrodissection techniques are useful because they separate anatomic planes while dissecting. The initial method for resection of a cyst consists of starting in the antimesenteric border with a small incision, after which the planes are dissected, the cyst is evacuated (except in the case of a dermoid cyst), cystoscopy is performed by directly inserting the laparoscope in the cyst's cavity, then by traction and countertraction the surrounding cortex is removed, hemostasis is achieved, and the cyst is removed.

The traction and countertraction maneuver helps in the dissection of decompressed cysts. Some surgeons prefer to suture them, but these incisions heal spontaneously if left alone. The use of sutures can predispose to the formation of adhesions, especially if the suture is of large caliber. If the ovary cannot be saved, a laparoscopic oophorectomy can be performed, particularly if only a small amount of healthy cortex is left or if complete hemostasis is not achieved.[54–56,80]

It is evident that many ovarian cysts in premenopausal women can be treated via laparoscopy; however, it is important to select patients carefully to avoid operating on one with a malignant tumor. Again, pre- and intraoperative evaluation is crucial when a cyst is to be approached laparoscopically. The patient and the physician should also be alert to the possibility of finding a malignancy in spite of the most meticulous analysis.[55–58,80]

In a study performed by Maiman et al,[59] 42 cases of malignant ovarian tumors were found to have been initially treated by laparoscopy. The laparoscopy was suspended or the cyst was aspirated in 38 of these cases, and a partial or complete resection was attempted in 33 and 29% of cases, respectively. Benign characteristics were found preoperatively and 31% turned out to be malignant. A laparotomy was performed at the time of the laparoscopy in 17% of these cases, and after the laparoscopy in 71% (after an average period of 4.8 weeks); no laparotomy was performed in 12%. At least 50% of the patients presented in stages 2 to 4. The authors concluded that the presence of benign characteristics does not rule out malignancy; attempts at partial or complete excision are common and often delay definitive treatment, and frequently the disease is in an advanced stage.

Most pelvic masses in premenopausal women are benign, and if strict criteria are applied and intraoperative evaluation is adequate, then the chances for operating on a malignant tumor will be reduced considerably, and if one is found accidentally, the appropriate treatment must be begun without delay, as long as the patient has been warned and adequately prepared for this contingency. These precautions make the laparoscopic method a suitable alternative to laparotomy for the treatment of selected cases of ovarian cysts. Laparoscopic surgery should not be just a modified laparotomy; it offers a different type of access to the operative field, and follows the same strict evaluation and handling methods used in laparotomy (Table 65–7).

Another procedure performed on the ovaries is coagulation and vaporization of endometrial implants, which is best performed with the CO_2 laser and offers accessibility and precision when done laparoscopically. Auxiliary abdominal ports can be used to mobilize and expose the ovarian surface. Modified segmental ovarian resection can also be performed in patients with polycystic ovaries

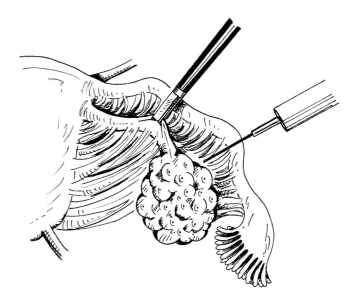

Figure 65–8. Ovarian perforation using the monopolar needle tip to treat resistant polycyistic ovaries.

who do not respond to hormonal treatment. Various instruments can be used to destroy the cortex of such lesions: via CO_2 laser microperforations, monopolar or bipolar energy, and endocoagulation (Fig. 65–8).[82]

Armar and Lochelin[60] reported 50 patients subjected to electrosurgical coagulation of the ovary by laparoscopy for treatment of refractory anovulatory infertility in the presence of polycystic ovarian syndrome. All had been treated unsuccessfully with antiestrogens, and more than half with gonadotrophins. Forty-three women (96%) ovulated after the treatment, with an average time for ovulation of 23 days (SD = 2). Three ovulated after antiestrogen treatment (having been resistant before), and 33 women conceived 58 pregnancies. Campo et al[61] reported 23 infertile patients with polycystic ovarian syndrome treated by laparoscopic ovarian resection, after which 55% had spontaneous ovulatory cycles and 13 pregnancies were achieved, 10 of which were spontaneous and 3 following treatment with clomiphene citrate. There is concern

TABLE 65–7. LAPAROSCOPIC MANAGEMENT OF ADNEXAL CYST-TYPE TUMORS DONE IN ACCORDANCE WITH THE PATHOLOGIC DIAGNOSIS

Definitive Pathologic Diagnosis	Total Cases	Laparoscopic Treatment		EAC*		IPC†		Oophorectomy		Biopsy via Puncture	Vaporization with Laser	
		n	(%)	n	(%)	n	(%)	n	(%)	n	(%)	n
Functional	96	95	99	9	9.4	16.7	1	1	69	71.9	—	—	—
Borderline and cancer	9	0	0	0	—	—	—	—	—	—	—	—	—
Paraovarian	61	58	95	12	19.7	43	70.5	—	—	3	4.9	—	
Endometrioma	100	90	90	8	8	50	50	1	1	25	25	6	6.6
Serosal	100	87	87	29	29	39	39	14	14	5	5	—	—
Mucinous	51	45	88	19	37.3	21	41.2	5	9.8	—	—	—	—
Teratoma	91	78	85	32	35.2	26	28.6	11	12.1	—	—	—	—

*EAC, Extra-abdominal cystectomy.

†IPC, Intra-peritoneal cystectomy.

From Mage et al.[53]

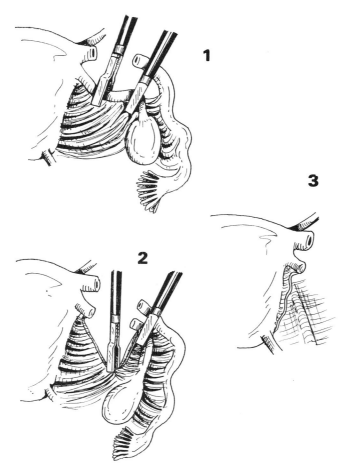

Figure 65–9. Laparoscopic salpingo-oophorectomy. **1.** The fallopian tube and the utero-ovarian ligament are severed with careful hemostasis. **2.** Dissection and hemostasis of the mesosalpinx and the infundibulopelvic ligament. **3.** View of lateral uterine wall after section of mesosalpinx and infundibulopelvic ligament and salpingo-oophorectomy.

about the formation of adhesions after these procedures, but a second laparoscopic exploration performed in some of these patients showed minimal adhesions. However, this method should not be reserved for patients with polycystic ovarian syndrome who do not respond to hormonal induction of ovulation.[62–64,82]

OOPHORECTOMY AND SALPINGO-OOPHORECTOMY

When the ovary is beyond repair, requires resection due to extensive adhesions, or when malignancy is suspected and a biopsy is required, oophorectomy can be performed laparoscopically (Fig. 65–9). If adhesions are present, they should be divided to liberate the ovary, including the abdominal walls and wide ligament. Sometimes, adhesions and a distorted anatomy can make identification of the ureter and the great vessels difficult, but it can be done with hydrodissection after entering the retroperitoneal space. Once the ovary is mobilized, it can be held with an atraumatic clamp, the ovarian ligament dissected with bipolar scissors, and its union to the uterus divided. The meso-ovary is cut into sections 1 to 2 cm

long, advancing from medially to laterally until the ovary is liberated.

If salpingo-oophorectomy is required, the isthmic portion of the fallopian tubes is coagulated and divided from the utero-ovarian ligament. Dissection is performed as for a simple oophorectomy, but includes the fallopian tube. The infundibulopelvic ligament can also be coagulated and divided, or simply ligated with a double loop, to remove the specimen. Staplers can be used to complete salpingo-oophorectomy, but when these automatic instruments are used, special care must be taken to identify the ureter and surrounding vasculature. The ovary must be included in its entirety within the specimen to avoid severe complications.

To extract the specimen, a bag is introduced through an accessory 10- to 12-mm trocar, and a cannula is used as a guide for extraction. The piece is placed in the bag, and both are removed through the trocar; if the specimen is too large, it can be morcellated in the bag to ease its extraction. All incisions over 10 mm should be sutured to avoid future herniation.[65–67]

FUNDAMENTALS OF LAPAROSCOPIC SURGERY

The main benefits that laparoscopic surgery offers over laparotomy for a number of gynecologic procedures are: shorter hospital stay, lower morbidity, less discomfort, and lower cost. Also, clinical statistics show that laparoscopic procedures offer effectiveness that is similar or even superior to laparotomy.

The performance of laparoscopic procedures requires special patient preparation compared to diagnostic laparoscopy. The instrumentation required is more extensive and anything that might be needed should be readily available to ensure that the procedure is done with ease and safety. The success of minimally invasive surgery is proportional to the degree of training that the surgeon has, the availability of instrumentation, the training of auxiliary personnel, and the clinical selection of patients.[1,4,6,68–70]

LAPAROSCOPIC TREATMENT OF GYNECOLOGIC CANCER

Despite the fact that laparoscopy is now widely accepted for the treatment of benign conditions affecting the ovary, its application in the diagnosis and treatment of gynecologic malignancies is still not well defined. With the introduction of minimally invasive surgery for oophorectomies, salpingo-oophorectomies and hysterectomies, it was inevitable that more ambitious dissections would be performed. New equipment for advanced procedures, including dissectors, staplers, scissors, and refined light sources, particularly for electrosurgery and laser, along with the use of new endoscopic cameras that provide excellent visualization have facilitated the performance of the extensive dissections required for surgery for gynecologic cancer.[81]

Lymphadenectomy

The ease and efficacy of pelvic and para-aortic lymphadenectomy has been demonstrated, and in the hands of an expert gynecologic oncologic surgeon, staging can be performed as well.[71–73] A recent study reported resection of an average of 19 lymph nodes with laparoscopic lymphadenectomy, comparable to the average 10 to 22 nodes removed with traditional laparotomy. However, these procedures require extensive knowledge of the anatomy and adequate oncologic training, which means that only gynecologists who are also oncologists can perform these procedures.

Ovarian Carcinoma

An early diagnosis of ovarian cancer is possible via laparoscopy, from staging through pelvic and para-aortic node sampling, following the same steps as for a staging laparotomy.[74] Laparoscopy allows systematic examination, intraperitoneal lavage, and biopsy sampling, including omentectomy, lymphadenectomy, appendectomy, and salpingo-oophorectomy with or without hysterectomy; the extraction of the specimens can be done vaginally.[75] In spite of this, laparoscopy is still investigational for ovarian malignancies, and should be reserved for groups in which expert oncologic gynecologists operate on selected patients.

Endometrial Carcinoma

Endometrial carcinoma has been treated via vaginal laparoscopically assisted hysterectomy. The procedure is useful for dissecting the adnexa and to perform selective lymphadenectomy when required. It also offers the advantage of extracting the specimen through the vagina, making it particularly useful in obese patients, and reduces hospital stay and morbidity.[76]

Cervical Cancer

The diagnosis of cervical cancer is simplified via laparoscopy, particularly in early stages of disease.[77] Lymphadenectomy can be performed via laparoscopy, and when required, radical hysterectomy can be accomplished combining the laparoscopic method with the radical vaginal route described by Schauta.[78–79]

To date only a few isolated series have been published that describe the use of operative laparoscopy in the treatment of gynecologic malignancies, and more investigation is required, particularly to determine the adequacy of the staging procedure, the contraindications of the endoscopic method, and the true complication rate.

These procedures should not be applied by general gynecologists, but their introduction as an alternative to treat selected patients will not only benefit the patients for whom the endoscopic method is appropriate, but gynecologic surgery as a whole, due to the easy access to pelvic organs they afford, and for the refinement of the endoscopic surgeon's technique that is attained. Laparoscopic surgery is still in the early stages for the treatment of gynecological malignancies but its future is brilliant.

SUMMARY AND CONCLUSIONS

Therapeutic laparoscopy has a growing place in gynecologic surgery, and when performed appropriately and for the proper indications, the benefits to the patient are significant, and the results are favorable, comparable to those obtained with laparotomy. The adnexa (fallopian tubes and ovary) can be safely treated by laparoscopy. Most surgical procedures that target the preservation and restoration of the fallopian tubes can be performed laparoscopically; however, when extensive disease is present, it is best to rec-

ommend in vitro fertilization and embryo transfer programs if fertility is desired.

The level of training of the gynecologic surgeon and the availability of appropriate instrumentation for performing these procedures are of the utmost importance, and the use of video systems should be advocated for teaching purposes as well as for documentation. Laparoscopic surgery of the tubes and ovaries can safely replace major abdominal surgery for most patients.[8–9]

Although it is still being evaluated, application of laparoscopy is becoming more widespread for the treatment of malignant conditions, including those affecting the ovary, the endometrium, and the cervix. Pelvic and para-aortic lymphadenectomy along with video-assisted vaginal hysterectomy are opening the door to the spread of minimally invasive treatment of gynecologic malignancies.

REFERENCES

1. Gomel V. Operative laparoscopy: A time for acceptance. *Fertil Steril.* 1989;52:1.
2. Semm K. *Operative Manual for Endoscopic Abdominal Surgery.* Year Book Medical Publishers:1987;175:184.
3. Sanfilippo JS, Levine RL, Buckhaum HJ. Operative gynecologic endoscopy. In: Bushbaum HJ (ed.). *Clinical Perspectives in Obstetrics and Gynecology.* Springer Verlag:1989.
4. Semm A, Mettler L. Clinical progress in pelvic surgery via operative laparoscopy. *Am J Obstet Gynecol.* 1980;138:121.
5. Murphy AA. Operative laparoscopy. *Fertil Steril.* 1987;47:1.
6. Nezhat C, Nezhat F. Operative laparoscopy (minimally invasive surgery): State of the art. *J Gynecol Surg.* 1992;8:111.
7. Sutton C. Lasers in infertility. *Hum Reprod.* 1993;8:133.
8. Nezhat C, Winer W, Cooper J, et al. Endoscopic infertility surgery. *J Reprod Med.* 1989;34:127.
9. Nezhat C, Crowgey SR, Nezhat F. Videolaseroscopy for the treatment of endometriosis-associated infertility. *Fertil Steril.* 1989;51:237.
10. Gomel V. *Microsurgery in Female Infertility.* Little Brown:1983.
11. Holtz G. Prevention and management of peritoneal adhesions. *Fertil Steril.* 1984;41:497.
12. Luciano AA, Whiteman G, Maier DB, et al. A comparison of formal injury, healing terms, and postoperative adhesion formation following CO_2 laser and electromicrosurgery. *Fertil Steril.* 1987;48:1025.
13. Luciano AA, Maier DB, Koch EI, et al. A comparative study of postoperative adhesions following laser surgery by laparoscopy versus laparotomy in the rabbit model. *Obstet Gynecol.* 1989;74:220.
14. Timbos-Keper TCM, Trimbos JB, Van Hall EV. Adhesion formation after tubal surgery: Results of the 8-day laparoscopy in 188 patients. *Fertil Steril.* 1985;43:395.
15. Tulandi T. Salpingo-ovariolysis: A comparison between laser surgery and electrosurgery. *Fertil Steril.* 1986;45:489.
16. Nezhat FR, Metzger DA, Luciano AA. Adhesion reformation after reproductive surgery by videolaseroscopy. *Fertil Steril.* 1990;53:1008.
17. Fayez JA. An assessment of the role of operative laparoscopy in tuboplasty. *Fertil Steril.* 1983;39:476.
18. Mettler L, Giesel H, Semm K. Treatment of female infertility due to tubal obstruction by operative laparoscopy. *Fertil Steril.* 1979;32:384.
19. Gomel V. Salpingo-ovariolysis by laparoscopy and infertility. *Fertil Steril.* 1983;40:607.
20. Bruhat JA, Mage G, Soualhat C, et al. Laparoscopy procedures to promote fertility, ovariolysis and salpingolysis: Results of 93 selected cases. *Acta Europeia Fertilitatis* 1983;14:113.
21. Reich H. Laparoscopic treatment of extensive pelvic adhesion, including hydrosalpinx. *J Reprod Med.* 1987;32:736.

22. Marana R, Muscatello P, Rizzi MG, et al. La salpingoscopia: Una nueva metodica per la valuatazione del fattore tubarico di sterilita. *Minerva Ginecologica* 1992;44:93.

23. Gomel V. Salpingostomy by laparoscopy. *J Reprod Med.* 1977;18:265.

24. Canis M, Mage G, Pouly JL, et al. Laparoscopic distal tuboplasty: Report of 87 cases and a 4-year experience. *Fertil Steril.* 1991;56:616.

25. Winston RML. Microsurgery of the fallopian tube: From fantasy to reality. *Fertil Steril.* 1980;24:251.

26. Watson AJ, Grupta JK, Donovan P, et al. The results of tubal surgery in the treatment of infertility in two non-specialist hospitals. *Br J Obstet Gynecol.* 1990;97:561.

27. Smalldridge J, Tait J. The results of tubal surgery in the treatment of infertility in Wellington: 1986–1990. *NZ Med J.* 1993;106:124.

28. Nederlof KP, Lawson HW, Safilas AF, et al. Ectopic pregnancy surveillance: United States, 1970–1987. *MMWR.* 1990;39:9.

29. Schwartz RO, Di Pietro DL. Beta-hCG as a diagnostic aid for suspected ectopic pregnancy. *Obstet Gynecol.* 1980;56:197.

30. Kadar N, Caldwell BV, Romero R. A method of screening for ectopic pregnancy and its indications. *Obstet Gynecol.* 1981;8:162.

31. Fossum GT, Davajan V, Kletzky OA. Early detection of pregnancy with transvaginal ultrasound. *Fertil Steril.* 1988;49:788.

32. Tait L. Five cases of extra-uterine pregnancy operated upon at the time of rupture. *Br Med J.* 1984;1:1250.

33. Stromme W. Salpingostomy for tubal pregnancy. *Obstet Gynecol.* 1953;1:472.

34. Timonen S, Nieminen U. Tubal pregnancy, choice of operative method of treatment. *Acta Obstet Gynecol Scand.* 1967;46:327.

35. DeCherney AH, Polan MI, Kort H, et al. Microsurgical technique in the management of tubal ectopic pregnancy. *Fertil Steril.* 1980;34:324.

36. Bruhat MA, Mamhes H, Mage G, et al. Treatment of ectopic pregnancy by means of laparoscopy. *Fertil Steril.* 1980;33:411.

37. Pouly JL, Mahmes H, Mage G, et al. Corrective laparoscopic treatment of 321 ectopic pregnancies. *Fertil Steril.* 1986;46:1093.

38. Vermesh M, Silva PD, Rosen GF, et al. Management of unruptured ectopic gestation by linear salpingostomy: A prospective, randomized, clinical trial of laparoscopy versus laparotomy. *Obstet Gynecol.* 1989;73:400.

39. Vermesh M, Presser SC. Reproductive outcome after linear salpingostomy for ectopic gestation: A prospective 3-year follow-up. *Fertil Steril.* 1992;57:682.

40. Pouly JL, Chapman C, Mamhes H, et al. Multifactorial analysis of fertility after corrective laparoscopic treatment of ectopic pregnancy in a series of 223 patients. *Fertil Steril.* 1991;56:453.

41. DeCherney AH, Romero R, Naftolin F. Surgical management of unruptured ectopic pregnancy. *Fertil Steril.* 1981;35:21.

42. DeCherney AH, Diamond MP. Laparoscopic salpingostomy for ectopic pregnancy. *Obstet Gynecol.* 1987;70:948.

43. Stoval TG, Ling FW, Buster JE. Outpatient chemotherapy of unruptured ectopic pregnancy. *Fertil Steril.* 1989;51:435.

44. Koosi S, Kock HCLV. A review of the literature on nonsurgical treatment in tubal pregnancies. *Obstet Gynecol Surv.* 1992;47:739.

45. Nezhat F, Winer W, Nezhat C. Salpingectomy with laparoscopy: A new surgical approach. *J Reprod Endoscop Surg.* 1991;1:91.

46. Di Saia DJ, Creasman WT. The adnexal mass and early ovarian cancer. In: Di Saia DJ, Creasman WT, eds. *Clinical Gynecologic Oncology.* Mosby:1989;292.

47. Luxman D, Bergman A, Sagy IJ, et al. Postmenopausal adnexal mass: Correlation between ultrasonic and pathologic findings. *Obstet Gynecol.* 1991;77:726.

48. Rustin GJS, Gennings JN, Nelstrop AE, et al. Use of CA-125 to predict survival of patients with ovarian carcinoma. *J Clin Oncol.* 1989;7:167.

49. Mongensen O, Mongensen B, Jacobsen A. CA-125 in the diagnosis of pelvic masses. *Eur J Cancer Clin Oncol.* 1989;25:1187.

50. Parker WH. Management of ovarian cysts by operative laparoscopy. *Contemp Ob/Gyn Now.* 1991;47:58.

51. Seltzer VL, Maiman M, Boyce J, et al. Laparoscopic surgery in the management of ovarian cysts. *Female Patient* 1992;17:16.

52. Hermann U, Locker G, Goldhirsch A. Sonographic patterns of malignancy—prediction of malignancy. *Obstet Gynecol.* 1987;69:777.

53. Mage C, Canis M, Manhes H, et al. Laparoscopic management of adnexal cystic masses. *J Gynecol Surg.* 1990;6:71.

54. Parker WH. Management of adnexal masses by operative laparoscopy. *J Reprod Med.* 1992;37:603.

55. Nezhat C, Winer WK, Nezhat F. Laparoscopic removal of demoid cysts. *Obstet Gynecol.* 1989;73:278.

56. Ballen N, Camus M, Toumaye H, et al. Laparoscopic removal of benign mature teratoma. *Hum Reprod.* 1992;7:429.

57. Reich H, McGlynn F, Sekel L, et al. Laparoscopic management of ovarian dermoid cysts. *J Reprod Med.* 1992;37:640.

58. Marrs RP. The use of potassium-titanyl-phosphate laser for laparoscopic removal of ovarian endometrioma. *Am J Obstet Gynecol.* 1991;164:1622.

59. Maiman M, Seltzer V, Boyce J. Laparoscopic excision of ovarian neoplasms subsequently found to be malignant. *Obstet Gynecol.* 1991;77:563.

60. Armar NA, Lochelin GC. Laparoscopic ovarian diathermy: An effective treatment for anti-oestrogen resistant anovulatory infertility in women with the polycystic ovary syndrome. *Br J Obstet Gynecol.* 1993;100:161.

61. Campo S, Felli A, Lamanna MA, et al. Endocrine changes and clinical outcome after laparoscopic ovarian resection in women with polycystic ovaries. *Hum Reprod.* 1993;8:359.

62. Ostrzenski A. Endoscopic carbon dioxide laser ovarian wedge resection in resistant polycystic ovarian disease. *Int J Fertil.* 1992;37:295.

63. Gurgan T, Urman B, Aksu T, et al. The effect of short interval laparoscopic lysis of adhesions on pregnancy rates following Nd:YAG laser photocoagulation of polycystic ovaries. *Obstet Gynecol.* 1991;80:45.

64. Gurgan T, Kisnisci HY, Arali H, et al. Evaluation of adhesion formation after laparoscopic treatment of polycystic ovarian disease. *Fertil Steril.* 1991;56:1176.

65. Perry CP, Upchurch JC. Pelviscopic adnexectomy. *Am J Obstet Gynecol.* 1990;162:79.

66. Nezhat F, Nezhat C, Silfen SL. Videolaseroscopy for oophorectomy. *Am J Obstet Gynecol.* 1991;165:1323.

67. Nezhat F, Nezhat C. Operative laparoscopy for the treatment of ovarian remnant syndrome. *Fertil Steril.* 1992;57:1003.

68. Levine RL. Economic impact of pelviscopic surgery. *J Reprod Med.* 1985;30:9.

69. Maruri F, Azziz R. Laparoscopic surgery for ectopic pregnancies: Technology assessment and public health implications. *Fertil Steril.* 1993;59:487.

70. Valle RF. Endoscopy: The impact on clinical practice in the U.S.A. In: Van Herendael B, Slaagen T, Martens P, eds. *Operative Endoscopy: Practical Aspects.* Gyntech Bvba.:1991;108.

71. Querleu D, Leblanc E, Castelain B. Laparoscopic pelvic lymphadenectomy in the staging of early carcinoma of the cervix. *Am J Obstet Gynecol.* 1991;164:579.

72. Childers JM, Hatch KD, Tran Ai-Nhi, et al. Laparoscopic paraaortic lymphadenectomy in gynecologic malignancies. *Obstet Gynecol.* 1993;82:741.

73. Boike GM, Sciarra JJ. Laparoscopic management of uterine malignancy. *Gynecologic Internationale.* 1996;5:108.

74. Reich A, McGlynn F, Wilkie W. Laparoscopic management of stage I ovarian cancer. *J Reprod Med.* 1990;35:601.

75. Nezhat C, Nezhat F, Burrel M. Laparoscopically assisted hysterectomy for the management of a borderline ovarian tumor: A case report. *J Laparoendosc Surg.* 1992;2:167.

76. Childers JM, Surwit EA. Combined laparoscopic and vaginal surgery for the management of two cases of stage I endometrial cancer. *Gynecol Oncol.* 1992;45:46.

77. Nezhat C, Burrel MO, Nezhat FR, et al. Laparoscopic radical hysterectomy with para-aortic and pelvic node dissection. *Am J Obstet Gynecol.* 1992;166:864.

78. Schauta F. Die operation des Gebarmutterkrebses mittels des Schuchardt'schen paravaginalschnittes. *Montsch f Geburtsch u Gynaek.* 1902;15:133.

79. Querleu D. Hysterectomies de Schauta-Amreich et Schauta-Stoeckel assistees par coelioscopie. *J Gynecol Obstet Biol Repr.* 1991;20:747.

80. Eltabbakh GH, Kaiser JR. Laparoscopic management of a large ovarian cyst in an adolescent. A case report. *J Reprod Med* 2000;45:231–234.

81. Classe JM, Mahe M, Moreau P, et al. Ovarian transposition by laparoscopy before radiotherapy in the treatment of Hodgkin's disease. *Cancer* 1998;83:1420.

82. Felemban A, Tan SL, Tulandi T. Laparoscopic treatment of polycystic ovaries with insulated needle cautery: a reapprisal. *Fertile Steril.* 2000;73:266.

83. Koh CH, Janik GM. Laparoscopic microsurgical tubal anastomosis. *Obstet Gynecol Clin North Am.* 1999;26:189.

84. Bissonnete F, Lapensee L, Bouzayen R. Outpatient laparoscopic tubal anastomosis and subsequent fertility. *Fertil Steril.* 1999;72:549.

Chapter Sixty-Six • • • • • •

Surgical Aspects of Endometriosis

MICHAEL R. SEITZINGER

Endometriosis is a condition that has been recognized for over 140 years. Rokitansky described this disease in the uterus, tubes, and ovaries in 1860.[1] Prior to the development of endoscopic techniques, treatment was total abdominal hysterectomy with bilateral salpingo-oophorectomy.[2] Since the 1960s, endoscopic diagnostic procedures have allowed for more conservative therapeutic options. Appropriate therapies were directed towards definitive goals—the relief of chronic pelvic pain, correction of infertility factors, and the restoration of anatomic relationships of pelvic structures. The adherence to strict microsurgical principles led to better postoperative results.[3] New instruments and ongoing refinement of techniques have led to marked reductions in disease recurrences, improved fertility rates and, perhaps most important, an enhanced quality of life for the patient.[4–6]

The purpose of this chapter is not to debate laparotomy versus laparoscopy for treatment of endometriosis. It has been well recognized that minimally invasive techniques have led to decreased postoperative pain, shorter hospital stays, and earlier return to work for the patient.[7,8] Endoscopic surgical therapies should be reserved for those surgeons who are skilled at these procedures and are comfortable in their knowledge of normal anatomic relationships. Recognition of various stages and presentations of endometriosis is critical for maximal results.[9] Classification of operative findings currently follow the revised system of the American Society for Reproductive Medicine (formerly the American Fertility Society).[10]

INCIDENCE

The incidence of endometriosis varies widely in published reports, from 5 to 10% in normal women and up to 60% of women who present with infertility or chronic pelvic pain.[11] Of all gynecologic office visits, 10 to 20% are for chronic pelvic pain.[12] Nearly 40% of all laparoscopies are for chronic pelvic pain.[13] Further, the number of hysterectomies for endometriosis is second only to those performed for leiomyomas.[14] Chronic pelvic pain is often related to pelvic or peritoneal adhesions. The adhesions may or may not be associated with endometriosis that is "active" or clearly visible. Deep fibrotic implants of the "gun-metal gray" appearance seem to represent "inactive" or old endometriosis, which may have led to the adhesion formation. In performing diagnostic laparoscopies, one must search diligently for the atypical as well as the typical appearance of endometriosis and treat both effectively.[9]

SURGICAL MANAGEMENT

Limiting the discussion to the endoscopic approach, management of endometriosis and/or pelvic adhesions will require instrumentation best suited for these purposes. In addition to a good video and light system, ancillary equipment depends on the availability to each hospital and physician. The goals are to enhance fertility, decrease pain, restore anatomic relations, and remove or destroy endometriosis. These can be accomplished using sharp dissection with scissors, monopolar or bipolar energy, or with a laser (preferably a CO_2 laser). If a laser is unavailable because of its high cost, a very effective instrument is the Seitzinger Tripolar Forceps. This enables the surgeon to bipolar coagulate the tissue, use the jaws to grasp, activate the knife to cut, and excise the implants with one instrument. The grasping abilities allow for the tissue to be removed for pathologic confirmation.

Other treatment modalities for endometriosis include bipolar or monopolar coagulation. This is reserved for superficial implants less than 5 mm in diameter. Thermocoagulation and sometimes laser coagulation may be appropriate depending on the wavelength used. Vaporization is also commonly employed for superficial implants. One must be cautioned that what appears on the surface as superficial endometriosis may actually be only the "tip of the iceberg"—that is, underlying deep fibrotic implants may actually be harboring active endometriosis.[15] If these are not completely excised, recurrence rates most certainly will be increased.[16–18]

ADHESIOLYSIS

Before attempting to surgically treat endometriosis, the surgeon will often be faced with a pelvis that is obliterated with adhesions. Familiarity with modalities of adhesiolysis and the prevention of their recurrence is of tantamount importance. The relationship of pelvic adhesions and chronic pelvic pain has been debated for years. A publication by Peters et al indicates a significant response to adhesiolysis in the reduction of chronic pelvic pain.[19]

Adhesions may be thin, avascular, thick, dense, fibrous, or vascular. An advantage of using the laparoscope and its afforded magnification is in assisting the surgeon in recognizing the type of adhesion. The specific instruments again will be monopolar, bipolar, laser, or sharp dissection with scissors. Most of these are 5 mm in diameter. Some may be 40 cm in length to allow their use through the channel of an operating laparoscope. The key to successful adhesiolysis is to apply traction and counter traction to identify the adhesion and separate it from critical structures such as bowel or bladder. Electrosurgery should be used with caution and reserved for known vascular tissue or bleeding after adhesiolysis has been performed. The risks of thermal or electrical damage to underlying structures are well known.[20] Reich described the use of high-pressure irrigating fluids delivered through a single-channel suction irrigating device to dissect tissue, or "aquadissection."[21] This not only aids in identifying tissue planes but provides a "backstop" for CO_2 laser energy, which will not penetrate the fluid, thus protecting underlying structures. Adhesive tissue should not simply be transected, but should be removed from the abdomen to aid in preventing recurrences. If dense adhesive disease is present in the rectovaginal septum, special instrumentation and digital examination will help delineate tissues. The prevention of adhesion recurrence includes the use of minimal thermal damage, meticulous hemostasis, and the prevention of post-operative infections. Underwater examination will decrease the tamponade effects of the CO_2 pneumoperitoneum. This provides visualization of oozing vessels or air from enterotomies that may have occurred during the adhesiolysis.[22] The use of 2 to 3 L of lactated Ringer's solution to float intraperitoneal tissue at the completion of laparoscopic adhesiolysis may assist in decreasing the recurrence of adhesions.[23]

TREATMENT OF ENDOMETRIAL IMPLANTS—PERITONEUM

Identification and complete visualization of all underlying or adjacent structures must precede destruction or excision of peritoneal implants. This may require mobilization and retraction of bowel through previously described adhesiolysis techniques. Ureterolysis may be aided by the introduction of ureteral stents (lighted stents are now available). A working knowledge of retroperitoneal anatomy including vascular structures is critical.

Excision of peritoneal implants begins by incising the peritoneum with scissors, bipolar or monopolar devices, or CO_2 laser at 20 to 40 W superpulse. The tissue is then separated from underlying structures with hydrodissection. A tissue margin of 2 to 4 mm should be included around the visible lesion. The depth of excision may be superficial (<5 mm) or deep (between 5 and 10 mm). The excision is completed using CO_2 laser energy, mechanical energy (scissors or Tripolar Forceps), or electrosurgical energy depending on the proximity of vital structures (Fig. 66–1).

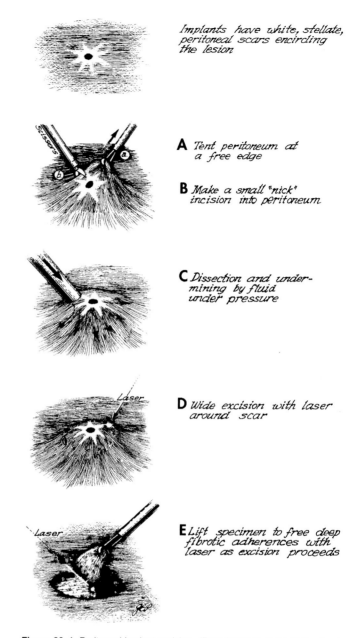

Implants have white, stellate, peritoneal scars encircling the lesion

A *Tent peritoneum at a free edge*

B *Make a small "nick" incision into peritoneum*

C *Dissection and undermining by fluid under pressure*

D *Wide excision with laser around scar*

E *Lift specimen to free deep fibrotic adherences with laser as excision proceeds*

Figure 66–1. Peritoneal implant excision. *(From Hulka X, Reich H: Textbook of Laparoscopy, 3rd ed. Saunders: 1998; Chapter 17. Reproduced with permission from Dr. Harry Reich and the publisher, W.B. Saunders Company.)*

Once underlying loose areolar tissue is identified, complete excision can be assured. Tissue that is not covered by loose peritoneum can be ablated or coagulated directly, provided adequate depth is achieved. Hemostasis must be obtained with minimal tissue damage (Fig. 66–2).[15]

TREATMENT OF OVARIAN ENDOMETRIOSIS

Superficial endometriotic implants on the ovarian capsule (<2 mm) may be successfully ablated or coagulated. Care must be taken to insure adequate depth of destruction. Hemosiderin deposits may

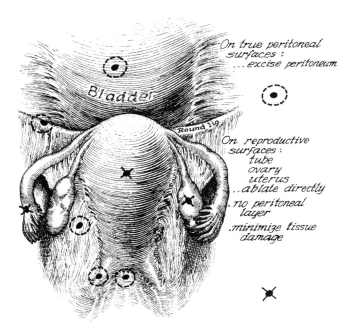

Figure 66–2. Excision versus ablation. *(From Hulka X, Reich H:* Textbook of Laparoscopy, *3rd ed. Saunders: 1998; Chapter 17. Reproduced with permission from Dr. Harry Reich and the publisher, W.B. Saunders Company.)*

be seen draining as the ablative procedure is performed. Irrigation of these deposits is continued until normal tissue is identified. One may need to pretreat patients after ovulation with a GnRH agonist (Depot Lupron 3.75 mg) intramuscularly to prevent the entrapment of an unruptured luteinized follicle. Once a cyst is entered either by purposeful incision or accidental rupture, the cyst wall must be carefully inspected. Biopsies of any papillary excrescences are taken to rule out an occult malignancy. Ovarian cystoscopy with a 5-mm laparoscope is invaluable at this juncture. Continuous irrigation during the inspection of the capsule provides excellent exposure. Small endometriomas may be destroyed with diathermy or ablated with CO_2 laser.

Once an endometrioma is decidedly benign, the capsule is grasped and is stripped from the underlying bed of ovarian tissue. If the cyst wall is incompletely excised, destruction of the remaining tissue is accomplished to prevent recurrence.[7,15] Coaptation of the incised ovarian tissue may be obtained by internal coagulation with bipolar or low-power CO_2 laser. This author has used the Tripolar Forceps at 10 to 15 W to grasp the edges and reapproximate them while applying bipolar energy. This has resulted in a well-approximated ovary. Postoperative adhesion formation appears to be greater if sutures are used to close the defect (Fig. 66–3).[24]

TREATMENT OF GASTROINTESTINAL ENDOMETRIOSIS

Samson described endometriosis of the intestine in 1922; he described obliteration of the cul-de-sac involving retrocervical and rectal deep fibrotic endometriosis.[25] Treatment of varying degrees of cul-de-sac obliteration demands a commitment from the surgeon

to spend hours completing the dissection and restoring the anatomy. It also requires surgical expertise that goes beyond most general gynecologists. However, the gastrointestinal tract may be involved with endometriosis in 3 to 37% of women with the disease.[26,27] Pain is the presenting factor that commands surgical excision of rectovaginal endometriosis.[28] This is not a condition amenable to adequate therapy by ablative techniques. Instruments that are useful for cul-de-sac dissection are shown in Figure 66–4. Figure 66–5 nicely depicts partial and complete cul-de-sac obliteration. The reader who is interested in Dr. Reich's technique of excision of cul-de-sac endometriosis is referred to Chapter 32 of Hulka and Reich, *Textbook of Laparoscopy,* third edition, published by Saunders in 1998. All patients who preoperatively are suspected to have involvement of the gastrointestinal system should undergo a bowel prep. The reader is referred to Chapter 11 of Nezhat et al, *Operative Gynecologic Laparoscopy—Principles and Techniques,* published by McGraw-Hill in 1995, for a comprehensive review of laparoscopy techniques for bowel resection and reanastamosis. These procedures are beyond the scope of this author and should be undertaken only by those physicians with expertise in these areas.

TREATMENT OF ENDOMETRIOSIS– INCISIONAL SCARS

Surgical scars are seen as the site for recurrent, cyclical pain. They may be from episiotomy repairs, cesarean sections, hysterectomies, or even trocar sites at laparoscopy.[29] Treatment should be local excision and pathologic examination of tissue. Ectopic endometrium may undergo malignant transformation.

INFERTILITY

There is an ongoing debate as to whether pregnancy rates are improved with laparoscopically treated endometriosis versus laparotomy. Rates have varied widely, from being equal to laparoscopy being superior.[30,31] The earlier studies were not prospective, randomized, and controlled. A 1997 study by Marcoux et al, performed in a randomized, controlled fashion, concluded that cumulative pregnancy rates in women treated surgically for endometriosis were 30.7% versus 17.7% in women who had diagnostic procedures alone.[32] As Gambone and DeCherney said, "if the results of this study are valid and can be generalized, women who undergo diagnostic laparoscopy for infertility should be treated by surgeons who are trained and prepared to perform ablation or resection even if the visualized endometriosis is minimal or mild."[33]

COMBINED MEDICAL AND SURGICAL TREATMENTS

There is an ongoing effort to attempt medical suppression of endometriosis prior to surgical intervention. This may result in a marked saving to the patient. There are no published randomized controlled studies showing the efficacy for this approach as compared to surgery.

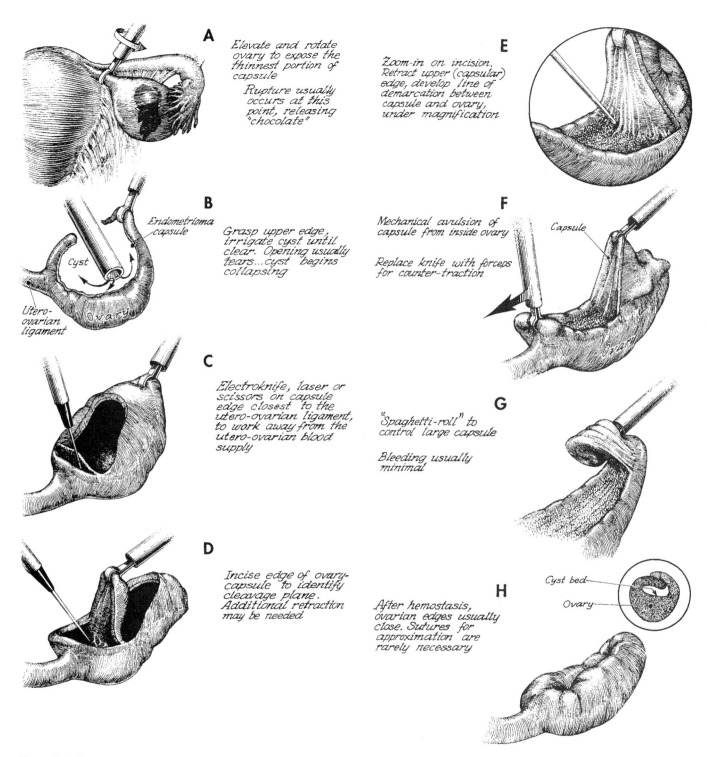

A Elevate and rotate ovary to expose the thinnest portion of capsule

Rupture usually occurs at this point, releasing "chocolate"

E Zoom-in on incision. Retract upper (capsular) edge, develop line of demarcation between capsule and ovary, under magnification

B Endometrioma capsule

Cyst

Utero-ovarian ligament

Ovary

Grasp upper edge, irrigate cyst until clear. Opening usually tears...cyst begins collapsing

F Mechanical avulsion of capsule from inside ovary

Capsule

Replace knife with forceps for counter-traction

Ovary

C Electroknife, laser or scissors on capsule edge closest to the utero-ovarian ligament, to work away from the utero-ovarian blood supply

G "Spaghetti-roll" to control large capsule

Bleeding usually minimal

D Incise edge of ovary-capsule to identify cleavage plane. Additional retraction may be needed

H After hemostasis, ovarian edges usually close. Sutures for approximation are rarely necessary

Cyst bed

Ovary

Figure 66–3. Dissection of endometrioma. *(From Hulka X, Reich H:* Textbook of Laparoscopy, *3rd ed. Saunders: 1998; Chapter 17. Reproduced with permission from Dr. Harry Reich and the publisher, W.B. Saunders Company.)*

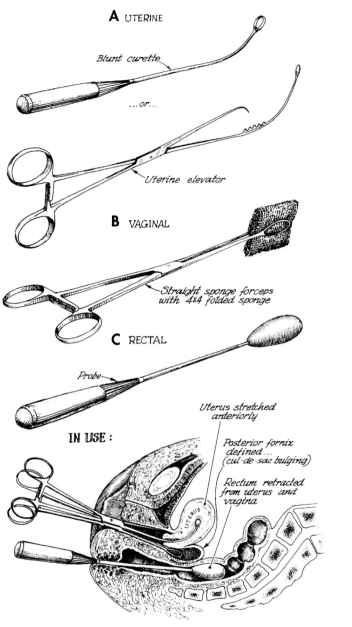

Figure 66–4. Probes for cul-de-sac dissection. *(From Hulka X, Reich H: Textbook of Laparoscopy, 3rd ed. Saunders: 1998; Chapter 17. Reproduced with permission from Dr. Harry Reich and the publisher, W.B. Saunders Company.)*

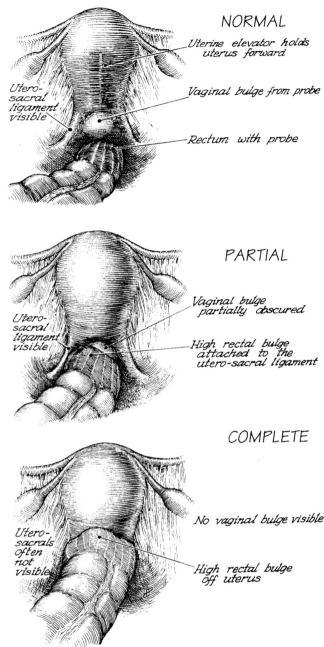

Figure 66–5. Staging of cul-de-sac obliteration. *(From Hulka X, Reich H: Textbook of Laparoscopy, 3rd ed. Saunders: 1998; Chapter 17. Reproduced with permission from Dr. Harry Reich and the publisher, W.B. Saunders Company.)*

Another approach is to perform cytoreductive surgery and follow with medical suppressive therapy. One such study, a randomized, prospective, placebo-controlled, multicenter clinical trial, compared the use of a GnRH agonist (nafarelin) versus a placebo after reductive laparoscopic surgery for symptomatic endometriosis. The major finding was that the nafarelin-treated group had a significantly prolonged length of time between surgery and the need for additional therapy. In addition, patients treated with nafarelin had significantly lower pain scores at the end of the 6-month treatment than placebo-treated patients.[34]

THE FUTURE

This author is presently evaluating the urinary bladders of patients suspected of having endometriosis by history and physical findings. A Stamey test is performed, at which time 400 to 500 mL of sterile saline is instilled in the bladder and allowed to remain for 2 minutes. Cystoscopy under anesthesia is concurrently performed. The bladder is drained and reevaluated. Patients with hemorrhagic areas or "glomerulations" have nearly a 100% correlation with active pelvic endometriosis. Since 1990, nearly 200 patients have been studied. Early findings were reported at the American Association of Gynecologic Laparoscopists 24th annual meeting in 1995. This study has been submitted for publication. If others can confirm these results, a method will be available by which active endometriosis can be diagnosed preoperatively and treatment options offered. Recurrences may be diagnosed with a simple office procedure requiring little or no sedation. This may result in tremendous financial savings if the patient can avoid diagnostic surgery.

REFERENCES

1. C. Ueber Uterusdrusen—Neubildung in uterus and ovarial sarcomen. *Z Gelellschaft Aertz Wein.* 1860;16:755.
2. Williams TJ. Endometriosis. In: Thompson JD, Rock JA, eds. *TeLinde's Gynecology*, 7th ed. Lippincott:1992;488.
3. Rokitansky Gomel V, McComb P. Microsurgery in gynecology. In: Silver JS, ed. *Microsurgery*. Williams & Wilkins:1979;43.
4. Cook AS, Rock JA. The role of laparoscopy in the treatment of endometriosis. *Fertil Steril.* 1991;4:663.
5. Nezhat C, Crowgey S. Nezhat F. Videolaseroscopy for the treatment of endometriosis associated with infertility. *Fertil Steril.* 1989;51:123.
6. Candiani GB, Fedele L, Vercellini P, et al. Presacral neurectomy for the treatment of pelvic pain associated with endometriosis: a controlled study. *Am J Obstet Gynecol* 1992;167:100.
7. Bateman BG, Kolp LA, Mills S. Endoscopic versus laparotomy management of endometriomas. *Fertil Steril.* 1994;62:690.
8. Luciano AA, Lowney J, Jacobs SL. Endoscopic treatment of endometriosis-associated infertility: therapeutic, economic and social benefits. *J Reprod Med.* 1992;37:573.
9. Martin DC, Hubert GD, Vander-Zwaag R, et al. Laparoscopic appearances of pelvic endometriosis. *Fertil Steril.* 1989;51:63.
10. American Fertility Society. Revised American Fertility Society classification of endometriosis: 1985. *Fertil Steril.* 1985;43:351.
11. Koninckx PR, Martin DC. Treatment of deeply infiltrating endometriosis. *Cur Opinion Obstet Gynecol.* 1994;6:231.
12. Reiter RC. Chronic pelvic pain. *Clin Obstet Gynecol.* 1990;33:117.
13. Howard F. Laparoscopic evaluation and treatment of women with chronic pelvic pain. *J Am Assoc Gynlaparosc.* 1994;1:325.
14. Williams TJ, Pratt JHL. Endometriosis in a 1000 consecutive celiotomies: Incidence and management. *Am J Obstet Gynecol.* 1977;129:245.
15. Redwine DB. Conservative laparoscopic excision of endometriosis by sharp dissection: Life table analysis of reoperation and persistent or recurrent disease. *Fertil Steril.* 1991;56:28.
16. Vernon MW, Beard JS, Graves K, et al. Classification of endometriotic implants by morphologic appearance and capacity to synthesize prostaglandin. *Fertil Steril.* 1990;53:984.
17. Cornillie FJ, Ooosterlynck D, Lauweryns JM, et al. Deeply infiltrating pelvic endometriosis: Histology and clinical significance. *Fertil Steril.* 1990;53:978.
18. Crain LJ, Luciano AA. Peritoneal fluid evaluation in infertility. *Obstet Gynecol.* 1983;61:1591.
19. Peters AA, Trimbos-Kemper GC, Admiraal C, et al. A randomized clinical trial on the benefit of adhesiolysis in patients with intraperitoneal adhesions and chronic pelvic pain. *Br J Obstet Gynaecol.* 1992;99:59.
20. Reich H, Vancaillie TG, Soderstrom RM. Electrical techniques. In: Martin DC, Holtz GL, Levinson CJ, et al, eds. Manual of Endoscopy. Santa Fe Springs, CA: American Association of Gynecologic Laparoscopists;1990:105.
21. Reich H. Aquadissection. In: Baggish MS, ed. Endoscopic Laser Surgery. The Clinical Practice of Gynecology, vol 2. Elsevier:1990;159.
22. Reich H. Endoscopic management of tuboovarian abscess and pelvic inflammatory disease. In: Sanfilippo JS, Levine RL, eds. *Operative Gynecologic Endoscopy*. Springer-Verlag:1989;118.
23. Sahakian V, Rogers RG, Halme J, et al. Effects of carbon dioxide-saturated normal saline and Ringer's lactate on postsurgical adhesion formation in the rabbit. *Obstet Gynecol.* 1993;82:851.
24. Nezhat C, Nezhat F. Postoperative adhesion formation after ovarian cystectomy with and without ovarian reconstruction. 47th annual meeting of the American Fertility Association, Orlando, October 1991. Abstract.
25. Sampson JA. Intestinal adenomas of endometrial type. *Arch Surg.* 1922;5:217.
26. Jenkinson EL, Brown WH. Endometriosis: A study of 117 cases with special reference to constricting lesions of the rectum and sigmoid colon. *JAMA.* 1943;122:349.
27. Samper ER, Sagle GW, Hand AM. Colonic endometriosis, its clinical spectrum. *South Med J.* 1984;77:912.
28. Koninckx PR, Meuleman C, Demeyere S, et al. Suggestive evidence that pelvic endometriosis is a progressive disease, whereas deeply infiltrating endometriosis is associated with pelvic pain. *Fertil Steril.* 1991;55:759.
29. Paull T, Tedeschi LG. Perineal endometriosis at the site of episiotomy scar. *Obstet Gynecol.* 1972;40:28.
30. Olive DL, Martin DC. Treatment of endometriosis associated infertility with CO_2 laser laparoscopy: The use of 1- and 2-parameter exponential models. *Fertil Steril.* 1987;48:18.
31. Chong AP, Luciano AA, O'Shaughnessy AM. Laser laparoscopy versus laparotomy in the treatment of infertility patients with severe endometriosis. *J Gynecol Surg.* 1990;6:179.
32. Marcoux S, Maheux R, Canadian Collaborative Group on Endometriosis. Laparoscopic surgery in infertile women with minimal or mild endometriosis. *N Engl J Med.* 1997;337:217.
33. Gambone JC, DeCherney AH. Surgical treatment of minimal endometriosis. *N Engl J Med.* 1977;337:269.
34. Hornstein MD, Hemmings R, Yuzpe AA, Heinrichs WL. Use of nafarelin versus placebo after reductive laparoscopic surgery for endometriosis. *Fertil Steril.* 1997;68:860.

Chapter Sixty-Seven • • • • • • •

*E*ctopic Pregnancy

JORGE KUNHARDT, CARLOS QUESNEL, VALENTÍN IBARRA,
ROBERTO NEVAREZ-BERNAL, and MÁXIMO CUNILLERA

The abnormal nidation of the fertilized ovum outside the uterus and subsequent implantation of trophoblastic tissue beyond the endometrial cavity represents a significant public health problem worldwide. The number of ectopic pregnancies has risen substantially not only in Mexico but all over the world, with current data showing increases every year.

In the United States, in 1970 nearly 17,800 cases were reported; 22 years later, in 1992, the number of cases was 108,800.[1] Up to 97% of all ectopic pregnancies are located in the fallopian tubes (Fig. 67–1). The present chapter will explain the surgical management of this pathology, placing special emphasis on the changes observed since the beginning of new techniques that allow minimal invasion in some cases.

DIAGNOSIS

Physical examination is still the basis for diagnosis, but the addition of new techniques, not only in the clinical area but also in the imaging field, have made ectopic pregnancy easier to diagnose and more frequently discovered in its early stages. The presence of elevated levels of the beta human chorionic gonadotropin (β-hCG), the use of vaginal ultrasound, and the high clinical suspicion of the physician, help to diagnose extrauterine pregnancy in the first weeks, allowing the use of a less aggressive and traumatic therapy, which is the ideal method whenever possible.

Current surgical management allows for short-term hospitalization with excellent results. This is particularly true in women with access to appropriate medical care.[2]

MANAGEMENT

Controversy still prevails concerning conservative surgical treatment, which involves a considerable risk of recurring ectopic pregnancy, making some authors think that radical treatment is the best choice if the fallopian tube on the opposite side is considered healthy. Figure 67–2 shows the management algorithm used for the diagnosis and treatment of ectopic pregnancy by the Instituto Nacional de Perinatologia, in Mexico City.[3]

Treatment options can be classified into two main categories: medical or surgical. Surgical treatment can be divided in two more categories: a conservative approach (lineal salpingostomy and salpingocentesis) and a radical approach (salpingostomy and salpingophorectomy).[4] Surgical treatment confirms the diagnosis of the extrauterine pregnancy, evaluates the affected and the opposite fallopian tubes, and also evaluates the presence of hemoperitoneum or tube rupture, representing an efficient and expeditious method of management regardless of gestational size.

Laparoscopic treatment offers significant advantages over laparotomy, especially in the short convalescent period and faster return to normal activities, less postoperative pain, and better aesthetic results.[5]

Surgical Alternatives

The treatment of ectopic pregnancy by laparoscopy began in the late 1970s but it was not until 1980 that it was chosen as the best treatment option.[6] This procedure is indicated when the diagnosis of ectopic pregnancy is made and the patient is hemodynamically stable with normal preoperative tests and hemoglobin levels exceeding 10 g/dL. No endoscopic surgery is advisable in patients with hypovolemic shock, hemoperitoneum exceeding 2000 mL, uncontrollable hemorrhage, interstitial pregnancy over 3 cm, or when unfavorable conditions prevail for the laparoscopic procedure.

Salpingostomy has gradually replaced salpingectomy as the surgical procedure of choice for an unbroken tubal pregnancy in women wishing to preserve fertility; nonetheless, recent publications disclose the incidence of a 5 to 8% persistent ectopic pregnancy risk after the procedure.

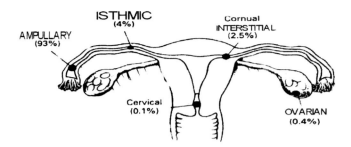

Figure 67–1. Frequent localization of ectopic pregnancies.

Salpingostomy

The patient is placed in a gynecologic position with a mechanical device that allows separation but no bending of the legs, and a uterine mobilizer like the Zumi type 4.5 or a Cohen tube is installed. The patient is held in a Trendelenburg position and the pneumoperitoneum established with the Veress needle. A 10 to 12-mm trocar is inserted in the abdominal cavity to explore it. Trocar placement depends on the localization of the ectopic pregnancy.

Two more trocars are inserted lateral to the umbilical scar; one port (10 mm) is used for aspiration/irrigation, or in a special case the camera can be changed here. A 5-mm reducer may be used to introduce additional instruments if necessary. The other trocar (5 mm) is used for electrocoagulation nippers and/or dissection. The initial step after locating the tube is injecting saline solution plus vasopressin in a 1:30 dilution into the mesosalpinx using a laparoscopic or spinal needle; 3 to 5 mL is enough to produce constriction of the tube vessels and to reduce the bleeding (Fig. 67–3). Then an incision is made with bipolar scissors or laser on antimesenteric edges not exceeding 1 to 2 cm (Fig. 67–4). Clots and trophoblastic tissue are removed with the help of a heparinized solution that is irrigated in the area. To avoid residual trophoblastic tissue, a nontraumatic nipper must be used; a sterile plastic bag for later removal may also be used (Figs. 67–5 and 67–6).

Finally, irrigation and aspiration must be repeated until the drained liquids come out clear. Careful hemostasia must be performed with electrocoagulation or laser. While controversy exists concerning closure of the salpingostomy with sutures, most authors suggest keeping the area open.[7]

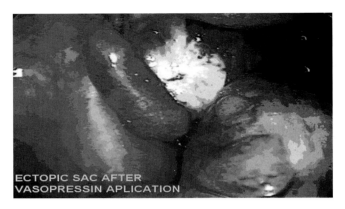

Figure 67–3. Ectopic sac after vasopressin application.

Follow-up of the patient is necessary by obtaining weekly β-hCG evaluations until these levels decline in order to avoid the possibility of a persistent ectopic pregnancy. If this is the case, a second laparoscopy may be necessary; another option is the use of methotrexate (explained later in the chapter).[8]

Salpingocentesis

The pioneers of salpingocentesis, Panski and Molina Sosa and their colleagues in Mexico, suggest salpingocentesis when the size of the ectopic pregnancy is smaller than 30 mm and the location is the isthmic portion, because in this area a lineal salpingostomy may cause stenosis.[9,10]

Once in the peritoneal cavity and after locating the affected tube, the first step is to irrigate the area. Then, with a nontraumatic nipper the tube is grabbed and the central portion is punctured with a long needle; the content is aspirated and 12 mg of methotrexate are instilled in the intraluminal portion. Finally, the process of irrigating is performed one more time before the end of the surgery.

In the postoperative stage, a β-hCG follow-up is done every 5 days in the beginning and complementary blood tests and ultrasound are performed before the patient is discharged from the hospital. The β-hCG levels decline over a period of 26 days after the surgery. The presence of persistent embryonic activity, free liquid, or an elevation in the β-hCG level can arouse the suspicion of

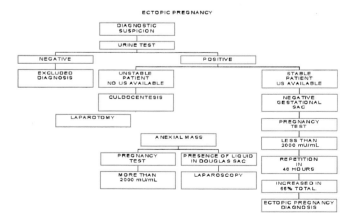

Figure 67–2. Ectopic pregnancy management scheme.

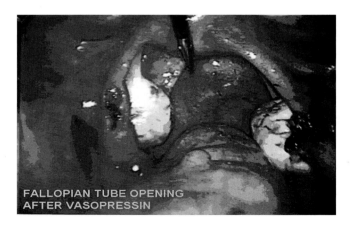

Figure 67–4. Fallopian tube opening after vasopressin application.

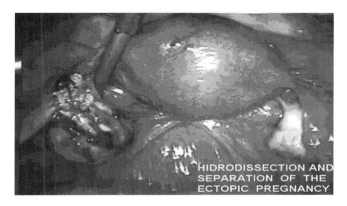

Figure 67–5. Hidrodissection and separation of the ectopic pregnancy.

persistent ectopic pregnancy, so application of systemic methotrexate or an open salpingo-oophorectomy is advised.

Salpingo-Oophorectomy

This operation may be partial or total. It is performed in cases of irreversible tube damage due to the ectopic pregnancy with the opposite tube being healthy. It is also performed in patients with previous pelvic illnesses or in patients with satisfied parity.

Partial Salpingo-Oophorectomy

Partial salpingo-oophorectomy is indicated when the compromised tube will require a reanastomosis in the future. The patient's position and conditions are the same as for a lineal salpingostomy. In such cases, the distal and proximal portions of the pregnancy are dissected with bipolar nippers; the mesosalpinx is cut with scissors and the segmented tube is removed. If there is a possibility of reanastomosis, the use of intra- and extracorporeal knots or prefabricated sutures for hemostasia is recommended instead of electrocautery.[11]

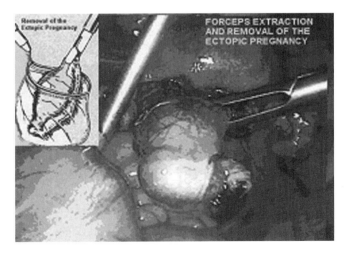

Figure 67–6. Extraction of ectopic pregnancy. *Insert:* Placement of ectopic pregnancy in a sterile plastic bag for removal.

Total Salpingo-Oophorectomy

In total salpingo-oophorectomy, a bipolar nipper and scissors are used in order to cut and coagulate the affected tube and the mesosalpinx. The dissected tube containing the ectopic pregnancy is retrieved in a sterile plastic bag through an 11-mm port placed in the umbilical area. The use of prefabricated sutures is recommended.

Fimbrial Evacuation of Ectopic Pregnancy

Fimbrial evacuation is quite controversial. It is designed to evacuate the conceptional product located in the fringe or nearby area. In 1980 Budowick and colleagues[12] mentioned that a substantial number of ectopic pregnancies occur in the extraluminal area, while Sherman and colleagues[13] reported this area as the most common in frequency.

Interstitial Ectopic Pregnancy

Cases of interstitial ectopic pregnancy may be treated by laparoscopy with corneal resection. Bipolar coagulation is needed to achieve hemostasis of the ascending uterine artery and the tuboovarian artery. The use of methotrexate is extremely helpful in this type of ectopic gestation.[14,15]

Broken Tubal Pregnancy

The laparoscopic approach is currently under dispute when the patient has unstable vital signs. In such instances, open surgery is preferred. If a laparoscopic procedure is to be done, the team should be experienced. Hemorrhage has to be controlled immediately and the affected tube removed. Ten-mm aspiration canulas to evacuate large clots are needed, as well as bipolar coagulation or prefabricated sutures.

Persistent Ectopic Pregnancy

The first case of persistent ectopic pregnancy was described in 1979 by Kelly and colleagues.[16] In order to detect persistent trophoblastic tissue after a salpingostomy, a β-hCG series must be ordered for a correct diagnosis. However, there are no uniform criteria about the number and frequency of such tests; the vast majority of cases are detected by elevated or stable levels of β-hCG in the first 30 days. However, these levels may persist up to 77 days until they disappear.[17] Some physicians perform the follow-up work every week until the levels decline.

The management of this diagnosis varies. If there is a possibility of a tubal collapse, a salpingectomy is performed. In asymptomatic patients with elevated β-hCG levels, the choice of surgical or medical approach (methotrexate) will depend on the progress and better outcome possibilities for the patient.

REPRODUCTIVE POSSIBILITIES

A group of studies concerning salpingostomy and salpingectomy compare the reproductive future of patients receiving radical or conservative procedures.[18] In both cases the success rate is very similar (70 and 80%, respectively). The incidence of recurrent ectopic pregnancies is about 6 to 8% regardless of the surgical approach (laparotomy or laparoscopy).

It is necessary to evaluate the fertility rate in patients with two ectopic pregnancies having at least one remaining fallopian tube;

that will allow us to evaluate the real advantage of salpingostomy in preventing sterility. It is accepted that after two tubal pregnancies up to 30% of patients may have intrauterine pregnancies. The condition of the opposite tube is very important, as it may affect subsequent pregnancies. Tuomivaara and Kauppila[18] reported an incidence of 87% of intrauterine pregnancies when the opposite tube was healthy. When diseased, the pregnancy rate dropped to 56% and the incidence of repeated ectopic pregnancy increased from 9 to 52%.

MEDICAL TREATMENT FOR ECTOPIC PREGNANCY

Since Tanaka and associates' report in 1982 that considers medical treatment the primary resource for treating ectopic pregnancies,[14] a great controversy remains. The current treatment regime is based on intramuscular methotrexate administration. Methotrexate is a folatum antagonist that inhibits the enzyme responsible for conversion of follinic acid into reduced cofactors, inhibiting DNA and to some degree RNA synthesis. This is particularly effective in tissues with a rapid cellular exchange, like trophoblastic tissue.

Toxicity levels of methotrexate depend on its serum concentration and the time of use. The use of follinic acid reduces toxicity; it is administered 24 hours after the methotrexate application. Various forms of administration have been proposed, and almost all schemes include methotrexate at 1 mg/kg per day and citrovorum on alternate days using 0.1 mg/kg per day.

Stovall and colleagues[19] use a sole dose of 50 mg/m² of body surface of methotrexate without citrovorum. With the aid of clinical and laboratory tests they watch over the undesirable effects, which are usually mild. They report a better therapeutic effect in reducing the β-hCG levels and in ultrasound imaging evolution. The β-hCG titers counts were made on days one, four and seven of treatment. The β-hCG levels on day four were sometimes found to be higher than on day one, but this was not considered abnormal. Tests were made each week until the β-hCG was reported as negative. In the situation when the β-hCG levels on day seven were higher than those on day four, a second dose of methotrexate was applied in the same dosage, and measurements from days four and seven were collected again. In fewer than 1% of all patients treated, the application of a third dose was needed.

The authors explain that the time of resolution of this condition was about 35.5 ± 11.8 days, which is about the same time that it takes the β-hCG levels to decline when patients undergo a salpingostomy.

The main advantage of medical treatment is the avoidance of an operation as well as the reduction of costs. Obviously, medical treatment is only suggested in hemodynamically stable patients with no signs of acute hemorrhage and with a tubal pregnancy whose maximum dimension is less than 3.5 cm. The disadvantages are the occasional need for hospitalization due to episodes of pain, the high risk of tubal rupture despite low β-hCG titers, long treatment periods causing an emotional burden on the patient, and the need for monitoring methotrexate levels to its toxic effects.

In selected patients, medical treatment appears to be extremely efficient, but it should not be used in cases when the β-hCG levels are extremely high (more than 6000 UT/liter), when the ultra-sonographic data reports fetal elements and/or cardiac activity, and when progesterone levels are higher than 10 ng/mL. In the case of a heterotopic pregnancy, medical treatment is not indicated.

MEXICAN INSTITUTIONAL EXPERIENCE

From June 1989 through December 1999, the National Institute of Perinatology in Mexico City received 374 patients with tubal ectopic pregnancy. The vast majority were treated by laparotomy due to the fact that most cases arrived in the emergency room in critical condition. The laparoscopic approach was used in stable patients with an unbroken tubal pregnancy.

Laparotomy was performed in 330 cases (88.23%) and laparoscopy in 44 (11.77%). Salpingectomy was used in 301 cases (80.48%) during laparotomy and in 20 laparoscopic cases (5.3%). Salpingostomy was done in 41 cases (10.96%) of laparotomies and only 2 cases (4.5%) were performed by laparoscopy. Partial salpingostomy was performed in 10 (2.67%) cases of laparotomies and in only one case by laparoscopy. Fringe evacuation was performed in 12 procedures by laparotomies (3.20%) and in only one case by endoscopy. Hospitalization stay on average was 3 days in the laparotomy group and one day in the laparoscopic group.

REFERENCES

1. Centers for Disease Control. *Ectopic Pregnancies: United States, 1990–1992. MMWR.* 1995;44:468.
2. Atrash HK, Friede A, Houge CJR. Ectopic pregnancy mortality in the United States, 1970–1983. *Obstet Gynecol.* 1987;70:817.
3. Instituto Nacional de Perinatología. *Normas de Endoscopia Quirúrgica Ginecológica.* Secretaría de Salud. México, D.F., 1996.
4. De Cherney A, Maheauxe R, Naftolin F. Salpingostomy for ectopic pregnancy in the sole patient oviduct: Reproductive outcome. *Fertil Steril.* 1982;37:619.
5. Bruhat M, Manhes H, Mage G, et al. Treatment of ectopic pregnancy by means of laparoscopy. *Fertil Steril.* 1982;37:619.
6. Pouly JL, Manges H, Mage C, et al. Corrective laparoscopic treatment of 321 ectopic pregnancies. *Fertil Steril.* 1986;46:1093.
7. Marvin C, Rulin M. Is salpingostomy the surgical treatment of choice for unruptured tubal pregnancy? *Obstet Gynecol.* 1995;86:1010.
8. S. Gomel V. *Microsurgery in Female Infertility.* Little-Brown: 1983.
9. Pansky M, Bukousky I, Golant A, et al. Methotrexate local injection for unruptured tubal pregnancy: An alternative to laparotomy? *Int J Gynecol Obstet.* 1992;37:265.
10. Molina S, Morales G. Tratamiento conservador del embarazo ectópico con methotrexate. *Rev Ginec Obstet Mex.* 1993;69:201.
11. Shapiro HJ, Adler DH. Excision of an ectopic pregnancy through the laparoscope. *Am J Obstet Gynecol.* 1987;117:290.
12. Budowick M, Johnson TRB Jr, Genandry B, et al. The histopathology of the developing tubal ectopic pregnancy. *Fertil Steril.* 1980;34:169.
13. Sherman D, Langer R, Herman A, et al. Reproductive outcome after fimbrial evacuation of tubal pregnancy. *Fertil Steril.* 1987;47:420.
14. Tanaka, Hayashi H, Kutsuzawa T, et al. Treatment of interstitial ectopic pregnancy with methotrexate: Report of a successful case. *Fertil Steril.* 1982;37:851.
15. Brandes MC, Youngs DD, Goldstein DP, et al. Treatment of cornual pregnancy with methotrexate: Case report. *Am J Obstet Gynecol.* 1986;155:655.

16. Kelly RW, Martin SA, Strickler RC. Delayed hemorrhage in conservative surgery for ectopic pregnancy. *Am J Obstet Gynecol.* 1979;133:225.

17. Bonatz G, Lehemann-Willenbrock G, Kunstaim P, et al. Management of patients with persistent β-hCG values following laparoscopic surgical and local drug treatment for ectopic pregnancy. *Int Gynecol Obstet.* 1994;47:33.

18. Tuomivara I, Kauppila A. Radical or conservative surgery for ectopic pregnancy? A follow-up study of fertility of 323 patients. *Fertil Steril.* 1988;50:580.

19. Stovall TC, Ling FW, Buster JE. Reproductive performance after methotrexate treatment of ectopic pregnancy. *Am J Obstet Gynecol.* 1990;162:1620.

Chapter Sixty-Eight ▪ ▪ ▪ ▪ ▪ ▪

*L*aparoscopic Hysterectomy

HARRY REICH

It is very dangerous to be right on a subject on which the established authorities are wrong.

—Voltaire

Laparoscopic hysterectomy (LH), defined as the laparoscopic ligation of the major vessels supplying the uterus, is an alternative to abdominal hysterectomy with more attention to ureteral identification.[1-3] First done in January 1988,[4] laparoscopic hysterectomy stimulated a general interest in the laparoscopic approach to hysterectomy as gynecologists not trained in vaginal or laparoscopic techniques struggled to maintain their fair share of the large, lucrative hysterectomy market. A watered-down version of LH, called LAVH (laparoscopic-assisted vaginal hysterectomy), was taught and became known as an expensive, overused procedure with indications for which skilled vaginal surgeons rarely found laparoscopic use necessary.

There are few reasons for the expert laparoscopic or vaginal surgeon to do an abdominal hysterectomy today. Abdominal hysterectomy should be done less frequently, worldwide, because laparoscopy can be used effectively to accomplish a less invasive laparoscopic or vaginal hysterectomy in most cases. In the United States, 600,000 hysterectomies are performed each year. The problem is that in the United States, Britain, and many other parts of the world, 70% of hysterectomies are still done with mutilating abdominal incisions. This has not changed in the 14 years since laparoscopic hysterectomy was invented. The only countries where more hysterectomies are done without these incisions—laparoscopically or vaginally—are places like Taiwan or India, in which doctors are reimbursed more if they do a hysterectomy without a major incision. In the United States, most gynecologists are trained to do abdominal hysterectomy. Then they go into a busy practice, usually as a junior partner, where they deliver babies for the next 20 years. Later, as their patients get older, they want to do some hysterectomies. Unfortunately, they do not go back to school to learn the most efficacious way to do a hysterectomy, but resort to the technique that they learned 20 years ago when they were residents, which means a large, mutilating

abdominal incision or, in some cases, a Pfannenstiel or a bikini cut. These incisions cause more adhesions, pain, and discomfort than if the operation were done with a laparoscope. Now we know that almost every case with an indication for hysterectomy can be done with a laparoscope.

In most specialties, innovative technology frequently separates a segment of the population into users and nonusers, and almost always the users have a clear advantage over the nonusers. This has been true with laparoscopic cholecystectomy, but not with laparoscopic hysterectomy.

Before 1988, laparoscopy was almost exclusively the domain of the gynecologist. It is ironic that though laparoscopic hysterectomy was introduced at the same time as laparoscopic cholecystectomy, it is done on a much more minor scale worldwide. The rapid acceptance of laparoscopic cholecystectomy by surgeons did not occur with laparoscopic hysterectomy probably because most gynecologists are not surgeons.

Soon after the technique of laparoscopic cholecystectomy was published, it became clear that the procedure represented a significant advance in clinical surgery and was rapidly accepted. General surgeons who became proficient with the method learned that, compared with open cholecystectomy, their patients were more comfortable postoperatively, required a shorter hospital stay, and experienced a more rapid convalescence and return to work and normal acts of daily living. Surgeons who did not learn the procedure found that few patients with gallbladder disease were referred to them, and many ceased performing operations on the biliary tract. Furthermore, they did not have the basic skills necessary to learn the new laparoscopic procedures that were subsequently developed.

Today laparoscopic hysterectomy, a highly practical and useful technique also associated with more postoperative comfort, a shorter hospital stay, and a more rapid convalescence and return to work and normal acts of daily living, has not been widely adopted primarily because many gynecologists have not exerted the effort to master it as they feel that they can function effectively with their current skills. Most women continue with the gynecologist who delivered their children for their gynecological operations. Contrary to the general surgeon's experience, most gynecologists do not feel any economic pressure to change even though it should be obvious that it is better for the patient.

Blame should not be placed entirely on the gynecologist. Laparoscopic hysterectomy is also unpopular with hospital administrations as it demands more operating room time and, in inexperienced hands, expensive disposable instrumentation. This combination, in a managed care environment, can result in a net loss for the hospital. The insurance industry has refused to compensate surgeons and hospitals with reasonable reimbursement for minimally invasive surgery done on women. Poor reimbursement for the time of surgery, and the time necessary to acquire the skill to do it, discourages gynecologists and surgeons from doing it. Certainly, women don't like large incisions and spend many millions of dollars on plastic surgery to reduce or correct them.

It is true that new techniques must be properly assessed. Is this possible in most cases? Are there fewer complications if the procedures are done by experts? Are patients generally satisfied? Are the procedures cost effective (if done with reusable instruments)? The answer to all of these questions is a resounding "yes."

COMPARISON TO OLDER TECHNIQUES

The first successful *vaginal hysterectomy* was done by the "patient" in 1670, as reported by Percival Willouby. A 46-year-old peasant woman named Faith Haworth was carrying a heavy load of coal when her uterus collapsed completely. Frustrated by this frequent occurrence, she grabbed her uterus, pulled as hard as possible, and cut the whole lot off with a short knife. The mighty bleeding stopped and she lived on for many years, water passing from her insensibly day and night (personal communication from S. Joel-Cohen). Conrad Langenbeck did the first planned vaginal hysterectomy in 1813.

Abdominal hysterectomy was done in 1843 by Clack, but the patient died of a pulmonary embolism. Walter Burnham did the first successful abdominal hysterectomy in 1853, by accident. When he opened the patient to remove a large ovarian cyst, she vomited, expelling a large fibroid uterus. As the surgeon was unable to put it back into the peritoneal cavity, he removed it supracervically. The first elective abdominal hysterectomy was by Clay and Koeberle in 1863.

Vaginal hysterectomy and abdominal hysterectomy techniques were progressively refined over the remainder of the 19th century, and by the early 20th century had become established as the "classic" techniques, to be passed down essentially unaltered to successive generations of gynecologists.

Most gynecologists believe that they know the correct indications for performing vaginal hysterectomy and abdominal hysterectomy, but after over 100 years of experience, there is still no consensus, as individual gynecologist may do close to 100% of their hysterectomies by either "classic" route. Though Querleu, Kovac, Grody, and Stovall report over 70% of their hysterectomies being done vaginally, most data from around the world suggest that over 70% of hysterectomies are abdominal hysterectomy, even in the absence of structural pathology.

Amazingly, vaginal hysterectomy and abdominal hysterectomy have never been subjected to a single class A evidence study (randomized controlled trial), and had attracted very few comparative studies until the recent introduction of laparoscopic hys-

terectomy. Most studies were single-center retrospective studies covering many years (class C: personal series by experts).[5] After a century of experience with the world's most commonly performed major operation, the gynecologic profession as a whole has no clear indication of the optimal method to perform it in differing situations. It is accepted that abdominal hysterectomy can be used for every indication and can be considered the "default operation."

Into this foray came laparoscopic hysterectomy in 1988. Laparoscopic hysterectomy stimulated a much greater interest in proper scientific evaluation of all forms of hysterectomy. Laparoscopic hysterectomy from its invention was considered a substitute for abdominal hysterectomy and not for vaginal hysterectomy. Yet unfavorable reports were published comparing laparoscopic hysterectomy to vaginal hysterectomy to further academic careers and hinder the acceptance of LH in the United States. Laparoscopic surgery has never been indicated for hysterectomy if the operation is feasible quickly and under good conditions by the vaginal route.

LH remains a reasonable substitute for abdominal hysterectomy. Its use, however, has presently plateaued because most managed care plans reimburse the surgeon poorly for using a laparoscopic approach. Hospitals may benefit if they are reimbursed by DRG's paying the same amount for a 2-day hysterectomy stay as for 7 days, but less if the hysterectomy patient is discharged within 24 hours (unbelievable). Unfortunately some plans, like Oxford, reward the hospital for additional postoperative days, discouraging both hospital administrator and surgeon from encouraging short hospital stay laparoscopic surgery over traditional laparotomy.

Most hysterectomies currently requiring an abdominal approach may be done with laparoscopic dissection of part, or all, of the abdominal portion followed by vaginal removal of the specimen. There are many surgical advantages to laparoscopy, particularly magnification of anatomy and pathology, easy access to the vagina and rectum, and the ability to achieve complete hemostasis and clot evacuation during underwater examination. Patient advantages are multiple and are related to avoidance of a painful abdominal incision. They include reduced duration of hospitalization and recuperation and an extremely low rate of infection and ileus.

The goal of vaginal hysterectomy, LAVH, or LH is to safely avoid an abdominal wall incision, with the resultant benefits just described. The surgeon must remember that if he or she is more comfortable with vaginal hysterectomy after ligating the ovarian ligaments, this should be done. Laparoscopic inspection at the end of the procedure will still permit the surgeon to control any bleeding and evacuate clots, and laparoscopic cuff suspension should limit future cuff prolapse. Unnecessary surgical procedures should not be done because of the surgeon's preoccupation with the development of new surgical skills. I emphasize, a laparoscopic hysterectomy is not indicated when vaginal hysterectomy can be easily and safely done.

DEFINITIONS

There are a variety of operations where the laparoscope is used as an aid to hysterectomy (Table 68–1). It is important that these different procedures are clearly delineated.

Diagnostic laparoscopy with vaginal hysterectomy indicates that the laparoscope is used for diagnostic purposes to determine if vaginal hysterectomy is possible when indications for a vaginal

TABLE 68–1. LAPAROSCOPIC HYSTERECTOMY CLASSIFICATION

1. Diagnostic laparoscopy with vaginal hysterectomy
2. Laparoscopic-assisted vaginal hysterectomy (LAVH)
3. Laparoscopic hysterectomy (LH)
4. Total laparoscopic hysterectomy (TLH)
5. Laparoscopic supracervical hysterectomy (LSH)—including CISH (classical interstitial Semm hysterectomy)
6. Vaginal hysterectomy with laparoscopic vault suspension (LVS) or laparoscopic pelvic reconstruction (LPR)
7. Laparoscopic hysterectomy with lymphadenectomy
8. Laparoscopic hysterectomy with lymphadenectomy and omentectomy
9. Laparoscopic radical hysterectomy with lymphadenectomy

approach are equivocal. It also assures that vaginal cuff and pedicle hemostasis is complete and allows clot evacuation.

Laparoscopic assisted vaginal hysterectomy (LAVH) is a vaginal hysterectomy after laparoscopic adhesiolysis, endometriosis excision, or oophorectomy. Unfortunately, this term is also used when the upper uterine ligaments (e.g., round, infundibulopelvic, or uteroovarian ligaments) of a relatively normal uterus are ligated with staples or bipolar desiccation. It must be emphasized that in most small uterus cases, the easy part of both an abdominal or vaginal hysterectomy is upper pedicle ligation.

Laparoscopic hysterectomy (LH) denotes laparoscopic ligation of the uterine arteries either by electrosurgery desiccation, suture ligature, or staples.[4] All surgical steps after the uterine vessels have been ligated can be done either vaginally or laparoscopically, including anterior and posterior vaginal entry by transection, cardinal and uterosacral ligament division, uterine removal (intact or by morcellation), and vaginal closure (vertically or transversely). Laparoscopic ligation of the uterine vessels is the *sine qua non* for laparoscopic hysterectomy. Ureteral identification often by isolation has always been advised.

Total laparoscopic hysterectomy (TLH) means that the laparoscopic dissection continues until the uterus lies free of all attachments in the peritoneal cavity. The uterus is then removed through the vagina, with morcellation if necessary. The vagina is closed with laparoscopically placed sutures. No vaginal surgery is done unless morcellation is necessary.[6]

Laparoscopic supracervical hysterectomy (LSH) has recently regained some support after suggestions that it offers physicians a less risky procedure than total hysterectomy performed through the laparoscope with decreased risk of dissection of the ureter and main division of the uterine artery. The uterus is removed by morcellation from above or below.[7]

Hysterectomy means removal of the uterus. Is the cervix a part of the uterus or not? If the cervix is left, better names would be partial hysterectomy, subtotal hysterectomy, or fundectomy, as these terms denote that the uterus was not completely removed.

The speculations regarding the cervical orgasm issue are groundless as there are no data. There are very few women who report a decrease in orgasmic ability with removal of the cervix.[8,9]

The other theory regarding the supracervical approach is that it is less likely to lead to future vault prolapse because of the preservation of the pelvic floor supports, with the cardinal and uterosacral ligaments remaining intact. Certainly, if the uterosacral–cardinal complex is attached to the upper vagina instead of the sides of the cervix and the endopelvic fascia is brought together with

underlying vagina across the midline, support should be better than before the operation.

Kurt Semm's version of a supracervical hysterectomy, often referred to as the CISH procedure (classical interstitial Semm hysterectomy), leaves the cardinal ligaments intact while eliminating the columnar cells of the endocervical canal. After perforating the uterine fundus with a long sound-dilator, a calibrated uterine resection tool (CURT) that fits around this instrument is used to core out the endocervical canal. Thereafter, at laparoscopy, suture techniques are used to ligate the utero-ovarian ligaments. An Endoloop is placed around the uterine fundus to the level of the internal os of the cervix and tied. The uterus is divided at its junction with the cervix and removed by laparoscopic morcellation.[10]

Laparoscopic pelvic reconstruction (LPR) with vaginal hysterectomy is useful when vaginal hysterectomy alone cannot accomplish appropriate repair for vaginal prolapse. Ureteral dissection and suture placement through the uterosacral ligaments near the sacrum, before the vaginal portion of the procedure, may be useful to achieve vaginal suspension (see below). Levator muscle plication vaginally or laparoscopically is often necessary. Retropubic Burch colposuspension can also be done laparoscopically.

I use the term *laparoscopic hysterectomy* to include all types of cases using the laparoscope. LAVH is just one type and is really a vaginal hysterectomy (almost all LAVH procedures can be done as completely vaginal hysterectomies; TLH implies that a vaginal hysterectomy would be difficult or impossible to perform, that is, TLH is a substitute for abdominal hysterectomy, not for vaginal hysterectomy).

INDICATIONS

Indications for laparoscopic hysterectomy include benign pathology such as endometriosis, fibroids, adhesions, and adnexal masses usually requiring the selection of an abdominal approach to hysterectomy. It is also appropriate when vaginal hysterectomy is not possible because of a narrow pubic arch, a constricted vagina with no prolapse, or severe arthritis that prohibits placement of the patient in sufficient lithotomy position for vaginal exposure. Laparoscopic procedures in obese women allow the surgeon to make an incision above the panniculus. Laparoscopic hysterectomy may also be considered for stage I endometrial, ovarian, and cervical cancer.[11-13] Pelvic reconstruction procedures including cuff suspension, retropubic colposuspension, and rectocele repair may also be simultaneously accomplished through the laparoscope.

The most common indication for laparoscopic hysterectomy is a symptomatic fibroid uterus (hypermenorrhea, pelvic pressure, and rarely pain). Almost all of these cases can be done laparoscopically as an outpatient or with a one to two day hospital stay. Morcellation is often necessary and is done laparoscopically and/or vaginally using a scalpel. Fibroids fixed in the pelvis or abdomen without descent are easier to mobilize laparoscopically. It is important to do current uterine size and weight measurements to confirm the appropriateness of the laparoscopic hysterectomy, because most small uteri can be removed vaginally. For example, the normal uterus weighs 70 to 125 g; a 12-week gestational age uterus weighs 280 to 320 g; a 24-week uterus weighs 580 to 620 g; and a term uterus weighs 1000 to 1100 g.

The other common indication is endometriosis. Endometriosis can involve the uterus and the areas around the uterus. The endometriosis often grows in the posterior cervix and causes painful periods and, in some people, pain all the time, 7 days a week. In all these cases, the endometriosis should be removed. Hysterectomy should not be done for stage IV endometriosis with extensive cul-de-sac involvement, unless the surgeon has the skill and time to resect all deep fibrotic endometriosis from the posterior vagina, uterosacral ligaments, and anterior rectum, and only then a hysterectomy to remove possible deep intrauterine endometriosis, which is called adenomyosis. Unfortunately, hysterectomy is commonly done using an intrafascial technique that leaves the deep fibrotic endometriosis behind to cause future problems. Later, when pain persists, it becomes much more difficult to remove deep fibrotic endometriosis when there is no uterus between the anterior rectum and the bladder. After hysterectomy, the endometriosis left in the anterior rectum and vaginal cuff frequently becomes densely adherent to, or invades into, the bladder and one or both ureters. In many patients with stage IV endometriosis and extensive cul-de-sac obliteration, it is preferable to preserve the uterus and prevent future vaginal cuff, bladder, and ureteral problems.[14] Obviously, this approach will not be effective when uterine adenomyosis is present. In these cases, after excision of cul-de-sac endometriosis, persistent pain will ultimately require a hysterectomy. Oophorectomy is not usually necessary at hysterectomy for advanced endometriosis, if the endometriosis is carefully removed. Reoperation for recurrent symptoms is necessary in less than 5% of my patients in whom one or both ovaries have been preserved. Bilateral oophorectomy is rarely indicated in women under age 40 undergoing hysterectomy for endometriosis.

Hysterectomy may be performed for abnormal uterine bleeding in women of reproductive age. Abnormal uterine bleeding is defined as excessive uterine bleeding, or irregular uterine bleeding, for more than 8 days during more than a single cycle or as profuse bleeding requiring additional protection (large clots, gushes, or limitations on activity). There should be no history of a bleeding diathesis or use of medication that may cause bleeding. A negative effect on quality of life should be documented. Physical examination, laboratory data, ultrasound, and hysteroscopy are frequently negative. Hormonal or other medical treatment should be attempted before hysterectomy, and its failure, contraindication, or refusal should be documented. The presence of anemia is recorded and correction with iron supplementation attempted. If hysterectomy is chosen, a vaginal approach is usually appropriate. Laparoscopic hysterectomy is done only when vaginal hysterectomy is not feasible, including history of previous abdominal surgery and lack of prolapse (nulliparous or multiparous). TLH is considered if the surgeon has little experience with the vaginal approach.

CONTRAINDICATIONS

Laparoscopic hysterectomy is not advised for the diagnosis and treatment of a pelvic mass that cannot be removed intact through a culdotomy incision or that is too large to fit intact into an impermeable sack, particularly in postmenopausal patients. The largest available sack for removal of intraperitoneal masses is the LapSac (Cook Ob/Gyn, Spencer, IN), which measures 11 × 8 inches. Although cyst aspiration is advocated by some investigators,[15,16] I feel that postmenopausal cystic ovaries should not be subjected to aspiration before oophorectomy because the inevitable

spillage may change the diagnosis from a stage Ia ovarian cancer to a stage Ic. Its effect on survival is unknown, but it may be detrimental. It must be emphasized that aspiration through a small-gauge needle placed through a thickened portion of the ovary and cyst aspiration devices with surrounding suction and endoloop placement (Cook) do not completely prevent spillage.

A history of extensive abdominal adhesions should not necessitate a laparotomy; remember that previous laparotomies are probably what caused the adhesions in the first place. The patient should be referred to an expert laparoscopic surgeon.

The medical status of the patient may prohibit surgery. Anemia, diabetes, lung disorders, cardiac disease, and bleeding diathesis should be excluded prior to surgery. Age alone should rarely be a deterrent.

Placenta accreta, uterine atony, unspecified uterine bleeding, and uterine rupture are relative contraindications to peripartum hysterectomy at present. However, laparoscopic hysterectomy may be considered for patients needing a postpartum hysterectomy.

Another contraindication is stage III ovarian cancer that requires a large abdominal incision. Finally, inexperience or inadequate training of the surgeon is a contraindication to the laparoscopic approach.

EQUIPMENT

Operating room tables capable of a 30-degree Trendelenburg position are extremely valuable for laparoscopic hysterectomy. Unfortunately these tables are rare, and this author has much difficulty operating when only a limited degree of body tilt can be attained. For the past 18 years, a steep Trendelenburg position (20 to 40 degrees), with shoulder braces and the arms at the patient's sides, has been used without adverse effects.

A Valtchev uterine mobilizer (Conkin Surgical Instruments, Toronto) is the best available single instrument to antevert the uterus and delineate the posterior vagina.[17] With this instrument, the uterus can be anteverted to about 120 degrees and moved in an arc about 45 degrees from the horizontal by turning the mobilizer around its longitudinal axis. Either the 100-mm long and 10-mm thick, or the 80-mm long and 8-mm thick, obturator may be used for uterine manipulation during hysterectomy. Placement of a #81 French rectal probe (Reznik Instruments, Skokie, IL) and intraoperative rectovaginal examinations remain important techniques for defining the rectovaginal space, even when the Valtchev uterine mobilizer is available whenever rectal location is in doubt.

Trocar sleeves are available in many sizes and shapes. For most cases, 5.5-mm diameter cannulas are adequate. Short trapless 5-mm trocar sleeves with a retention screw grid around the external surface (reusable: Richard Wolf Medical Instruments, Vernon Hills, IL; disposable: Apple Medical, Bolton, MA) are used to facilitate efficient instrument exchanges and evacuation of tissue while allowing unlimited freedom during extracorporeal suture tying.[18] With practice, a good laparoscopic surgical team will be able to make instrument exchanges fast enough so that little pneumoperitoneum is lost.

Self-retaining lateral vaginal wall retractors or Vienna retractors (Brisky-Navatril) are used for vaginal extraction of a large fibroid uterus without changing stirrups. Alternatively, after the abdominal portion of the procedure is completed, the stirrups are replaced with candy-cane stirrups to obtain better hip flexion, so that conventional vaginal sidewall retractors can be used.

Monopolar cutting current through electrosurgical electrodes that eliminate capacitance and insulation failures (Electroshield from Electroscope, Boulder, CO) is used. Bipolar forceps with high-frequency low-voltage cutting current (20 to 50 W) can coagulate vessels as large as the ovarian and uterine arteries. The Kleppinger bipolar forceps (Richard Wolf) are excellent for large vessel hemostasis. Microbipolar forceps contain a channel for irrigation and a fixed distance between the electrodes. Irrigation is used to identify bleeding sites before coagulation and to prevent sticking of the electrode to the eschar that is created. Irrigation is also used during underwater examination to dilute blood products surrounding a bleeding vessel so that it may be identified before coagulation. Disposable stapling instruments are rarely used for laparoscopic hysterectomy because of their expense. Suture and/or bipolar desiccation work better.

PREOPERATIVE PREPARATION

Surgical skill remains paramount. Ambidexterity separates the laparoscopic surgeon from those trained traditionally, as the surgeon must often hold the camera with the dominant hand.

The patient is optimized medically for coexistent problems. Patients are encouraged to hydrate and eat lightly for 24 hours before admission on the day of surgery. Fleet Phospho Soda prep kit #3 is administered the day before surgery to evacuate the lower bowel as follows: First Fleet Phospho Soda mixed into a half glass of cool clear juice in the late afternoon, then 4 Bisacodyl tablets in the early evening, and finally a Fleet Bisacodyl enema 1 to 2 hours before bedtime (10 mg). Lower abdominal, pubic, and perineal hair is not shaved. Antibiotics (usually cefoxitin or cefotetan) are administered preoperatively in all cases. A Foley catheter is inserted during surgery and removed in the recovery room or the next morning.

Patient Positioning

All laparoscopic surgical procedures are done under general anesthesia with endotracheal intubation. The routine use of an orogastric tube is recommended to diminish the possibility of a trocar injury to a gas-filled stomach and to reduce small bowel distension during the operation. The patient remains flat (0 degrees) on the operating table until the umbilical trocar sleeve has been inserted, and then is placed in a steep Trendelenburg's position (20 to 30 degrees). Lithotomy position with the hip extended (thigh parallel to abdomen) is obtained with Allan stirrups (Edgewater Medical Systems, Mayfield Heights, OH) or knee braces, which are adjusted for each individual patient before anesthesia. Examination under anesthesia is always performed prior to prepping the patient.

Laparoscopy was never thought to be a sterile procedure before the incorporation of video, as the surgeon operated with his head in the surgical field, attached to the laparoscopic optic. Furthermore, it is not possible to sterilize skin. Since 1983, I have maintained a policy of not scrubbing and not sterilizing or draping the camera or laser arm. Masking is optional. (Most surgeons in the United Kingdom don't mask for laparoscopic surgery.) Infection has been rare: less than 1%. The vertical intraumbilical incision is closed with a single 4-0 Vicryl suture opposing deep

fascia and skin dermis, with the knot buried beneath the fascia. This will prevent the suture from acting like a wick transmitting bacteria into the soft tissue or peritoneal cavity. The lower-quadrant incisions are loosely approximated with a Javid vascular clamp (V. Mueller, McGaw Park, IL) and covered with Dermabond (Ethicon) or Collodion (AMEND, Irvington, NJ) to allow drainage of excess Ringer's lactate solution.

TOTAL LAPAROSCOPIC HYSTERECTOMY

My technique for a total laparoscopic hysterectomy (TLH) is described in Figures 68–1 to 68–5. Other types of laparoscopic hysterectomy (e.g., LAVH or LH) are simply modifications of this more extensive procedure.

Incisions and Vaginal Preparation

Three laparoscopic puncture sites including the umbilicus are used: 10 mm umbilical, 5 mm right, and 5 mm left lower quadrant. The left lower quadrant puncture is the major portal for operative manipulation. The right trocar sleeve is used for retraction with atraumatic grasping forceps.

A recent study documented that most women prefer the cosmetic appearance of a 15-cm Pfannenstiel incision to multiple 12-mm high incisions required for stapling devices. Reduction in wound morbidity and scar integrity as well as cosmesis are enhanced using 5-mm sites.[19] The use of 12-mm incisions when a 5-mm incision will suffice is not an advance in minimally invasive surgery.

The endocervical canal is dilated to Pratt #25, and the Valtchev uterine mobilizer with blunt tip (Conkin Surgical Instruments, Toronto) is inserted to antevert the uterus and delineate the posterior vagina. When the uterus is in the anteverted position, the cervix sits on a wide pedestal, making the vagina readily visible between the uterosacral ligaments when the cul-de-sac is viewed laparoscopically.

Exploration

The upper abdomen is inspected, and the appendix is identified. If appendiceal pathology is present (dilatation, adhesions, or endometriosis), appendectomy is done by mobilizing the appendix,

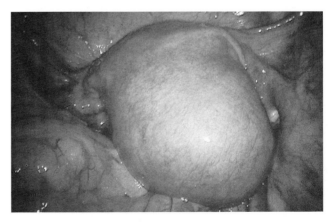

Figure 68–1. Large fibroid uterus fills the pelvis.

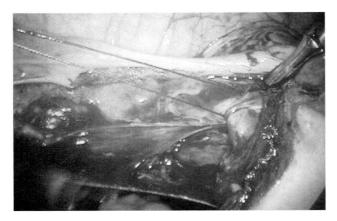

Figure 68–2. After dissection of the left uterine artery, 0 Vicryl on a CTB-1 needle is placed around the left uterine artery. See Color Section.

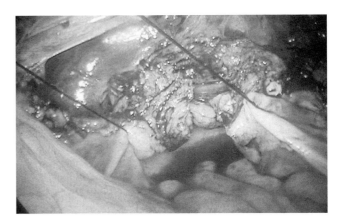

Figure 68–4. A single 0 Vicryl suture includes the uterosacral and cardinal ligaments along with the posterior vaginal wall. See Color Section.

isolating its blood supply by making a window in the mesoappendix near the cecum with reusable Metzenbaum-type scissors, passing a 2/0 Vicryl free ligature through this window, and securing it extracorporeally with the Clarke-Reich knotpusher. Three Endoloops [Endoloop (chromic gut ligature), Ethicon, Somerville, NJ] are then placed at the appendiceal–cecal junction, after desiccating the appendix just above this juncture. The appendix is left attached to the cecum; its stump is divided later in the procedure, after opening the cul-de-sac, so that removal from the peritoneal cavity is accomplished immediately after separation.

Ureteral Dissection

Three approaches have been used for laparoscopic ureteric identification, which may be called medial, superior, and lateral. Stents are not used as they cause hematuria and ureteric spasm in some patients. When the ureter is identified but not dissected, cystoscopy is done after vaginal closure to check for ureteral patency, 5 minutes after one ampule of indigo carmine dye is administered intravenously. The laparoscopic surgeon should dissect (skeletonize) either the ureter or the uterine vessels during the performance of a laparoscopic hysterectomy.

Medial Approach (Reich). If the uterus is anteflexed, the ureter can usually be easily visualized in its natural position on the medial leaf of the broad ligament provided there is no significant cul-de-sac or adnexal pathology. This allows the peritoneum immediately above the ureter to be incised to create a "window" in the peritoneum, which makes for safe division of the infundibulopelvic ligament or adnexal pedicle. Immediately after exploration of the upper abdomen and pelvis, each ureter is isolated deep in the pelvis, when possible. Ureteral dissection is performed early in the operation before the pelvic sidewall peritoneum becomes edematous and/or opaque from irritation by the CO_2 pneumoperitoneum or aquadissection and before ureteral peristalsis is inhibited by surgical stress, pressure, or the Trendelenburg position.[1]

The ureter and its overlying peritoneum are grasped deep in the pelvis. An atraumatic grasping forceps is used from the opposite-sided cannula to grab the ureter and its overlying peritoneum on the pelvic sidewall below and caudad to the ovary, lateral to the uterosacral ligament. Scissors are used to divide the peritoneum overlying the ureter and are inserted into the defect created and spread. Thereafter one blade of the scissors is placed on top of the ureter, its blade visualized through the peritoneum, and the peritoneum divided. This is continued into the deep pelvis where the

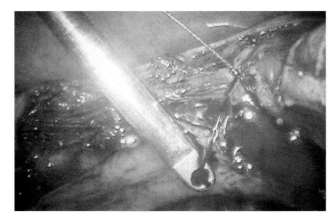

Figure 68–3. The suture around the left uterine artery is tied extracorporeally using a Clarke-Reich knot pusher. See Color Section.

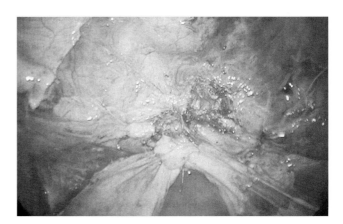

Figure 68–5. The vaginal closure is completed with a second interrupted midline suture. See Color Section.

uterine vessels cross the ureter, lateral to the cardinal ligament insertion into the cervix. Connective tissue between the ureter and the vessels is separated with scissors. Bleeding is controlled with microbipolar forceps. Often the uterine artery is ligated at this time to diminish backbleeding from the upper pedicles.

Superior Approach. The superior approach entails dissecting the colon (rectosigmoid on the left; caecum on the right) off of the pelvic brim and freeing the infundibulopelvic ligament vessels from the roof of the broad ligament to allow the ureter, which lies below it, to be identified. The ureter is then reflected off the broad ligament and traced into the pelvis.

Lateral Approach (Kadar). The lateral approach makes use of the pararectal space to identify the ureter, and the ureter does not have to be peeled off the broad ligament for its entire pelvic course to be visible. The tip of the laparoscope is often the best blunt dissector in this area, and may be inserted alongside and just lateral to the pelvic sidewall peritoneum into the loose areolar tissue already distended by retroperitoneal CO_2 until ureter and uterine vessels are identified.

By displacing the uterus to the contralateral side, a pelvic sidewall triangle is identified, formed by the round ligament, the lateral border by the external iliac artery, and the medial border by the infundibulopelvic ligament. The peritoneum in the middle of the triangle is incised with scissors and the broad ligament opened by bluntly separating the extraperitoneal areolar tissues. The infundibulopelvic ligament is pulled medially with grasping forceps to expose the ureter at the pelvic brim where it crosses the common or external iliac artery.[20]

The operator then searches for the ureter distal to the pelvic brim and lateral to the infundibulopelvic ligament. The dissection is carried bluntly underneath and caudad to the round ligament, until the obliterated hypogastric artery is identified extraperitoneally. If any difficulty is encountered, the artery is first identified intraperitoneally where it hangs from the anterior abdominal wall, traced proximally to where it passes behind the round ligament, and then with both its intraperitoneal portion and the dissected space under the round ligament in view, the intraperitoneal part of the ligament is moved back and forth. Once the obliterated hypogastric artery has been identified extraperitoneally, it is an easy matter to develop the paravesical space by bluntly separating the areolar tissue on either side of the artery. The obliterated hypogastric artery is next traced proximally to where it is joined by the uterine artery, and the pararectal space opened by blunt dissection proximal and medial to the uterine vessels, which lie on top of the cardinal ligament. Once the pararectal space has been opened, the ureter is easily identified on the medial leaf of the broad ligament, which forms the medial border of the pararectal space. The uterine artery and cardinal ligament at the distal (caudal) border of the space, and the internal iliac artery on its lateral border, also become clearly visible.

Retroperitoneal Dissection

At the start of most laparoscopic hysterectomies, the anterior broad ligament is stretched out by pulling the fallopian tube medially, and scissors are used to make an incision in it behind the round ligament for oophorectomy and in front of the round ligament for ovarian preservation. CO_2 from the pneumoperitoneum rushes into the retroperitoneum and distends it. The tip of the laparoscope is then used to perform "optical dissection" of the retroperitoneal space behind the uterus for oophorectomy and parallel to it for ovarian preservation.

Bladder Mobilization

The round ligaments are divided at their midportion using a spoon electrode (Electroscope) set at 150-W cutting current. Persistent bleeding is controlled with bipolar desiccation at 30-W cutting current. Thereafter scissors or the same electrode are used to divide the vesicouterine peritoneal fold starting at the left side and continuing across the midline to the right round ligament. The upper junction of the vesicouterine fold is identified as a white line firmly attached to the uterus, with 2 to 3 cm between it and the bladder dome. The initial incision is made below the white line while lifting the peritoneum covering the bladder. The bladder is mobilized off the uterus and upper vagina using scissors or bluntly with the same spoon electrode or a suction-irrigator until the anterior vagina is identified by elevating it from below with ring forceps.

Upper Uterine Blood Supply

When ovarian preservation is desired, the utero-ovarian ligament and fallopian tube pedicles are suture-ligated adjacent to the uterus with 2/0-Vicryl, using either a curved needle or a free ligature passed through a window created around the ligament. To create the window, the peritoneum is opened just lateral to the tubal cornua, and the Metzenbaum type scissors slid down lateral to the uteroovarian vessels until its tip can be seen through the broad ligament peritoneum, which is divided. Alternatively, the utero-ovarian ligament and fallopian tube may be coagulated until desiccated with bipolar forceps, at 25 to 35 W cutting current, and then divided.

When oophorectomy is indicated or ovarian preservation not desired, the anterior and posterior leaves of the broad ligament are opened lateral and below the infundibulopelvic ligament with a laparoscopic Metzenbaum-type scissors and a 2/0-Vicryl free ligature passed through the window thus created and tied extracorporeally using the Clarke-Reich knotpusher.[21] This is repeated twice around the ovarian vessels, so that two proximal ties and one distal one are placed, and then the ligament divided. I rarely desiccate the infundibulopelvic ligament today as it results in too much smoke early in the operation. While applying traction to the cut distal pedicle, the broad ligament is divided to the round ligament just lateral to the utero-ovarian artery anastomosis using cutting current through a spoon electrode.

If suturing skills are not developed and the tube and ovary are to be removed, the infundibulopelvic ligament is mobilized and Kleppinger bipolar forceps (Richard Wolf Medical Instruments, Vernon Hills, IL) are used to compress and desiccate its vessels or the Multifire Endo-GIA 30 (U.S. Surgical, Norwalk, CT) applied. The round ligament is desiccated and divided. If the ovary is to be preserved, the utero-ovarian ligament/round ligament/fallopian tube junction may be divided with the Endo-GIA stapler. This may be time saving for this portion of the procedure, thus justifying its increased cost.

Uterine Vessel Ligation

The uterine vessels may be ligated at their origin, at the site where they cross the ureter, or on the uterus. In most cases, the uterine vessels are suture-ligated as they ascend the sides of the uterus. The broad ligament on each side is skeletonized down to the uterine vessels. Each uterine vessel pedicle is suture-ligated with 0-Vicryl on a CTB-1 blunt needle (Ethicon JB260) (27″).[6] The needles are introduced into the peritoneal cavity by pulling them through a 5-mm incision.[22] The curved needle is placed around the uterine vessel pedicle at the side of the uterus. A short rotary movement of the Cook oblique curved needle holder brings the needle around the uterine vessel pedicle. The uterine artery is a sturdy structure and can be grasped and elevated carefully to avoid the uterine veins underneath. In some cases, the vessels can be completely skeletonized and a 2-0 Vicryl free suture ligature passed around them. Sutures are tied extracorporeally using a Clarke-Reich knot pusher.[21]

In some cases the curved needle is inserted on top of the unroofed ureter where it turns medially towards the previously mobilized bladder. A single suture placed in this manner on each side serves as a "sentinel stitch," identifying the ureter for the remainder of the procedure.

Division of Cervicovaginal Attachments and Circumferential Culdotomy

The cardinal ligaments on each side are divided with the CO_2 laser at high power (80 W) or with the spoon electrode at 150-W cutting current. Bipolar forceps are used to coagulate the uterosacral ligaments and are invaluable to control bleeding from vaginal branches. The vagina is entered posteriorly over the Valtchev retractor near the cervicovaginal junction. A 4-cm diameter vaginal delineator (R. Wolf) is placed in the vagina to outline circumferentially the cervicovaginal junction, serve as a backstop for laser work, and prevent loss of pneumoperitoneum. First, it identifies the anterior cervicovaginal junction and then the lateral fornices. They are incised using the laser with the delineator as a backstop to complete the circumferential culdotomy. The uterus is morcellated, if necessary, and pulled out of the vagina.

When the vaginal delineator is not available, a ring forceps is inserted into the anterior vagina above the tenaculum on the anterior cervical lip to identify the anterior cervicovaginal junction. The left anterior vaginal fornix is entered using the laser, so that the aquapurator can be inserted into the anterior vagina above the anterior cervical lip. Following the aquapurator tip or ring forceps, and using them as a backstop, the anterior and lateral vaginal fornices are divided. The aquapurator is inserted from posterior to anterior to delineate the right vaginal fornix, which is divided. The uterus can then be pulled out of the vagina.

Morcellation (Laparoscopic and Vaginal)

Morcellation can be done laparoscopically or vaginally. For the laparoscopic technique, a #10 blade on a long handle is introduced gently through the left 5-mm trocar incision after removing the trocar. With care the uterus and its enclosed large myoma can be bivalved with the blade. The surgeon's fingers in contact with the skin prevent loss of pneumoperitoneum.

Vaginal morcellation is done in most cases on a uterus free in the peritoneal cavity, but may be considered after securing the ovarian arteries from above and the uterine arteries from above or below. A #10 blade on a long knife handle is used to make a circumferential incision into the fundus of the uterus while pulling outwards on the cervix and using the cervix as a fulcrum. The myometrium is incised circumferentially parallel to the axis of the uterine cavity, with the scalpel's tip always inside the myomatous tissue and pointed centrally, away from the surrounding vagina. The knife is not extended through the serosa of the uterus. The incision is continued around the full circumference of the myometrium in a symmetrical fashion beneath the uterine serosa. Traction is maintained on the cervix, and the avascular myometrium is cut so that the endometrial cavity with a surrounding thick layer of myometrium is delivered with the cervix, bringing the outside of the uterus closer to the operator for further excision by wedge morcellation.

Wedge morcellation is done by removing wedges of myoma and myometrium from the anterior and posterior uterine wall, usually in the midline, to reduce the bulk of the uterus. After excision of a large core, the fundus is morcellated with multiple wedge resections, around either a tenaculum or an 11-mm corkscrew (WISAP, Sauerlach, Germany). The remaining fundus, if still too large for removal, can be bivalved so that one half can be pulled out of the peritoneal cavity, followed by the other half.

Morcellation of fibroids through anterior abdominal wall puncture sites is now practical when vaginal access is limited. The Steiner Electromechanical Morcellator (Karl Storz, Tuttlingen, Germany) is a 10-mm diameter motorized circular saw that uses claw forceps or a tenaculum to grasp the fibroid and pull it into contact with the trocar. Large pieces of myomatous tissue are removed piecemeal until the myoma can be pulled out through the trocar incision. With practice this instrument can often be inserted through a stretched 5-mm incision without an accompanying trocar.

Laparoscopic Vaginal Vault Closure and Suspension With McCall Culdoplasty

The vaginal delineator or a sponge in a glove pack is placed back into the vagina for closure of the vaginal cuff, occluding it to maintain pneumoperitoneum. The uterosacral ligaments are identified by bipolar desiccation markings or with the aid of a rectal probe. The left uterosacral ligament is elevated and a 0-Vicryl suture on a CT-1 needle is placed through it using an oblique Cook needle holder, then through the left cardinal ligament with just a few cells of posterolateral vagina just below the uterine vessels, and along the posterior vaginal epithelium with a few bites over to the right side. Finally, the same suture with needle is used to fix the right posterolateral vagina and cardinal ligament to the right uterosacral ligament.

This suture is tied extracorporeally and provides excellent support to the vaginal cuff apex, elevating it superiorly and posteriorly toward the hollow of the sacrum. The rest of the vagina and the overlying pubocervicovesicular fascia are closed vertically with one or two 0-Vicryl interrupted sutures. In most cases the peritoneum is not closed.

Cystoscopy

Cystoscopy is done after vaginal closure to check for ureteral patency, 10 minutes after intravenous administration of one ampule of indigo carmine dye. This is especially necessary when the ureter is identified but not dissected. Blue dye should be visualized through both ureteral orifices. The bladder wall should also be inspected for suture and thermal defects.[23]

Underwater Examination

At the close of each operation, an underwater examination is used to detect bleeding from vessels and viscera tamponaded during the procedure by the increased intraperitoneal pressure of the CO_2 pneumoperitoneum. The CO_2 pneumoperitoneum is displaced with 2 to 5 L of Ringer's lactate solution, and the peritoneal cavity is vigorously irrigated and suctioned until the effluent is clear of blood products. Any further bleeding is controlled underwater using microbipolar forceps to coagulate through the electrolyte solution, and at least 2 L of lactated Ringer's solution is left in the peritoneal cavity.

SPECIAL PROBLEMS RELATED TO LAPAROSCOPIC HYSTERECTOMY

My most recent technique involves isolation and ligation of the uterine artery on the side of the uterus early in the operation to limit backbleeding from the utero-ovarian ligament, especially if ovarian preservation is desired. The round ligament incision is extended into the ipsilateral portion of the vesicouterine peritoneal fold, and the pulsating uterine artery identified and ligated either with a CT-1 needle or a free ligature. In these cases, the ureter is not isolated because the uterine vessels on the side of the uterus are usually well above them; cystoscopy is done after cuff closure, 10 minutes after indigo carmine dye administration.

Endometriosis nodules in the muscularis of the anterior rectum can usually be excised laparoscopically. Full-thickness penetration of the rectum can occur during hysterectomy surgery, especially when excising rectal endometriosis nodules. Following identification of the nodule or rent in the rectum, a closed circular stapler [Proximate ILS Curved Intraluminal Stapler (Ethicon, Stealth)] is inserted into the lumen just past the lesion or hole, opened 1 to 2 cm, and held high to avoid the posterior rectal wall. The proximal anvil is positioned just beyond the lesion or hole, which is invaginated into the opening and the device closed. Circumferential inspection is made to insure the absence of encroachment of nearby organs and posterior rectum in the staple line and the lack of tension in the anastomosis. The instrument is fired, then removed through the anus. The surgeon must inspect and insure that the fibrotic lesion or a donut of tissue representing the excised hole is contained in the circular stapler. Once verified, anastomotic inspection is done laparoscopically underwater after filling the rectum with indigo carmine solution.

POSTOPERATIVE CONSIDERATIONS

Postoperatively, the vaginal cuff is checked for granulation tissue between 6 and 12 weeks, as sutures are usually absorbed by then and healing should be complete. Routine checks at 1 to 4 weeks are usually not indicated as a pelvic examination could impede healing. Examinations usually within 1 week are indicated for pain, pressure, or pyrexia. Patients usually experience some fatigue and discomfort for approximately 2 to 4 weeks after the operation, but may perform gentle exercise such as walking and return to routine activities between 2 and 6 weeks following the operation. Sexual activity may be resumed when the vaginal incision has healed, usually after 6 weeks.

COMPLICATIONS

Complications of laparoscopic hysterectomy are those of hysterectomy and laparoscopy: anesthetic accidents; respiratory compromise; thromboembolic phenomena; urinary retention; injury to vessels, ureters, bladder, and bowel; and infections, especially of the vaginal cuff (Table 68–2).[24–28] Ureteral injury is more common when staplers or bipolar desiccation are used without ureteral identification. Complications unique to laparoscopy include large-vessel injury, epigastric vessel laceration, subcutaneous emphysema, and trocar-site incisional hernias.[29]

Since the introduction of prophylactic antibiotics, vaginal cuff abscess, pelvic thrombophlebitis, septicemia, pelvic cellulitis, and adnexal abscesses are rare. Abdominal wound infection is rare.

Infection

The febrile morbidity rate associated with vaginal hysterectomy is about half that for the abdominal procedure. Laparoscopic evacuation of all blood clots, and sealing all blood vessels after the uterus has been removed, should reduce further the infection rate. Morcellation during laparoscopic or vaginal hysterectomy results in a slightly increased risk of fever, especially if prophylactic antibiotics are not used.

Since the introduction of prophylactic antibiotics, vaginal cuff infection is rare. This infection can result in pelvic cellulitis, septicemia, vaginal cuff abscess, adnexal abscesses, and pelvic thrombophlebitis. Abdominal trocar wound infection is also rare.

This author has experience with only 2 cases of pelvic cellulitis and 3 pelvic abscesses in over 400 laparoscopic hysterectomies.

TABLE 68–2. COMPLICATIONS OF 518 LAPAROSCOPIC HYSTERECTOMIES AND CONCOMITANT SURGERIES

	No. Patients		Percentage Rate	
Complication	**Subgroup Total**	**Group Total**	**Subgroup Total**	**Group Total**
Febrile morbidity		11		2.12
Pneumonia[1]	1		0.19	
Pelvic hematoma[2]	4		0.77	
Dehydration	1		0.19	
Transient febrile episodes	5		0.96	
Urinary tract system		7		1.35
Bladder injury	5		0.96	
Vesicovaginal fistula	1		0.19	
Ureterovaginal fistula	1		0.19	
Intestinal complications		6		1.15
Small bowel enterotomy	2		0.38	
Thermal injury of sigmoid colon	1		0.19	
Partial bowel obstruction	1		0.19	
Richter's hernia[3]	2		0.38	
Vaginal cuff bleeding		3		0.57
Blood transfusion		2		0.38
Pulmonary embolism		1		0.19
TOTAL		30		5.76

[1]This patient later developed ARDS (adult respiratory distress syndrome) and died.

[2]Two of the patients had second-look laparoscopy and the hematomas were evacuated.

[3]Richter's hernia occurred at the 12 mm trocar puncture sites.

The average surgical time was over 3 hours in this high-degree-of-difficulty population of extensive endometriosis and large uterus cases. In my first year at Columbia Presbyterian Medical Center, my 27 cases averaged 650 grams and involved extended morcellation.

The pelvic cellulitis cases presented with spiking pyrexia and pelvic pain and tenderness approximately one week postoperatively. Ultrasound examination was negative for a collection. They both responded to in-hospital intravenous antibiotics and one required multiple cuff treatments with silver nitrate sticks. All of the 3 abscess patients were treated during hospital readmission, and none responded to vaginal cuff drainage. One of the pelvic abscess patients was treated by laparoscopic drainage 16 days after her original surgery, another by ultrasound-guided aspiration with insertion of a drainage tube, and the third underwent laparotomy drainage 10 days postoperatively at a distant hospital after attempted vaginal drainage resulted in heavy bleeding. One other patient whose original hysterectomy surgery involved a pelvic abscess required rehospitalization.

I use one dose of a prophylactic antibiotic after induction of anesthesia in all cases. Interestingly, no antibiotic was administered in 4 of the 5 cases of infection. All of these cases involved a return to hospital and much patient dissatisfaction. I did not have any success with outpatient management that usually accompanies vaginal drainage after a vaginal hysterectomy.

To decrease postoperative infection, the surgeon should evacuate all large clots, obtain absolute hemostasis, and then do copious irrigation to dilute fibrin and prostaglandins arising from operated surfaces and bacteria. I believe that leaving at least 2 L of lactated Ringer's solution in the peritoneal cavity dilutes the peritoneal cavity bacterial and blood product counts and prevents fibrin adherences from forming by separating raw compromised surfaces during the initial stages of reperitonealization, especially after hysterectomy or bowel resection. No other antiadhesive agents are employed. No drains, antibiotic solutions, or heparin are used.

I have no experience with a serious wound infection after laparoscopic hysterectomy. I suspect this is because I rarely use more than two 5-mm lower trocar incisions, and I do not use suture to close them. The umbilical incision is placed vertically deep in the umbilicus where skin, deep fascia, and parietal peritoneum meet. This umbilical incision is closed with a single 4-0 Vicryl suture opposing deep fascia and skin dermis. The knot is buried beneath the fascia by catching first the fascia and then the skin closest to the surgeon with the needle and then taking skin and finally fascia on the other side.

Urinary tract infection, unexplained fever, and pneumonia likewise have rarely occurred. I doubt that early discharge is responsible, as all patients are followed with frequent phone calls during the postoperative period. Early cessation of both the Foley catheter and the IV within 2 hours of the end of the operation followed by early ambulation may reduce postoperative atelectasis and urinary tract infection.

Hemorrhage

Intraoperative hemorrhage occurs when a previously nonanemic patient loses more than 1000 mL of blood or requires a blood transfusion. By doing careful laparoscopic dissection, most profuse hemorrhage situations are avoided or controlled as they occur.

Postoperative hemorrhage is any bleeding event that requires therapy, either conservative or operative. In my experience, postoperative bleeding has occurred in only one case secondary to a hemorrhagic ovary stuck to the vaginal cuff. I treated it with Gelfoam and silver nitrate and family donor transfusion unsuccessfully before mobilizing it from the cuff with another laparoscopic procedure.

Postoperative hematomas were frequent with the early use of the Multifire Endo-GIA 30 (U.S. Surgical, Norwalk, CT) for the upper uterine pedicle during hysterectomy and oophorectomy. I have no experience with postoperative hematoma.

Transfusion rates are often misleading, as they usually include autologous blood, which may be given back to the patient on a routine basis. Presently I rarely obtain autologous blood because of the reluctance of most anesthesiologists to transfuse it. Nonautologous blood transfusion has been necessary in 6 of my cases (3%) for replacement of intraoperative blood loss.

Cuff Dehiscence

Cuff dehiscence is very rare following vaginal cuff closure using laparoscopic techniques to bring the endopelvic fascia together vertically in the midline. I am aware of some cuff breakdowns that my colleagues who use a transverse cuff closure have endured. I had one episode in 1991 of a peritoneovaginal fistula that was noted on routine cuff check 6 weeks postoperatively. The patient had been sexually active the day before and had experienced some pain. A laparoscopic closure was accomplished and again it broke down, again after coitus. Finally a vaginal repair using chromic catgut was successful.

Urinary Tract Complications: Prevention and Detection

Ureteral and bladder injuries may be expected with complicated cases but are less suspected in routine operations, and failure to recognize them during these cases or suspect them early postoperatively results in much patient dissatisfaction. These injuries most commonly are associated with the laparoscopic ligation of the uterine artery, but surgeons must be aware that both bladder and ureteral injury may occur during the "easy" vaginal part of a LAVH.

Although ureteral protection is advocated by all, how to best achieve it is hotly disputed. This author remains committed to prevention of ureteral injury intraoperatively by ureteral identification often with dissection and by cystoscopy at the conclusion of the procedure. Isolation by ureteral dissection has been criticized as unnecessarily adding time to the procedure. I find the time well spent if ureteral risk is diminished. My patients have not suffered any adverse sequela from this protective measure. Specifically, there has been no ureteral devascularization. My early technique of placing a single "sentinel" stitch around the uterine artery as it crosses just above the ureter to serve as a constant reminder of ureteral location is useful with the small uterus but is rarely used today.

Ureteral stents are not used routinely, though both lighted and infrared catheters are available. Most patients who have stent placement experience postoperative hematuria; anuria from ureteral spasm following surgery with a stent in place has been reported. Ureteral catheters are necessary when ureteral injury occurs during surgical dissection or the release of a ureteral stricture; in these cases the stent is left in place for at least 6 weeks. Ureteral stricture can be treated by dividing the stricture longitudinally and leaving the resultant ureterotomy open over a double J stent connecting the kidney to the bladder.

Cystoscopy is done in all hysterectomy cases after the vaginal cuff is closed to check for ureteral patency and bladder injury. Failure to see dye through a ureter can result from ureteral ligation (placement of a suture into or around the ureter), kinking from pulling endopelvic ureteral fascia towards the midline during the high McCall culdeplasty, or ureteral spasm if a ureteral stent was used. Cystoscopy also confirms bladder wall continuity and detects intravesicular suture placement and thermal injury, which will be seen as a patchy white area. I use suture instead of staples or bipolar desiccation for uterine artery ligation so that I can remove the suture if ureteral obstruction or a bladder suture is noted on cystoscopy. This has been necessary on more than one occasion.[23]

Preoperative IVP for patients with pelvic mass or suspected severe endometriosis is rarely recommended to avoid injury to the ureter.

This author has incurred ureteral injury during uterine vessel ligation with bipolar desiccation and has been close with the Endo-GIA. In 1988, a right ureterovaginal fistula occurred that was treated successfully with a stent. In that case, the injury was secondary either to bipolar desiccation of the right uterine vessels or to the performance of the vaginal portion of the procedure with the hip joint extended in Allan stirrups instead of converting to candy cane stirrups to flex the hip joint. On multiple occasions while using the Endo-GIA, inspection of the ureter after putting the Endo-GIA into position but before firing it revealed entrapment of the ureter. It is important to realize that the Endo-GIA is a straight device without staples in its distal 1 cm end and much wider than a Kelly clamp. In addition, during laparoscopic application, the uterine fundus is not usually put on upward traction as occurs in the open abdomen. The ureter at the level of the uterine artery is 15 mm lateral to the cervix. Stapling devices are 12 mm in width, leaving little room for error.

Careful techniques of bladder dissection are important. In difficult cases, the bladder may invaginate into a cesarean section scar and be surrounded by uterine myometrium. When bladder location is obscured, the surgeon should fill it intermittently during the procedure to check its position and keep the dissection at its junction with uterine muscle.

Urinary retention is a common undetected complication. Most people who undergo general anesthesia experience some degree of temporary inability to voluntarily contract their bladder musculature. It can take weeks for the bladder to regain normal tone if retention occurs. Postoperative urinary retention is more likely to occur with the use of large amounts of fluid for irrigation and hydroflotation. Urine can accumulate rapidly in the bladder in the drowsy patient who is recovering from anesthesia. The Foley catheter should not be removed at the end of operative procedures lasting longer than 2 hours until the patient is awake in the recovery unit and is aware that the catheter is in place, usually 1 hour postoperatively. In centers where IV fluids are not discontinued in the recovery room within 1 hour of the operation, the Foley catheter should be kept in longer.

A useful protocol if spontaneous voiding does not occur within 3 to 4 hours after the catheter is removed is to do straight catheterization and administer 25 mg of bethanechol chloride (Urecholine) every 4 hours until spontaneous voiding occurs. This

regimen has successfully reduced urinary retention during the past 6 years on our service.

Some endoscopically related injuries to the urinary tract may not become apparent for a few days following surgery. Although the incidence of these complications is low, the surgeon should nevertheless be aware of the risks and look for signs of such injuries that might have occurred. Unexplained fever, abdominal pain, back pain, or abdominal distention may be signs of some injury and should be investigated.

Any possible injury should be investigated as soon as suspected, identified immediately, and repaired. Potential postoperative problems that require prompt resolution include fever, CVA tenderness, low urine output relative to fluid intake, hematuria, abnormal vaginal discharge, hydronephrosis, and ureteral colic.

Postoperative recognition of insult to ureteral integrity is done early by obtaining a single-shot IVP on anyone reporting lateralized pain of any kind—abdominal, flank, or back. Uncontrollable loss of urine 1 to 2 weeks post-operatively requires an aggressive workup to determine if a ureterovaginal or vesicovaginal fistula is present. Treatment is with a Latzko operation for vesicovaginal fistula and long-term catheter placement or surgical reimplantation for ureterovaginal fistula.

The bottom line is that an aggressive approach to ureteral protection can reduce but not eliminate ureteral injury. However, prompt recognition and management can prevent multiple surgical procedures and significant patient morbidity including organ loss.

Ureteral Injury Management

The ureters are commonly injured at the level of the infundibulopelvic ligament, uterosacral ligament, or pelvic sidewall due to adhesions resulting from endometriosis, pelvic inflammatory disease, or previous abdominal surgery. During laparoscopic hysterectomy, ureteral injury may occur while cutting dense adhesions and fibrotic scar tissue, trying to stop bleeding close to the ureter with bipolar cautery, or in the process of ligating the uterine vessels with bipolar electrosurgery, staples, or suture. *Most ureteral injuries are not identified or even suspected without cystoscopy.* Without cystoscopic availability, one can expect problems. This is particularly true during TLH, even if the surgeon is visually able to identify the ureters. Normal peristalsis may occur in the damaged ureter.

In my experience, all but the grossest of ureteral injuries are discovered during the cystoscopic examination near the end of the operation. These injuries cannot usually be identified laparoscopically. If no dye is seen flowing from the ureter, the surgeon should first try to pass a ureteral catheter. If it passes without resistance, the ureter is fine. If it doesn't pass, the surgeon should systematically trace the ureter down into the deep pelvis. Previously ligated vessels must be isolated, skeletonized, and released from all ureteral attachments. Sometimes this entails release of the suture followed by religation. Continued attempts to pass the stent should be made while the laparoscopic dissection ensues. The dissection stops when the stent passes.

Ureteral injury at the level of or just below the infundibulopelvic ligament is usually recognizable early in the operation as urine oozes from it or a distally cut ureter becomes evident on the side of the uterus during dissection of the uterine vessels.

The avoidance of ureter-related complications requires a sophisticated familiarity with pelvic anatomy. When clamps or ligatures are required they should be placed and elevated high enough so that only targeted ligaments and vessels are caught in the clamp. Established operative techniques for skeletonizing the uterine arteries should be followed, so that the ureters will fall away from the operational field as the surgery proceeds. The location of the ureters within the retroperitoneal space should be identified, and a determination made where they and other structures are likely to move during the course of the TLH.

When severe pelvic adhesions are present, it is imperative to identify the ureter prior to ligation of the infundibulopelvic ligament. The cardinal ligament should be cut close to the cervix, after checking the panoramic view.

If a ureter is cut or coagulated, it is necessary to make the appropriate repair depending on the extent of injury: reanastomosis or ureteral reimplantation is indicated. When recognized during the surgery, a laparoscopic approach to these procedures can be considered.

Treatment Options for Ureteral Transection. When recognized, immediate repair of a transected ureter can be done using a combined laparoscopic–cystoscopic insertion of a pigtail double-J stent and laparoscopic end-to-end anastomosis using four 5-0 polyglactin extramucosal sutures. The proximal stump of the ureter is freed and checked for viability. A 5-0 Vicryl suture is placed in order to hold the two stumps together, allowing the urologist to insert a 6-French double J silicon catheter (pigtail) of 26 cm length through the cystoscope into the ureter crossing the site of the anastomosis. The anastomosis is then completed with four 5-0 polyglactin extramucosal sutures applied at the 12-, 3-, 6- and 9-o'clock positions. The knots are tied extracorporeally using a Clarke-Reich knotpusher. An adequate distance between sutures is mandatory to avoid ischemic damages. At the end of the operation, the anastomosis is checked for leakage by injecting IV indigo carmine dye and observing the anastomosis underwater, laparoscopically. The correct position of the stent is checked cystoscopically and radiologically.

Most surgeons use 4-0 absorbable suture (chromic, Vicryl, or Monocryl) on a small tapered atraumatic needle. Nonabsorbable suture is not used due to its propensity for stone and crust formation. A simple stitch is used, although occasionally a stay suture is required. Ideally a "no touch" technique is employed: the suture is placed to approximate mucosa to mucosa, without holding the ureter. If the ureter is transected, a half spatulated anastomosis is performed from the tip of one end to the apex of the other. Any kind of soft stent (Bard, Cook, Meditech, or Microvasive) can be placed cystoscopically and removed 6 weeks later. Patency is confirmed by either ureterogram or IVP. Ureteroneocystostomy is done if anastomosis is not possible.

Bladder Injury

Bladder laceration may result from a primary umbilical subcutaneous trocar puncture if the bladder is full. This condition is not easily diagnosed intraoperatively, as the surgeon perceives that he or she is in the preperitoneal space and tries again, and when in the true peritoneal cavity cannot see any injury. Leakage from the umbilicus, usually in the recovery room, may be the presentation. Treatment consists of placing an indwelling catheter for 7 to 10 days and prophylactic antibiotics.

The second-puncture trocar can perforate the bladder, especially in a patient who is obese and has had previous pelvic surgery, if the trocar is placed too low, especially if the bladder has

not been drained of urine. A reliable diagnostic sign is the sudden appearance of gas in the Foley catheter drainage bag. Injection of indigo carmine through a Foley catheter may identify the site of the injury.[26] When no bladder distention occurs during surgery without bladder drainage, consideration should be given to inserting a Foley catheter to observe for gas. If an injury is identified intraoperatively and is greater than 7 mm, the defect should be closed, in the majority of cases laparoscopically. Postoperatively, the insertion of an indwelling catheter for 7 to 10 days and prophylactic antibiotics are recommended.

The most important factor in treatment is early detection. If the defect is large from manipulation through the trocar sleeve during laparoscopic surgery, it should be closed with a figure-eight suture through the surrounding bladder muscularis and a second suture to close the overlying peritoneum. A watertight seal should be documented by filling the bladder with blue dye solution. Postoperative complications may include bladder atony and leaking of urine in the peritoneal cavity, which may also lead to peritonitis.

Bladder injury can occur during dissection of the bladder off the uterus and cervix or from an inflamed adnexa. In these cases the bladder is repaired using 3-0 Vicryl, usually in two layers.

Intravesicular thermal injury can be suspected by cystoscopic visualization of a white patch above the bladder trigone. The area should be reinforced with a laparoscopically placed suture into the bladder musculature surrounding the potential defect.

Bowel Injury

Bowel injury during laparoscopic hysterectomy is uncommon and is associated with extensive intraperitoneal adhesions. Two small bowel injuries during enterolysis occurred in 516 hysterectomies.[24]

Small bowel injuries can be suture repaired. Small bowel enterotomy may require mobilization from above, delivery through the umbilicus by extending the incision 1 cm, and resection as the injury frequently involves the small bowel mesentery. Alternatively, if the hole is confined to the antimesenteric portion, the bowel can be closed with interrupted 3-0 silk or Vicryl tied either externally or with intracorporeal instrument ties. Sterile milk or dilute indigo carmine is instilled into the bowel lumen prior to the closing of the last suture to assure the absence of leakage from the defect and to detect occult perforations near the small bowel mesentery. All enterotomies are suture repaired transversely to reduce the risk of stricture. If the hole involves greater than 50% of the bowel circumference, resection is done. An extracorporeal segmental enterectomy with side-to-side stapled anastomosis is preferred. The umbilical incision is enlarged to approximately 2.5 cm to permit extrusion and repair of the involved bowel. Using a GIA-60 fired twice, a segmental enterectomy encompassing the lesions is done. The involved mesentery is serially clamped, divided, and ligated with Vicryl 3-0. A functional side-to-side ileoileal anastomosis is constructed with the GIA-60 and a TA 35 used to close the antimesenteric opening. Patency is insured by palpation to assess proper luminal diameter equal to or greater than 2.5 cm; absence of leakage is confirmed by milking succus entericus through the anastomotic site. The bowel is then returned to the abdominal cavity. Pneumoperitoneum is reestablished, and laparoscopic inspection of the anastomosis should reveal no leakage.

Nodules in the muscularis of the anterior or lateral rectal wall can usually be excised laparoscopically.[27] Full-thickness penetrative injury to the rectum may occur during this surgery or accidentally during dissection or uterine morcellation. Following identification of the rent in the rectum, often surrounded by fibrotic endometriosis, a #29 or #33 French closed circular stapler [Proximate ILS Curved Intraluminal Stapler (Ethicon, Stealth)] is inserted into the lumen just past the hole, opened 1 to 2 cm, and held high to avoid the posterior rectal wall. The proximal anvil is positioned just beyond the hole, which is invaginated into the opening and the device closed. Circumferential inspection is made to insure the absence of encroachment of nearby organs and posterior rectum in the staple line and the lack of tension in the anastomosis. The instrument is fired, and then removed through the anus. The surgeon inspects the doughnut of tissue representing the excised hole contained in the circular stapler. Once verified, anastomotic inspection is done laparoscopically underwater after filling the rectum with indigo carmine solution.

Alternatively, a double-layer transverse repair is performed using 3-0 silk or Vicryl. Stay sutures are placed at the transverse angles of the defect and brought out through the lower quadrant incisions; the trocar sleeves are then placed again into the peritoneal cavity over the stay sutures. The suture is tied either inside the peritoneal cavity with two laparoscopic needle holders or outside as previously described. Suturing is facilitated by use of short self-retaining trocar sleeves without traps (Wolf or Apple).

Peritonitis After Unrecognized or Delayed Perforation

Delayed bowel injury can result from traumatic perforation that is not recognized during the procedure (Veress needle or trocar puncture or laceration during adhesiolysis or excision) or from thermal damage from any source. Rarely, delayed injuries can occur from perforation of mechanically devascularized bowel or from hemorrhagic ischemic necrosis after mesenteric venous thrombosis. Although the incidence of these complications is low, the surgeon should nevertheless be aware of the risks and look for signs of such injuries that might have occurred. Unexplained fever, abdominal pain, back pain, abdominal distention, altered bowel function, and elevated white blood cell count may all be signs of some injury and should be investigated.

Bowel perforation after thermal injury usually presents 4 to 10 days following the procedure. With traumatic perforation, symptoms usually occur within 24 to 48 hours. At surgery for delayed bowel perforation, gross appearance of traumatic and electrical injuries is the same; the perforation is usually surrounded by a white area of necrosis.[28] Microscopic examination of the lesions reveals the persistence of dead amorphous tissue without polymorphonuclear infiltrate following electrical burns. With puncture injuries, there is rapid and abundant capillary ingrowth, white cell infiltration, and fibrin deposition at the injury site.[28] The management of delayed bowel perforation with peritonitis consists of a bowel resection of all necrotic tissue with end-to-end anastomosis, copious lavage, antibiotics, and minidose heparin therapy (preferably supervised by a general surgeon).

Complications Unique to Laparoscopy

Subcutaneous Emphysema. Subcutaneous emphysema occurs when carbon dioxide is insufflated into the subcutaneous spaces. It may result from placement of the Veress needle into the extraperitoneal space of the abdominal wall and/or the omentum, a condition that is usually not discovered until the surgeon places the laparoscope for visualization. When this occurs, the gas should be disconnected, allowing the extraperitoneal gas to escape. Fortunately, carbon dioxide is absorbed rapidly and the subcutaneous emphysema begins to resolve by the time the patient is transferred to the recovery room. Subcutaneous emphysema may secondarily occur during prolonged laparoscopic procedures as gas gains access through enlargement of the trocar incision in the parietal peritoneum and extraperitoneal surgery. It is important for the surgeon to warn the patient's companions when fascial swelling is significant. Subcutaneous emphysema usually resolves in 12 to 24 hours.

Injury to Abdominal Wall Vessels. The incidence of trocar-induced vascular injuries to the abdominal wall during operative laparoscopic surgery is 2%. Though potentially avoidable, either the superficial or deep vessels of the anterior abdominal wall can cause bleeding and hematoma during or after laparoscopy.

The inferior epigastric vessels lie relatively deep in the rectus muscle in the lateral rectus sheath, and despite transillumination, these vessels often cannot be seen. Rupture of epigastric vessels may result from increasing use of multiple ancillary sites. These injuries can be minimized by placement of the trocar with laparoscopic visualization and transillumination lateral to the rectus muscles. Management depends on whether the injury is arterial or venous, the amount of bleeding, and the location of the injury. Use of bipolar desiccation through the operating channel of an operating laparoscope in front of the trocar and halfway between it and the medial portion of the inguinal ring is appropriate. Laparoscopic placement of a through-and-through loop of suture around the bleeding site is sometimes indicated. For moderate bleeding of epigastric vessels, pressures from the balloon of a Foley catheter may tamponade and stop the bleeding.

Injury to Large Vessels. Catastrophic severe vascular accidents during laparoscopic surgery, involving large vessels (aorta, vena cava, and iliac vessels) are fortunately rare. When they do occur, the surgeon and a vascular surgeon must usually perform immediate laparotomy and repair the vascular defects as soon as possible.

Shielded trocars should be avoided, as they give the surgeon a false sense of security and may cause additional "blunt trauma" from the shield itself as it blasts through the fascia.

On rare occasions a penetration injury to blood vessels at the time of insufflation may go unrecognized. This may lead to gas embolism and death. The classic mill wheel murmur over the pericardium may be heard by the anesthesiologist.

Trocar Site Incisional Hernias. The incidence of incisional hernias after operative laparoscopy is greatly increased if 10 mm or larger trocars are placed at extraumbilical sites. These sites should be closed. If the incision is lateral to the rectus muscle, the deep fascia is elevated with skin hooks and suture repaired. If the incision is through the rectus muscle, the peritoneal defect is closed with a laparoscopically placed suture.[29]

Incisional hernias present usually within 10 days of surgery. Postoperative discomfort with incisional swelling or distension should be cause for examination. If hernia is suspected, laparoscopic reduction should be considered. A patient of mine had one such hernia in 1991 during a short trial of 12-mm trocar sleeves for Endo-GIA application.

Instrument Failure. Occasionally instruments are faulty. Some, such as a grasper, dissectors, or scissors, can be immediately replaced. However, those that are electrically driven are often another matter and vary tremendously in reliability.

If the patient is not grounded appropriately and a monopolar electrosurgical instrument is used, burns to the patient at the return electrode contact sites from incomplete grounding may occur.

When multiple electronic instruments are activated by foot pedals, only one foot pedal should be used at any one time, to avoid activating the wrong instrument.

If an instrument breaks within the abdomen, all pieces should be extracted under direct visualization. If any instrument locks in an open position and won't retract into the trocar sheath, the trocar sheath along with the instrument should be withdrawn from the abdomen; it is rarely necessary to extend the incision.

CONCLUSIONS

In an editorial in the August 15, 1996 issue of *The New England Journal of Medicine*, it was suggested that, except for abortion, laparoscopic hysterectomy has generated more controversy and discussion than any other type of gynecologic surgery in recent times. The authors of this editorial would surely benefit from learning a little more about the procedure and its evolution before belittling it for the wrong reasons.[30]

It is difficult to extrapolate indications for the role of laparoscopy in hysterectomy from present publications, as the surgeons most skilled in the laparoscopic approach are referred the difficult cases and rarely see those that could be easily performed vaginally. The future place of laparoscopic hysterectomy will be determined by the increased familiarity and skill of surgeons with vaginal procedures, stimulated by doing the difficult part of a "laparoscopic assisted vaginal hysterectomy" vaginally. I suspect that over 50% of indicated hysterectomies can be performed using the vaginal route, without laparoscopy. The laparoscope may convert more than one half of the remaining cases to a vaginal procedure. I estimate that vaginal hysterectomy, after an initial diagnostic laparoscopy, will be possible in one half of those with some relative contraindication to the vaginal approach. One half of the remaining indicated hysterectomies will require laparoscopic oophorectomy or adhesiolysis of the upper portion to be removed, that is, an LAVH. Of the remaining hysterectomies, 12.5% of the total, the skilled laparoscopic surgeon will do a total laparoscopic hysterectomy and consider conversion to abdominal hysterectomy in fewer than 1% of cases.

REFERENCES

1. Reich H. Laparoscopic hysterectomy. In: *Surgical Laparoscopy & Endoscopy*. Raven:1992;85.
2. Liu CY. Laparoscopic hysterectomy: A review of 72 cases. *J Reprod Med.* 1992;37:351.
3. Liu CY. Laparoscopic hysterectomy. Report of 215 cases. *Gynaecol Endosc.* 1992;1:73.
4. Reich H, DeCaprio J, McGlynn F. Laparoscopic hysterectomy. *J Gynecol Surg.* 1989;5:213.
5. Garry R. Towards evidence-based hysterectomy. *Gynaecol. Endosc.* 1998;7:225.
6. Reich H, McGlynn F, Sekel, L. Total laparoscopic hysterectomy. *Gynaecol Endosc.* 1993;2:59.
7. Lyons TL. Laparoscopic supracervical hysterectomy. A comparison of morbidity and mortality results with laparoscopically assisted vaginal hysterectomy. *J Reprod Med.* 1993;38:763.
8. McGlynn F, Grabo TN, Reich H. Laparoscopic hysterectomy: Effect on perception of sexual behavior and pain relief. *Gynaecol Endosc.* 1995;4:269.
9. Rhodes JC. Sexual function improves following hysterectomy. *JAMA.* 1999;282:1934.
10. Mettler L, Lutzewitch N, Dewitz T, et al. From laparotomy to pelviscopic intrafascial hysterectomy. *Gynaecol Endosc.* 1996;5:203.
11. Reich H. Laparoscopic extrafascial hysterectomy with bilateral salpingo-oophorectomy using stapling techniques for endometrial adenocarcinoma. AAGL 19th annual meeting, Orlando, November 1990.
12. Reich H, McGlynn F, Wilkie W. Laparoscopic management of stage I ovarian cancer. *J Reprod Med.* 1990;35:601.
13. Canis M, Mage G, Wattiez A, et al. Does endoscopic surgery have a role in radical surgery of cancer of the cervix uteri? *J Gynecol Obstet Biol Reprod.* 1990;19:921.
14. Reich H, McGlynn F, Salvat J. Laparoscopic treatment of cul-de-sac obliteration secondary to retrocervical deep fibrotic endometriosis. *J Reprod Med.* 1991;36:516.
15. Reich H, McGlynn F, Sekel L, et al. Laparoscopic management of ovarian dermoid cysts. *J Reprod Med.* 1992;37:640.
16. Parker WH, Berek JS. Management of selected cystic adnexal masses in postmenopausal women by operative laparoscopy: A pilot study. *Am J Obstet Gynecol.* 1990;163:1574.
17. Valtchev KL, Papsin FR. A new uterine mobilizer for laparoscopy: Its use in 518 patients. *Am J Obstet Gynecol.* 1977;127:738.
18. Reich H, McGlynn F. Short self-retaining trocar sleeves. *Am J Obstet Gynecol.* 1990;162: 453.
19. Currie I, Onwude JL, Jarvis GJ. A comparative study of the cosmetic appeal of abdominal incisions used for hysterectomy. *Br J Obstet Gynaecol.* 1996;103:252.
20. Kadar N. A laparoscopic technique for dissecting the pelvic retroperitoneum and identifying the ureters. *J Reprod Med.* 1995;40:116.
21. Clarke HC. Laparoscopy: New instruments for suturing and ligation. *Fertil Steril.* 1972;23:274.
22. Reich H, Clarke HC, Sekel L. A simple method for ligating in operative laparoscopy with straight and curved needles. *Obstet Gynecol.* 1992;79:143.
23. Ribeiro S, Reich H, Rosenberg J, et al. The value of intra-operative cystoscopy at the time of laparoscopic hysterectomy. *Hum Reprod.* 1999;14:1727.
24. Liu CY, Reich H. Complications of total laparoscopic hysterectomy in 518 cases. *Gynaecol Endosc.* 1994;3:203.
25. Woodland MB. Ureter injury during laparoscopy-assisted vaginal hysterectomy with the endoscopic linear stapler. *Am J Obstet Gynecol.* 1992;167:756.
26. Reich H, McGlynn F. Laparoscopic repair of bladder injury. *Obstet Gynecol.* 1990;76:909.
27. Reich H, McGlynn F, Budin R. Laparoscopic repair of full-thickness bowel injury. *J Laparoendosc Surg.* 1991;1:119.
28. Levy BS, Soderstrom RM, Dail DH. Bowel injuries during laparoscopy: Gross anatomy and histology. *J Reprod Med.* 1985;30:168.
29. Kadar N, Reich H, Liu CY, et al. Incisional hernias after major laparoscopic gynecologic procedures. *Am J Obstet Gynecol.* 1993;168:1493.
30. Kadar N, Reich H, Liu CY, et al. Alternative techniques of hysterectomy. *N Engl J Med.* 1997;336:292. Letter, comment.

Chapter Sixty-Nine ● ● ● ● ● ●

*E*ndoscopic Approach to Female Infertility

ALBERTO KABLY

INTRODUCTION

Gynecologic endoscopy (laparoscopy and hysteroscopy) has provided gynecologists with a very useful tool for the diagnostic and therapeutic evaluation of many pathologies for more than three decades. Infertility is a public health problem that affects more than 15% of population and currently is the leading indication for endoscopy in gynecology, followed by adnexal and uterine surgery.[1]

As a method of treatment, the main limitation of laparoscopy was the fact that only the surgeon could see the internal anatomy, an inconvenience that ended with the arrival of video laparoscopy. Technology has made it possible for couples to actually have their infertility problem solved with the help of endoscopic surgery. Some examples of this include the surgical management of pelvic adhesions and endometriosis (Figs. 69–1 and 69–2).[2]

In this chapter we will describe how to perform a gynecologic endoscopy in an infertile woman and the efficacy of this method to solve specific problems related to female infertility.

WHEN TO PERFORM A LAPAROSCOPY FOR THE STUDY AND MANAGEMENT OF INFERTILITY

There are a variety of criteria used to decide when a laparoscopy should be performed to diagnose and treat an infertile couple (Table 69–1). These criteria can vary from center to center. With laparoscopy, the major factors that contribute to infertility can be evaluated: uterine, ovarian, and tubal. Tubal factors can be evaluated by inspection and confirmation of tubal patency, endometrial factors can be evaluated with hysteroscopy, and the male factor can be assessed by performing cervical insemination during the periovulatory period before surgery, and then taking a sample of peritoneal fluid to look for spermatozoa after introducing the laparoscope, at which time the presence of adhesions or endometriosis can also be determined.

Laparoscopy should be performed during the proliferative phase of the endometrial cycle, preferably immediately postmenses. At this time, the tissue is less vascularized, which makes ovarian, tubal, and pelvic adhesions easier to diagnose. Furthermore, at this point in the menstrual cycle, endometriosis can be seen more clearly, making treatment with electrical, thermal, or laser energy simpler. Also at this point in the cycle, hysteroscopic evaluation and surgical management of some endometrial problems (e.g., polyps, synechiae, myomata) is more practical due to the minimal growth of the endometrium and the absence of vascularity. The evaluation of the tubal ostia is more precise and tubal patency tests can be performed with less difficulty.

Before laparoscopy, nonsurgical tests should be performed to find the cause of infertility, and laparoscopy would be indicated in cases in which there is a normal sperm count, serum progesterone and prolactin are within normal limits, vaginal cultures (for chlamydia and *Mycoplasma*) are negative, and the hysterosalpingogram (HSG) and pelvic ultrasound are normal. Figure 69–3 shows an algorithm for determining if laparoscopy is indicated.

Every patient who has an abnormal HSG and is infertile must be evaluated by diagnostic and therapeutic laparoscopy, because HSG alone is inadequate to evaluate the uterine cavity, the morphology and patency of the fallopian tubes, or even to detect such pelvic pathologies as adhesions or endometriosis. As a matter of fact, HSG has a high positive predictive value when findings are abnormal, but it has a false negative rate of more than 50%. This is why direct visualization of the pelvis is mandatory when an HSG is normal.

Patients with more than 5 years of infertility, and women 35 years of age or older must be evaluated by laparoscopy. The fundamental objective of laparoscopy is to help a couple become pregnant, and other treatments such as assisted reproductive techniques

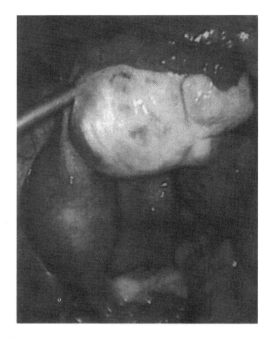

Figure 69–1. Large endometrioma located near the right ovary.

(ART) and in vitro fertilization (IVF) should also be considered in this group of patients, perhaps before laparoscopy is carried out.

Though our general indications for laparoscopy are listed above, if a couple has normal lab tests, the woman is younger than 35 years of age, and she has no history of pelvic surgery, before laparoscopy we offer 4 cycles of controlled ovarian hyperstimulation (COH) with recombinant gonadotropins. If after this period, adequate ovulation is proven by ultrasound, and the couple does not conceive, a laparoscopy is performed. In 1998 we published a study[3] in which we reported that if a couple has a normal fertility test and the woman has no history of pelvic surgery, pelvic disease was found via laparoscopy in 30% of cases, in contrast to the pregnancy rate of 60% seen when COH is performed before

TABLE 69–1. CRITERIA FOR PERFORMANCE OF LAPAROSCOPY IN AN INFERTILE PATIENT

- Perform the study during the proliferative phase of the endometrial cycle
- Perform a complete physical examination prior to the procedure
- *Always* perform a complementary hysteroscopy
- Use an intrauterine catheter to verify tubal patency
- Use an open insufflation technique
- Always have bipolar and laser instruments available
- Use gentle tissue management and continuous irrigation to prevent adhesions

laparoscopy. In other words, the possibility of finding pelvic disease in an infertile woman younger than 35 years of age, with a normal HSG and no history of pelvic surgery is lower than the pregnancy rate seen when COH is carried out before laparoscopy.[4]

Some studies have demonstrated that endometriosis can affect the ovarian response to induction of ovulation via ART, and that it reduces the quality and quantity of oocytes, as well as negatively affecting the segmentation, implantation, and pregnancy rates. Some authors consider laparoscopy mandatory to exclude or treat endometriosis before IVF; they also consider the use of adjuvant procedures such as tubal ligation to prevent ectopic pregnancies useful in increasing the success rate of ART.

A history of adnexal or uterine surgery such as ovarian tumor excision and myomectomy is an indication for laparoscopy because of the high possibility of formation of adhesions that can affect the anatomy and physiology of the fallopian tubes and ovaries. To sum up: we recommended endoscopic surgery as a first choice in patients 35 years of age and older, those with more than 5 years of infertility or a positive history of pelvic surgery, and in patients of any age and period of infertility with two or more pelvic surgeries.

We also recommend performing laparoscopy in patients in whom infertility was previously identified and treated and are still unable to achieve pregnancy. One common example of this is women with anovulation that have been treated, their problem solved, and yet they do not get pregnant within a defined period of time (e.g., 6 months). These patients must have a laparoscopy

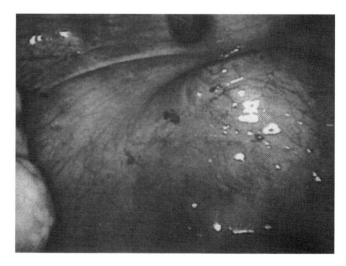

Figure 69–2. Pelvic endometriosis.

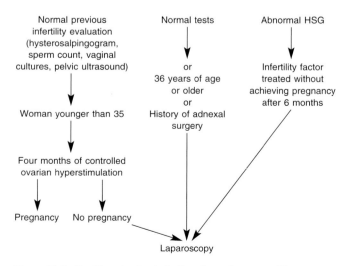

Figure 69–3. Algorithm showing indications for performance of laparoscopy in infertility.

and hysteroscopy performed, and the possibility of finding disease is over 30%.

PERFORMING A LAPAROSCOPY IN AN INFERTILE WOMAN

Without going into the technical details that are covered elsewhere in this book, we can point to some practical aspects to assure the successful performance of a laparoscopic procedure. First, a complete physical examination should be carried out prior to surgery. Then an intrauterine catheter (we prefer Jarcho or Humi) is inserted, which is useful in evaluating tubal patency. We prefer the open insufflation technique to avoid accidents related to the insertion of the Veress needle and the main trocar. For a laparoscopic procedure that is performed to assess an infertile patient, bipolar and laser instrumentation must be readily available. This is a requirement because the most common pathologic findings are adhesions and endometriosis.

For laparoscopic surgery of the ovaries and in other areas that are easily damaged, especially in the posterior cul-de-sac, there are some measures that may prevent adhesion formation. There is a wide variety of products available for this purpose. In our experience, the best way to prevent damage is to handle all these tissues gently, and we recommend facilitating this with the use of dehydrated cellulose.[5]

Regarding the use of electrical or laser energy, bipolar electrocautery is always preferable for hemostasis because the laser may present a hazard to other tissues when used to vaporize adhesions and treat endometriosis.[6] We have had a great deal of experience with various kinds of lasers, the most common being the CO_2 laser, and it is useful and efficient when the use of electocautery is inappropriate.

REFERENCES

1. Nezhat C, Gieofler A, Nezhat C. Operative Gynecologic Laparoscopy, 2nd ed. McGraw-Hill:2000.
2. Nezhat E. Adhesion formation after endoscopic surgery. *J Reprod Med.* 1993;38:534.
3. Kably AA, Garcia LE. The importance of controlled ovarian hyperstimulation prior to laparoscopy. *Ginec Obstet Mex.* 1998;66:320.
4. Campo S. Ovulatory cycles, pregnancy outcome and complications after surgical treatment of polycystic ovary syndrome (POS). *Obstet Gynecol Surv.* 1998;53:297.
5. Saravelos H, Li TC. Postoperative adhesions after laparoscopic electrosurgical treatment for polycystic ovary syndrome (POS). Use of Interceed. *Hum Reprod.* 1996;11:992.
6 Adamson GD, Pasta DJ. Surgical treatment of endometriosis-associated infertility: a meta-analysis. *Am J Obstet Gynecol.* 1994;171:1488.

Chapter Seventy ● ● ● ● ● ●

*H*ysteroscopy

LUCA MENCAGLIA, GIUSEPPE MARIO LENTINI, and ENNIO TISO

Hysteroscopy was one of the very earliest approaches to the direct study of the uterine cavity. Since the early 1980s, hysteroscopy has opened up new diagnostic vistas for the evaluation of the cervical canal and uterine cavity, revealing the limits of dilatation and curettage. A few years later, surgical interventions carried out through the hysteroscope demonstrated equivalent or better results than traditional laparotomic surgery of the uterus. Today it is possible to perform a comprehensive endoscopic examination of the uterine cavity in an office session without using any type of anesthetic or dilating the cervical canal. Surgical hysteroscopic interventions are regarded as the latest important step forward in gynecologic practice. Some indications, such as uterine malformations, intrauterine adhesions, and submucous and intramural myomas, which formerly were limited to conventional surgery, now fall within the domain of hysteroscopic techniques.[8] Also, management of abnormal uterine bleeding by means of hysterectomy has been largely replaced by endometrial ablation or resection through the hysteroscope, which is considered to more extensively preserve the integrity of the urogynecologic tract.[10,13]

HYSTEROSCOPY EQUIPMENT AND ROOM SET-UP

A good knowledge of the instruments is required of the surgeon, so that he or she can overcome a series of dysfunctions or malfunctions that occur quite frequently in hysteroscopy and may obstruct the intended purpose of the examination or surgical procedure.

To perform the hysteroscopy, the patient is placed in the gynecologic position, preferably on a table that permits ready modification of the patient's position to facilitate inclination of the telescope following the direction of the cervical canal and uterine cavity. In same cases preventive intramuscular or sublingual administration of atropine proves useful in preventing vagal reflexes.[19,22]

Distension Media

Several methods can be used to distend the uterine cavity. The choice of the method depends upon the type of procedure, surgical or diagnostic. In surgical hysteroscopy, the use of a hysteroresectoscope requires an electrolyte-free liquid distension medium to prevent the electricity from spreading.

The distension media are divided into two categories: gases, which are used exclusively in diagnostic hysteroscopy; and liquids, which are used both in diagnostic and surgical hysteroscopy.[12,18]

Gaseous Media

Distension of the uterine cavity with carbon dioxide is currently considered the method of choice in diagnostic hysteroscopy. The risk of gas embolism is easily avoided using proper insufflation criteria. Using an insufflation system able to keep the pressure within the 100 to 120 mm Hg range at a flow of 30 to 60 mL/min, the total dose of CO_2 is much lower than that required to induce the first signs of CO_2 intoxication. The use of CO_2 to perform diagnostic procedures permits an extremely fine, detailed evaluation of endometrial physiology because it does not distort the intrauterine view in any way.

The procedure requires an electronic hysteroflator with an insufflation gas flow of 30 to 60 mL per minute (corresponding to an intrauterine pressure of 40 to 80 mm Hg), insufflation pressure of 100 to 120 mm Hg, and an electronically controlled measuring/control system that ensures constant intrauterine pressure without exceeding the safety limit of 80 to 100 mm Hg.

Liquid Media

Hyskon is a 32% high-molecular-weight dextran solution (70,000 d) that is instilled using a 50-mL syringe; 100 mL is generally enough to distend the uterine cavity. Dextran transmits light well and is poorly miscible with blood, but its high viscosity makes it difficult to instill and requires prompt and thorough cleaning of the instruments in warm water to prevent crystallization. Furthermore, some authors report examples of dextran allergies and sometimes severe reactions with anaphylactic shock and even death.

Low-molecular-weight liquid media include electrolytic and nonelectrolytic solutions. Electrolyte solutions (5 and 10% dextrose, 4% and 6% dextran, and saline or physiologic solutions) can be used when no electricity is applied, and so these are mainly used in diagnostic hysteroscopy. The hypertonic, nonelectrolytic solutions (glycine and sorbitol/mannitol) are indicated in resectoscopic hysteroscopy because they are not very toxic, do not conduct electricity, and provide a good endoscopic view.

The low-molecular-weight liquids have the advantages of being physiologically reabsorbed by the peritoneum as well as low in cost. The disadvantages are that they are fairly miscible with blood and require constant perfusion of the liquid to maintain cavity distension. Possible complications associated with absorption of the hypertonic, nonelectrolytic solutions include hypervolemia with hyponatremia or the intravasation syndrome.

To maintain cavity distension, the continuous flow rate and the outflow pressure must be high enough to ensure rapid irrigation and an adequate distension of the cavity. If the pressure is too high, there is the risk of significant intravasation by the liquid distension medium.[5,6] To control pressure and flow a number of systems are available, including the following.

1. *Gravity fall system.* Raising the bag with the solution to an adequate height (90 to 100 cm above the patient's perineum is sufficient to achieve a pressure of 70 mm Hg) causes the liquid to flow down by gravity force. Irrigation is achieved by connecting the tubing of the resectoscope outflow connector to a collection basin.
2. *Pressure cuff.* These devices, similar to a sphygmomanometer, are inflated around the bag, exerting pressure on it.
3. *Electronic suction and irrigation pump.* These systems permit an automatically controlled suction and irrigation at preset flow rate, suction pressure, and irrigation pressure. Some systems also allow automatic monitoring and control of the preset volume difference in the inflow and outflow of the irrigation liquid and the change in this parameter per minute. The settings generally used are a flow rate of approximately 200 mm Hg, outflow pressure of 75 mm Hg, and suction pressure of 0.25 bar.

Light Source

High-quality sources are required, with xenon light sources giving the best results. In general, 175 W power is sufficient for routine interventions. For special interventions or when miniature telescopes are used, 300 W is recommended. Light is transmitted through cables containing glass fibers or fluid medium with diameters between 3.5 and 4.5 mm and lengths between 180 and 350 cm. Usually, light cables with a diameter of 5 mm and a length of 180 cm are used in hysteroscopy.

Camera Equipment

In modern hysteroscopy an endocamera should always be used. Actually several types of video cameras are available. The technical criteria for a good camera are resolution specified by the number of lines or pixels, sensitivity by units of lux, and a high quality of video output/images. Finally, a high signal-to-noise-ratio indicates that the changes in image quality in extreme situations, such as during hemorrhaging and all circumstances that involve a loss of luminous intensity, will only be minor. Recently, cameras have become available with three couple control device (CCD) chips, providing very high resolution and close-to-natural color reproduction.

Endoscope

Endoscopes can be either flexible or rigid. Because of their high operating cost and fragility, flexible hystero-fiberscopes are rarely used. Rigid telescopes are available with different directions of view: 0, 12, and 30 degrees. Usually the 30-degree telescope is indicated in performing diagnostic hysteroscopy, while the 12-degree telescope is used in conjunction with the resectoscope, thus keeping the loop always within the field of view.

Operating Hysteroscopes

In the case of operating hysteroscopes, the internal lumen must be of adequate size to allow passage of operating instruments. In fact, while the same types of telescopes are used in diagnostic hysteroscopy (2.9 to 4 mm in diameter), the external sheath diameter ranges between 3.5 and 7 mm to allow for passage of both operating instruments (scissors, biopsy forceps, catheters, and coagulation electrodes) and the liquid distension medium.

Diagnostic Hysteroscopes

Endoscopes of different diameters are available. Micro-hysteroscopy uses 2-mm telescopes. A powerful light source allows for close endoscopic observation of details. A telescope with a diameter of 2.9 mm can be used for diagnostic hysteroscopy with CO_2 insufflation. In the Bettocchi system, a single-flow operating sheath of 4.3 mm diameter can also be used as an inner sheath in conjunction with the continuous-flow outer tube of 5 mm diameter. The Hamou micro-hysteroscope, with a diameter of 4 mm and an examination sheath of 5 mm, offers a panoramic view of the uterine cavity and also optional microscopic contact vision after supravital staining of the cells.

Resectoscopes

The gynecologic resectoscope can be used to resect and remove intrauterine pathologic formations and/or for endometrial ablation. It consist of a classical 4-mm telescope, an electrical loop to perform passive cuts, and two sheaths for continuous-flow suction and irrigation of liquid distension medium. Besides the cutting loop, other instruments such as microknives or a series of coagulation or vaporization electrodes of various shapes can be connected to the resectoscope. There are essentially two types of resectoscopes, which differ in their outer diameter: 7.3 and 8.6 mm. The 8.6-mm resectoscope is generally used except when the uterine cavity is small.

Electrosurgery Unit

The resectoscope is connected to an electrosurgical generator. Two types of electrosurgical generators are available, unipolar and bipolar. The unipolar high-frequency electrosurgical generator represents the traditional system, which implies that the electrons flow from the electrosurgical generator to the active electrode (e.g., loop or knife electrode). From the electrode the current flows through the tissue to the neutral electrode and returns to the electrosurgical generator. Unipolar electrosurgery is potentially dangerous because part of the path traveled by the electrons is unknown and there is a risk of electrical burns at some distance from the active electrode. However, the new generators have an automatic cutting power regulation system depending on the tissue resistance, so the risk of electrical injury is very low. Unipolar electrosurgery can be used for coagulation, section, and a combination of coagulation and section using a modulated current (spray coagulation). Bipolar electrosurgery units have been recently introduced. They are theoretically safer than the traditional unipolar units, but at present the effectiveness of these electrodes is not comparable to that of the traditional resectoscope. Thus their use is indicated only in some specific cases such as septate uterus, small submucous fibroids, or polyps.

Hysteroscopic Laser Surgery

The most commonly used lasers in hysteroscopy are the argon, neodymium, YAG, and KTP lasers. They show good coagulation properties but poor vaporization characteristics.

BASIC PRINCIPLES OF DIAGNOSTIC HYSTEROSCOPY

Proper hysteroscopic examination requires accurate patient screening, selecting the right moment to perform the examination, and perfect knowledge of the technique.

In cases of almost total stenosis of either the cervical canal or isthmus (present in about 3% of patients), it may prove useful to administer preparatory drug treatment with estrogens (ethinylestradiol 0.01 mg/day po for 8 days), sulprostone (250 to 500 units IV or intracervical 2 to 3 hours prior to the examination), or laminaria tent intracervical 2 to 6 hours prior to the examination. Cervical dilatation can also be achieved using a Hegar probe to enable the examination.

In women of childbearing age, the best time to perform the examination is in the first half of the menstrual cycle, between the sixth and tenth days. During this period the isthmus is hypotonic, making the passage easier, and the endometrial mucosa is proliferative, lending itself to better endoscopic viewing. Moreover, during the proliferative phase of the cycle there is no risk of encountering an early, unexpected pregnancy. However the examination can be performed at any time in cases of emergency or in a patient using oral contraceptives. There are also some circumstances that do make one point in the cycle preferable over others. For example, functional exploration of the cervical canal or cervical endoscopy should be performed during the preovulatory phase, while differential evaluation of endometrial hyperplasia should be performed during the secretory phase.

There are many conditions where a diagnostic hysteroscopy is required. One of the most common situations where hysteroscopy should be used as a first choice is the presence of abnormal uterine bleeding, especially in perimenopausal and postmenopausal women.[21,27] In these cases, hysteroscopy in combination with endometrial biopsy permits identification of the pathologic conditions responsible for the bleeding.[19,22]

BASIC PRINCIPLES OF SURGICAL HYSTEROSCOPY

Surgical hysteroscopy is a true and proper operating technique and must therefore be performed on an inpatient or day-hospital basis, depending on the needs and type of surgery. However, it is unusual for surgical hysteroscopy to require hospitalization for more than 24 hours.

A through physical examination and careful analysis of the patient's history are essential prerequisites for selection of patients for surgical hysteroscopy. A recent history of pelvic inflammatory disease (PID) is an absolute contraindication to any form of hysteroscopic surgery, because there is the risk of reactivating the inflammatory process, making it acute. On the other hand, in the case of acute cervicovaginal infections, to prevent the infection from spreading to the endometrium and adnexa through the ascending canal, the lymphatic system, or the blood, it is best to postpone surgery until the infection has healed. Slight or moderate metrorrhagia does not in itself impede intrauterine endoscopic surgery. On the other hand, extremely abundant metrorrhagia must first be treated to enable intracavitary surgical interventions and to decrease the risk of the distension medium entering the bloodstream. Pregnancy itself must be considered a contraindication to hysteroscopy, although in some cases in early stages of pregnancy, a retained intrauterine device can easily be removed under hysteroscopy.

Equipment

Rigid hysteroscopes with an outer diameter of 7.5 mm, which are equipped with two channels, are normally used for surgery, one channel for the distension media and the other for introducing ancillary instruments including probes, catheters, miniature rigid or semirigid scissors, and various biopsy forceps. Currently, however, 95% of all hysteroscopic surgery is performed using a resectoscope. The distension media commonly used in hysteroscopic surgery are liquid media, in particular, sorbitol/mannitol and glycine solutions. Carbon dioxide and high-viscosity dextran solutions are not generally used in hysteroscopic surgery.

Surgical hysteroscopy does not require any particular preparation of the patient and can be performed both with local anesthesia administered by paracervical or epidural blocking or, particularly in the most complicated cases, under general anesthesia with orotracheal intubation. Epidural anesthesia is currently the method of choice, since the patient is awake and any symptoms of intravasation can quickly be recognized, as this is the worst possible complication encountered with this sort of surgery.

To date, no indications of serious infection have been found after intrauterine endoscopic surgery. Nor has it been proved that the fragments of endometrial mucosa released during surgery give rise to endometriotic foci at other sites. Finally, the concern regarding postoperative hemorrhage appears to have been reconsidered in light of experience now acquired. Bleeding has only occasionally been found after resecting submucous myomas. Under such circumstances, hemorrhage can be effectively controlled by inserting a Foley catheter into the uterine cavity. Perforation of the uterine fundus or creation of a false pathway are obviously intraoperative complications more closely related to the surgeon's experience. On the other hand, there are some rare case reports of intestinal lesions with severe peritonitis after surgery with an intrauterine electrocoagulator or electroresectoscope.

HYSTEROSCOPIC SURGICAL PROCEDURES

Endometrial Ablation

Endometrial ablation was introduced in the early 1980s as an operating technique for destroying the endometrium in patients with "abnormal uterine bleeding" with the aim of reducing or totally eliminating the bleeding. The main indication for endometrial ablation is abnormal drug-resistant bleeding when cancerous or precancerous endometrial lesions are not present. Endometrial ablation has also recently been proposed as treatment for recurrent endometrial hyperplasia that does not present any cytologic atypia. The procedure is currently indicated in patients at high risk for hysterectomy and in patients who for various reasons do not want to, or cannot, undergo traditional surgery. Various methods have been used with more or less success to totally destroy the endometrium:

1. *Chemical and radioactive substances.* For the most part, corrosive agents such as quinacrine, formaldehyde, oxalic acid, and adhesives such as methylcyanoacrylate or silicone have been tested. This type of procedure has been abandoned because of the potential damage these substances could cause when passing the peritoneum and because of poor results, often requiring multiple applications. While intracavitary radium applications did prove effective, the technique was subsequently abandoned because of the risks associated with the use of radioactive substances.

2. *Cryosurgery.* First proposed in 1987 by Droegemüller, cryosurgery never became widespread because of numerous technical difficulties.

3. *High-frequency radio waves.* Recently high-frequency radio waves have been proposed for endometrial ablation. However, this technique is still considered experimental.

4. *Resectoscopy.* The resectoscope allows for resection and coagulation. Endometrial "slices" of 3 to 5 mm thickness can be resected under direct endoscopic control with the instrument connected to an electrosurgical generator. This is the technique most widely used in Europe. The main advantage is that it enables histopathologic analysis of the material removed. However, it does require a fair amount of surgical skill to remove the entire endometrium without penetrating too deep into the myometrium. The 50 to 100 W unipolar electrosurgical generator can be connected to the resectoscope, the terminal portion of which is equipped with a U-shaped loop for endoscopy-guided resection.

5. *Roller bar coagulation.* This is a variation of the previous method. It is performed with an endoscopic resectoscope, but in this case the terminal loop is replaced with a roller bar. The roller bar electrode consists of a metal ball or bar connected to a unipolar electrosurgical generator and is used for systematic coagulation of the entire endometrium. Technically, this method is easier than resection, because the endometrium is simply coagulated and there is no risk of penetrating too deeply into the myometrium. However, the disadvantage is that it does not allow for postoperative histopathology. For this reason, many authors suggest an initial resection using the resectoscope followed by roller bar electrode to coagulate the vascular bed and access the corners of the tubes.

6. *Neodymium YAG laser coagulation.* This technique is similar to electrosurgical coagulation but performed with a laser.

7. *Thermal ablation techniques.* Recently introduced, thermal ablation techniques basically destroy the endometrium by inserting into the uterine cavity a balloon containing a liquid medium circulating at 90°C (balloon thermal ablation). An alternative to this technique is hot saline ablation, in which a liquid medium at 90°C is introduced directly into the uterine cavity to remain there for 10 minutes. These techniques are limited by the lack of any histologic or visual control during and after the procedure.

Surgery of Uterine Malformations

Muellerian malformations include a large group of congenital anomalies predominantly found in young women, which particularly involve the reproductive function. Uterine defects can affect fertility mainly by causing complications during pregnancy. In general, women with this pathology have no more difficulty than normal women in conceiving, whereas their gestational capacity may be compromised. The more common complications include abortion and premature delivery in 25% and 16% in patients, respectively. The didelphic and the bicornuate uterus are associated with increases in premature delivery. Since a fairly high number of pregnancies conclude at full term without requiring intervention, usually no therapy is recommended to correct these malformations. Septate uterus is apparently linked to a high rate of fetal loss generally occurring in the first half of pregnancy. Buttram and Gibbons reported 88% of pregnancy wastage in patients with completely septate uterus and 70% in patients with partially septate uterus. It may thus be concluded that septate uterus is a condition apt to present serious reproductive difficulty and that therefore almost always needs corrective management.

Several different procedures have been adopted for hysteroscopic management of septate uterus and yield more or less the same results. The basic concept involves hysteroscopic transcervical observation of the uterine septum followed by resection. All authors use operative hysteroscopes that permit the passage of operating instruments. The outer diameter of the endoscope ranges from 7 to 9 mm. Some authors suggest the use of scissors inserted separately in the uterine cavity along the cervical canal parallel to the hysteroscope; in our opinion this is not advisable, since we believe that the surgical procedure is cleaner and more accurate if all instruments are introduced through the operating sheath, as it may be extremely difficult in most cases to manipulate two separate instruments through the cervical canal. Of the numerous instruments that can be used to dissect the septum, the semirigid miniature scissors appear almost perfect for this type of surgery, as they produce the required force while being small enough to pass through the operating sheath of the hysteroscope and along the cervical canal without any difficulty or risk.

Special mention must be made of complete septa that also involve the cervical canal. This kind of malformation may take on different forms with one or two cervices and with or without isthmic communication. If a complete uterocervical septum with one cervix is found, we prefer to include the cervical part in the dissection. None of our patients treated with this technique experienced cervical incompetence in pregnancy.

Treatment of Intrauterine Adhesions

Asherman's syndrome, first described around 1920, is characterized by a decrease in fertility associated with menstrual disorders due to the presence of intrauterine synechiae of traumatic origin. The causal factor of Asherman's syndrome is the presence of scar tissue between the uterine walls, also known as "adhesions" or synechiae. Hysteroscopic surgery can be employed in virtually all cases of intrauterine synechiae except in some particular forms of total synechia where hysteroscopic surgery has proved ineffective and laparotomy may turn out to be more beneficial. In most cases, hysteroscopic treatment is performed under general anesthesia using a 7.5-mm operating sheath and semirigid scissors. We do not resect synechia with the distal end of the hysteroscope as proposed by some authors, except in cases of extremely thin, veil-like lesions that are often sectioned simply by distension of the uterine cavity. Recent use of the resectoscope has further simplified the procedure, making it possible to treat even the most severe cases in this manner.[15,25,26]

Myomectomy

Uterine leiomyomas are some of the most frequent benign neoplasms encountered in gynecologic practice. They occur in 20 to 30% of women of reproductive age and their frequency increases toward the end of the reproductive period. Hypermenorrhea with menorrhagia and abnormal uterine bleeding often accompanied by anemia is the most common cause for surgical removal of the leiomyoma. Symptoms are correlated more with the location than the size of the tumor except in extreme cases. Protrusion of the leiomyoma into the uterine cavity with anatomic distortion is associated with bleeding in almost all cases. Currently the main indication for hysteroscopic myomectomy in infertile patients or in candidates for hormone replacement therapy is the presence of abnormal uterine bleeding and submucous myomas, including asymptomatic cases.

Indications for hysteroscopic myomectomy include abnormal uterine bleeding, infertility (including asymptomatic cases), and candidates for HRT (including asymptomatic cases). For leiomyoma hysteroscopic resection, a 26 French resectoscope is normally used. Smaller resectoscopes are used if the uterine cavity and/or cervical canal is narrow. After cervical dilatation up to 10 mm, the resectoscope with the electrosurgical working element for control of the 90-degree cutting loop is introduced. Distension of the uterine cavity is obtained with glycine or sorbitol/mannitol solution. Irrigation is controlled with an electronic suction and irrigation pump (Hamou Endomat) that automatically controls both intrauterine pressure and flow rate. The system also ensures constant suction. A high-frequency generator is also required to supply the energy for electrosurgery through the resectoscope into the uterine cavity.[9,20,30,31]

Fallopian Tube Catheterization

Today there are essentially three indications for tubal catheterization:

1. Obstruction and occlusion of the tubal ostium and/or the proximal tract.
2. Transfer of gametes or embryos. This indication makes use of the positive effect the tubal factor has on gamete fertilization and embryo implantation in some assisted-fertilization techniques.
3. Placement of intratubal devices for reversible sterilization.

The traditional 4-mm diameter telescope with a 7-mm operating sheath is normally used for tubal catheterization. In cases in which the cervical canal is particularly narrow and the passage into the uterine cavity proves difficult, a 2.9-mm diameter telescope can be used with a 5-mm operating sheath. Fiberscopes can also be used, as they have proved particularly suitable, lining themselves up on the same directional axis as the tubal ostium, thus facilitating introduction of the catheter.

The choice of catheter is extremely important. To remove proximal tubal occlusions we use the Novy set (Cook), which includes a 9 French external catheter to reach the cornual area, a 3 French catheter to cannulate the orifice, and a guidewire to catheterize the fallopian tube. Confino et al,[32] on the other hand, presented their experience with the application of a 4 French angioplasty catheter in hysteroscopy. The most characteristic feature of this method is that after using an obturator to remove the obstruction, a balloon filled with a contrast medium is introduced to achieve a longer-lasting mechanical dilatation. Finally, Deaton et al[33] used a urologic catheter with a flexible obturator to achieve full recanalization in 7 of 10 cases of cornual fallopian tube occlusion.

A correct choice of the catheter is also important in the gamete or embryo tubal transfer through hysteroscopic catheterization. The basic requirements are a diameter ranging from 0.8 to 1 mm and adequate stiffness to enable cannulation of the tube without causing serious trauma. Simple catheters or special double catheters can be used, the latter serving to reduce contact with the CO_2 required to distend the uterine cavity.

Concerning the use of ITDs (intratubal devices) for reversible sterilization, we tried the Hamou ITD. It consists of a soft strand of surgical nylon 1 mm in diameter. At each end of the nylon strand (about 20 to 30 mm long) there is a loop made of self-retaining elastic material that makes it possible to remove the ITD. The loops prevent expulsion of the ITD into the uterine cavity and its migration along the fallopian tube. The ITDs are inserted under hysteroscopic control. The endoscope is 4 mm in diameter with an operative sheath that has a 6.5 mm outer diameter. The uterine cavity is distended by continuous CO_2 flow. Procedures are usually scheduled for the early proliferative phase of the menstrual cycle. After careful examination of the uterine cavity, the end of the insertion catheter is brought within about 3 mm of the tubal ostia and the ITD is inserted into the interstitial portion. The second ITD is placed in the other tube in the same manner without removing the hysteroscope from the uterus. The ITDs may be removed at any time by grasping and gently pulling, under hysteroscopic control, the proximal loop of the ITD.[16]

Removal of Foreign Bodies and IUDs

The term "lost IUD" is applied to those situations where the recovery filament is not visible from outside the cervix. The string may have ascended due to abnormal displacement, fragmentation of the device, perforation of the uterus, or unnoticed expulsion of the IUD itself and, finally, onset of a pregnancy.

Ultrasound is, in our view, the first method for diagnosis of IUD positioning; indeed this technique can detect a pregnancy that could increase the uterine cavity dimensions, causing the recovery filament to disappear from the external orifice. In these cases, dilatation of the cavity with gas must be carried out with great care in view of the reduced resistance of the walls. Frequently, the gestational sac presses the device against the uterine wall. Removal of the IUD must, in our opinion, always be performed no matter whether the pregnancy is to be interrupted or carried to term. Our experience is based on 15 cases of hysteroscopy-guided removal in patients wishing to continue the pregnancy. Only 2 cases of miscarriage occurred in the 2 days following IUD removal; the remaining pregnancies were successfully carried to term. Hysteroscopy is the method of choice for removal of the IUD or any fragments at all times, except in cases of total perforation of the uterine wall, with the IUD passing into the peritoneal cavity, and undetected expulsion. The IUD and/or fragments can be located and extracted by means of forceps, the procedure being performed on an outpatient basis without anesthesia or cervical canal dilatation.[3,12,26]

REFERENCES

1. Anastasiadis PG, Koutlaki NG, Skaphida PG, et al. Endometrial polyps: Prevalence, detection, and malignant potential in women with abnormal uterine bleeding. *Eur J Gynaecol Oncol.* 2000;21:180.
2. Bradley LD, Pasqualotto EB, Price LL, et al. Hysteroscopic management of endometrial polyps. *Obstet Gynecol.* 2000;95:S23.
3. Ben-Rafael Z, Bider D. A new procedure for removal of a lost intrauterine device. *Obstet Gynecol.* 1996;87:785.
4. Colacurci N, De Placido G, Perino A, et al. Hysteroscopic metroplasty. *J Am Assoc Gynecol Laparosc.* 1998;5:17.
5. Cooper JM, Brady RM. Late complications of operative hysteroscopy. *Obstet Gynecol Clin North Am.,* 2000;27:367.
6. Cooper JM, Brady RM. Intraoperative and early postoperative complications of operative hysteroscopy. *Obstet Gynecol Clin North Am.* 2000;27:347.
7. Gervaise A., Fernandez H, Capella-Allouc S, et al. Thermal balloon ablation versus endometrial resection for the treatment of abnormal uterine bleeding. *Human Reprod.* 1999;14: 247.
8. Gimpelson RJ. Hysteroscopic treatment of the patient with intracavitary pathology. *Obstet Gynecol Clin North Am.* 2000;27:327.
9. Hart R, Molnar BG, Magos A. Long term follow up of hysteroscopic myomectomy assessed by survival analysis. *Br J Obstet Gynaecol.* 1999;106:700.
10. Hidlebaugh DA. Cost of different types of surgical therapy for abnormal uterine bleeding: A review. *J Reprod Med.* 2000;45:163.
11. Homer HA, Li TC, Cooke ID. The septate uterus: A review of management and reproductive outcome. *Fertil Steril.* 2000;73:1.
12. Indman PD. Instrumentation and distension media for the hysteroscopic treatment of abnormal uterine bleeding. *Obstet Gynecol Clin North Am.* 2000;27:305.
13. Isaacson K. New developments in operative hysteroscopy. *Obstet Gynecol Clin North Am.* 2000;27:375.
14. Jourdain O, Dabysing F, Harle T, et al. Management of septate uterus by flexible hysteroscopy and Nd:YAG laser. *Int J Gynaecol Obstet.* 1998;63:159.
15. Katz Z, Ben.Arie A., Lurie S, et al. Reproductive outcome following hysteroscopic adhesiolysis in Asherman's syndrome. *Int J Fertil Menopausal Stud.* 1996;41:462.
16. Kitamura S, Miyazaki T, Iwata S, et al. Ultrastructural evaluation following catheterization of the fallopian tube with a hysteroscopic catheter. *J Assist Reprod Genet.* 1998;15:411.
17. Lin JC, Chen YO, Lin BL, et al. Outcome of removal of intrauterine devices with flexible hysteroscopy in early pregnancy. *J Gynecol Surg.* 1993;9:195.
18. Loffer FD, Bradley LD, Brill AI, et al. Hysteroscopic fluid monitoring guidelines. The ad hoc committee on hysteroscopic training guidelines of the American Association of Gynecologic Laparoscopists. *J Am Assoc Gynecol Laparosc.* 2000;7:167.
19. Loffer FD, Bradley LD, Brill AI, et al. Hysteroscopic training guidelines. The ad hoc committee on hysteroscopic training guidelines of the American Association of Gynecologic Laparoscopists. *J Am Assoc Gynecol Laparosc.* 2000;7:165.
20. Mencaglia L., Tiso E, Bianchi R., et al. Intramural myomectomy using a combination of hysteroscopy and laparoscopy. *J Am Assoc Gynecol Laparosc.* 1996;3:S30.
21. Mencaglia L, Perino A, Hamou J. Hysteroscopy in perimenopausal and postmenopausal women with abnormal uterine bleeding. *J Reprod Med.* 1987;32:577.
22. Pasqualotto EB, Margossian H, Price LL, et al. Accuracy of preoperative diagnostic tools and outcome of hysteroscopic management of menstrual dysfunction. *J Am Assoc Gynecol Laparosc.* 2000;7:201.
23. Porcu G, Cravello L, D'Ercole C, et al. Hysteroscopic metroplasty for septate uterus and repetitive abortions: Reproductive outcome. *Eur J Obstet Gynecol Reprod Biol.* 2000;88:81.
24. Preutthipan S, Linasmita V. Reproductive outcome following hysteroscopic lysis of intrauterine adhesions: A result of 65 cases at Ramthibodi Hospital. *J Med Assoc Thai.* 2000;83:42.
25. Romano S, Bustan M, Ben-Shlomo I, et al. Case report: A novel surgical approach to obstructed hemiuterus: Sonographically guided hysteroscopic correction. *Human Reprod.* 2000;15:1578.
26. Ross JW. Numerous indications for office flexible minihysteroscopy. *J Am Assoc Gynecol Laparosc.* 2000;7:221.
27. Serden SP. Diagnostic hysteroscopy to evaluate the cause of abnormal uterine bleeding. *Obstet Gynecol Clin North Am.* 2000;27:277.
28. Sheth SS, Sonkawde R. Uterine septum misdiagnosed on hysterosalpingogram. *Int J Gynaecol Obstet.* 2000;69:261.
29. Shushan A, Rojansky N. Should hysteroscopy be a part of the basic infertility workup? *Hum Reprod.* 2000;15:1650.
30. Varasteh NN, Neuwirth RS, Levin B, et al. Pregnancy rates after hysteroscopic polypectomy and myomectomy in infertile women. *Obstet Gynecol.* 1999;94:168.
31. Vercellini P, Zaina B, Yaylayan L, et al. Hysteroscopic myomectomy: Long-term effects on menstrual pattern and fertility. *Obstet Gynecol.* 1999;94:341.
32. Confino E. A system for simultaneous bilateral tubal cannulation. Int J Fertil Menopausal Stud. 1995;40:202–205.
33. Deaton JL, Gibson M, Riddick DH, Brumsted JR. Diagnosis and treatment of corneal obstruction using a flexible tip guidewire. Fertil Steril. 1990;53:232–236.

Chapter Seventy-One . . . . . .

Pregnancy and Laparoscopy

MYRIAM J. CURET

Laparoscopy has revolutionized the field of general surgery since the first laparoscopic cholecystectomy was done in the late 1980s. With this new technology has come questions about its limitations. Initially, pregnancy was considered an absolute contraindication to laparoscopic cholecystectomy.[1,2] Despite potential advantages of laparoscopic surgery in the pregnant patient, there were concerns about the effects of the carbon dioxide pneumoperitoneum on the mother and fetus. Obstetricians have performed laparoscopic procedures for many years in the pregnant patient to rule out suspected ectopic pregnancies, resulting in many normal deliveries after a negative exam.[3] These experiences have resulted in general surgeons attempting laparoscopic surgery in pregnant patients. Initial clinical reports have demonstrated the feasibility, advantages, and potential safety of laparoscopic cholecystectomy in the pregnant patient.[4–14]

Nongynecologic surgery occurs in 0.2% of all pregnancies.[15] The safest time to operate on the pregnant patient is during the second trimester when the risks of teratogenesis, miscarriage, and preterm delivery are lowest.[7,8,10–12,14,16] The miscarriage rate is highest in the first trimester (12%) and decreases by the third trimester to 0%. During the second trimester, there is about a 5 to 8% rate of preterm delivery that increases to 30% of all pregnant patients undergoing nongynecologic surgery in the third trimester.[9,11,16] Also, in the second trimester, the risk of teratogenesis seen during the first trimester is no longer present.[9] Finally, the gravid uterus in the second trimester is not yet large enough to obscure the operative field as occurs in the third trimester.[11,14] Pregnancy itself does not increase surgical maternal mortality; rather, morbidity and mortality are increased when the correct diagnosis is missed, when surgery is delayed, or when postoperative complications occur.[15] This can increase maternal mortality to as high as 15% and fetal loss up to 60%, which is usually caused by maternal hypoxia and hypotension.[15,17]

The most common surgical problems that general surgeons see in the pregnant patient are appendicitis and cholecystitis. Appendicitis occurs in 1 out of 1500 pregnancies.[15,16,18,19] The ability to correctly diagnose appendicitis preoperatively decreases as the pregnancy progresses. In the first trimester one should expect a 85% correct preoperative diagnosis, which decreases to 30 to 50% by the third trimester.[18,19] The reason for this is that the usual clinical signs of appendicitis such as leukocytosis, abdominal pain, anorexia, and nausea are already present in the patient in the third trimester and therefore are often not helpful. It has been suggested that the only laboratory value that is of significance in diagnosing appendicitis in the pregnant patient correctly is a total neutrophil count of greater than 80%.[18] The overall false diagnosis rate of appendicitis of 35 to 55% in pregnant patients leads to a 10% perforation rate. Fetal mortality has been shown to increase with perforation from 5 to 28% while preterm delivery can be as high as 40%.[15,18–20] Thus, the pregnant patient suspected of having acute appendicitis should be treated as if she were not pregnant. Immediate exploration after appropriate resuscitation is mandated regardless of gestational age.

Biliary tract disease is the second most common diagnosis requiring surgery during pregnancy. A cholecystectomy is performed in 3.8 out of every 10,000 pregnancies.[9,11,12,15,16,18] Gallstones are present in 12% of all pregnancies.[9,11,12,15,16,18] The majority of these patients are treated medically with a nonfat diet and pain medication to try to carry the patients to term or at least until the second trimester. However, more than one-third of patients will fail medical treatment and will require surgery.[7,9,11,16] An uncomplicated open cholecystectomy in a pregnant patient should be accompanied by a 0% maternal mortality with approximately 5% fetal loss and 7% preterm delivery.[8,14–18] Complications such as gallstone pancreatitis or acute cholecystitis will increase maternal mortality to 15% and fetal demise to 60%.[7,8,15–17] Patients with uncomplicated biliary colic should be treated medically with a nonfat diet and pain medication until after delivery. Patients with complications of biliary tract disease such as gallstone pancreatitis, acute cholecystitis, crescendo biliary colic, or persistent vomiting should be medically managed, if possible, until they are in the second trimester. If medical management fails, operative intervention should be attempted.[9,11,12]

Traditionally, appendicitis and cholecystitis in the pregnant patient have been treated with open laparotomy. There are complications of open laparotomy that would be preferable to avoid in the pregnant patient. For example, it is well known that a large abdominal incision leads to respiratory splitting and an increased rate of atelectasis. Likewise, laparotomy can lead to decreased gastrointestinal function. This is especially important in the pregnant patient in whom gastrointestinal function may already be depressed.[15] There have also been concerns about an increased rate of incisional hernia as the uterus expands. Obviously, a laparotomy is associated with more postoperative pain than a laparoscopy, which can lead to increased narcotic usage and fetal depression. These are some of the problems that could potentially be decreased by the use of laparoscopic surgery instead of open laparotomy. In addition, the proven advantages of laparoscopy seen with nonpregnant patients such as shortened hospital stay, earlier ambulation, and quicker return to regular activity should also be enjoyed by the pregnant patient.[2,5,10,12]

Gynecologists have used laparoscopy for many years. Its overall mortality is less than 4 in 100,000 with an overall complication rate of 2%. The most commonly quoted complications include vascular and visceral injury from needle or trocar insertion.[5,6,10,12,14] There have been reports of cardiovascular depression, respiratory acidosis, gas embolism, and thromboembolic events.[5,14,20] These data quoted in the gynecologic literature lead one to believe that laparoscopy is safe. In the last 7 years the use of laparoscopic general surgery has expanded rapidly. Laparoscopic cholecystectomy is now the gold standard for treatment of biliary tract disease in nonpregnant patients.[2] Likewise, laparoscopic Nissen-type fundoplication, laparoscopic colectomy, and laparoscopic appendectomy are widely accepted surgical treatment for certain medical diseases. The major advantages of laparoscopic surgery that have been demonstrated in the literature are earlier return of GI function, earlier return to ambulation, decreased hospital stay, and a faster return to routine activity.[2,5,10,12] All of these would clearly benefit the pregnant as well as the nonpregnant patient. Likewise, there have been reports of decreased incidence of thromboembolic events, lower rates of wound infections and hernias, and decreased pain and narcotic usage in patients undergoing laparoscopic surgery rather than laparotomy.[5,6,10–12,14] Again, these would clearly benefit the pregnant patient and her fetus. Another potential advantage of therapeutic laparoscopy in the pregnant patient includes the fact that there is less manipulation of the uterus in attempting to obtain intra-abdominal exposure. This could potentially lead to decreased uterine irritability and decreased premature labor and spontaneous abortion.[5,13]

Despite these potential advantages, there are concerns that laparoscopic surgery could have serious negative effects on the pregnant patient and her fetus. Increased intra-abdominal pressure can lead to decreased inferior vena cava return resulting in a decrease in cardiac output.[21–25] The fetus is dependent on maternal hemodynamic stability and the primary cause of fetal demise is maternal hypotension or hypoxia.[15] Clearly, a drop in maternal cardiac output could result in fetal distress. There have also been concerns that increased intra-abdominal pressure could lead to decreased uterine blood flow and increased intrauterine pressure, both of which could result in fetal hypoxia.[5,6,14] Finally, it has been demonstrated that carbon dioxide is absorbed across the peritoneum and can lead to respiratory acidosis in both mother and fetus.[10,21,22,25,26] Fetal acidosis could be potentiated by the decreased vena cava return seen during laparoscopy.[27] These concerns about laparoscopic surgery in the pregnant patient initially led surgeons to consider laparoscopy a contraindication to laparoscopic cholecystectomy during pregnancy.[1,2]

As surgeons became more familiar with laparoscopic surgery and could complete it in shorter operative times, there began to be reports in the literature of pregnant patients undergoing laparoscopic cholecystectomies. A review of the literature through June 1999 reveals data on 202 pregnant patients who underwent laparoscopic cholecystectomy.[4–14,28–63] The majority of operations took place in the second trimester (130) with 28 in the first and 24 in the third. Gestational age was unknown in the remaining 22 patients. Operative times ranged from 30 to 106 minutes (average, 66) while length of stay ranged from 1 to 7 days (average, 1.8). Two studies retrospectively compared pregnant women undergoing laparoscopy to pregnant women undergoing laparotomy and found that the patients in the laparoscopy group resumed a regular diet earlier, required less pain medication, were discharged sooner, and had a lower rate of preterm labor.[5,30] These differences were statistically significant. One article reported a maternal and a fetal death 15 days after a laparoscopic cholecystectomy was performed at 20 weeks' gestation, caused by intra-abdominal hemorrhage.[30] No other reports of maternal complications or deaths or intraoperative fetal deaths or complications have been published. At the time of publication, 166 babies had been delivered. Five were premature,[12,32,38,57,60] one born at 37 weeks' gestation had hyaline membrane disease,[11] and the remainder were healthy infants delivered at full term gestation. An additional 5 patients experienced preterm labor, which was controlled prior to term delivery.[30,32,34,36,39] A total of 6 fetal deaths have been reported, including the previously described maternal-fetal death.[4,28,30,45] One series reported 3 patients who underwent laparoscopic cholecystectomy that experienced postoperative fetal loss.[28] The deaths occurred during the first postoperative week. The gestational age at the time of surgery ranged from 12 to 15 weeks.[30] The causes of the deaths are unknown but may have been due to prolonged operative time. The operative time in these 3 patients was 106 minutes while the average for the remaining patients was 55 minutes. The laparoscopic procedure was performed for pancreatitis, and it is possible that fetal loss was the result of the inflammatory process rather than the laparoscopy itself. In another report one fetal death occurred 9 weeks after laparoscopic cholecystectomy was performed in the second trimester of pregnancy.[45] The final fetal death occurred in a woman who underwent a laparoscopic cholecystectomy in the 16th week of gestation, needed a bowel resection for obstruction 4 weeks later, then delivered an immature infant at 24 weeks' gestation.[4]

There are an additional 199 pregnant patients who underwent laparoscopic cholecystectomy discussed in an article detailing the results of a survey sent to members of the Society of Laparoendoscopic Surgeons regarding their experiences with laparoscopic procedures in pregnant patients.[54] There were 2 spontaneous abortions, both in patients who had surgery in the first trimester. Further information on these fetal deaths is not available. A 2 to 5% fetal death rate as demonstrated in Reedy's study[54] and calculated from published reports compares favorably to the 5% fetal mortality rate seen with open cholecystectomies.[4,16,17,18] In addition, Graham et al[40] reviewed the literature on laparoscopic cholecystectomy in pregnancy to correlate adverse outcome with gestation at surgery. In all three trimesters, the rates of spontaneous abortion or premature delivery were equal to or less than those seen with open cholecystectomy for the same trimester. These data on 11 cases suggest that laparoscopic cholecystectomy is safe in all three trimesters of pregnancy with no increase in fetal morbidity or mortality.

The problems with these clinical studies are that they are anecdotal, only two-thirds have followed the patients long term, and they are all retrospective. It has become clear that what is needed are prospective animal studies evaluating the use of laparoscopy in pregnant animals. There have been several such studies done. Reedy et al[64] studied four pregnant baboons at an intra-abdominal pressure of 10 mm Hg for 20 minutes followed by 20 mm Hg for 20 minutes.[64] This study found that at the end of 20 minutes at 20 mm Hg there was an increase in pulmonary capillary wedge pressure, pulmonary artery pressure, and central venous pressure. Cardiac output, blood pressure, systemic vascular resistance, and heart rate remained stable. End-tidal CO_2 and P_{CO_2} increased, and there was a decrease in pH despite controlled ventilation and an increase in respiratory rate resulting in maternal respiratory acidosis. There were no changes in the umbilical artery Doppler flow studies. One fetus developed severe bradycardia, which corrected with desufflation. The authors' conclusions were that a CO_2 pneumoperitoneum in baboons caused maternal respiratory acidosis. An intra-abdominal pressure of 20 mm Hg may result in significant fetal morbidity, and they recommended further investigation before concluding that laparoscopy during pregnancy is safe. Unfortunately, this study looked at the endpoints of pressure of 10 mm Hg (which is lower than what is used clinically) and 20 mm Hg pressure (which is more than is used clinically). Also, the authors presented no data on whether or not the young delivered with problems, therefore there were no data on the long-term effects of CO_2 pneumoperitoneum in the gravid baboon.

Another study by Barnard et al[27] studied the effects of CO_2 pneumoperitoneum in 8 gravid ewes that were near term. These animals were placed under general endotracheal anesthesia and a CO_2 pneumoperitoneum was established at 13 mm Hg. Study measurements were made after 60 minutes and after 120 minutes both in the supine and lateral positions. Placental blood flow was then measured with radioactive microsphere techniques. This study found no change in maternal placental blood flow. There was an increase in maternal P_{CO_2} and fetal P_{CO_2}, resulting in maternal and fetal respiratory acidosis. Their conclusions were that maternal placental blood flow was unaffected by increased abdominal pressure, and that fetal well being did not seem to be adversely affected by an intra-abdominal pressure of 13 mm Hg. This study is very helpful because it was done at intra-abdominal pressures that are used clinically, and over a time period that is normally seen in both laparoscopic appendectomy and cholecystectomy. Unfortunately, this study does not address whether an increased abdominal pressure has any long-term negative effects on fetal well being.

Hunter et al[65] addressed the physiologic consequences of a pneumoperitoneum for the fetus in a pregnant sheep model. They investigated the effects of both carbon dioxide and nitrous oxide as the insufflating gas. Fetal and maternal respiratory acidosis occurred with carbon dioxide pneumoperitoneum but not with nitrous oxide. This difference was statistically significant. There was also a greater prevalence of fetal tachycardia and hypertension during carbon dioxide pneumoperitoneum than with nitrous oxide insufflation. In the animals that developed maternal respiratory acidosis, changes in maternal end-tidal CO_2 lagged behind changes in maternal P_{CO_2} determined by blood gases. Altering the ventilator settings based on end-tidal CO_2 results resulted in late and incomplete correction of maternal respiratory acidosis. This study indicated that there is significant fetal respiratory acidosis with carbon dioxide pneumoperitoneum and the authors recommended that alternative gases such as nitrous oxide be considered when performing laparoscopy in pregnant patients. In addition, they felt that insertion of an arterial line was necessary in pregnant patients undergoing laparoscopic surgery because the end-tidal CO_2 results lagged behind acidosis measured by arterial blood gas, making the end-tidal CO_2 monitor untrustworthy.

Maternal and fetal respiratory acidosis and fetal hypertension and tachycardia are constant findings in all studies investigating the effects of a CO_2 pneumoperitoneum on a pregnant animal.[27,29,65-67] Typically, the fetal acidosis is not completely corrected by maternal hyperventilation. In addition, two studies found that intrauterine pressure is increased with increased intra-abdominal pressure.[66,67] One series found that uterine blood flow also decreased by 40% with increased intra-abdominal pressure.[66] Despite these intraoperative changes, one study investigating the long-term effects of a CO_2 pneumoperitoneum found that all ewes delivered full-term healthy lambs, suggesting that short-term fetal acidosis may not lead to long-term deleterious effects.[66]

Several guidelines should be followed when performing laparoscopic surgery in the pregnant patient to ensure the safety of the mother and fetus. The patient should be placed in the left lateral decubitus position as in open surgery to prevent uterine compression of the inferior vena cava. Minimizing the degree of reverse Trendelenburg position may also further reduce possible uterine compression of the vena cava.[9,12,14] Antiembolic devices should be used to prevent deep venous thrombosis. Stasis of blood in the lower extremities is common in pregnancy and levels of fibrinogen and factors VII and XII are increased during pregnancy, leading to an increased risk of thromboembolic events.[5,12] These changes, coupled with the decreased venous return seen with increased intra-abdominal pressure and the reverse Trendelenburg position used during laparoscopic surgery, significantly increase the risk of deep venous thrombosis.

An open Hasson technique for gaining access to the abdominal cavity is safer compared to a percutaneous access in the pregnant patient. Although several authors have used a closed percutaneous route for abdominal access without complications, the potential for puncture of the uterus or intestines still exists, especially with increasing gestational age. It is recommended that routine continuous intraoperative fetal monitoring be used so that if fetal distress is noted, the pneumoperitoneum can be released. Intravaginal ultrasound may be necessary for fetal monitoring as the pneumoperitoneum can decrease fetal heart tones if ultrasound is performed transabdominally.[11] The intra-abdominal pressure should be as low as possible while still achieving adequate visualization. A pressure of 10 to 12 mm Hg is probably safest and pressure should not be above 15 mm Hg until concerns about the effects of high intra-abdominal pressure on the fetus are answered.

It is important to monitor end-tidal CO_2 continuously, maintaining it between 25 and 33 mm Hg by changing the minute ventilation. Prompt correction of maternal respiratory acidosis is critical as the fetus is typically slightly more acidotic than the mother.[10,11,65,66] If intraoperative cholangiography is to be performed, the fetus should be protected with a lead shield. Several studies have demonstrated a correlation between the duration of a CO_2 pneumoperitoneum and an increase in Pa_{CO_2}.[28] Thus it is important to minimize operative times whenever possible. Finally, tocolytic agents should not be administered prophylactically but are appropriate if there is any evidence of uterine irritability or contractions.[5,9,11]

In conclusion, clinical studies have indicated pregnant patients can successfully undergo nongynecologic laparoscopic surgery in all three trimesters with no apparent perioperative or long-term maternal or fetal harm. The advantages of laparoscopic surgery such as decreased hospital stay, decreased narcotic usage, and earlier return to diet and ambulation apply to the pregnant patient as well as the nonpregnant patient. Animal studies indicate possible perioperative deleterious effects including maternal and fetal respiratory acidosis and hemodynamic changes; however, animal studies demonstrate no long-term harm to the fetus. It may be safest to consider an alternative to CO_2 pneumoperitoneum in order to achieve the advantages of laparoscopic surgery in the pregnant patient while decreasing the potential for complications.

REFERENCES

1. Gadacz TR, Talamini MA. Traditional vs. laparoscopic cholecystectomy. *Am J Surg.* 1991;161:336.
2. Soper NJ, Stockmann PT, Dunnegan DL, et al. Laparoscopic cholecystectomy: the new "gold standard"? *Arch Surg.* 1992;127:917.
3. Samuellson S, Sjovall A. Laparoscopy in suspected ectopic pregnancy. *Acta Obstet Gynecol Scand.* 1972;51:31.
4. Abuabara SF, Gross GWW, Sirinek KR. Laparoscopic cholecystectomy during pregnancy is safe for both mother and fetus. *J Gastrointest Surg.* 1997;1:48.
5. Curet MJ, Allen D, Josloff RK, et al. Laparoscopy during pregnancy. *Arch Surg.* 1996;131:546.
6. Arvidsson D, Gerdin E. Laparoscopic cholecystectomy during pregnancy. *Surg Laparosc Endosc.* 1991;1:193.
7. Elerding SC. Laparoscopic cholecystectomy in pregnancy. *Am J Surg.* 1993;165:625.
8. Wilson RB, McKenzie RJ, Fisher JW. Laparoscopic cholecystectomy in case reports. *Aust N Z J Surg.* 1994;64:647.
9. Lanzafame R. Laparoscopic cholecystectomy during pregnancy. *Surgery* 1995;118:627.
10. Soper NJ, Hunter JG, Petri RH. Laparoscopic cholecystectomy during pregnancy. *Surg Endosc.* 1992;6:115.
11. Comitalo JB, Lynch D. Laparoscopic cholecystectomy in the pregnant patient. *Surg Laparosc Endosc.* 1994;4:268.
12. Morrel DG, Mullins JR, Harrison PB. Laparoscopic cholecystectomy during pregnancy in symptomatic patients. *Surgery* 1992;112:856.
13. Bennett TL, Estes N. Laparoscopic cholecystectomy in the second trimester of pregnancy: a case report. *J Reprod Med.* 1993;38:833.
14. Constantino GN, Vincent GJ, Mukalian GG, et al. Laparoscopic cholecystectomy in pregnancy. *J Laparoendosc Surg.* 1994;4:161.
15. Kammerer WS. Nonobstetric surgery during pregnancy. *Med Clin North Am.* 1979;63:1157.
16. McKellar DP, Anderson CT, Boynton CJ, et al. Cholecystecomy during pregnancy without fetal loss. *Surg Gynecol Obstet.* 1992;174:465.
17. Printen KJ, Ott RA. Cholecystectomy during pregnancy. *Am Surg.* 1978;44:432.
18. Kort B, Katz Vl, Watson WJ. The effect of nonobstetric operation during pregnancy. *Surg Gynecol Obstet.* 1993;177:371.
19. Schreiber JH. Laparoscopic appendectomy in pregnancy. *Surg Endosc.* 1990;4:100.
20. Ostman PL, Pantle-Fisher FH, Faure EA, et al. Circulation collapse during laparoscopy. *J Clin Anesth.* 1990;2:129.
21. Motew M, Ivankovich AD, Bieniarz J, et al. Cardiovascular effects and acid-base and blood gas changes during laparoscopy. *Am J Obstet Gynecol.* 1973;113:1002.
22. Ivankovich AD, Miletich DJ, Albrecht RF, et al. Cardiovascular effect of intraperitoneal insufflation with carbon dioxide and nitrous oxide in the dog. *Anesthesiology* 1975;42:281.
23. McKenzie R, Wadhwa RK, Bedger RC. Noninvasive measurement of cardiac output during laparoscopy. *J Reprod Med.* 1980;24:247.
24. Westerband A, Van de Water JM, Amzallag M, et al. Cardiovascular changes during laparoscopic cholecystectomy. *Surg Gynecol Obstet.* 1992;175(6):535.
25. El-Minawi MF, Wahbi O, El-Bagouri ES, et al. Physiologic changes during CO_2 and N_2O pneumoperitoneum in diagnostic laparoscopy. *J Reprod Med.* 1981;26:338.
26. Fitzgerald SD, Andrus CH, Baudendistel LJ, et al. Hypercarbia during carbon dioxide pneumoperitoneum. *Am J Surg.* 1992;163:186.
27. Barnard JM, Chaffin D, Droste S, et al. Fetal response to carbon dioxide pneumoperitoneum in the pregnant ewe. *Obstet Gynecol.* 1995;85:669.
28. Amos JD, Schorr SJ, Norman PF, et al. Laparoscopic surgery during pregnancy. *Am J Surg.* 1996;171:435.
29. Andreoli M, Sayegh SK, Hoefer R, et al. Laparoscopic cholecystectomy for recurrent gallstone pancreatitis during pregnancy. *South Med J.* 1996;89:1114.
30. Barone JE, Bears S, Chen S, et al. Outcome study of cholecystectomy during pregnancy. *Am J Surg.* 1999;177:233.
31. Chandra M, Shapiro SJ, Gordon LA. Laparoscopic cholecystectomy in the first trimester of pregnancy. *Surg Laparosc Endosc.* 1994;4:68.
32. Davis A, Kiatz VL, Cox R. Gallbladder disease in pregnancy. *J Reprod Med.* 1995;40:759.
33. Edelman DS. Alternative laparoscopic technique for cholecystectomy during pregnancy. *Surg Endosc.* 1994;8:794.
34. Eichenberg BJ, Vanderlinden J, Miguel C, et al. Laparoscopic cholecystectomy in the third trimester of pregnancy. *Am Surg.* 1996;62:874.
35. Friedman RL, Friedman IH. Acute cholecystitis with calculous biliary duct obstruction in the gravid patient: Management by ERCP, papillotomy, stone extraction, and laparoscopic cholecystectomy. *Surg Endosc.* 1995;9:910.
36. Gadacz T, Jamal A, Gorski TF, et al. Laparoscopic cholecystectomy during pregnancy. *Surgical Rounds* 1997;20:209.
37. Geisler JP, Rose SL, Mernitz CS, et al. Nongynecologic laparoscopy in second and third trimester pregnancy: Obstetric implications. *J Soc Laparoendosc Surg.* 1998;2:235.
38. Glasgow RE, Visser BC, Harris HW, et al. Changing management of gallstone disease during pregnancy. *Surg Endosc.* 1998;12:241.
39. Gouldman JW, Sticca RP, Rippon MB. Laparoscopic cholecystectomy in pregnancy. *Am Surg.* 1998;64:93.
40. Graham G, Baxi L, Tharakan T. Laparoscopic cholecystectomy during pregnancy: A case series and review of the literature. *Obstet Gynecol Surg.* 1998;53:566.
41. Gurbuz AT, Peetz ME. The acute abdomen in the pregnancy patient: Is there a role for laparoscopy? *Surg Endosc.* 1997;11:98.
42. Hart RO, Tamadon A, Fitzgibbons RJ, et al. Open laparoscopic cholecystectomy in pregnancy. *Surg Laparosc Endosc.* 1993;3:13.
43. Iafrati MD, Yarnell R, Schwaitzberg SD. Gasless laparoscopic cholecystectomy in pregnancy. *J Laparoendosc Surg.* 1995;6:127.
44. Jackson SJ, Sigman HH: Laparoscopic cholecystectomy in pregnancy. *J Laparoendosc Surg.* 1995;5:399.
45. Jamal A, Gorski TF, Nguyen HY, et al. Laparoscopic cholecystectomy during pregnancy. *Surgical Rounds* 1997;468.
46. Lemaire BMD, van Erp WFM. Laparoscopic surgery during pregnancy. *Surg Endosc.* 1997;11:15.

47. Liberman MA, Phillips EH, Carrol B, et al. Management of choledo-cholithiasis during pregnancy: A new protocol in the laparoscopic era. *J Laparoendosc Surg.* 1995;5:399.

48. Martin IG, Dexter SPL, McMahon MJ. Laparoscopic cholecystectomy in pregnancy: A safe option during the second trimester? *Surg Endosc.* 1996;10:508.

49. O'Connor LA, Kavena CF, Horton S. The Phoenix Indian Medical Center experience with laparoscopic cholecystectomy during pregnancy. *Surg Laparosc Endosc.* 1996;6:441.

50. Panton ON, Nagy AG, Scudamore CH, et al. Laparoscopic cholecystectomy: A continuing plea for routine cholangiography. *Surg Laparosc Endosc.* 1995;5:43.

51. Paternoster DM, Floreani A, Sacco NA, et al. Chronic recurrent pancreatitis in pregnancy. *Minerva Ginecol.* 1997;47:561.

52. Posta CG. Laparoscopic surgery in pregnancy: Report on two cases. *J Laparoendosc Surg.* 1995;6:203.

53. Pucci RO, Seed RW: Case report of laparoscopic cholecystectomy in the third trimester of pregnancy. *Am J Obstet Gynecol.* 1991;165:401.

54. Reedy MB, Galan HL, Richards WE, et al. Laparoscopy during pregnancy: A survey of laparoendoscopic surgeons. *J Reprod Med.* 1997;42:33.

55. Rusher AH, Fields B, Henson K. Laparoscopic cholecystectomy in pregnancy: Contraindicated or indicated? *J Ark Med Soc.* 1993;899:383.

56. Schorr RT. Laparoscopic cholecystectomy and pregnancy. *J Laparoendosc Surg.* 1993;3:291.

57. Schwartzberg BS, Conyers JA, Moore JA. First trimester of pregnancy laparoscopic procedures. *Surg Endosc.* 1997;11:216.

58. Shaked G, Twena M, Charuzi I. Laparoscopic cholecystectomy for empyema of gallbladder during pregnancy. Surg Laparosc Endosc 1997;4:65.

59. Steinbrook RA, Brooks DC, Datta S. Laparoscopic cholecystectomy during pregnancy: Review of anesthetic management, surgical consideration. *Surg Endosc.* 1996;10:511.

60. Thomas SJ, Brisson P. Laparoscopic appendectomy and cholecystectomy during pregnancy: Six case reports. *J Soc Laparoendosc Surg.* 1998;2:41.

61. Weber AM, Bloom GP, Allan TR, et al. Laparoscopic cholecystectomy during pregnancy. *Obstet Gynecol.* 1991;78:958.

62. Williams JK, Rosemurgy AS, Albrink MH, et al. Laparoscopic cholecystectomy during pregnancy: A case report. *J Reprod Med.* 1995;40:243.

63. Wishner JD, Zolfaghari D, Wohlgemuth SD, et al. Laparoscopic cholecystectomy in surgery: A report of 6 cases and review of the literature. *Surg Endosc.* 1996;10:314.

64. Reedy MB, Galan HL, Bean JD, et al. Laparoscopic insufflation in the gravid baboon: maternal and fetal effects. *J Am Assoc Gynecol Laproscopists.* 1995;2:399.

65. Hunter JG, Swanstrom L, Thornburg K. Carbon dioxide pneumoperitoneum induces fetal acidosis in a pregnant ewe model. *Surg Endosc.* 1994;4:268.

66. Curet MJ, Vogt DM, Schob O, et al. Effects of CO_2 pneumoperitoneum in pregnant ewes. *J Surg Res.* 1996;63:339.

67. Cruz AM, Southerland LC, Duke T, et al. Intraabdominal carbon dioxide insufflation in the pregnant ewe. Uterine blood flow, intraamniotic pressure, and cardiopulmonary effects. *Anesthesiology.* 1996;85:1395–1402.

Chapter Seventy-Two • • • • • • •

*U*rinary Incontinence in Females

JAMES ROSS

Urinary incontinence is a common condition having significant medical, social, and psychological ramifications in women. Many women think it is a natural circumstance following childbearing and with aging, while others are too embarrassed to discuss the problem.[1] Regrettably, many who seek medical help are told by their physician that leaking is normal.[2] Fifty-eight percent of healthy, noninstitutionalized women, age 42 to 50, report urine loss at some time, and 31% have incontinence at least once a month.[3] Fifty-two percent of nulliparous college students reported stress incontinence, although only 5% had urine loss on a regular basis.[4] There are many causes of urinary incontinence and it is necessary to know which type a patient has.

DEFINITION AND TYPES OF INCONTINENCE

The International Continence Society (ICS) defines urinary incontinence as involuntary urine loss that is severe enough to constitute a social or hygienic problem and that is objectively demonstrable.[5] By this definition, urinary incontinence can be a symptom (patient's report of urine loss), a sign (objective demonstration of urine loss), or a diagnosis (established with urodynamic testing). There are four major types of incontinence: genuine stress incontinence (GSI), detrusor instability (DI), mixed incontinence (GSI and DI), and overflow incontinence. GSI is the most prevalent form of urinary incontinence, followed by mixed and DI. Unfortunately, signs and symptoms of urinary loss do not accurately differentiate the different types of incontinence.[6-8]

Genuine Stress Incontinence

Genuine stress incontinence (GSI) is defined as the involuntary loss of urine in the absence of a detrusor contraction. With GSI, the intravesical pressure exceeds the maximum urethral pressure and urine is lost. Normally, intra-abdominal pressure is transmitted to the urethra and bladder neck, which is supported by the pubocervical fascia (PCF) "hammock." Firm support by the hammock aids in compression of the urethra (extrinsic system) and urethral

muscle contraction (intrinsic system) acts as a urethral sphincter.[9] A weakened PCF permits hypermobility of the bladder neck and urethra, allowing intra-abdominal pressure to be fully transmitted to the bladder. Lack of urethral compression overcomes the intrinsic system, resulting in urine loss.

GSI occurs when the urethral sphincter muscles cease to function as sphincters, independent of bladder support. Type III incontinence, intrinsic sphincter deficiency (ISD), and low-pressure urethra are examples of this. Terminology for these conditions has not been clearly defined by the ICS, leading to confusion in the literature. Generally, a fixed, lead pipe urethra with a low valsalva leak point pressure and low urethral closure pressure is termed ISD or type III incontinence. Etiologic causes consist of multiple incontinence procedures, age, or trauma. Low-pressure urethra has the same urodynamic findings, but the urethra is hypermobile. It is imperative to diagnose these conditions prior to surgery because of their high failure rate with conventional colposuspension.[10,11] ISD is more appropriately treated by a sling procedure.[12-14]

Detrusor Instability

Detrusor instability (DI) is a condition in which the bladder is objectively shown to contract spontaneously or with provocation, during the filling phase in a neurologically intact female, while the patient is attempting to inhibit micturition. These contractions can be asymptomatic or they can cause urgency, frequency, and urge incontinence.[15] DI is urodynamic diagnosis and urge incontinence is a physical condition. DI increases with age and does not respond to surgery, making the preoperative diagnosis important.[16] Following incontinence surgery, de novo DI can occur.[17]

Mixed Incontinence

A patient with a combination of GSI and DI has mixed incontinence. Successful surgical outcome is lower than with GSI alone. This condition increases with age and possibly multiple incontinence surgeries.[17]

Overflow Incontinence

Overflow incontinence is any involuntary loss of urine associated with overdistension of the bladder.[18] Signs and symptoms include stress incontinence, intermittent dribbling, constant wetness, difficulty voiding, or increased postvoid residual. It can be due to urinary retention, infections, neurologic lesions, urethral obstruction, or pharmacologic effects. Many women are unable to feel an overdistended bladder and their leaking is diagnosed as GSI. Overflow incontinence is often seen in women following a delivery, due to overdistension secondary to trauma. The overdistension causes leaking similar to GSI, making differentiation important.

ETIOLOGY OF GENUINE STRESS INCONTINENCE

The etiology of all types of urinary incontinence is beyond the scope of this chapter. Only factors related to the development of GSI and the laparoscopic treatment of this condition will be discussed.

Pregnancy and vaginal delivery have been associated with GSI.[19,20] Shearing and stretching mechanical forces on pelvic muscles and pelvic neuropathy have been implicated as etiologic factors.[21,22] Neurodiagnostic studies in women with GSI have revealed dennervation patterns in the anal sphincter, pubococcygeus, and urethral sphincter muscles.[23–26] Single-fiber EMG recordings have revealed a dennervation and reennervation pattern with both GSI and pelvic organ prolapse.[27,28] Chronic cough and constipation cause increased intra-abdominal pressure that stretches the pudendal nerve, leading to neuropathy.

Gilpin et al performed muscle biopsies of the pubococcygeus in patients with and without GSI.[29] He found pathologic changes in the muscles fibers of patients with GSI. Muscle degeneration results in weakness of the pelvic floor.[30] Poor contractility of pelvic floor muscles leads to decreased bladder neck and urethral support. In addition to muscle changes, a decrease in collagen content and makeup has been demonstrated in patients with GSI.[31–34]

Incidence of GSI increases with aging, multiparity, hard labor, menopause, and estrogen deficiency.[3,16,35,36] The atrophic changes secondary to estrogen deficiency result in decreased coaptation of the urethral mucosa, which can affect incontinence.[37] GSI is multifaceted and is associated with pelvic organ prolapse and fecal incontinence.[38–40] The physician must be ready to evaluate patients with these problems in evaluating GSI.

PATIENT EVALUATION

A thorough patient evaluation is essential to achieve maximum surgical outcome. Missed preoperative diagnosis can lead to inappropriate surgery, undertreatment, or poor success.

History

The history should note onset, duration, severity, associated symptoms, and precipitating conditions of the incontinence. Frequency, urgency, frequent urinary tract infections, and nocturia must be documented. Prior urinary evaluations and bladder or pelvic prolapse surgeries should be noted. Other disease processes such as diabetes and systemic or neurologic diseases can play a role in GSI. Common medications, like diuretics, can increase symptoms of urinary incontinence.

Physical Examination

A general physical examination is mandatory. Attempts to reproduce the incontinence, assess pelvic support, and exclude pelvic pathology and neurologic disorders are the goals of examination.

Careful visual and manual examination of the pelvis and perineum must be done. Is there a gaping introitus, bulging vaginal wall at maximal straining, or atrophic changes of the mucosa? Is there good vaginal tone with contraction of the pelvic floor? A careful site-specific examination of the vagina is required to answer these questions. A single-bladed speculum is used to evaluate the vaginal wall. Any type of prolapse (uterine, anterior, posterior, or apical vaginal wall) must be described and graded. The grade of prolapse is made during maximal vaginal straining. The type of vaginal defect is determined (paravaginal, transverse, or central cystocele, enterocele, apical vault prolapse). The presence or absence of vaginal fistula or palpable urethral diverticulum is determined.

Fecal incontinence (FI) is common with GSI.[41–43] The history of obstetrical tears, anorectal surgery, or inflammatory bowel disease must be noted. It is necessary to document loss of flatus, diarrhea, or solid stool. The office evaluation for FI includes sigmoidoscopy, anal manometry, anal ultrasound, and pudendal nerve terminal motor latency studies.[44–46]

Neurologic Examination

Several common neurologic diseases, such as multiple sclerosis and Parkinson's disease, can begin with a loss of bladder control. The neurologic exam must evaluate the cortical function down to the peripheral nerves that innervate the bladder. First, mental status, balance, and gait are tested. Since the sacral cord is important, the neurologic evaluation concentrates on the innervation of the lower extremities and sacral reflexes. Strength and deep tendon reflexes in the extremities are estimated. Sensation in the distribution of the pudendal nerve (S2-S4) is tested. Bulbocavernosus and anal wink reflexes test the sacral nerve roots.

Voiding Diary

A patient's history of voiding and leaking patterns is often inaccurate. A 24-hour or 7-day urolog documents frequency, fluid intake, and voiding patterns. The patient notes urinary incontinence episodes and associated events or symptoms such as laughing, coughing, or urgency. The maximum voided volume gives a fair estimate of maximum bladder capacity.

Q-Tip Test

Urethral hypermobility is an important component of GSI. With a patient in the supine position, a sterile, lubricated Q-tip is passed through the urethra into the bladder and then gently pulled back until resistance is met. During cough or maximal Valsalva maneuver, the excursion of the Q-tip from horizontal is measured and a measurement greater than 30° is considered abnormal. The test has poor specificity and continent women can have a positive test.[47] The sensitivity is good and most patients with GSI have a positive test.[48] Urinary incontinence and negative Q-tip test are associated with a high colposuspension failure rate.[49] These findings should alert the physician to the possibility of ISD. The Q-tip test is not diagnostic, but the results will give important early information.

Cough Stress Test

A standardized protocol is used for the cough stress test (CST) in our clinic. After filling the bladder to 300 mL, the patient is asked to cough vigorously several times while standing over a disposable pad. Patients with GSI tend to lose spurts of urine with each cough, while those with DI often leak a second or two after coughing and tend to leak a larger volume. CST is an objective test to identify the presence of urinary incontinence. It does not diagnose the type of incontinence.

Ultrasound

Ultrasound examination can be used to evaluate several conditions of the urinary system. Postvoid residual is often measured by ultrasound.[50] It can be used to assess the status of the bladder neck in GSI.[51,52] Several ultrasound techniques have been developed to quantitatively measure bladder neck and urethral hypermobility associated with GSI.[53–55] A transperineal ultrasound technique is used in our clinic to document preoperative urethral hypermobility. It is the first test done to determine if bladder neck hypermobility has recurred after colposuspension.[56]

Cystourethroscopy

A thorough examination of the bladder and urethra can identify several factors causing urinary symptoms. In our clinic, a 2.5-mm (7.5 French) flexible hysteroscope (Karl Storz, Storz Endoscopy, Culver City, CA) is used for cystoscopy, requiring no anesthesia. With the patient in the supine position, the bladder is carefully examined for stones, tumors, chronic inflammation, and detrusor trabeculations. The bladder neck is examined for chronic urethritis (shaggy fronds, erythema, and polyps) or atrophic changes, conditions that can cause urgency. To identify discharge from urethral diverticula the scope is slowly withdrawn, while massaging the urethra through the anterior vaginal wall. Urethral diverticula can mimic GSI symptoms.[57]

Dynamic cystourethroscopy consists of placing the scope 1 cm from the urethrovesical junction and instructing the patient to cough or strain maximally. An intact urethra will remain closed, but with GSI, it will open. When the bladder neck opens with valsalva, the patient is asked to stop her urinary stream (hold command). The bladder neck will close with the hold command if the urethral sphincter is intact. Inability to close the urethra could indicate peripheral neuropathy or a frozen urethra, signs consistent with ISD.[58]

Multichannel Urodynamics

The causes of urinary incontinence can be complex and multiple in nature. The basic indications for urodynamic testing are seen in Table 72–1. Many clinics suggest routine urodynamic testing,[12] but a complete discussion of this procedure is beyond the scope of this chapter. Essential measurements include filling cystometrics, urethral pressure profiles, pressure transmission ratios, surface EMG, valsalva leak point pressure, and uroflowmetry. The patient should be tested supine, sitting, and standing. Maneuvers such as coughing, maximal straining, heel jounces, and handwashing, should be carried out. The goal of these studies is to reproduce

TABLE 72–1. INDICATIONS FOR URODYNAMIC TESTING

History
  Prior or failed incontinence surgery
  Elderly patient
  Prior radiation or radical surgery
  Symptoms of severe incontinence
  Suspected neurologic disease
Clinical or Physical Findings
  High postvoid residual
  Abnormal neurologic exam
  Abnormal bladder capacity (high or low)
  Leaking with a negative Q-tip test
  Severe symptoms of urgency, frequency, or urge incontinence
  Absent bladder sensation

symptoms and leaking. After achieving the correct diagnosis from a complete evaluation, an adequate treatment plan can be devised.

LAPAROSCOPIC BURCH COLPOSUSPENSION

Technique

After making the diagnosis of GSI, the surgeon must decide on the desired incontinence procedure. The general categories of incontinence surgeries include colposuspension, needle suspension, and sling procedures. Most gynecologists consider the Burch colposuspension the gold standard. A laparoscopic Burch colposuspension employing the same technique as an open Burch will be presented here.

Pelvic reconstructive surgery often requires the repair of several defects in the same setting. It is unusual for a patient to require only a Burch procedure. It is important to consider the order of repairs to achieve maximum benefit. In general, our order starts with the posterior pelvic compartment, moving to the middle and anterior compartment, and doing the Burch last. The colposuspension is dependent on achieving the correct height of the bladder neck and doing the Burch last insures correct bladder elevation.

The patient is placed in the supine position in Allen stirrups. After establishing a pneumoperitoneum, four trocars are put in place. The infraumbilical and left lateral suprapubic trocars are 11 mm in diameter. The midline supra-pubic and right lateral trocars are 5 mm in diameter. After trocar placement, the patient is placed in moderate Trendeleburg position. Approximately 150 mL of methylene blue solution is placed in the bladder through a three-way 20-French Foley catheter to outline the bladder under the pubic arch. A circumscribing semilunar incision is made around the lateral pubic arch through the peritoneum. It is very important to find the correct plane when entering the space of Retzius, which should appear as fine areolar tissue with very little vascularity (Fig. 72–1). The entire paravaginal area and Cooper's ligament can be seen with the space of Retzius open. On the lateral pelvic sidewalls, the right and left arcus white line is identified. The pubocervical fascia (PCF) is part of the endopelvic fascia that forms a taut sheet from the right to the left arcus white line. The bladder and urethra rest on the PCF. Lateral (paravaginal) cystoceles occur when the PCF is pulled free of the arcus, allowing the bladder to bulge into this potential space. Paravaginal defects are repaired by suturing the PCF to the arcus white line with permanent sutures.

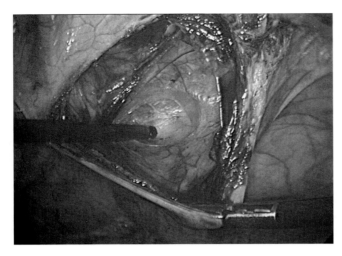

Figure 72–1. Opening the space of Retzius. Note the filmy areolar tissue. See Color Section.

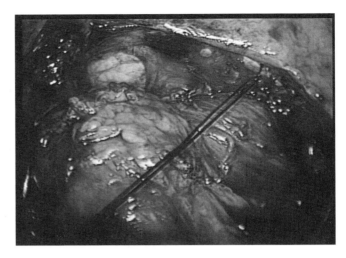

Figure 72–3. Suture placed through the right Cooper's ligament. See Color Section.

The surgical principles developed by Tanagho[59] are followed for the Burch colposuspension. First, the paravaginal fat is removed all the way to the pelvic sidewalls, staying 2 cm lateral to the urethra and bladder neck. The two Burch sutures are placed on the right and left side. The two distal sutures are 2 cm lateral to the midurethra and the proximal two sutures are 2 cm lateral to bladder neck. If the vaginal hand is used to elevate the PCF, suture placement is greatly aided (Fig. 72–2). With a delayed absorbable or permanent suture, a large needle is used to insure a substantial purchase on the PCF. All four sutures are passed through Cooper's ligament, and while the bladder neck is elevated with the vaginal hand, extracorporeal knots are tied (Fig. 72–3). Seven to eight knots are used. At the finish, a classic "dog-ear" repair can be seen (Fig. 72–4), which indicates the establishment of a hammock of PCF under the bladder neck to the midurethra (Fig. 72–5).

The patient is given indigo carmine intravenously as the last Burch sutures are being tied. Cystoscopy is performed to visualize the entire bladder mucosa, rule out perforation by sutures, and insure ureteral integrity. It is important to see dye coming from

both ureteral orifices, insuring no obstruction. As the cystoscope is removed, the urethra is checked carefully for possible crimping or perforation.

Following cystoscopy, the space of Retzius is closed, preventing peritoneal contents from pushing directly on the Burch hammock (Fig. 72–6). The weight of the abdominal contents could possibly tear the Burch sutures from the PCF. Closure also prevents pressure on paravaginal repairs, allowing healing and scarring to take place. If the correct surgical plane in the space of Retzius is entered, the Burch colposuspension is almost a bloodless procedure. It is rare for surgical drains to be necessary.

Postoperative Care

Postoperative catheterization can be by a Foley or suprapubic catheter. Because the catheter can often be removed in 24 to 48 hours, a Foley catheter is used in our clinic, primarily for expense. Our criterion for removal is that the patient must be able to void 80%

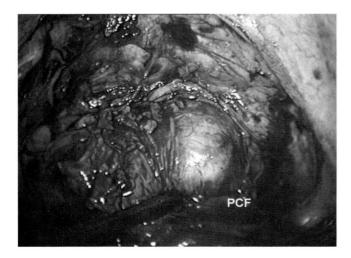

Figure 72–2. Elevation of the right pubocervical fascia with the vaginal hand. See Color Section.

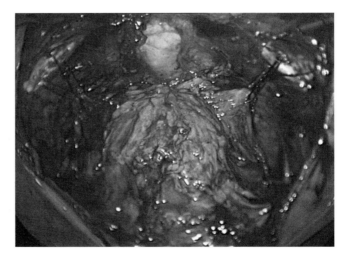

Figure 72–4. Completed Burch procedure. Note the "dog ears" formed as the pubocervical fascia is used to form a hammock under the bladder neck and urethra. See Color Section.

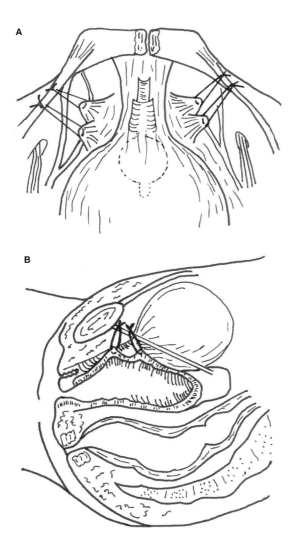

Figure 72–5. A. Anterior view of a completed Burch colposuspension. Note the elevation of the pubocervical fascia lateral to the bladder neck and urethra. **B.** Lateral view of Burch colposuspension demonstrating formation of the supporting hammock.

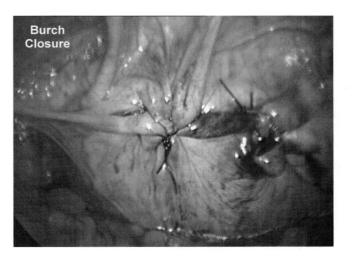

Figure 72–6. Closure of the space of Retzius. See Color Section.

of her intravesical volume. For an adequate test, the patient should have at least 200 mL of urine in the bladder before voiding. When postvoid residuals are 20% or less, catheter replacement is rare.

Patients are active on postoperative day one. Length of stay is less than 24 hours with laparoscopic Burch alone and some clinics report it as an outpatient procedure. A two-night stay is common when the Burch is combined with a laparoscopic hysterectomy. Most authors report less pain medication required by patients following laparoscopic surgery, which is in agreement with a shortened length of hospital stay.

Several postoperative instructions are important for patient recovery. Patients are instructed against heavy lifting (maximum of 10 pounds) or straining for 8 weeks. The liberal use of stool softeners and bulk laxatives should be prescribed and patients should be instructed to increase their fluid intake to prevent constipation. Cough suppression is important during recovery time.

Complications

Complications can be divided into short and long term. Reported rates range from zero to 24%. In most classical surgical procedures, bleeding and infection are usually the most common problems. In the initial reports on laparoscopic Burch, both of these problems appear to be low. The majority of studies report less blood loss with laparoscopic Burch than with open procedures. Because of the superior visualization, it seems hemostasis is easier to achieve. After several hundred procedures in our series, a small number of seromas in the space of Retzius have been found. None were infected or drained, resolving spontaneously. All of these occurred in patients with prior bladder surgery, which made dissections in the space of Retzius more difficult.

Complications inherent to laparoscopy can include trocar injury (bowel and vascular) and energy-related problems (mono- or bipolar burns). Bowel injuries most commonly occur at the time of entry. There is much debate on whether open or closed entry is safer. Most large series have not found any statistical difference in the two techniques, although the open technique decreases the chance of vascular injury. A thorough understanding of monopolar energy sources is mandatory for laparoscopic surgeons. Fortunately, with better equipment and more education, energy-related injuries seem to be on the decline.

A major criticism by some concerns a purported increase in bladder injuries with laparoscopy. In our experience, bladder perforation has not been common (less than 1%). The incidence is highest in patients with prior bladder surgery, and the injuries have been tears in the dome of the bladder. These tears are recognized immediately, because of the methylene blue installation, and are easily repaired. The defects are usually small and laparoscopic suturing adequately corrects the problem. Small bladder tears do not require prolonged catheterization.

Damage to ureters can occur with both laparoscopic and open Burch procedures, making intraoperative cystoscopy imperative. Harris et al[60] have shown overcorrection can obstruct the ureters by a kinking effect. It appears that placement of a suture around a ureter is less common.[61] Visualization of indigo carmine from both ureteral orifices guarantees ureteral integrity.

Long-term complications are the same for the laparoscopic Burch as with the open procedure. Recurrent urinary incontinence is the most common. This can be secondary to suture breakage, suture pull-through, or improper suture placement. Other predisposing factors influencing long-term failure include age, prior incontinence surgery, incorrect preoperative diagnosis, low-pressure urethra, de novo detrusor instability, chronic urinary retention, and posterior compartment defects (enterocele and rectocele). In one 5-year report,[62] no specific differences between open or laparoscopic procedures were reported. In our clinic, preliminary data suggest that prophylactic apical vault repair significantly decreases middle and posterior compartment defects commonly reported following Burch colposuspension.

Outcome

The first attempted laparoscopic incontinence procedure was by Vancaillie and Schuessler.[63] They attempted a Marshall-Marchetti-Krantz procedure in a small number of patients. Many early studies reported as Burch procedures had significant modifications, usually attempting to eliminate suturing. With these modifications, it is questionable whether these procedures should be called Burch colposuspensions. Modifications included surgical mesh,[64] staples,[65] and automatic suturing devices.[66] Liu and Paek[67] reported on laparoscopic Burch using the traditional Tanagho technique through an intraperitoneal approach, while others developed an extraperitoneal entry.[68,69] The extraperitoneal approach is limited by prior surgery and does not allow concomitant pelvic support procedures, which are usually necessary.

To adequately evaluate the effectiveness of the laparoscopic Burch-procedure long-term objective, preferably randomized studies are needed. Short-term data suggest similar objective cure rates between the open and laparoscopic colposuspension.[70,71] One 5-year objective study reported a similar cure rate to open Burch technique.[62] In this report, 87 women with GSI by objective and urodynamic testing had a laparoscopic Burch colposuspension using the evaluation and operative technique described in this chapter. Thirty-three had prior bladder surgery, 63 were menopausal, and 61 had prior hysterectomies. Patients with detrusor instability, intrinsic sphincter deficiency, or low-pressure urethra were excluded. Testing at 6 weeks and 1 and 5 years included cough stress tests and bladder neck ultrasound. Any symptom or sign of leaking resulted in repeat urodynamic testing. Cure rates of 95, 92, and 84% were obtained at 6 weeks, 1 year, and 5 years, respectively. These rates are comparable to three long-term studies seen in Table 72–2.[62,72–74] The adjusted cure rate represents patients lost to follow-up being considered as either all failures or all successes. All four of these studies had similar patient demographics, study criteria, urodynamic studies, and objective long-term follow-up.

Some studies suggest short and long-term outcome is poor with the laparoscopic Burch procedure.[75–77] Burton[75] had 60 patients randomized to the laparoscopic or open procedure. The laparoscopic cure rates were considerably worse than open rates at 1 year (73% versus 97%) and continued to decline at 3 years (60% versus 93%). The criticism of this trial is that Burton used absorbable suture with a very small needle. Reconstructive surgery requires a large purchase on tissue when suturing. In addition, Burton did not have sufficient experience with advanced laparoscopic surgery before starting this trial.

TABLE 72–2. LONG-TERM AND ADJUSTED CURE RATES FOR BURCH COLPOSUSPENSION[1]

	Objective 5-Year Cure (%)	All Failures (%)	All Successes (%)
Ross	84	74	87
Bergman	82	71	84
Stanton	79	69 plateau at 10 years	
Eriksen	82	66	84

[1]Objective cures represent patients seen at 5 years. All failures represent cure rate if all patients lost to follow-up had recurrent incontinence at 5 years. All successes represent cure rate if all patients lost to follow-up were continent.

Su et al[76] randomized 92 patients to laparoscopy versus laparotomy, with cure rates of 80% versus 96% at one year. There are significant differences in technique between their two procedures. The open technique consisted of three absorbable sutures on each side. The majority of the laparoscopic procedures had only one suture per side. The reason stated for using a single suture was that there was not sufficient room in the laparoscopic procedure for multiple sutures. In our experience, the paravaginal space is much easier to visualize and work in via the laparoscope than in open cases, which suggests operative inexperience by the Su et al group. Persson and Wolner-Hanssen[78] demonstrated, in a randomized study of 161 women, that a two-suture technique is superior to a one-suture technique. At one year the objective cure rate of two sutures was 83% versus 58% for single suture. Lobel and Davis[77] reported poor long-term data at 3 years with laparoscopy. Their procedure was a modified type of colposuspension more closely related to a needle suspension and is difficult to compare to a laparoscopic Burch-Tanagho colposuspension.

In the studies in Table 72–2, the incidence of de novo detrusor instability was 3% in the laparoscopic group, as compared to 15 and 25% in two of the laparotomy groups.[73,74] This low incidence has been constant in several hundred patients at our center and superior visualization with laparoscopy could play an important role. The video camera allows very precise dissection and placement of sutures, which possibly results in less chance of overcorrection of the bladder angle and urethra[79] or possible urethral muscle or nerve damage.[26] These possibilities are currently being investigated.

In several laparoscopic series, patients have been able to void spontaneously in 24 hours or less.[71,80,81] The reason for this finding is unknown. It could be due to less dissection close to the urethra, less overcorrection of urethral support, or less pain from smaller abdominal incision sites. Shorter hospital stays and returning to normal activities sooner is related to less pain with laparoscopic surgery.[81–83]

SUMMARY

There are conflicting reports as to the effectiveness of the laparoscopic Burch procedure, with some authors reporting significantly poorer outcomes and others reporting results similar to laparotomy. In the majority of studies with poor outcomes, several modifications have been made to the classical Burch-Tanagho procedure. The most common causes of failure relate to different suture technique, small needles, or single sutures on each side. Many studies that have closely followed the Burch-Tanagho technique have excellent results. Better laparoscopic outcomes are possible with careful patient selection, evaluation, and following the classic two-suture Burch technique. More long-term studies are necessary to confirm early reports and objective results must be reported. There is no reason that good outcomes cannot be achieved when the laparoscopic Burch colposuspension mirrors the open procedure, both in patient selection and in operative technique.

REFERENCES

1. Goldstein M, Hawthorne ME, Engeberg S, et al. Urinary incontinence. Why people do not seek help. *J Gerontol Nurs.* 1992;18:15.
2. Flood C, Drutz HP. Physicians' perception of urinary incontinence as a health care problem in women. *Int Urogynecol J.* 1995;6:89.
3. Burgio K, Matthews KA, Engel BT. Prevalence, incidence, and correlates of urinary incontinence in healthy, middle-aged women. *J Urol.* 1991;146:1255.
4. Nemar A, Middleton RP. Stress incontinence in young nulliparous women: Statistical study. *Am J Obstet Gynecol.* 1954;68:1166.
5. Abrams P, Blavias JG, Stanton SL, et al. Standardisation of terminology of lower urinary tract function. *Neurourol Urodynam.* 1988;7:403.
6. Sand PK, Hill, RC, Ostergard, DR. Incontinence history as a predictor of detrusor stability. *Obstet Gynecol.* 1988;71:257.
7. Berstein I, Sejr T, Able I, et al. Assessment of lower urinary tract symptoms in women by a self-administered questionnaire: Test-retest reliability. *Int Urogynecol J.* 1996;7:37.
8. Ramsay I, Ali HM, Heslington K, et al. Can scoring the severity of symptoms help to predict the urodynamic diagnosis? *Int Urogynecol J.* 1995;6:267.
9. DeLancey J. Structural support of the urethra as it relates to stress urinary incontinence: The hammock hypothesis. *Am J Obstet Gynecol.* 1994;170:1713.
10. Koonings P, Bergman A, Ballard CA. Low urethral presure and stress urinary incontinence in women: Risk factor for failed retropubic surgical procedure. *Urology.* 1990;36:245.
11. Sand P, Bowen LW, Panaganiban R, et al. The low pressure urethra as a factor in failed retropubic urethropexy. *Obstet Gynecol.* 1987;69:399.
12. Amaye-Obu FA, Drutz HP. Surgical management of recurrent stress urinary incontinence: A 12-year experience. *Am J Obstet Gynecol.* 1999;181:1296;discussion,1307.
13. Horbach N, Blanco JS, Ostergard DR. A suburethral sling procedure with polytetrafluoroethylene for treatment of genuine stress incontinence in patients with low urethral closure pressure. *Obstet Gynecol.* 1988;71:648.
14. Summitt R, Bent AE, Ostergard DR. Suburethral sling procedure for genuine stress incontinence and low urethral closure pressure: A continued experience. *Int Urogyn J.* 1992;3:18.
15. Kjolhede P, Ryden G. Clinical and urodynamic characteristics of women with recurrent urinary incontinence after Burch colposuspension. *Acta Obstet Gynecol Scand.* 1997;76:461.
16. Collas D, Malone-Lee JG. Age-associated changes in detrusor sensory function in women with lower urinary tract symptoms. *Int Urogynecol J.* 1996;7:24.
17. Cardozo L, Stanton SL, Williams JE. Detrusor instability following surgery for genuine stress incontinence. *Br J Urol.* 1979;51:204.
18. Abrams P, Blaivas JG, Stanton SL, et al. The standardization of lower urinary tract function recommended by the International Continence Society. *Int Urogynecol J.* 1990;1:45.
19. Sampselle C, Miller JM, Mims BL, et al. Effect of pelvic muscle exercise on transient incontinence during pregnacy and after birth. *Obstet Gynecol.* 1998;91:406.
20. Abu-Heija AT. Long-term results of colposuspension operation for genuine stress incontinence. *Asia Oceania J Obstet Gynaecol.* 1994;20:179.
21. Kjolhede P, Lindehammer H. Pelvic floor neuropathy in relation to the outcome of Burch colposuspension. *Int Urogynecol J.* 1997;8:61.
22. Parys B, Woolfenden KA, Parsons KF. Bladder dysfunction after simple hysterectomy: Urodynamic and neurological evaluation. *Eur Urol.* 1990;17:129.
23. Smith AR, Hosker GL, Warrell DW. The role of partial denervation of the pelvic floor in the aetiology of genitourinary prolapse and stress incontinence of urine. A neurophysiological study. *Br J Obstet Gynaecol.* 1989;96:24.
24. Anderson R. A neurogenic element to urinary stress incontinence. *Br J Obset Gynecol.* 1984;91:41.
25. Snooks S, Swash M. Abnormalities of the innervation of the urethral striated sphincter musculature in incontinence. *Br J Urol.* 1985;56:401.
26. Benson J, Lucente V, McClellan E. Vaginal versus abdominal reconstructive surgery for the treatment of pelvic support defects: A prospective randomized study with long-term evaluation. *Am J Obstet Gynecol.* 1996;175:1418.
27. Snooks S, Badenoch DF, Tiptaft RC, et al. Perineal nerve damage in genuine stress urinary incontinence: An electrophysiological study. *Br J Urol.* 1985;57:422.
28. Smith A, Hosker GL, Warrell DW. The role of partial denervation of the pelvic floor in the aetiology of genitourinary prolapse and stress incontinence of urine. A neurophysical study. *Br J Obstet Gynaecol.* 1989;96:24.
29. Gilpin S, Gosling JA, Smith AR,et al. The pathogenesis of genitourinary prolapse and stress incontinence of urine. A histological and histochemical study. *Br J Obstet Gynaecol.* 1989;96:15.
30. Fischer W, Pfister C, Tunn R. Comparison between histological, histochemical and clinical findings from musculature of pubococcygeal repair (pcr) in urinary incontinence. *Int Urogynecol J.* 1992;3:124.
31. Bergman A, Elia G, Cheung D, et al. Biochemical composition of collagen in continent and stress urinary incontinent women. *Gynecol Obstet Invest.* 1994;37:48.
32. Falconer C, Ekman G, Malmstrom A, et al. Decreased collagen synthesis in stress incontinent women. *Obstet Gynecol.* 1994;84:583.
33. Ulmsten U, Ekman G, Giertz G, et al. Different biochemical composition of connective tissue in continent and stress incontinent women. *Acta Obstet Gynecol Scand.* 1987;66:455.
34. Versi E, Cardozo L, Brincat M, et al. Correlation of urethral physiology and skin collagen in postmenopausal women. *Br J Obstet Gynaecol.* 1988;95:147.
35. Cosimo O, Pierluigi P, Angelo ZM, et al. A clinical and urodynamic study of patients with varying degrees of cystocele. *Maturitas.* 1997;27:125.
36. Harrison G, Memel DS. Urinary incontinence in women: Its prevalence and its management in a health promotion clinic. *Br J Gen Pract.* 1994;44:149.
37. Bhatia N, Bergman A, Karram MM. Effects of estrogen on urethral function in women with urinary incontinence. *Am J Obstet Gynecol.* 1989;160:176.
38. Nakanishi N, Tatara K, Naramura H, et al. Urinary and fecal incontinence in a community-residing older population in Japan. *J Am Geriatr Soc.* 1997;45:215.
39. Thorpe A, Roberts JP, Williams NS, et al. Pelvic floor physiology in women with faecal incontinence and urinary symptoms. *Br J Surg.* 1995;82:173.
40. Jackson SL, Weber AM, Hull TL, et al. Fecal incontinence in women with urinary incontinence and pelvic organ prolapse. *Obstet Gynecol.* 1997;89:423.
41. Jackson S, Weber AM, Hull TL, et al. Fecal incontinence in women with urinary incontinence and pelvic organ prolapse. *Obstet Gynecol.* 1997;89:423.

42. Peet S, Castleden CM, McGrother CW. Prevalence of urinary and faecal incontinence in hospitals and residential and nursing homes for
older people. *BMJ.* 1995;311:1063.

43. Nakanishi N, Tatara K, Naramura H, et al. Urinary and fecal incontinence in a community-residing older population in Japan. *J Am Geriatr Soc.* 1997;45:215.

44. Sultan A, Kamm MA, Hudson CN, et al. Anal-sphincter disruption
during vaginal delivery. *N Engl J Med.* 1993;329:1905.

45. Sangwan Y, Coller JA, Barrett RC, et al. Unilateral pudendal neuropathy impact on outcome of anal sphincter repair. *Dis Colon Rectum.* 1996;39:686.

46. Wexner S, Marchetti F, Salanga VD, et al. Neurophysiologic assessment of the anal sphincters. *Dis Colon Rectum.* 1991;34:606.

47. Montz F, Stanton SL. Q-tip test in female urinary incontinence.
Obstet Gynecol. 1986;67:258.

48. Bergman A, McCarthy TA, Ballard CA, et al. Role of the Q-tip test
in evaluating stress urinary incontinence. *J Reprod Med.* 1987;32:273.

49. Bergman A, Koonings PP, Ballard CA. Negative Q-tip test as a risk
factor for failed incontinence surgery in women. *J Reprod Med.* 1989;
34:193.

50. Bent A, Nahhas DE, McLennan MT. Portable ultrasound determination of urinary residual volume. *Int Urogynecol J.* 1997;8:200.

51. Versi E. The significance of an open bladder neck in women. *Br J
Urol.* 1991;68:42.

52. Schaer G, Koechli OR, Schuessler B, et al. Perineal ultrasound for
evaluating the bladder neck in urinary stress incontinence. *Obstet Gynecol.* 1995;85:220.

53. Bergman A, Vermesh M, Ballard CA, et al. Role of ultrasound in urinary incontinence evaluation. *Urology.* 1989;33:443.

54. Creighton S, Clark A, Pearce JM, et al. Perineal bladder neck ultrasound: Appearances before and after continence surgery. *Ultrasound
Obstet Gynecol.* 1994;4:428.

55. Demirci F, Kuyumcuoglu U, Uludogan M, et al. Evaluation of urethrovesical junction mobility by perineal ultrasonography in stress urinary incontinence. *J Pak Med Assoc.* 1996;46:2.

56. Ross J. Transperineal ultrasound measurement of urethro-vesical descent in genuine stress incontinence. *J Ultrasound Med.* 1995;14:72.

57. Scotti RJ, Ostergard DR, Guillaume AA, et al. Predictive value of urethroscopy as compared to urodynamics in the diagnosis of genuine
stress incontinence. *J Reprod Med.* 1990;35:772.

58. Robertson JR. Gynecologic urethroscopy. *Am J Obstet Gynecol.* 1972;
115:986.

59. Tanagho E. Colpocystourethropexy: The way we do it. *J Urol.* 1976;
116:751.

60. Harris R, Cundiff GW, Theofrastous JP, et al. The value of intraoperative cystoscopy in urogynecologic and reconstructive pelvic surgery.
Am J Obstet Gynecol. 1997;177:1367.

61. Virtanen HS, Kiilholma PJ, Makinen JI, et al. Ureteral injuries in conjunction with Burch colposuspension. *Int Urogynecol J.* 1995;6:114.

62. Ross J. 5-Year outcome of laparoscopic Burch for stress incontinence.
J Am Assoc Gynecol Laparosc. 1999;6:48 S.

63. Vancaillie T, Schuessler W. Laparoscopic bladder neck suspension.
J Laparoendosc Surg. 1991;13:169.

64. Ou C, Presthus J, Beadle E. Laparoscopic bladder neck suspension using hernia mesh and surgical staples. *J Laparoendosc Surg.* 1993;3:563.

65. Lyons T. Minimally invasive treatment of urinary stress incontinence
and laparoscopically directed repair of pelvic floor defects. *Clin Obstet Gynecol.* 1995;38:380.

66. Gunn G, Cooper RP, Gordon NS, et al. Use of a new device for en-
dospcoic sutureing in the laparoscopic Burch prodedure. *J Am Assoc
Gynecol Laparosc.* 1994;2:64.

67. Liu C, Paek W. Laparoscopic retropubic colposuspension (Burch procedure). *J Am Assoc Gynecol Laparoscp.* 1993;1:31.

68. Frankel G, Knatipong M. Sixteen-month experience with video-
assisted extraperitoneal laparoscopic bladder neck suspension.
J Endourol. 1995;9:259.

69. Gunn G. Laparoscopic versus preperitoneal Burch. *J Am Assoc Gynecol Laparosc.* 1995;2:S18.

70. Ross J. Laparoscopic Burch repair compared to laparotomy Burch for
cure of urinary stress incontinence. *Int Urogynecol J.* 1995;6:323.

71. Lam AM. Laparoscopic Burch colposuspension for stress incontinence.
Med J Aust. 1995;162:18.

72. Bergman A, Giovanni E. Three surgical procedures for genuine stress
incontinence: Five year follow-up of a prospective randomized study.
Am J Obstet Gynecol. 1995;173:66.

73. Gillon G, Stanton SL. Long-term follow-up of surgery for urinary incontinence in elderly women. *Br J Urol.* 1984;56:478.

74. Eriksen B, Hagen B, Eik-Nes SH, et al. Long-term effectiveness of the
burch colposuspension in female urinary stress incontinence. *Acta Obstet Gynecol Scand.* 1990;69:45.

75. Burton G. A randomized comparison of laparoscopic and open colposuspension. *Neurourol Urodyn.* 1993;13:497. Abstract.

76. Su T, Wang KG, Hsu Cy, et al. Pospective comparison of laparoscopic
and traditional colposuspensions in the treatment of genuine stress incontinence. *Acta Obstet Gynecol Scand.* 1997;76:576.

77. Lobel R, Davis G. Long-term results of laparoscopic Burch urethropexy. *J Am Assoc Gynecol Laparosc.* 1997;4:341.

78. Persson J, Wolner-Hanssen P. Laparoscopic Burch colposuspension
for stress urinary incontinence: A randomized comparison of one or
two sutures on each side of the urethra. *Obstet Gynecol.* 2000;95:151.

79. Rosenzweig BA, Pushkin S, Blumenfeld D, et al. Prevalence of abnormal urodynamic test results in continent women with severe genitourinary prolapse. *Obstet Gynecol.* 1992;79:539.

80. Liu C. Laparoscopic retropubic colposuspension (Burch procedure). A
review of 58 cases. *J Reprod Med.* 1993;38:526.

81. Ross J. Multichannel urodynamic evaluation of laparoscopic Burch colposuspension for genuine stress incontinence. *Obstet Gynecol.* 1998;91:55.

82. Miannay E, Cosson M, Lanvin D, et al. Comparison of open retropubic and laparoscopic colposuspension for treatment of stress urinary
incontinence. *Eur J Obstet Gynecol Reprod Biol.* 1998;79:159.

83. Malone-Lee J. Is detrusor instability and hypertrophy a smooth-
muscle disease of the lower urinary tract? *Lancet.* 1996;348:1395.

*L*aparoscopic Procedures
in Urology

Chapter Seventy-Three •••••••

Laparoscopic Prostatectomy

ROBERT N. CACCHIONE and GEORGE S. FERZLI

Laparoscopy had its origins in 1867, when Desormeaux examined the lower urinary tract using a rigid hollow tube and an alcohol lamp for illumination.[1] A decade later Nitze, who was a general practitioner, used a 7-mm telescope to examine the lower urinary tract.[2] The twentieth century witnessed a greatly expanded role for laparoscopy in all areas, including the management of urologic problems. These included kidney biopsy,[3] nephrectomy,[4] partial nephrectomy,[5] management of renal cysts,[6] pyeloplasty,[7] ureterolithotomy,[8] ureterolysis,[9] ligation of varices,[10] management of undescended testes,[11] bladder neck suspension,[12] and pelvic lymph node dissection.[13] It was thus only a matter of time before laparoscopy would be applied to prostatectomy.

Our own experience began with extraperitoneal laparoscopic inguinal hernia repair. As we gained more experience with the technique, we realized the ease with which pelvic lymph node dissection and bladder neck suspension could be performed. We also began to perform more sigmoid and rectal procedures through the laparoscope, which brought the necessary experience in the pelvis to begin to approach the prostate.

In this country approximately 180,000 men are diagnosed with prostate cancer each year, and 35,000 die of it. It has become the most prevalent cancer in American men and the second leading killer. Suspicion of the disease is based on history, digital rectal exam, and prostate specific antigen (PSA) level with transrectal ultrasound and biopsy confirming the diagnosis and further characterizing the cancer.

Options for treatment of localized prostate cancer range from watchful waiting, through radiation therapy, to surgical excision. The choice of therapy is based on disease stage, comorbidities, age, life expectancy, and patient preference. The decision to proceed with surgical management is a culmination of both the art and the science of urology, and is beyond the scope of this chapter.

SELECTION OF PATIENTS

Because the laparoscopic procedure differs primarily in its means of access, the indications for it are identical to those for open prosta-

tectomy. Patients should have localized disease, minimal comorbid conditions, and a life expectancy of more than 10 years. A history of prior abdominal surgery might make the procedure more demanding, and should be considered a relative contraindication.

PREOPERATIVE PREPARATION

The procedure, alternatives, risks, and possible complications are discussed with the patient and family prior to surgery, as is the possibility that it may be necessary to convert to an open procedure. We typically have our patients complete a mechanical bowel prep to reduce the risk of infectious complications should injury to the rectum occur. Preoperative antibiotics are administered.

Patients undergoing radical prostatectomy are at risk of developing deep venous thrombosis (DVT). This is because (1) the creation of a pneumoperitoneum to 15 mm Hg pressure impedes venous return; (2) the dissection sometimes requires manipulation of the iliac veins, particularly if a pelvic lymph node dissection is performed; and (3) hematologic factors related to the cancer favor thrombogenesis. Prophylaxis against DVT is thus required until the patient is ambulatory. We usually use sequential compression stockings, but an alternative is subcutaneously administered heparin or low-molecular-weight heparin.

EQUIPMENT AND ROOM ARRANGEMENT

The anesthesiologist and anesthesia machine are stationed at the head of the operating table during the entire procedure, with the monitor at the foot of the table. The surgeon and assistant stand opposite each other, and the scrub nurse is beside the assisting surgeon, toward the patient's feet.

The patient is placed supine on the operating table with both arms well padded and tucked securely at his sides. He should be positioned so that the break in the operating table falls between the umbilicus and the anterior superior iliac spine. The table can then be flexed to open a view of the pelvis (Fig. 73–1). The area to be

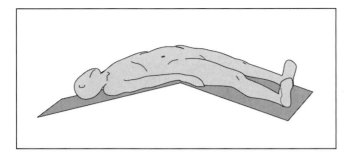

Figure 73–1. The patient is positioned supine with his arms at his sides. The table can be flexed to open the view to the pelvis.

exposed extends from the xyphoid process to the upper thigh, and should be shaved and prepped appropriately. A Foley catheter is manipulated, removed, and reinserted during the procedure. For this reason, the penis and scrotum are prepped in the operating field, and a sterile Foley catheter and collection bag are placed once the sterile drapes have been arranged. A nasogastric tube is also inserted to ensure adequate decompression and drainage of the stomach.

STEPS OF THE PROCEDURE

For those unfamiliar with excision of the prostate, we like to present it as being analogous to the dissection of a tumor at the esophagogastric junction (Fig. 73–2). In this analogy, the esophagus and urethra are equivalent structures, as are the stomach and bladder. The esophagogastric tumor represents the prostate. The vagus nerves travel alongside the esophagogastric tumor just as the cavernous nerves travel beside the prostate. The goal of these operations is to remove the tumor (prostate), while preserving the integrity of the nerves, and then to restore esophagogastric (vesicourethral) continuity. The operation proceeds in the tight confines of the subdiaphragmatic space (pelvis), sandwiched between the liver (pubic symphysis) anteriorly and the aorta (rectum) posteriorly.

The operation begins on the posterior surface of the bladder, where the seminal vesicles are dissected from their close approximation to the bladder (Fig. 73–3). The prostate is separated from the rectum, which is posterior to it. The anterior surface is

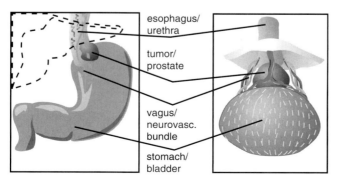

esophagus/
urethra

tumor/
prostate

vagus/
neurovasc.
bundle

stomach/
bladder

Figure 73–2. Prostatectomy can be viewed figuratively as analogous to resecting an esophagogastric junction tumor.

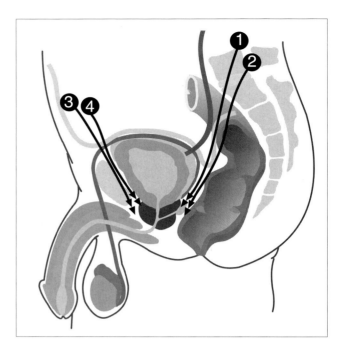

Figure 73–3. The anterior and posterior steps of the procedure. **1.** Liberation of the seminal vesicles. **2.** Development of the plane between the prostate and rectum. **3.** Anterior dissection to the prostatic apex and transection of the urethra. **4.** Excision of the prostate from the bladder neck.

approached, and the dorsal venous complex found and secured. The urethra is divided below the prostate, and the prostate is then excised from its connection to the bladder. Finally, the anastomosis is created.

Trocar Placement

The operation is accomplished through five operating ports, arranged in a line level with the umbilicus (Fig. 73–4). The umbilical port is 10 mm in size. A 10-mm, zero-degree laparoscope is inserted at this site and remains there through most of the procedure. The next two ports are 5 mm in size and are placed along the lateral rectus borders. These are used to introduce operating instruments and sutures. If needed, one or both may be enlarged to accommodate a 10-mm clip applier. The most lateral ports are also 5 mm in size and are placed just medial and superior to the anterior superior iliac spines. These are used to introduce operating and retracting instruments, as well as the suction-irrigation cannula.

An alternative arrangement for placement of the five operating ports is in the shape of a diamond with its highest point at the umbilicus (Fig. 73–5). The outer ports are placed a few centimeters lateral to the rectus borders in the iliac fossa. The lowermost port is placed just above the superior extent of the bladder. We have found this arrangement useful in thin patients, in whom the pelvis is very narrow.

Exposure and Dissection of the Seminal Vesicles

The seminal vesicles are located posterior to the bladder, and are covered by peritoneum. This peritoneum is opened over the vasa deferentia bilaterally. Both vasa are divided and traced medially and inferiorly toward the seminal vesicles. Care must be taken

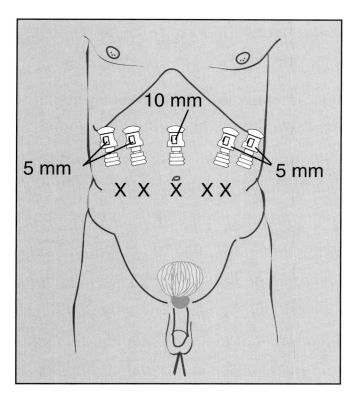

Figure 73–4. Trocar placement.

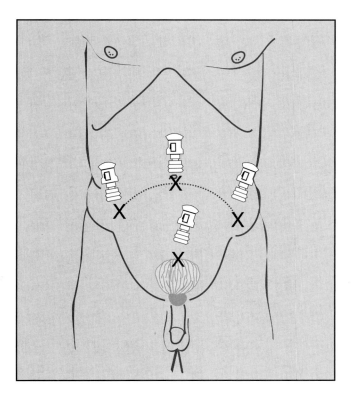

Figure 73–5. Alternative trocar placement.

during this first portion of the procedure to avoid injury to the ureters, which pass posteriorly and inferiorly to the vasa deferentia as they enter the posterior bladder (Fig. 73–6). The distal vasa deferentia and seminal vesicles are completely dissected from the posterior bladder.

Posterior Dissection of the Prostate

The seminal vesicles lead directly to the prostate in the midline superiorly. The dissection continues posteriorly and inferiorly through Denonvilliers' fascia, separating the prostate anteriorly from the rectum posteriorly. Once the urogenital diaphragm is reached, the dissection proceeds laterally. The cavernous nerves are located just lateral to the prostate, and are encountered for the first time during this part of the dissection.

Anterior Dissection

The peritoneum is opened anteriorly between the dome of the bladder and the pubic symphysis. This space of Retzius is opened bluntly. The pubic symphysis is cleared, and Cooper's ligaments and the superior rami of the pubis are identified.

The obturator nerve is located deep to Cooper's ligaments and the superior rami, and the external iliac veins are located laterally as they pass through the femoral ring. The lymph nodes are located just medial to the external iliac veins and anterior to the obturator nerves. The boundaries of nodal dissection are the circumflex iliac vein distally, the obturator nerve posteriorly, and the internal iliac vessels superiorly. When lymph node dissection is performed in conjunction with prostatectomy, it is performed at the beginning of the procedure.

The anterior dissection continues beyond the pubic symphysis to the prostatic apex. The puboprostatic ligaments are transected. Care must be taken to avoid cutting the dorsal venous plexus of Santorini before it is ligated, as major bleeding will result. The veins are ligated with sutures (Fig. 73–7) and then divided. The lateral dissection of the prostate then leads to the second view of the cavernous nerves, this time from the anterior aspect.

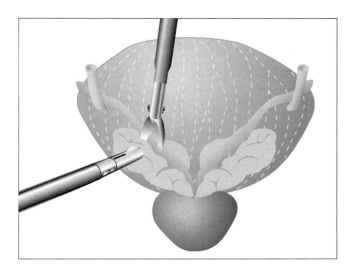

Figure 73–6. Arrangement of seminal vesicles, vasa deferentia, and ureters.

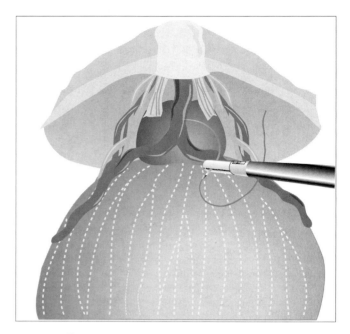

Figure 73–7. Ligation of the dorsal venous complex.

Excision of the Prostate

The urethra is transected at the prostatic apex (Fig. 73–8). As the urethra is being divided, the Foley catheter becomes visible. After the prostate is detached from the urethra, the catheter can be used as a handle to provide cephalad traction on the prostate for better visualization of the junction between bladder and prostate. Additionally, the balloon of the Foley catheter can be inflated to

30 cc, which may further improve visualization of the bladder–prostate junction. The bladder neck is then divided, and the catheter removed. If the bladder neck is opened too far from the junction between bladder and prostate, injury to the ureteral orifices on the posterior aspect of the bladder can occur. The prostate and attached seminal vesicles are placed in a retrieval bag. After the specimen is moved out of the pelvis, a diligent search for potential bleeding points in the operative field must be undertaken. The rectum is examined carefully for inadvertent injury; this may require digital rectal examination to be complete.

The Anastamosis

The final goal is to connect the bladder neck to the urethra. This is accomplished by careful placement of six interrupted sutures, using absorbable suture material. It may be necessary to narrow the opening of the bladder neck if there is a mismatch in size between it and the urethra. This is also done using absorbable sutures, in either a running or interrupted fashion. Sutures for the anastamosis are planned so that the posterior ones are placed first, and so that knots are tied on the outside of the bladder (Fig. 73–9). These are some of the most challenging and technically demanding sutures to place. During the course of suturing, a large-bore Foley catheter with a 30-cc balloon is placed through the anastamosis into the bladder.

Once this process is completed, a closed suction drain is placed through one of the lateral ports and directed near the suture line. Finally, inflating the bladder with saline tests the anastamosis for potential leaking points. The operating ports are removed, and all ports 1 cm or larger are closed with suture at the fascial level.

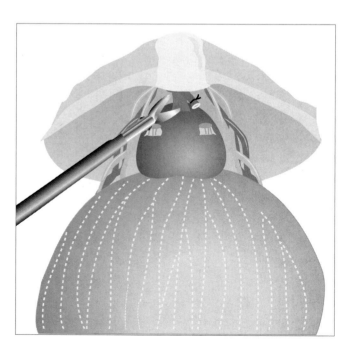

Figure 73–8. Transecting the urethra.

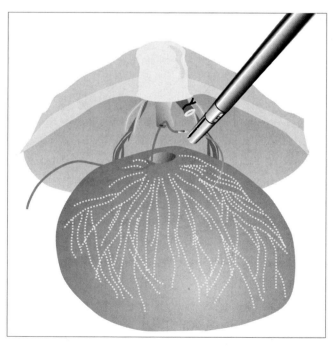

Figure 73–9. The anastamosis.

POSTOPERATIVE CARE

The nasogastric tube is removed in the recovery room after postoperative nausea has subsided. A normal diet is resumed on the first postoperative day. Patients are encouraged to sit in a chair on the night of surgery, and to ambulate on the first postoperative day. Once ambulatory status is achieved, DVT prophylaxis is discontinued. Most patients are ready for discharge from the hospital by the third postoperative day; the Foley catheter is left in place for 5 to 7 days.

RESULTS

Schuessler et al reported the first laparoscopic radical prostatectomy in 1992.[14] Then in 1997 they described 9 patients who had undergone the procedure, with operative times averaging 9.4 hours.[15] All of these men remained continent postoperatively, and there was a 50% postoperative potency rate. However, based on this small series, the authors concluded that the laparoscopic procedure offered no real advantage over the open approach for length of stay, postoperative pain, or cosmetic result, which have generally been considered the major advantages of laparoscopic techniques applied to other surgical procedures.

Also in 1997, Raboy and Ferzli reported on their technique for laparoscopic radical prostatectomy performed with a totally extraperitoneal approach.[16] A later report on two patients by these authors[17] was encouraging in that operative time was reduced to an average of just under 5 hours.

In 2000, Abbou et al reported on their experience with 43 patients.[18] Using a reproducible standardized technique, they showed a reduction in operative time to 4.3 hours. Short-term oncologic results were similar to the open procedure, with a positive margin rate of 27.9% and a 1-month postoperative PSA level of less than 0.1 ng/mL in all patients. Of these, 84% were fully continent.

Most encouraging has been the experience of Guillonneau and Vallancien from Paris.[19] In their experience with 260 patients, operative time has been reduced to 3 hours, hospital stay to 3 days, and the Foley catheter was removed prior to discharge. For the most recent 120 patients in their series, operative blood loss was 250 mL, and none required blood transfusion.

COMPLICATIONS

As with most surgical procedures, the associated risks can be categorized as general complications, which can occur during or as a result of any surgical procedure; and procedure-specific complications, which in this case are related to the use of laparoscopy or the performance of prostatectomy. The general complications associated with laparoscopic prostatectomy are intraoperative or postoperative hemorrhage that might require transfusion, wound infection that might develop at the port site incisions, port site hernias, and anesthesia-related complications. The procedure-specific complications are intraoperative injury to the ureters or rectum, postoperative leak at the vesicourethral anastamosis, deep venous thrombus formation, incontinence, and impotence. Although port-site tumors have been reported following laparoscopic pelvic lymphadenectomy, this has not yet been reported following laparoscopic prostatectomy. The true rate of complications following laparoscopic prostatectomy is not yet known, as even the largest patient series are still rather small.

CONCLUSION

The laparoscopic approach to radical prostatectomy has been shown to be a safe although technically difficult procedure. Once the learning curve is surmounted, the available data suggest that it is comparable to the open procedure in terms of operating time and short-term oncologic and functional results. Further data on large patient groups are still lacking regarding the procedure's long-term oncologic efficacy and functional outcome. Furthermore, there are as yet no studies available comparing laparoscopic radical prostatectomy and open retropubic techniques.

The laparoscopic approach to radical prostatectomy differs from other minimally invasive techniques in that the potential benefit lies not in shorter hospital stays or in improved cosmetic results. These benchmarks appear to be the same with laparoscopic and open procedures. The expected benefits are anticipated to result from the greater magnification afforded by the laparoscope. It is reasonable to expect that reduced operative blood loss will result. Additionally, this elegant dissection may well avoid injury to the neurovascular bundles, ultimately preserving potency.

ACKNOWLEDGMENT

The authors would like to acknowledge the artistic work of William Koslosky, MD, who created the illustrations appearing in this chapter.

REFERENCES

1. Desormeaux A. The endoscope and its application to the diagnosis and treatment of urinary affections. *Chicago Med J.* 1867;24:177.
2. Berci G. History of laparoscopy. In: Andrus CH, Cosgrove JM, Longo WE, eds. *Minimally Invasive Surgery: Principles and Outcomes.* Amsterdam: Harwood Academic Publishers, 1998;1–12.
3. Healey D, Newman R, Choen M, et al. Laparoscopically assisted percutaneous renal biopsy. *J Urol.* 1993;150:1218.
4. Kavoussi L, Kerbl K, Capelouto C, et al. Laparoscopic nephrectomy for renal neoplasia. *Urology.* 1993;42:603.
5. Winfield H, Donovan J, Godet A, et al. Laparoscopic partial nephrectomy: Initial case report for benign disease. *J Endourol.* 1993;7:521.
6. Sidney R, John H, Daniel P, et al. Laparoscopic ablation of symptomatic renal cysts. *J Urol.* 1993;150:1103.
7. Schuessler W, Grune M, Tecuanhuey L, et al. Laparoscopic dismembererd pyeloplasty. *J Urol.* 1993;150:1795.
8. Raboy A, Ferzli G, Ioffreda R, et al. Laparoscopic ureterolithotomy. *Urology.* 1992;39:223.
9. Kavoussi L, Clayman R, Brunt L, et al. Laparoscopic ureterolysis. *J Urol.* 1992;147:426.
10. Donovan J, Winfield H. Laparoscopic varix ligation. *J Urol.* 1992;147:77.
11. Lowe D, Brock W, Kaplan G. Laparoscopy for localization of nonpalpable testes. *J Urol.* 1984;134:728.
12. Albala D, Schuessler W, Vancaille T. Laparoscopic bladder neck suspension. *J Endourol.* 1992;6:137.
13. Ferzli G, Trapasso J, Raboy A, et al. Extraperitoneal endoscopic pelvic lymph node dissection. *J Laparoendosc Surg.* 1992;2:39.

14. Schuessler W, Kavoussi L, Clayman R, et al. Laparoscopic radical prostatectomy: Initial case report. *J Urol* 1992;147(suppl): 246A.

15. Schuessler W, Schulam P, Clayman R, et al. Laparoscopic radical prostatectomy: Initial short term experience. *Urology.* 1997;50:849.

16. Raboy A, Ferzli G, Albert P. Initial experience with extraperitoneal endoscopic radical retropubic prostatectomy. *Urology.* 1997;50:849.

17. Raboy A, Albert P, Ferzli G. Early experience with extraperitoneal endoscopic radical retropubic prostatectomy. *Surg Endosc.* 1998;12: 1264.

18. Abbou C, Salomon L, Hoznek A, et al. Laparoscopic radical prostatectomy: Preliminary results. *Urology.* 2000;55:630.

19. Guillonneau B, Vallancien G: Laparoscopic radical prostatectomy: The Montsouris technique. *J Urol.* 2000;163:1643.

Chapter Seventy-Four • • • • • •

*L*aparoscopic Pelvic Lymphadenectomy in Prostate Cancer

ROBERT G. MOORE, DONALD MEHAN, and RAUL O. PARRA

Prostate cancer is the most common malignancy in the male patient. Many new medical advances have been used to diagnose, stage, and treat prostate cancer. Laparoscopic pelvic lymphadenectomy (LPLD) has been employed since 1989 to stage prostate cancer.[1]

Current radiographic imaging techniques (computed tomography and magnetic resonance imaging) have proven to be ineffective in predicting lymph node involvement by prostate cancer.[2–4] The addition of fine-needle aspiration does not improve the diagnostic accuracy of these imaging techniques. Pathologic assessment of nodal tissue is the only method to accurately predict involvement of pelvic lymph nodes by prostate cancer.

INDICATIONS

The incidence of pelvic lymph node involvement with prostate cancer in the pre-prostate specific antigen (PSA) era is reported to be greater than 20%.[4] Contemporary reviews (since 1987) have demonstrated a 5 to 10% incidence of pelvic lymph node metastases at the time of radical prostatectomy.[5]

Histologic involvement of pelvic lymph nodes in a patient with otherwise clinically localized prostate cancer dramatically changes the prognosis and treatment in this group of patients. In order to better predict micro-metastases, clinical models based on serum PSA, Gleason's score/grade, and clinical stage have been developed; indications for laparoscopic pelvic lymph node dissection include patients with greater than 20% predicted probability of having micro-metastases based on the models.[6] Elevated PSA greater than 20 ng/mL and a Gleason's score of 8 or greater are specific indications for LPLD.

Contraindications to laparoscopic pelvic lymphadenectomy are similar to contraindications for general laparoscopy. Absolute contraindications include bleeding disorders and severe cardiopulmonary disease. Relative contraindications include prior pelvic surgery, prior hip prosthesis, and a history of diverticulitis.

OPERATIVE TECHNIQUE

Laparoscopic Pelvic Lymphadenectomy

Only routine preoperative anesthesia care is needed (a bowel preparation is not necessary). All patients undergoing interventional laparoscopic procedures should have general anesthesia. The patient is placed in supine position with both arms adducted and secured to the operative table via 2-inch cloth tape across the chest. The bladder and stomach are decompressed with a Foley catheter and an orogastric tube, respectively. The patient is positioned in the Trendelenburg position to move the bowels out of the pelvis for trocar placement. The entire anterior abdominal wall is prepped and draped.

Intraoperitoneal access can be obtained by two techniques: open and closed. For the closed technique, a pneumoperitoneum is obtained via a Veress needle prior to initial trocar placement. The abdominal wall is retracted upward by placing a Kocker clamp on the inferior portion of the umbilicus. With counter-traction from the upward pull of the Kocker clamp, a Veress needle is introduced into the peritoneal cavity through the base of the umbilicus. After intraperitoneal access is confirmed, insufflation is initiated at a low flow rate (1 L/min). Opening pressures for intraperitoneal insufflation are less than 5 mm Hg. When intra-abdominal inflation is confirmed, insufflation is increased to 4 to 5 L/min.

The open technique of intra-abdominal access involves the direct placement of a Hasson cannula into the abdominal cavity. A 10-mm infraumbilical incision is made. The rectus fascia is exposed and a vertical fascial incision is made. In addition, the posterior sheath of the rectus fascia and peritoneum are incised vertically. Two stay sutures (2-0 vicryl) are placed on each side of all layers. A 10-mm laparoscopic cannula is backloaded onto a zero-degree laparoscopic lens and placed into the peritoneal cavity under direct vision.

The fan trocar configuration (Fig. 74–1a) is used when performing laparoscopic pelvic lymphadenectomy. During placement of secondary trocars, the intraperitoneal pressure is increased to 20 mm Hg. After placement of secondary trocars, the intra-abdominal pressure is decreased to 15 mm Hg.

Midline intraperitoneal orientation can be readily obtained by pulling on the Foley catheter. The Foley catheter balloon is seen in the midline. Additional intraperitoneal landmarks include the urachus, vas deferens, iliac vessels, internal inguinal ring, and gonadal vessels (Fig. 74–2).

The node dissection is initiated on the side with the greatest chance of being histologically positive (based on previous biopsies or radiographic abnormalities). The operative table is repositioned with this side up. Any intraperitoneal adhesions are taken down by sharp dissection with laparoscopic scissors.

A peritoneotomy is performed lateral and parallel to the medial umbilical ligament starting just medial to the internal inguinal ring and stopping at the bifurcation of the common iliac vessels.[7] The vas deferens is divided with electrocautery by using 5-mm laparoscopic scissors. The external iliac vein is exposed by gently spreading tissue under the incised vas. The external iliac vein is the lateral extent of the lymphadenectomy. Nodal tissue is swept off the medial and inferior surfaces of external iliac vein and pelvic side wall (Fig. 74–3).

The medial extent of the pelvic lymphadenectomy is the medial umbilical ligament. This structure is grasped and retracted medially. All nodal tissue is dissected off the medial umbilical ligament and bladder. The inferior extent of the node dissection is the pubic ramus. This structure is easily identified by following the nodal package inferiorly. Using a combination of blunt dissection, laparoscopic clips, and electrocautery, the inferior portion of the nodal tissue is detached from the pubic bone.

The obturator vessels and nerves are exposed by retracting the distal nodal packet upward and superiorly (Fig. 74–4). With blunt dissection the package is dissected off the nerve and pelvic side

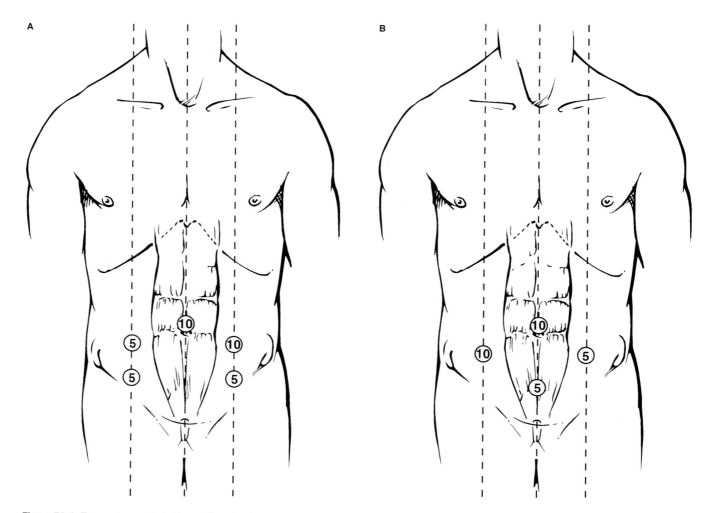

Figure 74–1. Trocar placement. **A.** Fan configuration for laparoscopic lymphadenectomy. **B.** Diamond configuration for extraperitoneal endoscopic pelvic lymph node dissection. The circled numbers denote trocar size.

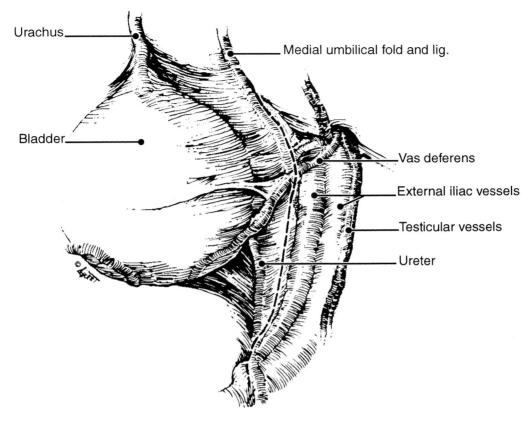

Figure 74–2. Pelvic anatomic intraperitoneal landmarks. Dotted line demonstrates the initial peritoneotomy.

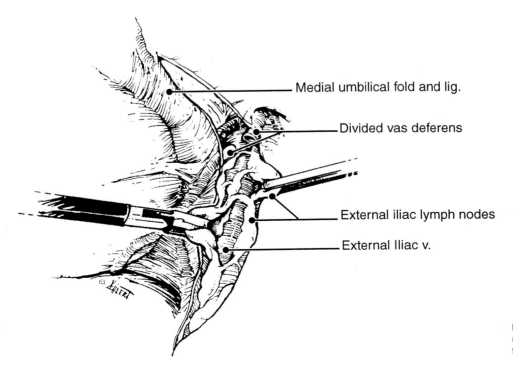

Figure 74–3. The later border of the laparoscopic pelvic lymphadenectomy is the external iliac vein.

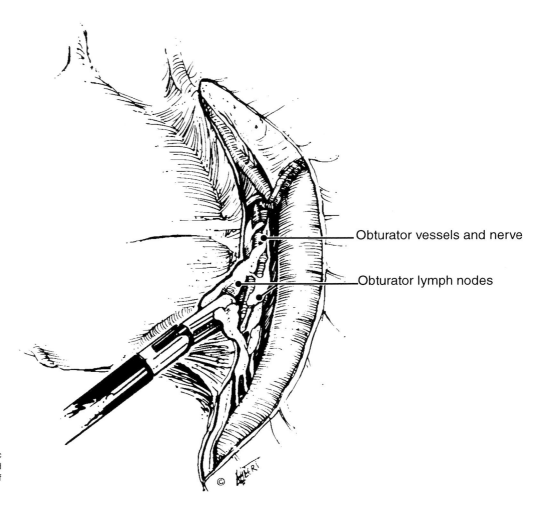

Figure 74–4. Completion of pelvic lymphadenectomy is accomplished by rolling the lymph node packet off the obturator vessels and nerve.

Obturator vessels and nerve

Obturator lymph nodes

wall up to the common iliac bifurcation. The ureter is identified crossing the common iliac vessels. The superior portion of the nodal packet is freed with sharp dissection and clips. The nodal package is removed through a 10-mm cannula via a spoon-billed grasper. If the lymph node packet is felt to be suspicious for malignancy, a frozen section is performed prior to proceeding with the contralateral lymphadenectomy. After completion of both sides of the pelvic lymphadenectomy, the obturator space is inspected for signs of hemorrhage with the peritoneal pressure at 5 to 8 mm Hg.

Extraperitoneal Endoscopic Lymphadenectomy

Preoperative preparation and anesthesia are the same as used for laparoscopic pelvic lymphadenectomy. A 1.5-cm vertical skin incision is made 2 to 3 cm inferior to the umbilicus. The anterior rectus fascia is exposed and incised vertically just off the midline. Stay sutures (2-0 vicryl) are placed on each side of the fascia. Digital dissection is performed deep in the anterior rectus fascia and rectus muscle but superficial to the posterior rectus sheath and peritoneum.

The extraperitoneal space can be developed with either balloon dilation or blunt dissection with the zero-degree laparoscope. Two different types of balloon dilators have been used. A commercially available balloon (Origin Medical Systems, Laguna Hills, CA) has the distinct advantage of allowing direct visualization of the space being dilated. Unfortunately this balloon is very expensive. A cheaper alternative is a balloon fashioned from the middle finger of a latex surgical glove and attached to an 18 French red rubber catheter by 2-0 silk. After creation of an adequate extraperitoneal working space a 10-mm laparoscopic cannula is placed at the infraumbilical site.

A second trocar (5 mm) is placed 2 cm above the pubic ramus. A 5-mm scissor is introduced through this port and the lateral aspects of the extraperitoneal space are developed (laterally toward the anterior superior iliac spine). Two additional trocars (one 5 and one 10 mm) are placed on the right and left sides in the midclavicular line (diamond trocar configuration, Fig. 74–1B).

Extraperitoneal landmarks are identified by pulsation of the external iliac artery laterally and the Foley balloon in the midline. Nodal dissection is performed in a manner similar to the transperitoneal approach. The fascia on all 10-mm trocars is closed to prevent hernia formation.

OUTCOMES

Outcomes of new surgical procedures are assessed by comparing them to established procedures. The gold standard for pelvic lymph node extraction for prostate cancer is open pelvic lymphadenectomy (OPLD). Comparisons should be made in terms of nodal tissue removed, operative time, and postoperative morbidity.

Several investigators have performed a direct comparison with OPLD and have demonstrated that laparoscopic pelvic lymphadenectomy (LPLD) was equal with regard to lymph node yield.[9,10] Laparoscopic pelvic lymphadenectomy has been shown to cause less postoperative morbidity. Narcotic requirement was decreased (1.55 versus 47 mg of morphine). Hospital stay (1.7 versus 5.37 days) and return to full activity (10.8 versus 65.5 days) were shorter for LPLD compared to OPLD.[10] With regard to operative time, LPLD takes approximately 1 hour longer but experience can decrease this by 30 minutes.[11]

Comparison of LPLD to extraperitoneal endoscopic pelvic lymphadenectomy (EEPD) in a randomized trial demonstrated EEPD to require significantly less operative time (117.3 versus 86.9 minutes).[12] The complication rate for EEPD was greater than that for LPLD, with a higher conversion rate to open procedure, epigastric artery injury, and lymphocele formation.

The complication rate for LPLD during early experience is 15%.[13] Increased surgeon experience decreases the complication rate to 4%.[14]

NEW DEVELOPMENT

New advances in laparoscopic instruments and lenses have recently been introduced. Several instrument companies have successfully manufactured minilaparoscopic ($\leq$4 mm) instruments. Prospective randomized trials comparing minilaparoscopic instruments to traditional laparoscopic instruments (5 to 12 mm) used in performing laparoscopic pelvic infertility procedures have demonstrated equivalence between both sets of instruments.[15] Our group at Saint Louis University has successfully performed LPLD with minilaparoscopic instruments. These new instruments eliminate three 5-mm and one 10-mm laparoscopic ports. Three 4-mm instrument cannulas are used for LPLD, while only one 10-mm cannula is needed for removal of lymph nodes. The elimination of larger cannulas can potentially decrease postoperative morbidity.

CONCLUSION

With the advent of new minimally invasive methods (cryotherapy and brachytherapy) to treat prostate cancer, the importance of accurate histologic staging of pelvic lymph nodes is always important. Minimally invasive technique should be used to assess pelvic nodal tissue when there is a greater than 20% chance of micrometastasis.[16]

REFERENCES

1. Schuessler WW, Vancaillie TG, Reich IT, et al. Transperitoneal endosurgical lymphadenectomy in patients with prostate cancer. *J Urol.* 1991;145:988.
2. Benson KH, Watson RA, Sprihg DB, et al. The value of computerized tomography in evaluation of pelvic lymph nodes. *J Urol.* 1981;126:63.
3. Hricak H. Noninvasive imaging for staging of prostate cancer: Magnetic resonance imaging, computerized tomography and ultrasound. *NCI Monogram.* 1988;7:31.
4. Fowler JE Jr, Whitmore WH Jr. The incidence and extent of pelvic lymph node metastases in apparently localized prostate cancer. *Cancer.* 1981;47:2941.
5. Partin AW, Pound CR, Clemens JQ, et al. Serum PSA after anatomical radical prostatectomy: The Johns Hopkins experience after 10 years. *Urol Clin North Am.* 1993;20:713.
6. Partin AW, Yoo J, Carter HB, et al. The use of prostate specific antigen, clinical stage, and Gleason's score to predict pathological stage in men with localized prostate cancer. *J Urol.* 1993;150:110.
7. Moore RG, Kavoussi LR. Laparoscopic lymphadenectomy in genitourinary malignancies. *Surg Oncol.* 1993;2:51.
8. Raboy A, Adler H, Albert P. Extraperitoneal endoscopic pelvic lymph node dissection: A review of 125 patients. *J Urol.* 1997;158:2202.
9. Parra RO, Andrus C, Boullier J. Staging laparoscopic pelvic lymph node dissection: Comparison of results with open pelvic lymphadenectomy. *J Urol.* 1992;147:875.
10. Kerbl K, Clayman RW, Petros JA, et al. Staging pelvic lymphadenectomy for prostate cancer: A comparison of laparoscopic and open techniques. *J Urol.* 1993;150:396.
11. Winfield HN, See WA, Donovan JF, et al. Comparison effectiveness and safety of laparoscopic vs open pelvic lymph dissection for cancer of the prostate (abstract). *J Urol.* 1992;147:244A.
12. Persson BE, Haggman M. Minimally invasive techniques for prostate cancer pelvic lymph node dissection: A randomized trial of trans and extraperitoneal methods (abstract). *J Urol.* 1996;155:658A.
13. Kavoussi LR, Josa E, Chandohoke P, et al. Complications of laparoscopic pelvic lymph node dissection. *J Urol.* 1993;149:322.
14. Lang GS, Ruckle HC, Hadley HR, et al. One hundred consecutive laparoscopic pelvic lymph node dissections: Comparing complication of the first 50 cases to the second 50 cases. *Urology.* 1994;44:221.
15. Faber BM, Coddington CC. Microlaparoscopy: A comparative study of diagnostic accuracy. *Fertil Steril.* 1997;67:952.
16. LPLND or mini-laparotomy for evaluating pelvic nodal tissue: Laparoscopic pelvic lymphadenectomy. *Contemp Urol.* 1997;9:39.

Chapter Seventy-Five ......

*L*aparoscopic Varicocelectomy

JUAN MANUEL MARINA and RAÚL JOSÉ SALGUEIRO

INTRODUCTION

Varicocele (dilatation or tortuosity of the veins of the pampiniform plexus) is a disease related to infertility and pain. Since 1952 it has been widely recognized as a correctable cause of male infertility.[1] It is currently accepted that 39% of cases of infertility have a vascular origin.[2]

In 1885, Barwell reported decreased testicular size associated with the disease. He also mentioned that the testis regained its normal size and consistency following ligation of the spermatic vein.[3] A few years later Bennett described varicocele as a congenital malformation difficult to diagnose before puberty, primarily affecting the left side, and added that after successful surgical correction the pain disappeared and the sperm count normalized.[4]

INCIDENCE

The reported incidence of varicocele in the general and subfertile populations varies depending on the method of evaluation and diagnosis. In the general population the incidence is between 15 and 18% on physical examination,[5] and 18% and 35% on scrotal sonography and color flow Doppler imaging, respectively.[6] Varicocele is considered the most identifiable cause of male infertility.[7] The incidence of varicocele in prepubertal individuals ranges from 10 to 15% in various series and the importance of treatment early in childhood to prevent testicular damage is widely accepted.[8]

DIAGNOSIS

Varicoceles generally develop during adolescence. The diagnosis of a varicocele is based primarily on a careful physical examination. We recommend that our patients stand for 10 to 15 minutes in a warm room prior to examination. We inspect and palpate the scrotum for varicocele at a point just superior to the testes. This pathology is graded with respect to size and/or appearance: grade I—a small varicocele is palpable only during a Valsalva maneuver; grade II—a medium-sized varicocele is palpable without a Valsalva maneuver; and grade III—a large varicocele is visible upon inspection.[9] Small varicoceles can be difficult to detect on physical examination, but they may be as significant for reducing male reproductive function as medium or large varicoceles.[10] The treatment of subclinical varicocele remains controversial. However, McClure et al[11] reported greater improvements in sperm motility in response to treatment of patients with subclinical varices compared with patients with clinically obvious varices. Other modalities are often used to assist in confirming the diagnosis of varicocele,[12–14] including contact thermography, Doppler sonography, radionuclide angiography, color Doppler sonography, and venography. Each of these tests has intrinsic limitations.

TREATMENT

There are four indications for surgical treatment of the varicocele: (1) male subfertility, as demonstrated by abnormal seminal fluid analysis and failure to impregnate a partner who is free of demonstrable female factor infertility; (2) pain that is not attributable to other intrascrotal pathologic conditions; (3) adolescent testicular growth retardation that persists for at least 6 months; and (4) the cosmetic appearance of the scrotum, specially in larger varicoceles. There is no medical treatment for varicoceles; it is treated surgically and/or invasively with variceal ablation. Treatment options include spermatic vein sclerotherapy or embolization; open surgical treatment via the scrotal, high retroperitoneal, or inguinal approach; microsurgical bypass; and most recently by laparoscopy.[15–18] The first attempt was reported by Dr. Sanchez de Badajoz in 1988,[19] who performed high varix ligation of the spermatic veins.

This technique has several advantages over the classic surgical approach: (1) the use of magnifying lenses allows better visualization of the vascular structures, so identification of the spermatic veins and the spermatic artery is simpler, helping to prevent damage to these structures; (2) a more thorough surgical dissection is performed and accessory spermatic veins are ligated, decreasing the rate of recurrence; and (3) for bilateral varicoceles the endoscopic procedure obviates the need for a second surgical incision and decreases the operative time.

Contraindications to laparoscopic variceal ligation include previous surgical exploration for peritonitis, multiple intraperitoneal operations, a large umbilical hernia, or coagulation disorders.

PATIENT PREPARATION

This procedure can be done as outpatient surgery. The patient should be informed about the risks of vascular, intestinal, or other visceral injury that may require open surgical repair. We perform laparoscopic varix ligation exclusively under general anesthesia. There is a report of the use of local anesthesia during laparoscopic varix ligation in which no attempt was made to preserve the testicular artery,[20] but we believe that preservation of the spermatic artery is one of the advantages of this procedure. Prior to the induction of general anesthesia the patient should empty his bladder. Once the patient is under anesthesia, the skin is scrubbed and a topical antiseptic solution is applied. Drapes are placed to provide access to the entire abdomen and genitals. Manual retraction of the testes during laparoscopy assists in identifying the spermatic vessels and collateral veins that traverse the internal ring.

TECHNIQUE

The patient is placed in the Trendelenburg position (30°). We use a Veress needle to insufflate the peritoneal cavity with CO_2 using a small incision in the inferior arch of the umbilicus, and in instances in which the patient has had previous intra-abdominal surgery, a Hasson cannula is introduced through a 2- to 3-cm vertical midline skin incision inferior to the umbilicus. Next, a 2-cm incision is made in the linea alba. Horizontal mattress sutures are placed into the rectus fascia on both sides of the linea alba. Lateral traction is placed on these stay sutures to expose the underlying traversalis fascia and the peritoneum, which are then incised sequentially under direct vision. The use of the Hasson cannula may decrease the likelihood of intra-abdominal injury to several organs during the establishment of the pneumoperitoneum. When the pneumoperitoneum reaches 15 mm Hg of intra-abdominal pressure, a 5-mm incision is made in the same place where the Veress needle was inserted and a 5-mm trocar is introduced. A 5-mm laparoscope is inserted through the subumbilical port, and the peritoneal contents are inspected. Other two additional operative ports are placed, 3 to 5 cm cephalad to the internal ring.[21] This site can be identified by transilluminating the abdominal wall at the internal ring from inside the abdomen. This site is more cephalad than McBurney's point. The abdominal wall is transilluminated at the site of trocar insertion and subcutaneous vessels are identified. A 3- or 5-mm skin incision is made for trocar insertion. The 3-mm ports may be used for scissors and/or dissectors when such mini-laparoscopic instruments are available; otherwise a 5-mm port is used for the standard instruments.

Once the laparoscope and instruments are placed, attention is directed to the identification and dissection of the spermatic veins. A 3- to 4-cm peritoneal incision is made parallel and lateral to the spermatic vascular bundle. If the sigmoid colon is fixed over the spermatic veins cephalad to the internal ring, it is mobilized to expose the underlying spermatic vessels. At the middle of this incision a second perpendicular incision is made running medially through the peritoneum overlying the spermatic vessels. This T-shaped incision provides ample exposure for access to the spermatic veins. The entire spermatic vascular bundle is dissected free from the underlying psoas muscle. Once the spermatic vessels have been mobilized, one may find from 3 to 8 veins. The bundle is separated carefully into lateral and medial portions to identify the site of the spermatic artery where pulsations can be seen in either side. Care must be taken to distinguish true spermatic artery pulsations from those transmitted from the iliac artery. Generally speaking, the artery may be found in the medial bundle, and if identification of the artery is difficult, a laparoscopic Doppler probe and/or a papaverine or lidocaine 2% drip over the bundle will facilitate the identification and dissection of the artery. Once the artery is located, the nonarterial tissue is clipped and divided. When a 5-mm port is used, a 5-mm hemoclip applier is introduced through the contralateral side to the bundle being dissected. When a 3-mm port is used, a 3-mm laparoscope is exchanged for the 5-mm one and inserted through the ipsilateral port, and the 5-mm hemoclip applier can be inserted through the site of the subumbilical port. Monopolar electrocautery is not used to avoid damage to the spermatic artery.

After varix ligation is completed, a systematic intraperitoneal inspection is done, particularly near the operative area. On occa-

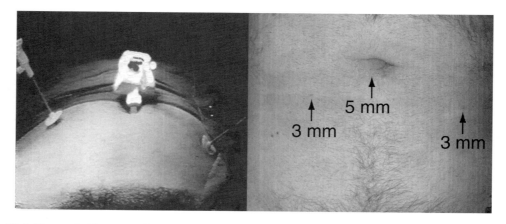

Figure 75–1. Placement of the trocars: A 5-mm one in the umbilicus and two more lateral and 3–5 cm cephalad to the internal ring.

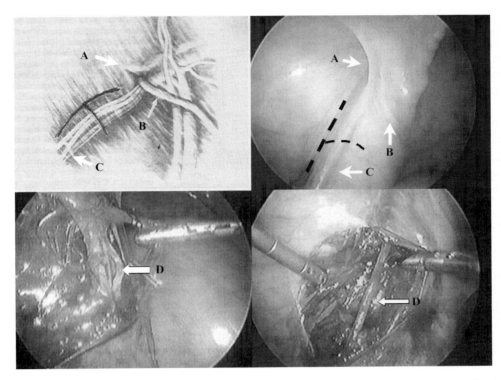

Figure 75–2. A "T" incision (A, B, C) is made in the peritoneum. Identification of the spermatic arteries (D) and clippage of the spermatic veins. See Color Section.

sion the patient may also have an inguinal hernia that can be repaired using a laparoscopic approach.[22]

The operative site is inspected following reduction in the intraperitoneal pressure to 5 mm Hg. Careful hemostasis is done using electrocautery, preferably bipolar. The patient is returned to the horizontal position and irrigation and aspiration of the pelvis is done. Lower quadrant trocars are removed under direct vision and these sites are inspected for abdominal wall bleeding. The subumbilical port is the last one to be removed. The laparoscope should be inserted through this port prior to its removal to prevent entrapment of small bowel in the fascia defect. When a Hasson trocar is used, the stay sutures are divided prior to its removal. These sutures are then tied across the wound to approximate the fascia.

POSTOPERATIVE CARE

All patients resume oral intake after recovery from anesthesia and are discharged on the day of surgery and instructed to increase their activity ad libitum. Oral analgesics are used to control postoperative pain. Patients return for an office visit 1 week after surgery. For infertile males, an assessment of response to varix ablation using a semen analysis is done 4 months postoperatively and at 3-month intervals thereafter.

DISCUSSION AND CONCLUSIONS

The development of laparoscopic surgical skills requires training in basic laparoscopic techniques and accumulation of operative experience to refine the use of instruments and techniques spe-

cific to laparoscopy.[23,24] Initially, the use of laparoscopy for varicocelectomy required a prolonged operating time and the authors required 125 minutes to perform a careful dissection and preservation of the spermatic artery for bilateral varicoceles. As our surgical experience has grown, the duration of the procedure has been reduced to 60 to 70 minutes for bilateral varicoceles, a time comparable to microscopic inguinal or subinguinal varix ligation with spermatic artery preservation or to a Palomo's bilateral procedure.[25] This technique appears to be as safe and effective as the more traditional operative procedures for treatment of varicocele. A particular advantage of this procedure is the rapid postoperative recovery, particularly when the 3-mm instruments are used. (See Figs. 75–1 and 75–2.)

We believe that every urologist must be trained to perform this type of surgery given its many advantages, and that performing it will provide experience that will be useful for more advanced urologic endoscopic operations.

REFERENCES

1. Tolloch WS. A consideration of sterility factors in the light of subsequent pregnancies: Subfertility in the male. *Trans Edinb Obstet Soc.* 1952;104:29.
2. Dubin L, Amelar RD. Etiologic factors in 1294 consecutive cases of male infertility. *Fertil Steril.* 1971;22:469.
3. Barwell R. One hundred cases of varicocele treated by the subcutaneous wire loop. *Lancet* 1885;1:978.
4. Bennet WH. Varicocele, particularly with reference to its radical care. *Lancet* 1889;1:261.
5. Jarow JP, Coburn M, Sigman M. Incidence of varicoceles in men with primary and secondary infertility. *Urology* 1966;47:73.

6. Meacham RB, Townsend RR, Rademacher E, et al. The incidence of varicoceles in general population when evaluated by physical exam, Gray scale sonography and color Doppler sonography. *J Urol.* 1994; 151:1535.

7. Kass EJ, Reitelman C. Adolescent varicocele. *Urol Clin North Am.* 1995;22:151.

8. Kass EJ, Freitas JE, Bour JB. Adolescent varicocele: results. *Acta Urol.* 1989;142:579.

9. Nagler HM, Zippe CD. Varicocele: Current concepts and treatment. In: Lipshultz LI, Howards SS, eds. *Infertility in the Male.* Mosby-Year Book:1991;313.

10. Dubin L, Amelar RD. Varicocele size and results of varicocelectomy in selected subfertile men with varicocele. *Fertil Steril.* 1970;21:606.

11. McClure RD, Khoo D, Jarvi K. Subclinical varicocele: The effectiveness of varicocelectomy. *J Urol.* 1985;145:789.

12. World Health Organization. Comparison among different methods for the diagnosis of varicocele. *Fertil Steril.* 1985;43:575.

13. Petros JA, Andriole GL, Medleton WD. Correlation of testicular color Doppler ultrasonography, physical examination and venography in the detection of left varicoceles in men with infertility. *J Urol.* 1991;145:785.

14. Horstman WG, Middleton WD, Melson GL. Color Doppler US of the scrotum. *Radiographics* 1991;11:941.

15. Frangi I, Keppenne V, Coppens L, et al. Antegrade scrotal embolization of varicocele: results. *Acta Urol Belg.* 1998;66:5.

16. Puleo S, Trombatore G, Lombardo R, et al. Microsurgery and varicocele: state of the art. *Microsurgery* 1998;18:479.

17. Abdulamaaboud MR, Shokeir AA, Garage Y, et al. Treatment of varicocele: a comparative study of conventional open surgery, percutaneous retrograde sclerotherapy, and laparoscopy. *Urology* 1998;52: 294.

18. Kass EJ, Bodgan M. Results of varicocele surgery in adolescents: a comparison of techniques. *J Urol.* 1992;148:694.

19. Sanchez de Badajoz E, Diaz Ramírez R. Tratamiento endoscópico del varicocele. *Arch Esp Urol.* 1988;135:286.

20. Matsuda T, Horii Y, Takeuchi H. Laparoscopic varicocelectomy. *J Urol.* 1991;2145:325A.

21. Donovan JF Jr., Winfield HN. Laparoscopic varix ligation. *J Urol.* 1992;147:73.

22. Schultz L, Graber J, Pietrafitta J. Laser laparoscopic herniorrhaphy. *J Laparendosc Surg.* 1990;1:41.

23. See WA, Winfield HN, Fisher R, et al. Laparoscopic surgical training: Effectiveness and impact of urological surgical practice patterns. *J Urol.* 1993;149:1054.

24. See WA, Cooper CS, Fisher RJ. Predictors of laparoscopic complications after formal training in laparoscopic surgery. *JAMA.* 1993;270: 2689.

25. Marina-Gonzalez JM, Salgueiro RJ. Varicocele. In: Cueto J, Weber A, eds. *Laparoscopic Surgery.* McGraw-Hill Interamericana:1994;289.

Chapter Seventy-Six ● ● ● ● ● ●

Laparoscopic Live-Donor Nephrectomy

MICHAEL EDYE and VALERIU EUGEN ANDREI

In addition to better graft survival, advantages of live donor renal transplantation over cadaver donor transplantation include decreased waiting time, lower incidence of delayed function, the opportunity to optimize the recipient's medical condition,[1–3] and the positive emotional and physiologic impact on both donor and recipient.[4,5] Yet despite better outcomes, there have traditionally been an insufficient number of available kidneys from living donors. In 1995, United Network for Organ Sharing (UNOS) reported that live donors accounted only for 27% of kidney transplants, a number that had not changed significantly since 1988 (20%). Increasing the number of kidneys from living donors would reduce the deficit of organs and make kidneys from cadaver donors available to patients who are unable to obtain the organ from a living donor.

More people would consider kidney donation if the recovery period were shorter so they could resume their financial, social, and family responsibilities.[5,6] Accordingly to increase the live kidney donor pool, a laparoscopic approach was developed with a view towards fewer postoperative complications and a faster recovery.

HISTORICAL PERSPECTIVE

Clayman et al performed the first laparoscopic nephrectomy for a benign lesion in 1990.[7] After this, the introduction of laparoscopic donor nephrectomy was just matter of time. The laparoscopic approach with a living kidney donor was first reported in an animal experiment by Gill et al in 1994.[8] Ratner et al performed the first laparoscopic live-donor nephrectomy in humans in 1995,[9] reporting good recoveries by donor and recipient, and thus ushering in a new chapter in transplant surgery. Two series (25 and 70 cases) of laparoscopic live-donor nephrectomies, have subsequently been reported[10,11] that showed the feasibility of the procedure and equivalence of graft function.

PATHOPHYSIOLOGY OF PNEUMOPERITONEUM

One important theoretical concern raised in connection with laparoscopic nephrectomies involves the variety of physiologic changes that occur after the induction of carbon dioxide pneumoperitoneum. Elevated IAP causes an elevation in intracranial pressure,[12] decreased abdominal wall blood flow,[13] and increased end-inspiratory pressure.[14] Increased IAP has also been associated with a reduction in visceral perfusion. Blood flow to the abdominal organs, including kidneys, is affected with reduction in flow occurring with IAP as low as 10 mm Hg.[15–17]

It is known that a decrease in urinary output can be produced experimentally in animal models by increasing the IAP without a significant drop in systemic blood pressure. Urinary output returns to normal once abdominal decompression is achieved.[18,19] The significance of reduction in renal blood flow at the pressure used during laparoscopic nephrectomies is of concern.

The underlying mechanism of transient renal dysfunction secondary to an increase in IAP observed in experimental and clinical settings, however, is not known. A high level of antidiuretic hormone accompanies a decrease in blood flow to the kidney. This phenomenon, associated with preferential perfusion of renal medulla over renal cortex, may explain the transient impairment in renal function.[18–21]

In addition, carbon dioxide pneumoperitoneum may lead to local vasoconstriction by local absorption.[22] Moreover, low-flow anesthesia[23] and decreased cardiac output secondary to the reverse Trendelenburg position may also decrease splanchnic blood flow.[20] These physiologic consequences are well compensated in patients with normal respiratory and cardiovascular systems but may become clinically significant in patients with known cardiorespiratory dysfunction.[24] Live donors for kidney transplant have few comorbid conditions and should experience minimal deleterious effects from laparoscopy. We conclude that using the lowest possible pneumoperitoneum pressure necessary for good visualization should minimize the reduction of renal blood flow. In addition to better splanchnic blood flow, low IAP (6 to 8 mm Hg) would result in better postoperative pulmonary function and less pain.[25]

COMPARISON OF OPEN AND LAPAROSCOPIC LIVE-DONOR NEPHRECTOMY

The outcomes observed after laparoscopic nephrectomy for benign and malignant lesions are comparable, and to some extent better, than those observed after open procedures. There is reduced morbidity and postoperative pain with a shorter hospitalization, faster recovery, and more rapid return to regular activity.[9,26] Currently laparoscopic nephrectomy is offered as an alternative to the open procedure for benign and malignant diseases in certain centers where advanced laparoscopic surgery is performed.[26,27]

These encouraging results led to the development of laparoscopic transperitoneal donor nephrectomy as an alternative to open live donor kidney harvesting on the theory that a laparoscopically harvested kidney should function as well as a conventionally harvested kidney. Yet for laparoscopic donor nephrectomy (LDN) to become an alternative approach to open donor nephrectomy (ODN), it must be shown that donors undergoing laparoscopic nephrectomy, with its attendant benefits of quicker rate of recovery and return to regular activity, experience no additional morbidity compared to donors undergoing open procedures.

Due to the recent introduction of LDN, there is no long-term follow-up data; however there are at least two significant studies published.[10,11] In 1997, Flowers et al[11] compared the results of 70 cases of LDN to the results of 65 cases of ODN using a prospective longitudinal database, medical record review, and patient interviews. A conversion rate of 6% (3 vascular injuries and one for morbid obesity and inability to sustain pneumoperitoneum) was reported. The mean warm ischemia time in the LDN group was 3 minutes (range, 1.9 to 6.9 minutes). The mean follow-up was 7 months (range, 2 to 12 months). The graft function and survival data did not show a statistically significant difference between the two groups and were comparable to results reported elsewhere.

A faster postoperative recovery was reported in LDN group. Less pain (significantly less use of parenteral narcotics in the LDN group) and the ability to resume regular activities earlier may explain this.

There were no statistically significant differences in postoperative complication rates and no mortality was reported in either group. In the LDN group, the avoidance of pneumothorax, ileus and wound complications may account for the faster recovery. A higher incidence of vascular injuries during LDN may be explained by the operative experience of the surgeon and is expected to approach the same figures as seen in ODN as the experience with LDN increases. The results related to ODN are comparable to those in the largest series of ODN with mortality of 0.07% and morbidity as high as 20%.[1,28]

Since October 1996 we have performed 87 LDN at Mount Sinai Medical Center (MSMC). The same surgeon (ME) performed all cases, with radioimaging workup and operative strategy evolving as our experience with this new approach grew (described later). The operative data and postoperative morbidity are given in Tables 76–1 and 76–2.

TABLE 76–1. OPERATING ROOM DATA

Operating room time (min)[1]	268
Estimated blood loss (mL)[1]	255
Warm ischemia time (min)[1]	4.5
I/O (ml/mL)[1]	5000/1800
Conversions	2

[1]Mean values.

Early graft survival rate for kidneys harvested via laparoscopic nephrectomy at MSMC is 95.4% (83 out of 87). Delayed graft function, defined as slow correction of creatinine clearance (e.g., ATN) in the early postoperative period, was found in 6 of 87 recipients (6.9%). However, at long-term follow-up (up to 12 months) the graft function normalized. There were no statistical differences in creatinine levels in open or laparoscopic groups postoperatively (e.g., at 1 week, and at 1, 3, 6, and 12 months postoperatively) (Fig. 76–1).

ADVANCED LAPAROSCOPIC TRAINING

For success with LDN, it is essential to assemble a team with advanced laparoscopic skills.[29] Complete familiarity with laparoscopic surgical physiology and anatomy is mandatory. Before the procedure is carried out on humans it is important to develop and perfect skills and steps of the procedure in the laboratory.[29,30] Henkel et al described a step-by-step technique for teaching LDN involving graded exposure to the procedure in laboratory and operating room settings.[29] Developing proper bimanual instrument coordination and familiarity with angled telescopes is necessary to perform LDN. It is difficult to overestimate the whole range of advanced laparoscopic skills necessary to perform this operation safely.

RENOVASCULAR ANATOMY AND IMAGING WORKUP

The left kidney is usually used for donor nephrectomies because its vein is longer. The purpose of renovascular imaging before harvesting the kidney is to identify anatomic anomalies that would lead the transplant surgeon to use the right kidney and exclude donors with significant renovascular disease or horseshoe kidney.

An important part of the radioimaging workup includes conventional angiography and, more recently, computed tomographic

TABLE 76–2. POSTOPERATIVE MORBIDITY

	LDN (n = 87)
Hemorrhage[1]	3 (3.45%)
Incidental splenectomy	1 (1.14%)
Pulmonary complication[2]	3 (3.45%)
Urinary retention[2]	1 (1.14%)
Ileus	2 (2.3%)

[1]One patient required blood transfusion and was laparoscopically reexplored for extraction site bleeding.
[2]Atelactasis (1), pneumonia (1), pulmonary edema (1).

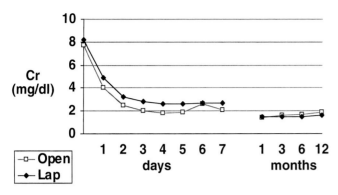

Figure 76–1. Serum creatinine level at 1 week and 1, 3, 6, and 12 months postoperatively. (Recipients from LDN group, 87 patients; recipients from ODN group, 27 patients.)

(CT) angiography. Studies show that CT angiography provides results comparable to renal angiography regarding renal artery anatomy and also offers valuable preoperative information about the renal venous system and parenchyma.[31,32] Both tools provide a comprehensive anatomic depiction of the renal arterial and venous supplies that aids in surgical kidney harvest selection. We currently still prefer conventional angiography because of its ability to identify small lower pole arteries which, when present, may be the main supply to the proximal ureter (Fig. 76–2). Although negligible lower pole renal ischemia may result from thrombosis of such a small vessel, the ureter may necrose, leading to urinary leaks.

Of the 87 LDN cases performed at MSMC, the transplant surgeon opted to harvest 21 right kidneys mainly as a result of angiographic demonstration of vascular anomalies found in the left kidney (Table 76–3).

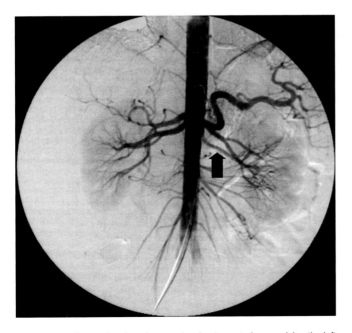

Figure 76–2. Conventional angiogram showing two arteries supplying the left kidney. The lower vessel (*arrow*) would probably remain patent after anastomosis, but smaller vessels thrombose more readily with the risk of proximal ureteral necrosis. The donor's right kidney was used in this case.

TABLE 76–3. INDICATIONS FOR RIGHT KIDNEY HARVEST

	Anatomic Anomalies (n = 21)
Left renal artery anomaly	13[1]
Left renal vein anomaly	2
Unequal kidney size (L > R)	4
Other (ptotic right kidney)	2

[1]Two patients had small accessory arteries to lower pole of the kidney; 11 patients had multiple renal arteries.

ESSENTIAL LAPAROSCOPIC EQUIPMENT

Telescope

A good-quality high-resolution video camera with high-intensity light source is essential for clear operating conditions. For non-obese donors, a 5-mm 45-degree telescope provides an excellent image while minimizing the size of the abdominal puncture. Three-chip or the latest generation electronically enhanced single-chip cameras are ideal.

Ports

During left-sided laparoscopic nephrectomy, four ports are necessary for mobilization of the kidney (three ports of 5-mm size and one larger port of 10 or 12-mm size). An extra epigastric 5-mm cannula is necessary during right nephrectomy for liver retraction.

A 15-mm cannula inserted through the extraction incision for the retrieval device is needed to insert the extraction device. Use of the PneumoSleeve (Dexterity, Inc.) may play a role in reducing operating time but necessitates a longer, more proximal extraction site than the Pfannenstiel incision we prefer.

Instruments

Good-quality insulated grasping instruments of the fenestrated, atraumatic type are useful for handling delicate structures. A narrow pointed grasper is needed for accurate dissection around vessels. A right-angled dissector is also necessary for vascular dissection and looping vein and artery. Colored silicone vascular loops are used to tag artery, vein, and ureter and allow gentle retraction of these structures. Ultrasonic shears are very effective for both dissection and hemostasis and are available in both 5 and 10-mm versions. Veins of 3 to 4 mm and arteries of 2 to 3 mm diameter can be coagulated and divided with a single application of this instrument.[33]

Staplers

A clip applier is usually sufficient for the artery. Alternatively, large vessels can be divided after ligation with an extracorporeally tied slip knot of Gore-Tex® or 2-0 silk. An endoscopic linear cutter stapler requires a 12-mm cannula. We remove the row of staples on the kidney side which allows the kidney to empty and preserves vessel length.

OPERATIVE STRATEGY

General Considerations

Although the left kidney is the preferred donor side, our experience with right donor nephrectomy has proved this to be a feasible alternative if the anatomy on the left is unsuitable. Mannitol (25 g) is administered intravenously at the commencement of dissection of the vessels to promote renal parenchymal perfusion and free radical protection.

Left Nephrectomy

Donor Position and Port Site Planning. While the donor is supine after induction of general anesthesia and endotracheal intubation, a urinary catheter is inserted. The skin crease and midline for Pfannenstiel or periumbilical extraction incision are marked with an indelible pen, as the correct site is impossible to judge when the donor is positioned. The donor is placed in standard right lateral decubitus position so that if conversion to an open nephrectomy is necessary there will be adequate distraction of the costal margin from the iliac crest achieved by breaking the table, use of bolsters and axillary roll, and so forth. Port 1 situated 8 cm above and 8 to 10 cm lateral to the umbilicus for the laparoscope (preferably a 45-degree optic) gives an excellent viewing angle of the renal pedicle. This site still allows visualization of the ureter as distal as the pelvic brim on each side, and the upper pole of the spleen on the left. The tip of the 12th rib is marked and a line carried forward to the umbilicus. The point of intersection of this line with the lateral border of the rectus is a good position for a 12-mm cannula (port 2) for the clip applier, ultrasonic shears, or stapler used in the right hand of the surgeon. Eight cm above port 1, the 5-mm cannula for the surgeon's left hand is placed (port 3). Ten or 12 cm laterally on the line marked is a fourth puncture for a 5-mm cannula for suction and retraction (port 4).

Procedure. Pneumoperitoneum is induced by Veress needle puncture directly through the abdominal wall at the costal margin in the midclavicular line. The laparoscope cannula (port 1) is inserted first. By rotating the telescope to look upwards at the abdominal wall, the three subsequent cannulas are inserted under vision. The most comfortable position for the operator is to stand facing the donor's abdomen viewing the monitor positioned behind the donor's back. Dissecting instruments are introduced on either side (ports 2 and 3) of the laparoscope that is held by the first assistant standing to surgeon's right side. This assistant also

holds the suction cannula positioned at port 4, an invaluable aid for countertraction and aspiration of smoke.

The splenic flexure is frequently adherent to the abdominal wall, and this is divided by sharp dissection using shears or scissors. Neither splenic parenchyma nor colonic wall is handled. Rather, the peritoneal attachments to them are picked up for traction during the subsequent mobilization. The peritoneum of the splenorenal ligament is opened sharply and the cut carried down just lateral to the colon. Afterwards this line of incision is carried superiorly, enabling the surgeon to reflect the colon and the spleen medially out of the operative field. The bulge of the kidney within Gerota's fascia is easily seen below the lower pole of the spleen and behind the colon. If the peritoneum overlying the kidney is elevated it will be seen to move separately from Gerota's fascia deep to it. By elevating this layer, the colon and spleen are further reflected to the midline. The tail of the pancreas rolls forward with the spleen, and the splenic vein is exposed on its posterior aspect.

Directly posterior to the splenic vein, but within Gerota's fascia, is the left renal vein seen as a darkening in the fat medial to the mound of the kidney. The mesocolon is very thin at this point, and perforating it will expose loops of proximal jejunum. The inferior mesenteric vein (IMV) ascends in the mesocolon and can be visualized here. Running very close and roughly in the same cephalad direction, but in a more posterior plane, is the gonadal vein, with no medial branches, which makes it possible to distinguish it from the IMV if clean anatomic planes have been breached. The gonadal vein (or veins) up to 8 mm in diameter course just deep to Gerota's fascia to drain multiply or as a single trunk into the left renal vein, and can thus be used to locate the latter if still obscured by fat. The gonadal vein is divided between clips, superomedial to the ureter, and the dissection carried superiorly to its junction with the renal vein. A long gonadal vein stump is used as a handle to rotate the back of the renal vein forward when cleaning its lower border (Fig. 76–3a). In about three fourths of left kidneys, one or more posterior communicating veins (commonly called *lumbar veins*) may enter the gonadal vein, or the confluence of the gonadal and renal vein. With upward traction on the gonadal vein these branches will come into view and can be cleanly dissected with the right-angle instrument (Fig. 76–3). The lumbar vein is treacherous if not tightly secured because it is short, broad, and

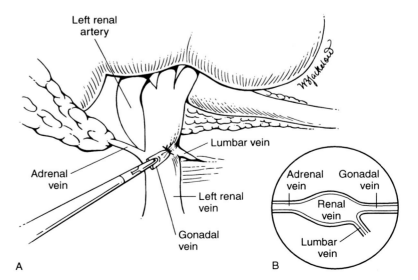

Figure 76–3. A. Exposure of the lumbar vein(s) using medial traction on the stump of the gonadal vein to gain access to the area behind the renal vein. **B.** Anteroposterior section of the renal vein at the level of adrenal, gonadal, and lumbar veins.

there is little to grasp. Bleeding from it is brisk, and attempts to control this risk injury to the main renal trunk and even renal ischemia. A 2-0 silk tie passed around the lumbar vein is tied extracorporeally and the knot snugged down on the side that will remain with the kidney. Clips can be applied on the muscle side but should be avoided near the main renal vessels as they may prevent proper firing of the stapler during the extraction phase (Fig. 76–4). When small (1 to 1.5 mm), the lumbar vein is often multiple. Indeed, any vessel of this size is too small to safely hold a clip and can be divided with the ultrasonic shears.

The left adrenal vein is the most constant feature of the venous anatomy. We found it present and single in all (66 of 66) left kidneys. Ligating firmly with fine thread flush with the renal vein, clipping flush with the adrenal tissue, and dividing between with scissors is our preferred method (Fig. 76–5). By hugging the lower pole of the adrenal, any vessels passing to it from the renal artery can be seen and secured.

After the posterior aspect of the renal vein is cleared with care, the right-angle instrument is passed behind the vein to grasp a short length (about 3 inches) of blue Vessel loop, which is secured with a clip after encircling the vein. The vein is freed as far medially as possible over the front of the aorta. This dissection is limited by the superior mesenteric artery medially and the pancreas superiorly. If the spleen and the pancreas seem to be in the way, this is probably because the splenophrenic ligament has not been divided high enough to enable the spleen to fall forward.

Because of the decubitus position of the donor and the laparoscopic view, the artery must be imagined as running vertically behind the vein. To do this, accurate maintenance of the video horizon by correct orientation of the camera is vital. Disorientation may lead to mistaken dissection of the anterior aspect of the aorta or the superior mesenteric artery. A lateral prolongation of the superior mesenteric ganglion covers the origin of the left renal artery (LRA), unless the artery is lower than normal. In about two thirds of cases it is easier to access it by depressing the upper border of the LRV, usually by gently retracting the adrenal vein stump. However, for much of its course it is better accessed and cleaned from its posterior aspect, after medial reflection of the kidney. Nonrenal branches of the LRA are very rare. Fibrofatty tissue, lymphatics, and autonomic nerves surrounding the artery are divided with ultrasonic shears. It is not uncommon to see chyle in the tissue fluid accumulating in the operative field during this dissection. The adventitia of the artery should be sharply dissected on the upper and lower aspect to expose the shiny white arterial wall. Thus displayed, the right-angle instrument will pass behind the artery with gentle side-to-side rocking movements, causing little deformation of the arterial wall. The jaws should not be spread unless both tips are visible. The artery is encircled with a white Vessel loop secured with a clip. The areolar tissue proximal to this is gently pushed away with a peanut dissector to the point where the origin of the artery appears to flare onto the aortic wall. This completes dissection of the artery from the medial aspect.

If Gerota's fascia is thin, it may be possible to find the ureter easily as it crosses the iliac vessels and start to mobilize it from the pelvic brim upwards. Another technique is to dissect the triangular block of tissue lateral to the gonadal vein from the lower border of the renal vein above and the psoas muscle posteriorly. This contains the ureter and its blood supply and should be looped for ease of identification and retraction. Avoiding dissection or handling of tissues in this region lowers the chance of proximal ureteral ischemia. The contents of this triangle (ureter, fat) are freed from the psoas muscle posterior to it, creating an avascular plane

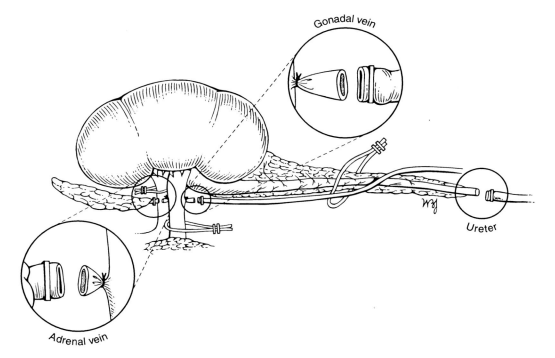

Figure 76–4. The left kidney is ready to be removed after the looped renal vein and artery are transected. Once the renal vein has been clipped or stapled, the warm ischemia time is recorded until the specimen is removed and placed in the iced saline container. The adrenal and gonadal vein stumps at the side of the renal vein are tied using silk. Clips are not used on the renal vein to avoid interference with the stapling line.

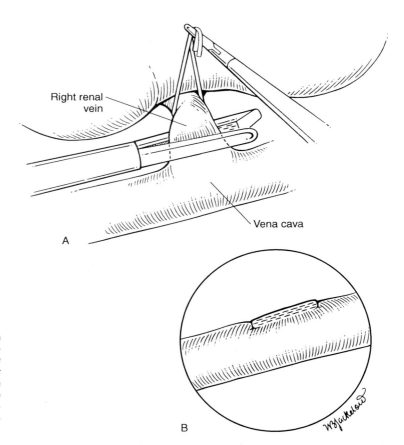

Figure 76–5. A. Transection of the right renal vein using the Ethicon Endopath linear cutter stapler. The three rows of staples on the kidney side of the vascular-sized cartridge have been removed to allow the kidney to empty of blood and to preserve length on the donor vein side. The stapler must be applied so that it extends beyond the edge of the vein. The stapler has been marked so as not to confuse the correct orientation of the cartridge. **B.** The staple line on the inferior vena cava after renal vein transection is slightly retracted, indicating a maximum length of vein has been harvested.

that leads up behind the kidney. At about the point where the ureter passes behind the gonadal vein, Gerota's fascia is cut directly upwards toward the lower pole of the kidney to expose the capsule. This cut is carried toward the upper pole and avoids the hilar structures. Countertraction is provided by an instrument in the flank trocar, and after complete clearance of the lower pole of the kidney, the surgeon's left-handed instrument can be used to elevate the lower pole as it is shelled out of Gerota's fascia. This mobilization of the front, back, and lateral border of the kidney proceeds cephalad till the upper pole is free. The kidney will fold further forward. As dissection is carried further medially toward the back of the hilum, the loop on the renal artery may be seen from the posterior aspect among perivascular fat.

Circumferential mobilization of the kidney is completed by ensuring that Gerota's entire fascia on the back of the upper pole and between the ureter and psoas muscle is cleared. For extraction, see the later section on removal of the donor kidney.

Right Nephrectomy

Donor Position and Port Site Planning. The donor is placed in left lateral decubitus position. Lines are marked between the 12th rib and umbilicus, and in the infraumbilical site. Port placement differs from the left side. A 12-mm Hasson cannula (port 3) is situated in the right lower quadrant over the lateral border of the rectus, about 3 cm above McBurney's point, and pneumoperitoneum is induced. Instruments inserted through this are parallel to the long axis of the cava, at an elevation of 15 to

20 degrees to it; thus this is the ideal site for insertion of a stapler. The 5-mm laparoscope and flank ports are inserted according to the landmarks for the left (ports 1 and 4). An epigastric 5-mm port is sited for a toothed grasper used to retract the liver cephalad (port 6). Port 2, located between the laparoscope (port 1) and epigastric (port 6) ports, should be the correct size for a right-handed surgeon using the 5 or 10 mm ultrasonic shears.

Procedure. First the liver is elevated from Morrison's pouch. This may require division of the right triangular ligament of the liver if there is not enough mobility of the right lobe. A toothed grasper inserted through the epigastric port, under the liver and clamped high on the lateral abdominal wall, will keep the liver elevated until the end of the procedure. The hepatic flexure of the colon is reflected medially to expose the second portion of the duodenum. Inferiorly, enough mobilization of the colon to allow access to the ureter as it crosses the iliac vessels is necessary. The duodenum is partly reflected medially (Kocher maneuver) by incision of the posterior peritoneum to expose the vena cava, right renal vein, and gonadal vein origin. Dissection as high as the adrenal vein is not necessary. Gerota's fascia over the origin of the renal vein is incised longitudinally, staying lateral to the gonadal vein, and the ureter identified and looped as described earlier. It is not necessary to divide the vein close to the cava. The junction of right gonadal vein and cava is very fragile and easily torn by rough handling. The triangle of fat below the lower pole, lateral to the ureter and anterior to the psoas muscle, is preserved to ensure good ureteral blood supply. Dissection proceeds superiorly along the upper border of the renal vein and upper pole separating the fat containing the right adrenal from that surrounding the kidney. This is carried laterally over the top of the upper pole. The renal vein is dissected circumferentially, looped, and gently retracted in search of pulsations of the renal artery. Usually the vein is too short to expose an artery running behind it unless it is close to the upper border. However, once the kidney has been fully mobilized from within the perirenal fat, it can be flopped medially and the arterial dissection performed from the posterior aspect. The artery is looped and dissected as far as possible posterior to the cava to include early upper or lower pole branches.

Removal of the Donor Kidney

The kidney will be ready for explantation when both vein and the artery have been skeletonized, there are no peripheral attachments to the kidney, and the ureter is mobilized to the pelvic brim and divided (Fig. 76–4 for the left side). It is important that the ureter not be divided till the last moment, as this helps to prevent torsion of the kidney, which could occur inadvertently. It may be difficult to rapidly untwist the kidney, leading to disastrous intraoperative ischemia.

If a Pfannenstiel incision is to be used for extraction, this is prepared now. A skin incision approximately equal to the diameter of the waist of the kidney (5 to 7 cm) is made through the fat to the muscle fascia, which is incised horizontally through the midline. The midline attachments to this anterior layer are divided with electrocautery as far inferiorly as the pubic symphysis and superiorly a similar distance. A 15-mm diameter trocar is inserted in the midline under direct vision from within. The only layer ensuring maintenance of the pneumoperitoneum will thus be the peritoneum posterior to the lower rectus muscles. The extraction bag device (EndoCatch II, US Surgical, Norwalk, CT) is advanced through the trocar under vision and fixed to the drapes so that it will not interfere with subsequent maneuvers.

An absorbable ligature is inserted through the 12-mm trocar, looped around the ureter, tied extracorporeally, and snugged down around the ureter as far distally as possible, preferably at the pelvic brim. The scissors is introduced through the same trocar to divide the ureter and the ligating thread. Clips are an acceptable alternative. A jet of urine establishes that the kidney is making urine. The ureteral loop is retrieved and discarded. The donor is now heparinized.

Vascular Division. Testing the positioning of the clip applier and/or stapler before the extraction sequence will demonstrate which works best. On the left, the kidney is firmly retracted laterally through port 4, and while stretching the artery with the loop, it is doubly clipped through port 3 and divided with scissors. Sometimes better access on the left is achieved by flipping the kidney medially and clipping from the posterior aspect. This is the best approach for the right kidney.

A stapler is used to transect the renal vein after a row of staples is removed (described earlier). Lateral traction on the kidney straightens the pedicle. Upward or downward traction with the vein loop allows the stapler to be positioned over the vein, which is divided as medial as possible. On the right, where length is critical, it is possible to draw some of the caval wall into the jaws of the stapler. When the jaws are closed around the vein and caval wall, they should project a few millimeters beyond the vessel wall (Fig. 76–5) to avoid producing a defect at the top of the staple line with potential major hemorrhage.

The kidney is scooped into the fully deployed retrieval bag. Two fingers are plunged through the Pfannenstiel incision on each side of the trocar to stretch the peritoneal layer, and the kidney is rapidly withdrawn and chilled. The warm ischemia time is recorded. A slow infusion of protamine is commenced to reverse the heparin (1 mg per 100 units of heparin).

Aftercare

Once the donor returns to the ward, oral analgesia is usually adequate (e.g., compound paracetamol/opioid formulations). Oral liquids can begin the evening after surgery. There will be a substantial overnight diuresis from volume loading and intraoperative diuretics, so the indwelling urinary catheter is removed at 6 AM on the first postoperative day. The donor's abdomen is usually soft and nontender, and there should be no hemodynamic instability. A normal diet is commenced then as ileus is rare. Simple analgesics should suffice from the second postoperative day (NSAIDS, such as ibuprofen). The hematocrit should reflect intraoperative blood loss and hemodilution, so serial estimations are not necessary if the donor is stable. It is common for the serum creatinine to be approximately double the preoperative level. The first bowel movement may not occur until the third of fourth postopertative day. Therefore these are not reasons to delay discharge on the second postoperative day. The donor is examined in the office at 2 weeks, when serum creatinine and urea levels are measured.

CONCLUSION

Since its emergence, laparoscopic nephrectomy has proven to be a safe and valuable approach for living renal donors in the hands of a surgeon who masters advanced laparoscopic technique. Because of lower morbidity and quicker recovery rates when compared with open donor nephrectomy, the laparoscopic approach has become an attractive option for live kidney donors.

The advantages of LDN are thus an incentive for prospective kidney donors, potentially increasing the number of kidneys from live donors, which in turn would address the shortage of organs. On a more cautionary note, although overall graft function and survival appear comparable, longer-term follow-up is necessary for full validation of the laparoscopic operation.

REFERENCES

1. Bay WH, Hebert LA. The living donor in kidney transplantation. *Ann Intern Med.* 1987;106:719.
2. Beekman GM, van Dorp WT, van Es LA, et al. Analysis of donor selection procedure in 139 living-related kidney donors and follow-up results for donors and recipients. *Nephrol Dial Transplant.* 1994;9:163.
3. Johnson EM, Remucal MJ, Gillingham KJ, et al. Complications and risks of living donor nephrectomy. *Transplantation.* 1997;64:1124.
4. Binet I, Bock AH, Vogelbach P, et al. Outcome in emotionally related living kidney donor transplantation. *Nephrol Dial Transplant.* 1997; 12:1940.
5. Hiller J, Sroka M, Holochek MJ, et al. Functional advantages of laparoscopic live-donor nephrectomy compared with conventional open-donor nephrectomy. *J Transpl Coord.* 1997;7:134.
6. Ratner LE, Hiller J, Sroka M, et al. Laparoscopic live donor nephrectomy removes disincentives to live donation. *Transplant Proc.* 1997; 29:3402.

7. Clayman RV, Kavoussi LR, Soper NJ, et al. Laparoscopic nephrectomy: Initial case report. *J Urol.* 1991;146:278.

8. Gill IS, Carbone JM, Clayman RV, et al. Laparoscopic live-donor nephrectomy. *J Endourol.* 1994;8:143.

9. Ratner LE, Ciseck LJ, Moore RG, et al. Laparoscopic live donor nephrectomy. *Transplantation.* 1995;60:1047.

10. Ratner LE, Kavoussi LR, Sroka M, et al. Laparoscopic assisted live donor nephrectomy—a comparison with the open approach. *Transplantation.* 1997;63:229. See comments.

11. Flowers JL, Jacobs S, Cho E, et al. Comparison of open and laparoscopic live donor nephrectomy. *Ann Surg.* 1997;226:483;discussion, 489.

12. Josephs LG, Este-McDonald JR, Birkett DH, et al. Diagnostic laparoscopy increases intracranial pressure. *J Trauma.* 1994;36:815;discussion,818.

13. Diebel L, Saxe J, Dulchavsky S. Effect of intra-abdominal pressure on abdominal wall blood flow. *Am Surg.* 1992;58:573;discussion,575.

14. Richardson JD, Trinkle JK. Hemodynamic and respiratory alterations with increased intra-abdominal pressure. *J Surg Res.* 1976;20:401.

15. Caldwell CB, Ricotta JJ. Changes in visceral blood flow with elevated intraabdominal pressure. *J Surg Res.* 1987;43:14.

16. Diebel LN, Wilson RF, Dulchavsky SA, et al. Effect of increased intra-abdominal pressure on hepatic arterial, portal venous, and hepatic microcirculatory blood flow. *J Trauma.* 1992;33:279;discussion,282.

17. Diebel LN, Dulchavsky SA, Wilson RF. Effect of increased intra-abdominal pressure on mesenteric arterial and intestinal mucosal blood flow. *J Trauma.* 1992;33:45;discussion,48.

18. Caldwell CB, Ricotta JJ. Evaluation of intra-abdominal pressure and renal hemodynamics. *Curr Surg.* 1986;43:495.

19. Barnes GE, Laine GA, Giam PY, et al.Cardiovascular responses to elevation of intra-abdominal hydrostatic pressure. *Am J Physiol.* 1985;248:R208.

20. Junghans T, Bohm B, Grundel K, et al. Does pneumoperitoneum with different gases, body positions, and intraperitoneal pressures influence renal and hepatic blood flow? *Surgery.* 1997;121:206.

21. Savino JA, Cerabona T, Agarwal N, et al. Manipulation of ascitic fluid pressure in cirrhotics to optimize hemodynamic and renal function. *Ann Surg.* 1988;208:504.

22. Ishizaki Y, Bandai Y, Shimomura K, et al. Changes in splanchnic blood flow and cardiovascular effects following peritoneal insufflation of carbon dioxide. *Surg Endosc.* 1993;7:420.

23. Murray JM, Rowlands BJ, Trinick TR. Indocyanine green clearance and hepatic function during and after prolonged anaesthesia: Comparison of halothane with isoflurane. *Br J Anaesth* 1992;68:168.

24. Hebebrand D, Menningen R, Sommer H, et al. Small-bowel necrosis following laparoscopic cholecystectomy: A clinically relevant complication? *Endoscopy.* 1995;27:281.

25. Wallace DH, Serpell MG, Baxter JN, et al. Randomized trial of different insufflation pressures for laparoscopic cholecystectomy. *Br J Surg.* 1997;84:455.

26. Doehn C, Fornara P, Fricke L, Jocham D. Comparison of laparoscopic and open nephroureterectomy for benign disease. *J Urol.* 1998;159:732.

27. Gill IS, Clayman RV, McDougall EM. Advances in urological laparoscopy. *J Urol.*1995;154:1275.

28. Shaffer D, Sahyoun AI, Madras PN, et al. Two hundred one consecutive living-donor nephrectomies. *Arch Surg.* 1998;133:426.

29. Henkel TO, Potempa DM, Rassweiler J, et al. Experimental studies for clinical standardization of transabdominal laparoscopic nephrectomy. *Eur Urol.* 1994;25:55.

30. De Canniere L, Lorge F, Rosiere A, et al. From laparoscopic training on an animal model to retroperitoneoscopic or coelioscopic adrenal and renal surgery in human. *Surg Endosc.* 1995;9:699.

31. Cochran ST, Krasny RM, Danovitch GM, et al. Helical CT angiography for examination of living renal donors. *AJR Am J Roentgenol.* 1997;168:1569. See comments.

32. Smith PA, Ratner LE, Lynch FC, et al. Role of CT angiography in the preoperative evaluation for laparoscopic nephrectomy. *Radiographics.* 1998;18:589.

33. Helal M, Albertini J, Lockhart J, et al. Laparoscopic nephrectomy using the harmonic scalpel. *J Endourol.* 1997;11:267.

Chapter Seventy-Seven ● ● ● ● ● ●

*L*aparoscopic Techniques Used to Treat Testicular Ectopia

ROBERT G. MOORE, DONALD MEHAN, and RAUL O. PARRA

Testicular ectopia (cryptorchid testis) is defined as a testis that is not in the scrotum. In a review of several series on undescended testes Kleintech et al established the frequency of undescended testes by anatomic location.[1] The following estimations were found: intra-abdominal testicle, 8%; inguinal position, 62.5%; ectopic, 11%; and high scrotal or low inguinal, 24%. The cryptorchid testis is more common on the right (70% incidence) compared to the left (30%). Thirty percent of the cryptorchid testes in this cumulative series were bilateral.

This chapter is a review of laparoscopic techniques used to treat and evaluate the undescended testis. The cryptorchid testis is divided into two specific types based on physical examination: palpable and nonpalpable. Laparoscopy is only applied to the non-palpable testis. The percentage of nonpalpable testes ranges from 9 to 54% of all undescended testes,[2–8] but the incidence is generally accepted to be 20%.[9]

Contraindications to laparoscopy in the pediatric patient are similar to adult patients. Absolute contraindications include severe cardiopulmonary disease and bleeding disorders. Relative contraindications include extensive prior abdominal pelvic surgery.

Interventional techniques described in this chapter will deal with the intra-abdominal or emergent/peeping testicle. In these conditions, foreshortening or fixation of the gonadal vascular structures can cause maldescent into an intra-abdominal location. Multiple series on cryptorchid testes have described increased association of inguinal hernias and testicular ductal abnormalities.[10–12] Because of the circumstances described, these testicles can be challenging to mobilize into the scrotum by traditional open operative techniques.

Bilateral nonpalpable testicles must be thoroughly evaluated to rule out either anorchidism or intersex disorders prior to surgical intervention. Intersex syndromes can be excluded when a karyotype analysis reveals 46XY. Anorchidism can be diagnosed when a human chorionic gonadotropin stimulation test fails to increase serum testosterone and when basal serum gonadotropin levels have been elevated on at least two occasions.[13] If the diagnosis of anorchidism is made, surgical exploration is not warranted.

In reference to a unilateral undescended testicle that is not palpated on physical examination, endocrine testing is of no value. Human chorionic gonadotropin (hCG) has been used in several series in an effort to enlarge the undescended testicle in hopes of making it palpable. The results of hCG localization of the nonpalpable testicle are controversial, and this technique is ineffective for localization of the high undescended testis.[14,15]

Several radiographic imaging modalities have been used to identify the nonpalpable testes. Ultrasound has been successful in diagnosing some of the canalicular nonpalpable testes, but has difficulty localizing canalicular testicular remnants or intra-abdominal testes.[16,17] Both computed tomography and magnetic resonance imaging cannot reliably localize a nonpalpable testicle or prove its absence.[18,19] In addition, children younger than 5 years have to be sedated to obtain a reliable study. Venography is invasive and requires considerable technical expertise to perform on children younger than 5 years.[20]

Diagnostic laparoscopy has been used to identify the location of the nonpalpable testis since the 1970s.[21] Since this time, several articles have demonstrated that the diagnostic accuracy of laparoscopy for localizing the undescended testis approaches 100%, making it the most accurate modality for assessment of nonpalpable testes.[11,12]

DIAGNOSTIC LAPAROSCOPY

The patient is positioned in the supine position. All laparoscopic procedures should be conducted under general anesthesia. Reexamination after induction of anesthesia is essential to rule out a palpable testis. General anesthesia can often relax the abdominal wall, making examination easier. Occasionally a preoperative nonpalpable testis can become a palpable testis under anesthesia, in which case laparoscopic localization would not be needed.

In all laparoscopic procedures the potential for an open laparotomy exists. For this reason, the whole abdominal wall must be prepared and draped and open instrumentation must be available. The stomach and bladder are decompressed with an orogastric tube and bladder catheter, respectively.

The initial step in diagnostic laparoscopy is obtaining intraperitoneal access to the abdominal cavity. Two techniques, open and closed (Veress needle), can be used. For the closed technique, the surgeon must be conscious of the decreased space between the abdominal wall and vital organs/structures in a child. The abdominal wall is elevated by placing a pediatric Kocker clamp or towel clamps on the inferior margin of the umbilicus. The Veress needle is introduced into the peritoneal cavity through the base of the umbilicus. Localization studies are performed to confirm intraperitoneal placement of the Veress needle. Insufflation is initiated at low flow rates (1 L/min). Opening pressures should be less than 5 mm Hg. After confirmation of intra-abdominal placement of the Veress needle, the insufflation is increased to 4 to 5 L/min until an intraperitoneal pressure of 20 mm Hg is reached. Placement of a 5-mm trocar through an infraumbilical incision is facilitated by pulling laterally with towel clamps. After initial trocar placement, the intra-abdominal pressure is decreased to 10 to 15 mm Hg.

Intraperitoneal access via the open technique is initiated by making a 5-mm infra-umbilical incision. The rectus fascia is exposed by blunt dissection. A 5-mm fascial and peritoneal incision is made in the midline. Stay sutures are placed on the edge of both the fascia and peritoneum. A 5-mm laparoscopic cannula is backloaded onto a zero-degree laparoscope and placed in the peritoneal cavity under direct vision.

The surgeon will immediately visualize intra-abdominal structures. Orientation of the midline can be readily obtained by putting gentle traction on the Foley catheter. Other midline structures are easily identified: the urachal remnant superiorly and the sigmoid colon inferiorly. The paired medial umbilical ligaments are seen on each side of the bladder (Fig. 77–1).

The internal inguinal ring is visualized lateral to the medial umbilical ligament. If the inguinal region is not clearly observed, additional maneuvers, such as pulling on the respective hemiscrotum or putting pressure on the external inguinal ring, can be helpful.

For unilateral undescended testes the normal side should be visualized first. The testicular vascular pedicle is noted transversing the internal inguinal ring (Fig. 77–1). An inguinal hernia may or may not be present (Fig. 77–2). The vas deferens is noted as it crosses the external iliac vessels (medial to lateral) and courses toward the internal inguinal ring.

After depicting the normal anatomy on the side of the descended testicle, attention is turned to the undescended side. Possible findings include (1) canalicular vas and vessels (normal gonadal artery and vein, and vas deferens entering the internal inguinal ring; Figs. 77–1 and 77–2); intra-abdominal testis (Fig. 77–3); (3) intra-abdominal blind-ending vessels and vas (vanishing gonad); and (4) blind-ending vas with proximal testicular dissociation.

When a surgeon identifies canalicular vas and vessels, he or she has to rule out an emerging/peeping testis. A peeping testis can be diagnosed by placing gentle pressure over the internal ring. If an emerging testis is present, optimal management is primary laparoscopic orchiopexy. These testes are often palpable after induction of general anesthesia and can also be managed by primary laparoscopic orchiopexy.[22]

When a peeping testis is not present, an open inguinal exploration must be performed. Possible inguinal findings include high inguinal gonad or ectopic testis with or without (50%) inguinal hernia, remnant testis, or canalicular vanishing testis (blind-ending vas and vessels).[11] All gonadal remnants should be excised because viable seminiferous tubules have been found in several series.[11,12]

Intra-abdominal vanishing testis (blind-ending vas and vessels) is found in 7 to 17% of nonpalpable testes.[11,12] If no gonadal tissue is found in the area of the blind-ending vas and vessels, the patient can with absolute diagnostic accuracy be declared to have a vanishing testis on that side.[11] With this finding, no additional exploration is needed. If remnant gonadal tissue is present, it can

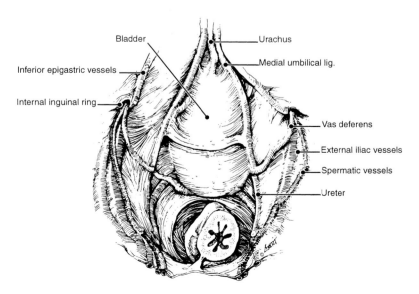

Figure 77–1. Normal intraperitoneal anatomy of the pediatric pelvis and internal inguinal ring region.

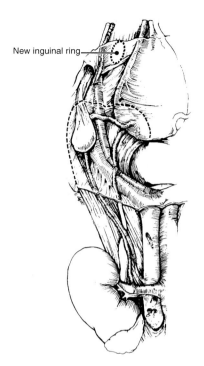

New inguinal ring

Figure 77–2. Intraperitoneal view of a left intra-abdominal testis. A patent processus (hernia) is seen at the internal ring. The dotted lines demonstrate where peritoneotomy is performed for both primary and staged laparoscopic orchiopexy. For first stage of the staged laparoscopic orchiopexy, the spermatic vessels are clipped at level of the iliac bifurcation.

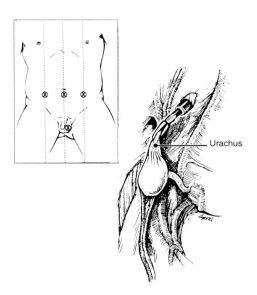

Urachus

Figure 77–3. Laparoscopic port sites are demonstrated for both primary laparoscopy orchiopexy and second stage laparoscopic staged orchiopexy. The scrotal port is placed by back-loading a 5-mm cannula over a straight laparoscopic grasper. The internal view demonstrate the transfer of the testis from an intra-abdominal location through the new internal inguinal ring into the dependent portion of the scrotum.

be easily excised using laparoscopic techniques and removed through a 4 to 5-mm cannula. However, if only a blind-ending vas is found, the gonadal remnant is superior (proximal) to the blind-ending vas. When remnant gonadal tissue or blind-ending vessels are not found in the pelvis, secondary trocars must be placed and the exploration carried proximally by reflection of the respective colonic flexure. The dissection proceeds superiorly up to the kidney. A viable gonad has been found as high as the right lobe of the liver (personal communication, Craig A. Peters, Boston).

When an intra-abdominal testis is found, therapeutic options depend on the location of the intra-abdominal testis (below or at/above external iliac vessels) and the length of spermatic vessels. If the gonad is located at the internal ring and is associated with an inguinal hernia, a primary laparoscopic orchiopexy is almost universally successful in bringing the testis into the scrotum.[23] When a testis located at the internal ring is not associated with an inguinal hernia, the spermatic vessels can often be short. Surgical options include laparoscopic orchiectomy, primary laparoscopic orchiopexy, or staged laparoscopic orchiopexy.[23]

High (at/above external iliac vessels) intra-abdominal testes are described in approximately one-third of all intra-abdominal testes.[11] The testes often have severe epididymal dissociation. If the high intra-abdominal testis is unilateral and a viable contralateral descended testis is present, a laparoscopic orchioectomy is the treatment of choice. If the high intra-abdominal testis is the only viable gonad present, the therapeutic options include laparoscope-assisted testicular autotransplantation or staged laparoscopic orchiopexy.

PRIMARY LAPAROSCOPIC ORCHIOPEXY

The primary objective of orchiopexy is to bring the undescended testis into a scrotal location. The treatment of the intra-abdominal testis is challenging, with the open technique having suboptimal outcomes.[24] Laparoscopic orchiopexy has several advantages over its open counterpart, including (1) the ability to achieve extensive dissection of the testicular vascular pedicle up to its origin, (2) dissection of the proximal vessels without disturbing the peritoneum between the vas and distal testicular vessels (thus not precluding a Fowler–Stephens orchiopexy), (3) magnification (10 to 15 times normal), and (4) laparoscopic creation of a neo-internal ring medial to the inferior epigastric vessels (to increase spermatic cord length).[22]

After intra-abdominal access is achieved (see the earlier diagnostic laparoscopy section) and the diagnosis of intra-abdominal testis has been made, two additional 5-mm trocars are placed in the midclavicular line at the level of the anterior superior iliac spine on both the right and left side of the abdominal wall (Fig. 77–3). All cannulas are secured to the skin with 2-0 silk suture to prevent inadvertent dislodgment from the abdominal wall.

The technique for primary laparoscopic orchiopexy is initiated by incising the peritoneum lateral to the gonadal vessels and distal to the patent processus vaginalis (Fig. 77–2). Additional peritoneotomy is performed medial and distal to the vas. The goal of this dissection is to allow mobilization of the plane behind the whole cord.

If the testis is peeping, mild pressure is applied to the abdominal wall to deliver the testis into the abdominal cavity. The gubernaculum is identified and grasped and the anterior portion of the processus vaginalis is incised. Next, the distal vas deferens ("looping vas") is identified and the distal gubernaculum is divided with electrocautery (Fig. 77–4).[22] The posterior attachments of the testis and spermatic vessels are freed. Additional cord length is provided by extending the peritoneotomy over the iliac vessels superiorly up to its origin at the great vessels. By gentle lateral traction on the spermatic cord, the vessels are dissected away from the surrounding colonic mesentery. Incision of the lateral peritoneal reflection of the colon is rarely needed. Adequate length of the cord can be demonstrated by retracting the testis to the contralateral internal inguinal ring. Every attempt should be made to spare the triangle of peritoneum between the spermatic vessels and vas deferens.

An incision is made in the dependent portion of the respective anterior hemiscrotum. A standard subdartos pouch is created. In order for the undescended testis to be brought into the scrotum, a new internal inguinal ring must be made. A neo-internal ring is created by passing a straight 5-mm laparoscopic grasper through the ipsilateral midclavicular cannula and then directing it either laterally or medially to the inferior epigastric vessels. The new internal inguinal ring is passed medially to the epigastric vessels if the spermatic cord length is marginal. The straight grasper is directed over the pubic ramus (via bimanual palpation of the external inguinal ring) and then guided through the scrotal incision (Fig. 77–3). During this maneuver, the bladder is retracted medially with the contralateral grasper. A 5-mm cannula is back-loaded over the grasper until it is laparoscopically visualized at the new internal inguinal ring. A laparoscopic locking atraumatic grasper is placed through the scrotal trocar and the gubernaculum is grasped. Using a slow backward twisting motion, the grasper and cannula are drawn backwards until the testis is delivered into the created subdartos pouch. Attention is then directed back to the neo-inguinal ring to rule out iatrogenic torsion of the spermatic vessels. The testis is transfixed to the hemiscrotum using a Prolene suture through the junction of the testis and gubernaculum. The prolene suture is secured and tied over a button on the external scrotal wall. No attempt is made to close the peritoneal defect at the internal inguinal area. The inguinal ring will

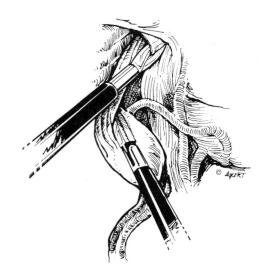

Figure 77–4. Dissection of the internal ring begins by incising the patent processus anteriorly and medially. The gubernaculum is mobilized superiorly and is divided distal to vasal structures.

TALE 77–1. PRIMARY LAPAROSCOPIC ORCHIOPEXY

Series	No. of Testes	Success Rate	Follow-Up (months)
Jordon et al[25]	13	100%	6
Docimo et al[26]	2	100%	4
Lindgren et al[27]	35	100%	3–4
Docimo et al[22]	12	100%	1–9
Peters et al[28]	8	87% (7/8)	—
Bogaert et al[29]	2	100%	9
Poppas et al[30]	10	90% (9/10)	3.5
Janetschek et al[31]	4	100%	—
Figenshau et al[32]	9	78% (7/9)	1.5

rapidly reperitonealize (2 to 5 days). Using this technique in over 30 cases, no postoperative inguinal hernia was found after 6 months or more (personal communication, S. G. Docmo, Baltimore). The scrotal button is removed after one week.

Outcomes of Primary Laparoscopic Orchiopexy

In order to properly evaluate a new surgical procedure, three critical categories must be assessed: outcome, postoperative morbidity, and operative time. Outcome must be compared to the "gold standard," in this case, open orchiopexy. Successful outcomes are measured by placement of the undescended/nonpalpable (nonatrophied) testes in the dependent position of the scrotum. Using this criterion for success, 95.8% (91 of 95) of the primary orchiopexies in the literature were successful (Table 77–1).[22,25–32] Follow-up of these patients ranged from 1 week to 9 months. Docimo used a meta-analysis to assess the successful outcome of open orchiopexy.[33] Success rates by anatomic position were 74% for abdominal and 82% for peeping (internal inguinal ring location) testes. Although this comparison is to historical open orchiopexies, preliminary results for primary laparoscopic orchiopexy are superior to its open counterpart.

Complications occurred in 2 patients (2.7%) undergoing primary laparoscopic orchiopexy. Operative time for primary laparoscopic orchiopexy was prolonged, at a mean operative time of 2.5 hours for unilateral and 3.0 hours for bilateral. Recently, several surgeons have reported a decrease in operative time for unilateral cases to 1.5 hours. The majority of these surgeries were performed as outpatient procedures.

LAPAROSCOPIC STAGED (FOWLER–STEPHENS) ORCHIOPEXY

Laparoscopic staged orchiopexy is indicated when the intra-abdominal testis is located at or above the iliac vessels or there are shortened spermatic vessels. One accessory cannula (5 mm) is needed for this procedure. A 5-mm laparoscopic clip applier (U.S. Surgical) can be used to occlude the gonad vessels. Alternatively, electrocautery or laser has been used to transect the spermatic vessels.[29,34]

The spermatic vessels must be ligated as high as possible (above the external iliac vessels). This maneuver is necessary in order to preserve the distal triangle of peritoneum between the vessels and vas deferens, which can potentially enhance collateral circulation.

The second stage of staged (Fowler–Stephens) orchiopexy can be performed with either open or laparoscopic techniques. This stage is deferred for at least 6 months after spermatic vessel clipping. Both approaches employ the same surgical concepts and principles: to preserve a wide band of peritoneum between the vas deferens and distal spermatic vessels, thus insuring adequate blood flow to the transposed testis.

Access for the open second stage of the Fowler–Stephens orchiopexy has been achieved via a lower midline or Jones incision (muscle splitting incision medial to the anterior superior iliac spine).[35,36] Laparoscopic intraperitoneal access is obtained as previously described in this chapter. Two additional 5-mm trocars are placed on the right and left sides in the midclavicular line at the level of the anterior superior iliac spine (Fig. 77–3).

After intra-abdominal access is accomplished, the previously placed clips are identified and the spermatic vessels are transected. A peritoneotomy is performed on the lateral aspect of the spermatic vessels (distal clips) and around the intra-abdominal testis. A V-shaped peritoneal flap is completely created by making a peritoneotomy from the clips over the iliac vessels toward the vas. The peritoneal flap and testis are dissected away from the retroperitoneum. Transposition of the intra-abdominal testis is accomplished as described earlier in the primary laparoscopic orchiopexy section. All abdominal wall trocar sites ($\geq$4 mm) are closed to prevent hernia formation. Alternatively, the Fowler–Stephens orchiopexy can be performed laparoscopically in one operation.

Outcomes of Laparoscopic Staged Orchiopexy

Successful surgical outcomes of the staged orchiopexy (Fowler–Stephens) are judged by the same criterion as primary laparoscopic orchiopexy. Using this standard for successful outcome, 98% of laparoscopic (both first and second-stage) staged orchiopexies were successful (Table 77–2). Eighty-eight percent of laparoscopic first-stage (clipping spermatic vessels) and open second-stage orchiopexy were successful. Follow-up ranged from 1 to 54 months. A review by Docimo found a success rate of 77% for open staged Fowler-Stephens orchiopexy.[33] Comparison between laparoscopic and open staged Fowler–Stephens orchiopexy

is beyond the scope of this chapter, but preliminary data favor the laparoscopic technique.

In addition to having a higher success rate, laparoscopy potentially can cause fewer postoperative adhesions. Moore and coauthors[41] evaluated the incidence of adhesion formation after urological laparoscopy. Adhesions formed in 9.8% (4 of 41 cases) of the laparoscopic procedures. The incidence of adhesion formation after staged laparoscopic orchiopexy was 2.9% (34 of 35 cases). The actual rate of postoperative adhesion formation after open staged orchiopexy is unknown, but similar open procedures form adhesions in half of the cases.[42]

LAPAROSCOPIC ORCHIECTOMY

Laparoscopic removal of an intra-abdominal testicle is not technically challenging. The gonad is freed from the adjacent peritoneum. Electrocautery or 5-mm clips are used to secure the vascular pedicle and vas deferens. A small Lap Sac is introduced through a 5-mm port. After placing the testis in the Lap Sac, it is removed from the peritoneal cavity by slightly extending the skin and fascial incision.

An inguinal hernia is often associated with an intra-abdominal testis and should be repaired at the time of orchiectomy. A laparoscopic herniorrhaphy is performed by incision and clipping the patent processus. The peritoneum is then reapproximated.[31]

CONCLUSION

Laparoscopic techniques used to treat the nonpalpable testis have proven to be more successful than comparable open procedures. The nonpalpable testis is an excellent indication for the use of laparoscopy in pediatric urology.

REFERENCES

1. Kleintech B, Hadziselimovic F, Hessi V, et al. *Kongenital Hodendystopien.* Stuttgart: Georg Thieme; 1989.
2. Redman JF. Impalpable testis: Observations based on 208 consecutive operations for undescended testes. *J Urol.* 1980;124:379.
3. Campbell HE. Incidence of malignant growth of the undescended testicle. A critical and statistical study. *Arch Surg.* 1942;44:353.
4. Tibbs DJ. Unilateral absence of the testis. Eight cases of true monorchism. *Br J Surg.* 1961;48:601.
5. Jones PG. Undescended testes. *Aust Paediatr J.* 1966;2:36.
6. Lach A. *Maldescensus Testis.* Colloquium at Tübingen, West Germany. Baltimore: Urban & Schwarzenberg; 1977.
7. Illig R, Exner GU, Kollmann F, et al. Treatment of cryptorchidism by intranasal synthetic luteinizing-hormone releasing hormone. Results of a collaborative double-blind study. *Lancet* 1977;2:518.
8. Smolko MJ, Kaplan GW, Brock WA. Location and fate of the nonpalpable testis in children. *J Urol.* 1983;129:1204.
9. Levitt SB, Kogen SJ, Engel RM, et al. The impalpable testis: A rational approach to management. *J Urol.* 1978;120:515.
10. Scorer CG, Farrington GH. *Congenital Deformities of the Testis and Epidymis.* Appleton-Century-Crofts: 1971;56.
11. Moore RG, Peters CA, Bauer SB, et al. Laparoscopic evaluation of the nonpalpable testis: A prospective assessment of accuracy. *J Urol.* 1994;151:728.
12. Tennenbaum SY, Lerner SE, McAleer IM, et al. Preoperative

TABLE 77–2. STAGED (FOWLER-STEPHENS) ORCHIOPEXY

Laparoscopic First and Second Stage			
Series	No. of Testes	Success Rate	Follow-Up (months)
Poppas et al[30]	1	0%	3.5
Bogaert et al[29]	3	100%	9.0
Jordan & Winslow[25]	3	100%	12.0
Caldamone & Amaral[37]	5	100%	5–17
Esposito & Garipoli[38]	33	100%	5–54
Figenshau et al[32]	2	100%	—
Humphrey & Najmaldin[40]	10	100%	24.0
Janetschek et al[31]	4	100%	—
Lindgren et al[27]	3	100%	1–11
Laparoscopic First Stage and Open Second Stage			
Bogaert et al[29]	5	100%	9.0
Esposito & Garipoli[38]	2	50%	5–54
Bloom[39]	7	85.7%	6–36

laparoscopic localization of the nonpalpable testis: A critical analysis of a 10-year experience. *J Urol.* 1994;151:732.

13. Levitt SB, Kogan SJ, Schneider KM, et al. Endocrine tests in phenotypic children with bilateral impalpable tests can reliably predict "congenital anorchism." *Urology.* 1978;11:11.

14. Rajfer J. Congenital anomalies of the testis. In: Walsh PC, Retik AB, Stamey TA, et al, eds. *Campbell's Urology*, 6th ed, vol. 2. Saunders: 1992;1543.

15. Naslund MJ, Gearhart JP, Jeffs RD. Laparoscopy: Its selected use in patients with unilateral nonpalpable testis after human chorionic gonadotropin stimulation. *J Urol.* 1989;142:108.

16. Madrazo BL, Klugo RC, Parks JA, et al. Ultrasonographic demonstration of undescended testes. *Radiology.* 1979;133:181.

17. Weiss RM, Carter AR, Rosenfield AT. High resolution real-time ultrasonography in the localization of the undescended testis. *J Urol.* 1986;135:936.

18. Wolverson MK, Jagannadharao B, Sundaram M, et al. CT in localization of impalpable cryptorchid testes. *AJR.* 1980;134:725.

19. Fritzsche PJ, Hricak H, Kogan BA, et al. Undescended testis: Value of MR imaging. *Radiology.* 1987;164:169.

20. Weiss RM, Glickman MG, Lytton B. Clinical implication of gonadal venography in the management of the non-palpable undescended testis. *J Urol.* 1979;121:745.

21. Cortesi N, Ferarri P, Zambarada E, et al. Diagnosis of bilateral abdominal cryptorchidism by laparoscopy. *Endoscopy.* 1976;8:32.

22. Docimo SG, Moore RG, Adams J, et al. Laparoscopic orchiopexy for the high palpable undescended testis: Preliminary experience. *J Urol.* 1995;154:1513.

23. Jordan GH. Management of the abdominal nonpalpable undescended testicle. In: Resnick MI, Winfield HN, eds. *Atlas of the Urologic Clinics of North America.* Saunders: 1993;49.

24. Docimo SG. The results of surgical therapy for cryptorchidism: A literature review and analysis. *J Urol.* 1995;154:1148.

25. Jordan GH, Winslow BH. Laparoscopic single stage and staged orchiopexy. *J Urol.* 1994;152:1249.

26. Docimo SG, Moore RG, Kavoussi LR. Laparoscopic orchidopexy in the prune belly syndrome: A case report and review of the literature. *Urology.* 1995;45:679.

27. Lindgren BW, Darby EC, Faiella L, et al. Laparoscopic orchidopexy: Procedure of choice for the non-palpable testis (abstract). *J Urol.* 1997;157(suppl 4):90.

28. Peters PA, Kavoussi LR, Retik AB. Laparoscopic management of intraabdominal testis (abstract). *J Endourol.* 1993;7(suppl 1):S170.

29. Bogaert GA, Kogan A, Mevorach RA. Therapeutic laparoscopy for intraabdominal testes. *Urology.* 1993;42:182.

30. Poppas DP, Lemack GE, Mininberg DT. Laparoscopic orchiopexy: Clinical experience and description of technique. *J Urol.* 1996;155:708.

31. Janetschek G, Corvin S, Radmayr C, et al. Laparoscopic approach to pathology of the internal inguinal ring: Hernia, hydrocele, cryptorchidism (abstract). *J Endourol.* 1997;11(suppl 1):S135.

32. Figenshau R, Elbahnasy A, Shalhan A, et al. Laparoscopic management of children with an impalpable testis: The Washington University experience (abstract). *J Endourol.* 1997;11(suppl 1):S135.

33. Docimo SG. The results of surgical therapy for cryptorchidism: A literature review and analysis. *J Urol.* 1995;154:1148.

34. Walschmidt J, Scher F. Surgical correction of abdominal testes after Fowler-Stephenson's using the neodymium:YAG laser for preliminary vessel dissection. *Eur J Pediatr Surg.* 1991;1:54.

35. Gheiler EL, Barthold JS, Gonzalez R. Benefits of laparoscopy and the Jones technique for the nonpalpable testis. *J Urol.* 1997;158:1948.

36. Koota DH, Rushton HG, Belma AB. Management of the intraabdominal testis: The open approach revisited (abstract). *J Urol.* 1997;157(suppl 4):90.

37. Caldamone AA, Amaral JF. Laparoscopic stage 2 Fowler-Stephens orchiopexy. *J Urol.* 1994;152:1253.

38. Esposito C, Garipoli V. The value of 2-step laparoscopic Fowler-Stephens orchiopexy for intra-abdominal testis. *J Urol.* 1997;158:1952.

39. Bloom DA. Two-step orchiopexy with pelviscopic clip ligation of the spermatic vessels. *J Urol.* 1991;145:1030.

40. Humphrey G, Najmaldin AS. Laparoscopy for the impalpable testis. *J Endourol.* 1997;11(suppl 1):S135.

41. Moore RG, Kavoussi LR, Bloom DA, et al. Postoperative adhesion formation after urological laparoscopy in the pediatric population. *J Urol.* 1995;153:792.

42. Weibel MA, Majno G. Peritoneal adhesions and their relation to abdominal surgery. A postmortem study. *Am J Surg.* 1973;126:345.

Chapter Seventy-Eight ● ● ● ● ● ■

*L*aparoscopic Nephrectomy for Benign and Malignant Renal Disease

RALPH V. CLAYMAN, ARIEH SHALHAV, and DAVID HOENIG

It has been more than a century since the first nephrectomy was performed by Gustav Simon. At that time, Dr. Simon had failed to correct a ureteral vaginal fistula in an older woman, despite five attempts. Following a successful nephrectomy in the animal laboratory, Dr. Simon subsequently offered this procedure to his patient. On August 2, 1869 in a 40-minute operation, he was successful in removing the kidney. Of interest, while the intraoperative time was short, the postoperative course was lengthy, requiring 6 months' hospital stay before drainage from the wound ceased.[1] Despite significant advances during the past 100 years in anesthesia, antibiotics, analgesia, and surgical instrumentation, the basic open approach to nephrectomy has not changed significantly since Dr. Simon's initial report.

In 1990, Clayman et al began animal studies to see if the trend in laparoscopic surgery could be applied to the removal of a normal-sized kidney.[2] After development of an entrapment sack and a tissue morcellator system (Cook Urological, Spencer, IN), they were successful in perfecting a technique for laparoscopic nephrectomy. In June 1990, their laboratory work was brought into the clinical realm, when they removed a right tumor-bearing kidney in an 85-year-old woman. The surgical time was lengthy, 6 hours and 15 minutes, but her hospital stay was relatively brief: 6 days.[3] Since that time, the technique for laparoscopic nephrectomy has spread worldwide. Indications for laparoscopic nephrectomy have now mirrored the basic indications for open surgical nephrectomy. As such, these techniques are employed for the removal of kidneys with benign as well as malignant disease.

Laparoscopic simple nephrectomy for benign disease has now been accomplished by both transperitoneal and retroperitoneal approaches. The transperitoneal approach is preferred when the estimated renal weight is over 200 g or when the retroperitoneum is scarred due to prior renal inflammation,

perirenal abscess, or earlier retroperitoneal open surgery. As such, ideal candidates for the retroperitoneal approach are patients with renovascular hypertension, end-stage ureteropelvic junction obstruction without associated pyelonephritis, or renal failure due to noninfectious causes.

Today, laparoscopic simple nephrectomy has been performed for all situations in which a nephrectomy is required; however, this procedure is particularly difficult in patients undergoing donor nephrectomy, nephrectomy for polycystic kidney disease, or nephrectomy for xanthogranulomatous pyelonephritis (XGP). The last is the most challenging situation; as with open surgery, this condition, makes renal dissection difficult and is fraught with potential complications such as vascular injury or trauma to neighboring structures.[4,5]

LAPAROSCOPIC SIMPLE NEPHRECTOMY FOR BENIGN RENAL DISEASE

Transperitoneal Approach

Preoperative Preparation

Twenty-four hours prior to a laparoscopic nephrectomy, the patient is placed on a clear liquid diet and also given a laxative. No formal mechanical or antibiotic bowel preparation is given. Food and drink are stopped after midnight on the day of the planned procedure.

Preoperative procedures are rarely indicated. A ureteral stent is placed only if there is a history of significant perirenal or periureteral scarring. Likewise, there is no need for arteriography in these patients prior to their laparoscopic nephrectomy, regardless of the benign or malignant nature of their underlying disease.

Methods

General. Transperitoneal laparoscopic nephrectomy involves eight steps:

1. Lateral insufflation with placement of four or five ports.
2. Retroperitoneal incision of the colonic peritoneal reflection (base of the "triangle").
3. Incision in peritoneum overlying the kidney and in Gerota's fascia (sides of the "triangle").
4. Securing the ureter.
5. Dissection of the renal hilum.
6. Incision of the ureter.
7. Entrapment and morcellation of the specimen.
8. Exiting the abdomen.

Transperitoneal Technique. Under a general anesthetic, the patient is placed in a lateral decubitus position. Padding is placed under all dependent bony prominences. A Veress needle is passed via a 12-mm incision, two finger breadths medial to and two finger breadths superior to the anterior superior iliac spine. This is facilitated by grasping the fascia of the external oblique muscle with two atraumatic clamps, thereby stabilizing the abdominal wall while passing the Veress needle. Alternatively, an open cannula (Hasson) technique can be used.

After obtaining a pneumoperitoneum, a 12-mm port is placed through the initial incision; two more 12-mm ports are placed, both under endoscopic control: one in the midclavicular line subcostal and another port in the pararectus area just lateral and superior to the umbilicus (Fig. 78–1).

For simple nephrectomy, on the *right* side, the concept is one of creating a "triangle" around the kidney (Fig. 78–2). The line of Toldt is incised from the level of the cecum up to the level of the liver, thereby forming the base of the triangle. Next, off of the incision in the line of Toldt, at its lowermost extent, a second incision is made traveling cephalad and medial; this incision lies approximately 1 to 2 cm above the ascending colon, and parallels the colon up to the hepatic flexure. This incision releases the colon, which then can be bluntly dissected away from Gerota's fascia. As the colon is mobilized medially, the duodenum is identified lying deep to the colon and immediately juxtaposed to the medial aspect of the kidney; a Kocher maneuver is performed on the duodenum. As the duodenum is rolled medially, the inferior vena cava is seen lying deep to the duodenum. The medial extent of this lower incision in the peritoneum now overlies the inferior vena cava at the level of the insertion of the gonadal vein into the vena cava. This incision forms one side of the triangle. From this point overlying the inferior cava, the incision in the peritoneum is then continued cephalad and lateral until the line of Toldt is again encountered, usually at the level of the liver, thereby completing the triangle. Dissection along this line and through Gerota's fascia exposes the upper pole of the kidney, thereby allowing the surgeon to push the adrenal gland cephalad, away from the kidney. As such, the apex of the triangle is centered over the inferior vena cava. With these three incisions in the peritoneum, a triangular patch of peritoneum is left on the kidney.

On the *left*, the triangle concept does not apply, because the mesentery of the large bowel is more easily separated from the surface of Gerota's fascia. On the left, the approach is one of creating two parallel lines of dissection. Accordingly, the line of Toldt is incised from just above the iliac vessels to just above the upper pole of the kidney; the latter point lies just opposite to the lower edge of the spleen. The medial peritoneal edge of the line of Toldt can be elevated and the plane between the colonic mesentery and Gerota's fascia is identified and entered. This plane is most easily found just inferior to the kidney. Once entered, the dissection along this plane is continued cephalad, thus completing a second and roughly parallel vertical line of dissection. The colon is rolled medially away from Gerota's fascia all the way up to the splenic flexure of the colon. Further medial dissection in this plane leads the surgeon directly to the aorta. The surgeon must be extremely wary

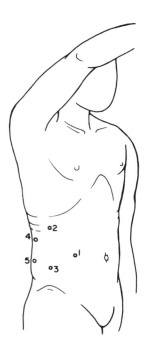

Figure 78–1. Port placement for a transperitoneal laparoscopic nephrectomy. The patient is in a full lateral decubitus position. Ports 1 to 3, 12 mm; ports 4 and 5, 5 mm. Port 3 is at the location where the Veress needle was initially passed to perform a lateral insufflation. *(Reprinted with permission from Clayman RV, McDougall E, eds. Laparoscopy Urology. St. Louis, Quality Medical Publishers, 1993.)*

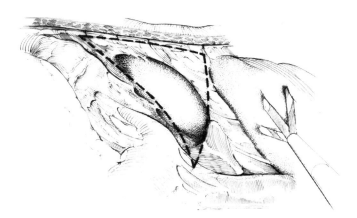

Figure 78–2. The "triangle" concept for right-sided, simple laparoscopic nephrectomy. The patient is in a lateral decubitus position.

at this juncture in the procedure, as this plane can inadvertently be developed too deeply, thus moving medial to the aorta; indeed, if this dissection is carried too far medially, the third portion of the duodenum or small bowel may be encountered. There is no need to develop the plane beyond the lateral border of the aorta. Once the splenic flexure of the colon is rolled somewhat medially, the tissue lying between the upper pole of the kidney and the edge of the spleen can be undermined going between the overlying tissue and the upper part of Gerota's fascia. This plane is developed laterally until the initial incision in the line of Toldt is reached. Within the overlying tissue is the splenocolic and splenorenal ligaments; these ligaments, and all of the overlying pararenal fatty tissue, can be rapidly secured and divided with a GIA tissue stapler, directed from the superior extent of the more medial vertical incision (the one separating the colonic mesentery from the medial extent of Gerota's fascia) toward the incised line of Toldt.

Two additional 5-mm ports are usually placed at this time. One port is placed in the posterior axillary lines subcostally and another 5-mm port can be placed in the anterior axillary line just above the iliac crest.

The ureter is next identified. On the right side, it is often necessary to identify, dissect, and clip the gonadal vein, following which the ureter can be identified just beneath it. The ureter is then carefully dissected and secured. On the left side, the gonadal vein likewise crosses the ureter and can be identified, dissected, and clipped and the ureter identified and secured. A helpful technique is to pass a Carter–Thomasson device through the lower abdomen with a 1-0 Vicryl suture on it. The suture can then be passed around the ureter and then retrieved with the Carter-Thomasson device and delivered onto the abdominal wall. The two ends of the suture can then be drawn up to the abdominal wall and secured with a mosquito clamp in order to place tension on the ureter.

Now, using a small grasping forceps through the two 5-mm ports, the kidney within Gerota's fascia can be retracted laterally. The medial edge of Gerota's fascia can then be incised vertically just lateral to the inferior vena cava on the right side and just lateral to the aorta on the left side. Dissection along the vena cava will soon reveal the right renal vein. On the left side, the left renal vein will be noted as it crosses over the aorta. *It is most helpful to follow the left gonadal vein cephalad until it enters the renal vein; this will prevent the surgeon from dissecting too far medially.* A horizontal incision in Gerota's fascia can then be made over the renal vein and continued upward, thereby exposing the midportion of the anterior renal surface. At this point, Gerota's fascia and the perirenal fat can be cleared from the anterior surface of the kidney. The grasping forceps, via the two lateral 5-mm ports, can then be repositioned on the upper and lower poles of the kidney, thereby retracting the kidney laterally and placing some mild tension on the renal hilum. This will greatly facilitate the dissection of the renal vessels. The hilar dissection is completed by the surgeon working through the two midclavicular-line ports, with the camera in the most medial 12-mm port. The hilar dissection can be done with a grasping forceps and the scissors, although the authors much prefer to use a hook electrode, which allows for a very fine and controlled dissection along the vessels.

The renal vein is first identified and carefully dissected, following which the renal artery is then identified. On the right, the vascular hilum to the kidney usually lies beneath the edge of the liver. As such, this liver edge needs to be retracted cephalad. If need be, an additional 5-mm port can be placed, in the area of the

xiphoid, in order to retract the liver edge. The right renal artery usually lies directly posterior, or posterior and slightly superior, to the right renal vein. On the left side, the gonadal and ascending lumbar veins need to be carefully dissected and separately occluded with 9-mm clips, in order to free the left renal vein. It is best to place these clips approximately 1 cm away from the left renal vein, so that they will not interfere with the subsequent placement of the GIA vascular stapler on the left renal vein. At this point, the upper edge of the left renal vein should also be carefully dissected and the left adrenal vein identified and preserved. Gerota's fascia can be entered, and the dissection can be continued along the medial and superior surface of the renal capsule, thereby widely separating the left adrenal gland from the kidney. Once the left renal vein is dissected, the left renal artery, which usually lies directly posterior or posterior and slightly inferior to the left renal vein, can be identified and dissected.

Following this, five 9-mm clips are placed across the artery and the artery is incised such that three of the 9-mm clips remain on the aortic side of the artery (Fig. 78–3). Next, the renal vein can be taken with a 12-mm GIA 3-cm long vascular stapler. This stapler places six rows of staples and cuts between the third and fourth row (Fig. 78–4). The rest of the renal hilar is dissected and the kidney is completely freed such that its only attachment is the ureter. In this regard, for a simple nephrectomy, it is important for the surgeon to stay directly on the renal capsule, as the remainder of the kidney is freed from the perirenal fat.

Next, the ureter is secured with four 9-mm clips. A locking grasping forceps is placed on the ureter proximal to the clips via the upper and lateral-most port. The ureter is then cut between the second and third clip, thereby completing the dissection (Fig. 78–5).

The now-free right or left kidney is moved into the respective upper abdominal quadrant such that it rests on the liver or

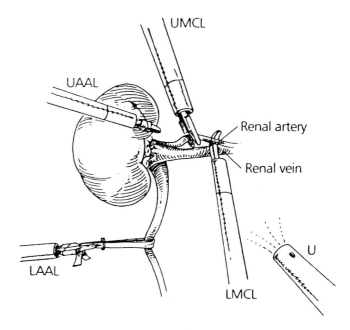

Figure 78–3. Clip placement on the renal artery after dissection of the renal hilum. *(Reprinted with permission from Clayman RV, McDougall E, eds. Laparoscopy Urology. St. Louis, Quality Medical Publishers, 1993.)*

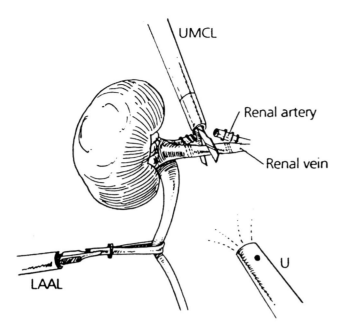

Figure 78–4. The use of a vascular EndoGIA stapler for simultaneous stapling and cutting of the renal vein. *(Reprinted with permission from Clayman RV, McDougall E, eds. Laparoscopy Urology. St. Louis, Quality Medical Publishers, 1993.)*

spleen. Following this, a laparoscopic entrapment sack is passed into the abdomen (Fig. 78–6). The newer entrapment sacks (such as Endocatch, U.S. Surgical, Stamford, CT) have spring-wire attached to the mouth of the sack such that upon deploying the sack into the abdomen, it immediately opens to its full size. This type

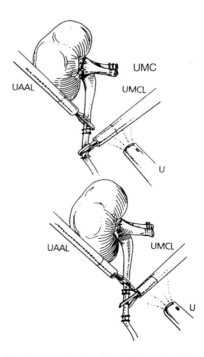

Figure 78–5. Clip placement and cutting of the ureter. *(Reprinted with permission from Clayman RV, McDougall E, eds. Laparoscopy Urology. St. Louis, Quality Medical Publishers, 1993.)*

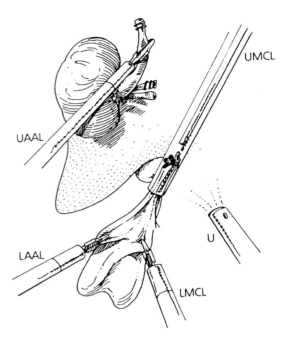

Figure 78–6. Entrapment sack insertion. Note that the proximal ureter has been secured with a locking grasping forceps. This is used to move the kidney cephalad until it rests on the surface of the liver. *(Reprinted with permission from Clayman RV, McDougall E, eds. Laparoscopy Urology. St. Louis, Quality Medical Publishers, 1993.)*

of sack is best introduced via a lower 12-mm port such that the mouth of the sack faces cephalad and is positioned under the inferior edge of the liver or spleen; it is then quite easy to scoop the specimen into the opened sack. If a nonself-expanding sack is used (such as LapSac, Cook Urological, Spencer, IN), then the sack is introduced via the upper medial 12-mm port. The sack is unfurled in the abdomen using atraumatic grasping forceps. Next, the camera port is moved to the upper midclavicular line port, following which the lower three ports are used for the passage of grasping forceps that can be used to further unfurl the sack. Traumatic locking grasping forceps are then introduced, through the three lowermost ports, and are used to grasp the tabs on the sack and *triangulate* it open. The middle grasper is used to pull the sack upward against the underside of the abdominal wall, thereby forming the apex of the triangle, while the lateral and medial graspers are used to stretch the sack laterally and medially and thereby form the base of the triangle. The base of the triangle in the sack is then moved until it lies underneath the lower lip of the liver or spleen. The laparoscope is introduced into the sack to further open it (Fig. 78–7). Now, the specimen is placed into the sack by moving the locking grasping forceps on the ureter towards the grasping forceps that is at the apex of the sack (Fig. 78–8). The kidney is thus moved deeply into the sack. Once the kidney appears to have entered the sack, the person holding the two grasping forceps on the base of the sack can then lift the forceps upward, further trapping the kidney and pushing it deeper into the sack (Fig. 78–9).

Now the entrapment sack is closed by pulling on the drawstring of the sack; this string is retrieved via one of the 12-mm port sites, usually the upper midclavicular-line port. Once the drawstring has been pulled through the port, the port itself is removed and the entire neck of the sack is delivered through the port site

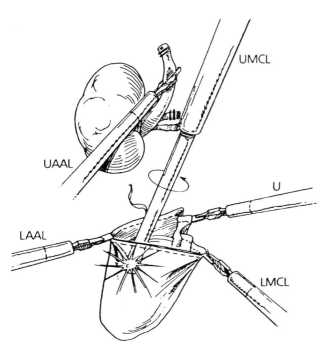

Figure 78–7. The laparoscope is inserted into the sack and moved in a widening circular motion to help open the sack. *(Reprinted with permission from Clayman RV, McDougall E, eds. Laparoscopy Urology. St. Louis, Quality Medical Publishers, 1993.)*

incision (Fig. 78–10). The specimen is morcellated with a Kelly clamp and ring forceps and the pieces of the kidney are removed from the sack; the now empty sack is pulled from the abdomen.

Lastly, the port sites are closed. Any port larger than 5 mm requires closure of the fascia; the skin of these larger sites is also

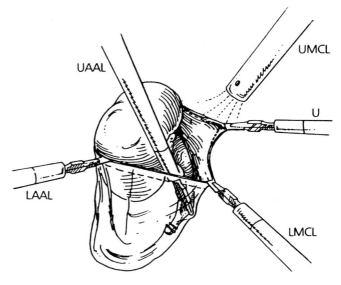

Figure 78–9. Elevation of the lower edge of the sack by the medial and lateral grasper completes delivery of the specimen deep into the sack. *(Reprinted with permission from Clayman RV, McDougall E, eds. Laparoscopy Urology. St. Louis, Quality Medical Publishers, 1993.)*

closed with a subcuticular absorbable suture. All skin sites are also closed with adhesive strips.

Retroperitoneal Approach

Preoperative Preparation. The preparation of the patient for retroperitoneoscopy is the same as for the transperitoneal approach.

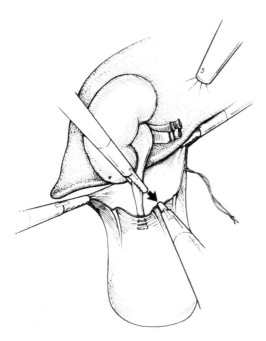

Figure 78–8. Specimen is inserted into the sack; the grasper on the ureter is directed towards the top grasper on the sack, which forms the apex of the triangular opening in the sack.

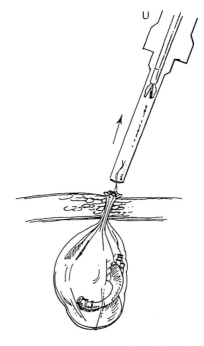

Figure 78–10. The neck of the sack is delivered through a 12-mm port site by pulling on the drawstrings. The 12-mm cannula has already been removed. *(Reprinted with permission from Clayman RV, McDougall E, eds. Laparoscopy Urology. St. Louis, Quality Medical Publishers, 1993.)*

The only difference is that early in one's experience it is extremely helpful to place an external ureteral stent, to help identify the ureter. This is especially valuable in the obese patient. Usually for the ureteral stent, the authors prefer to place a 7 Fr., 11.5-mm occlusion balloon catheter under fluoroscopic control. The balloon can then be inflated in the renal pelvis, and a 0.035 Amplatz super-stiff guidewire can be advanced through the catheter to further stiffen the shaft of the balloon catheter. This external ureteral stent is then prepared and draped into the operative field, allowing the surgeon to easily access the catheter and move it back and forth, thereby facilitating identification of the ureter.

Methods

General. There are seven steps to performing a laparoscopic retroperitoneal nephrectomy:

1. Retroperitoneal access.
2. Identifying and securing the ureter.
3. Incision of Gerota's fascia.
4. Hilar dissection.
5. Incision of the ureter.
6. Entrapment and morcellation.
7. Exiting the retroperitoneum.

Retroperitoneal Technique. Entry into the retroperitoneum can either be with a Veress needle or by an open cannula technique. For Veress needle entry, the Veress needle is passed either at the inferior or superior lumbar triangle. The usual signs for entering the peritoneal cavity apply to entering the retroperitoneum, as the Veress needle will spring forward readily once the retroperitoneal fat is entered. After obtaining a pneumoretroperitoneum, a 12-mm port is placed in either of the two places mentioned. After laparoscopic inspection, to visually confirm entry into the retroperitoneum (that is, visualization of retroperitoneal fat), balloon dilation of the retroperitoneum can be performed. This can be done with a commercial balloon or with a very simple homemade balloon using a 16 Fr. catheter and the excised middle finger of a size 8 latex surgeon's glove (Fig. 78–11). Using two 1-0 silk sutures, the glove finger is affixed to the shaft of the 16 Fr. catheter, just proximal to the sideholes in the catheter. This apparatus is then backloaded through a 30 Fr. Amplatz sheath, which in turn is

passed through the 12-mm port. The balloon is pushed out of the sheath and into the retroperitoneum. It is then filled with 1 L saline, following which it is left in place for several minutes, drained, and removed through the Amplatz sheath. The sheath is then removed (Fig. 78–12).[4,6]

A quicker and easier route to the retroperitoneum is by an open cannula placement. A 2-cm incision is made in the superior lumbar triangle, which lies just posterior to the tip of the twelfth rib. The incision is deepened until the retroperitoneal fat is encountered. The surgeon's finger is used to dissect the pararenal fat lying outside of Gerota's fascia. If desired, the dilating balloon can be used at this point, or alternatively the surgeon can use his or her finger to develop the retroperitoneal space. In the latter circumstance, additional ports can be placed into the retroperitoneum using the surgeon's finger as a guide. This manual digital method allows for the rapid development and placement of all of the ports, usually within a span of only a few minutes.[7]

Following placement of 12-mm cannulas in the inferior and superior lumbar triangles, the peritoneum is dissected anterior and a 5-mm port is placed in the anterior axillary line subcostal. Additional ports are placed, posterior to the superior lumbar triangle (12-mm port) and sometimes in the anterior axillary line just above the superior iliac spine (5-mm port) (Fig. 78–13). The latter port may be eliminated if a Carter–Thomasson device is used to secure the ureter, as previously described.

Upon first passing the laparoscope into the retroperitoneum, the psoas muscle can usually be clearly seen. Next, the ureter is sought. Moving the ureteral catheter at the urethral meatus rapidly reveals the ureter, which lies just medial and slightly deep to the medial edge of the psoas muscle. The Carter–Thomasson device, armed with a 1-0 silk suture, is passed via a separate stab wound incision; this incision is usually superior and slightly lateral to the anterior superior iliac spine. The silk suture is passed around the ureter, following which the two ends of the suture are grasped by the Carter–Thomasson device and delivered onto the abdominal wall. The suture is secured on the abdominal wall with a small clamp; the ureter is thus placed under slight tension. Following

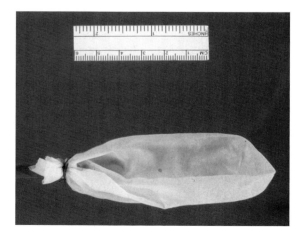

Figure 78–11. The homemade balloon for retroperitoneal space creation; the middle finger of a #8 latex glove has been affixed to the end of a 16 Fr. catheter with two 1-0 silk sutures.

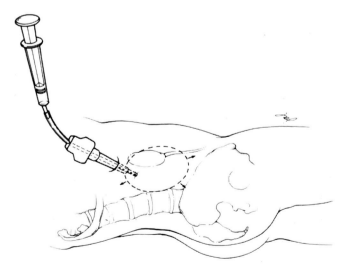

Figure 78–12. Positioning and inflation of the balloon in the retroperitoneal space. *(Reprinted with permission from Clayman RV, McDougall E, eds. Laparoscopy Urology. St. Louis, Quality Medical Publishers, 1993.)*

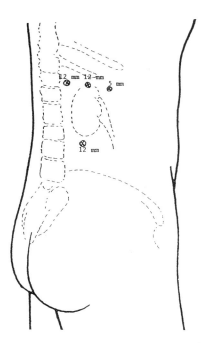

Figure 78–13. Port placement for retroperitoneal laparoscopic nephrectomy in full lateral position. *(Reprinted with permission from Clayman RV, Mc-Dougall E, eds. Laparoscopy Urology. St. Louis, Quality Medical Publishers, 1993.)*

this, Gerota's fascia is further incised posterior, and the perirenal fat is cleared from the kidney down to the surface of the renal capsule.

The medial edge of the ureter can be followed cephalad to the renal pelvis and renal hilum. On the right side, the renal artery is seen first, dissected and secured with five clips. However, on the left side, the ascending lumbar vein may be seen first; it should be divided between clips. The left renal artery can then be seen. Also on the left side, the gonadal and sometimes adrenal veins need to be taken separately prior to securing the renal vein. Also of note, after taking the renal artery, the renal vein is often 5 to 10 mm deep to the site of the arterial dissection. It is important to carefully dissect the hilar tissue anterior to the artery in order to identify and not injure the renal vein.

Following the hilar dissection, the remaining renal attachments are freed by dissecting the kidney directly on the renal capsule. Once this is done, the ureter is secured with a locking grasping forceps via the uppermost medial port; distal to this site the ureter is clipped (four 9-mm clips) and divided.

Now, the kidney, which is usually of a small size, can either be extracted through the initial 2-cm incision if an open access was performed, or a small 4 by 5-inch entrapment sack can be introduced and opened with two clamps, and the specimen can then be placed deep within the sack and retrieved via one of the 12-mm port sites. The specimen can then be morcellated and the empty sack removed.

With regard to exiting the retroperitoneum, the 12-mm port sites are closed with a subcuticular 4-0 absorbable suture. The skin of all port sites is reapproximated using adhesive strips. There is no need to close the fascia on the 12-mm ports after retroperitoneoscopy.

Results

To date there have been over 500 laparoscopic simple transperitoneal nephrectomies performed worldwide for benign disease. The average operative time has been 3.6 hours and the rate of conversion to open surgery has been 9%. Hospital stay has averaged 4.3 days, with a convalescence requiring 1.8 weeks. Overall major and minor complications have been 11% and 7%, respectively.[8–10]

One of the largest series comparing open and laparoscopic transperitoneal nephrectomy has been completed at Washington University: 55 laparoscopic simple nephrectomies versus 60 open simple nephrectomies, performed between June 1990 and June 1995. In this study, the operative time for the laparoscopic procedure was 2.4 hours longer than for the open procedures. However, the use of analgesics decreased by 77% in the laparoscopic group. The hospital stay was reduced from 7.5 days to only 3.2 days. In addition, return to normal activity occurred in 2.3 weeks in the laparoscopic group versus 7 weeks in the open group, while full recovery was accomplished in 3.7 weeks as opposed to 40 weeks in the open group. Complications occurred in 24% of the laparoscopic and 13% of the open group. However, because of the lengthy operative time, the overall cost for the laparoscopic procedure was $2000 to $3000 more than for an open nephrectomy.[8–10]

With regard to the *retroperitoneal* approach, to date there have been over 150 laparoscopic retroperitoneal nephrectomies reported. The average operative time has been 3.1 hours, with a hospital stay of 3.8 days. The conversion rate has only been 8% and convalescence has taken 1.5 weeks. Major and minor complications have occurred in only 4% and 3%.

A retrospective comparison of the laparoscopic transperitoneal and retroperitoneal approaches for simple nephrectomy of kidneys weighing less than 200 g was performed by McDougall and Clayman.[4] In their study, the retroperitoneal approach resulted in only a 5-minute decrease in operative time; however, a trend toward decreased analgesics and decreased hospital stay was noted in the retroperitoneal group. The retroperitoneal approach was approximately $900 less expensive than the transperitoneal method.

Ono et al[12] reviewed 32 transperitoneal nephrectomies and compared them with 6 retroperitoneal nephrectomies for benign disease. In their experience, greater time savings were realized with the retroperitoneal approach: operative time decreased from 4.4 hours to 2.7 hours. Hospital stay decreased from 9 days to 8 days. Overall it would appear that the retroperitoneal approach is best for the small noninflamed kidney of a size less than 9 cm or an expected weight of less than 200 g.[4,11,12]

The boundaries for laparoscopic simple nephrectomy are continually being tested. For example, in patients with renal failure and associated renovascular hypertension, bilateral simultaneous laparoscopic nephrectomies have been reported.[13] Also, polycystic kidneys, despite their large size, have now been removed laparoscopically, following meticulous aspiration of cyst fluid in order to reduce the volume of the kidney.[4] In addition, Ratner et al have initiated laparoscopic donor nephrectomy.[14] To date they have done over 90 cases of laparoscopic donor nephrectomy. In their initial report of 22 patients, among 5 right donor nephrectomies there were 2 failures secondary to renal vein thrombosis. Among 17 left donor nephrectomies there were 2 failures: one for rejection and one for cholesterol embolus. Further reports regarding an extensive experience with donor nephrectomy have also come from Jacobs at the University of Maryland. Currently, both groups recommend using only the left kidney for laparoscopic donor nephrectomy.

One area of renal disease remains in which laparoscopic nephrectomy is extremely difficult to perform: xanthogranulomatous pyelonephritis (XGP). Indeed, in the Washington University series the only death among over 100 patients undergoing laparoscopic nephrectomy for benign disease was an elderly woman with XGP who postoperatively developed hepatic failure. In addition, this group of patients also accounts for the only 2 conversions in the laparoscopic simple nephrectomy series at Washington University.[9,15]

LAPAROSCOPIC RADICAL/ TOTAL NEPHRECTOMY

There is much controversy regarding the extension of laparoscopic technology to treating malignant diseases. However, these concerns have been shown to be largely unfounded. Over the past 7 years, neither port site seeding nor intraperitoneal seeding has occurred. Likewise, adequate tumor resection has been achieved. With regard to the subsequent course of the patient, recent work by Cadeddu et al has shown that the 5-year survival rate of patients undergoing laparoscopic nephrectomy for localized renal cell cancer is identical to the course of those patients having an open procedure.[16] Nonetheless, continued scrutiny of the outcome of the procedure is needed until 5-year data become available in a large number of patients (more than 100).

Indications. To date, laparoscopic nephrectomy for renal cell cancer has been performed for lesions up to 8 cm in size. As such, T1 and T2 lesions have been successfully removed. In addition, there has been one report of removal of a T3b lesion (involving the renal vein). In all of these procedures, a total or radical nephrectomy has been performed.

Preoperative Preparation. Preparation of the patient for a laparoscopic radical nephrectomy is identical to the preparation for a transperitoneal nephrectomy for benign disease. In addition, a chest x-ray, staging CT scan of the abdomen and pelvis, and serum alkaline phosphatase value are obtained to assess for metastatic disease. If the alkaline phosphatase is elevated, then a bone scan is completed. If the patient presented with macroscopic hematuria, then cystoscopy is performed immediately prior to the planned nephrectomy, in order to rule out any bladder pathology. Of course, a serum creatinine value is obtained and the contralateral kidney is evaluated on both the CT scan and IVP, to be certain that the patient's renal function is sufficient to permit a radical nephrectomy.

During a surgeon's initial experience, it maybe valuable to consider embolization of the renal artery immediately prior to the planned laparoscopic procedure. However, if one has had significant experience with laparoscopic simple nephrectomy, this is certainly not necessary. Likewise, it is unnecessary to place a ureteral catheter in these patients.

Methods

General. There are basically seven steps for performing a laparoscopic radical nephrectomy:

1. Lateral insufflation—three-port placement.
2. Incision into the retroperitoneum—two-port placement.
3. Securing the ureter.

4. Hilar and adrenal dissection.
5. Incision of the ureter.
6. Specimen retrieval.
7. Exiting the abdomen.

Specific. As previously described for a transperitoneal laparoscopic simple nephrectomy, the pneumoperitoneum is obtained with the patient in a lateral position. This is usually done by lateral insufflation with a Veress needle, although an open Hasson cannula technique can be used. The port placement for the laparoscopic radical nephrectomy is identical to that for the laparoscopic simple nephrectomy (Fig. 78–1).

Likewise, the initial incision of the colonic peritoneal reflection (line of Toldt) on the right side is similar for the simple and radical nephrectomy. However, when doing a radical nephrectomy, this incision in the line of Toldt is carried well above the liver edge such that the triangular ligament of the liver is completely incised up to the diaphragm. The incision in the line of Toldt is then extended medially just beneath the liver such that the posterior coronary ligament of the liver is incised. This incision is continued medially until the supra-adrenal inferior vena cava is identified. Next, the incision in the line of Toldt is again continued medially, only this time at a point 1 to 2 cm above the colon. After the ascending colon and hepatic flexure are mobilized medially, the duodenum comes into view at the level of the lower half of the kidney. It too is mobilized medially (a Kocher maneuver), thereby exposing the infrarenal portion of the inferior vena cava. A fourth incision is now made connecting the upper and lower medial corners of the earlier incisions over the vena cava (Fig. 78–14). As such, a large "trapezoidal" piece of peritoneum is left on the kidney. With this approach, a wide expanse of the inferior vena cava from the supra-adrenal portion to below the renal vein is exposed; the inferior portion of the incision can then be continued caudal along the anterior border of the inferior vena cava, thereby exposing the entry of the gonadal vein into the cava. The gonadal vein can then be dissected and divided between a pair of 9-mm clips. This approach insures that any pericaval lymph node tissue will be included with the en bloc specimen.

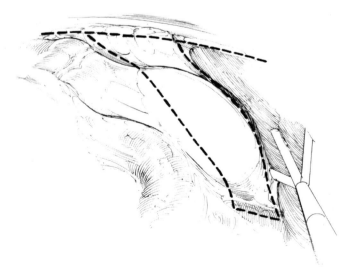

Figure 78–14. The "trapezoid" incision in the peritoneum and hepatic ligaments defines the limits of an "en bloc" right radical nephrectomy. The patient is in a lateral decubitus position. A retractor is pushing the liver cephalad.

On the left side, the incision is made along the line of Toldt and carried up to include the splenophrenic ligament. Next, the plane between the descending colonic mesentery and Gerota's fascia is identified over the lower half of the kidney; this plane is developed in a vertical line paralleling the initial incision in the line of Toldt; thus the colon is moved medially, well away from Gerota's fascia. The area of the renal hilum is exposed. This maneuver also serves to move the tail of the pancreas well away from the area of the dissection. Lastly, blunt dissection is used to separate Gerota's fascia overlying the upper pole of the kidney from the overlying splenocolic and splenorenal ligaments. This horizontal plane, extending from the upper extent of the dissection along the colonic mesentery, toward the line of Toldt, lies just beneath the inferior edge of the spleen. The tissue comprising this plane can be secured and divided with one or two loads of a GIA tissue stapler, thereby dividing and securing the splenocolic and splenorenal ligaments.

With this approach, all of the pararenal fat along with Gerota's fascia and the perirenal fat are included in the specimen. Indeed, all of the pararenal fat underneath the liver and spleen on the right and left sides, respectively, is removed.

The rest of the hilar dissection is identical to that for a simple nephrectomy. Again, in order to expose the vessels, a deliberate incision in Gerota's fascia, where it overlies the vessels, is necessary. On the right side, this will have already been done when the medial corners on the incision over the vena cava are connected. On the left side, it is best to make this incision as a direct extension of the course of the gonadal vein as it enters the renal vein. The importance of the gonadal vein as a landmark to follow to access the left renal vein cannot be overstressed. Again, on the left side, it is recommended to take the adrenal, gonadal, and ascending lumbar veins between pairs of clips, early in the hilar dissection. This will allow the left renal vein to become more mobile, thereby facilitating the dissection of the left renal artery; the left renal artery should always be secured prior to securing and dividing the renal vein. At this point, the left renal artery is secured with five 9-mm clips and divided such that three clips remain in the aortic stump; then, the left renal vein is taken with a vascular GIA stapler.

For the adrenalectomy, the adrenal vein on the *right* side is approached after taking the right renal artery and right renal vein, thereby allowing excellent exposure of the inferior and superior medial aspects of the adrenal gland. The right adrenal vein may be quite short, allowing for the placement of only two or three clips. If this is the case, the incision of the adrenal vein is made such that at least two clips stay on the caval side. At times, it is easier to place a vascular GIA across the pedicle of the adrenal vein; this is a safe maneuver as long as the area alongside the inferior vena cava and superior to the adrenal gland has been cleanly dissected, thereby allowing a clear view of the tips of the GIA stapler. On the *left* side, the adrenal vein is more easily secured, as previously described.

At this point, the entire kidney, Gerota's fascia, and the adrenal gland, exist as an en bloc specimen, attached only by the ureter. The ureter is secured with four clips. Via the uppermost lateral port, a 5-mm traumatic locking grasping forceps is passed and affixed to the ureter proximal to the clips; the ureter is then cut between the pairs of clips, thereby freeing the specimen from the retroperitoneum.

Placement of an entrapment sack (LapSac, Cook Urological, Spencer, IN) and renal entrapment are the same as for a simple nephrectomy. If the specimen appears large, then an 8 by 10-inch entrapment sack should be used.

With regard to a lymph node dissection with a radical nephrectomy, this is really up to the discretion of the surgeon. Certainly, all of the hilar lymph nodes are included with the specimen. On the right side, due to the approach, any pericaval lymph nodes are included with the en bloc dissection; an effort to separate this tissue from the larger specimen and send it separately can be made just prior to entrapment of the specimen. On the left side, the periaortic lymph nodes are not routinely removed; however, if desired, this can be undertaken just before entrapping the renal specimen, so that these second-tier lymph nodes can be sent as a separate specimen. As a routine, a periaortic lymph node dissection is not performed.

With regard to the actual removal of the kidney, there are two methods available: intact removal and morcellation. For intact removal, a 7 to 10-cm incision is made, either subcostal by connecting the two upper ports, or midline. The neck of the sack, once delivered, allows one to pull up very firmly on the sack and deliver the specimen intact via the incision. At times, it is helpful to use a pair of Army-Navy retractors to help open the full thickness of the incision in order to facilitate specimen retrieval.

Alternatively, for morcellation, once the neck of the sack is delivered via one of the 12-mm ports, the neck of the sack is triply draped: a nephrostomy drape, a separate adhesive drape, and a fenestrated absorbent towel. This is done in an effort to prevent any fluid from coming over the lip of the sack and contaminating the port site. A high-speed electrical tissue morcellator (Cook Urological, Spencer, IN) is used to fragment and evacuate the entrapped kidney (Fig. 78–15). None of the specimen is pulled directly from the sack, thereby potentially decreasing any chance of contamination of the port site (Fig. 78–16). Once the sack is completely empty of all tissue, it is pulled out of the port site and passed from the operating room table. The surgeon then proceeds to remove the three additional drapes and then changes gloves and gown.

Nuances. If the planned approach for laparoscopic radical nephrectomy includes intact removal, then the surgeon may wish to perform an "assisted" laparoscopic procedure in which the surgeon

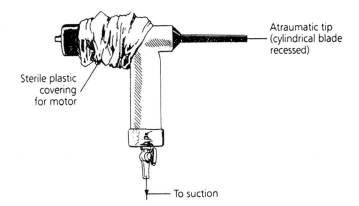

Figure 78–15. The high-speed tissue morcellator (Cook Urological, IN). *(Reprinted with permission from Clayman RV, McDougall E, eds. Laparoscopy Urology. St. Louis, Quality Medical Publishers, 1993.)*

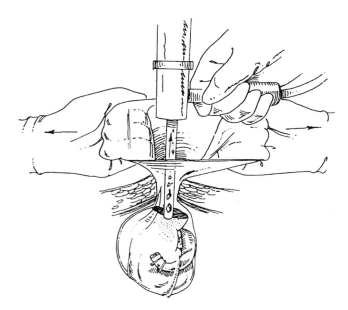

Figure 78–16. Morcellation of the specimen within the entrapment sack. Note that the surgeon and assistant forcefully pull the sack upward until it is taut, thereby eliminating any folds in the sack, which could potentially be caught up in the morcellator and shredded. *(Reprinted with permission from Clayman RV, McDougall E, eds. Laparoscopy Urology. St. Louis, Quality Medical Publishers, 1993.)*

is able to place his or her hand in the abdomen to facilitate the procedure. In this case, the incision for intact removal is made at the outset of the procedure and a sleeve type device is placed into the wound. With this device (for example, Pneumosleeve, Intromit), the pneumoperitoneum can be maintained during the procedure. For a right-handed surgeon, this would mean that when doing a left nephrectomy, the left hand would be inserted via a subcostal incision; whereas during a right nephrectomy, the left hand would be inserted via a lower midline incision. Reports have shown that with an assisted laparoscopic technique, the operative time can be reduced by upwards of 2 hours; indeed, with this approach, the operative time is similar to the time needed to do a standard open radical nephrectomy.[17,18]

Results

Presently, over 200 laparoscopic radical nephrectomies have been reported in the world literature.[19,20] The average operative time has been 5 hours, and the average hospital stay has been 4.7 days. However, with experience, this operative time has been reduced at some centers to only 3.0 hours.[21,22] Convalescence has occurred over a 3.5-week period. Major and minor complications have occurred in 12% and 18% of patients, respectively.

In order to assess the value of laparoscopic radical nephrectomy, the group at Washington University compared 21 patients undergoing laparoscopic radical nephrectomy to 20 patients undergoing open nephrectomy between June 1990 and April 1996, for clinical T1 or T2 renal cell carcinoma less than 7 cm in diameter.[23,24] The average operative time for the laparoscopic procedure was 6 hours versus only 2.3 hours for the open procedure. The estimated blood loss was similar in both groups: 240 to 250 mL. Of interest, the laparoscopic specimens outweighed the open

specimens: 520 versus 290 g. In addition, the laparoscopic patients required only one third as much parenteral analgesics as the open group. The hospital stay for the laparoscopic group was 3.8 days versus 8.5 days for the open procedure. Complications were similar between the open and laparoscopic patients: 5% major and 26 to 30% minor complications. Convalescence occurred in 3.1 weeks in the laparoscopic group and 3.7 weeks in the open group. The average cost for the laparoscopic procedure was $400 more than for the open procedure, at a total of $17,000. Given these results, the operative time for laparoscopic radical nephrectomy will need to fall to 4 hours or less in order for it to become equivalent in total cost to open radical nephrectomy. Indeed, this has already occurred in some centers.[21,22]

Also in the Washington University series, intact, not "assisted" laparoscopic specimen removal was compared with entrapment and morcellation. Patients having morcellation of the specimen required significantly less parenteral pain medications: 10 mg versus 34 mg morphine sulfate equivalents; they also experienced fewer minor complications: 17% versus 33%. Also, in the intact removal group there were 2 late incisional hernias, resulting in an 11% delayed complication rate versus 0% for the morcellation group. However, the overall operative time, convalescence, and hospital stay were similar in the two groups, as was the incidence of major complications. Our current policy is to morcellate all of our radical nephrectomy specimens.

The major concerns over laparoscopic radical nephrectomy center on two issues. First, will there be late intraperitoneal or port site seeding? Although such has been the case with colon cancers approached laparoscopically, to date there have been no reports of seeding of renal cell cancer either intraperitoneally or at any of the port sites despite follow-up in the earliest laparoscopic patients up to 6 years. The fact that these tumors are removed "en bloc" and never exposed likely has contributed to this favorable outcome. Second, will the overall patient survival after laparoscopic total/radical nephrectomy be equal to the survival after open total/radical nephrectomy for renal cell cancer? Recently, Cadeddu et al reviewed over 150 laparoscopic radical nephrectomy patients collected from five major laparoscopic centers. The survival rate based on clinical stage and pathologic grade was identical between the open and laparoscopic groups; indeed, the survival trend favored the laparoscopic patients. While follow-up data among these patients is still far from the 10-year maturity that is needed, these results strongly support the contention that the laparoscopic and open approaches yield equivalent cancer survival results.[16]

CONCLUSIONS

Laparoscopic nephrectomy for benign and malignant renal disease has become an everyday reality at many laparoscopic centers throughout the world. Almost all forms of benign renal disease can be successfully treated in this manner. The only exceptions are xanthogranulomatous pyelonephritis and polycystic kidney disease, which remain relative contraindications given the fibrotic scarring of the former and the huge size of the latter. For renal malignancy, the laparoscopic approach has gained favor at many minimally invasive centers worldwide. Present indications include all T1 and T2 disease of a diameter less than 10 cm. Long-term follow-up is needed to determine the risk for intraperitoneal or port site seeding and to evaluate the long-term efficacy of the laparoscopic approach. Finally, laparoscopic donor nephrectomy remains a most exciting procedure, which at this time is limited to only a few centers.

Minimally invasive urology continues to grow. It is anticipated that the horizons for the application of laparoscopy to renal surgery will only continue to expand provided that urologists are willing to become more knowledgeable and experienced with this approach. To this end, it is hoped that this chapter will serve as a valuable step-by-step guide to the novice and as a source of stimulation to those urologists already experienced with other laparoscopic urological procedures.

REFERENCES

1. Murphy LJT. The kidney. In: *The History of Urology.* Thomas: 1972; 251.

2. Clayman RV, Kavoussi LR, Long SR, et al. Laparoscopic nephrectomy: Initial report of pelviscopic organ ablation in the pig. *J Endourol.* 1990;4:247.

3. Clayman RV, Kavoussi LR, Soper NJ, et al. Laparoscopic nephrectomy. *N Engl J Med.* 1991;324:1370. Letter.

4. McDougall EM, Clayman RV. Laparoscopic nephrectomy for benign disease: Comparison of the transperitoneal and the retroperitoneal approaches. *J Endourol.* 1996;10:45.

5. Elashry OM, Nakada SY, Wolf JS Jr, et al. Laparoscopy for adult polycystic kidney disease: A promising alternative. *Am J Kid Dis.* 1996;27: 224.

6. Gaur DD. Laparoscopic operative retroperitoneoscopy: Use of a new device. *J Urol.* 1992;148:1137.

7. Rassweiler JJ, Stock C, Frede T, et al. Transperitoneal and retroperitoneal laparoscopic nephrectomy in comparison with conventional nephrectomy. *Urologe A.* 1996;35:215.

8. Eraky I, El-Kappany H, Shamaa MA, et al. Laparoscopic nephrectomy: An established routine procedure. *J Endourol.* 1994;8:275.

9. Kerbl K, Clayman RV, McDougall EM, et al. Laparoscopic nephrectomy: The Washington University experience. *Br J Urol.* 1994; 73:231.

10. Katoh N, Kinukawa T, Hirabayashi S, et al. Review of laparoscopic nephrectomy in 26 patients. *Jpn J Endourol ESWL.* 1992;6:129.

11. Guillonneau B, Ballanger P, Lugagne PM, et al. Laparoscopic versus lumboscopic nephrectomy. *Eur Urol.* 1996;29:288.

12. Ono Y, Ohshima S, Hirabayashi S, et al. Laparoscopic nephrectomy using a retroperitoneal approach: Comparison with a transabdominal approach. *Int J Urol.* 1995;2:12.

13. Fornara P, Doehn C, Fricke L, et al. Laparoscopic bilateral nephrectomy: Results in 11 renal transplant patients. *J Urol.* 1997;157:445.

14. Ratner LE, Ciseck LJ, Moore RG, et al. Laparoscopic live donor nephrectomy. *Transplantation.* 1995;60:1047.

15. Tolia BM, Iloreta A, Freed SZ, et al. Xanthogranulomatous pyelonephritis: Detailed analysis of 29 cases and a brief discussion of atypical presentations. *J Urol.* 1981;126:437.

16. Cadeddu JA, Ono Y, Clayman RV, et al. Laparoscopic nephrectomy for renal cell cancer: Evaluation of efficacy and safety. A multicenter experience. *Urology.* 1998;52(5)773–777.

17. Coptcoat MJ, Rassweiler JJ. The future of laparoscopic surgery in urology. *Urologe A.* 1996;35:226.

18. Wolf JS Jr, Nakada SY, Moon TD. Hand-assisted laparoscopic nephrectomy: Comparison to standard laparoscopic nephrectomy. *J Endourol.* 1997;11:S128.

19. Clayman RV, McDougall EM. Laparoscopic radical nephrectomy for renal tumor. *J Urol.* 1995;153:480A.

20. Ono Y, Kinukawa T, Hattutori R, et al. Laparoscopic radical nephrectomy: Nagoya experience. *J Endourol.* 1997;11:S127.

21. Barrett PH, Fentie DD, Taranger L. Laparoscopic radical nephrectomy with morcellation. *J Endourol.* 1997;11:S128.

22. Joual A, Gasman D, Salomon L, et al. Laparoscopic radical nephrectomy by retroperitoneal approach. *J Endourol.* 1997;11:S127.

23. McDougall EM, Clayman RV, Elashry OM. Laparoscopic radical nephrectomy for renal tumor: The Washington University experience. *J Urol.* 1996;155:1180.

24. Clayman R, Elbahnasy A, Elashry O, et al. Laparoscopic vs. open radical/total nephrectomy for renal cell carcinoma. *J Urol.* 1997; 157(suppl):328.

Chapter Seventy-Nine ● ● ● ● ● ●

*L*aparoscopic Retroperitoneal Lymph Node Dissection in Testicular Cancer

OCTAVIO CASTILLO

INTRODUCTION

Testicular cancer has an incidence of almost 3 per 100,000 males, and it has become one of the most curable solid tumors in the past decade because of important advances in staging and follow-up, improvement in surgical technique, and the development of effective chemotherapy regimens based on the use of cisplatin.

Currently, the disease-free rates are close to 100% for patients in stage I (disease limited to the testis), and more than 95% for those in stages IIa and IIb (retroperitoneal lymph node disease). Even for patients with massive retroperitoneal disease (stage IIc) or pulmonary disease or disease of other organs (stage III) survival rates are around 85%.[1]

For patients with nonseminomatous germ cell tumors in clinical stage I, the surveillance protocols constitute an acceptable alternative of management. Their purpose is to avoid the risks and morbidity of retroperitoneal lymph node dissection (RPLND) in patients with a low risk of progression. The most important objection to this follow-up protocol is that modern methods of staging, such as physical examination, the use of serum markers, and radiologic studies such as lymphography and CT scanning, do not identify cases with microscopic lymph node disease that could benefit from a diagnostic RPLND.

The rapid development of laparoscopic surgery in recent years has permitted its application in many surgical subspecialties, including urology. The author's wide experience in laparoscopic urologic surgery[2,3] has allowed him to prospectively perform via videolaparoscopy a theoretically more complex procedure, RPLND for nonseminomatous testicular cancer (NSTC), the results of which are presented in this chapter.

INDICATIONS

The procedure is primarily indicated for patients with NSTC in clinical stage I, (disease limited to the testis), whose serum markers (alpha-fetoprotein and chorionic gonadotropin) and imaging studies of the thorax and abdomen (conventional radiography and CT scanning) are normal.

Though these patients in stage I could have been selected for a surveillance protocol, RPLND allows early identification of 30% of patients that will present with a retroperitoneal relapse, and thereby permits faster and more accurate staging.

Although once considered a contraindication, we have also applied this technique to patients with a retroperitoneal residual mass after chemotherapy. We select for this procedure patients with retroperitoneal masses less than 5 cm in diameter. Although it is feasible to resect larger metastases, we are performing a laparoscopic unilateral dissection, and it is unknown whether the extent of the dissection would be oncologically adequate for larger tumors.

PREOPERATIVE PREPARATION

Each patient is informed of the procedure and its risks. They are also informed of the possibility of conversion to open surgery in the event complications such as a vascular or intestinal injury develop.

All patients are hospitalized the night before the operation and are subjected to the common preoperative blood tests done prior to any surgical procedure. Bowel preparation is by intake of clear fluids only the evening before surgery. We no longer use mechanical bowel preparation or oral laxatives. A prophylactic dose of antibiotic is given intravenously 1 hour before surgery.

After the induction of general anesthesia, an orogastric tube is placed. A Foley catheter is placed in the bladder and antiembolism compression stockings are used. The patient is positioned in the standard full flank position (Fig. 79–1); rotation of the surgical table allows moving the patient into a supine or lateral position.

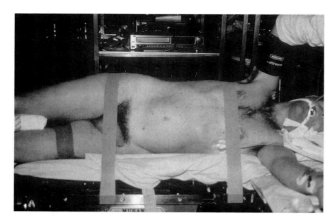

Figure 79–1. Full flank position for right laparoscopic retroperitoneal lymph node dissection (RPLND).

SURGICAL TECHNIQUE

We use the standard dissection previously described by Weissbach and Boedefeld in 1987 for open RPLND.[4] For right-sided tumors, the boundaries of laparoscopic RPLND are the ureter laterally, the left aspect of the aorta medially, the renal hilum superiorly, and the origin of the inferior mesenteric artery inferiorly (Fig. 79–2). For left-sided tumors the boundaries are the ureter laterally, the left aspect of the inferior vena cava medially, the renal hilum superiorly, and the origin of the inferior mesenteric artery inferiorly (Fig. 79–3). On both sides, the dissection is carried out to the level of the bifurcation of the common iliac vessels.[5,6]

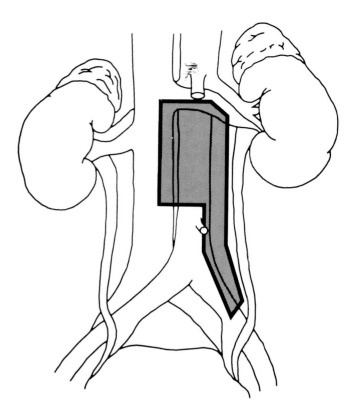

Figure 79–3. Extent of surgical excision for left-sided tumors.

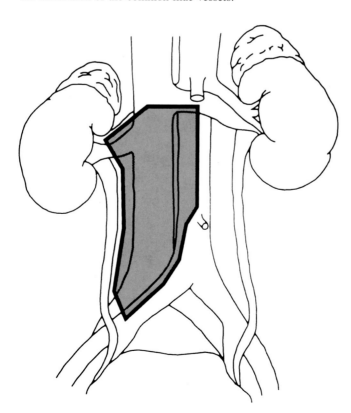

Figure 79–2. Extent of surgical excision for right-sided tumors.

Abdominal access may be achieved using a Veress needle, which we employ in nearly every case, or the open technique with the Hasson cannula, which is useful for patients with previous abdominal surgery. The peritoneum is insufflated with carbon dioxide to 15 mm Hg of pressure. A standard three-port technique is used (Fig. 79–4), with an additional flank port added which is especially useful for retraction of the liver. The first 10-mm trocar is placed in the umbilicus if we are using the 30° scope. In cases in which we use a zero degree scope, we prefer to place the first trocar in the ipsilateral midclavicular line at the level of the umbilicus to provide better visualization of the retroperitoneum. The secondary trocars are placed in subcostal and iliac positions (Fig. 79–5). One prerequisite for an adequate laparoscopic RPLND is wide exposure of the retroperitoneum.

For a right RPLND, the white line of Toldt is completely incised from the cecum to the hepatic flexure of the colon. A Kocher maneuver is done, retracting the colon and duodenum. This exposes the vena cava and aorta, and the left renal vein is seen crossing the aorta. The first step is to excise the gonadal vessels from the internal inguinal ring (the site of previous radical orchidectomy) up to the level of the vena cava. The spermatic vein is transected and clipped at the surface of the vena cava, and the spermatic artery is clipped where it crosses the vena cava. The lymphatic tissue is dissected according to the extent of disease for a right RPLND, starting at the level where the ureter crosses the iliac vessels (Fig. 79–6), medial to the ureter, and making a split-roll maneuver over the vena cava. The dissection proceeds in a cephalad manner, avoiding the inferior mesenteric artery and along the left border of the aorta, removing all the ventral lymphatic tissue in the interaortocaval zone up to the level of the left renal vein (Fig. 79–7).

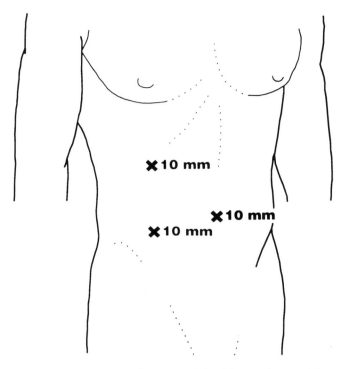

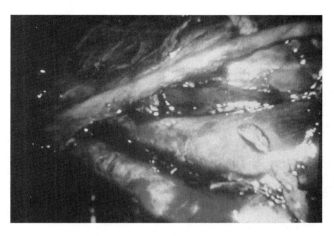

Figure 79–6. Inferior postoperative view of a right-side dissection. The ureter crosses over the iliac vessels.

Figure 79–4. Port placement (three-port technique) for ventral approach to a right-sided tumor.

The specimen is always placed in a plastic bag before retrieval. The colon is not sutured in its original position and we do not use retroperitoneal drains.

The orogastric tube and the Foley catheter are removed before leaving the operating room. Oral fluids are normally started 6 hours after surgery and patients are discharged within 48 hours of surgery.

CLINICAL EXPERIENCE

Between May 1993 and December 2000, laparoscopic RPLNDs were performed on 82 consecutive patients. Stage I testicular tumors were diagnosed in 64 patients, and stage II tumors in 18 patients (5 patients in stage II had postchemotherapy residual masses). Right RPLNDs were performed in 49 patients and left RPLNDs in 33. The clinical characteristics of this group of patients are shown in Table 79–1.

The operative time ranged from 65 to 260 minutes (average time, 140 min). There were no significant differences in operative time between left-sided versus right-sided tumors; however, our

For a left RPLND, the white line of Toldt is incised from the splenic colic flexure to the pelvic rim. It is helpful to also incise the phrenicolic ligament. The spermatic vein is removed from the internal inguinal ring to its opening into the left renal vein. The dissection proceeds caudally to cranially, resecting the lymphatic tissue from the ureter laterally and from the crossing of the ureter and the iliac vessels distally. The lymphatic tissue is removed from the medial border of the aorta, preserving the inferior mesenteric artery, up to the level of the left renal vein.

We do not perform retrocaval or retroaortic dissection because it has been proven that the primary location for metastases from NSTC is invariably anterior to the lumbar vessels.[7]

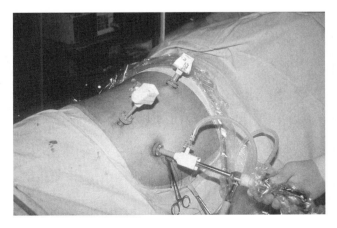

Figure 79–5. Ventral approach in a right laparoscopic RPLND.

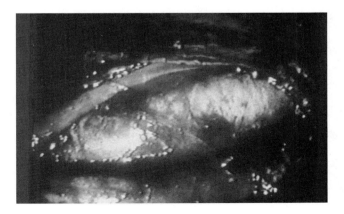

Figure 79–7. Postoperative view after a right-side dissection. The excised lymphatic tissue has been removed over the anterior surface of the vena cava and the aorta.

group considers that surgery is relatively easier on the left side. All patients were started on a liquid diet on the first postoperative day. The shortest hospital stay was less than 23 hours in 27 patients (32.9%) and the average hospitalization was 40 hours (Table 79–2). In four patients, minor bleeding occurred, which was controlled with a clip-applier. In two patients bleeding from the lumbar veins could not be managed laparoscopically, so they were converted to open surgery. However, the incision was a transversal paramedian laparotomy, and this accident did not affect the early discharge and it was not associated with other morbidity.

There were no early postoperative complications, and no patients required blood transfusions. The average number of lymph nodes obtained was 12, with a range of 4 to 25 nodes. The number of microscopic lymph node metastases was 14 in 64 patients with clinical stage I disease (22%).

On long-term follow-up, one patient with a stage I left-sided tumor developed a small asymptomatic lymphocele. Another patient having a laparoscopic RPLND for a postchemotherapy residual mass developed massive chylous ascites. He required a laparoscopic ligation of lymphatic vessels at the level of the cisterna chyli and intravenous hyperalimentation and had a successful outcome. Antegrade ejaculation was preserved in all patients.

Of 64 patients with stage I disease, 2 developed retroperitoneal and concurrent pulmonary metastases. Both were submitted to standard chemotherapy with complete resolution.

Since there is no other series that can serve as a valid comparison—given the meticulousness of the author's laparoscopic technique of dissection—with conventional open surgery, all patients having pathological stage II disease (microscopic lymph node metastases) were subjected to two cycles of adjuvant chemotherapy after retroperitoneal lymphadenectomy. In this group of patients there were no recurrences after long-term follow-up.

DISCUSSION

Before the development of effective chemotherapy schemes using cisplatin, the open RPLND was the only truly efficient means of treating metastatic cancer of the testis. At that time, the RPLND necessarily involved a bilateral radical dissection, with excision of all lymphatic tissue, from the renal suprahilar area to the bifurcation of the iliac arteries, and from one ureter to the other. Lumbar veins and arteries were sectioned, allowing the elevation of the great vessels on a frontal plane in order to remove all the

TABLE 79–1. CHARACTERISTICS OF A SERIES OF 82 PATIENTS TREATED WITH LAPAROSCOPIC RETROPERITONEAL LYMPH NODE DISSECTION

Average age: years (range): 29 years (15–45)	
Histology of testicular tumor:	
Embryonal carcinoma	38
Teratocarcinoma	24
Mixed histology	19
Unknown	1
Clinical stage:	
Stage I	64
Stage II	18
Side of tumor:	
Right	49
Left	33

TABLE 79–2. RESULTS OF LAPAROSCOPIC RETROPERITONEAL LYMPH NODE DISSECTION

Average operative time (range):	140 min (65–260 min)
Average blood loss (range):	103 mL (30–500 mL)
Average number of lymph nodes excised (range):	12 (4–25)
Number of metastases:	12/64 (22%)
Average hospital stay (range):	40.7 h (24–96 h)
Conversion to open surgery:	2/84
Average follow-up (range):	44 mo (6–92 mo)

retrovascular retroperitoneal tissue, including lymphatic and neural tissue. Due to the radical nature of the surgery, virtually all patients lost ejaculatory capacity due to the damage to the efferent sympathetic fibers. This form of RPLND allowed a disease-free rate of 65% without the need for any complementary treatment.[6]

The survival of patients with early-stage NSTC has increased in recent decades (and is currently over 90%), due to multidisciplinary management that uses a combination of chemotherapy and surgery. The improvement in the efficacy of this type of treatment produced an increase in survival, and has been associated with the additional benefit of a notable reduction in morbidity.

The morbidity of RPLND is low in centers in which the procedure is done frequently, and mortality approaches zero.[8,9] The most significant morbidity after RPLND is the loss of ejaculation, with secondary infertility, which is present in almost 90% of patients.[10] Preservation of fertility is very important in this young population, and although sperm can be preserved in semen banks, the altered fertility in these patients will limit the success of the procedure to approximately 40%.

Although the global morbidity of classic RPLND is low, infertility secondary to ejaculatory dysfunction is common. The efficacy of chemotherapy has led some physicians to promote protocols of surveillance only in patients with nonseminomatous germ cell tumors (NSGCT) in clinical stage I, but even though 99% of patients are free of disease, relapse may occur in 32% of patients, mainly at the retroperitoneal level.[11] The efficacy of RPLND in producing a prolonged survival is unquestionable. Rates of recurrence in stage I, after retroperitoneal lymphadenectomy, varies between 10 and 13%, and are close to the rates of extra-abdominal recurrence seen in patients in whom only a surveillance protocol is done. In most series of RPLND reported, the retroperitoneal relapse rate after surgery is low (less than 2%), and most of them occur outside the abdomen, mainly in the lungs.

The low risk of retroperitoneal recurrence after RPLND makes follow-up of these patients simpler. The serum markers and pulmonary imaging allow easy detection of serological or pulmonary relapse, which are more frequent than recurrence in the abdomen.

Another benefit of RPLND is the achievement of adequate staging, since nearly 30% of patients that present in clinical stage I actually have pathological stage II disease,[12] which means the only option is to rapidly and effectively diagnose and treat patients with metastatic retroperitoneal disease. They are candidates for complementary chemotherapy, since the probability of recurrence in patients in stage II subjected only to RPLND varies between 30 and 50%.[13]

A careful analysis of the retroperitoneal pattern of metastasis has led to modification of the extent of excision in RPLND. The

TABLE 79–3. PUBLISHED LITERATURE ON LAPAROSCOPIC RETROPERITONEAL LYMPH NODE DISSECTION

Author	Patients	Clinical Stage I	Clinical Stage II	No. Complications (%)	No. Conversions (%)	Relapse	Follow-up (mo)
Rassweiler[17]	26	17	9	5/26 (19.2%)	Est. 1: 1/17 (5.8%) Est. 2: 7/9 (77.7%)	Pulmonary (2)	27
Janetschek[18]	29	29	0	6/29 (20.6%)	1/29 (3.4%)	None	16
Janetschek[19]	73	73	0	5/73 (6.8%)	2/73 (2.7%)	Retroperitoneal (1)	42.3
Rassweiler[20]	34	34	0	5/34 (14.7%)	1/34 (2.9%)	Pulmonary (2)	40
Nelson[22]	29	29	0	4/29 (13.7%)	2/29 (6.8%)	Pulmonary and biochemical (2)	1 to 65 in range
Castillo (current series)	82	64	18	6/82 (7.3%)	2/82 (2.4%)	Pulmonary and retroperitoneal (2)	44

pioneering work of Weissbach and Boedefeld[4] established the precise anatomic location of lymph node metastases most frequently seen in NSTC. They showed that testicular tumors disseminate through lymph nodes in a predictable manner (right tumors in the interaortocaval superior zone and the left ones in the left paraaortic and preaortic zones), which has permitted development of a modified retroperitoneal lymphadenectomy in a smaller area compared to that of the classic dissection.

The reduction of the boundaries of the RPLND and the preservation of sympathetic nerve fibers have allowed the preservation of ejaculation in 88 to 100% of patients, while maintaining the therapeutic efficacy of the lymphadenectomy.[5,6]

In this context, another theoretical advantage of laparoscopic RPLND is that it can achieve results equivalent to those of an open procedure while also reducing postoperative recovery time.[14–16] In addition, the excellent visualization of the sympathetic chain produced by magnification of the operative field allows preservation of the hypogastric nerve plexus in the aortic bifurcation, and by limiting distal dissection allows normal postsurgical ejaculation.

Laparoscopic RPLND has been developed as a staging procedure for patients with clinical stage I NSTC. These patients have a risk of almost 30% of developing metastatic retroperitoneal disease in the follow-up period. In this regard, accurate staging can be very important in planning early and effective adjuvant chemotherapy. The pathological staging of lymph nodes in clinical stage I NSTC offers the opportunity to identify patients with metastatic disease that can be treated successfully, and simplifies surveillance of patients without involvement of retroperitoneal lymph nodes.

Several studies have shown that laparoscopic RPLND for clinical stage I NSTC is feasible.[17–22] The experience of the author in Santiago, Chile is summarized in Table 79–3. This series is probably one of the largest ever accumulated and reported, and the results are very encouraging, underlining the shorter surgical time (average, 140 min) and the absence of major complications. It must be emphasized that these results were obtained after extensive laparoscopic experience, especially in retroperitoneal dissection.

Laparoscopic RPLND was initially considered to be contraindicated in patients with known metastatic disease, bulky adenopathy, or previous chemotherapy. In particular, prior chemotherapy increases the difficulty of dissection because of the dense scar tissue surrounding the great vessels of the retroperitoneum. Our experience shows that in well-selected patients laparoscopic dissection can be carried out without major morbidity in cases of retroperitoneal residual mass after chemotherapy for testicular cancer.

Today, the standard treatment for patients with clinical stage I NSTC following orchidectomy is either primary RPLND or close surveillance with cisplatin-based chemotherapy in cases of relapse. Both treatment modalities provide excellent overall survival rates of nearly 100%. For this reason, selection of the most effective management option must not be guided by survival considerations alone. On the contrary, it should be based on consideration of treatment morbidity, patient preference, physician expertise in surgical treatment, and other prognostic factors.

Our experience and that of other groups clearly shows that laparoscopic retroperitoneal lymph node dissection is an effective and safe alternative for the management of patients with stage I nonseminomatous testicular germ cell tumors (Table 79–3). It is also an alternative surgical approach for selected cases of retroperitoneal stage II disease of residual retroperitoneal mass after chemotherapy.

CONCLUSION

RPLND continues to be an alternative treatment for patients with testicular tumors of the nonseminomatous type. It allows differentiation of patients with stage I disease (limited to the testis) from those with stage II disease (in the retroperitoneal lymph nodes), leading to more accurate assignment of each patient to surveillance only or to systemic chemotherapy.

The improved knowledge of the anatomic distribution of lymph node metastases has permitted more focused retroperitoneal dissection, thus maintaining diagnostic sensitivity and postsurgical ejaculation. This same procedure, when done by video laparoscopy, affords staging accuracy that is equivalent to that attained with classic surgery, but has lower morbidity and faster patient recovery. We must emphasize that this approach has a long learning curve, and its use should be limited to urologists with laparoscopic expertise. Once the learning curve has been overcome, laparoscopic RPLND is superior to open surgery.

REFERENCES

1. Richie JP. Complications of retroperitoneal lymph node dissection. AUA Updates Series Vol. XII, 1993, Lesson 16:122.
2. Castillo O, Wöhler C. Cirugía laparoscópica en Urología. In: Hepp J, Navarrete C, eds. *Cirugía Laparoscópica*. Sociedad de Cirujanos de Chile:1993;177.
3. Castillo O, Van Cauwelaert R, Wöhler C, et al. Cirugía laparoscópica urológica. *Cuad Chil Cir (Santiago)* 1993;37:264.
4. Weissbach L, Boedefeld EA. Localization of solitary and multiple metastases in stage II nonseminomatous testis tumor as a basis for a modified staging of lymph node dissection in stage I. *J Urol.* 1987;138:77.
5. Donohue JP. Primary retroperitoneal lymph node dissection in clinical stage A testicular cancer. *Brit J Urol.* 1993;71:326.
6. Foster RL, Donohue JP. Nerve-sparing retroperitoneal lymphadenectomy. *Urol Clin North Am.* 1993;20:117.
7. Höltl L, Hobisch A, Knapp R, et al. Where are the primary landing sites for retroperitoneal metastases from testicular tumor? *J Urol.* 1997;157:303A.
8. Donohue JP. Controversies in testis cancer management. In: De Kernion J, Paulson D, eds. *Genitourinary Cancer Management*. Lea and Febiger:1987;161.
9. Donohue JP. Management of low clinical stage testis cancer (Editorial comment). *Urol Clin North Am.* 1987;14:729.
10. Richie JP. Modified retroperitoneal lymphadenectomy for patients with clinical stage 1 testicular cancer. *Sem Urol.* 1988;6:216.
11. Sturgeon JFG, Jewett MAS, Alison RE, et al. Surveillance after orchiectomy for patients with clinical stage 1 nonseminomatous testis tumors. *J Clin Oncol.* 1992;10:564.
12. Freedman L, Parkinson M, Jones W, et al. Histopathology in the prediction of relapse of patients with stage 1 testicular teratoma treated by orchidectomy alone. *Lancet* 1987:II;294.
13. Williams SD, Stablein DM, Einhorn LH, et al. Immediate adjuvant chemotherapy versus observation with treatment at relapse in pathological stage II testicular cancer. *N Engl J Med.* 1987;317:1433.
14. Hulbert JC, Fraley EE. Laparoscopic retroperitoneal lymphadenectomy: New approach to pathologic staging of clinical stage I germ-cell tumor of the testis. *J Endourol.* 1992;6:123.
15. Rutkstalis DB, Chodak G. Laparoscopic retroperitoneal lymph node dissection in a patient with stage I testicular carcinoma. *J Urol.* 1992;148:1907.
16. Castillo O, Azócar G, Van Cauwelaert R, et al. Laparoscopic retroperitoneal lymph node dissection in testicular cancer. *J Urol.* 1995;153:516A.
17. Rassweiler JJ, Seeman O, Henkel TO, et al. Laparoscopic retroperitoneal lymph node dissection for nonseminomatous germ cell tumors: indications and limitations. *J Urol.* 1996;156:1108.
18. Janetschek G, Hobisch A, Höltl L, et al. Retroperitoneal lymphadenectomy for clinical stage I nonseminomatous testicular tumor: laparoscopy versus open surgery and impact of learning curve. *J Urol.* 1996;156:89.
19. Janetschek G, Hobisch A, Peschel R, et al. Laparoscopic retroperitoneal lymph node dissection for clinical stage I nonseminomatous testicular carcinoma: long-term outcome. *J Urol.* 2000;163:1793.
20. Rassweiler JJ, Frede T, Lenz E, et al. Long-term experience with laparoscopic retroperitoneal lymph node dissection in the management of low-stage testis cancer. *Eur Urol.* 2000;37:251.
21. Janetschek G, Hobisch A, Peschel R, et al. Laparoscopic retroperitoneal lymph node dissection. *Urology* 2000;55:136.
22. Nelson JB, Chen RN, Bishoff JT, et al. Laparoscopic retroperitoneal lymph node dissection for clinical stage I nonseminomatous germ cell testicular tumors. *Urology* 1999;54:1064.

Chapter Eighty ● ● ● ● ● ●

*I*nterventional Radiology in the Urinary Tract

RICARDO DI SEGNI, BEATRIZ LOSCERTALES, W. RICARDO CASTAÑEDA, MARCOS HERRERA, and DANIEL VALLE

Interventional uroradiology started as a method of expediently decompressing the obstructed kidney. The field of interventional uroradiology has evolved in the hands of the interventional radiologist as a means of addressing a myriad of problems in the urinary tract and has dramatically changed the practice of uroradiology. The foundation of interventional uroradiology is the creation of an appropriate, percutaneous access into the urinary system.

Percutaneous nephrostomy (PN) has been the essential primary procedure for the development of interventional techniques in the urinary tract. Goodwin et al[1] reported the use of percutaneous trocar nephrostomy in the management of hydronephrosis in 1955. PN has virtually replaced surgical nephrostomy for the relief of supravesical obstruction, because it is simple to perform and has lower morbidity and mortality. Percutaneous nephrostomy very rapidly replaced other techniques for the treatment of ureteral strictures, stenting of ureteral fistulas, biopsies of the collecting system and ureters, intrarenal surgery, and the local infusion of drugs. Its most important impact has been in the removal of urinary tract calculi. In 1979 Smith et al[2] reported the use of percutaneous nephrostomy in the management of ureteral and renal calculi. This gave birth to what came to be known as endourology, and the new procedure was termed percutaneous nephrolithotomy (PNL). In 1984 Clayman et al[3] described the extraction of calculi with the use of a fiber-optic nephroscope. The golden age of percutaneous stone removal by interventional procedures reached its climax very fast and started to fade away with the approval by the Food and Drug Administration of the first device for the performance of extracorporeal shock wave lithotripsy (ESWL) in 1984. This new modality took the place of PNL as the primary method of treatment for most upper urinary tract stones. As experience was gained with ESWL, the limitations of the extracorporeal technique were defined. Percutaneous techniques still play an important role as primary or supplemental therapy in some specific cases.

Currently, the primary indications for percutaneous nephrostomy are (1) urinary diversion for supravesical obstruction and urinary fistula management, (2) adjunct therapy for complex infections, (3) renal calculus as a primary therapy or as coadjuvant with ESWL, (4) nephroscopy and ureteroscopy for diagnosis or therapy, and (5) ureteral interventions. Most of the percutaneous procedures are currently performed for complex urinary tract stones.[4] The same basic interventional techniques are applied with excellent results to the transplanted kidney and bladder. Self-expandable metallic stents have been used in the management of malignant obstruction with variable success, with a patency rate of 75 to 94% with a follow-up ranging from 2 to 48 months with a mean of 25 months.[5–9] Lopez-Martinez et al recommended the placement of a double J catheter across the metallic stent until the reactive edema caused by the placement of the metallic stent disappeared.[6]

PERCUTANEOUS NEPHROSTOMY

The success of interventional uroradiologic procedures is based in the creation of an appropriate nephrostomy tract. Knowledge of the renal anatomy and familiarity with its common variations is essential to avoid major complications and to achieve a successful outcome.

Hemorrhage is the most important complication, and accidental puncture of major arteries is of great concern. The ideal renal access should be created along the posterolateral margin of the kidney, between the anterior and posterior renal artery divisions. Because of the orientation of the kidneys in the body, entry through a posterior calyx often provides the best path through this relatively avascular area of the kidney (Brödel's bloodless line of incision).[10] This entry is accomplished easily by using rotational fluoroscopy at an angle of approximately 25 to 35 degrees from the sagittal plane, ipsilateral to the kidney to be entered. The first step to identify the anatomy and site of entrance into the collecting system is the introduction of a fine 21 to 22-gauge needle into the renal pelvis. Once the fine needle is introduced, urine samples are obtained for culture, and opacification of the collecting system is obtained by the injection of contrast medium under fluoroscopy. A definitive puncture is then made into a posterolateral calyx through which the remaining steps of the procedure are performed. An alternative and accurate method for primary approach that some prefer is entrance of the collecting system with ultrasound guidance. This only requires a single puncture directly into the selected calyx.[11–13] The use of ultrasound guidance is particularly indicated during pregnancy for manipulations in the collecting system.[14]

Recent studies on human volunteers and animals have proven the feasibility of using MRI guidance for the placement of percutaneous access into the urinary tract.[15–18] Hagspiel et al reported the first successful percutaneous nephrostomy performed under MRI guidance.[18]

Puncture under fluoroscopy using the straight-down-the-barrel technique holding the 18-gauge needle with a plastic handle, is the technique preferred by the authors to enter the collecting system. With this technique, a precise site of entrance can be selected in the calyx of choice, and with oblique fluoroscopy, a through-and-through puncture of the collecting system is avoided. With this technique, the selected calyx is placed in the center of the x-ray field, and a diamond-tip needle held by a plastic handle is advanced under continuous fluoroscopy towards the target point. After advancing the needle for 7 to 8 cm, the image intensifier is rotated to verify the position of the needle and to control the entrance of the needle into the calyx. The position of the needle within the collecting system is confirmed by the aspiration of urine. Under fluoroscopy, a guidewire is then advanced and is coiled into the renal pelvis, or if possible, it is advanced into the ureter for added safety. A second wire is placed as a working wire. Over this guidewire, dilatation of the nephrostomy tract is performed with Teflon dilators or with a dilating balloon. Jackman et al described the use of a 13 Fr. "mini-perc" technique using a ureteroscopy sheath for PNL. They claimed this technique minimized the trauma to the kidney without any loss of the ability to remove the stones.[19]

Morsy et al reported the use of telescopic metal dilators to dilate the percutaneous access in patients with previous surgery.[20] Once the procedure is completed, a drainage catheter is advanced over the guidewire for decompression of the collecting system. The sideholes of the catheter have to be carefully placed inside the urinary tract to avoid extravasation and urinoma formation. Recently released nephrostomy tubes are coated with a hydrophilic material; this eliminates the need to overdilate the tract for the introduction of the drainage catheter. A self-retaining drainage catheter is preferred such as the Cope-loop or Tegtmeyer catheters. In a small-volume collecting system, a Malecot-type catheter may be more appropriate. When pyonephrosis is present, larger tubes need to be placed due to the high viscosity of the fluid.

When the indication for the PN is removal of stones, the tract needs to be dilated using large-bore dilators (up to 30 Fr.). When severe areas of stenosis or obstruction are found, angiographic catheters need to be used to manipulate a guidewire across the obstruction. The procedure is facilitated by the use of hydrophilic-coated guidewires (Glidewire, Boston Scientific, Nadick, MA). In experienced hands, successful creation of an appropriate tract can be accomplished in more than 98% of cases. The rate of major complications that require alternative therapy or hospitalization is about 4%.[21]

Major Complications

Renal hemorrhage (4%) and sepsis (2.5%) are the most common complications. They may be prevented with adequate technique and with the administration of antibiotics. Considered also as a major complication but with lesser frequency is adjacent organ injury such as spleen, bowel, or pneumothorax (0.1%). Mortality secondary to the procedure occurs in 0.046 to 0.3%.

Obstruction

Percutaneous nephrostomy for decompression is performed most commonly in patients with malignancy. Essentially in this type of patient, PN has replaced the surgical procedures.

In patients with acute urinary tract infections, the primary procedure is retrograde ureteral stent placement. PN is indicated only when the retrograde attempt has failed. In those patients with known large tumors localized to the bladder, cervix, or prostate and with a long segment of ureteral obstruction, PN is the procedure of choice (Figs. 80–1 and 80–2). Generally after several days of decompression of the collecting system, passage of the obstruction can be easily accomplished. Once the area of obstruction is crossed, the external drainage can be replaced by the placement of internal ureteral stents. If the obstruction cannot be crossed, an external drainage catheter is left in place. The problem in patients with external catheter drainage is dislodgement or obstruction with risk of infection.

Stone Disease

The primary therapeutic modality for treatment of upper urinary tract stones is ESWL. Although ESWL can be used as an effective monotherapy in 70 to 80% of the cases, PNL can be used as a primary alternative or in conjunction with ESWL (Fig. 80–3). PNL has traditionally provided better results than ESWL, although with a higher morbidity.[22,23]

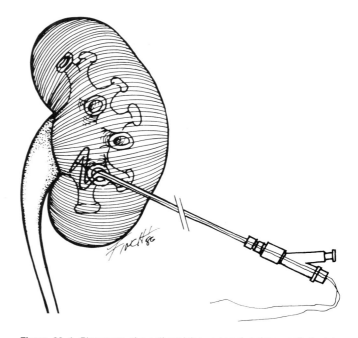

Figure 80–1. Placement of a self-retaining, external drainage catheter into the renal pelvis.

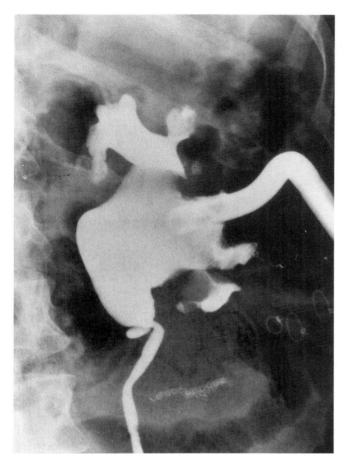

Figure 80–2. Nephrostogram after placement of a 24 Fr. Councill catheter into the renal pelvis following stone removal.

The indications for the use of PN with ESWL are large stone volume, complicated renal anatomy, suboptimal results with ESWL, or unique patient characteristics.[24] In those patients with a single stone measuring 2.5 cm in diameter, or an aggregated diameter of several stones of more than 3 cm, the volume of stone fragments produced by ESWL causes a high incidence of urinary tract obstruction. PNL is a more effective approach in these cases.[25] A classic example of this situation is a large staghorn calculi. In these cases percutaneous stone debulking or complete percutaneous removal or placement of a percutaneous nephrostomy for drainage of the fragments after ESWL is preferred. The complete clearance of all fragments is essential because of the higher incidence of urinary tract infections and rapid recurrence of stones if residual fragments are left.

A special case is patients with a horseshoe kidney in whom stone formation has an incidence of 50%. In these cases, PN is only possible through an upper-pole posterior calyx.[26] The reason for this is that the lower pole is more medially and ventrally located than in the normal kidney. Another indication is cystine calculi, which when treated with ESWL, produce large calculi that are difficult to pass.[24] Additionally, cystine stones have a high tendency to recur.[27] Ultrasonic lithotripsy performed via a percutaneous access can clear even the larger stones. In some cases, if necessary, chemolysis can be used to dissolve the stones.[28] In those

cases where strictures of the collecting system exist or in the presence of caliceal diverticuli, PNL is preferred over ESWL.

PNL has been successfully used in pediatric patients. Modifications to the technique have been used to minimize trauma to the kidney, including the use of the "mini-perc" technique.[29–31]

Ureteral obstruction during pregnancy is electively treated with the placement of a retrograde ureteral stent; however, sometimes patients cannot tolerate the stents. In these cases, with limited fluoroscopy and with the help of US, PN is undertaken. Granados Loarca described the use of finger guidance to create percutaneous access into the kidney. This technique has potential application in pregnant women.[32] Some patients with unusual body habitus such as morbid obesity are not candidates for ESWL, because they may exceed the weight limits for the x-ray table. In patients with skeletal deformities due to myelodysplasias or other pathologies, stone targeting may be impossible with ESWL and PNL is indicated.[33,34]

Joshi et al described the emergent use of ESWL in patients with acute ureteric obstruction caused by stones, with a mean success rate of 81%, compared with 70% in those treated with a double J stent and 54% success in those treated with PN.[35]

Other Indications

Other indications for PN include the treatment of ureteropelvic junction obstruction (UPJ). Successful results have been achieved in pediatric and geriatric patients, particularly in patients who have had previous operations.[36–38]

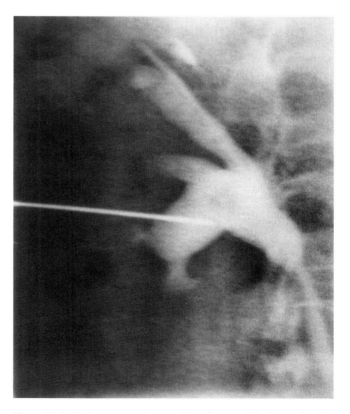

Figure 80–3. Nephrostogram shows position of stone within the renal pelvis. An 18-gauge needle has been passed through a posterior calyx in the lower pole of the kidney into the infundibulum.

When a radiolucent defect is found in the collecting system and its etiology is unknown, PN can help in the diagnosis and treatment, as in the case of transitional cell carcinoma (TCC), fibroepithelial polyps, blood clots, sloughed papillae, aberrant papillae, or some inflammatory-associated conditions like fungus ball, pyeloureteritis cystica, or inflammatory debris. Through PN, inspection of these defects can be accomplished and biopsy or removal is possible. In patients with fungus balls, direct intrarenal instillation of amphotericyn can be done.

Ureteral Interventions

Strictures. The initial approach in extrinsic compression causing ureteral strictures is the placement of a double J ureteral stent in a retrograde fashion. When retrograde ureteral manipulation fails, an antegrade approach is undertaken. Additionally, if the ureteral course is tortuous, the antegrade approach could be considered initially. After the creation of a PN, manipulations through the stricture or obstruction are performed with a success rate of

A

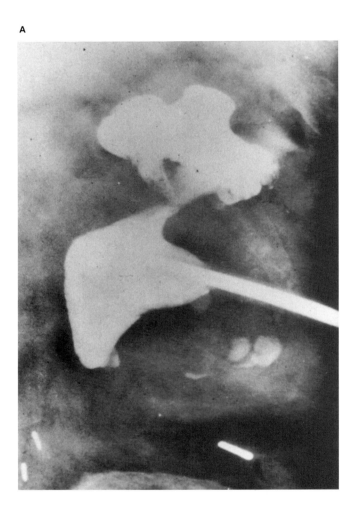

B

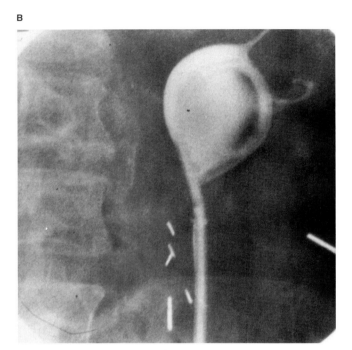

C

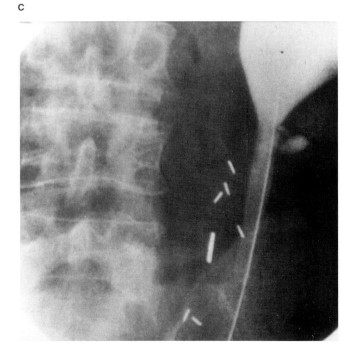

Figure 80–4. A. Nephrostogram through an external drainage catheter shows complete obstruction of the ureteropelvic junction in a patient with chronic obstruction. Patient has had external drainage for 3 years. **B.** Nephrostogram shows that the obstruction has been crossed and a double-J catheter is now in place following dilatation. **C.** The double-J catheter has been replaced by a metallic stent, which has remained patent.

more than 80%.[38] When obstructions or stenosis of unknown etiology are found, biopsy may be performed. In case of a malignant obstruction a permanent stent is placed. Internalization of the external drainage is preferred (Fig. 80–4). In cases of benign stenosis, balloon dilatation is performed with long-term ureteral stenting. If the stricture is recent and short, dilatation constitutes the definitive therapy in 50% of patients.[39] Chronic and long strictures are more refractory and frequently stricture dilatation fails.[40,41] Obstructions caused by the presence of clots due to renal trauma can be managed with ureteral stents.[42]

A

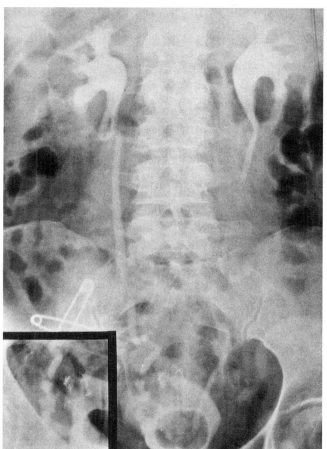

B

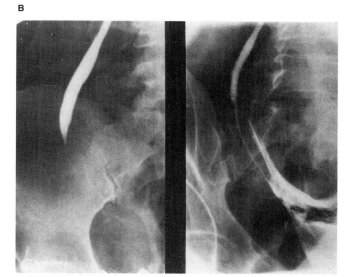

C

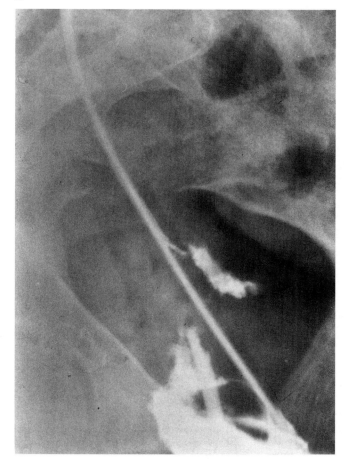

Figure 80–5. A. Intravenous pyelogram shows extravasation of contrast medium from the distal right ureter in a patient with accidental laceration of the ureter during pelvic surgery. **B.** Close-up view following placement of a percutaneous nephrostomy catheter in the right kidney shows extravasation from a localized site in the distal right ureter. **C.** A drainage catheter has been advanced into the urinary bladder. Note persistent extravasation of contrast medium adjacent to the catheter.

Urinary Fistulas. Urine leaks can be managed successfully by urinary diversion and ureteral stent placement.[43]

A small volume of urine leak can be easily treated by the placement of a percutaneous nephrostomy. Uretal stenting is required for a longer period of time in malignant fistulas or when there is incomplete healing after radical surgery. Placement of a stent across the site of leakage is beneficial in many ways; the presence of the stent accelerates healing of the segment, because it reduces the flow through the defect and also prevents ureteral strictures (Fig. 80–5). External drainage is provided until the fistula is healed, and then conversion to internal drainage with preservation of the external access is performed.

In those patients in whom conservative management has failed and with high-output fistulas, more radical interventions are needed. Methods of permanent occlusion include detachable balloons,[44] tissue adhesives,[44] electrocautery,[45] the combination of a "nest of coils" and gelfoam,[46] and ureteral clipping.[47] A permanent outside catheter is placed in those patients undergoing permanent ureteral occlusion.

Renal Transplants

The same basic techniques for PN are applied in cases of problems with transplanted kidneys. Urologic complications in renal transplanted kidneys occur in about 10% of cases. The most common early complication is urinary leak or urinary obstruction, which can appear early or late.[48] The procedures in the transplanted kidney are facilitated by the fact that the graft is superficial and extraperitoneal. External drainage and stenting of the ureter can therefore be easily accomplished.[49,50] Although uncommon, stones can form in transplanted kidneys, sometimes due to anatomic problems; ESWL is contraindicated. In these cases, PNL through a nephrostomy tract is indicated.[52]

CONCLUSIONS

In 40 years, since the first attempt to gain access into the collecting system, interventional uroradiology has dramatically changed the diagnosis and treatment of urologic patients. After a PN is performed, the therapeutic possibilities are multiple. Most of the procedures performed today have passed the test of time and are widely accepted. The field is still open for the development of new methods.

REFERENCES

1. Goodwin WE, Casey WC, Woolf W. Percutaneous trocar (needle) nephrostomy in hydronephrosis. *JAMA.* 1955;157:891.
2. Smith AD, Reinke DB, Miller RP, et al. Percutaneous nephrostomy in the management of ureteral and renal calculi. *Radiology.* 1979;133:49.
3. Clayman RV, Surya V, Miller RP, et al. Percutaneous nephrolithotomy: Extraction of renal and ureteral calculi from 100 patients. *J Urol.* 1984;131:868.
4. Irby PB, Schwartz BF, Stoller ML. Percutaneous access techniques in renal surgery. *Tech Urol.* 1999;5:29.
5. Barbalias GA, Siablis D, Liatsikos EN, et al. Metal Stent: A new treatment of malignant ureteral obstruction. *J Urol.* 1997;158:54.
6. Lopez-Martinez RA, Singireddy S, Lang EK. The use of metallic stent to bypass ureteral strictures secondary to metastatic prostate cancer: Experience with 8 patients. *J Urol.* 1997;158:50.
7. Wakui M, Takeuchi S, Isioka J, et al. Metallic stents for malignant and benign ureteric obstruction. *BJU Int.* 2000;85:227.
8. Diaz-Lucas EF, Martinez-Torres JL, Fernandez Mena J, et al. Self-expanding wallstent endoprosthesis for malignant ureteral obstruction. *J Endourol.* 1997;11:441.
9. Burgos Revilla FJ, Gomez Dosantos V, Carrera Puerta C, et al. Treatment of ureteral obstruction with auto-expandable metallic endoprosthesis. *Arch Esp Urol.* 1999;52:363. Discussion, 371.
10. Brödel M. The intrinsic blood vessels of the kidney and their significance in nephrotomy. *John Hopkins Hosp Bull.* 1901;12:10.
11. Montanri E, Serrafo M, Expsosito N, et al. Ultrasound-fluoroscopy guided access to the intrarenal excretory system. *Ann Urol* (Paris). 1999;33:168.
12. Chisena S. Echoguided percutaneous nephrostomy. *Arch Ital Urol.* 1998;70:133.
13. Gupta S, Gulati M, Suri S. Ultrasound guided percutaneous nephrostomy in nondilated pelvicaliceal system. *J Clin Ultrasound.* 1998;26:177.
14. Fabrizio MD, Gray DS, Feld RI, et al. Placement of ureteral stents in pregnancy using ultrasound guidance. *Tech Urol.* 1996;2:121.
15. Robert M, Maubon A, Roux JO, et al. Direct percutaneous approach to the upper pole of the kidney: MRI anatomy with assessment of the visceral risk. *J Endourol.* 1999;13:17.
16. Mekle EM, Hashim M, Wendt M, et al. MR-guided percutaneous nephrostomy of the nondilated upper urinary tract in a porcine model. *AJR.* 1999;172:1221.
17. Nolte-Ernsting CC, Bucker A, Neuerburg JM, et al. MRI-guided percutaneous nephrostomy of the contrast-enhanced, nondilated upper urinary tract: Initial experimental results. *Rofo Fortschr Geb Rontgenstr Neuen Bildgeb Verfahr.* 1998;168:616.
18. Hagspiel KD, Kandarpa K, Silverman SG. Interactive MR-guided percutaneous nephrostomy. *JMRI.* 1998;8:1319.
19. Jackman SV, Docimo SG, Cadeddu JA, et al. The "mini-perc" technique: A less invasive alternative to PNL. *World J Urol.* 1998;16:371.
20. Morsy A, el Gammal M, Abdel-Razzak OM. Modified technique for dilation in difficult nephrostomy tracts. *Tech Urol.* 1998;4:148.
21. Ferral H, Stackhouse DJ, Bjarnason H, et al. Complications of percutaneous nephrostomy tube placement. *Semin Intervent Radiol.* 1994;11:198.
22. Gerber GS. Combination therapy in the treatment of patients with staghorn calculi. *Tech Urol.* 1999;5:155.
23. Havel D, Saussine C, Fath C, et al. Single stone of the lower pole of the kidney. Comparative results of extracorporeal shock wave lithotripsy and percutaneous nephrolithotomy. *Eur Urol.* 1998;33:369.
24. Banner MP. Extracorporeal shock wave lithotripsy: Selection of patients and long-term complications. *Radiol Clin North Am.* 1991;29:543.
25. LeRoy AJ. Diagnosis and treatment of nephrolithiasis: current perspectives. *AJR.* 1994;163:1309.
26. Stening SG, Bourne S. Supracostal percutaneous nephrolithotomy for upper pole caliceal calculi. *J Endourol.* 1998;12:359.
27. Gupta M, Bolton DM, Stoller ML. Etiology and management of cystine lithiasis. *Urology.* 1995;45:344.
28. Sheldon CA, Smith AD. Chemolysis of calculi. *Urol Clin North Am.* 1982;9:121.
29. Fraser M, Joyce AD, Thomas DF, et al. Minimally invasive treatment of urinary tract calculi in children. *BJU Int.* 1999;84:339.
30. Desai M, Ridhorkar V, Patel S, et al. Pediatric percutaneous nephrolithotomy: Assessing impact of technical innovations on safety and efficacy. *J Endourol.* 1999;13:359.
31. Jackman SV, Hedican SP, Peters CA, et al. Percutaneous nephrolithotomy in infants and preschool age children: Experience with a new technique. *Urology.* 1998;52:697.
32. Granados Loarca EA. Percutaneous extraction of renal lithiasis without radiological assistance. *Arch Esp Urol.* 1995;52:505.
33. Issa MM, McNamara DE, Myrick SE, et al. Surgical challenge of

massive bilateral staghorn calculi in a spinal cord injury patient. *Urol Int.* 1998;61:247.

34. Golijanin D, Katz R, Verstanding A, et al. The supracostal percutaneous nephrostomy for treatment of staghorn and complex kidney stones. *J Endourol.* 1998;12:403.

35. Joshi HB, Obadeyi OO, Rao PN. A comparative analysis of nephrostomy, double J stent and urgent in situ extracorporeal shock wave lithotripsy for obstructing ureteric stones. *BJU Int.* 1999;84:264.

36. Jorgan JD, Maidenberg MJ, Smith AD. Endopyelotomy in the elderly. *J Urol.* 1993;150:1107.

37. Kavoussi LR, Meteryk S, Dierks SM, et al. Endopyelotomy for secondary ureteropelvic obstruction in children. *J Urol.* 1991;145:345.

38. Rickards D, Jones SN. Percutaneous interventional uroradiology. *Br J Radiol.* 1989;62:573.

39. Lang EK, Glorioso LW III. Antegrade transluminal dilation of benign ureteral strictures: Long-term results. *AJR.* 1988;150:131.

40. Lang EK. Percutaneous management of ureteral strictures. *Semin Intervent Radiol.* 1987;4:79.

41. Bechman CF, Roth RA, Bihrle W III. Dilatation of benign ureteral strictures. *Radiology.* 1989;172:437.

42. Haas CA, Reigle MD, Selzman AA, et al. Use of ureteral stents in the management of major renal trauma with urinary extravasation: Is there a role? *J Endourol.* 1998;12:545.

43. Druy EM, Gharib M, Finder CA. Percutaneous nephroureteral drainage and stenting for post-surgical ureteral leaks. *AJR.* 1983;141:389.

44. Scheld HH, Günther R, Thelen M. Transrenal ureteral occlusion: Results and problems. *JVIR.* 1994;5:321.

45. Reddy PK, Moore L, Hunter D, et al. Percutaneous ureteral fulguration: A known surgical technique for ureteral occlusion. *J Urol.* 1987;138:724.

46. Gaylord GM, Jonhsrude IS. Transrenal ureteral occlusion with Gianturco coils and gelatin sponge. *Radiology.* 1989;172:1047.

47. Cragg AH, Castañeda F, Amplatz K, et al. Percutaneous ureteral clipping: Technique and results. *Semin Intervent Radiol.* 1989;6:176.

48. Streem SB. Endourological management of urological complications following renal transplantation. *Semin Urol.* 1994;12:123.

49. Yong AA, Ball ST, Pelling MX, et al. Management of ureteral strictures in renal transplants by antegrade balloon dilatation and temporary internal stenting. *Cardiovasc Intervent Radiol.* 1999;22:385.

50. Trapeznikova MF, Urenkov SB, Kulachkov SM, et al. Use of stent-nephrostomy in the treatment of renal transplant urologic complications by percutaneous surgical techniques. *Urol Nefrol.* 1998;1:3–7.

51. Bhagat VJ, Gordon RL, Osorio RW, et al. Ureteral obstruction and leaks after renal transplantation: Outcome of percutaneous antegrade ureteral stent placement in 44 patients. *Radiology.* 1998;209:159.

52. Hulbert JC, Reddy P, Young AT, et al. The percutaneous removal of calculi from transplanted kidneys. *J Urol.* 1985;134:324.

Endocrine Surgery

Chapter Eighty-One ・ ・ ・ ・ ・ ・

Endoscopic Thyroid and Parathyroid Surgery

WILLIAM B. INABNET AND MICHEL GAGNER

INTRODUCTION

With the first endoscopic parathyroidectomy in 1995, endoscopic neck surgery moved from the animal laboratory to clinical practice.[1] Although the results of conventional thyroid and parathyroid surgery have withstood the test of time, there were few major refinements in these techniques during most of the twentieth century. Conventional neck exploration requires a centrally located incision (Kocher incision), the creation of myocutaneous flaps, and the separation or division of the strap muscles in order to gain access to the thyroid/parathyroid basin. The conventional approach is well tolerated by most patients but leaves a scar in a cosmetically unappealing location. In addition, some patients experience significant pain and impaired neck mobility following bilateral neck exploration, particularly in the immediate postoperative period.

When developing a new, minimally invasive technique, the results of conventional open surgery must be equaled or surpassed. Early reports of video-assisted and endoscopic neck surgery have demonstrated equal cure rates with superior cosmesis and less pain compared to conventional neck surgery.[2,3] In addition, an endoscopic approach offers high magnification of cervical anatomy including the recurrent laryngeal nerve, parathyroid glands, and the external branch of the superior laryngeal nerve, a fact that may ultimately lead to less morbidity. In this chapter, the techniques of endoscopic thyroidectomy and parathyroidectomy will be reviewed, paying particular attention to patient selection and operative technique.

ENDOSCOPIC THYROIDECTOMY

Patient Selection

Multiple factors influence patient selection for endoscopic thyroidectomy. The type and size of pathology, body habitus, the age of the patient, and patient preference all play a role in patient selection. The presence of a solitary nonfunctioning thyroid nodule that is less than or equal to 3 cm in diameter is one of the best indications for endoscopic thyroidectomy. Accordingly, the preoperative evaluation should include a thorough history and physical examination, indirect laryngoscopy, thyroid function tests, and fine-needle aspiration. Ultrasonography provides useful information on the size and location of thyroid nodules and permits evaluation of the contralateral thyroid lobe. Other indications for endoscopic thyroidectomy include solitary toxic nodules, small multinodular goiters with a dominant nonfunctioning nodule, and recurrent thyroid cysts.

Endoscopic thyroidectomy should not be offered in certain clinical conditions. Since a virtual space is created during endoscopic neck surgery, endoscopic thyroidectomy is not recommended for patients with nodules greater than 3 cm in diameter, as exposure may be compromised by larger thyroid nodules. Other relative contraindications include a large multinodular goiter, a history of prior neck surgery, and the presence of thyroiditis and/or morbid obesity, as a wide, short neck will limit maneuverability. In Graves' disease, the thyroid gland is highly vascular and diffusely enlarged, which increases the chance of bleeding during surgery. For this reason, open conventional thyroidectomy is preferred in patients with Graves' disease. Finally, elderly patients with comorbid medical problems may not tolerate CO_2 insufflation; therefore these patients are not considered good candidates for endoscopic thyroidectomy.

Surgical Technique

The patient is placed on the operating table in the supine position with the neck slightly extended.[4] Anatomic landmarks are outlined with a marking pen, including the sternal notch, the midline, the anterior border of the sternocleidomastoid muscle (SCM), and the external jugular veins. The head is slightly rotated to maximize access to the ipsilateral neck.

A 0.5-cm incision is made at the sternal notch and the cervical fascia is opened under direct vision. The subplatysmal space is developed along the anterior border of the ipsilateral SCM. A purse-string suture is placed in the subcutaneous tissue and a 5-mm trocar is inserted. Alternatively, the first incision may be placed in the superolateral quadrant of the neck where the space medial to the carotid artery and lateral to the strap muscles is developed using blunt dissection. Carbon dioxide is insufflated to a pressure of 12 mm Hg, but once an adequate working space has developed, the insufflation pressures are decreased to 8 to 10 mm Hg for the remainder of the procedure. A zero-degree 5-mm endoscope is used to perform the initial dissection in the avascular space along the anteromedial border of the ipsilateral SCM.

After the initial dissection, a 30° or 45° 5-mm endoscope is used for the remainder of the procedure. Additional trocars are inserted under direct vision, including a 2- or 3-mm trocar at the midline, a 2- or 3-mm trocar in the lower quadrant of the neck, and a 5- or 10-mm trocar superolaterally along the anterior border of the SCM (Fig. 81–1). The latter trocar site, which is located in a cosmetically favorable location, is used to extract the specimen at the conclusion of the operation.

The carotid artery is identified and the space between the lateral border of the strap muscles and the medial edge of the carotid artery is developed. The strap muscles are retracted anteromedially and the thyroid gland is approached laterally. The thyroid lobe is visualized and mobilized using a combination of sharp and blunt dissection. The middle thyroid vein is ligated using 5-mm clips or the 5-mm ultrasonic scalpel. Using blunt dissection, the recurrent laryngeal nerve and parathyroid glands are identified and carefully dissected free of their attachments to the thyroid gland (Fig. 81–2). The inferior thyroid artery is mobilized at its junction with the recurrent laryngeal nerve and ligated with the 5-mm clip-applier or ultrasonic scalpel (Fig. 81–3).

The superior pole vessels are dissected and divided with the ultrasonic scalpel. An effort is made to identify the external branch of the superior laryngeal nerve. The inferior pole vessels are di-

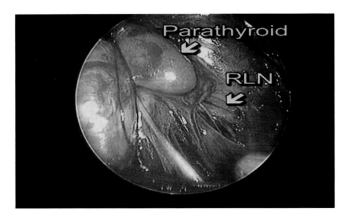

Figure 81–2. Recurrent laryngeal nerve (RLN) and a normal superior parathyroid gland.

vided in a similar manner. After releasing the anteromedial attachments of the recurrent laryngeal nerve by blunt dissection, the 5-mm ultrasonic scalpel is used to divide the ligament of Berry. The recurrent laryngeal nerve must be in full view during this maneuver. Finally, the isthmus is divided using the ultrasonic scalpel.

A small sac is constructed by removing the thumb portion of a large surgical glove and a purse string suture is fashioned (Fig. 81–4). The specimen is placed in the sac and extracted through the superolateral trocar site, which may need to be slightly enlarged to accommodate the specimen (Fig. 81–5). By placing the thyroid lobe in an extraction sac direct contact with the edges of the incision is avoided. Steri-Strips™ are used to close the incisions.

Results

To date, we have performed endoscopic thyroidectomy on 28 patients. There were 26 females and 2 males with a mean age of 42 years (range, 17 to 66 years). Indications for surgery included follicular neoplasm (n = 12), indeterminate/inadequate cytology (n = 10), recurrent thyroid cyst (n = 2), Hürthle cell neoplasm (n = 1), and toxic thyroid nodule (n = 3).

Twenty-five of 28 cases were successfully completed endoscopically with a mean operating time of 200 minutes (range, 100

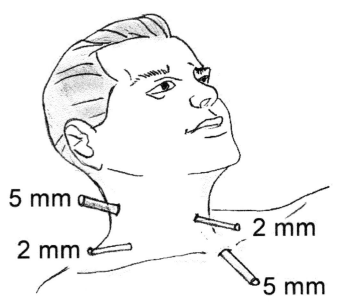

Figure 81–1. Trocar placement for endoscopic thyroidectomy.

5 mm

2 mm

2 mm

5 mm

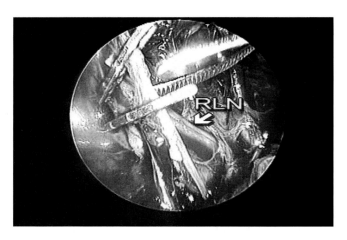

Figure 81–3. Ligation with titanium clips and division of the inferior thyroid artery.

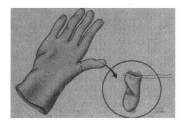

Figure 81–4. A small sac is fabricated from the thumb of a surgical glove and a purse-string suture.

to 330 min). In the last 6 cases, however, the mean duration of surgery decreased to less than 150 minutes. In 3 patients thyroidectomy was accomplished through a small ipsilateral incision for two indications: an inadequate working space (n = 2), and bleeding that occurred during ligation of the inferior thyroid artery (n = 1). Operative procedures included left thyroid lobectomy (n = 11), left subtotal thyroidectomy (n = 2), right thyroid lobectomy (n = 9), right subtotal thyroidectomy (n = 2), and isthmusectomy (n = 4).

Final pathology yielded diagnoses of follicular adenoma (n = 16), Hürthle cell adenoma (n = 1), oncocytic adenoma (n = 1), thyroid cyst (n = 1), multinodular goiter (n = 6), and papillary thyroid carcinoma (n = 3). Two patients with papillary carcinoma (one with the follicular variant) underwent open completion thyroidectomy without evidence of residual disease. In the third patient a small focus of papillary carcinoma was detected incidentally. All patients were highly satisfied with their cosmetic result (Fig. 81–6).

During surgery 3 patients developed mild hypercarbia that was successfully controlled by increasing the minute ventilation. One patient developed a temporary recurrent laryngeal palsy that completely resolved after 3 weeks.

ENDOSCOPIC PARATHYROIDECTOMY

Patient Selection

Unilateral neck exploration for primary hyperparathyroidism was first suggested by Tibblin et al in 1982.[5] Advantages of a unilateral exploration include a shorter operating time, a quicker

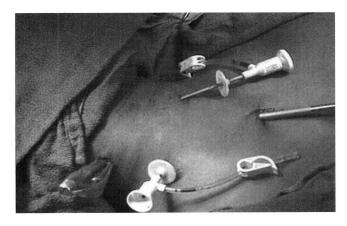

Figure 81–5. Extraction of the specimen, external view

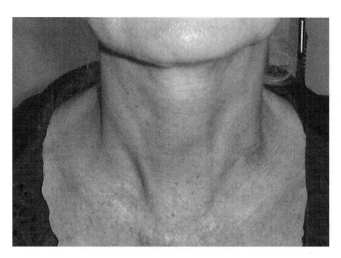

Figure 81–6. Cosmetic result 3 weeks following endoscopic left thyroidectomy.

recovery, and avoidance of surgical dissection around the normal parathyroid glands. Over the last decade, minimally invasive parathyroidectomy has gained acceptance among most endocrine surgeons. Several factors have contributed to the development of these targeted surgical techniques, such as improved preoperative localization with high-resolution ultrasonography and/or 99mTc sestamibi scanning and the availability of intraoperative parathyroid hormone (PTH) monitoring. These advances have permitted the use of local anesthesia during parathyroidectomy as well as the development of video-assisted and solely endoscopic techniques.[1,6–8]

Endoscopic parathyroidectomy is offered to patients with a solitary parathyroid adenoma visualized on preoperative imaging who have a biochemical diagnosis of primary hyperparathyroidism. Although an endoscopic approach is ideally suited for most patients with a solitary adenoma, it is especially indicated for lesions that are located in deep or ectopic locations, including the mediastinum. Exclusion criteria include familial hyperparathyroidism, multiple endocrine neoplasia, prior neck surgery, and a history of thyroiditis.

Surgical Technique

Endoscopic parathyroidectomy is performed under general anesthesia with the patient in the supine position. Intraoperative PTH monitoring is used in all cases, with levels being taken at the following times: baseline, pre-excision, and 5, 10, and 30 minutes following parathyroidectomy. Cervical access is similar to that for endoscopic thyroidectomy, however in most cases the procedure can be performed with three trocars (Fig. 81–7). The first trocar, which

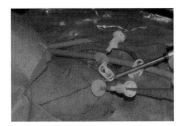

Figure 81–7. Trocar placement for endoscopic parathyroidectomy.

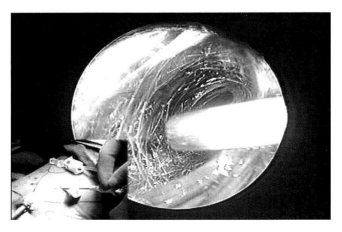

Figure 81–8. Creation of the subplatysmal space.

is 5-mm in size, is placed at the sternal notch for superior adenomas, whereas for inferior adenomas it is placed along the anterior border of the SCM. The remaining trocars are 2 to 3 mm in size.

The carotid artery is identified and the space between the lateral border of the strap muscles and the medial edge of the carotid artery is developed. Strap muscles are retracted anteromedially in order to expose the lateral aspect of the thyroid lobe (Fig. 81–8). The thyroid is then gently retracted medially in order to provide further exposure of the area, exposing the loose connective tissue posterolateral to the thyroid.

Enlarged parathyroid glands may sometimes be easily identified without the need for extensive dissection of other structures. When parathyroid glands are not immediately visualized, classic anatomic landmarks are used during the dissection. The recurrent laryngeal nerve is identifiable in most cases. The superior parathyroid glands will be found most often at the level of the upper two-thirds of the posterior thyroid capsule. The inferior thyroid artery or its branches lead in most cases to the inferior parathyroid glands. An endoscopic approach also allows excellent visualization of glands in the tracheoesophageal groove and superior mediastinum.

Once the parathyroid adenoma has been carefully mobilized, the vascular pedicle is dissected and ligated with a 2-mm vessel loop. Alternatively, a 2-mm endoscope can be inserted through one of the smaller trocars so that a 5-mm clip-applier can be used through the 5-mm trocar. The adenoma is placed in a small retrieval bag and extracted. If there is a greater than 50% reduction of the highest baseline PTH value, the operation is concluded. If the PTH level remains elevated, the operation is continued until all hyperfunctioning glands have been removed.

Results

Over a 3-year period, 64 parathyroidectomies were performed in 56 patients, including 53 patients with a single adenoma and 3 with hyperplasia. There were 14 males and 42 females with an average age of 51.5 (range, 37 to 70). All patients had successful localization on preoperative sestamibi scanning, and in addition 18 patients underwent ultrasonography. There were six conversions to open parathyroidectomy for the following reasons: large gland size (5.7

g) (n = 1), an intrathyroidal adenoma (n = 1), and inability to locate the gland (n = 4).

Two patients had 4-gland hyperplasia and underwent 3½-gland excision. Another patient with secondary hyperparathyroidism underwent 3-gland excision. Mean operative time for single gland removal was 121 minutes (range, 60 to 300 min) whereas the multiple gland excisions took an average of 270 minutes (range, 240 to 300). There were no other complications.

Mean preoperative calcium was 11.4 mg/dL (range, 7.8 to 12.8 mg/dL) which decreased to a mean of 8.6 mg/dL (range, 7.5 to 10.4) following surgery. Average preoperative PTH was 268 pg/mL (range, 41 to 1877), compared to 34 pg/mL after surgery. The mean weight of the gland removed was 1105 mg (range, 240 to 5700). All patients have remained normocalcemic following surgery.

DISCUSSION

Endoscopic thyroid and parathyroid surgery is a new frontier in endocrine surgery that offers numerous advantages over conventional endocrine neck surgery. Although conventional open thyroid and parathyroid surgery can be performed with few complications, this approach leaves a visible scar on the anterior surface of the neck in a cosmetically unappealing location. The endoscopic approach provides a superior cosmetic result when compared to conventional surgery and results in a quicker return to normal activity. Endoscopic neck surgery provides superior magnification of thyroid anatomy, including the recurrent laryngeal nerve, superior laryngeal nerve, and the parathyroid glands. In addition, since muscle is not divided, there is less tissue trauma, resulting in a quicker return to normal activity. The long duration of surgery is the primary disadvantage to endoscopic thyroidectomy; however, this should decrease as additional experience is gained. Prior experience with endoscopic parathyroidectomy is recommended prior to attempting endoscopic thyroidectomy.

REFERENCES

1. Gagner M. Endoscopic subtotal parathyroidectomy in patients with primary hyperparathyroidism. *Br J Surg.* 1996;83:875.
2. Gagner M, Inabnet WB. Endoscopic thyroidectomy for solitary thyroid nodules. *Thyroid* 2001;11:161.
3. Miccoli P, Bendinelli C, Berti P, et al. Video-assisted versus conventional parathyroidectomy in primary hyperparathyroidism: a prospective randomized study. *Surgery* 1999;126:1117.
4. Inabnet WB, Gagner M. How I do it: endoscopic thyroidectomy. *J Otolaryngol.* 2001;30:1.
5. Tibblin S, Bondeson AG, Ljungberg O. Unilateral parathyroidectomy in hyperparathyroidism due to single adenoma. *Ann Surg.* 1982;195:245.
6. Inabnet WB, Fulla Y, Luton LP, et al. Unilateral neck exploration under local anesthesia: The approach of choice for asymptomatic primary hyperparathyroidism. *Surgery* 1999;126:1004.
7. Miccoli P, Bendinelli C, Vignali E, et al. Endoscopic parathyroidectomy: report of an initial experience. *Surgery* 1998;124:1077.
8. Cougard P, Goudet P, Bilosi M, et al. Video-endoscopic parathyroidectomy. *Ann Chir.* 2001;126:314.

Section Thirteen . . . . . .

Vascular Surgery

Chapter Eighty-Two • • • • • •

Aortobifemoral Bypass

CARLOS R. GRACIA and IVES-MARIE DION

INTRODUCTION

Minimally invasive surgical (MIS) techniques have been evolving over the past decade. The ability to remotely access various body parts through tiny incisions has revolutionized the practice of surgery. Laparoscopic surgery has been recognized as beneficial in the performance of a growing number of surgical procedures. The development of superior optics, video imaging equipment, and design of instrumentation to work remotely, have enabled numerous advances which have centered predominantly on gastrointestinal, gynecologic, urologic, and general thoracic procedures, and more recently coronary bypass surgery.

The field of vascular surgery has now also been experiencing new advances in operative procedures. Minimally invasive techniques utilizing scopes and specialized instrumentation have been evolving for saphenous vein harvesting and for subfascial endoscopic perforator vein surgery (SEPS).[1] While the proclaimed advantages of laparoscopic surgery such as diminished postoperative pain, shorter hospital stay, and earlier return to work have been documented,[2-5] this often high-risk group of patients for vascular surgery would seem to benefit greatly from other techniques for minimally invasive surgery. Vascular surgeons, however, have been slow in their adoption of MIS operative developments such as laparoscopy for other vascular conditions such as aortoiliac disease.

In aortoiliac disease, arteriosclerosis is usually segmental in distribution, despite its widespread nature. This makes it amenable to effective treatment. A wide range of options for therapeutic management of aortoiliac disease have emerged which, and they can be categorized as: (1) anatomic (direct reconstructive procedures on the aortoiliac vessels); (2) extra-anatomic (indirect bypass grafts that avoid normal anatomic pathways); and (3) nonoperative catheter-based endoluminal therapies that emphasize treatment of occlusive lesions by a remote, often percutaneous access site (minimally invasive approach) to the arterial system.[6]

The slowness of the adoption of operative MIS to aortoiliac disease may in part be due to three factors. First is the fact that laparoscopy has grown predominantly within nonvascular circles, limiting the laparoscopic experience of vascular surgeons to date. Second,

the technical challenges imparted by the fundamentals of vascular surgery (e.g., exposure, vascular control, vascular occlusion, anastomosis of vessels and/or grafts, and hemostasis) are not readily accomplished in laparoscopic surgery with currently available instruments. Advancements in MIS technology for application of laparoscopy to vascular reconstruction have lagged significantly behind those that have helped spread its application in gastrointestinal laparoscopy. Advances in MIS technology have centered attention on MIS cardiac surgery and not peripheral vascular reconstruction. Finally, the ongoing technological developments and focus of MIS have revolved around endoluminal therapies by both industry and surgeon.

The current minimally invasive vascular techniques for arterial disease are endoluminal and include angioplasty, stent placement, and angioscopy. Experience is also being reported with stent grafts, not only for aneurysmal disease, but also for aortoiliac occlusive disease.[7] These modalities have grown due to an investment in the technology to enable their reproducibility and applicability. However, confusion exists due to differences in reported early and late results of the various options for the various therapeutic modalities. No one single option for inflow revascularization is ideal or applicable to all cases.

Standard bypass procedures for aortoiliac disease have achieved excellent long-term patencies.[8] For most patients with diffuse aortoiliac occlusive disease, aortobifemoral (ABF) bypass grafts remain the most durable and functionally effective means of revascularization and should continue to be rightfully regarded as the gold standard with which other options must be compared.[6]

Although still in its infancy, the laparoscopic aortoiliac vascular procedure has been performed on patients. We will review the experimental and developmental aspects of this and its current successful application in clinical settings.

FEASIBILITY OF LAPAROSCOPY FOR TREATING AORTOILIAC OCCLUSIVE DISEASE

Early experimental work led to the conclusion that exposure and surgery of the aorta via laparoscopy was feasible. From 1991

589

through 1992 work was done to evaluate the possible access and exposure of the aorta utilizing a new abdominal wall lifting device (Laborie Surgical, Ltd.) by Dion et al in Quebec, Canada. This represents one of the earliest applications of applying laparoscopic experience to vascular surgery. A porcine model was selected. The abdominal wall lifting device was chosen due to concerns of not being able to suction while working on vascular structures under pneumoperitoneum. Development of venous air embolism while working near the major venous structures in the retroperitoneum under insufflation also was a concern. The gasless approach eliminated these concerns. As early instrumentation was also nonexistent, this model allowed for conventional vascular instrumentation (particularly occlusive clamps and needle-drivers) to be utilized. In this model, they could be inserted through blunt ports without concerns for leakage of pneumoperitoneum. Early successes with exposure and surgery in the animal model led to new instrument design with adaptation of standard vascular instrumentation onto remote handles for laparoscopic application.

The result of this developmental work was the first application of laparoscopy to major vascular reconstructive surgery (ABF bypass) in humans, performed in March of 1993, by a surgical team led by Dr. Yves Dion of Quebec.[9] Four more ABF bypasses followed this early case.[10] These cases were laparoscopically assisted with all of the dissection, control, insertion, and tunneling of graft done laparoscopically. However, a small mini-laparotomy was performed in order to construct an end-to-side proximal anastomosis. This allowed for the use of traditional occlusive clamps and needle-drivers. Operative details include the use of a transperitoneal approach under pneumoperitoneum to accomplish this. All patients demonstrated improved postoperative courses characterized by early ambulation with less pain and need for analgesics.

Clinical work by Berens and Herde[11] ensued with a variety of cases being performed, including one ABF bypass, one aortoiliac endarterectomy, and two iliofemoral bypasses. Although similar in utilization of a transperitoneal route, an abdominal wall lift was used in this experience to maintain the working cavity, as opposed to insufflation. Again, a mini-laparotomy was utilized for the vascular suturing and occlusion. It was also used as an avenue for insertion of more conventional retractors and packing pads for small bowel retraction. Therefore this experience is also more appropriately termed laparoscopic-assisted surgery. These patients also experienced a faster postoperative recovery with less pain.

Although time consuming and lengthy, these early experiences demonstrated reproduction of the standard operative approach for aortoiliac arteriosclerotic occlusive disease in each circumstance. The reason for the mini-laparotomy was to perform a continuous sutured vascular anastomosis, a task considered tedious and difficult with current endoscopic instrumentation. Not only were occlusive devices inserted through these small incisions, they were necessary for retraction of abdominal viscera. By applying MIS in place of the standard traditional incisional approach, patients enjoyed improved and shortened postoperative courses.[10,11] It now seemed feasible to apply laparoscopy to vascular reconstruction.

LABORATORY AND DEVELOPMENTAL WORK

These pioneering experiences had identified important issues. Experience was obtained with both a gasless and a traditional gas-insufflation technique. Frustrations were present with both techniques. Were these difficulties the result of problems intrinsic to either of these techniques or to the transperitoneal route common to both experiences? The early human clinical experience of Dion et al confirmed the difficulty of the transperitoneal route with respect to bowel retraction. Due to these difficulties, aortic dissection and end-to-side aortoprosthetic anastomosis remained quite tedious. The solution may be a retroperitoneal approach. It was felt that the peritoneal sac would function as an organ "container" and provide improved exposure to the major vessels.

Dion et al[12] in 1995 reported the first work in an animal series using a retroperitoneal approach. Initially, the anterior approach of Schumaker[13] was used, but it was abandoned for a lateral approach to access the retroperitoneum. Piglets were placed in a right lateral decubitus position. Balloon dissectors aided in retroperitoneal dissection to create a retroperitoneal space. After dissection, visualization of the aorta from the left renal artery distally was possible. Abdominal wall suspension (Laparolift, Origin Medsystems, Menlo Park, CA) was then utilized due to the aforementioned concerns of using suction with pneumoperitoneum. Also, there was the need to use instrumentation not designed to work in a sealed gas environment. Totally laparoscopic aortoprosthetic anastomoses were performed. In order to complete the aortobifemoral bypass procedure, the animals had to be turned onto a supine position for exposure of the femoral vessels and tunneling of the prosthetic graft to the groins. Bowel retraction became less of a problem now.

Despite the success of the previous experience, to completely translate this model to actual human application would require the undesirable task of having to turn the patient from a lateral position. Turning the patient would not allow access for proximal control once the patient was repositioned and could allow for breaks in the sterile technique. Considering the consequences of aortic prosthetic infection and bleeding, it would be important to avoid these risks. This approach would need to be modified in order for the patient to remain in a supine rather than lateral position.

In this experience, the issue of a laparoscopically-assisted approach was also being addressed. Completely endoscopic anastomoses were now constructed in contrast to the laparoscopically-assisted anastomoses used in the clinical experience. This is significant in that the limitations of a laparoscopic-assisted approach became apparent. The variability of the thickness of the abdominal wall in patients of different sizes would be problematic. With increased abdominal wall thickness, the incisions must increase in size in order to maintain exposure. It is difficult to make small incisions in obese patients or those with thick abdominal walls. At some point you begin to lose any advantages sought by minimizing trauma from the access. Therefore, a completely laparoscopic approach may ultimately be more reproducible and overcome limitations imposed by small incisions. This would require resolution of other technical challenges, as well as development of appropriate instrumentation for these tasks.

Additional work by Dion between 1993 and 1994 had demonstrated the feasibility of a totally laparoscopic approach to the tasks required for aortic surgery. A canine model was utilized under CO_2 insufflation with a 2-cm aortotomy performed with a side-biting Satinsky-style clamp (adapted for laparoscopy). A Hemashield™ (Bard) vascular prosthesis was sutured into this aortotomy as a hemostatic patch with running monofilament suture performed totally laparoscopically under pneumoperitoneum.

These previous two experiences confirmed that standard vascular maneuvers, such as occlusion, opening of the vessel, and its direct suturing, could be successfully performed in a totally laparoscopic environment. In one, a gasless environment was utilized while in the other pneumoperitoneum was successfully utilized.

Other investigators were also looking at the challenges of applying laparoscopy to vascular surgery. Jones et al[14] reported in 1996 on evaluation of both transperitoneal and retroperitoneal approaches. Ten aortofemoral procedures were performed with five animals used for each approach. Mini-laparotomy was utilized in their transperitoneal approach with an abdominal wall lift. Serial balloon dissection was used to open the retroperitoneum while the abdominal wall lift device again maintained the retroperitoneal working space. The anastomoses were performed via the mini-laparotomy with overall experience demonstrating acceptable clamp times and overall operative times. The complications related to laparoscopic technique in this experience pertained to retraction of small bowel, occurring only in the transperitoneal group. These investigators reported both approaches effective for gasless laparoscopic-assisted exposure of the aorta, but noted that the retroperitoneal approach facilitated bowel retraction by using the intact peritoneal sac.

Two concepts were developing from these works. The first is that a totally endoscopic approach was feasible, as was used in other laparoscopic procedures. The other is that a retroperitoneal approach did indeed seem to have advantages over a transperitoneal approach. However, there was no benefit of either a gasless environment or a traditional insufflation approach. A gasless approach seemed promising for the ability to suction with impunity and to insert a variety of traditional instrumentation. Although gasless technique would represent an alternative to pneumoperitoneum when surgery is performed in localized regions of the abdomen, such as the pelvis or upper abdomen, its application to the peritoneal cavity at large can become problematic. The compressing effect of carbon dioxide under normal working pressures (12 to 15 mm Hg) is not present under a gasless environment. Therefore the small bowel tends to occupy more space in the abdominal cavity. Variation in body size and morphology of patients could make working under a gasless environment more difficult. The three-dimensional compressing effect of working with gas insufflation was known, workable, and potentially desirable. The safety of its use would require further investigation.

Since carbon dioxide embolization during laparoscopy is a recognized and potentially lethal complication,[15,16] the potential for pulmonary embolization following major venous laceration was evaluated under laparoscopic conditions by Dion et al.[17] A model with anesthetized dogs and hemodynamic monitoring via an arterial line and Swan-Ganz catheter was evaluated under carbon dioxide pneumoperitoneum. Transesophageal echocardiography was used to evaluate the status and amount of embolism within the heart chambers. Euvolemic dogs were submitted to a 1-cm longitudinal incision made into the vena cava while maintaining a carbon dioxide pneumoperitoneum with pressures between 12 and 15 mm Hg. No gas embolism was seen in 82% of the cases after exposure of the venotomies to the pneumoperitoneum. Only 18% had gas bubbles visible in the right heart cavities by transesophageal echocardiography. In contrast, direct intravenous bolus injection of only 15 mL of carbon dioxide led to visualization of many more gas bubbles in the right heart cavities. Massive IV injections of CO_2 (>300 mL) led to the appearance of gas bubbles in the left heart cavities and death.

These experiments also identified transesophageal echocardiography as more precise than relying on elevation of pulmonary artery pressure to detect gas embolism. A bolus of 15 mL of CO_2 was easily visualized by the transesophageal echocardiography probe without concomitant elevation of pulmonary artery pressure. The routine use of transesophageal echocardiography has not been clinically encouraged since in clinical practice very few episodes of gas embolism have been reported. In three studies, the incidence of gas embolism was 1 in 63,845 patients, 15 in 113,253 patients, and 8 in 50,247 patients, respectively.[18] Because of these studies, it was felt that it would be safe to proceed in this area under routine pneumoperitoneum if it were deemed necessary and/or helpful.

An anterolateral laparoscopic approach with the subject supine was subsequently performed and reported by the authors Dion and Gracia.[19] With the advantages of a retroperitoneal approach, it would be desirable to allow for simultaneous access to proximal aortic control or maneuvering and access to the groins. This necessitates a standard supine position to provide access to the groins for exposure of the femoral arteries and to tunnel the limbs of the vascular graft. The goal was to reproduce the exposure and control obtained by the lateral approach and also to completely expose and control the distal aorta, iliac arteries, and the inferior mesenteric artery. Uncontrolled lumbar vessels at the time of incision or division of the aorta could result in significant bleeding and their exposure and control was necessary.

In the technique of Dion and Gracia, attention was given to approach the aorta in models for occlusive disease as well as aneurysmal disease. After proximal occlusion and oversewing of the distal aorta, the aorta was transected and an end-to-end aorto-prosthetic anastomosis performed for an occlusive model. In the aneurysmal model, the aorta was opened longitudinally, with the lumbar arteries controlled not only from outside of the aorta, but oversewn intraluminally while bleeding, as in open repair. As in the open technique of aneurysmorraphy, the anastomosis was constructed in end-to-end fashion by suturing from within the aorta and incorporating an intact posterior wall. All anastomoses were constructed with standard running monofilament 4-0 polypropylene suture with curved vascular needles.

Construction of aortobifemoral bypass was consistently performed in less than 4 hours with blood loss never exceeding 550 mL. Bleeding most commonly occurred at the time the aorta was opened and flushed. On occasion bleeding came from the oversewn aortoiliac stump after the limbs of the grafts were opened, which was corrected with additional suture as necessary. The totally laparoscopic aortic anastomosis did not take more than 60 minutes to perform. No operative mortality was encountered in this series, as well as in the previous one, which together account for 34 consecutive totally laparoscopic aortobifemoral bypasses.

In these experiments, piglets were selected for several reasons. Their anatomy in the retroperitoneal aorta and surrounding structures is comparable to that of the human. The abdominal wall of the piglet is composed of the same muscles as that of humans.[12] The large size of this animal model (Yorkshire piglets, 75 to 80 kg) also makes comparison with human surgery more realistic. It allows performance of an aortobifemoral bypass in conditions similar to those in humans. The surgeon and assistant can work in the same fashion as if the abdomen were opened. The anterolateral retroperitoneal approach possesses numerous advantages over a transabdominal technique and is better than a lateral approach.

One must acknowledge that despite these similarities and advantages, the actual end organs, the human aorta and iliac arteries, are considerably different from those in the porcine model. Despite the enormous size of the Yorkshire-cross piglet torso and similarity to that of the human torso, it has an aorta that typically measures 7 to 8 mm in diameter. The aortic prosthesis is custom made from 6-mm-diameter grafts sewn in end-to-side fashion to form an appropriate bifurcated prosthesis for aortobifemoral bypass. In addition, the porcine aorta contains no atheromata. Finally, an aneurysmal mass and the resultant difficulties that it would generate are obviously absent. The commonplace destruction of the posterior wall of the aorta in aneurysmal disease is not available in the nonatheromatous porcine aorta.

Once consistent exposure and anastomosis could be constructed in the laboratory animal model without excessive blood loss, excessive surgery times, or operative mortality, it seemed appropriate to begin to offer patients the option of laparoscopic aortobifemoral bypass. Based on the completed animal experiments in which a retroperitoneal approach solved many of the exposure and retraction difficulties, this was felt to be the best approach for clinical application. It was believed it would solve the troublesome problem of small bowel retraction, which had proven problematic in the first human transperitoneal work. A totally endoscopic approach was also selected based on laboratory successes.

Evaluation in the human cadaver lab was also appropriate before embarking on further clinical work. A series of experiences were collected by recreating the retroperitoneal working space in human cadavers. Application of balloon technology (General Surgical Innovations, Cupertino, CA) allowed rapid and reproducible dissection of the retroperitoneum from a virtual space to actual space. This space was maintained with CO_2 insufflation with pressures of 12 to 14 mm Hg. Thus the space maintained was a pneumo-retroperitoneum. This allowed for placement of the other working trocars for dissection, retraction, tunneling, occlusion, and anastomosis.

EARLY CLINICAL EXPERIENCE

Dion et al[9] completed the first human aortic vascular experience in 1993, as previously noted. A laparoscopically-assisted aortobifemoral bypass graft was performed in a 63-year-old male with a history of myocardial infarction. He had developed ischemic rest pain due to aortoiliac occlusive inflow disease. Four additional such procedures were performed and reported.[10] The only intraoperative complication was a small bowel perforation due to retraction difficulties in this transperitoneal route. Postoperatively, patients felt less pain and were able to cough better and walk more easily. There were no postoperative complications.

A second series, with a variety of procedures, was reported in 1995 by Berens and Herde.[11] Their experience included one left iliofemoral bypass, one aortobifemoral bypass, one right iliofemoral bypass, and one aortoiliac endarterectomy. The two iliac patients were ambulating early and taking a diet within 24 hours with discharge in 24 hours. The aortic procedure patients were taking a diet at 48 hours postoperatively and discharged on the third postoperative day. There were no complications.

Details were previously noted of both Dion's experience and Berens and Herde's work. Both approaches used a transperitoneal route, whereas Dion utilized gas insufflation for the working space and Berens used an abdominal wall lift device (Origin Medsystems, Menlo Park, CA). The authors of both also noted the difficulties of retraction of intra-abdominal organs that renders aortic dissection and end-to-side aortoprosthetic anastomosis tedious.

A third experience was reported by Fabiani et al[20] in 1997. A combination of procedures and access were used. Aortobifemoral bypass was completed in three patients by a transperitoneal approach, while unilateral aortofemoral bypass was performed by a retroperitoneal approach in four patients. Two other patients had been attempted but converted to open laparotomy due to inadequate aortic exposure in one and extensive aortic calcification in the other. The procedures were completed in a fashion that was termed "video-assisted." Dissection, vascular control, tunneling, and placement of graft were all accomplished under laparoscopic view. A small 3-cm median mini-laparotomy allowed for insertion of a Satinsky clamp, at which time the aortotomy and anastomosis were performed through this route with video guidance of the laparoscope. Patient experience was once again favorable. Short postoperative ileus was noted with enteral diets started 48 hours postoperatively. Lengths of stay in the hospital ranged from 4 to 7 days.

As a result of our own laboratory experiences[19,21–24] and the evaluation of the retroperitoneal approach for a completely laparoscopic aortobifemoral bypass in human cadavers, we began our clinical experience in March of 1995. Four patients underwent successful aortobifemoral bypass (2) or iliofemoral graft (2) using a completely endoscopic and retroperitoneal approach. Ages of patients ranged from 62 to 71 years, and all four were male. The indications for surgery were rest pain in one (ankle-brachial index [ABI] <0.20) and severe claudication in 3 (ABI <0.60), all with aortoiliac occlusive disease. All patients were candidates for standard open surgery based on routine preoperative cardiopulmonary evaluation. Patients were not considered ideal candidates for endoluminal procedures based on the extent and distribution of the arteriosclerotic disease on arteriography. All were given the option of endoluminal interventions.

The first clinical case to use a completely retroperitoneal approach was a right iliofemoral bypass graft for a completely occluded right external iliac artery. The application of the retroperitoneal dissection established a satisfactory working space. Gas insufflation was utilized to maintain the space, as it did not need to extend up to the infrarenal aorta. At this time there was a concern that pneumoretroperitoneum would not be successful for exposure of the infrarenal aorta. An end-to-end anastomosis was constructed without difficulty. This patient required minimal analgesics and was discharged from the hospital in 48 hours. A second case of right iliofemoral bypass was performed with similar technique and results using an end-to-side anastomosis.

We then moved on to our first patient for ABF bypass by the same technique. Based on our extensive laboratory work we used the gasless space with abdominal wall suspension we were so familiar with. There were difficulties in maintaining the working space and exposure for dissection and proximal anastomosis, resulting in a lengthy operation about 12 hours long. Cross-clamp time approached 240 minutes. The patient developed compartment syndromes, which were readily identified and treated. A lengthier hospital stay was also experienced due to myoglobinuria, before the patient was ready for discharge.

Valuable experience had been gained from these first two cases. The iliofemoral bypass proceeded smoothly with insufflation. Instrumentation appeared to be the biggest obstacle, requiring adaptation of some endoscopic bulldogs as occlusive devices. In the aortobifemoral bypass, the gasless environment was significantly more difficult to maintain in the human torso than the porcine model, despite their similarities. The advantages of working under insufflation were not easily dismissed from our experiences. If exposure could be consistently performed and maintained better with insufflation, then adaptation of basic vascular instrumentation for laparoscopy should allow vascular anastomosis to be constructed in this totally laparoscopic environment. For these reasons, we began to work with insufflation on the next aorta and all subsequent cases.

The second aortobifemoral bypass was performed under insufflation with much improved visibility. Surgical time remained long at ~10 hours, but improved overall. Aortic cross-clamp time, however, dropped to 70 minutes due to the improved exposure and visibility. Most of the operative time was spent in orientation and dissection in the retroperitoneum. The patient required minimal analgesics postoperatively. Intraoperatively, minute ventilation was adjusted to cope with rising end-tidal CO_2. There were no major pH shifts and no postoperative problems with subcutaneous emphysema. The patient ambulated and started a diet within 48 hours of surgery. Although he could have been discharged in 72 hours, he was observed for an additional day. This was now more in line with the recovery expected for MIS procedures.

The surgical time remained lengthy, but it should be evaluated in light of learning curve issues. Many of the early applications of laparoscopy to gastrointestinal procedures were commonly several hours long. Technology and experience improved the reproducibility and ability to do laborious tasks in shorter times. Patient disease and morphology will also affect overall operative times as well. Surgery times are difficult to compare overall due to many variables and lack of documentation in the literature. However, for the application of laparoscopy to be successful in the reproduction of aortobifemoral or iliofemoral bypass grafting, further improvement and evolution of what has been learned would be necessary. Surgical times would need to improve and attention applied to the technology and instrumentation that would not only improve operating times, but also contribute to the reproducibility of the procedure.

In review of the first cases, more isolated procedures such as iliofemoral bypass lent themselves to rapid extraperitoneal dissections under insufflation. With the larger exposures and spaces needed for aortic exposure and control, insufflation appeared to work better. However, pneumoretroperitoneum created three problems. First, with the larger space, there is more peritoneum that can be violated and allow for intraperitoneal leak and collapse of the retroperitoneal working space. Second, with time it was noted that there would be competitive insufflation of the peritoneal cavity across thinned out areas of the peritoneum. The most susceptible area for this was the anterior portion of the peritoneum. Even without violation of the peritoneal lining, we would experience competitive insufflation and a gradual decrease of the retroperitoneal working space. The third problem was that the volume of the retroperitoneal working cavity was small and very sensitive to suctioning. These difficulties were significant and dealing with

them accounted for a large part of the operative time. There would need to be solutions to these challenges to improve on time, reproducibility, and patient safety.

A potential problem area based on our laboratory experience included concerns over the size of the aorta. However, the larger human aorta (a 16-mm-diameter prosthesis being utilized) had proven technically easier to work with because of this larger size, which facilitates many of the maneuvers utilized in laparoscopic suturing in a confined space such as the retroperitoneum. The human iliac artery was more accurately approximated by the porcine aorta, allowing for an adequate re-creation of operating on the actual iliac vessel. The tactile feedback critical to a surgeon working with instruments is just as palpable with the laparoscopic tools as it is with open tools. Assessment of the calcified plaque with the needle tip to determine how and where to place the graft was comparable between open and laparoscopic needle-drivers.

TECHNIQUE

These experiences were taken back to the laboratory to evaluate how the difficulties in exposure might be solved. The solution lay in working with the vulnerable area of anterior peritoneum rather than avoiding it. By incising this area anteriorly under the left rectus sheath, a peritoneal "apron"[25] could be constructed. This could be suspended with transabdominal sutures towards the right of the abdomen. This served several purposes. There was no longer concern regarding a leak in the peritoneal lining. It eliminated problems between the two compartments and avoided competitive insufflation and collapse of the retroperitoneum. It allowed the entire volume of the peritoneal cavity to be insufflated, creating a larger work space. The field was now stable despite aggressive suctioning, when modern 20 to 30 L/min insufflators were used. It also succeeded in view of the primary reason for the retroperitoneal approach, that of containment of abdominal viscera.

General anesthesia is induced with hemodynamic monitoring as necessary. Patients are placed supine with a padded gel roll under the patient's left flank to elevate it and provide for adequate access to the lateral abdominal wall. The patient is then prepped and draped in the usual standard fashion to expose the entire abdomen and groins. A 10-mm trocar is then introduced at the umbilicus after a CO_2 pneumoperitoneum is instituted to an intraperitoneal pressure of 14 mm Hg. The abdominal cavity is then inspected in the routine fashion. The second and third trocars are then inserted under direct vision into the peritoneal cavity. The table is then tilted to the right with a 10° to 20° Trendelenburg position.

A muscle splitting 1.5 cm opening, located 1.5 cm both medial and superior to the anterior-superior iliac crest, is made through the various layers of the lateral abdominal wall to identify the preperitoneal space. A small retroperitoneal space is created directed at the psoas muscle with gentle blunt dissection with the index finger. The left iliac artery is commonly palpated and is a useful landmark. Retroperitoneal dissection is then begun at the site of the fourth trocar. The retroperitoneal space is now insufflated after insertion of a 12-mm trocar into the previously dissected opening to the retroperitoneum. By utilization of the pneumoretroperitoneum and gentle blunt scope dissection with a zero-degree laparoscope, to gently dissect the now crepitant retroperitoneal areolar tissue, a very large hemostatic retroperitoneal space can be rapidly created. It is best to find the left external iliac artery and follow it up to the common iliac artery and ureter, leaving the ureter on top of the psoas muscle. As this continues medially, the aorta is commonly seen pulsating, surrounded by its retroperitoneal connective layers. Blunt dissection is finally carried cephalad and laterally under the lateral aspect of Gerota's fascia to mobilize the kidney.

The creation of the apron begins approximately 3 cm above the left internal inguinal ring. The midline ports are used to place the laparoscope with a grasping forceps and laparoscopic scissors. The appropriate line of incision of the peritoneum is just under, or lateral to, the lateral edge of the rectus abdominis muscle. The cephalad extent of the dissection is to ~6 cm above the costal margin. Dissection in the correct plane between the peritoneum and the posterior fascia will proceed quickly and hemostatically. The cut edge of the peritoneum is mobilized to connect the intraperitoneal cavity with the previous retroperitoneal dissection. Once the peritoneum has been freed from its lateral attachments, the fifth and sixth trocars are inserted. This peritoneal apron will be used as the internal retractor of the intestines.

In order to function as a retractor, the peritoneal apron must now be suspended at its incised upper edge at the three sites corresponding to the three midline trocars. A suture of 0 nylon on a straight needle is placed through and through the abdominal wall behind each of the midline trocars. This needle is grasped using the lateral trocar sites and sutured through the cut edge of the peritoneum before being passed back through the abdominal wall. This creates a suspension suture that will suspend the peritoneal apron behind each midline trocar. The resulting compartmentalization of the peritoneal cavity creates a larger working space. This eliminates the threat of competitive insufflation as the spaces are connected. The larger volume of insufflated CO_2 will allow the more aggressive use of suction if necessary, without a compromise in the working space. Most importantly, it removes any concerns regarding retraction of the intestines, as they are securely and gently held back in their own natural environment without manipulation.

Retraction is provided by the upper two midline trocars. Fan retractors are placed behind the apron to support the bulk of the intestinal contents. An external retractor holder secures them to the operating table. The upper retractor brings the kidney cephalad and the lower retractor maintains the bulk of the intestines off of the aorta. The surgeon will work from the patient's left side via ports four, five, and six, while the assistant will work from the inferior midline third trocar to provide suction, additional retraction, or to assist in completion of the anastomosis. Dissection begins by identifying the left common iliac artery and ureter and proceeding to identify the aortic bifurcation and the right common iliac artery. Dissection continues up the aorta to the inferior mesenteric artery. Division of the inferior mesenteric artery, if occluded, will facilitate further exposure. If it is patent or if there is a question regarding dividing it, leaving it intact will not compromise the exposure. It is divided or left intact based on the usual indications.

Dissection is continued cephalad to expose the remaining infrarenal aorta and the left renal vein. Care must be taken to not injure the left gonadal vein where it joins the left renal vein. In the process of dissecting the aorta, it is also important to identify retroaortic renal veins and other venous anomalies as it is in the standard open exposure. The proximal site of aortic cross-clamping is carefully dissected, inspected, and palpated to evaluate for calcification. It has proven useful to obtain preoperative CT scans

to evaluate for venous anomalies and aortic calcifications. Posterior dissection is completed to identify the lumbar arteries. The final seventh trocar, which is for the aortic cross-clamp, is inserted in its transrectus position for end-to-end anastomosis. In the case of an end-to-side anastomosis, a laparoscopic Satinsky clamp is inserted through the lower abdominal wall by puncturing it with a 10-mm trocar. This allows the direct insertion of the laparoscopic Satinsky clamp through the abdominal wall without CO_2 leakage.

This left anterolateral approach provides excellent visualization of the posterior aorta allowing the lumbar arteries to be clipped and/or divided as necessary to mobilize the aorta for the site of anastomosis. Generally, no more than one or two pairs require clipping and/or division. The preoperative arteriogram is also useful in predicting the site and number of lumbar arteries to contend with. It is important to be certain that the vena cava is neither injured when the aorta is transected nor interfered with during the anastomosis. Also, during the posterior dissection for the lumbar arteries, one must take care to identify lumbar veins, which may be torn or injured if unrecognized. These maneuvers are particularly important for an end-to-end anastomosis. In the case of an end-to-side anastomosis, only satisfactory mobilization of the right side of the aorta is necessary to place a Satinsky clamp on the aorta. Posterior control of the lumbar arteries is not necessary for end-to-side anastomosis.

Groin incisions are now made bilaterally to perform a conventional dissection of the femoral vessels. Upon completion of the groin dissection, the aorta is sized and the appropriately-sized conventional bifurcated vascular graft (Hemashield™, Meadox Medical, Oakland, NJ) is selected. The aortic graft is readily introduced into the abdomen through a lateral trocar. Large blunt dissection maneuvers under the inguinal ligament to tunnel into the retroperitoneum must be avoided. These maneuvers may result in bleeding or leakage of the pneumoperitoneum through an excessively patulous tunnel. A malleable grasper with a blunt tip (Karl Storz Endoscopy of America, Culver City, CA) is designed to tunnel easily and atraumatically. Laparoscopically the limbs of the grafts are carefully oriented and care taken to avoid any rotation as they are delivered into the groins. The limbs are clamped after they are tunneled to prevent leakage of the pneumoperitoneum. The right limb of the graft is tunneled first. The graft is completely positioned as described before aortic occlusion in order to limit cross-clamp time. The patient is then systemically heparinized.

The aorta is cross-clamped with a laparoscopic DeBakey clamp (Karl Storz Endoscopy of America, Culver City, CA) inserted through the seventh trocar. In the case of an end-to-end anastomosis, the previously mobilized aorta above the inferior mesenteric artery is transected with a laparoscopic Endo-GIA 30 stapler (Tyco-U.S. Surgical, Norwalk, CT). The aorta is then transected at a suitable location ~1.5 cm below the aortic cross-clamp. The transected aorta is evaluated for plaque and thrombus directly. Appropriate instrumentation in the form of DeBakey style grasping forceps and endarterectomy instruments (Karl Storz Endoscopy of America, Culver City, CA) enable endarterectomy of the aortic cuff as necessary. Because we now have the appropriate instrumentation available, we approach the proximal cuff as we do in open surgery in order to prepare it for the best possible anastomosis. In the case of an end-to-side anastomosis, transection of the aorta is not done. The laparoscopic Satinsky clamp is placed from below and an aortotomy is then made with a laparoscopic scalpel and laparoscopic Potts scissors (Karl Storz Endoscopy of America, Culver City, CA).

Anastomosis is now completed with two running 3-0 polypropylene sutures. This is done using intracorporeal laparoscopic suturing technique. The first suture is started posteriorly at the seven o'clock position and run up the right side of the anastomosis. Once the anastomosis is half completed, the second suture is placed adjacent to the previous posterior suture. It is now run across the remaining back wall and around the left side of the anastomosis and across the anterior portion. The two sutures are tied anteriorly. Conventional flushing techniques are used both after the aortic anastomosis is complete and upon completion of the distal anastomosis to the femoral arteries

Once satisfactory hemostasis is identified throughout, the peritoneal apron sutures are removed and the peritoneum is allowed to fall back into place. As the pneumoperitoneum is released the peritoneum comes back to lie in its normal position and completely covers the prosthetic graft material. Trocar sites are either closed with a one layer of 0 polyglactin or with through-and-through strands of 0 polyglactin placed with an EndoClose™ (Tyco-U.S. Surgical, Norwalk, CT) device. The groin incisions are closed in the conventional manner.

RESULTS

Sixteen patients have undergone totally laparoscopic aortobifemoral bypass since June 1995. From March 1996 to May 1998, a total of 14 patients (11 men and 3 women, 42 to 76 years of age, mean = 58 years) were operated on with the apron technique. The first three cases with this technique were reported[25] and an additional seven cases, all completed with end-to-end anastomoses, were also reported.[26] Indications for surgery in all cases were incapacitating claudication (ABI <0.60) with aortoiliac occlusive disease. The total 14 patients had a completely laparoscopic aortobifemoral bypass with 10 end-to-end anastomoses and 4 end-to-side anastomoses. Improvement in overall surgical times continued, with a range of 245 to 510 minutes (average = 367). Mean aortic cross-clamp time was 111 minutes (range = 65 to 189). Cross-clamp times also varied depending on whether additional reconstruction was required at the femoral or profunda femoris vessels. Aortic anastomotic times ranged from 22 to 155 minutes (mean = 65). All anastomoses were completed with intracorporeal laparoscopic suturing using continuous running monofilament suture. The average amount of fluid administered was 6482 mL (range = 4000 to 8500).

Intraoperative complications occurred in four patients with three requiring conversion. Intraoperative conversions was never hurriedly performed for a life-threatening situation. In two of these three patients, they occurred for anastomotic difficulties related to heavily calcified atheromata at the proximal aorta. The first female developed a disruption of a calcified plaque by the aortic clamp, which led to graft occlusion immediately after unclamping. A minilaparotomy of 4 to 5 cm was performed to explore the anastomosis and endarterectomize the site of cross-clamping and; the anastomosis had to be redone. Small renal vein retractors could be inserted behind the retroperitoneal apron to readily expose the infrarenal anastomotic area without interference or difficulties in bowel retraction. The second conversion was necessary in a patient in whom the anastomosis was redone after having to

endarterectomize the proximal aortic cuff. This was accomplished laparoscopically. However, it was felt that due to lack of prior experience with laparoscopic endarterectomy, it would be best to cautiously inspect the anastomosis. Although the utilization of the apron allowed for excellent exposure in this case as well, cross-clamp time was 189 minutes (the longest of all patients). The final conversion was due to trauma to the graft during insertion, which resulted in two holes in the graft which were not recognized until the anastomosis was flushed. It was elected to replace it. This was done via the same technique as the previous conversions, by using the apron for containment of the intestines for a true 4- to 5-cm incision to replace the graft. The limbs of the new graft were tied to the cut limbs of the old graft, allowing them to be pulled into correct position via the small 4- to 5-cm incision. This resulted in a cross-clamp time of 179 minutes.

Conversions in these cases certainly affect the overall times of surgery and cross-clamping. However, only the second patient (cross-clamp time of 189 minutes) experienced any difficulty from this, developing a mild compartment syndrome of the right leg, which did not require intervention. It should be noted that as a result of growing experience in handling proximal aortic disease, along with custom-built instrumentation to handle the vessel wall and atheromata, overall times have consistently improved and should continue to approximate that of open surgery.

Bleeding difficulties occurred in two cases. The patient with injury to the graft requiring replacement also had a retroaortic left renal vein, which was not recognized on preoperative CT scan. Blood loss (3050 mL) was the highest in this group of patients. He did develop thrombosis of the left renal vein and an edematous left kidney, which had recovered upon follow-up duplex ultrasonography 6 weeks later. A second patient had lost ~2000 mL due to postoperative bleeding from a trocar injury to the superior epigastric artery.

The most serious postoperative complication occurred in a male patient who required reoperation for an acute false aneurysm of the aortic anastomosis. This was identified as having eroded into the left ureter. He presented via the emergency room 2 weeks after surgery with hematuria and renal colic. Evaluation identified an anastomotic aneurysm and angiography revealed an aortoureteral fistula. At laparotomy the apron was noted to have regained its original position, covering the graft completely. The origin of the false aneurysm measured only 2 mm and was located proximal to the actual anastomosis. It was concluded that the sutures from the laparoscopically-constructed anastomosis were placed too closely and may have torn or caused necrosis of a portion of the aortic wall. This was repaired by excision of the old anastomosis and revision with a short interposition piece of graft. The ureter was repaired by a urologist over a J wire with healthy edges of ureter. CT scan at 1 month and ultrasonography at 6 months were normal.

The mean postoperative hospital stay was 7 days (range = 4 to 23). Patients with uncomplicated aortobifemoral bypasses were discharged between the fourth and eighth days. The oldest patient was discharged on the seventh day while a younger patient with a mitral valve prosthesis was not discharged until the eighth day due to the need to regulate her anticoagulant therapy for her cardiac prosthesis. The patient staying 23 days was mostly to follow the status of his edematous left kidney. This was done in the hospital rather than as an outpatient due to a distance of his home from the hospital of greater than 300 miles.

The key to the successful completion of the bypass was in the careful creation of the retroperitoneal cavity, aided by the apron. This allowed for the necessary exposure to have adequate room to work. Most of the operative time involved in the earliest cases was spent primarily in the careful creation of the retroperitoneal cavity. In contrast, the aortic anastomosis was generally completed within 50 to 60 minutes, having been facilitated by the excellent exposure made possible by the apron. The remaining improvement in decreasing surgical time was due to: (1) overall increased familiarity with the retroperitoneal anatomy as seen laparoscopically, (2) improved surgical instrumentation to accomplish vascular-specific tasks, and (3) increasing familiarity and confidence that the same techniques used to deal with atheromatous plaque in open surgery also applied in the laparoscopic approach. The time required to establish the retroperitoneal work space and complete the dissection had decreased from over 4 to 5 hours to less than 2 hours

This series of patients demonstrates that laparoscopic aorto-bifemoral bypass is feasible. As with open surgery, both types of anastomotic methods should be possible depending on the clinical needs of the patient and surgeon preference. Operative times and parameters have continued to improve. The duration of the procedures is now is comparable to that of some other procedures (e.g., laparoscopically-assisted colectomy), and shorter than other laparoscopic procedures, such as esophagectomies

ABDOMINAL AORTIC ANEURYSMS

The gold standard for aortic aneurysm repair was described by Creech in 1966 with the technique of endo-aneurysmorrhaphy.[27] Until that time, mortality rates had remained high. Continued improvements in modern anesthetic techniques and critical care have continued to contribute to the decreased mortality rates of 2 to 4%.[28] The surgical approach to infrarenal aortic aneurysm requires a long xiphopubic incision, which is associated with considerable postoperative pain. The surgical treatment for abdominal aortic aneurysm involves the placement of a prosthetic graft in the involved area. Postoperative care requires a critical care stay, which adds cost and an additional 5 to 10 days in the hospital. MIS techniques used with other abdominal laparoscopic procedures may give similar advantages to patients if applied to aortic aneurysm repair. The challenges to the successful application of MIS techniques to aneurysms are significant. Despite these challenges, efforts have been made to pursue this goal.

The earliest work on laparoscopic aortic aneurysm repair was reported by Chen et al.[29] In these experiments, there were 15 successful graft insertions in 21 pigs undergoing transabdominal dissection of the aorta. Six were unsuccessful because of technical, anatomic, or bleeding difficulties. A retroperitoneal approach was attempted in two cases, but only one was successful due to a tear in the peritoneum of the other. There were other complications noted, including injuries to the bladder, ureter, renal vein, inferior vena cava, aorta, and lumbar vessel. Operative time decreased from 6 to less than 2 hours with a concomitant decrease in estimated blood loss from 1000 mL to less than 150 mL with increased experience. Chen and coworkers secured endoluminal grafts with extraluminal umbilical tapes after insertion by aortotomy. In the experience of the authors[19] we attempted to reproduce the endo-aneurysmhorrhaphy technique of suturing a graft in place with an intact back wall. Lumbar vessels were controlled intraluminally

as well as extraluminally. In these attempts to develop MIS techniques to approach an aneurysm, one must recognize the limitation of the animal models (i.e., the lack of an aneurysmal mass or calcification in the wall). Without this mass, the dissection is simpler and without the calcification there is no risk of distal embolization.

The result of the work of Chen et al[30] has been the successful completion of laparoscopic-assisted repair of infrarenal abdominal aortic aneurysm in humans. An asymptomatic 6-cm abdominal aortic aneurysm in a 62-year-old male was successfully repaired. This first case was performed with 10 trocars and a 10-cm mini-laparotomy. The approach was transabdominal and bowel retraction was facilitated by a modified "fish" retractor for the special task. Total operative time was 4 hours and estimated blood loss was 1000 mL. Decreased operative fluid requirement with early mobilization of fluids was observed. A more rapid return of bowel function with an earlier discharge on postoperative day 6 was reported. Kline and coworkers[31] have since simplified the approach, reducing the number of trocars and the operative times. This and the work of others contributes to determining the feasibility of performing laparoscopic aortic surgery, whether totally laparoscopic or laparoscopic-assisted. Recent studies[32,33] confirmed that laparoscopic abdominal aortic aneurysm repair is a feasible technique. They also suggest that the benefits of laparoscopy seen in general surgery could be translated to abdominal aortic aneurysm repair.

Percutaneous placement of endoluminal stent-grafts is directed at avoiding the morbidity and mortality associated with major abdominal surgery. Despite the technical success achieved in the majority of cases, endovascular grafts require great skill for implantation[34] and are subject to complications themselves. May et al[35] report in a phase 1 trial, a vascular complication rate of 10% for a tube graft, which rises to 43% for a bifurcated endovascular graft. In another phase 1 trial with 46 patients, Moore and Rutherford[36] reported contrast enhancement outside the graft but within the aneurysmal sac in 17 grafts (44%), of which 9 (51%) resolved spontaneously. Hospital stay varied between 1 and 14 days.[35,36] Uncontrolled lumbar vessels and endo-leaks have raised concern over continued aneurysmal growth and risk of rupture.

Continued technological improvements and increasing clinical experience with endoluminal graft placement have provided improved results with endoluminal stent grafts. Recent FDA approval for use of endoluminal devices in the United States has also changed the landscape for minimally invasive aortic aneurysm repair. The subsequent numbers of patients undergoing repairs with endo-prostheses will steadily rise, providing more data for follow-up on these patients. An interesting approach to the treatment of abdominal aortic aneurysm may be to combine laparoscopic and endovascular techniques. This may help in solving many of the challenging problems encountered during the performance of one of these two described techniques.

We have initiated work in the laboratory to begin to explore this possibility. The application of the "apron" approach for a totally laparoscopic repair of an infrarenal aortic aneurysm was reported by the authors.[37] A 67-year-old female with rest pain in the right leg (ABI .35 on the right and .65 on the left) was operated on. Angiography demonstrated an occlusion of the right common and external iliac arteries. The CT scan revealed a moderately calcified aorta and a 4.6 cm infrarenal abdominal aortic aneurysm with mural thrombus. A totally laparoscopic aortobifemoral bypass and abdominal aortic aneurysm resection was completed. Surgery lasted 230 minutes with an aortic cross-clamp time of 76 minutes and the aortic anastomosis requiring 22 minutes to complete. Intraoperatively the patient received a total of 4500 mL of crystalloid. No intraoperative transfusion was required with a blood loss of 450 mL. Postoperatively the patient recovered with no complications and was discharged home on the seventh postoperative day. As laparoscopic instrumentation and experience improves and grows, totally laparoscopic abdominal aortic aneurysm repair could be offered in selected patients.

CONCLUSIONS

The authors feel that laparoscopic aortic surgery is now feasible. It has been developed in the laboratory,[12,19,21–24] and performed on a few well-selected patients.[25,26,36] The totally laparoscopic approach to the aortoiliac segment in our experience and evaluation remains more appealing than a laparoscopic-assisted method utilizing an 8- to 10-cm incision or a purely mini-laparotomy approach.[38]

The development of minimal access vascular aortoiliac surgery must follow accepted rules.[39] In order to promote the further development, safety, efficacy, reproducibility, and ability to teach the procedures, many areas require improvement. Thus far, it has been safely performed with primarily "off the shelf" instrumentation. This has included conventional open and laparoscopic instrumentation. Recently, dedicated and custom-built prototype laparoscopic vascular instrumentation (Karl Storz Endoscopy, Culver City, CA) has become available to the authors and has greatly aided in the safe completion of the most recent procedures, also enabling shorter surgery times. For further application of laparoscopy to aortoiliac surgery, additional developments are necessary and are clearly on the way. The instrument design is critical. Not only will standard vascular instruments need to be adapted to work laparoscopically, but also new technology and concepts will be required. An example would be in the area of occlusion devices, where they should be designed to work extracorporeally or intracorporeally. Finally, the anastomosis will require instrumentation that will allow the consistent construction of a safe and durable anastomosis. A number of technologies are under evaluation for this express purpose. One can certainly envision an automated anastomotic device. Stapling technology has certainly revolutionized the way in which gastrointestinal anastomoses are performed.

Vascular surgeons have a wide range of exposure and experience in laparoscopy, from none to extensive, for those who also do laparoscopic gastrointestinal surgery. Over the next several years, experience should be more uniform as many of tomorrow's vascular surgeons come from training programs with laparoscopic training and experience. As for venous disease, other procedures are exposing more vascular surgeons to nonendoluminal minimally invasive techniques, skills, and instrumentation. Increasing development of anterior spinal fusion using laparoscopic technique requires an increasing need for the vascular surgeon to provide anterior exposure so the orthopedist may acquire laparoscopic knowledge, experience, and skills. With growing understanding of the importance of the need for increased skills and experience in laparoscopy, the ability to perform laparoscopic suturing will become more prevalent.

Laparoscopic vascular surgery of the infrarenal aortoiliac segment holds many potential benefits for the patient. In occlusive disease, it differs only by the approach (laparoscopic vs. open), therefore the long-term results are expected to be similar. Performing laparoscopic surgery for occlusive disease is currently easier than attempting to treat abdominal aortic aneurysms completely laparoscopically. The role of laparoscopy in the ultimate treatment of aortic aneurysm requires further definition and investigation, and will depend on the continued interest in and the fate of endoluminal stent grafts. Ongoing experience supports the continued investigation and development of these techniques with laparoscopic aortoiliac surgery clearly in the feasibility stage. Controlled multicenter feasibility studies including preceptorship are presently being conducted to evaluate the reproducibility of the technique. This approach is ethical and workable for new surgical procedures.

REFERENCES

1. Bergan J, Murray J, Greason K. Subfascial endoscopic perforator vein surgery: a preliminary report. *Ann Vasc Surg.* 1996;10:211.
2. Périssat J, Collet D, Belliard R. Traitement laparoscopique par lithotripsie intra-corporelle suivi de cholécystostomie ou de cholécystectomie. *Chirurgie* 1990;116:243.
3. Peters JH, Ortega A, Lehnerd SL, et al. The physiology of laparoscopic surgery: pulmonary function after laparoscopic cholecystectomy. *Surg Laparosc Endosc.* 1993;3:370.
4. Poulin EC, Mamazza J, Breton G, et al. Evaluation of pulmonary function in laparoscopic cholecystectomy. *Surg Laparosc Endosc.* 1993;2: 292.
5. Svenberg T. Pathophysiology of pneumoperitoneum. In: Ballantyne GH, Leahy PF, Modlin IM, eds. *Laparoscopic Surgery.* W.B. Saunders:1994;61.
6. Brewster DC. Current controversies in the management of aortoiliac occlusive disease. *J Vasc Surg.* 1997;25:365.
7. Marin M, Veith F, Cynamon J. Transfemoral endovascular stented graft treatment of aortoiliac and femoropopliteal occlusive disease for limb salvage. *Am J Surg.* 1994;168:156.
8. Veith F, Gupta S, Wengerter K, et al. Changing arteriosclerotic disease patterns and management strategies in lower-limb-threatening ischemia. *Ann Surg.* 1990;212:402.
9. Dion YM, Katkhouda N, Rouleau C, et al. Laparoscopy-assisted aortobifemoral bypass. *Surg Laparosc Endosc.* 1993;3:425.
10. Dion YM, Rouleau C, Aucoin A. Laparoscopy-assisted aortobifemoral bypass. *Surg Endosc.* 1994;8:438.
11. Berens E, Herde JR: Laparoscopic vascular surgery: four case reports. *J Vasc Surg.* 1995;22:73.
12. Dion YM, Chin AK, Thompson TA. Experimental laparoscopic aortobifemoral bypass. *Surg Endosc.* 1995;9:894.
13. Schumaker HB. Midline extraperitoneal exposure of the abdominal aorta and the iliac arteries. *Surg Gynecol Obstet.* 1972;135:791.
14. Jones DB, Thompson RW, Soper NJ, et al. Development and comparison of transperitoneal and retroperitoneal approaches to laparoscopic-assisted aortofemoral bypass in a porcine model. *J Vasc Surg.* 1996;23:466.
15. Chui PT, Gin T, Oh TE. Anaesthesia for laparoscopic general surgery. *Anaesth Intensive Care.* 1993;21:163.
16. McQuaide JR. Air embolism during peritoneoscopy. *S Afr Med J.* 1972;46:422.
17. Dion YM, Levesque C, Doillon CJ. Experimental carbon dioxide pulmonary embolization after vena cava laceration under pneumoperitoneum. *Surg Endosc.* 1995;9:1065.
18. De Plaizer RMH, Jones ISC. Non-fatal carbon dioxide embolism during laparoscopy. *Anaesth Intensive Care.* 1989;17:359.
19. Dion YM, Gracia CR. Experimental laparoscopic aortic aneurysm resection and aortobifemoral bypass. *Surg Laparosc Endosc.* 1996;6:184.

20. Fabiani JN, Mercier F, Carpentier A, et al. Video-assisted aortofemoral bypass: results in seven cases. *Ann Vasc Surg*. 1997;11:273.

21. Dion YM, Gaillard F, Demalsy JC, et al. Experimental laparoscopic aortobifemoral bypass for occlusive aortoiliac disease. *Can J Surg*. 1996;39:451.

22. Dion YM, Gracia CR, Demalsy JC, et al. Laparoscopic aortic surgery: animal and human clinical evaluation. *Minimally Invasive Therapy* 1995;4(Suppl. 1):40.

23. Dion YM, Gracia CR. A reproducible animal model for laparoscopic retroperitoneal aortobifemoral bypass in aortoiliac occlusive disease. *Surg Endosc*. 1996;10:270.

24. Dion YM, Gracia CR, Demalsy JC, et al. Laparoscopic and laparoscopy-assisted aortoiliac surgery: animal and clinical evaluation. *J Endovasc Surg*. 1996;3:114.

25. Dion YM, Gracia CR. A technique for laparoscopic aortobifemoral grafting in occlusive aortoiliac disease. *J Vasc Surg*. 1997;26:685.

26. Dion YM, Gracia CR, Estakhri ME, et al. Totally laparoscopic aortobifemoral bypass: a review of 10 patients. Accepted for publication. *Surg Laparosc Endosc*. 1998;8(3):165.

27. Creech Jr. O. Endo-aneurysmorrhaphy and treatment of aortic aneurysm. *Ann Surg*. 1966;164:936.

28. Cambria RP, Brewster DC, Abbott WM, et al. Transperitoneal vs. retroperitoneal approach for aortic reconstruction: a randomized prospective study. *J Vasc Surg*. 1990;11:314.

29. Chen HM, Murphy EA, Levison J, et al. Laparoscopic aortic replacement in the porcine model: a feasibility study in preparation for laparoscopically assisted abdominal aortic aneurysm repair in humans. *J Am Coll Surg*. 1996;183:126.

30. Chen HM, Murphy EA, Halpern V, et al. Laparoscopic-assisted abdominal aortic aneurysm repair. *Surg Endosc*. 1995;9:905.

31. Kline RG, D'Angelo AJ, Chen MH, et al. Laparoscopically assisted abdominal aortic aneurysm repair: first 20 cases. *J Vasc Surg*. 1998;27:81.

32. Jobe BA, Duncan W, Swanstrom LL. Totally laparoscopic abdominal aortic aneurysm repair. *Surg Endosc*. 1999;13:77.

33. Edoga JK, James KV, Resnikoff M, et al. Laparoscopic aortic aneurysm resection. *J Endovasc Surg*. 1998;5:335.

34. Veith FJ, Marin ML. Endovascular surgery and its effect on the relationship between vascular surgery and radiology. *J Endovasc Surg*. 1995;2:1.

35. May J, White JH, Yu W, et al. Results of endoluminal grafting of abdominal aortic aneurysms are dependent on aneurysm morphology. Ann Vasc Surg 1996;10:254–261.

36. Moore WS, Rutherford RB. Transfemoral endovascular repair of abdominal aortic aneurysm: results of the North American EVT phase 1 trial. *J Vasc Surg*. 1996;23:543.

37. Dion YM, Gracia CR, Demalcy JC. Laparoscopic aortic surgery. *J Vasc Surg*. 1995;23:539.

38. Weber G, Jako GJ. Retroperitoneal "mini" approach for aortoiliac reconstructive surgery. *Vasc Surg*. 1995;29:387.

39. Schrock TR: The endosurgery evolution: no place for sacred cows. *Surg Endosc*. 1992;6:163.

Chapter Eighty-Three ▪ ▪ ▪ ▪ ▪ ▪ ▪

*H*arvesting of Saphenous Vein for Bypass Using Minimally Invasive Surgery

JESÚS MERELLO-GODINO

INTRODUCTION

The extraction of a saphenous vein is a procedure necessary to perform a coronary bypass, whether associated with use of the internal mammary artery or not. Normally a large incision from the groin to the malleolus is required, although it can be done through discontiguous incisions.

To avoid these large incisions, three minimally invasive systems to reduce the problems that arise from conventional surgery have been developed; they employ retraction systems combined with endoscopic elements, or use completely endoscopic systems to extract the saphenous vein.[1]

In light of the results of saphenous vein extraction using conventional methods, and in the search for the advantages that minimally invasive systems can provide, we must first ask if the extraction of the vein by endoscopic methods is possible, evaluate the advantages and disadvantages of the procedure, and prove that veins harvested by this means are in good condition and useful for coronary bypass, as well as evaluate whether the surgical time and cost justify this approach.

HISTORICAL BACKGROUND

In 1984 the first minimally invasive system, the subcutaneous vein extractor, was presented. It could only be used in the thigh and was a blind and traumatic system that caused frequent hemorrhagic complications because the tributary veins were not ligated. In the late 1980s, with the development of new endoscopic techniques beginning with cholecystectomy and followed by other procedures, vascular surgery saw great advances as well, with application of endoscopic technique to ligation of incompetent veins in the leg (Linton's technique) and to perform aortofemoral bypass surgery. Each of the three systems for the extraction of saphenous veins discussed here has its own particular characteristics.

The Mini Harvest System is a procedure that reduces the incisions in the leg to three or four, and does not employ endoscopy. Through small incisions and using the retraction system with the aid of fiberoptic light, the saphenous vein is isolated, and the tributary veins are ligated using standard open techniques. A small tunnel is then made using digital subcutaneous dissection, maintaining the space open with the retraction system until the saphenous vein can be completely removed.

The Endopath Subcu-Dissector and Subcu-Retractor are employed in conjunction with an endoscopic system, including an endoscope, endo-camera, endoscopic instruments, and a monitor. Dissection of the anterior wall is accomplished by direct endoscopic vision, then the tributaries are ligated and the vein is exposed in its entire circumference to allow its extraction to complete the procedure. This method requires some endoscopic experience to accomplish, but it is not an entirely endoscopic procedure.

The Vasoview system, which is a completely endoscopic system, uses a 5-mm transparent dissector with a conical tip which allows visualization of the operative field, and has a balloon which is filled to create a space to isolate the saphenous vein, ligate the tributaries, and extract the vein. It requires a complete endoscopic system with a CO_2 insufflator. The gas distends the space made by the Vasoview, exposing the entire circumference of the vein, leaving it suspended only by small fibrous bands. The procedure is performed with endoscopic video control in a closed system and requires smaller incisions; however, the subcutaneous space created is sufficient due to the dissection and the gas insufflation.

All of these systems allow extraction of the saphenous vein in a condition suitable for coronary bypass. The least invasive system, which requires smaller incisions and provides total control of the vein while extracting it, is the Vasoview system. This system does, however, require endoscopic training.

SURGICAL TECHNIQUE

With the patient in the supine position with a slight external rotation, a 1-cm incision is made above the knee, and dissection is done until the saphenous vein is identified (Fig. 83–1), as for conventional surgery. A tunnel is then made by blunt dissection over

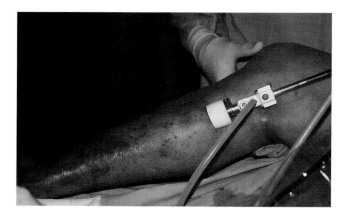

Figure 83–1. The Vasoview is inserted through a 1-cm incision to create the tunnel. The tip and balloon can be seen by transillumination.

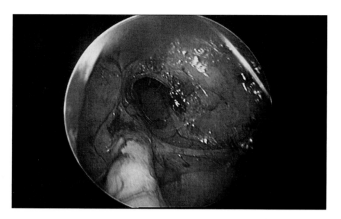

Figure 83–3. Once the CO_2 is insufflated, the tunnel distends and the saphenous vein is seen suspended from fibrous elements and tributaries. See Color Section.

the vein for the Vasoview. This instrument has a transparent conical tip with an inflatable balloon behind it that provides a clear image up to 1 cm in front of the tip with a 5-mm endoscope. The instrument is placed over the anterior wall of the saphenous vein, which under endoscopic vision has a pearly white color. The instrument is slowly advanced cephalically in small movements of less than 2 cm, inflating the balloon to create the tunnel (Fig. 83–2). The vein will always be below the instrument (between 4 and 8 o'clock). The tributary veins encountered should be avoided once the space is completely dissected. The Vasoview is removed, and a 10-mm trocar is placed, sealing the incision with a balloon. CO_2 insufflation to a pressure of 12 mm Hg is performed, producing an effect similar to that produced in the retroperitoneal space. The gas diffuses and the saphenous vein is left suspended from its fibrous elements (Fig. 83–3). Now the saphenous vein can be completely detached by ligating the tributaries using an orbital dissector, which is inserted through the trocar along with a 10-mm endoscope. The dissector has a **C**-shaped rod at its end, which is slid along the entire length of the vein, liberating it from its fibrous elements and avoiding the tributaries (Fig. 83–4). Another 5-mm trocar is placed laterally, to allow insertion of coagulators, staplers, and scissors (Fig. 83–5), which are used to ligate and section the tributaries.

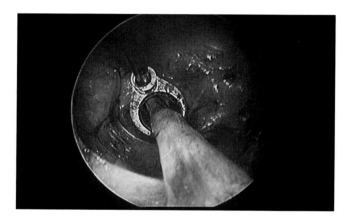

Figure 83–4. The saphenous vein is completely detached from its tributaries with the orbital dissector. See Color Section.

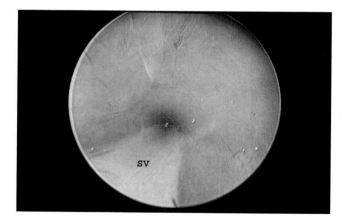

Figure 83–2. The saphenous vein is identified with a 5-mm endoscope through the Vasoview, and the balloon is inflated every 2 cm over it to create the tunnel. See Color Section.

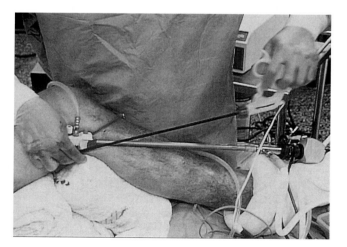

Figure 83–5. External view. Under endoscopic vision a 5-mm trocar is placed to allow the bipolar scissors to be inserted.

Another small incision is made in the groin to identify the proximal end of the saphenous vein and ligate it, allowing extraction through the incision near the knee. The procedure is repeated caudally, making another incision near the malleolus and extracting the rest of the saphenous vein.

DISCUSSION

One reason to consider using endoscopy to extract the vein is the fact that the conventional method has a high complication rate (between 1 and 15%), owing mainly to the large incision or to multiple small incisions made from the groin to the ankle, which cause pain, erythema, edema, cutaneous necrosis, induration, hematoma, infection, and wound dehiscence. It is common for coronary bypass patients to have complications of saphenous harvesting as their only postoperative problem. If we also consider additional complications such as diabetes, obesity, other vascular diseases, and skin diseases, we can affirm that these new techniques can improve the outcome.[2–8]

An obvious benefit of reducing the number and size of the incisions is that there is less postoperative pain, as is the case for all minimally invasive procedures, allowing earlier ambulation and avoiding the complications mentioned above, which in turn also reduces length of hospital stay and cost.

The extracted vein is in suitable condition for use for a bypass, because throughout the procedure the vein is in view of the surgeon, and the ligature of the collaterals and the coagulation of the tributaries is done at a safe distance from the vein.

As for any new surgical technique, especially an endoscopic one, one must consider the operative time of the procedure. Also a new procedure requires overcoming a learning curve, which initially means increased surgical time, but once experience is gained the time becomes reduced, approaching that needed for conventional surgery. It should also be kept in mind that though use of endoscopic technique increases the time needed to extract the vein, closing the wounds takes very little time, unlike the case for the large incisions required for conventional surgery.

The overall cost of the procedure is reduced if the hospital stay is reduced, and the rate of complications is lower than that of the large incision, although this is difficult to evaluate precisely.

This technique requires training in endoscopic surgery. General surgeons have steadily gained experience in this field in recent years, first in the laboratory, then by performing more complex procedures, so when a new technique is discovered, most surgeons should have little difficulty in adapting to it. In cardiovascular surgery there are no endoscopic techniques currently in use, so endoscopic saphenous vein harvesting has not become widespread and is still considered to be in the developmental phase. However, the results obtained thus far are quite satisfactory, so our mission as general surgeons is to support and collaborate with cardiovascular surgeons as they learn to use endoscopic techniques.[8] Today some groups utilize endoscopic techniques to harvest the saphenous vein for coronary bypass, as well as for saphenectomy required due to saphenous vein diseases.[9,10]

CONCLUSION

At the beginning of this chapter, the author pondered the necessity, advantages, disadvantages, cost, and benefit of this technique, and there is no doubt that the minimally invasive approach as applied to any surgical procedure is advantageous. The only difference between our technique and conventional technique is the reduced incisions needed to access the site of interest. This reduces pain and surgical trauma, and causes fewer inflammatory reactions. The complications inherent in the use of large incisions are avoided, and this is a great advantage, reducing the overall cost of the procedure and hospital stay. Due to the endoscopic training required, there is a learning curve that at first increases the duration of the procedure, but once this is overcome it appears that the operative time is comparable to that of a conventional procedure.

The author believes that these procedures are effective and their use will become more widespread, and their continued development will undoubtedly change surgeon attitudes towards minimally invasive surgery.

REFERENCES

1. Lee J. Minimally invasive vein harvesting. *Surg Physician Assistant.* 1996;Nov.–Dec.:25.
2. Farrington M, Webster M, Fenn A, et al. Study of cardiothoracic wound infection at St. Thomas Hospital. *Br J Surg.* 1985;72:759.
3. Baddour LM, Bisno AL. Recurrent cellulitis after saphenous venectomy for coronary bypass surgery. *Ann Intern Med.* 1982;97:493.
4. Baddour LM. Delayed soft tissue infections in saphenous venectomy limbs of coronary bypass patients. *Infect Surg.* 1985;1:243.
5. Reifsnyder T, Bandyk D, Seabrook G, et al. Wound complications of the in situ saphenous vein bypass technique. *Vasc Surg.* 1992;15:843.
6. Kent KC, Bartek S, Kuntz KM, et al. Prospective study of wound complications in continuous infrainguinal incisions after lower limb arterial reconstruction: Incidence, risk factors and cost. *Surgery* 1996;119:378.
7. Utley JR, Thomason ME, Wallace DJ, et al. Preoperative correlates of impaired wound healing after saphenous vein excision. *J Thorac Cardio Surg.* 1989;98:147.
8. Greenberg J, DeSanctis RW, Mills RM. Vein donor leg cellulitis after coronary artery bypass surgery. *Ann Intern Med.* 1982;97:565.
9. Personal communication. Charles Simonsz, Cape Town, South Africa.
10. Personal communication. Marco Vianni, Hospedale Abbiategraso, Milano, Italy.

Chapter Eighty-Four · · · · · · ·

*I*nterruption of Perforating Veins for Postphlebitic Syndrome Using Minimally Invasive Surgery

JESÚS MERELLO-GODINO

The development of minimally invasive techniques in general surgery, applied initially to cholecystectomy, opened up the possibility of its application to other procedures. Laparoscopic surgical instruments have been improved, new technology has been developed, and it has been used successfully to treat a number of diseases. In the beginning, the original surgical technique was reproduced as closely as possible, and then new techniques were devised.

Linton in 1938,[1] Cockett and Jones in 1955,[2] and Boyd in 1960[3] described the disease state that results from incompetent perforating veins in the leg, and each of them proposed different forms of surgical treatment. All of them include identifying the perforating veins, then ligating and cutting them. Later, Edward in 1976, Palma in 1979, and Hide-Lim in 1981 proposed new forms of therapy that were aimed at avoiding the problems described by most authors, notably the morbidity of these procedures due to the large incisions that are needed over sites with severe skin damage, and the difficult approaches required to avoid sites that would sustain serious scarring.

Incompetence of the perforating veins in the leg (Cockett's system) produces a typical picture in the lower extremities that is characterized by severe cutaneous ulcers, trophic skin changes, and dermatosclerosis contingent on the degree of vascular damage sustained. This is a common disease of the elderly, and it is not unusual to see situations in which the entire extremity is affected, complicated by the presence of other conditions such as diabetes, obesity, immunosuppression, and other vascular diseases.

The surgical approach to these lesions carries a high morbidity rate, which is related to the large incisions that are made in poorly vascularized tissue and ulcerous plaques that may produce serious scars, infection, and wound dehiscence.

Despite technological advances in diagnosis, especially Doppler which allows precise localization of the perforating veins, the surgical approach still requires large incisions over compromised sites, leading to ulcers, sclerosis, and edema, and forcing long hospital stays with close postoperative observation. This produces long recuperation times and long periods before return to everyday activities, and in the elderly can create infirmity so great that the patients are no longer able to take care of themselves.

New videoendoscopic techniques as applied to vascular surgery have created the need for new types of endoscopes (Fig. 84–1) and instruments designed specifically to perform these procedures with a minimally invasive approach. Hauer was the first to describe this new approach in 1987.[4]

The keys to successful treatment lie in making a small incision, away from the affected skin, and under endoscopic guidance to locate, isolate, ligate, and interrupt the incompetent perforating veins. This is done with the patient in the supine position in the classic position for a saphenectomy, with general or regional anesthesia. An incision is made in the groin to locate the saphenofemoral union, the collateral veins are ligated, and the saphenous vein is stripped down the thigh.

A tourniquet is placed over the knee to cut off blood flow. The endoscopic procedure is begun with a 1-cm incision on the anterior surface of the leg, about 2 cm behind the tibia, opening all the way to the sural fascia. Dissection is done digitally and caudally to make space to insert a 10-mm blunt tip trocar with a fixing balloon, which is inflated in the subfascial space. A zero degree 10-mm straight endoscope is inserted (Fig. 84–2) to perform the dissection of the subfascial space under visual control, and is connected to a CO_2 insufflator to create pressure of 15 to 20 mm Hg, which aids in dissecting the space and locating the veins. This step can be done using Hauer's instrument without CO_2, but the gas is of great help despite the small space its creates, leaving the vascular elements "hanging" from their fibrotic structural elements. The procedure can sometimes be done through an endoscope with

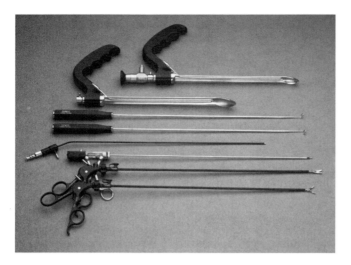

Figure 84–1. Instrumentation needed for the endoscopic approach to postphlebitic interruption of perforating veins.

a work channel, but we recommend making another 5-mm incision slightly more distally and posteriorly. The dissection of the subfascial space is sometimes difficult due to the presence of adhesions between the muscle and fascia, and may require scissors for removal. Once the veins have been identified, careful separation of them must be carried out, and then according to their caliber, clips are applied or they are cut, or bipolar coagulation is used if they are smaller than 2 mm. This should be done from the ankle to the knee to avoid accidentally moving a clip with the endoscope due to the small work space created. The distal zone near the malleolus is markedly difficult because the anatomy only allows a very small work space, and areas of dermatosclerosis and ulceration are common. Here it is recommended to remove the adhesions and fibrotic areas to allow the dermis to recover more quickly. Also in places where dermal induration is marked and distensibility reduced, fasciotomies can be performed under endoscopic vision, contributing to the success of the procedure. On average, three incompetent perforating veins can be interrupted. The procedure is completed by suturing the sural fascia in the first in-

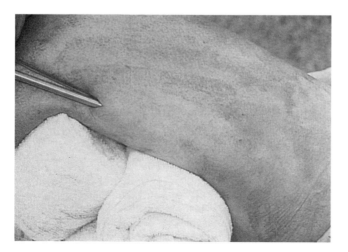

Figure 84–2. An endoscope is introduced into the work channel and used to identify the perforating veins. The work channel is seen by transillumination.

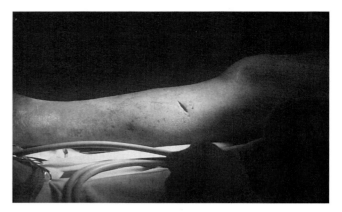

Figure 84–3. Final appearance of the leg after endoscopic interruption of perforating veins. See Color Section.

cision and applying a compressive bandage for the next few hours. This procedure can be done on an outpatient basis, but complete postsurgical bedrest is recommended. Over the next several days the ulcerated zones should undergo curettage until their complete resolution.

This endoscopic approach affords several advantages over the conventional method. First, the use of small incisions over unaffected skin helps ensure adequate closure of the wounds without infection (Fig. 84–3). Dehiscence only rarely affects the borders of the wounds, and edema and scarring are rare. This avoids one of the most severe complications of the procedure, namely wound necrosis, which is a cause of major morbidity. All of these factors foster faster recuperation, earlier mobilization of the lower extremities, and reduction of pain, factors that are especially important for the elderly patient who is at greatest risk.[5–7]

However, the approach does have some negative aspects that must be noted. The primary one is the learning time needed to adapt to the endoscopic technique, especially for vascular surgeons who have used endoscopic approaches for other procedures. The work space is very limited in spite of thorough exposure of the subfascial space, especially in the region near the malleolus. Handling the instruments is therefore difficult, and inadequate trocar placement will make the effort impossible. As with conventional surgery, the formation of a subfascial hematoma as well as damage to the tibial nerve are possible, but rare, complications.[8]

There are no advantages to using disposable materials for the extraction of the saphenous vein using minimally invasive technique. Space-creating systems that employ balloons are not useful either, because the space created disappears quickly due to tension of the muscle and sural fascia, even when CO_2 is used at high pressures.

In conclusion, it is clear that in spite of the short time the procedure has been in use, the short-term results are satisfying. This is encouraging many surgeons to use the minimally invasive approach for this disorder. The reduction in wound complications, morbidity, and long recuperation times makes the endoscopic approach an effective one, despite the technical expertise required to perform it successfully.

REFERENCES

1. Linton R. The communicating veins of the lower leg and the operative technique for their ligation. *Ann Surg.* 1938;107:582.

2. Cockett F, Jones B. The ankle blow-out syndrome; A new approach to the varicose ulcer problem. *Lancet* 1955;1:17.

3. Boyd AM. Treatment of varicose veins. *Proc R Soc Med.* 1961;41:633.

4. Hauer G, Borkun J, Wigger I, et al. Endoscopic subfascial dissection of perforating veins. *Surg Endosc.* 1988;2:5.

5. O'Donnell TF. Surgical treatment of incompetent communicating veins. In: Bergan JJ, Kistner RL. *Atlas of Venous Surgery.* WB Saunders: 1992;111.

6. Gloviczic P, Cambria RA, Rhee RY, et al. Surgical technique and preliminary results of endoscopic subfascial division of perforating veins. *J Vasc Surg.* 1996;23:517.

7. Wittens CHA, Plerik RGL, Van Urk H. The surgical treatment of incompetent perforating veins. *Eur J Vasc Endovasc Surg.* 1995;9:19.

8. Paraskeva PA, Darzi AW. Endoscopic subfascial division of incompetent perforating calf veins. In: Darzi AW, ed. *Retroperitoneoscopy.* Oxford Isis Medica:1996;65.

*T*horacic and Lumbar Spinal Disc Surgery

Chapter Eighty-Five ∎ ∎ ∎ ∎ ∎ ∎

*M*inimally Invasive Endoscopic Approach to the Spine

JEFFREY A. GOLDSTEIN and PAUL C. McAFEE

The usefulness of endoscopic techniques in orthopedics as well as in general surgical, gynecologic, urologic, and thoracic procedures is well established. The development of the minimally invasive endoscopic approach to the thoracic and lumbar spine is a technique prompted by the surgeon's desire to increase access to the spine while decreasing morbidity. In this chapter, we will address video-assisted thoracic surgery (VATS) of the spine and the laparoscopic approach to the lumbar spine. Discussion will focus on indications and applications of the procedures as well as operative setup. Finally, personal experience will also be reviewed.

VIDEO-ASSISTED THORACIC SPINAL SURGERY

The traditional approach to the thoracic spine is performed through a posterolateral thoracotomy or a thoracolumbar incision.[1–3] The use of thoracoscopy for intrathoracic procedures for the lysis of tuberculous lesions was first reported in 1910.[4] Lewis et al emphasized the importance of the video-assisted technology for evaluation of the thoracic cavity.[5,6] Video-assisted thoracic surgery (VATS) has since been applied to several thoracic procedures including sympathectomy,[7] lung biopsy and resection,[8,9] pericardiectomy,[10] mediastinal tumor excision,[11,12] and esophageal procedures.[13]

Landreneau et al[14] studied 106 patients undergoing VATS for lung lesions and reported reduced postoperative pain, improved shoulder girdle function, and decreased hospital stays compared with patients who underwent conventional thoracotomy. The technique of VATS for spinal disease or injury was first described in 1993 by Mack et al.[15] In vivo porcine experience led to the development of specialized equipment that was used clinically in 1991 to perform diagnostic tissue biopsy and subsequent drainage of a thoracic paravertebral abscess. Subsequent work applied VATS to numerous cases of thoracic disk herniation,[15–17] spinal deformity requiring anterior release,[18] osteotomy and bone grafting,[13] infection,[19] and corpectomy for vertebral body tumor. McAfee et al[20] have reported the incidence of complications in 100 consecutive endoscopic spinal procedures.

The purpose of this section is to review the indications as well as the contraindications for video-assisted thoracic spine surgery. We will then discuss the operative setup and technical procedures. These procedures have been well illustrated in a recently published atlas by Regan et al.[21] Surgical judgment and experience, including complications, will then be discussed.

Indications

VATS is the technique of choice for a thoracic herniated nucleus pulposus. A 30-degree thoracoscope offers the greatest visualization with a high degree of magnification. Enhanced visualization makes it possible to minimize vertebral body resection. Access is between the ribs and therefore rib excision is not needed. Rib retraction is not necessary. Minimally invasive surgery therefore provides less postoperative pain that leads to diminished postoperative atelectasis and respiratory problems.

In a prospective evaluation, patients usually required only an overnight stay in the intensive care unit, with chest tubes for less than 1.5 days on average.[20]

In general, VATS should be considered for the patient requiring an anterior approach to the thoracic spine. Compared to open thoracotomy, VATS patients have significantly less postoperative pain and require less narcotics. Postoperative shoulder girdle dysfunction is also diminished using VATS. Furthermore, early pulmonary impairment is reduced when compared with that experienced in traditional thoracotomy.[14]

Patients undergoing thoracotomy are subjected to several physiologic sequelae including a decrease in functional residual capacity as well as postoperative atelectasis secondary to chest wall splinting from painful respirations. Minimizing incision length can reduce postoperative pain.

An outline of indications for VATS of the spine is presented in Table 85–1.[21] As mentioned, the first VATS spine procedure was a diagnostic biopsy. After failure of a computed tomography-guided percutaneous attempt, endoscopy allowed direct visualization of the lesion as well as the entire hemithorax.

In reviewing a multicenter prospective study of 95 patients, the most common indication for VATS spinal surgery was thoracic discectomy and spinal canal decompression (57 patients). Spinal deformity represented the next most common surgical indication. In this multicenter series, 20 patients underwent multilevel anterior discectomy for correction of scoliosis. Anterior releases for kyphosis were performed in 4 patients and hemivertebrae excision in 3 patients. Decompression of pyogenic vertebral osteomyelitis was performed in 2 patients. Nine patients had decompressive corpectomy for neurologic compromise.[22]

Between 1991 and 1996 we have performed 15 thoracoscopic corpectomies. Eight patients presented with pathologic fractures from tumor, 5 with traumatic fractures and fracture dislocations, and 2 patients had vertebral osteomyelitis. Fourteen of 15 presented with incomplete neurologic deficits (Frankel grading system)[22,23] with MRI and/or CT evidence of anterior spinal cord compression. The last patient had a radiculopathy secondary to a neurofibroma involving the origin of the left T3 nerve root. Successful anterior spinal canal decompression was documented using MRI after VATS corpectomy. The indications for minimally invasive decompression are the same as those for traditional open procedures.

Following surgery, 12 of the 15 patients demonstrated improvement in their Frankel grade of neurologic function. Two patients did not show improvement despite MRI evidence of successful spinal canal decompression. In 13 patients, stabilization was provided using a variety of techniques.

Minimally invasive VATS of the spine, in general, is contraindicated for patients who cannot tolerate single-lung ventilation or high airway pressures with positive pressure ventilation, and in patients with pleural diseases. Relative contraindications include previous chest tube placement and previous thoracotomy.

The Surgical Procedure

Anesthesia. An anesthesiologist skilled in single-lung ventilation is a prerequisite. A double-lumen endotracheal tube is used. This tube is always placed with the aid of a fiber-optic bronchoscope down the left mainstem bronchus regardless of which lung is to be collapsed. Preoperative planning by the anesthesiologist must consider all central and peripheral access that may be needed. After patient positioning, it will not be possible to access the extremities. Unlike laparoscopic procedures, a carbon dioxide pneumoperitoneum is not necessary. The rigidity of the thoracic cage and single-lung ventilation of the contralateral lung provide excellent visualization.

Patient Positioning. The patient is placed on a standard operating table. With unilateral surgical pathology, the operative side is placed up in the lateral decubitus position.[24] We are presently working on the adaptation of a radiolucent table to be used in minimally invasive surgery (Jackson Table; OSI Medical, Union City, CA).

The patient's back must be perpendicular to the floor. If the pathology does not dictate the surgical approach, then it is preferable to place the right side up, since performing the procedure in the right hemithorax allows a wider working space. The patient is then elevated on two longitudinally placed blanket rolls. With this elevation, a separate axillary roll is not usually necessary. We place 3-inch-wide adhesive tape, fixed with Benzoin, across the patient at the level of the greater trochanter and near the axilla, well cephalad with respect to the operative field.

Before prepping and draping the patient, it is imperative to make sure that adequate fluoroscopic visualization of the spine can be achieved. The C-arm is brought in from below. A good-quality cross-table anteroposterior image is necessary. Experienced radiology technicians are required, as well as high-quality fluoroscopic units. Placing the operative table in the reverse Trendelenburg position, and rotating the table towards the operative surgeon, will allow the deflated lung to fall away from the field. After positioning the patient, the anesthesiologist should recheck the position of the endotracheal tube.

Thoracoscopic Anatomy. Because of differences in the anatomy of the two hemithoraxes, special attention is needed when approaching the vertebral interspace. The hemithorax is divided into upper, middle, and lower operative fields. In the upper field, the intercostal veins from the second, third, and fourth levels empty into the superior intercostal vein before emptying into the azygos vein on the right side. In the middle and lower fields, the intercostal veins empty directly into the azygos vein. The first intercostal vein empties into the brachiocephalic vein.

In the upper and middle fields, the rib head articulates with

TABLE 85–1. INDICATIONS FOR THORACOSCOPIC SPINAL PROCEDURES

Infection	Tumor	Degenerative Disc Disease	Spinal Deformity	Trauma
Biopsy, debridement	Biopsy, tumor excision	Excision of thoracic herniated disc	Anterior release for scoliosis >75 degrees	Decompression, fusion
Drainage of spinal abscess	Corpectomy and grafting Internal fixation	Fusion for discogenic pain Interbody instrumentation	Anterior release, fusion for Scheuermann's kyphosis >90 degrees	Internal fixation
			Anterior epiphysiodesis in skeletally immature patients at risk of developing crankshaft phenomenon.	
			Congenital spinal anomalies requiring anterior arthrodesis	
			Neuromuscular deformity requiring anterior arthrodesis	

Adapted from Regan JJ, McAfee PC, Mack MJ, eds. *Atlas of Endoscopic Spine Surgery.* St. Louis, Quality Medical Publishing, 1995.

the bodies above and below the interspace. The 9th rib articulates with the 8th and 9th vertebral bodies as well as the intervening disc space. In the lower field, the rib head articulates with its respective vertebral body. Therefore, in order to approach the T11–12 disc space there is no intervening rib head to be excised. The minimally invasive approach provides access from T2 to L1.

Operating Room Setup. Before starting the procedure, consideration should be given to the appropriate placement of surgical personnel as well as monitors for video and fluoroscopy. The operating spine surgeon stands along the ventral aspect of the patient near the axilla. The first assistant, generally a thoracic surgeon, stands just caudal to the spinal surgeon. These two surgeons look across the OR table at their monitor. A second assistant stands along the dorsum of the patient and looks across the field to the monitor. The C-arm monitor is placed next to the surgeon's video monitor. In the room, also, there should be equipment for open thoracotomy in case quick access is required. We also use spinal cord monitoring.

Operative Approach: Right-Sided T7 Corpectomy. For illustrative purposes we will describe the approach for VATS spinal surgery for a right-sided T7 corpectomy.

For a thoracoscopic corpectomy, we recommend four portals 10 mm in diameter. We have exclusively adopted the flexible Endopath (Ethicon, Somerville, NJ) trocars with an aim of reducing the incidence of intercostal neuralgia. We enter the chest at the 6th or 7th intercostal space in the midaxillary line for the first portal and then we explore the pleural cavity and release chest wall adhesions. At this point, it may be possible to visualize the pathologic level directly—either hemorrhage beneath the parietal pleura in the case of a fracture, or a paraspinal mass in the case of infection or neoplasm. It is helpful to place a small Steinmann pin in the midaxillary line directly through the chest wall into the spinal pathology. A confirmatory cross-table anteroposterior radiograph is obtained, and this also demonstrates the optimum location for the "working portal." Actually, as the corpectomy decompression progresses, it is often helpful to switch the camera and working portal around to get alternative angles for Kerrison rongeurs and other fixed-angle instruments. When the working portal is identified, the two other portals can be placed. Four ports are required to perform the procedure: one for a 30-degree thoracoscopic camera, one working port directly overlying the pathologic vertebral level, one port for a fan retractor for retraction of the lung, and one port for dissecting instruments and suction/irrigation. It is usually helpful to have the camera anterior and the suction posterior to the working portal. The surgeon tries to triangulate as much as possible within the constraints of the particular vertebral level being approached. There is some flexibility that can be used with the approach. We always find it helpful to use a 30-degree angled thoracoscope rather than a 0-degree scope because it allows "a straighter shot" for the working instruments without "sword fighting" the scope.

Once the vertebral level is identified, the lung is retracted anteriorly and the fluoroscopic image is taken to confirm the vertebral level. We use electrocautery to mark the intervertebral discs adjacent to the involved lesion. It is important to always locate the aorta and vena cava in the preoperative CT scan and MRI.

The next phase of the T7 corpectomy is identical to that for a T6–7 discectomy. The head of the seventh rib is osteotomized and the proximal 3 to 4 centimeters are resected. A complete T6–7 discectomy is then performed using curettes, pituitary rongeur, and a Cobb elevator. It is important to perform a meticulous and thorough discectomy cephalad (T6–7) and caudad (T7–8) to the involved vertebrae before starting the corpectomy.[24,25] These discs are avascular, so there should be very minimal hemorrhage. The surgeon should now be well oriented to the anterior and posterior extent of the vertebral bodies, the posterior longitudinal ligament, and the extent of the posterior annulus fibrosus; completion of a thorough discectomy clearly identifies and removes the soft tissue from the vertebral endplates (inferior endplate at T6 cephalad and the superior endplate at T8 caudad), which will be the anchoring point of the spinal fusion.

After the T6–7 and T7–8 discectomies, the surgeon needs to have access to three methods of hemostasis before starting the corpectomy: (1) Endoavitene (MedChem Products, Woburn, MA); (2) Gelfoam (Upjohn, Kalamazoo, MI) soaked in thrombin; and (3) bipolar endoscopic electrocautery. The T7 segmental vessels are now dissected from the underlying bone and elevated with a right-angled clamp. It is important to use two vascular clips on the high-pressure side of the vessels, and they are divided with Endoshears (Ethicon, Somerville, NJ). The surgeon may prefer to use an Endoloop (Ethicon, Somerville, NJ) or Surgitie (U.S. Surgical Corp., Norwalk, CT) on the proximal cut end of the vessels. The segmental vessels are ligated and divided in the anterior half of the vertebral body to allow the maximum potential for collateral circulation to the neuroforamina and spinal cord. If the lesion is a tumor or infection, then both a culture and frozen section are obtained.

A 45-degree 4-mm wide endoscopic Kerrison rongeur is used to resect the right T7 pedicle. Starting cephalad, the instrument is pointed caudad in order to protect the exiting spinal roots. After resection of the T7 pedicle on the right, the right T7 nerve root should be well visualized. It is helpful to remove a wedge of bone from the T7 vertebral body anterior to the posterior longitudinal ligament. The key is to debulk the T7 vertebral body going from disc space to disc space, rather than to head straight back towards the spinal canal. The surgeon should conceptualize "shelling out" the T7 vertebral body, so that the posterior bone compressing the spinal cord posteriorly can be curetted or displaced anteriorly into the hollowed-out T7 vertebral body. Either Kaneda heavy-duty rongeurs or high-powered 5-mm burrs, such as the Zimmer (Warsaw, IN) Ultra-power or Anspach Black Max (West Palm Beach, FL) with long extensions, can be used to hollow out the T7 vertebral body. Curettes and 2 to 3 mm Kerrison rongeurs are used to complete the corpectomy. It is important to thoroughly decompress the spinal cord across to the base of the opposite pedicle (in this case, the left T7 pedicle). It is only after palpating or visualizing the opposite pedicle that the objective of the decompression will be accomplished.

Hemostasis is achieved, and the endoscope can be placed directly into the T7 corpectomy defect and the entire anterior aspect of the dura is visualized. It is important to see the smooth glistening surface of the dura and epidural vessels. It is important to ensure removal of possible epidural extensions of tumors or bone fragments visualized at this point. A traumatic free-fragment disc herniation can be very adherent to the anterior aspect of the dura, and epidural loculated abscesses need to be removed at this point in the procedure. Gelfoam soaked in thrombin is placed over the anterior aspect of the thecal sac. The T6 and T8 vertebral bodies can be prepared for a strut fusion according to the preference of the surgeon. Either the resected portions of the 8th rib or an iliac strut graft is placed to fill the anterior portion of the corpectomy defect. Postoperatively, the patient is placed in a TLSO brace for 8 weeks or until radiographic evidence of fusion is obtained.

Complications

In a multicenter study evaluating the first 100 consecutive endoscopic anterior thoracolumbar spinal reconstructive procedures, there were 78 patients.[19] The complications are listed in Table 85–2. The most common complication was postoperative intercostal neuralgia. The etiology was thought to be due to multiple factors including monopolar electrocauterization of the rib before excision; the use of rigid, as opposed to flexible, 10-mm thoracoports; and compression of a spinal nerve with a Kerrison rongeur. This neuralgia resolved in all 6 patients by 6 weeks postoperatively. We now use only flexible thoracoports. The trade-off is that these ports may collapse upon themselves after an instrument is removed.

An 84-year-old woman with a previous empyema that caused extensive pleural adhesions had a thoracoport penetrate an elevated right hemidiaphragm. The perforation was repaired, without sequelae, using endoscopic staples. We now emphasize that the first port be placed in the 6th intercostal space, above the level of the diaphragm, and that all subsequent ports be placed under direct vision. All instruments must be visualized when entering or exiting the hemithorax.

There were no permanent iatrogenic spinal neurologic injuries. One scoliosis patient undergoing a thoracic release from T5 to T10 developed transient leg weakness from occult spinal stenosis at T12–L1. To avoid this complication, we no longer "jackknife" the operative table.

There were no dural tears that required repair in this series. Repair of a dural tear would be tedious. We have used CSF shunt drainage according to the techniques described by Kitchel et al in 2 patients.[26]

TABLE 85–2. COMPLICATIONS OF VIDEO-ASSISTED THORACIC SURGERY

Procedure Type	No. Patients
Thoracoscopic	
Intercostal neuralgia (all transient)	6
Atelectasis	5
Excessive epidural blood loss, more than 2500 mL	2
Conversion to open thoracotomy caused by previous costotransversectomy	1
Penetration of right hemidiaphragm from the thoracoport in patient with previous empyema	1
Transient paraparesis related to spinal stenosis at a different vertebral level and operative positioning	1
Laparoscopic	
Conversion to open laparotomy for repair of left common iliac vein	1
Bone graft donor site infection	2
Postoperative upper gastrointestinal bleed in patient anticoagulated with coumadin up to 2 weeks before surgery	1

No cases of permanent iatrogenic neurologic deficit.

No cases of spinal wound infection.

Future applications of the endoscopic technique include its use for stabilization of the spine following endoscopic corpectomy. Vertebral body removal after resection for infection or tumor, or for spinal cord compression after fracture, leads to thoracic instability. McAfee et al[24] found, in a series of 185 patients undergoing anterior spinal decompression, that instability caused the majority of complications. There was an overall complication rate of 20%. In McAfee's series of endoscopic corpectomies, 3 patients had undergone spinal stabilization before corpectomy and one patient had posterior instrumentation 4 days following the endoscopic procedure. We are currently evaluating endoscopic placement of fusion cages (Spine-Tech, Minneapolis, MN) and anterior Z-plates. (Sofamor-Danek, Memphis, TN).

LAPAROSCOPIC APPROACH TO THE LUMBAR SPINE

Laparoscopic approaches have been used for cholecystectomy, splenectomy, hernia repair, colectomy, Nissen fundoplication, discectomy, and appendectomy. Successful use of endoscopic techniques has resulted in decreased patient morbidity and hospital costs as well as improved cosmesis. The chief benefit of laparoscopic cholecystectomy is a more rapid return to work.[6–10,27–29]

Endoscopic management of degenerative lumbar disc herniation has been performed using posterior percutaneous techniques for foraminal disc herniations and contained herniations. One of the benefits of endoscopic spinal techniques is reduced epidural scarring, which is a potential problem with open posterior techniques. Laparoscopic approaches to the disc space provide a more direct approach. Controlled prospective randomized outcome studies will determine which approach to a specific pathology provides maximized patient outcome.

Patients with previous peritoneal or pelvic infections, or previous laparotomy, are poor candidates for laparoscopic approach to the spine. Lower abdominal or pelvic procedures, appendectomies, or herniorrhaphies may present areas of scarring that will need to be addressed during the laparoscopic approach.

The Surgical Procedure

Anesthesia. One advantage, from an anesthetic standpoint, of laparoscopy compared to thoracoscopic surgery is that single-lung ventilation is not necessary. However, the use of CO_2 pneumoperitoneum provides a different set of anesthetic considerations. An anesthesiologist must be comfortable with the resultant effects of CO_2 pneumoperitoneum and patient positioning on mean arterial blood pressure, cardiac output, changes in venous return, and ventilation.

Patient Positioning. As in the thoracoscopic approach, proper positioning of the patient before commencing with the procedure will help to diminish later frustration. The patient is placed supine on a standard operating table. A Foley catheter and nasogastric tube are placed. The nasogastric tube is removed at the completion of the procedure. All peripheral access required by the anesthesiologist is placed preoperatively because the extremities will not be accessible during the procedure. Intermittent pneumatic compression devices are placed on the lower extremities. The rationale for this is to help increase venous flow, which is diminished with pneumoperitoneum. We also place a 2-inch mat beneath the patient's buttocks. This serves two purposes. The patient's arms will be tucked at his or her sides during the procedure. It is important to tuck the arms so that they are below the trunk of the patient. Otherwise the extremities will obstruct your fluoroscopic image. Second, elevation of the buttocks will help to increase the Trendelenburg position of the patient. Three-inch tape is placed using Benzoin along the patient's shoulders to the operating table to help secure the patient. Maximal use of the Trendelenburg positioning will allow gravity to help the small intestines and omentum to fall cephalad, away from the operative field. Use of the Foley catheter and nasogastric tube diminish the imposition of an enlarged bladder or stomach upon the operative field.

Prior to prepping and draping of the patient, the surgeon should verify that adequate lateral fluoroscopic images can be obtained along the operative length of the spine and that the upper extremities of the patient do not obstruct the image.

Operating Room Setup. After proper positioning of the patient, consideration should next be given to the appropriate placement of operative personnel and equipment. This will be described for right-handed spine and laparoscopic access surgeons. Each surgeon must have an unobstructed view of a monitor across from the patient. Because the camera visualizes from cephalad to caudad, "mirroring" is not as much of a concern with surgeons on opposite sides of the patient compared to thoracoscopy. As an alternative, we have recently begun to place a single monitor that provides 3-D images (Carl Zeiss) at the foot of the table for use by all surgical personnel. C-arm and monitor as well as spinal cord monitoring are also appropriately positioned. A robotic arm is placed to facilitate video imaging. The robotic arm is able to track the operation smoothly while holding the camera steady. Furthermore, one of the assistants is freed up to perform other tasks such as retraction. The scrub nurse must have rapid access to instruments for conversion to an open laparotomy in case of a vascular complication.

Operative Approach

Portal Strategy. The key to portal placement is to have the exposure ports placed first and then to place the appropriate working ports. Initially, however, CO_2 pneumoperitoneum must be established. We use a closed technique. The umbilicus is elevated with two towel clips and the Veress needle is placed percutaneously. Pneumoperitoneum to 15 mm Hg is obtained. Analogous to the thoracoscopic approach, the first portal is 10 mm and is for the 0-degree laparoscope. All subsequent portals are placed under direct visualization. Unlike thoracoscopy, all trocars must have an airtight seal. Instruments must fit through the trocar without allowing loss of CO_2. The portals are placed in sequence. A 10-mm portal is placed by the access surgeon for use of the harmonic scalpel. Once the working portals are established, the abdomen is explored. Any adhesions preventing access to the operative site are gently taken down using Endoshears (Ethicon, Somerville, NJ).

Before incising the sigmoid mesentery, the great vessels and ureters are identified. The sigmoid mesentery is approached from the right side and incised longitudinally and elevated towards the left lower quadrant. We have found it helpful to use the mesentery as a sling to suspend the sigmoid colon. The mesentery is gently elevated and suspended to the abdominal wall with a 2-0 nylon suture. The median sacral vessels are identified and ligated. The parietal peritoneum between the iliac vessels is now visualized. In male patients, this is dissected bluntly. The harmonic scalpel is used to help diminish the risk of retrograde ejaculation. At this point, the L5–S1 interspace is exposed.

Approach to the L4–5 interspace is often impeded by the bifurcation of the aorta, thus making exposure more difficult. For this reason we are presently concentrating on retroperitoneal endoscopic access at this level.

LAPAROSCOPIC DISCECTOMY AND INTERBODY FUSION

Several groups are developing prospective series of laparoscopic discectomy and interbody fusion for discogenic back pain. Special instrumentation has been developed for laparoscopic placement of bone dowels (Sofamor-Danek, Memphis, TN and Spine-Tech, Minneapolis, MN). The technique for placement of autograft or a fusion cage is well described and illustrated.[30-34] In 1995, a prospective multicenter study described the complications of 22 procedures performed at four institutions[20] using the Spine-Tech BAK fusion cage protocol for an FDA-approved study evaluating its use for anterior laparoscopic insertion at L4–5 and L5–S1.

The average length of stay was 5.6 days (range, 1 to 23 days); intraoperative blood loss 194 mL (range, 50 to 800 mL); and mean operative time 4 hours and 17 minutes (range, 2 hours and 40 minutes to 9 hours). No patient required blood transfusion.

Complications are listed in Table 85–2. There were no complications from pneumoperitoneum or CO_2 insufflation. During the second BAK implantation, vascular injury occurred when a retractor tore an edge of the left iliac vein. Hemorrhage was controlled using direct pressure and the vein repaired after gaining access through a 4-inch Pfannenstiel incision.

In order to decrease the risk of infection of the iliac crest donor site, we now harvest the graft and close the wound before beginning the laparoscopic procedure.

Following successful completion of the laparoscopic procedure, patients are allowed to advance their diet as tolerated. Physical therapy is initiated on the first postoperative day, and patients ambulate using a lumbosacral support such as a "warm and form" or corset.

RETROPERITONEAL APPROACH TO THE LUMBAR SPINE

Recently the minimally invasive approach to has been adapted for retroperitoneal exposure to the lumbar spine.[35] Retroperitoneal surgery does not require CO_2 insufflation, Trendelenburg positioning, entrance into the peritoneal cavity, or anterior dissection near the great vessels.

The approach uses a combination of video-assisted thoracoscopic and laparoscopic methods. The patient is placed under general anesthesia and placed in the lateral decubitus position on a radiolucent Jackson Table (OSI Corporation, Union City, CA). A 1-cm incision is made at the anterior portion of the 12th rib for approaching from L1 to L2. Below L2, a lateral C-arm fluoroscopic image is obtained with a marker overlying the skin in the midaxillary line. The retroperitoneum is dissected using balloon insufflation, an optical dissecting trochar, and finger dissection.

Once the spine is reached, discectomy or corpectomy can be performed. Fusion can be augmented using a cage or bone dowels in a mediolateral direction. Lordosis may be dialed in using implants of different diameters.

CONCLUSION

The endoscopic approach to the spine provides the surgeon with a means of approaching complex pathology with a minimally invasive approach. There is a learning curve, and laboratory practice and instructions are necessary before attempting clinical use. The procedures may reduce iatrogenic neurologic sequelae. Prospective randomized clinical trials will determine patient success and outcome. Development of appropriate instrumentation will be of extreme importance.

REFERENCES

1. Anderson TM, Mansour KA, Miller JI. Thoracic approaches to anterior spinal operations. Anterior thoracic approaches. *Ann Thorac Surg.* 1993;44:1447.
2. McElvcin RB, Nasca RJ, Dunham WK, et al. Transthoracic exposure for anterior spinal surgery. *Ann Thorac Surg.* 1988;45:278.
3. Naunheim KS, Barnett MG, Crandall DG, et al. Anterior exposure of the thoracic spine. *Ann Thorac Surg.* 1994;46:1436.
4. Jacobaeus HC. Possibility of the use of cystoscope for the investigation of the serous cavities. *Munch Med Wochenschr.* 1910;57:3090.
5. Lewis RJ, Caccavale RJ, Sisler GE. Special report: Video-endoscopic thoracic surgery. *NJ Med.* 1991;88:473.
6. Lewis RJ, Caccavale RJ, Sisler GE. Imaged thoracoscopic surgery: A new thoracic technique for resection of mediastinal cysts. *Ann Thorac Surg.* 1992;53:318.
7. Landreneau RJ, Mack NJ, Hazelrigg SR, et al. Video-assisted thoracic surgery: Basic technical concepts and intercostal approach strategies. *Ann Thorac Surg.* 1992;54:800.
8. Ferson PF, Landreneau RJ, Dowling RD, et al. Thoracoscopic versus open lung biopsy for the diagnosis of diffuse infiltrative lung disease. *J Thorac Cardiovasc Surg.* 1993;105:194.
9. Landreneau RJ, Hazelrigg SR, Ferson PF, et al. Thoracoscopic resection of 85 pulmonary lesions. *Ann Thorac Surg.* 1992;54:415.
10. Krasna MJ, Mack MJ. *Atlas of Thoracoscopic Surgery.* St. Louis, Quality Medical Publishing, 1994.
11. Landreneau RJ, Dowling RD, Castillo WM, et al. Thoracoscopic resection of an anterior mediastinal tumor. *Ann Thorac Surg.* 1992;54:142.
12. Landreneau RJ, Dowling RD, Ferson PF. Thoracoscopic resection of a posterior mediastinal neurogenic tumor. *Chest.* 1992;102:1288.
13. Regan JJ, Mack MJ, Picetti GD, et al. A comparison of video-assisted thoracoscopic surgery (VATS) with open thoracotomy in thoracic spinal surgery. *Today's Ther Trends* 1994;11:203.
14. Landreneau RJ, Hazelrigg SR, Mack MJ. Postoperative pain-related morbidity: Video-assisted thoracic surgery versus thoracotomy. *Ann Thorac Surg.* 1993;56:1285.
15. Mack MJ, Regan JJ, Bobechko WP, et al. Applications of thoracoscopy for diseases of the spine. *Ann Thorac Surg.* 1993;56:736.
16. Horowitz MB, Moossy JJ, Julian T, et al. Thoracic diskectomy using video assisted thoracoscopy. *Spine.* 1994;19:1082.
17. Mack MJ, Aronoff RJ, Acuff TE, et al. Present role of thoracoscopy in the diagnosis and treatment of diseases of the chest. *Ann Thorac Surg.* 1992;54:403.
18. Regan JJ, Mack MJ, Picetti GD. A technical report on video-assisted thoracoscopy in thoracic spinal surgery. *Spine.* 1995;20:831.
19. Parker LM, McAfee PC, Fedder IL, et al. Minimally invasive surgical techniques to treat spine infections. *Orthop Clin North Am.* 1996;27:183.
20. McAfee PC, Regan JJ, Picetti GD, et al. The incidence of complications in endoscopic anterior thoracic spinal reconstructive surgery: A prospective multicenter study comprising the first 100 consecutive cases. *Spine.* 1995;20:1624.
21. Regan JJ, McAfee PC, Mack MJ, eds. *Atlas of Endoscopic Spine Surgery.* St. Louis, Quality Medical Publishing, 1995.
22. Mack JM, Regan JJ, McAfee PC, et al. Video-assisted thoracic surgery for the anterior approach to the thoracic spine. *Ann Thorac Surg.* 1995;5:1100.
23. Frankel HL, Hancock DO, Hysop G. The value of postural reduction in the initial management of closed injuries of the spine with paraplegia and tetraplegia. Part I. *Paraplegia.* 1969;7:179.
24. McAfee PC, Bohlman HH, Yuan HA. Anterior decompression of traumatic thoracolumbar fractures with incomplete neurological deficit using a retroperitoneal approach. *J Bone Joint Surg.* 1985;67A:89.
25. McAfee PC, Zdeblick TA. Tumors of the thoracic and lumbar spine. Surgical treatment via the anterior approach. *J Spinal Disord.* 1989;2:145.
26. Kitchel SH, Eismont FJ, Green BA. Closed subarachnoid drainage for management of cerebrospinal fluid leakage after an operation on the spine. *J Bone Joint Surg.* 1989;71-A:984.
27. Reddick EJ, Olsen DO. Laparoscopic laser cholecystectomy. A comparison with mini-lap cholecystectomy. *Surg Endosc.* 1989;3:131.
28. Pier A, Gortz F, Bacher C. Laparoscopic appendectomy in 625: From innovation to routine. *Surg Laparosc Endosc.* 1991;1:8.
29. Scott TR, Graham SM, Flowers JL, et al. An analysis of 12,397 laparoscopic cholecystectomies. *Surg Laparosc Endosc.* 1992;2:191.
30. Sachs BL, Schwoitzberg SD. Lumbosacral (L5–S1) discectomy and interbody fusion technique. In: Atlas of Endoscopic Spine Surgery, Quality Medical Publishing, Inc., St. Louis, MO., page 275.
31. Kuslich SD, McAfee PC, Regan JJ. Spinal instrumentation. In: Regan JJ, McAfee PC, Mack MJ, eds. *Atlas of Endoscopic Spine Surgery.* St. Louis, Quality Medical Publishing, 1995;293.
32. McAfee PC. Laparoscopic fusion and BAK stabilization of the lumbar spine. In: Regan JJ, McAfee PC, Mack MJ, eds. *Atlas of Endoscopic Spine Surgery.* St. Louis, Quality Medical Publishing, 1995;306.
33. Regan JJ. Endoscopic application of the BAK System (L4–5). In: Regan JJ, McAfee PC, Mack MJ, eds. *Atlas of Endoscopic Spine Surgery.* St. Louis, Quality Medical Publishing, 1995;321.
34. Zuckerman JF, Zdeblick TA, Bailey SA, et al. Instrumented laparoscopic spinal fusion—Preliminary results. *Spine.* 1995;20:2029.
35. McAfee PC, Regan JJ, Geis WP, et al. Minimally invasive anterior retroperitoneal approach to the lumbar spine—Emphasis on the lateral BAK. *Spine.* 1998;23:1476.

Hand-Assisted Laparoscopy

Chapter Eighty-Six ● ● ● ● ● ● ●

*H*and-Assisted Laparoscopy

J.J. JACKIMOWICZ

INTRODUCTION

Several restrictions on performing major operations laparoscopically have limited the spread of use of advanced endoscopic procedures. In particular, laparoscopic colorectal surgery, pancreatic surgery, gastric surgery, liver surgery, splenectomy, and many other procedures have spread slowly.[1] The restrictions of the laparoscopic approach include inadequate exposure during complex dissection, lack of tactile information, particularly in oncologic patients, resulting in difficulties in localizing the pathology, inadequate assessment of lymph nodes, and tumor spread. Laparoscopic instruments are traumatizing to tissue, potentially resulting in exfoliation of tumor cells or trauma to organs. The necessity of using multiple access ports and different instrumentation results in a more complex and time-consuming procedure, which also discourages surgeon use of laparoscopy. The well-known problem of port side metastasis is related to the technical aspects of the standard laparoscopic approach to colorectal surgery for malignant disease. Problems with wound contamination due to traumatic manipulations of the resected bowel segment may occur when extracting organs through the small incisions or the small laparotomy sometimes used at the end of the procedure. Morcellation of the resected specimen inside a bag is not applicable to cancerous tissues since it precludes histologic staging. When done entirely laparoscopically, tissue approximation and anastomosis necessitates the use of laparoscopic stapling devices as well as special instruments and techniques used in open surgery. The ongoing development and improvement of devices for HALS (hand-assisted laparoscopic surgery) is promising and should solve many of the technical difficulties that restrict the widespread use of laparoscopic procedures.

DEVICES

Currently there are five devices available that allow HALS, but there are significant differences between the devices. Conceptually, the devices can be divided into three groups:

- Devices that are connected to the skin surface of the abdominal wall by an adhesive flange (e.g., the Dexterity device and the Intromit device);
- The HandPort device, which utilizes two mating balloons; and
- One-piece devices (e.g., the Lapdisc and the Omniport device).

The pros and cons of different devices have been reviewed by Meijer et al.[2] Here we will briefly describe one of the most recently developed devices, the HandPort, and the way it is applied.

The HandPort system (Smith & Nephew Inc., Boston, MA) consists of the following components: base retractor, sleeve, cap, bracelet, and sterile lubricant. The base retractor is composed of a ring that is placed intraperitoneally below the insertion site, and an inflatable ring that is placed on the skin. The rings are connected by a wound protector. The hand-powered insufflation pump, connected to the inflatable ring, enables insufflation of the ring, providing nonadhesive attachment of the device in the incision. The bracelet allows easy attachment of the sleeve, eliminating any pressure on the surgeon's arm. The cap can be placed on the base retractor and allows maintenance of pneumoperitoneum and performance of the laparoscopic part of the procedure. A minilaparotomy incision corresponding to the surgeon's glove size is placed in the selected spot and the peritoneal cavity is entered. The principle of triangulation of instruments should be kept in mind, provided the surgeon's (nondominant) hand is one of the instruments. If suitable for the procedure at hand, a muscle-splitting incision is recommended, but a medial or Pfannenstiel type of incision may also be used. The distance from the insertion site to the target area should be adequate to avoid interference with the laparoscope and allow free movements of the hand. After making the incision that enables passage of the surgeon's hand, the lower ring of the base retractor is carefully inserted into the peritoneal cavity such that neither omentum nor bowel are entrapped under the ring. Subsequently the outer ring of the device is inflated using the hand pump or another pump. The bracelet is now placed on the wrist of the nondominant hand of the surgeon under the cuff of the glove. Use of dark gloves is recommended to avoid reflection of light from the laparoscope, which may reduce illumination of the site. Sterile lubricant is rubbed on the back of the surgeon's hand, and the wide end of the sleeve is then pulled over the surgeon's gowned forearm, and the ring on the narrow end of the sleeve is clicked into the groove of the bracelet. The wide end of the sleeve is inverted over the surgeon's hand, and the ring on the wide end is attached to the base retractor. Now the surgeon's hand can be inserted through the retractor into the abdominal cavity while the pneumoperitoneum is maintained. Detailed descriptions of the device and preliminary experience with its application have been reported by several authors.[3,4,5]

Development of new devices is ongoing. A new device called Omniport, which is based on the balloon principle, has been introduced most recently. Initial experience with this device has been reported by Cushieri for applications such as liver resection, pancreatic resection, and drainage of pancreatic cysts.[6]

ERGONOMIC CONSIDERATIONS FOR HALS

When placing the device, some ergonomic considerations are important to enable efficient performance of the procedure. Location of the access incision is dependent on the specific procedure to be performed, and on the body morphology of the individual patient. Nonetheless, basic rules for ergonomic placement of the instruments in laparoscopic surgery have to be fulfilled. The size of the mini-laparotomy needed to place the access port varies from 6 to 8 cm, depending on the surgeon's hand size, and if possible it should be a muscle-splitting incision. Location of the incision is dependent on the anatomic region of the intended operation, the position of the surgeon at the operating table, and the way the patient is positioned. The incision should be placed far enough from bony structures such as the costal margin or pelvis to enable adequate deployment of the device.

The distance from the incision to the target area must not be too short, or the surgeon's hand may restrict the view of the target area. The wrist of the surgeon must be inserted into the abdomen to provide maximum freedom of movement.

When choosing the location of the incision, one should keep in mind that in case of conversion to an open procedure, the incision can be potentially extended and used to complete the operation.

The rules of triangulation of instruments as for laparoscopic surgery should be honored, with the hand considered to be an instrument. The video port should be located at equal angles between the two operating ports. In some situations it may be necessary to place the video port next to the access incision where the Hand-Port device is placed, which places it on one side or the other of the surgeon's hand. This positioning of the video port does not create major problems, because the surgeon's proprioception will enable compensation for the somewhat awkward positioning of the scope. Placement of the video port and the additional instrument port next to the HandPort device should be far enough from the device so they do not damage its internal ring.

APPLICATIONS OF HALS

HALS has been successfully applied to a wide range of surgical procedures, such as gastric resection, gastric bypass, vertical banded gastroplasty, transhiatal esophagectomy, pancreatic resection, drainage of pancreatic cysts, liver resection, splenectomy, and nephrectomy, including live-donor nephrectomy. Its use in colorectal surgery (Hartmann's procedure), rectopexy, right hemicolectomy, left and right total colectomy, sigmoid resection, and even proctocolectomy has been reported.[4–16]

DISCUSSION

A decade after the introduction of laparoscopic cholecystectomy, many other advanced laparoscopic procedures had not yet gained widespread acceptance. When performed entirely laparoscopically, these procedures are technically complex and difficult to perform, requiring special laparoscopic skills and much experience to master. The need for an additional incision to remove the resected specimen at the end of the laparoscopic procedure stimulated surgeons to seek new techniques and solutions. In 1994, the first use of HALS was reported, describing a hand-assisted Hartmann procedure. In the same year, Dunn[8] suggested digital-assisted laparoscopic surgery, and Meijer et al[9] reported a laparoscopic hand-assisted sigmoid resection in a porcine model, using the Dexterity sleeve. O'Reilly et al[10] reported a hand-assisted low anterior resection using a Dexterity sleeve soon thereafter. Jakimowicz et al[11] presented several applications of HALS, for procedures such as splenectomy, colon resection, and small bowel resection, among others. These reports were followed by development of different HALS devices for endoscopic surgery, such as Intromit and EPAB (Extracorporeal Pneumoperitoneum Access Bubble), HandPort, and most recently OmniPort.

The increasing acceptance of hand-assisted surgery is confirmed by the experience of several investigators, providing evidence of its usefulness.[2,4–18] The continuing improvement of HALS devices and development of new ones, as well as their efficiency and effectiveness of use, are discussed in an overview by Meijer et al.[2] HALS appears to retain most of the advantages of the laparoscopic approach. It simply facilitates the procedure so that it is executed more expeditiously and with greater safety. The ability to immediately control any major bleeding with the internal hand considerably reduces the stress level of the surgeon during complex major operations in anatomically crowded regions.[6] The benefits of HALS are presented in an editorial in the October 2000 issue of *Surgical Endoscopy*,[19] and the major advantages are listed as enhanced exposure, safe blunt digital dissection, atraumatic tissue handling, immediate control of major bleeding, restoration of tactile feedback, and compensation for the loss of normal stereoscopic vision by restored proprioception. In addition, it offers distinct advantages for the conduct of laparoscopic resections for cancer, and may indeed reduce the risk of tumor dissemination and port-site metastasis. The reduction in operative time using the HALS approach is well documented for live donor nephrectomy, especially with regard to warm ischemia time.

In all these respects HALS is superior to the totally laparoscopic approach, particularly for colon surgery. Studies using motion analysis have demonstrated the superior efficiency of HALS versus a totally laparoscopic approach, thus confirming the potential benefit of HALS for advanced major laparoscopic procedures. This is strongly supported by the outcome of a prospective randomized trial comparing HALS to standard laparoscopic surgery for colorectal disease, in a study by Litwin on behalf of the HALS

Study Group.[20] The conclusion of this study is that HALS is safe for benign and noncurative malignant disease, and preserves the benefits of the laparoscopic approach, allowing the surgeon to perform complex operations more easily and quickly. It provides ample evidence that will spur further development and exploration of the HALS approach, especially for colon surgery.[20]

The October and November 2000 issues of *Surgical Endoscopy* contain several papers on HALS, and editorials further illuminate the current status of hand-assisted surgery. The recent literature leads one to the conclusion that HALS is a promising hybrid of laparoscopic and open surgery that is worth further development and evaluation.

REFERENCES

1. Jakimowicz JJ. Current state and trends in minimal access surgery in Europe. *J R Coll Surg Edinburgh.* 1995;40:397.
2. Meijer DW, Bannenberg JJG, Jakimowicz JJ. Hand-assisted laparoscopic surgery—An overview. *Surg Endosc.* 2000 14(10):891.
3. Jakimowicz JJ, Darzi A, Meijer DW. A new device for hand-assisted laparoscopic surgery. *J Laparoendosc Adv Surg Tech A.* 1999;16–20.
4. Litwin D. Hand-assisted laparoscopic surgery versus standard laparoscopic surgery for colorectal disease: A prospective, randomized trial. *Surg Endosc.* (in press).
5. Bleier JI, Krupnick AS, Kreisel D, et al. Hand-assisted vertical banded gastroplasty: early results. *Surg Endosc.* 2000 14(10):902.
6. Cuschieri A. laparoscopic hand assisted surgery for hepatic and pancreatic disease. *Surg Endosc.* 2000;14(11):991.
7. Gorey TF, O'Conell PR, Waldron D, et al. Laparoscopically assisted reversal of Hartmann's procedure. *Br J Surg.* 1993;80:109.
8. Dunn DC. Digitally assisted laparoscopic surgery (letter). *Br J Surg.* 1994;81:474.
9. Bemelman WA, Ringers J, Meijer DW, et al: Laparoscopic-assisted colectomy with the Dexterity Pneumo Sleeve. *Dis Colon Rectum.* 1996;39:S59.
10. O'Reilly MJ, Sarge WB, Mullins SG, et al. Techniques of hand-assisted laparoscopic surgery. *J Laparoendosc Surg.* 1996;6:239.
11. Jakimowicz JJ, Rutten H, Meijer D. Video-assisted surgery using dexterity device. *Surg Endosc.* 1995;9:631.
12. Gorey TF, Bonadio F. Laparoscopic-assisted surgery. *Semin Laparosc Surg.* 1997;4:102.
13. Kusminsky RE, Boland JP, Tiley EH, et al. Hand-assisted laparoscopic splenectomy. *Surg Laparosc Endosc.* 1995;5:463.
14. Mooney MJ, Elliott PL, Galapon DB, et al. Hand-assisted laparoscopic sigmoidectomy for diverticulitis. *Dis Colon Rectum.* 1998;41:630.
15. Naitoh T, Gagner M. Laparoscopically assisted gastric surgery using Dexterity Pneumo Sleeve. *Surg Endosc.* 1997;11:830.
16. Naitoh T, Gagner M, Garcia-Ruiz A, et al. Hand-assisted laparoscopic digestive surgery provides safety and tactile sensation for malignancy or obesity. Surg Endosc 1999;13(2):157.
17. Gossot D, Meijer D, Bannenberg J, et al. La splénectomie laparoscopique revisitée. *Ann Surg.* 1995;49:487.
18. Ravizzini PI, Shulsinger D, Guarnizo E, et al. Hand-assisted laparoscopic donor nephrectomy versus standard laparoscopic donor nephrectomy: a comparison study in the canine model. *Tech Urol.* 1999;5:174.
19. Jakimowicz JJ. Will advanced laparoscopic surgery go hand-assisted? *Surg Endosc.* 2000 14(10):881.
20. Litwin D. Hand-assisted laparoscopy versus standard laparoscopy for colorectal resection. HALS Study Group. Submitted to *Dis Colon Rectum.* (personal communication).

*E*ndoscopy

Chapter Eighty-Seven • • • • • • •

Role of Endoscopy as an Adjunct to Laparoscopic Surgery

MOISÉS JACOBS, EDDIE GOMEZ, and ALEXIS BOLIO

The specialty of general surgery has recently undergone a revolution. The application of video-assisted surgery to cholecystectomy led to the greatest postgraduate training effort in the history of general surgery. Just a few years after the first successful case in 1987, laparoscopic cholecystectomy has become the preferred technique for cholecystectomy throughout the world. Many surgeons felt that this revolution was patient-driven, and most were forced reluctantly to learn the technique. Now, virtually any intra-abdominal procedure can be accomplished using laparoscopic guidance.[1]

With the ever-growing trend toward minimally invasive procedures, endoscopy has become an integral part of laparoscopic procedures. Improvement in technology and advances in video visualization have been vital to the integration of these expanding modalities. Endoscopy as applied to laparoscopic surgery began with the work of John C. Ruddock and his publication "Peritoneoscopy" in 1937. Ruddock describes the technique of using laparoscopy and endoluminal intubation with a special tube fitted with a light that allowed inflation and visualization of the stomach or colon during laparoscopy.[2]

Also in 1937 E.T. Anderson published a report entitled "Peritoneoscopy," published in the *American Journal of Surgery* that described similar methods of endoscopic transillumination during laparoscopy.[3]

The advent of newer technology, camera equipment, and smaller scopes has facilitated the use of endoscopy during laparoscopic procedures.

LOCALIZATION OF TUMORS AND LESIONS

One of the most important roles of endoscopic intervention during laparoscopy is the localization of tumors that would otherwise require resection or open laparotomy for identification. Gastroscopy and colonoscopy, procedures once only performed in the GI suite, now are commonplace in the operating room during laparoscopic procedures. Another important aspect of endoscopy is the ability

not only to localize, but to tag or tattoo lesions prior to or during procedures (Fig. 87–1). During laparoscopic procedures, or open procedures for that matter, tumor localization is one of the most important aspects of the procedure, first for anatomic location of the tumor or lesion, and second for the determination of adequate margins. This is especially important in colon surgery, a procedure in which localization previously had been done by the gastroenterologist in a different setting. Due to the lack of tactile sensation during laparoscopic procedures, such localization of the lesion is of utmost importance. In colon surgery, the terminal ileum is identified and pressure is applied to prevent insufflation of the small bowel. This can be done using atraumatic graspers or laparoscopic Babcock clamps. Once complete occlusion has been attained, a complete colonoscopy can be done. The lesion is located via colonoscopy, then the laparoscope is used to visualize it via transillumination through the bowel wall (Fig. 87–2). Once the lesion has been found, the area can be localized laparoscopically by placing a suture or endo-loop on the pericolonic fat in the area of the lesion. This simple procedure can help avoid an inadequate resection and assist in attaining ample surgical margins. Intraoperative tumor localization also avoids conversion to an open procedure in cases in which a tumor cannot be found.

LAPAROSCOPIC BILIARY SURGERY

Biliary surgery is another field that has been most drastically affected by minimally invasive surgery.[4-6] Using the choledochoscope during laparoscopic cholecystectomy has become a useful means to retrieve common duct stones and explore the duct.[7,8] During the procedure a choledochoscope can be passed via a trocar and directed into the cystic duct. Under direct visualization it is directed into the common bile duct in search of stones or other source of occlusion.[9] Once a stone is found, extraction can be attempted using a basket. If efforts to extract the stone fail, it can be pushed or flushed distally into the duodenum under direct visualization.

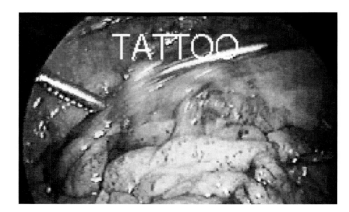

Figure 87–1. Tattoo of colonic region.

A

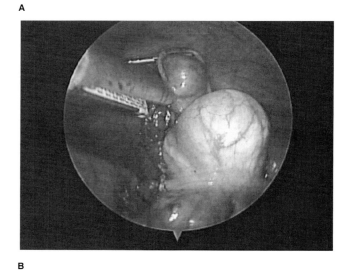

B

Figure 87–2. Colonoscopic assisted localization and transection of cecal lesion.

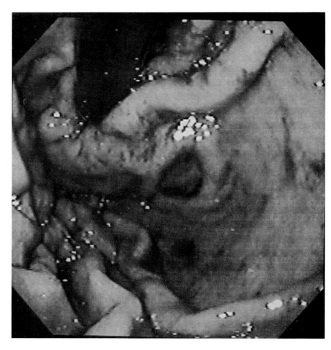

Figure 87–3. Endoscopic view of Nissen fundoplication.

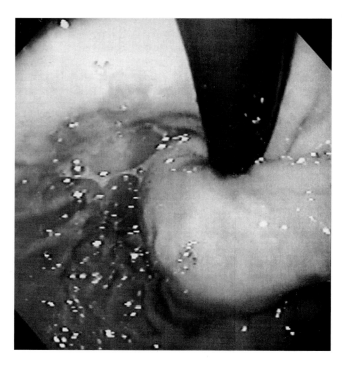

Figure 87–4. Endoscopic view of LAGB.

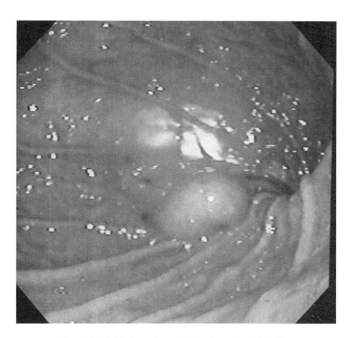

Figure 87–5. Endoscopic indentification of gastric lesion.

Using this technique may avoid the need for endoscopic retrograde cholangiopancreatography (ERCP) in patients in whom the procedure would be technically impossible, or the need for open common bile duct exploration. In patients in whom preoperative ERCP has failed, a guidewire can be passed via the open cystic duct through the papilla into the duodenum. This gives the endoscopist a visible guide to the ampulla and into the common bile duct, fa-

cilitating papillotomy and removal of stones without the added risk of iatrogenic perforation. A multidisciplinary approach is the most effective way to treat these patients.[10,11]

CONTROL AND LOCALIZATION OF UPPER GASTROINTESTINAL BLEEDING

Localization of gastrointestinal bleeding is one of the more clinically challenging tasks of the laparoscopic surgeon due to the difficulty of locating the exact point of bleeding. Two approaches have been described for localizing the bleeding lesion or vessel. One describes an external approach in which the bowel is transilluminated using the endoscope, thereby visualizing the bleeding vessel so that laparoscopic bowel resection can be done with confidence that the bleeding vessel will be contained in the resected segment. The second method involves the transgastric approach with the laparoscope. Once transgastric laparoscopic visualization of the bleeding vessel has been made, direct cauterization or ligation can be done via a transgastric trocar.[12,13] This method is effective without the need for resection of gastric tissue. After localizing the gastric bleeding by endoscopy, laparoscopic ligation of the bleeding vessel can be done from the abdominal cavity, avoiding a gastrotomy. Prior to resection of colon or duodenal vascular malformations, localization can be made to ensure that adequate resection margins leave no vascular lesions in the residual segment.

Another use for intraoperative endoscopy is for duodenal ulcer microperforation, in which case the duodenum is insufflated to confirm the leakage of air, and laparoscopic repair is done with a Graham patch to assure adequate closure of the perforation.[14] Any leakage can be detected by filling the place where the patch was placed with saline to confirm adequate sealing of the lesion.

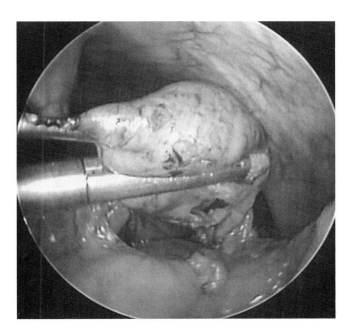

Figure 87–6. Transection of a gastric mass.

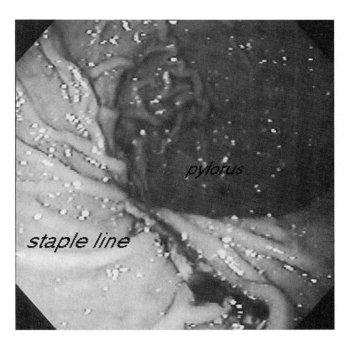

Figure 87–7. Gastroscopic control post-transection.

PERIOPERATIVE SURVELLIANCE DURING LAPAROSCOPIC PROCEDURES

During laparoscopic procedures one of the most worrisome concerns is the patency and adequate sealing of the anastomosis. This concern can arise in colon, small bowel,[15] and gastric surgeries. With the aid of the endoscope, after a low anterior resection the anastomosis can be checked for bleeding under direct vision and for small leaks by placing the anastomosis under water in the pelvis to look for bubbles with minimal distention. Air escaping from the rectum indicates that sufficient air has been applied. This serves not only to detect leaks, but also prevents diversion procedures in cases in which an intact anastomosis cannot be confirmed. During Nissen fundoplication, endoscopy serves to visualize a complete wrap around the lower esophagus and correct wrap placement, and also allows visualization of the esophagus for early detection of traumatic perforation (Fig. 87–3). This is useful in all upper GI surgeries in which a bougie[16] or balloon has to be placed during or prior to surgery. In patients with achalasia in which the esophageal muscular layers are resected leaving the mucosa without protection, endoscopy is useful to ascertain the total separation of the muscular layers. Confirmation of correct wrap placement and detection of leakage can be done via this method as well. During laparoscopic upper gastrointestinal resections, endoscopy can be used to pass feeding tubes into or through an anastomosis under direct vision, avoiding damage from blind passage of these tubes after a procedure, and preventing bleeding in the region of the anastomosis. When a laparoscopic adjustable gastric band (LAGB)[17,18] is placed for the treatment of morbid obesity, intraoperative endoscopy can be done to assure the correct size of the gastric pouch and adequate placement of the band by performing a **J** maneuver (Fig. 87–4). By visualizing the band, the sites where the sutures have been placed can be checked to assure that the band will stay in place and will not migrate. In a laparoscopic gastric bypass for the treatment of morbid obesity, an intraoperative upper endoscopy can be done to assure that there is no air leakage, no bleeding of the anastomosis, and that the size of the pouch is adequate. Another use for endoscopy in a surgical procedure is the use of insufflation to check for patency of small bowel anastomoses. One example of this is during a Roux-en-Y gastric bypass, in which the patency of the jejunal anastomosis is in question, and for insufflation of the gastrojejunostomy to check for leaks in the anastomosis. During insufflation the patency can be checked by the flow of air into the Roux limb by distention of the bypassed stomach and into the distal jejunum as well. These methods are used selectively in cases in which concerns of leakage or patency are present.

COMBINED LAPAROSCOPIC AND ENDOSCOPIC EXCISION OF GASTRIC MUCOSAL LESIONS

With the introduction of gastric endoscopy the treatment of gastric pathology has changed significantly. Routine endoscopy has led to the early detection of mucosal gastric lesions. And the combined use of laparoscopy and endoscopy has permitted the treatment or excision of these lesions with decreased morbidity and excellent results.

In a patient with a gastric lesion the excision can be completed via this combined approach. Pneumoperitoneum is achieved in the usual fashion. A Penrose drain is placed around the pylorus to avoid insufflation of the small intestine. The endoscope is then passed into the stomach and insufflation of the stomach is attained. Two radial expanding trocars are placed into the gastric lumen while observing via the laparoscope and the endoscope. Once access into the stomach is achieved, CO_2 is attached to the gastric trocars to maintain gastric dilatation. The position of the trocars varies according to the location of the lesion.[19] Once the lesion is localized, a submucosal plane is infiltrated with adrenaline solution to raise the mucosa and decrease bleeding.[20] Using a grasper, the lesion is elevated and the harmonic scalpel is used to excise the lesion. One or two sutures can be used to approximate the mucosa and further attain hemostasis. The lesion is removed via one of the trocar sites and the gastrotomies are sutured closed.[21] This method of combined endoscopic/laparoscopic approach is another modality available for excisions of gastric lesions without major resection.

Another approach to gastric tumors is to endoscopically localize them (Fig. 87–5) and under endoscopic control a stapled partial gastric resection is done, making sure the lesion is completely excised (Fig. 87–6). Then, after tumor localization a gastrotomy can be done and an excision can be done directly from the gastric lumen using endostaples. Staples are also used to close the gastrotomy, and the endoscope can check for hemostasis and air tightness (Fig. 87–7).

REFERENCES

1. Berici G, Nyhus LM. Problems in general surgery. *Laparosc Surg.* 1991;8:442.
2. Ruddock JC. Peritoneoscopy. *Surg Gynecol Obstet.* 1937;65:623.
3. Anderson ET. Peritoneoscopy. *Am J Surg.* 1937;35:136.
4. Berici G, Shore JM, Morgenstern L. An improved rigid choledochoscope. *Am J Surg.* 1971;122:567.
5. Yamakawa T, Mieno K. An improved choledochofibrescope. *Gastrointest Endosc.* 1975;17:459.
6. Jakimowicz JJ, Carol EJ, Haeck L, et al. A new improved flexible choledochoscope: preliminary experience. *Dig Surg.* 1985;2:49.
7. McIver MA. An instrument for visualisation of the interior of the common bile duct at operation. 1941;9:112.
8. Jakimowicz J, Mark B, Carol EJ, et al. Post-operative choledochoscopy. A five year experience. *Arch Surg.* 1983;188:810.
9. Stark ME, Loughry CW. Routine operative cholangiography with cholecystectomy. *Surg Gynaecol Obstet.* 1980;151:657.
10. Wheeler BR, Anigian G, Stephens G, et al. Choledochoscopy and common bile duct exploration. *Am Surg.* 1990;56:182.
11. Apelgren KN, Zambos JM, Vargish T. Intraoperative flexible videocholedochoscopy. An improved technique for evaluating the common duct. *Am Surg.* 1990;56:178.
12. Kitano S, Kawanaka H, Tomikawa M, et al. Bleeding from gastric ulcer halted by laparoscopic suture ligation. *Surg Endosc.* 1994;8:405.
13. Mixter CG III, Sullivan CA. Control of proximal gastric bleeding; combined laparoscopic and endoscopic approach. *J Laparoendosc Surg.* 1992;2:105.
14. Branicki FJ, Nathanson LK. Minimal access gastroduodenal surgery. *Aust NZ J Surg.* 1994;64:589.
15. Jacobs M, Verdeja JC, Goldstain HS. Minimally invasive colon resection (laparoscopic colectomy). *Surg Laparosc Endosc.* 1991;1:144.
16. Edelman DS, Jacobs M, Lopez-Penalver C, et al. Safe esophageal bougie placement for laparoscopic hiatal hernia repair. *JSLS.* 1998;2:31.
17. Betachew M, Legrand M, Vincent V, et al. Laparoscopic adjustable gastric banding. *World J Surg.* 1998;22:955.
18. O'Brien PE, Brown WA, Smith A, et al. Prospective study of a laparoscopically placed adjustable gastric band in the treatment of morbid obesity. *Br J Surg.* 1999;85:113.
19. Takekoshi T, Baba V, Ota H, et al. Endoscopic resection of early gastric carcinoma: results of a retrospective analysis of 308 cases. *Endoscopy* 1994;26:352.
20. Phillips EH, Rosenthal RJ. *Operative Strategies in Laparoscopic Surgery.* Springer-Verlag:1995;141.
21. Ohashi S. Laparoscopic intraluminal surgery for early gastric cancer. *Surg Endosc.* 1995;9:169.

Complications of Laparoscopic Surgery

Chapter Eighty-Eight ▪ ▪ ▪ ▪ ▪ ▪

Anesthetic Complications

CARLOS HURTADO

The secret to face and solve any complication is summarized in two Latin words: "pracmonitus pracmunitus"—forewarned is forearmed.[1] The goal is to review the possible complications, prevent them, and to manage them on a timely basis.[2] This can be achieved only by keeping them in mind, having close communication between surgical team members, and training paramedics for emergency situations. Just as in any other type of procedure, these complications are related to the learning curve and may be associated with the operation itself or with the pneumoperitoneum, which may alter the effects of anesthesia.

A morbidity rate of 2% and mortality rate of 0.04% have been reported in 77,604 laparoscopic cholecystectomies. In expert hands laparoscopic surgery is a safe procedure.[3]

COMPLICATIONS DUE TO THE PLACEMENT OF THE VERESS NEEDLE AND TROCARS

One of the complications which may show up when the Veress needle or trocars are placed is bleeding. This complication is due to the perforation of large vessels (e.g., vena cava, iliac artery, or aorta) and occurs in 3 out of every 10,000 procedures.[3] A liver laceration may cause hypovolemia unrelated to the vasodilating effect of the anesthetic agents, a decrease in O_2 saturation as measured by oximetry readings, or a decrease in end-expiratory CO_2 because of diminished pulmonary perfusion. When this happens, we recommend deflation of the pneumoperitoneum, placing the patient in a neutral position, performing fluid infusion, a decrease in anesthetic agents, and conversion to an open procedure.

Uncontrolled CO_2 dissection of soft tissues and the subsequent subcutaneous emphysema and continued absorption during anesthesia may cause a progressive increase in CO_2 as measured by capnography. While this may be difficult to manage, it can be avoided if trocar placement is done carefully, if low intra-abdominal pressures are used, and if changes are made in the respiratory variables at the beginning of the operation.

A lesion of the epigastric vessels can generate significant bleeding that may dissect the abdominal wall and produce hypovolemia, primarily if the surgical time is prolonged. In such a case we suggest that the surgeon inhibit the bleeding from the very beginning.

Retroperitoneal hematoma may cause hypovolemia without any visible evidence of bleeding. This possibility must be kept in mind and should be communicated to the surgical group if hemodynamic changes suggest it.

COMPLICATIONS OF INSUFFLATION

Subcutaneous Emphysema

This complication may occur if the placement of the Veress needle is improper and insufflation is done within the abdominal wall. The CO_2 will then dissect the soft tissue planes and crepitation will be palpable in the area. The risk is of hypercarbia (produced by the very high diffusibility of the CO_2 in the blood) that shows up during the first 15 minutes after surgery has begun.[13] The same thing can happen in retroperitoneal procedures with CO_2 insufflation.[14]

Embolism

Gas embolism was described in 1667 by Francisco Redi. He wrote: "animals die when air is insufflated into their veins." Since then, this has been the subject of extensive research and it remains a threat lurking in every type of surgery; endoscopic surgery is no exception.[1]

Gas embolism[5] occurs when CO_2 leaks into the venous system through a vessel or an open vascular bed in a fashion similar to that seen with open surgery. A gravitational gradient of 5 cm H_2O between the right atrium and the exposed area is enough to cause it to occur.[1] Due to the pneumoperitoneum required for laparoscopic surgery, larger pressure gradients are produced, so the risk of embolism is increased. The factors that can potentially cause gas embolism are the position of the body, depth of ventilation, the central venous pressure, and the gas volume reaching the circulation.[1] When the amount of gas is small, there are rarely any adverse effects because of its great solubility.[6] Small gas embolisms are common and generally go unnoticed.[7] However, large amounts of gas may establish an air trap in the right ventricle, precluding pulmonary flow and causing cardiovascular collapse.

If dispersion of the gas occurs, it passes in boluses into the pulmonary circulation producing an increase in pulmonary pressure. This may result in right heart failure with hypotension, jugular distension, tachycardia, hypoxemia, cyanosis, and sudden and transient increase of CO_2 as seen in capnography, a complication noted by several authors.[6,8–10] Treatment consists of immediate evacuation of the pneumoperitoneum and placing the patient in the Trendelenburg position with left lateralization (Durant's position) to prevent entry of gas into the outgoing tract of the right ventricle. Hyperventilation and suction of gas through a central atrial catheter should also be performed.[3]

Hypercarbia

During anesthesia, hypercarbia caused by excessive CO_2 absorption from the peritoneal cavity and tissues (generally at insufflation pressures of over 30 mm Hg)[11] or by inadequate management of ventilatory parameters may develop. This may cause the patient to develop a compromised acid-base status which can trigger cardiac arrhythmias and even myocardial acidosis, making cardiopulmonary resuscitation difficult if it is needed.[12]

In trying to determine which ventilating pattern is most effective in eliminating the excess CO_2, Hirvonen—in a study performed during laparoscopic hysterectomy—observed that the increase in volume was larger when respiratory rate was modified than when tidal volume was modified.[11]

There may be a higher level of CO_2 absorption during preperitoneal procedures such as surgery for inguinal hernias, since the absorptive surface is increased. In these cases, CO_2 absorption and a decrease in blood pH appear during the first 15 minutes of the procedure.[13] This phenomenon also occurs in retroperitoneal procedures with CO_2 insuflation.[14]

Pneumothorax and Pneumomediastinum

These complications occur as a consequence of passive diffusion of CO_2 through a patent pleuroperitoneal duct (congenital remnant), a diaphragmatic lesion, a direct pleural lesion, or a bronchopleural communication (e.g., rupture of the emphysematous bulla, ventilatory barotrauma). Pneumothorax should be suspected when there is a sudden decrease in saturation as seen on pulse oximetry with an increase in both airway pressure and end-expiratory CO_2 without a decrease in blood pressure.[3,15]

In a tension pneumothorax, treatment is carried out according to the cardiopulmonary status of the patient and the course of the surgery. If the patient is unstable and the procedure is going to be a long one, a pleural tube must be placed. When the patient is stable, positive airway pressure may be applied to improve oxygenation.[13] If the problem was caused by a direct laceration, it must be repaired. This sort of injury is most commonly caused during dissection of the esophageal hiatus or during a cholecystectomy when multiple adhesions have to be dissected.

CARDIAC COMPLICATIONS

Ischemia and Heart Failure

We should always keep in mind that an imbalance between the heart's oxygen supply and demand will result in ischemia that may become evident in different ways during anesthesia or as late as 1 week after surgery. The manifestations vary, and include cardiac arrhythmias, a depressed ST level, and even intraoperative cardiac arrest. For this reason, patients with significant cardiovascular disease should be observed as closely as possible, including the use of invasive monitoring if necessary. This will help provide the required treatment and reduce the incidence of later complications.

In these patients, fluids should be given carefully because if a large load is given with the goal of decreasing the hemodynamic response to the pneumoperitoneum (as recommended by some authors), full-blown heart failure can appear even before the operation has begun. If the patient is also placed in the Trendelenburg position, the situation becomes hard to compensate (especially if the patient is ischemic or has valvular disease) because increasing pressure in the left ventricle wall, increased myocardial oxygen consumption, and diminishing coronary perfusion might result in myocardial ischemia or left ventricular failure with acute pulmonary edema.[16]

Hypertension

Hypertension may become apparent in patients with undiagnosed hypertension or in those who are adequately treated for it, but in whom the pneumoperitoneum triggers an excessive sympathetic response. Continuation of antihypertensive medication even on the day of surgery should induce an adequate cardiovascular status for the operation.

If a hypertensive crisis should occur during the operation, treatment may be carried out with calcium channel blockers, short-acting beta blockers such as esmolol, or intravenous vasodilators such as nitroglycerin or nitroprusside.

Cardiac Arrhythmias

When CO_2 is used, arrhythmias may occur in up to 17% of cases. Most are ventricular extrasystoles that may be generated by acidosis and sympathetic stimulation. Bradycardia may develop in up to 30% of patients, as may sudden asystole during insufflation due to a vasovagal reaction.[3] This is why we recommend the use of atropine before insufflation. It is also recommended that $PaCO_2$ be kept at normal levels and that the pneumoperitoneum be established slowly (1 L/min).[3]

Venous Stasis and Thrombosis

Since the intra-abdominal CO_2 pressure obstructs the flow of the inferior vena cava by increasing venous pressures and decreasing the flow in large veins, there is an increased risk of deep venous thrombosis and pulmonary thromboembolism. Beebe et al[17] reported on a group of patients who had laparoscopic cholecystectomy with a pneumoperitoneum of 14 mm Hg. They found an increase in femoral pressure from 10.2 ± 4.4 mm Hg to 18.2 ± 5.1 mm Hg and a decrease in the speed of flow from 24.9 cm/s to 18.5 cm/s and a reduction of pulsatility in 75% of patients. These changes disappear at the end of the surgical procedure. We always suggest the use of external compression stockings to decrease the risk of this complication.[17]

NEUROPATHY IN EXTREMITIES

This complication may occur in any type of surgery unless careful protection of areas of bone compression, folds, and plexuses is performed with soft pads or water bags. There are patients who are more prone to neuropathy, such as are diabetics, patients with morbid obesity, and those subjected to prolonged operations.[19]

ORGANIC COMPLICATIONS

During prolonged operations cerebral edema may occur, mainly in gynecologic operations with a forced Trendelenburg position because of increases in brain perfusion due to the effect of gravity, which is exacerbated by the vasodilating effect of CO_2. Increases in intraocular pressure are also observed when the patient is placed in this position.

If these occur, rupture of intracranial aneurysms is an ever-present risk that may show up during brain vessel stimulation with CO_2 and sudden hemodynamic changes.

HYPOTHERMIA

This complication is most commonly seen in procedures of long duration, in which there may be a temperature loss of .05°C for every 4 L of CO_2 insufflated, in addition to the vasodilation caused by anesthetic agents. Under these conditions, a prolonged period of CO_2 exchange may cause metabolic acidosis caused by hypothermia in addition to the respiratory acidosis caused by CO_2 retention, both of which can cause arrhythmias.

EXPLOSION

The use of electrocautery during CO_2 pneumoperitoneum carries a risk of explosion when N_2O is used as a part of the anesthesia.[5] This gas diffuses into the peritoneal cavity, and in the presence of methane, which may leak through an intestinal perforation, may create a potentially explosive mixture.[20]

POSTOPERATIVE PAIN

For the pain that follows laparoscopic surgery, the variability of the threshold of each individual must be taken into account. This variability is more marked in laparoscopic procedures.[21] The pain is not comparable to that seen with laparotomy; the duration is shorter and intensity is lower in laparoscopy, but still it can be quite uncomfortable. For its evaluation, we have divided it into three types: shoulder, parietal, and visceral.

Shoulder pain, which has late onset, presents most commonly on the second postoperative day.[22] It can be unilateral or bilateral and is frequently seen in gynecologic procedures.[23] It is attributed to peritoneal irritation caused by the CO_2 and some authors believe that the residual volume remaining after closure of the cavity may contribute. Shoulder pain is present in 35 to 60% of cases.[22]

Visceral pain shows up in the immediate postoperative period and diminishes quickly after the first 24 hours. This sort of pain is not affected by mobilization, but cough can increase the discomfort.

Parietal pain is less intense, and only occurs in the small incisions of the abdominal wall. It increases with contractions of the abdominal wall.

To avoid this complication, several studies were carried out using instillation of local anesthetics such as bupivacaine in the abdominal surface of the diaphragm. Results vary, some with good results[24] and others less so. These differences have been attributed to the doses[25] and dilutions used.[21,23] Analgesia has also been attempted with local opiates, but is ineffective due to the inadequate penetration of the macromolecules into the peritoneum of intact intercostals.[21]

Adverse effects after the intraperitoneal administration of 0.25% bupivacaine have also been reported, such as periods of hypoxemia with an O_2 saturation of less than 92%.[26]

Several IV or IM analgesics such as ketorolac and tromethamine have also been used to decrease pain, particularly in the immediate postoperative period, and these have enjoyed good acceptance.[27] Some authors suggest the use of preoperative ibuprofen (800 mg by mouth) as an alternative in outpatient surgery.[28] Preoperative naproxen has been also used successfully in gynecologic laparoscopy.[29]

Multimodal analgesia is also becoming popular. It consists of preoperative administration of IM meperidine at a dose of 0.6 mg/kg, ketorolac at 0.5 mg/kg, and the infiltration of local anesthetic agents 10 minutes before the surgical incisions are made. Results have been excellent.[30,31]

POSTOPERATIVE NAUSEA AND VOMITING

Nausea and vomiting are still the most common postoperative complications related to anesthesia and may be increased after laparoscopy.[31,34,35] The degree of nausea and vomiting depends on several variables, including the anesthetic technique used and the use of opioids,[33] the duration of pneumoperitoneum, and the susceptibility of each patient. Age, sex, obesity, anxiety, and gastroparesis are also involved, as well the presence of nausea and vomiting with previous anesthesia.[32] Sung and Wetchler[34] recommend the administration of ondansetron (8 mg) before the laparoscopic procedure to avoid this complication. Dodner and White agree, and add that it does not cause cardiorespiratory depression or sedation.[37] Antiemetic effects have been attributed to ephedrine (0.5 mg/kg IM) when used at the end of the operation.[38] Also, recent studies have reported the same effect with good results when propofol is used in subhypnotic doses.[39]

COMPLICATIONS DURING HYSTEROSCOPY

As in every procedure in which solutions are infused into the body, there is a risk of absorption of these solutions and subsequent hemodilution. This may result in hyponatremia, hypocalcemia, embolization, anaphylaxis, and encephalopathy. Other complications are perforation of the uterus, rupture of the fallopian tubes, and hydrosalpinx.[40]

Hemodynamic surveillance in prolonged procedures, the use of diuretics, and close monitoring to determine the need for emergency intubation will help avoid delays in treatment. The aforementioned risk must be kept in mind for urologic procedures in which intravesical solutions are used.

CONCLUSION

Laparoscopy has revolutionized surgery, and in the process influenced the practice of anesthesiology. It is crucial for the anesthesiologist to understand the physiologic stresses of pneumoperitoneum and the nuances of laparoscopic surgery.

REFERENCES

1. Albin M. Embolia gaseosa; embolia II. *Clin Anest NA.* 1993;1.
2. Wolf SJ, Stoeller M. The physiology of laparoscopy: Basic principles, complications and other considerations. *J Urol.* 1994;152:294.
3. Crist DW, Gadacz TR. Complications of laparoscopic surgery. *Surg Clin North Am.* 1993;73:265.
4. Noguchi J, Takagi H, Konishi M. Severe subcutaneous emphysema and hypercapnia during laparoscopic cholecystectomy. *Masui* 1993;42:602.
5. Witgen M, Andrus CH, Fitzgerald D. Analysis of hemodynamic and ventilatory effects of laparoscopic cholecystectomy. *Arch Surg.* 1991;126:997.
6. Yacuob O, Cardona I, Coveler L. Carbon dioxide embolism during laparoscopy. *Anesthesiology* 1982;57:533.
7. Derouin M, Couture P, Boudreault D. Detection of gas embolism by transesophageal echocardiography during laparoscopic cholecystectomy. *Anesth Analg.* 1996;82:119.
8. Schindler E, Muller M, Kelm C. Cerebral carbon dioxide embolism during laparoscopic cholecystectomy. *Anesth Analg.* 1995;81:643.
9. Gilliart T, Etienne B, Bonnard M. Pulmonary interstitial edema after probable carbon dioxide embolism during laparoscopy. *Surg Laparosc Endosc.* 1995;4:327.
10. Moskop R, Lubarsky D. Carbon dioxide embolism during laparoscopic cholecystectomy. *South Med J.* 1994;87:414.
11. Hirvonen A, Nuutinen S, Kauko M. Ventilatory effects, blood gas changes and oxygen consumption during laparoscopic hysterectomy. *Anesth Analg.* 1995;80:961.
12. Maldonado F, Weill H, Tang W, et al. Myocardic hyperbaric acidosis reduces cardiac resuscitability. *Anesthesiology* 1993;78:343.
13. Liem M, Kallewaard JW. Does hypercarbia develop faster during laparoscopic herniorrhaphy than during laparoscopic cholecystectomy? Assessment with continuous blood gas monitoring. *Anesth Analg.* 1995;81:1243.
14. Giebler R, Walz M, Peitgen K. Hemodynamic changes after retroperitoneal CO_2 insufflation for posterior retroperitoneoscopic adrenalectomy. *Anesth Analg.* 1996;82:827.
15. Joris J, Chiche J, Lamy M. Pneumothorax in laparoscopic fundoplication: Diagnosis and treatment with positive end expiratory pressure. *Anesth Analg.* 1995;81:993.
16. Kaplan J. Treatment of perioperative left heart failure. In: Kaplan J. *Cardiovascular Anesthesia.* Grune and Stratton:1963.
17. Beebe DS, McNevin MP, Crain JM. Evidence of venous stasis after abdominal insufflation for laparoscopic cholecystectomy. *Surg Gynecol Obstet.* 1993;171:443.
18. Ortega A, Peters J, Ungson G, et al. Las bases fisiológicas de la cirugía laparoscópica. *Cir Gen.* 1995;17:123.
19. Johnston RD, Lawston NW, Nealon WH. Lower extremity neuropathy after laparoscopic cholecystectomy. *Anesthesiology* 1992;77:835.
20. Neuman CC, Sidebotham S, Nagoianu E. Laparoscopy explosion hazards with nitrous oxide. *Anesthesiology* 1993;70:875.
21. Joris J, Thirty E, Paris P, et al. Pain after laparoscopic cholecystectomy: Characteristics and effect of intraperitoneal bupivacaine. *Anesth Analg.* 1995;81:379.
22. Smith Y, Ding Y, White PF. Muscle pain after outpatient laparoscopy; influence of propofol versus thiopental and enflurane. *Anesth Analg.* 1993;76:1101.
23. Schultz-Steinberg H, Weninger E, Jokisch D. Intraperitoneal versus intrapleural morphine or bupivacaine for pain after laparoscopic cholecystectomy. *Anesthesiology* 1995;82:634.
24. Weber A, Muñoz J, Garteiz D, et al. Use of subdiaphragmatic bupivacaine instillation to control postoperative pain after laparoscopic cholecystectomy. *Surg Laparosc Endosc.* 1997;7(1):6.
25. Rademaker BMP, Kalkman J, Odoom I. Intraperitoneal local anesthetics after laparoscopic cholecystectomy: Effects on postoperative pain, metabolic responses and lung function. *Br J Anesth.* 1994;72:263.
26. Raetzell M, Maier C, Schroeder D. Intraperitoneal application of bupivacaine during laparoscopic cholecystectomy: Risk or benefit? *Anesth Analg.* 1995;81:967.
27. Ding Y, White PF. Comparative effects of ketorolac, dozocine and fentanyl as adjuvants during outpatient anesthesia. *Anesth Analg.* 1992;75:566.
28. Rosemblum M, Weller RS, Contad PL. Ibuprofen provides longer lasting analgesia than fentanyl after laparoscopic surgery. *Anesth Analg.* 1991;73:255.
29. Dunn TJ, Clark VA, Jones G. Preoperative oral naproxen for pain relief after day-case laparoscopic sterilization. *Br J Anesth.* 1995;75:12.
30. Michaloliakou C, Chung F, Sharma S. Preoperative multimodal analgesia facilitates recovery after ambulatory laparoscopic cholecystectomy. *Anesth Analg.* 1996;82:44.
31. Smith I. Anesthesia for laparoscopy with emphasis on outpatient laparoscopy. *Anesthesiol Clin North Am.* 2001;19:21.
32. Watcha M, White P. Postoperative nausea and vomiting. Its etiology, treatment and prevention. *Anesthesiology* 1992;77:162.
33. Okum SS, Colonna R, Horrow JC. Vomiting after alfentanil anesthesia: Effect of dosing method. *Anesth Analg.* 1992;75:550.
34. Sung YF, Wetchler DV. A double blind placebo controlled pilot study examining the effectiveness of intravenous ondansetron in the prevention of postoperative nausea and emesis. *J Clin Anesth.* 1993;5:22.
35. Cunningham AJ. Anesthetic implications of laparoscopic surgery. *Yale J Biol Med.* 1999;71:551.
36. McKenzie R, Kovac A, O'Connor T. Comparison of ondansetron versus placebo to prevent postoperative nausea and vomiting in women undergoing ambulatory gynecologic surgery. *Anesthesiology* 1993;78:21.
37. Dodner M, White PF. Antiemetic efficacy of ondansetron after outpatient laparoscopy. *Anesth Analg.* 1991;73:250.
38. Rothenberg DM, Parnass SM, Litwack K. Efficacy of ephedrine in the prevention of postoperative nausea and vomiting. *Anesth Analg.* 1991;72:58.
39. Borgeat A, Wilde R, Smith S. Subhypnotic doses of propofol possess direct antiemetic properties. *Anesth Analg.* 1992;74:539.
40. Palahniuk R. Clinical pearls. The patient for o'scopy surgery. International Anesthesia Research Society (Suppl.). *Anesth Analg.* 1995;103.

Chapter Eighty-Nine ● ● ● ● ● ●

*P*neumoperitoneum-Related Complications

ALEJANDRO WEBER-SÁNCHEZ, SALVADOR VALENCIA-REYES, and DENZIL GARTEIZ-MARTÍNEZ

INTRODUCTION

In 1938, János Veress published a paper entitled "New device for thoracic and abdominal puncture and for pneumothorax treatment."[1] Since then, the Veress needle has been used for pneumoperitoneum induction in a variety of clinical settings and every surgeon that performs laparoscopic techniques is well acquainted with this device.

Laparoscopic surgery has evolved considerably over the years and new procedures are constantly being developed using this approach. As might be expected, the types of complications encountered vary according to the procedure performed, but one risk factor remains constant for all laparoscopic interventions: pneumoperitoneum-related complications. As a direct result of this, many modifications and techniques for pneumoperitoneum induction have been developed in an attempt to decrease morbidity and mortality.[2–9]

Induction of pneumoperitoneum is an essential part of most laparoscopic interventions. With it, the surgeon is able to convert the virtual intra-abdominal space into a true cavity (Fig. 89–1) in which other instruments can be introduced and maneuvered in order to perform the desired surgical procedure. Problems related to pneumoperitoneum induction have existed ever since laparoscopy was created, and the most likely explanation for these problems is that it is a blind procedure. It involves penetration of the abdominal wall with a fine needle, without the ability to see what structures lie beneath. The most obvious consequence is the possibility of a variety of mechanical injuries to intra-abdominal organs and major blood vessels.

Pneumoperitoneum-related complications are not solely due to induction. The maintenance of an adequate surgical field during the procedure requires a constant flow of gas into the abdominal cavity, which results in changes of intra-abdominal pressure that may affect circulatory and ventilatory functions. The constant exposure of the peritoneal surface to CO_2 leads to alterations in blood-gas constitution, and thus several physiologic changes can be seen. If these changes are not adequately controlled and monitored, severe complications may arise during the procedures that are discussed at length elsewhere in this book.

Pneumoperitoneum-related complications may be divided into two main categories: mechanical and physiologic. Some of the most common problems are shown in Table 89–1 and will be described in this chapter. The fact that these complications may be serious and even fatal in some cases has led many authors to describe different preventive measures for use in induction and maintenance of pneumoperitoneum.

Mechanical Complications

Induction of pneumoperitoneum can be performed with open, partially open, or closed techniques, all of which have been described by various authors. The latter is the one most commonly used, but it is also the one with the highest risk of intra-abdominal injury due to the fact that it is a blind procedure. All of these methods have been associated with injury to underlying structures, and thus no single technique is complication-free. As in open surgery, the likelihood of producing an injury to an intra-abdominal organ is higher when abdominal adhesions are present. For this reason this classification of mechanical lesions has been proposed: Type 1—injuries to normally situated structures (e.g., all major vascular injuries, injuries to normally situated bowel, bladder, and stomach, among others); and Type 2—injuries to structures adherent to the abdominal wall. It is important to differentiate between injuries caused by the Veress needle (Fig. 89–2) and those caused by the primary trocar (Fig. 89–3), because the seriousness of the injury is different for each.

The presence of adhesions should be anticipated when the patient has a history of previous abdominal surgery or peritonitis. It has been reported that up to 34% of patients with a surgical scar

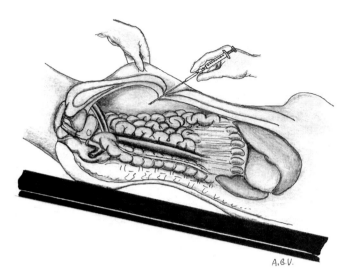

Figure 89–1. Conversion of the virtual intra-abdominal space into a true cavity by the induction of pneumoperitoneum.

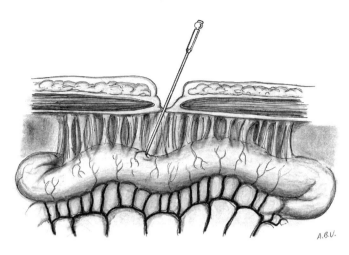

Figure 89–2. Puncture of an intestinal loop with the Veress needle.

near the umbilicus will have adhesions at that site.[10] Some authors have reported adhesions in 21% of patients with Pfannenstiel incisions and in 0.7% of patients with no surgical scars at all.[11] Another study found adhesions in 5% of more than 2000 laparoscopies and of these, only one case had a history of previous laparotomy.[12] What these results show is that closed pneumoperitoneum technique may cause type 2 injuries when adhesions are not suspected.

It is important to mention that injury to intra-abdominal organs is also a problem with conventional open surgery. A study by Krebs of 5700 open gynecologic procedures showed an entry-related injury rate of 0.84%, while analysis of 3700 laparoscopies showed a 0.15% rate of the same problem.[13] As Weston[10] points out, other authors have shown even lower injury rates with closed pneumoperitoneum techniques (Table 89–2).[14–19]

While these reports are mainly of gynecologic procedures, analysis of several large series has reported an overall incidence of visceral injury with needle and first trocar ranging from 0.05 to 0.2%.[20] Clinically significant stomach or intestinal injury rates range from 0.01 to 0.4%,[20,21] but these low figures must be considered with skepticism since many small or insignificant injuries may not be routinely reported or may even go undetected. The ability of the stomach and intestine to heal small lesions spontaneously means that such

cases have no clinical significance. On the other hand, undetected bowel injury may be a major contributor to postoperative mortality and morbidity.[22,23] Such patients may present with postoperative sepsis, peritonitis, intra-abdominal abscesses, and enterocutaneous fistulas. A survey of more than 75,000 laparoscopic cholecystectomies reported a 4.6% mortality rate in patients with gastrointestinal injuries.[24] Adequate nasogastric suction and Trendelenburg position during needle introduction can prevent such injuries. It is

TABLE 89–1. THE MOST COMMON COMPLICATIONS OF PNEUMOPERITONEUM

Mechanical Complications	Physiologic Complications
Abdominal wall bleeding and hematomas	Hypercarbia
Subcutaneous emphysema	Cardiac arrhythmias
Bowel injury	Hypothermia
Major vascular injury	Postoperative emesis
Genitourinary injury	Postoperative drowsiness
Air embolism	
Pneumothorax	
Hypotension due to excess intra-abdominal pressure	
Ventilatory restriction	

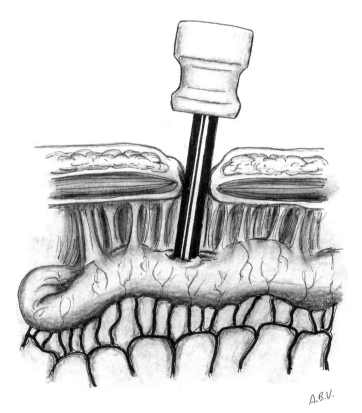

Figure 89–3. Perforation of an intestinal loop with a trocar.

TABLE 89–2. BOWEL AND MAJOR VASCULAR INJURY RATES

Author	Total Laparoscopies	Bowel Injury Rate (%)	Vascular Injury Rate (%)
Mintz[14]	99,204	0.03	0.05
Loeffer[15]	32,719	0.07	
Bergquist[16]	75,035	0.07	
Querleu[17]	17,521	0.04	0.02
Chapron[18]	29,996	0.05	0.02
Harkki-Siren[19]	102,812	0.03	0.01
Total	357,257	0.04	0.02

advisable to carry out the maneuvers described elsewhere in this book to verify that the needle is in the proper position.

The occurrence of complications with the closed technique has led surgeons to develop partially or totally open methods thought to be useful in reducing the incidence of these complications. Nonetheless, the open approach (Hasson's technique) has not proved to completely prevent entry injuries, especially type 2 lesions. The American Association of Gynecologic Laparoscopists[25] presented a report of 80,000 laparoscopies with a bowel injury rate of 1.2% using this approach, although the major vascular injury rate was zero in this series. From these results, Weston[10] concludes that the open technique may be useful in preventing type 1 but not type 2 lesions. If adhesions are suspected near the umbilicus, a different entry site should be considered. Statistically, the least likely site to have adhesions is at the tip of the 9th rib at the costal margin in the left upper quadrant (Palmer's point).[26] In some instances, once access to the abdominal cavity has been achieved at a different site, lysis of adhesions can be performed under direct laparoscopic vision, and additional trocars can be placed with careful dissection (Fig. 89–4).

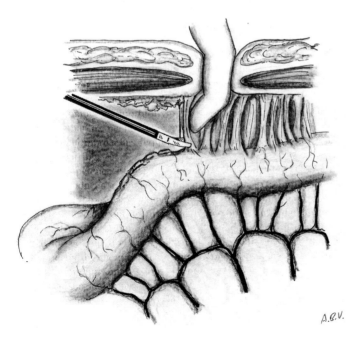

Figure 89–4. Lysis of adhesions under direct laparoscopic vision. In some instances this can be digitally assisted.

Abdominal wall bleeding and hematomas due to needle insertion have been reported but are rare, especially if the needle is introduced at the midline and at the base of the umbilicus. A more serious problem may be encountered when epigastric vessels are injured during trocar placement lateral to the umbilicus. These lesions may cause significant hemorrhage and large abdominal wall hematomas, particularly in elderly patients. If bleeding at these sites cannot be controlled with conventional measures, the trocar should be removed and a Foley catheter inserted. The catheter's balloon is inflated and pulled upward against the abdominal wall, compressing the bleeding site. Direct ligation and/or electrocautery may be used for hemostasis in some instances. The trocar is then placed at a different site. Small lesions of omental or mesenteric blood vessels may be insignificant, but must be observed for progression and inspected carefully at the end of the procedure before the trocars are removed.

On the other hand, the most serious life-threatening laparoscopic complications associated with pneumoperitoneum induction are hemorrhage and air embolism due to large vessel injury. It has been estimated that needle introduction is responsible for approximately 36% of vascular injuries and primary trocar placement for another 32%.[27] A survey of 77,604 laparoscopic cholecystectomies found that 0.05% of major vascular injuries were injuries to the aorta, inferior vena cava, or iliac vessels.[24] The mortality in these patients was 8.8%. Another series of 16 major vascular injuries reported a mortality rate of 13%.[28] An emergency laparotomy should be performed if a major vessel is injured.

Inadequate introduction of the needle into the abdominal cavity leads to tissue insufflation and emphysema. The most common sites of emphysema of this type are in the subcutaneous, preperitoneal, and omental spaces, but retroperitoneal emphysema has also been reported.[29] If detected promptly, these complications have little clinical significance except perhaps for increased postoperative pain and crepitation of the affected area. Resolution is spontaneous and usually takes 24 to 48 hours. Introduction of the tip of the needle into intra-abdominal structures such as the falciform ligament, hollow organs, or major blood vessels may lead to more serious complications. Mechanical injury with the needle tip can be managed by simple observation during the procedure, whereas intramural insufflation into an organ may cause severe damage. Primary repair or resection of the affected organ segment may be necessary and can be performed laparoscopically (Fig. 89–5) or by conversion to laparotomy (Fig. 89–6), according to the surgeon's choice and experience.

Little information has been published with respect to laparoscopic-related genitourinary injuries. Bladder injuries generally occur during needle or trocar insertion, whereas ureteral injury is usually a consequence of a thermal burn, ligation, or laceration caused by inadequate exposure or poor dissection techniques. Bladder catheterization and emptying decreases the risk of needle puncture. Management of bladder injury is similar to that of bowel injury. Veress needle punctures may be managed conservatively with bladder decompression.

Physiologic Complications

Carbon dioxide is the most commonly employed gas for pneumoperitoneum induction in laparoscopic procedures. It is innocuous, easily available, and inexpensive. Its ability to diffuse and dissolve as well as its rapid metabolism in the lungs give it the

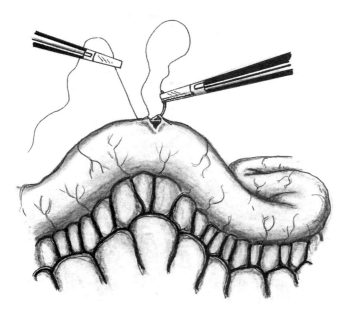

Figure 89–5. Laparoscopic repair of intestinal lesion.

advantage when compared to other gases. The anesthesiologist can "flush" it from the bloodstream by increasing the ventilatory rate and thus its side effects are better controlled.[30] Its uncontrolled absorption through the peritoneum or subcutaneous tissue causes acidosis and hypercarbia, which may lead to cardiac dysrhythmias.[31] These effects are not seen with nitrous oxide pneumoperitoneum,

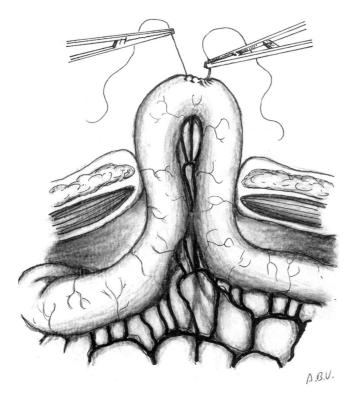

Figure 89–6. Repair of intestinal lesion performed via a small laparotomy.

but it is flammable and may ignite with only a small spark, and may explode when electrocautery or laser devices are used during the procedure.[32,33]

Because of the systemic effects of absorbed CO_2, continuous capnographic monitoring during laparoscopic surgery is mandatory. When CO_2 saturation reaches high levels (the level is variable, but is usually around 45 mm Hg), the anesthesiologist must increase the patient's ventilatory rate or the pneumoperitoneum must be evacuated momentarily. The cardiopulmonary effects of hypercarbia are due to sympathetic reflexes, and may include an increase in heart rate, cardiac contractility, and vasoconstriction, all of which lead to an increase in cardiac output and arterial blood pressure.

Overdistention of the abdomen due to high pneumoperitoneum pressure can interfere with venous blood return and pulmonary compliance. Cautious surveillance of these parameters during the entire procedure is thus important.[34] When the pressure is abnormally high the gas should be evacuated and the anesthesiologist should verify the patient's homeostasis.

A specific intra-abdominal pressure setting for adequate visibility does not exist. Most surgeons currently work at pressures below 15 mm Hg, because at these levels there are fewer problems with mechanical ventilation or the dissection of anatomic planes by the gas. The authors prefer lower pressures, around 10 to 12 mm Hg, especially in patients with restrictive pulmonary problems, those in whom hiatal surgery is being performed, and during pregnancy. The maintenance of low pressures is very important when laparoscopic procedures are performed under regional anesthesia because abdominal distention greatly increases the ventilatory workload and patients can develop respiratory complications. Our group routinely employs and recommends general endotracheal anesthesia. Although initially surgeons were unwilling to perform laparoscopy in sedated patients, enthusiasm for diagnostic laparoscopic procedures in ambulatory patients has increased, particularly for gynecologic procedures, and insufflation pressures between 8 to 10 mm Hg are recommended in these situations.

Pneumothorax may occur during upper abdominal procedures when injury occurs to the diaphragm, resulting in a sudden collapse of the lung on the affected side. Occasionally, however, pneumothorax may develop without diaphragmatic injury, possibly as a result of retroperitoneal dissection of CO_2. This may have a subtler onset manifested by increased ventilatory pressures and arterial oxygen desaturation. Treatment in either instance is by insertion of a thoracostomy tube.

Reports of gas embolism are unusual and have ranged from 0.002 to 0.0016%. The etiology is presumably venous injury combined with high insufflation pressures. Signs of gas embolus include circulatory collapse, an abrupt increase in end-tidal CO_2, a so-called millwheel cardiac murmur, and flash pulmonary edema. Cardiac arrhythmias may also occur, and electrocardiographic alterations including a widened QRS complex may be evident. Treatment consists of placing the patient in Trendelenburg position with the left side down (the Durant position) to prevent the gas from entering the pulmonary outflow tract, aspiration of the gas with a central venous catheter, and external cardiac massage to break up large bubbles.[31]

Drowsiness and emetic sequelae have been found to have a close relationship with the amount of CO_2 used, so this fact should always be kept in mind when planning postoperative management.[35]

CONCLUSIONS

After reviewing the different pneumoperitoneum-related complications and analyzing the results with different techniques, it can be concluded that no single method, open or closed, can claim to be overwhelmingly superior. Laparoscopists should therefore acquaint themselves with most of these procedures and use them appropriately on an individualized basis with each patient. The presence of previous surgical scars or the suspicion of intra-abdominal adhesions warrants special care when deciding the type and site of entry. Open techniques do not prevent type 2 injuries although they may be useful in preventing type 1 lesions and are particularly useful in preventing major vascular injuries. These methods should be reserved for very thin patients without previous surgical scars. Closed techniques should be performed far from the site of surgical scars and if the umbilicus is selected, the incision should be in the base of the umbilicus.

Intra-abdominal pressure should be kept at a level low enough to allow adequate visibility and safe maneuvering. Constant capnographic, ventilatory, and circulatory monitoring is essential in any laparoscopic procedure, and both anesthesiologists and surgeons must be well acquainted with methods of prompt detection and management of potential physiologic and mechanical complications.

REFERENCES

1. Sandor J, Ballagi F, Nagy A, et al. A needle-puncture that helped to change the world of surgery: Homage to János Veress. *Surg Endosc.* 2000;14:201.
2. Weber SA, Serrano BF, Cueto GJ. Puntos claves para facilitar la técnica en cirugía endoscópica. *Cirujano General* 1994;16:25.
3. Weber SA, Serrano BF, Cueto GJ. Puntos claves para facilitar la técnica en cirugía endoscópica. *Cirujano General* 1994;17:88.
4. Rosen DM, Lam AM, Chapman M, et al. Methods of creating pneumoperitoneum: a review of techniques and complications. *Obstet Gynecol Surv.* 1998;53:167.
5. Jacobson MT, Helmy M, Smith KS, et al. Transumbilical direct trocar entry for operative videolaparoscopy. *Obstet Gynecol.* 2000;95(4 Suppl 1):S33.
6. Galen DI. Improved patient outcomes using a radially expandable access device for laparoscopic surgery. *Obstet Gynecol.* 2000;95(4 Suppl 1):S27
7. Santala M, Jarvela I, Kauppila. A transfundal insertion of a Veress needle in laparoscopy of obese subjects: a practical alternative. *Hum Reprod.* 1999;14:2277.
8. Schiavaon CA, Schaffa TD. Avoiding complications in closed pneumoperitoneum (umbilicus lifting) insufflation, retaining good cosmetic results. *Surg Endosc.* 1995;9:543(letter).
9. Weber SA, Serrano BF, Cueto GJ. Técnicas de neumoperitoneo. In: Sepúlveda AC, ed. *Cirugía Laparoscópica.* Ediciones Video Cirugía 1993;1:121.
10. Weston UJ. Personal communication received via e-mail via SURGINET.
11. Audebert AJM. The role of microlaparoscopy for safer wall entry: Incidence of umbilical adhesions according to past surgical history. *Gynaecological Endosc.* 1999;8(6):363.
12. Bateman BG, Kolp LA, Hoeger K. Complications of laparoscopy—operative or diagnostic. *Fertil Steril.* 1996;66:30.
13. Krebs HB. Intestinal injury in gynecologic surgery: a ten-year experience. *Am J Obstet Gynecol.* 1986;155:509.
14. Minz M. Risks and prophylaxis in laparoscopy: A survey of 100,000 cases. *J Reprod Med.* 1977;18:269.
15. Loffer FD, Pent D. Indications, contraindications and complications of laparoscopy. *Obstet Gynecol Surv.* 1975;30:407.
16. Bergqvist D, Bergqvist A. Vascular injuries during gynaecological surgery. *Acta Obstet Gynecol Scand.* 1987;66:19.
17. Querleu D, Chevallier L, Chapron C, et al. Complications of gynecological laparoscopic surgery. A French collaborative study. *Gynaecological Endosc.* 1993;2:3.
18. Chapron C, Querleu D, Bruhat MA, et al. Surgical complications of diagnostic and operative gynaecological laparoscopy: a series of 29,966 cases. *Human Reprod.* 1998;13:867.
19. Harkki-Siren P. Kurki T. A nationwide analysis of laparoscopic complications. *Obstet Gynecol.* 1997;89(1):108.
20. Crist DW, Gadacz TR: Complications of laparoscopic surgery. *Surg Clin North Am.* 1993;73:265.
21. Flowers JL, Zucker KA, Bailey RW: Complications. In: Ballantyne GH, Leahy PF, Medlin IM, eds. *Laparoscopic Surgery.* Saunders:1994;77.
22. Broten M. *Laparoscopic Complications: Prevention and Management.* BC Decker:1980.
23. Erickson LD. Insufflation needle insertion techniques: management of perforation of bowel and bladder. In: Corfman RS, Diamond MP, DeCherney A, eds. *Complications of Laparoscopy and Hysteroscopy.* Blackwell Scientific:1993;22.
24. Deziel DJ, Millikan KW, Economou SG, et al. Complications of laparoscopic cholecystectomy: A national survey of 4292 hospitals and an analysis of 77,604 cases. *Am J Surg.* 1993;165:9.
25. Levy BS, Hulka JF, Peterson HB, et al. Operative Laparoscopy: American Association of Gynecologic Laparoscopists, 1993 survey. *J Am Assoc Gynecologic Laparoscopists.* 1994;1:301.
26. Garry R. Complications of laparoscopic entry. *Gynaecological Endosc.* 1997;6:319.
27. Yuzpe AA. Pneumoperitoneum needle and trocar injuries in laparoscopy: a survey on possible contributing factors and prevention. *J Reprod Med.* 1990;35:485.
28. Baadsgaard SE, Bille S, Egeblad K. Major vascular injury during gynecologic laparoscopy: Report of a case and review of published cases. *Acta Obstet Gynecol Scand.* 1989;68:283.
29. Smith S. Minimizing, recognizing and managing laparoscopic complications. In: Azziz R, Alvarez MA, eds. *Practical Manual of Operative Laparoscopy and Hysteroscopy.* Springer:1996;248.
30. Liu S, Leighton T, Davis I, et al. Prospective analysis of cardiopulmonary responses to laparoscopic cholecystectomy. *Laparoendosc Surg.* 1991;1:241.
31. Scott DB, Julian DG. Observation on cardiac arrhythmias during laparoscopy. *Br Med J.* 1972;1:411.
32. Hunter JG, Staheli J, Oddsdottir M, et al. Nitrous oxide pneumoperitoneum revisited. *Surg Endosc.* 1995;9:501.
33. Staheli J, Bordelon B, Hunter JG. Nitrous oxide pneumoperitoneum: No need to fear. *Surg Endosc.* 1991;1:26(abstract).
34. Hirvonen EA, Poikolainen EO, Paakkonen ME, et al. The adverse hemodynamic effects of anesthesia, head-up tilt, and carbon dioxide pneumoperitoneum during laparoscopic cholecystectomy. *Surg Endosc.* 2000;14:272.
35. Koivusalo AM, Kellokumpu I, Lindgren L. Postoperative drowsiness and emetic sequelae correlate to total amount of carbon dioxide used during laparoscopic cholecystectomy. *Surg Endosc.* 1997;11:42.

Chapter Ninety • • • • • •

Complications of Electrosurgery

TOMÁS BARRIENTOS-FORTES

INTRODUCTION

There are many beneficial aspects of electrosurgical cutting and co-agulating techniques. The major contribution of electrosurgery has been to drastically reduce both blood loss and operative time, resulting in reduced morbidity and mortality.

In 1928 Harvey Cushing published one of the first articles on the use of an electrosurgical unit designed by William. T. Bovie for the removal of cranial tumors.[1] Today, electrogenerators have become finely tuned instruments that offer many versatile ways for the contemporary surgeon to harness and deliver electric energy to tissue in a precise or broad manner to obtain a desired effect. A knowledge of the biophysics of electrical energy's effect on tissues and safety considerations related to these devices are the places to begin understanding these surgical tools.

For optimal results with these techniques, the surgeon carrying out the procedure should use highly technical equipment, and have formal training in its use. Above all, the surgeon must adhere rigidly to guidelines for appropriate technique. Deviation from these will most assuredly result in complications and even death.

Electrophysics and its application to surgery, in particular endoscopic surgery, is a unique science. Usually there is little attention paid to the principles of the physics involved with electrosurgery when surgeons receive their formal training in the technical aspects of its use. Most training programs consider the discipline of electrosurgery as a skill that is left for the student to learn first-hand on the job, and the skills and knowledge of the average professor have been gained over a process of learning how to use them over a period of years.[2] As a result, many myths have been perpetuated over the years since William Bovie introduced the first electrosurgical diathermy machine that used high-frequency radio waves instead of heat to destroy human tissue.

An awareness of the hazards of diathermy together with an understanding of the mechanisms of injury should enable the surgeon to dissect tissue and achieve hemostasis, while at the same time decreasing the risk of serious complications to the patient.

Surgical diathermy performs its function by the application of high-density radio frequency current, which can be used to cut or coagulate tissue. Its improper use can result in electrical burns and even electrocution.[3]

Surgical diathermy (electrocoagulation) operates on the principle that high-frequency current can be passed through the body with no effects other than the production of heat. The amount of heat produced by the current is inversely proportional to the electrode area.

TYPES OF ELECTROSURGICAL INSTRUMENTS

There are two types of diathermy electrodes in widespread use: monopolar and bipolar. Their principles of action, risk factors, and benefits are somewhat different. Their properties will be addressed separately. Ultrasonic scalpels will be discussed in a later section (Table 90–1).

Monopolar Diathermy

The use of monopolar electrosurgical energy has been the gold standard for the past 50 years. It has diverse capabilities, such as fulguration, precise vaporization, and coaptation of large vessels.

With a monopolar diathermy probe, one electrode (the return electrode or ground plate) is large, with an average area of about 100 cm^2. The other electrode is small, usually less than 1 cm^2 in size. The small one is also known as the **active electrode** and it controls the current density. The current density is expressed as the current per unit area. The rate of heat production and the resulting therapeutic effect are a direct function of the current density and depend on: (1) the applied voltage, (2) the area of the active electrode in contact with the tissue, and (3) the tissue resistance.

Electrical current enters the patient through the active electrode and exits through the return electrode. It is important for the latter to have a large surface area in order to shield the patient against high current flow. A continuous high-frequency current produces a cutting effect, while an intermittent high-frequency current causes coagulation of vessels with little or no cutting. Hemostasis alone is accomplished when the waveform is pulsed (or

TABLE 90–1. ADVANTAGES AND DISADVANTAGES OF THE DIFFERENT INSTRUMENTS USED IN ELECTROSURGERY

Instrument	Advantages	Disadvantages
Monopolar electrocautery	Diverse effects, fulguration, cutting, coagulation, etc. Less expensive, widespread availability	Electrical energy is quickly diffused in the surrounding tissue. There is evidence of tissue damage, mainly due to poor trocar insulation. Works poorly in the presence of blood and saline solution. Possible interaction with pacemakers.
Bipolar electrocautery	Functions at a much lower power output. Current is largely concentrated at the tip of the instrument (up to 2 mm). Cells are instantly charred and dehydrated. Safe to use around pacemakers and excitable tissues.	The instrument has to be changed in order to dissect, cut, or coagulate. Its low energy output is insufficient to coagulate larger blood vessels. Expensive.
Harmonic scalpel	The same instrument is able to cut, dissect, and coagulate. Tissue denaturation with production of water vapor and and cell debris is accomplished in a clean, bloodless manner with limited penetration of the ultrasonic wave.	Decreased availability and increased expense. Coagulates vessels up to 5 mm in diameter.

Adapted from Redenbach HD, Buess G, Keckstein J. Ancillary technology: Electrocautery, thermocoagulation and laser. In: Cuschieri A, Buess G, Perissat J, eds. *Operative Manual of Endoscopic Surgery.* Springer-Verlag: 1992:43.

damped) on and off, with the on times being one-fifth to one-tenth as long as the off times. A modified or blended effect of cutting and coagulation is produced by greater on and off time ratios.

In a monopolar electrode, electrical energy is relatively quickly diffused into the surrounding tissue. Monopolar electrosurgery works better in dry conditions than bipolar electrosurgery. The monopolar electrode works poorly in blood and saline solution because of the low resistance it presents to the current, and the alternate paths divert much of the current away from the tissue directly under the electrode.

Monopolar methods tend to favor hemostasis in deeper tissues, which makes them ideal for hemostasis in submucosal and muscular areas. This penetration is also one of its disadvantages, as it is a significant cause of complications associated with its use.

The introduction of laparoscopic surgery has led to new developments in electrosurgical instrumentation and operative technique. The monopolar hook electrode is a device specially created for laparoscopic surgery. Its safety has been proven for organ dissection, mainly in cholecystectomy.[4]

Bipolar Diathermy

The availability of newly developed bipolar and multipolar surgical instruments for cutting and coagulating without changing instruments and at low or high frequency power opened up a new dimension in laparoscopically assisted electrosurgery.[5]

Bipolar electrodes function at a much lower power output than monopolar electrodes.[6] They are also safer and should be used in preference to monopolar diathermy, especially in anatomically crowded areas. With the bipolar electrode, current density is largely concentrated at the tip because tissue contact completes a circuit between two wires 3 mm apart. In bipolar diathermy the cells are instantly charred and dehydrated, obstructing the passage of current to adjacent tissue, avoiding damage to it.

COMPLICATIONS OF ELECTROSURGERY

As a source of high energy in the operating theatre, there are hazards attendant to the use of electrosurgery.[50] To minimize the potential for complications it is essential to have an in-depth knowledge of their operating principles.[7] Moreover, since high-frequency signals are involved, the nature of machine-patient interactions can create a potentially hazardous situation that is not easily identifiable. Stray electric and magnetic fields have been measured near therapeutic and surgical diathermy equipment. The fields associated with electrosurgical units operating at frequencies of 0.3 to 0.5 MHz only approach reference levels within 20 to 30 cm of the cables, and because of the relatively short duration of the emissions, precautions are considered unnecessary.[8]

The significant hazards of electrosurgery while in use include explosion of combustible mixtures including anesthetic gases and bowel gas; interference with instruments and pacemakers; stimulation of excitable tissues, which on occasion has caused ventricular fibrillation; and accidental radio frequency burns.[9]

Though the rate of incidents is low in terms of the number per 100,000 procedures, individual accidents can be catastrophic and traumatic to both the patient and surgical team. The overall incidence of recognized injuries is between 1 and 2 patients per 1000 operations. The majority go unrecognized at the time of the electrical insult, and commonly present 3 to 7 days afterward with fever and pain in the abdomen. Also, not surprisingly the majority of injuries are caused by monopolar diathermy.

Lack of knowledge and insufficient attention on the part of laparoscopic surgeons and operating room personnel may result in electrosurgical accidents. Electrical burns sustained during laparoscopy have long been recognized as a serious problem.[10]

Electrosurgical injuries occur during laparoscopic operations and are potentially serious. Frequently, litigation results from these accidents. Though the hazards cannot be eliminated, the probability of an incident can be minimized by using careful technique. Because of the safety benefits of bipolar electrosurgical devices as opposed to monopolar, their use is advocated, particularly in view of the anticipated increase in litigation costs.[11]

A common factor in all burns is that the user is not sufficiently familiar with electrosurgery, its power, and its possible dangers. The simplest way to avoid burns is to educate those engaged in electrosurgery about these matters.

PATHOPHYSIOLOGY OF ELECTROSURGICAL COMPLICATIONS

The pathophysiology of electrosurgical complications in real-time laparoscopic procedures remains speculative. From the physics of electrosurgery and heat production, it can be shown that a residual voltage across the neutral electrode plays a dominant role. Monitoring this voltage and processing it appropriately will open up new possibilities in avoiding burns.[12]

Capacitive coupling between unipolar instruments and 10-mm operating laparoscopes requires relatively high generator output to cause serosal injury. Lower generator output settings may cause injury with electrosurgical generators capable of higher voltages.[13] In 1978 and 1979, two women in the United States were reported to have died from electrical complications following sterilization with unipolar coagulating devices.[14]

In the early phases of therapeutic laparoscopy, complication rates secondary to the use of monopolar diathermy were reportedly as high as 7.7% in some series.[15] More recently these frequencies have significantly decreased to less than 1%.[16,17] There is a low but real potential for inadvertent serious electrical burns during laparoscopic procedures.[18–22]

To decrease the frequency of complications, some innovative safety features have been devised. The addition of an autostop feature to some monopolar diathermy units has made them safer to use. This circuit detects the rising impedance as the tissues are desiccated and automatically shuts off the power.[23]

Burns Related to the Port Site

Direct and capacitive coupling of diathermy current has been reported to be a cause of occult injury during surgical laparoscopy. Plastic cannulas afforded no greater protection from skin burns than metal cannulas. Burns may result from direct or capacitive coupling to metal cannulas or capacitive coupling to the skin edge across plastic cannulas. There is potential for burns to other tissues that are also in close proximity to a cannula used for electrosurgery.[24] The adaptation of active electrode monitoring for stray energy as a result of insulation failure or capacitive coupling and the use of completely metal trocar cannulas will increase the confidence of the surgeon and the safety of the patient.[25]

The two factors that probably contributed most to the bowel burns that have occurred during monopolar laparoscopy were the use of higher-than-necessary voltages and the electrical isolation of the treated organ. To minimize the risk of port-site burns the surgeon should use low peak voltages.[26]

By using monopolar electrosurgery during laparoscopy the surgeon decreases the risk of secondary sparking. Under some conditions, the chances for distal burns may increase by forcing the entire electric current through narrow structures.[27] Another potential problem of monopolar electrosurgery relates to unrecognized energy transfer (stray current) outside the view of the laparoscope.

Capacitive coupling poses the greatest risk for injury when the outer conductor (trocar cannula or irrigation cannula) is electrically isolated from the abdominal wall by nonconducting plastic. The risk of capacitive coupling is increased by use of the coagulation mode (versus cutting mode), an open circuit (versus tissue contact with the electrode), 5-mm cannulas (versus 11-mm cannulas), and higher-voltage generators.[28] Thus metal trocar sleeves are recommended for use with the monopolar, single-puncture technique only.[26]

The safety of electrosurgery can be improved by educating surgeons about the biophysics of radio frequency electrical energy, technical choices in instruments using all-metal cannula systems, and engineering developments including dynamically monitored systems to detect insulation failure and capacitive coupling.

Mechanisms of stray current and unrecognized tissue injury include: (1) insulation breaks in electrodes; (2) capacitive coupling, or induced currents through the intact insulation of the active electrode to surrounding cannulas or other instruments; and (3) direct coupling (or unintended contact) between the active electrode and other metal instruments or cannulas within the abdomen.

Tissue Injury

Irreversible tissue damage because of protein denaturation occurs in the temperature range of 55 to 60°C.[29]

Ramsay et al[30] compared the intraluminal tissue heat from both types of electrodes applied to rabbit bladders. They found an average increase of 19.9°C above core temperature in the lumen adjacent to the monopolar electrode, which was probably sufficient to cause protein denaturation. In contrast, the bipolar technique produced a maximum temperature rise of only 3.5°C under similar circumstances.[30]

Because tissue damage is a delayed phenomenon, severe complications may take days to become apparent. Intervals from time of injury to onset of symptoms vary from 18 hours to 14 days.[31] It is very important to realize that monopolar burns can occur at a site distant from the application, particularly in the presence of staples or metal clips.

At laparotomy, the appearance of both traumatic and electrical injuries is the same: a white area of necrosis usually surrounds the perforation. Microscopic examination of thermal injuries shows persistence of necrotic tissue without a leukocytic infiltrate.[32]

Histologic analysis (in pigs and dogs) showed characteristics of electrosurgical damage that included areas of complete necrosis and coagulation, perivascular changes, endothelial damage, and hyperchromic pyknotic nuclei. White cell infiltration was seen only at the margin of necrotic zones of coagulation.[33]

The wide spectrum of histology from electrosurgical burns is primarily a result of the area that is sampled. The diameter of injury with either technique may be more closely related to the electrode diameter than the amount of current passed. The tissue necrosis resulting from misuse of diathermy varies directly with the duration, energy, and force of electrode application.

There are certain advantages of bipolar over monopolar diathermy: it operates at lower current levels, thereby reducing nerve and muscle stimulation; there is no possibility of sparking; it can operate in normal saline solutions; and there is no capacitance effect, possibly because of a canceling of the waveform. Bipolar diathermy also significantly reduces the production of smoke.

The main criticism of bipolar diathermy is that it is more difficult to use. Its low energy output may be insufficient to coagulate larger blood vessels, a fact contested by some neurosurgeons. A further drawback is the adherence of coagulated tissue to the bipolar forceps, which may require repeated cleaning.

OTHER COAGULATION DEVICES

Electrosurgical burns are said to be the most common electrical hazards in operating rooms,[34] so the search for innovations in electrosurgical dissectors and coagulators is a vast field for research. New devices with safer and more sophisticated ways to use energy for surgical purposes are being continuously added to the surgical armamentarium.

Laparoscopic procedures often require an energy source to provide hemostatic dissection. The safety of the argon beam coagulator makes it an acceptable alternative to electrosurgical coagulation, and it allows the surgeon to operate in a smokeless field. Hemostatic tissue electrocoagulation is rapidly achieved without the coagulator contacting the tissue, and it is easy to apply laparoscopically.[35] The prototype 10-mm argon beam delivery probe is cumbersome, and the argon gas flow rate of 4 L/min when in use requires constant venting of the peritoneum with close monitoring of intraperitoneal pressures.

The ultrasonic scalpel (harmonic scissors) may be another good alternative to conventional electrosurgical techniques. The basic physics behind the ultrasonically-activated scalpel and shears have been carefully analyzed to demonstrate the disadvantages and hazards of other energy modalities.[36] The experience reported in common clinical settings will determine its place in surgical practice.

ISSUES RELATED TO ULTRASONIC SURGERY

The harmonic scalpel is one of the greatest recent innovations for the laparoscopic surgeon. It combines in a single instrument the ability to cut, coagulate, and dissect, and it accomplishes these tasks in a clean, bloodless, and noncharring manner.

The first reports of the use of ultrasonic energy applied to surgical procedures date back to 1996.[37] The biophysics of this type of energy indicates that the transfer of heat is produced by the rapid motion (55,000 cycles per minute) of the tip of the instrument.[38]

The ultrasonic scalpel has three main parts. The first is a piezoelectric device. It produces dynamic motion that is transmitted through a cable to the moving parts that do the cutting. The second part is a detachable cable through which energy is dispatched to the surgical field. The third piece is a disposable tip that can be fitted with instrument tips of different shapes and sizes.

According to the task at hand, the surgeon can choose the tip that will enhance the efficacy of the procedure he or she intends to perform. If the technique requires fine dissection, the surgeon can choose to use a fine hook or a beveled tip. These tips are ideal for the dissection of anatomic planes, facilitating the detachment of organs such as the stomach, spleen, gallbladder, pancreas, adrenal glands, or uterus.[39-44]

The physical interaction between the fast-moving tip and the loose connective tissue will facilitate plane dissection. Cells and fibers are instantly affected, and the products of tissue denaturation are water vapor and cellular debris. These products will flow through the pathways of least resistance. The surgeon can see an active process that will automatically separate planes with ease and safety. This phenomenon is known as a **cavitation effect** and is characteristic of the use of this kind of energy.[45]

As tissues separate, capillaries that travel within the connective tissue also undergo denaturation. As a result, the blood within their lumen coagulates, producing a bloodless dissection field. The energy sent into tissue travels only a few millimeters away from the surgical plane. The penetration of the ultrasonic waves is restricted, limiting the necrotic effect to tissue that is in direct contact with the scalpel tip.[46]

If the technique requires severance of ligaments or large blood vessels, there is a clipping tip that resembles a pair of jaws. One of the jaws is connected to the moving cable through a disposable tip, while the other jaw is fixed, containing a hard plastic piece. The moving jaw closes against the plastic piece mounted on the opposite jaw, holding the tissue in between. The energy travels between these two parts of the scalpel tip, and denatures tissue by the process explained above.

There are several different harmonic scissors on the market. They vary according to manufacturer, but all follow the same basic principles. Their differences lie in the size and shape of their jaws. There are 10-mm and 5-mm instruments, and the tips can be straight or slightly curved. They are designed to fit different surgeons' preferences and needs.

With the harmonic scalpel one can coagulate and cut any kind of tissue. The instrument has variable energy output of different levels. Primarily, there are five different settings that correlate more or less with the different settings used for electrosurgery. With the ultrasonic device one can coagulate by utilizing low energy levels. The lower the level, the more intermittent the delivery of energy, and thus the more coagulating effect produced. As the energy level increases, tip motion is more continuous, increasing the cutting effect of the instrument. The surgeon can change the level by setting it ahead of time, or by using foot pedals during the procedure.

The tension applied to the tissue by grasping it with the instrument determines the degree of energy that flows into it. The tighter it is held, the faster the energy gets transmitted, producing more denaturation.

With the harmonic scalpel one can coagulate and cut small and medium-sized vessels. Kanehira et al[47] determined that a blood vessel cut with a harmonic scissors can withstand pressures as high as 353 mm Hg before bursting. These are pressures far above physiological ranges. This also makes it possible to use the harmonic scalpel for cutting blood vessels without sutures, ligation, or clips. We have described a cholecystectomy technique in which a single ligation of the cystic duct is the entire ligation requirement for the procedure.[48] The utilization of this kind of ultrasonic energy will enhance the surgeon's capability to minimize the use of foreign material needed for the accomplishment of hemostasis.

A large percentage of complications described from use of laparoscopic techniques occur because of improper tissue dissection and control of bleeding with clips and electrosurgical techniques.[49] The design of novel laparoscopic surgical techniques that replace the clips and electrocautery with ultrasonic scalpels will likely diminish the complication rate seen in today's laparoscopic practice.

Laparoscopic techniques will continue to improve. There will always be new additions and better ways to deliver surgical care for our patients. However, there will always remain risks that will require technical solutions.

REFERENCES

1. Cushing IL. Electrosurgery as an aid to the removal of intracranial tumors. Surg Gynecol *Obstet.* 1928;17:751.

2. Soderstrom RM. Electrosurgical injuries during laparoscopy: prevention and management. Curr Opin Obstet Gynecol. 1994;6:248.

3. Watson AB, Loughman J. The surgical diathermy: principles of operation and safe use. Anaesth Intensive Care. 1978;6:310.

4. Metzger A, Z'graggen K, Klaiber C. Monopolar current, with particular attention to hook dissection in laparoscopic cholecystectomy. Endosc Surg Allied Technol. 1994;2:172.

5. Mueller W. The advantages of laparoscopic assisted bipolar high-frequency surgery. Endosc Surg Allied Technol. 1993;1:91.

6. Tucker RD, Kramolowsky EV, Bedell E, Platz CE. A comparison of urologic application of bipolar versus monopolar: five French electrosurgical probes. J Urol. 1989;141:662.

7. Cali RW. Laparoscopy. Surg Clin North Am. 1980;60:407.

8. Tzima E, Martin CJ. An evaluation of safe practices to restrict exposure to electric and magnetic fields from therapeutic and surgical diathermy equipment. Physiol Meas. 1994;15:201.

9. Pearce J. Current electrosurgical practice: hazards. J Med Eng Technol. 1985;9:107.

10. Neufeld GR, Johnstone RE, Garcia CR, et al. Letter: Electrical burns during laparoscopy. JAMA. 1973;226:1465.

11. Tucker RD, Hollenhorst MJ. Bipolar electrosurgical devices. Endosc Surg Allied Technol. 1993;1:110.

12. Nduka CC, Super PA, Monson JR, et al. Cause and prevention of electrosurgical injuries in laparoscopy. J Am Coll Surg. 1994;179:161.

13. Grosskinsky CM, Ryder RM, Pendergrass HM, et al. Laparoscopic capacitance: a mystery measured. Experiments in pigs with confirmation in the engineering laboratory. Am J Obstet Gynecol. 1993;169:1632.

14. Peterson HB, Ory HW, Greenspan JR, et al. Deaths associated with laparoscopic sterilization by unipolar electrocoagulating devices, 1978 and 1979. Am J Obstet Gynecol. 1981;15;139.

15. Lane GE. Lathrop JC. Comparison of results of KTP/532 laser versus monopolar electrosurgical dissection in laparoscopic cholecystectomy. J Laparoendosc Surg. 1993;3:209.

16. Baggish MS, Lee WK, Miro SJ, et al. Complications of laparoscopic sterilization. Comparison of 2 methods. Obstet Gynecol. 1979;54:54.

17. Galbinski S, Varela MAS, Garcia F. Electrosurgical injuries in gynecologic laparoscopy. J Am Assoc Gynecol Laparosc. 1996;3(4, Suppl):S13.

18. Koetsawang S, Srisupandit S, Cole LP. Laparoscopic electrocoagulation and tubal ring techniques for sterilization: a comparative study. Int J Gynaecol Obstet. 1978;15:455.

19. Seow-Choen F, Cheah LK, Eu KW, et al. Bladder injury during laparoscopic abdominoperitoneal resection. Br J Surg. 1996;83:426.

20. Winslow PH, Kreger R, Ebbesson B, et al. Conservative management of electrical burn injury of ureter secondary to laparoscopy. Urology. 1986;27:60.

21. Martin RF, Rossi RL. Bile duct injuries. Spectrum, mechanisms of injury, and their prevention. Surg Clin North Am. 1994;74:781.

22. Horvath KD. Strategies for the prevention of laparoscopic common bile duct injuries. Surg Endosc. 1993;7:439.

23. Phillips AG. Lateral heat spread with bipolar diathermy during laparoscopic hysterectomy. J Am Assoc Gynecol Laparosc. 1995;2(4, Suppl):S42.

24. Willson PD, Van der Walt JD, Moxon D, et al. Port site electrosurgical (diathermy) burns during surgical laparoscopy. Surg Endosc. 1997; 11:653.

25. Odell RC. Electrosurgery: principles and safety issues. Clin Obstet Gynecol. 1995;38:610.

26. Harris FW. Electrosurgery in laparoscopy. J Reprod Med. 1978;21:48.

27. Saye WB, Miller W, Hertzmann P. Electrosurgery thermal injury. Myth or misconception? Surg Laparosc Endosc. 1991;1:223.

28. Voyles CR, Tucker RD. Education and engineering solutions for potential problems with laparoscopic monopolar electrosurgery. Am J Surg. 1992;164:57.

29. Beisand HO, Stranden F. Rectal temperature monitoring during neodymium-YAG laser irradiation for prostatic carcinoma. Urol Res. 1984;12:257.

30. Ramsay JW, Shepard NA, Buttler M, et al. A comparison of bipolar and monopolar diathermy probes in experimental animals. Urol Res. 1985;13:99.

31. Loffler FD, Pent D. Indications, contraindications and complications of laparoscopy. Obstet Gynecol Surv. 1975;30:407.

32. Levy BS, Soderstorm RM, Dali DH. Bowel injuries during laparoscopy: gross anatomy and histology. J Reprod Med. 1985;30:168.

33. Tucker RD, Platz CE, Landas SK. Histologic characteristics of electrosurgical injuries. J Am Assoc Gynecol Laparosc. 1997;4:201.

34. Irnich W. How to avoid surface burns during electrosurgery. Med Instrum. 1986;20:320.

35. Daniell J, Fisher B, Alexander W. Laparoscopic evaluation of the argon beam coagulator. Initial report. J Reprod Med. 1993;38:121.

36. Miller CE, McCarus SD. Ultrasonic cutting and coagulation in gynecologic surgery. J Am Assoc Gynecol Laparosc. 1995;2(4, Suppl):S33.

37. Geis WP, Kim HC, McAfee PC, et al. Synergistic benefits of combined technologies in complex, minimally invasive surgical procedures. Clinical experience and educational processes. Surg Endosc. 1996;10:1025.

38. Lee SJ, Park KH. Ultrasonic energy in endoscopic surgery. Yonsei Med J. 1999;40:545.

39. Walther MM, Herring J, Choyke PL, et al. Laparoscopic partial adrenalectomy in patients with hereditary forms of pheochromocytoma. J Urol. 2000;164:14.

40. Barron-Vallejo J, Jurado-Jurado M, Almanza-Marquez R. Methods of pedicle ligation in laparoscopically assisted vaginal hysterectomy: analysis of results. Obstet Gynecol. 2000;95(Suppl 1):S33.

41. Stanton CJ. Laparoscopic splenectomy for idiopathic thrombocytopenic purpura (ITP). A five-year experience. Surg Endosc. 1999;13: 1083.

42. Kusunoki M, Shoji Y, Yanagi H, et al. Current trends in restorative proctocolectomy: introduction of an ultrasonically activated scalpel. Dis Colon Rectum. 1999;42:1349.

43. Vezakis A, Dexter SP, Martin IG, et al. Laparoscopic cholecystectomy after pancreatic debridement. Surg Endosc. 1998;12:865.

44. Helal M, Albertini J, Lockhart J, et al. Laparoscopic nephrectomy using the harmonic scalpel. J Endourol. 1997;11:267.

45. Ott DE, Moss E, Martinez K. Aerosol exposure from an ultrasonically activated (harmonic) device. J Am Assoc Gynecol Laparosc. 1998;5:29.

46. McCarus SD, Miller CE. Tissue effects of ultrasonic cutting and coagulation in gynecologic laparoscopic surgery. J Am Assoc Gynecol Laparosc. 1995;2(4, Suppl):S73.

47. Kanehira E, Omura K, Kinoshita T, et al. How secure are the arteries occluded by a newly developed ultrasonically activated device? Surg Endosc. 1999;13:340.

48. Barrientos-Fortes T, Barragan R, Gonzalez A. Ultrasonic retrograde cholecystectomy. A new simplified technique. Surg Endosc. 2000; 14(Suppl 1):S5.

49. Cooper MJ, Cario G, Lam A, et al. Complications of 174 laparoscopic hysterectomies. Aust N Z J Obstet Gynaecol. 1996;36:36.

50. Villalobos MA, Gutierrez L. Complicaciones de la electrocirugia. In: Cueto J, Weber A, eds. Cirugia Laparoscopica, 1st ed. Interamericana-McGraw-Hill:1994;341.

Chapter Ninety-One • • • • • • •

Morbidity and Mortality of Laparoscopic Cholecystectomy

JACQUES PERISSAT

Laparoscopic cholecystectomy (LC) became the gold standard treatment in widespread use and paved the way for other minimally invasive procedures in only a few years. The reasons for this are that the patient can eat, drink, and walk around on the day after surgery, and can resume his previous physical, personal and professional activities less than a week postsurgery. But if the postoperative course is anything less than uneventful, the slightest symptom should be taken seriously and trigger a number of investigations and should be diagnosed and treated as quickly as possible.

The specific complications of laparoscopic cholecystectomy are usually the result of lesions accidentally inflicted on the anatomic structures near the gallbladder. These complications are always the same, but their clinical appearance may vary depending on their initial presentation, the seriousness of their pathologic effect, and their evolution. We classify complications based on the length of time between the operation and appearance of symptoms:

- Immediate complications: complications that develop on the first postoperative day (within 24 hours of surgery);
- Early postoperative complications: complications that appear between postoperative days 2 and 15; and
- Late postoperative complications: complications that appear after postoperative day 15, with some occurring much later, sometimes even months or years later.

INJURY TO STRUCTURES NEAR THE GALLBLADDER

Although laparoscopic surgery has been termed "minimally invasive," which is indeed the case during its initial stages, it can be dangerously invasive for the deep organs, especially if the surgeon is inexperienced.

Accidental injuries during surgery may cause vascular and/or biliary lesions, lesions to the hollow viscera (duodenum, colon, and stomach), to solid organs (liver), and the abdominal wall. These injuries may have a mechanical origin (tearing, partial or complete division), or they may be caused indirectly due to improper application of electric current during cutting or coagulation. They can cause hemorrhages, biliary leakage or stenosis, hollow organ perforation, and abdominal wall lesions. There may be one or several lesions on the same structure or concomitant isolated or multiple lesions on different structures. They may jeopardize the patient's life and always generate large increases in cost.[1] Moreover, they often lead to litigation and lawsuits.[2]

VASCULAR LESIONS

Cholecystectomies always involve hemostatic control through ligation and division of the cystic artery, the nutrient artery of the gallbladder. Its anatomy was described in detail for the first time by François Calot in 1892. In his thesis, he defined an area, subsequently called Calot's triangle, whose upper limit is the cystic artery, its proximal limit is the common bile duct (CBD), and the lower limit is the cystic duct, and whose center is the junction of the cystic artery and cystic duct, where a lymph node described by Mascagni is normally found. Since that time, surgeons have extended the area of Calot's triangle, moving its upper edge to the area where the parietal peritoneum inserts itself in the lower edge of the hepatic parenchyma.[3] The cystic artery thus becomes the central element of this extended triangle of Calot, as it branches off from the common hepatic artery. However, major anatomic variations are sometimes found.[4] The surgeon should be able to locate it, detach it through careful dissection, and divide it between two ligatures or staples. Accidental injury or inadequate hemostatic control causes an immediate massive hemorrhage, which obscures the operative field. This causes the proximal end of the artery to retract and position itself at the level of the CBD, making it dangerous and difficult to perform hemostatic control.

Cystic arteries in unusual locations may also be inadvertently injured. Some originate from the posterior and superior pancreaticoduodenal artery. The cystic artery in its shorter version may branch off directly from a branch of the right hepatic artery, immediately below the liver. Accidental injury or ligation of the right hepatic artery has been described, when it was mistaken for the cystic artery. Some anomalies, although exceptional, do exist. Twice in our experience we have discovered an artery of the same caliber as the cystic artery, that originated directly from the liver parenchyma and supplied the gallbladder fundus.

As far as accidental ligation is concerned, nothing is impossible, and even the most incredible accidents may happen, such as the ligation of the hepatic artery proper at the foot of the hepatic pedicle. A number of cases of liver necrosis following such mistakes have been described.

Venous injuries of the portal axis have been reported, once by laser, and in another case by electrocoagulation, but this is rare. On the other hand, venous hemorrhages should be a concern, because they are extremely dangerous in patients with portal hypertension. The latter was once listed as an absolute contraindication to laparoscopic cholecystectomy. Today, portal hypertension is still considered a contraindication, but only a relative one. However, it is advisable to preoperatively explore patients with suspected portal hypertension carefully, with Doppler sonography or magnetic resonance imaging (MRI). Whenever portal thrombosis of a periportal cavernomatous malformation is discovered, the patient should be informed that the risk of conversion to laparotomy exceeds 50%. The procedure should nevertheless begin with a laparoscopic exploration. We have sometimes found a slightly inflamed gallbladder hanging from the liver by a kind of meso-gallbladder consisting of hypervascular connective tissue, but whose hemostasis was in fact quite simple.

BILIARY LESIONS

These complications have such serious consequences that they represent a serious concern for the surgeon who performs laparoscopic cholecystectomy.

Common Bile Duct Injuries

These injuries are invariably caused by confusion of the cystic duct with the CBD. This confusion may be facilitated by the presence of anatomic congenital anomalies (Fig. 91–1).[4] Most of the time, a mistake is made due to inadequate exposure of the area, or to the dissection of inflamed surrounding tissues, the result of inadequate control of hemorrhage. There are two kinds of mechanism of injury: direct trauma caused by surgical instruments and inadequate application of electrical current during division or coagulation.

Direct trauma is caused by accidental opening of the bile duct, partial lateral opening, or complete division. The accidental ligation of the CBD may be total or subtotal. In some cases, excessive upward traction is applied to the gallbladder, causing the hepatocystic junction to bend. Clip application at this level partly occludes the lumen of the CBD.

There are also combined lesions, consisting of a lateral injury over a complete stricture. This type of lesion is the most difficult to diagnose and to treat.

Lesions due to the use of electric current for hemostasis seldom appear as clean openings in the CBD, but rather as electric burns. They can occur during dissection of Calot's triangle, either because a vessel has been mistaken for a bile duct and coagulated with bipolar forceps or, as in most cases, they occur far from the CBD from the use of monopolar current that is too strong and diffuses through the tissues. Most of the time, this electric burn is not immediately visible, but is revealed when the scab falls off, creating a bile leak or progressive stenosis some distance from the surgical site. One must remember that the view through the laparoscope is magnified, and that the maneuvering space is in fact less than 3 cm². There is a high risk for the monopolar current to diffuse toward the CBD.

The presence of a biliary or arterial anomaly in the area of Calot's triangle by no means accounts for all the complications seen. In most cases these are found during laborious dissection in this area, which is made more difficult by the presence of inflamed fibrosis more often than acute infection. The conjunctive tissue is difficult to separate mechanically, and is marbled with small capillaries that represent a source of hemorrhage. Hence the confusion

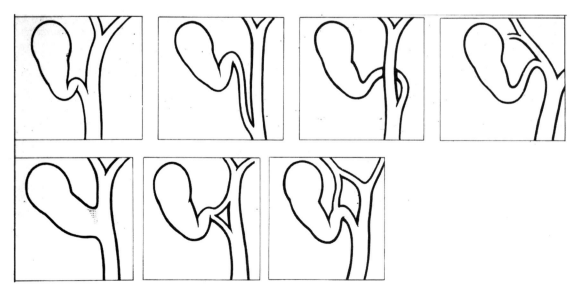

Figure 91–1. Cystic duct variations.

between a cystic duct, a CBD, a cystic artery, and a hepatic artery, which is made even worse by the untimely use of hemostasis via monopolar electrocoagulation. The latter should never be used during the dissection of Calot's triangle.

The pathologic consequences of these injuries are well known. The presence of bile inside the peritoneum immediately causes an extensive inflammatory and necrotic reaction through a kind of chemical peritonitis. It destroys the ends of the divided or injured bile ducts, with a tendency to extend upward toward the mucosa over several millimeters. The peritoneal leaf becomes edematous within a few hours. Within 4 to 5 days, the edema turns into hypervascularized inflamed tissue. Cicatricial sclerosis appears after postoperative day 25, which alters the positions of the pedicle and the neighboring organs (duodenum, stomach, transverse colon, and greater omentum). The peritoneal leaf turns into a strong sheath of fibrotic tissue that is very similar to the vitrification caused by nuclear explosions. Experience shows that although proper dissection is still possible at the edematous stage, it becomes very difficult if not impossible at the stage of acute inflammation, due to hemorrhage. Dissection again becomes possible after 2 months, although it remains extremely difficult. Surgeons have also described this phenomenon after conventional surgery.[5] Bismuth et al[5] described several types of this lesion after open surgery, and the laparoscopic approach has not changed it. The best way to successfully perform biliary repair is to restore either biliary or bilioenteric mucosal continuity. The optimal periods are the immediate (before the end of the fourth postoperative day) or late (after the thirtieth postoperative day) postoperative periods. The intermediate period is the most risky. The harmful consequences of this chemical peritonitis become even worse when the bile is infected, thus causing local collections or general dissemination of pus that leads to biliary peritonitis, with the risk of death from septicemia.

The lateral injuries affected by the posttraumatic inflammatory sclerosis may eventually close completely, thus effecting complete stenosis, with the same clinical features as subtotal or total blockage of the bile ducts. CBD blockage entails immediate hepatic consequences in the form of jaundice and cholestasis. The biliary origin of this postoperative complication then becomes obvious, and it has serious consequences that can jeopardize the patient's life either immediately from infection, or later from intrahepatic sclerosis that can lead to secondary biliary cirrhosis.

These biliary complications are more common in laparoscopic than open surgery. The areas with the highest risk of injury go from the cystocholedochal junction to the intrahepatic entrance of the right duct; lateral lesions of the right hepatic duct and its aberrant locations led to a special classification by Strasberg et al.[6] Finally, catastrophic mistakes have been described, such as a virtually complete resection of the CBD, from the liver hilum to the duodenum. Vascular lesions are often associated with such injuries. Such catastrophes are rare but do occur, which emphasizes the necessity of thorough training of surgeons who practice laparoscopic surgery (Figs. 91–2 and 91–3). Whenever an abdominal plain film taken in a patient who is not feeling well after laparoscopic cholecystectomy shows more than 4 clips, one should suspect complications. If there are more than 4, this means that the surgeon encountered difficulties during the procedure, and re-exploration needs to be done.

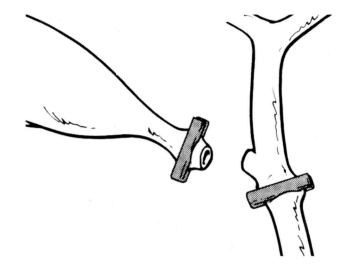

Figure 91–2. Example of improper clip placement.

Gallbladder Injuries

The gallbladder wall may rupture during dissection, either from tearing with the grasping forceps, or through accidental rupture during its detachment from the hepatic bed. The rupture may also take place during extraction through the abdominal wall. The contents of the gallbladder spill in the peritoneal cavity or onto the abdominal wall, and this may induce secondary infection, but it may also cause scattering of gallstones, which sooner or later may cause intraperitoneal or parietal suppuration. In cases of undetected cancer of the gallbladder, such ruptures may lead to intraperitoneal or intraparietal seeding of malignant cells. To avoid such an occurrence, use a plastic bag when extracting the gallbladder. The bag should also be placed under the gallbladder whenever dissection turns out to be difficult, and it should always be used for the extraction of the specimen.

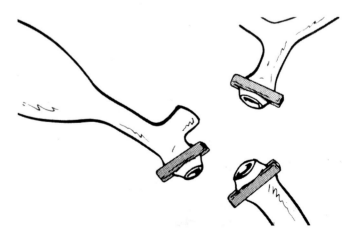

Figure 91–3. Broad resection of the common bile duct.

LESIONS TO NEIGHBORING ORGANS

Liver

In some cases of inflamed chronic cholecystitis, the gallbladder may adhere strongly to the liver parenchyma, and in some cases it may be embedded in it, with no distinct line between its wall and the liver parenchyma. It may also be congenitally joined to the liver, either partially or totally. Detaching it from the liver parenchyma may cause immediate or secondary hemorrhage significant enough to call it a complication. Some cases of ischemia and abscess of segments of the liver have been described, and these are caused by improper ligation of a major branch of the hepatic artery.

Hollow Organs

Other organs near the gallbladder include the duodenum and the right angle of the colon. Both organs may be damaged during dissection of a gallbladder surrounded with particularly dense, fibrotic, and hemorrhagic adhesions. The cause may be mechanical perforation that goes unnoticed during the procedure, or an electric burn from diffusion of monopolar current during coagulation. The perforation will be revealed later on, when the scab comes off during the first 15 postoperative days. The consequences may be serious: peritonitis, either general or local, in the form of a subhepatic abscess.

PARIETAL LESIONS

By definition, the laparoscopic approach minimizes parietal complications. However, one must keep in mind that apart from epigastric artery injury during trocar placement, minor vessels may bleed at the level of the trocar ports, especially if the ports are 10 mm or more in diameter. A lengthy operation also increases local musculoaponeurotic trauma. It may cause postoperative intraparietal hematoma and incisional hernia, a source of subsequent strangulation. Cases of detachment of the parietal peritoneum have also been described. This artificial space is due to misalignment of the transmusculoaponeurotic orifice with the peritoneal trocar orifice. This allows CO_2 insufflation to intrude in the preperitoneal space. This space may be contaminated by septic fluid from the gallbladder and cause early phlegmons or secondary abscesses. The transcutaneous and transmusculoaponeurotic points of insertion of the trocars may be the sites of secondary or late complications. Cases of early suppuration of trocar ports at the extraction site of an infected gallbladder have been described. Secondary suppuration does occur, due to the presence of residual stones, as does cancer cell seeding of the extraction site of the specimen.

CLINICAL FEATURES, DIAGNOSIS, AND TREATMENT

All the complications linked to laparoscopic cholecystectomy are generated during the surgical procedure. They may be discovered early or late, depending on the quality of postoperative surveillance, the significance of the lesions, and the point at which the major clinical features appear.

COMPLICATIONS OCCURRING DURING THE FIRST 24 POSTOPERATIVE HOURS

Complications Discovered Intraoperatively

Hemorrhage. Hemorrhage obscures the operative field, infiltrates conjunctive tissues, and makes it difficult to distinguish the planes of dissection and to locate the two major anatomic landmarks represented by the arterial and biliary trees. If these hemorrhages cannot be definitively controlled by laparoscopy and the origin identified, the surgeon should abandon the laparoscopic approach and convert to open surgery. By the beginning of 1989, we had established a simple rule, the 30-minute rule, which states that if 30 minutes pass without significant progress in laparoscopic dissection, one must convert to open surgery. These bleeding mishaps can be avoided by obeying a few simple rules. First, precise identification of the different elements of Calot's triangle must be done. This is the key to success. Adequate exposure of the area should first be achieved, then traction is applied to the gallbladder in order to open the triangle as wide as possible. This is achieved through use of the French technique (Figs. 91–4 and 91–5). The liver should be lifted out of the way, and we use a washing/aspiration cannula introduced through a 5-mm trocar inserted subcostally near the midclavicular line for this purpose. This instrument is positioned above the field of dissection to allow a clear view of the surgical site by alternating irrigation and aspiration. In patients with a large or friable liver, this instrument may be replaced with retractors introduced in the same port through a 10-mm trocar. The lower edge of the gallbladder neck is held with grasping forceps introduced through a 5-mm trocar inserted in the right upper quadrant on the anterior axillary line so it can apply slightly downward and right lateral traction (Fig. 91–4). The anterior aspect of Calot's triangle is thus opened and exposed.[11] A vertical incision is made with scissors in the anterior peritoneal leaf as closely as possible to the gallbladder. This opens the way for the blunt dissector, which is used to gently incise the connective tissue and isolate the cystic artery (upper element) and the cystic

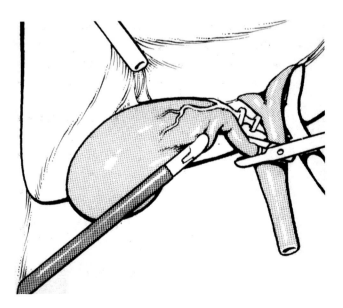

Figure 91–4. Proper exposure of Calot's triangle.

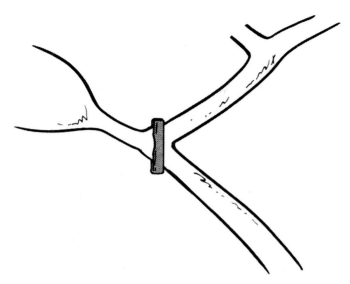

Figure 91–5. Excessive traction placed on the gallbladder bends the common bile duct so the clip is applied to the cystohepatic junction instead of the cystic duct.

duct (lower element). The grasping forceps are then used to seize the gallbladder neck, and it is lifted in order to expose the posterior aspect of Calot's triangle, and an opening is made similarly to that in the front. This maneuver allows positive identification of the cystic artery, cystic duct, CBD, and cysticocholedochal junction. This posterior approach reveals the route followed by the right hepatic artery, which enters into the liver. Because it sometimes curves toward the gallbladder, it may be mistaken for the cystic artery. The latter is always dissected over a length sufficient to allow application of two clips, between which a clear division is performed. Should this maneuver fail, one must resort to tamponade, using a forceps fitted with a tampon, to wash and aspirate the operative field until the retracted arterial stump becomes visible. Its end is grasped with a grasping forceps and a clip is applied in the correct position. The surgeon should not try to apply a clip in an approximate position or apply monopolar electrocoagulation in this area. Such attempts can lead to the most serious lesions of the CBD. These maneuvers can be difficult to perform, and sometimes require an additional trocar. If no satisfactory repair can be achieved, this is an indication for conversion to open surgery.

Primary dissection of Calot's triangle is sometimes impossible. This is the case when the gallbladder has undergone numerous recurrences of acute infection that were treated medically. Inflammatory reactions take place around the gallbladder, which develop into sclerosis. The triangle of Calot may disappear completely, and the upper edge of the gallbladder comes into contact with the CBD. Some surgeons have advocated the laparoscopic performance of anterograde cholecystectomy, a procedure common in open surgery, in which the dissection begins with the gallbladder fundus, between the gallbladder and the liver. We strongly advise against attempting this laparoscopically, because it can lead to injury of the CBD. When the Mirrizzi syndrome is discovered, we advise conversion to open surgery.

Inflammatory sclerosis around the gallbladder may also extend to the duodenum, the right angle of the colon, and the greater omentum. In such circumstances major hemorrhaging may occur.

All these organs should be lowered, while precise dissection is performed along the gallbladder, with immediate coagulation of each vessel with the bipolar forceps. After doing so, one can lower the great omental flap, the duodenal bulb, then the right angle of the colon. These maneuvers may require insertion of an additional trocar, usually in the left paraumbilical area. This helps prevent diffuse hemorrhaging, which obscures visibility and exposes the neighboring hollow organs to potential injury.

The last source of intraoperative hemorrhage is the gallbladder bed. The more inflamed and sclerotic the gallbladder wall, the more difficult (or impossible) it is to find an adequate cleavage plane between the gallbladder and the liver parenchyma. One should therefore proceed patiently, taking great care to avoid two major pitfalls, the accidental opening of the gallbladder and the deep tearing of the liver bed. All techniques available to the surgeon must be used, including hydrodissection and the use of monopolar current for division and coagulation. In this case, because the anatomic connections between the gallbladder and the CBD have been severed, the risk of diffusion of electric current no longer exists, so monopolar coagulation can be used extensively. An argon laser can be used to cauterize superficial capillary bleeders over a large area. It is wise to devote whatever time is necessary to achieve thorough hemostasis of the gallbladder bed after a cholecystectomy, even a difficult one. An uneventful postoperative course depends on it.

Visceral Perforation. We have seen how injuries to the right angle of the colon and the junction of the first and second duodenums may occur. If such an injury is detected during the operation, one must try to repair it laparoscopically. Concerning the duodenum, provided it is a lateral injury without excessive loss of tissue, the edges should be trimmed and sutured with interrupted stitches using absorbable suture material and covering the suture with an omental patch whenever possible. Nasogastric aspiration should be left in place during the postoperative period until resumption of bowel movements, and a gastrograffin test performed before the tube is removed (usually on postoperative day 4). Regarding the colon, if the lesions are punctiform and without inflammation, one can perform direct suturing in interrupted stitches using absorbable suture material. On the other hand, if the tear is jagged and the tissue inflamed, the tear's edges must be trimmed, and the neighboring inflamed tissue resected to create conditions that will allow stapling of the colon. Once repaired, any perforation requires drainage through a right side trocar port. If the drainage is not productive, the drain can be removed on postoperative day 4. In some circumstances, the adhesions between the gallbladder and the neighboring hollow organs turn out to be impossible to take down. One must then deliberately open up these organs. It is preferable to leave a piece of gallbladder wall attached to the colon if necessary. If this is impossible, one can try to open up the colon or the duodenum, taking care to create conditions amenable to secondary closure as described above. Of course, these laparoscopic maneuvers can only be performed by an experienced surgeon, one familiar with laparoscopic suturing technique. Otherwise one must convert to laparotomy.

Biliary Complications

Gallbladder Injuries. We have already described the circumstances under which the gallbladder wall may be torn or accidentally opened during the procedure. Such tearing may occur when stones are present in the gallbladder neck that make it difficult to hold with the grasping forceps, or when the gallbladder is overdistended due to bile or pus retention. Tearing may also be due to a gangrenous and therefore fragile gallbladder wall. A distended gallbladder must be punctured under visual control in order to evacuate the contents. This provides the opportunity to perform bacteriologic analysis of the fluid collected. The puncture site is then closed, either with a ligation or a clip, or through placement of a broader grasping forceps. When the stone is located in the infundibulum, the surgeon must try and push it back into the gallbladder body. If this is not possible, one can make an incision over the impacted stone, extract it, put it into a bag previously inserted under the liver. The bag is then closed with a clip or an endo-loop. In case of gangrene, the 5-mm grasper should be replaced with the broader 10-mm fenestrated forceps, which allow broader grip on the tissues. If the tissues are too brittle to allow adequate exposure of the elements of Calot's triangle, the laparoscopic approach should be abandoned and the procedure converted to open surgery. Only after identification of the cystic artery and cystic duct, and after x-ray examination of the CBD to make sure that it is intact, can one open the gallbladder lengthwise, drop the stones into a plastic bag previously positioned under the liver, and resect the gallbladder walls. If the cleavage plane would involve too much intrahepatic damage, some parts of the gallbladder wall may be left attached to the liver parenchyma. The mucous aspect is carefully destroyed by fulgurizing electrocoagulation or argon laser. In such cases, the patient should be informed that should pathologic examination of the specimen reveal signs of malignancy, laparotomy will be required to complete the removal of the remaining gallbladder wall.

We have also seen the gallbladder rupture during extraction. The consequences can be disastrous, as the calculi spill in the abdominal cavity. One must try to immediately retrieve all the stones because they can quickly slip away into the right coloparietal fossa or scatter among the intestinal loops. Late abscesses and bowel obstruction have been described, proving that stone spillage is far from harmless. Tolerance of the stones depends on the degree of infection present. This can be prevented by always placing the gallbladder in an extraction bag before removal. This should be a compulsory maneuver, because it also prevents the spread of infection and the seeding of malignant cells along the route followed by the trocar used for specimen extraction.

Common Bile Duct Injuries. These lesions are all the more serious because they often go unnoticed during surgery, so one should always try to avoid them. At the end of the procedure, one should always inspect the CBD for injury. Potential findings include complete ligation of the CBD, a minor lateral cut or opening of variable length, or complete division of the CBD.

Intraoperative Preventive Measures

As is the case with vascular injuries, the key to a successful operation lies in the careful dissection of the elements of Calot's triangle combined with the performance of intraoperative cholangiography. The operative field should be clear and free of bleeding, so the biliary elements can easily be identified. A small lateral opening is made in the cystic duct to allow passage of a catheter and performance of intraoperative cholangiography. This procedure is done under endoscopic control, showing the gradual filling of the downstream bile ducts as well as filling of the upper part of the biliary tree. This map must be complete. Some pictures are selected and analyzed, making sure that no part of the biliary tree is missing, up to and including the intrahepatic level. Such imaging is reassuring and is a key element in the patient's file in case postoperative complications develop and/or there are medicolegal issues. We strongly recommend routine use of intraoperative cholangiography, as the surgeon can use it as protection against any suspicion of technical defects in the procedure if postoperative complications occur. It is also perfectly safe. If a lateral opening has been made in a duct other than the cystic duct, x-ray examination allows detection of the error and the map of the biliary tree can be used to assist in identification of the proper duct. The small opening made in the bile duct to allow catheter introduction can then be closed, and an external biliary drain is inserted that is left in place for a few days after the operation. The drain should be checked on postoperative day 4 and removed if imaging studies are normal. If a bile leak is detected, the drain is left in place for another week. Correct identification of the bile ducts depends on the quality of the surgeon's dissection. In case of misinterpretation, intraoperative cholangiography can be performed that allows detection of the error without irreparable damage being done. One of the basic rules is never to ligate or divide a nonpulsating duct before making a small incision to check if bile flows out, and before having introduced a catheter for an intraoperative radiograph. However, despite these precautions taken during dissection, in some cases (such as seriously inflamed or dense connective tissues), accidental opening may occur, even before the bile duct has been identified. Such a lesion may be complete or incomplete. The solution is once again to introduce a catheter through this opening and make a map of the biliary tree above and below the injury via x-ray examination. The course of action that follows depends on the assessment. The bile leak may remain undetected during the operation, so at the end of the procedure, one has to systematically search for it through careful inspection of the operative field using irrigation and aspiration, and the application of light ascending pressure on the hepatic pedicle with a surgical instrument. Here again, whenever a leak is discovered, one must look for the hole and take a radiologic inventory. If the procedure has been uneventful, one must always be careful about cystic duct ligation. The portion of cystic duct to be saved should be long enough to allow cholangiography followed by ligation or clip application without encroaching on the cysticocholedochal junction (Fig. 91–5). This might cause secondary suture rupture, stenosis with fistula, or partial stenosis of the CBD. At the end of the procedure, the operative specimen should be carefully inspected immediately after extraction, to make sure that another biliary structure adjoining the area around the gallbladder neck and the cystic duct has not been accidentally resected. If this happens, laparoscopic intraabdominal exploration must be immediately resumed in order to locate the injury, which obviously must be found. If laparoscopic exploration fails, conversion to an open procedure is mandatory.

Complete Division of the Common Bile Duct

A clean division, without loss of substance, can be repaired with an end-to-end anastomosis using separate stitches of absorbable suture material, under cover of a **T**-tube inserted below the suture, and whose upper branch is used to bridge it. But this is rare, because in most cases an end-to-end anastomosis is contraindicated, due to a bile duct less than 4 mm in diameter, loss of substance, or a highly inflamed environment. Under such conditions, an end-to-end anastomosis is not worth attempting, and a Roux-en-Y bilio-enteric anastomosis must be performed. Whatever the technique chosen, it should approximate the two healthy mucous membranes. It may be too difficult for the inexperienced surgeon, and if so, conversion to open surgery is required.

Lateral Injuries

Lateral injuries may be small, such as a simple puncture similar to that which is made in the cystic duct for intraoperative cholangiography. In this case the hole can be repaired with one or two stitches made with 5-0 or 6-0 absorbable suture, provided the bile duct wall is not inflamed and the surrounding area is not infected. Following repair it is advisable to install a temporary external drain as well as a subhepatic drain at the end of the procedure. The lateral injury may be accompanied by a large or small loss of substance. If the loss of substance is less than half the circumference of the bile duct, suturing should not be attempted, and a T-tube type drain of adequate caliber should be introduced through this accidental opening. If the loss of substance is more than half the circumference of the bile duct, simple drainage is not enough and a more complex type of repair is necessary. The extended lateral injury of the bile duct must be trimmed so as to create tissues suitable for the performance of a Roux-en-Y hepaticojejunostomy of healthy tissues. Although simple repairs can be done by a laparoscopic approach, if the lesions are significant, one must revert to open surgery.

Complex Cases

These combine total ligation of the CBD with an underlying lateral injury. One of the most frequently reported but exceptional examples is CBD ligation associated with lateral injury of the right edge of the right hepatic duct. In such cases a Roux-en-Y bilioenteric anastomosis must be performed. The lateral injury is sutured under cover of a Völker-type drainage or a T-tube inserted into the area with lateral loss of substance, and the lower branch goes through the bilioenteric anastomosis. For such complex maneuvers conversion to open surgery is always necessary.

POSTOPERATIVE COMPLICATIONS THAT DEVELOP ON POSTOPERATIVE DAY 1

Apparently the operation has been a complete success, and the patient leaves the operating room. Now the immediate postoperative follow-up begins. During the first 24 hours, in the absence of complications, the scenario is quite simple: after an average of 6 hours, vomiting and sleepiness due to the anesthetics wear off. In most cases, the patient feels a stinging sensation at the trocar sites and slight discomfort in the right upper quadrant that does not affect breathing. To relieve this slight discomfort, some advocate infiltration of the trocar sites with lidocaine. In some cases, patients complain about sharp pain in the right shoulder, the exact cause of which is unknown. But this is rare if one takes care to carefully evacuate the pneumoperitoneum after trocar removal, and warms the gas used for pneumoperitoneum insufflation. However, the shoulder pain is usually only a problem when the operation lasts several hours, which is not the case with cholecystectomy. Twelve hours after leaving the operating room, the patient can move and

sit on the edge of his bed without experiencing pain. The patient can take liquids, or be given a light meal upon request. At 24 postoperative hours, the patient is smiling and can walk around the room without pain, and quickly recovers a normal level of ambulation and may resume some normal activities. At this point, if the postoperative course has remained uneventful, the patient is discharged from the hospital.

During this period, there are signs that warn of developing complications, mainly pain and symptoms of shock, that can lead to two different pictures, depending on the cause of the complication.

Hemorrhage

The patient has taken a little longer than expected to awaken, and he is agitated, with signs of tachypnea. The patient then begins to sweat, the patient's face and conjunctivae are pale, and the pulse rate quickens. One must not wait for a drop in blood pressure or for diuresis before treating hemorrhagic shock. Clinical examination is unremarkable, and there is no pain in the right upper quadrant. This clinical picture obviously points to a major early postoperative hemorrhage. In case of doubt, immediate sonography performed at the patient's bedside confirms the diagnosis. The patient must be taken back to the operating room without delay. Unless extreme collapse occurs, which would require emergency laparotomy, these premonitory symptoms of shock must be explored by another laparoscopic examination. Pneumoperitoneum insufflation helps to temporarily control the hemorrhage. The same port sites can be used again. An inspection of the operative field allows location of the source of the hemorrhage. In most cases, the hemorrhage is located in the gallbladder bed or it is due to clip slippage on the cystic artery. In rare cases, it is a secondary hemorrhage of a vessel to a neighboring organ, such as a major vessel of the greater omentum. Secondary hemostasis must be carried out following the same principles as previously described. The procedure ends with the installation of an alarm suction drain in the gallbladder bed that will warn the surgeon in case of early recurrence.

Perforation

Another clinical picture is that of septic shock. There is intense pain in the abdomen with guarded inspiration, which is soon accompanied by a rise in body temperature. Clinical examination reveals a contracted right upper quadrant and resonance of the entire abdomen exceeding that normally seen after laparoscopic pneumoperitoneum. These symptoms reveal the existence of a hollow organ perforation that went unnoticed during the operation. A plain film of the abdomen reveals a major pneumoperitoneum. The patient must be quickly returned to the operating room, the trocars reinserted, and laparoscopic exploration repeated. The perforating lesions must be located and repaired as described above if they are located in the duodenum or right colon. If no perforation is discovered there, one should suspect a perforation some distance from the operative field, and carefully explore the stomach, colon, and loops of the small intestine. We know how difficult thorough laparoscopic exploration of these viscera can be, so when laparoscopy does not reveal any obvious perforation, a control laparotomy is performed.

These complications, both immediate hemorrhage and perforation within the free peritoneal space, are exceptional. Because they seldom occur, it is unnecessary to keep most patients in the surgical ward for the first 24 postoperative hours. For this reason, it has been correctly determined that uncomplicated laparoscopic cholecystectomy should usually be an outpatient procedure. Patients are discharged and sent home when the conditions for follow-up are adequate at home, or they may be sent for 24 hours to a facility that allows close follow-up outside the hospital. However, if the operation has been difficult, it is logical that the first 24 postoperative hours be spent in a surgical ward. In such cases, we recommend the installation of a drain in the right upper quadrant, which allows quick confirmation of the diagnosis of a complication, whether bleeding or perforation, by revealing passage of blood or digestive fluid.

SECONDARY COMPLICATIONS OCCURRING BETWEEN POSTOPERATIVE DAYS 2 AND 15

The operated patient is now at postoperative hour 24. The patient is smiling, enjoys drinking and eating, and is relaxed and physically active. It is time to discharge him from the hospital or from close follow-up and send him home, or he may be already there if the protocol followed was that of uneventful ambulatory surgery. This state of well being will continue, and after 8 days the patient will feel as if he had not been operated on at all. What disorders are there that might disrupt this harmony? They fall into 2 categories: functional disorders and general disorders.

Included in functional disorders are right upper quadrant pain, digestive disorders (nausea, vomiting, and abdominal bloating with constipation and diarrhea), and the onset of jaundice that may develop into severe jaundice with gradual darkening of urine and stools that gradually become discolored. The symptoms seen may consist mainly of a rise in temperature, with deep asthenia and clinical signs of anemia. The association of these symptoms creates syndromes that indicate complications due to perivesical lesions as described previously. Precise clinical examination of the patient and additional tests must be carried out without delay. For both simple and complex cases, one must prescribe laboratory tests including CBC to check for anemia and hyperleukocytosis, hepatic function tests to detect cholestasis including total conjugated and nonconjugated bilirubin, cholesterol, alkaline phosphatase, gamma globulin, and a coagulation screen.

Morphologic assessment consisting of a plain film of the entire abdomen and another focusing on the right upper quadrant, and sonography of the area around the liver and the biliary tree. If a collection is revealed, an even more detailed examination must be performed via a CT scan, or even better via MRI cholangiography. Only if the latter is impossible to perform should one resort to endoscopic retrograde cholangiopancreatography (ERCP).

Biliary Complications

As soon as a biliary complication is suspected, the morphologic assessment described above must be performed. Three questions must be answered:

- Does the biliary lesion cause a bile leak into the peritoneal cavity (in other words, is the biliary lesion a closed [stenotic] or open wound)? If it is an open lesion, emergent mandatory interventional treatment is required.

- Has the injured CBD retained its anatomic axis? If the answer is yes, minimally invasive treatments are suitable; otherwise one must resort to open surgery.
- Is the junction of the left and right bile ducts within the liver hilum involved in the lesion? If the answer is yes, the patient must be referred to a practitioner that specializes in biliary surgery.

Common Bile Duct Stenosis

This may be due to complete ligation of the CBD. This situation is the easiest to diagnose, and the clinical history is very simple. It consists of the onset of jaundice with dark colored urine and discolored stools with no other symptoms, neither pain nor elevated temperature. The operated patient still feels well, but he or she is becoming yellower and yellower. Concern soon spreads to the family and these symptoms should also alarm the surgeon. The physical examination is otherwise normal. Laboratory tests show that signs of cholestasis are on the rise as the jaundice develops. Sonography shows gradual dilation of the intrahepatic bile ducts and of the biliary tree. However, one should be aware that the obvious signs do not become visible until postoperative day 4 or 5. CT scan shows that the biliary tree is dilated up to the level of a complete blockage. MRI cholangiography is even more convincing, as it shows the dilated biliary tree and its contents above the stenosis, and the normal bile duct below. It even shows whether there is a solution of continuity, which allows differentiation between a simple ligation and a ligation associated with an underlying transection. This precise map supplies all the necessary elements to devise a therapeutic course: a Roux-en-Y hepaticojejunostomy is clearly indicated. When should the operation be performed? There is no emergency, since there is no infection, so it is better to wait. The elective surgery is performed 2 weeks later on a bile duct dilated to 8 to 10 mm. The biliary mucosa are normal. It is now possible to perform the bilioenteric anastomosis under optimal conditions with the best chance for long-term success. The operation's degree of difficulty depends on the level of the stenosis. At the level of the pedicle, it is within the abilities of the average gastrointestinal surgeon. At the level of the hilum, when the lesion involves the biliary junction, the operation is more difficult, and we advise referral to a center that specializes in hilar surgery. The reason is that the secondary repair must be successful with the first attempt. The more often one operates, the worse the results become, with increasing risk of recurrence of a postoperative fistula or stenosis higher and higher up the biliary tree.

Subtotal Stenoses

These are usually caused by a clip partially blocking the CBD. This type of stenosis is often asymptomatic and may remain so indefinitely. However, the clip may ulcerate the CBD wall and create a secondary leak. It may also cause a less acute but lasting inflammatory reaction, leading to total stenosis after several months. As soon as the diagnosis has been confirmed by morphologic examination, we recommend reoperating to remove the clip responsible for the subtotal stenosis. The procedure may first be attempted by laparoscopy. Some titanium clips are easily removed. If the part of the CBD caught in the clip's jaws is fragile or if it breaks, the loss of substance is always moderate. It should not be sutured, but instead filled with a T-tube for bile drainage. If these maneuvers are too difficult to perform laparoscopically, one must convert to open surgery.

Intraperitoneal Bile Leaks

This is when the second question must be answered: Has the CBD retained its anatomic axis? If it has, one must give priority to minimally invasive techniques, namely endoluminal endoscopy and interventional radiology. If the biliary axis has been destroyed, the only solution is open surgery. This last resort surgery is all the more effective because it is performed early (before postoperative day 4). Beyond this limit, it becomes rescue surgery.

The clinical picture becomes clear after the twenty-fourth postoperative hour, after a symptom-free interval of variable length. Right subcostal pain reappears and tends to increase, with impaired deep breathing, and sometimes an irritating cough. From a digestive point of view, the patient feels nauseous again, and may even vomit due to abdominal bloating. Conversely, there may be irritating diarrhea. The body temperature rises, the patient's general condition deteriorates, he looks anxious, and the jaundice reappears. Blood tests reveal hyperleukocytosis without anemia and a variable increase in bilirubin. There are no clear signs of cholestasis at this early stage. Sonography shows a subhepatic collection. All these symptoms are enough to make a quick decision: The patient must be reoperated. The best thing to do is to refer the patient to a center that specializes in the treatment of hepatobiliary disorders, where all the necessary means of investigation will be available to obtain an accurate biliary map. The best examination is MRI cholangiography, and if this cannot be performed one should ask for an endoscopic retrograde cholangropancreatography (ERCP) without hesitation. The origin of the leak and its exact nature will be pinpointed. There are three therapeutic aims: (1) vacuation of the subhepatic collection; (2) stoppage of the bile leak; and (3) restoration of bile flow to the digestive tract.

In view of the rapid development of chemical peritonitis, extremely urgent action needs to be taken. On postoperative day 4, one may hope to enter the edematous stage. All three objectives can be attained with a single procedure. The course of action is the same as for intraoperative discovery of a biliary lesion. Beyond day 4, it is usually impossible to achieve all three aims in a single stroke. The first objective is to save the patient's life by completing the first two objectives, then one must try to postpone fulfilling the third until after postoperative day 30. During this period of peritoneal reaction, necrosis, and hemorrhage when elective surgery is risky, one should use all the resources afforded by the other minimally invasive interventional techniques, namely interventional radiology and endoluminal flexible endoscopy. Also not to be overlooked is the excellent information that can be obtained with another exploratory laparoscopy. We advise performing it, even if reoperation has been chosen as the best treatment, and conversion to open surgery if the lesion appears to be beyond the capacity of laparoscopy to repair.

Slippage of Cystic Stump Ligation

This is the least serious biliary complication. It should be suspected whenever a plain abdominal film shows that the clip applied to the cystic duct has migrated far from the biliary area. Alternatively, MRI cholangiography or even ERCP can also show the lesion. The treatment is simple: a repeat laparoscopy using the same trocar ports as the original cholecystectomy, evacuation of the bile col-

lection, cleansing of the subhepatic region, repositioning of the cystic duct ligation (this time using thread instead of a clip), then temporary subhepatic drainage. If no radiologic check was performed during the cholecystectomy or during the search for the source of the bile leak, a control cholangiography must be carried out intraoperatively. In fact, some cases of cystic duct slippage are due to excess pressure in the bile ducts caused by the presence of a residual stone in the CBD. If this is the case, one should not attempt laparoscopic stone extraction in this context at the onset of chemical peritonitis. A transcystic drain must be installed, properly fastened to the cystic duct by ligation, and the stone must be extracted via an endoscopic sphincterotomy. In order to avoid failure in sphincterotomy (the failure rate is 5%, even for the best surgeons), we recommend installation of a transcystic transpapillary drain during the laparoscopic procedure. Thanks to this guide, sphincterotomy is feasible in 100% of cases.[12]

Lateral Injuries

If the lesion is discovered before postoperative day 4, laparoscopic examination must be repeated to complete lesion assessment. Suturing should never be attempted, even if the lesion is small; instead, a T-tube should be inserted. If the injury is located below the cysticocholedochal junction, one may even use a transcystic transpapillary drain, which is the equivalent of stent placement through endoscopic sphincterotomy.

The advantage of laparoscopy is that it allows elimination of the subhepatic collection of bile and pus through careful cleansing of the entire area and removal of the false membranes in a single procedure. Beyond postoperative day 4, one must attempt a combination of minimally invasive procedures. The ERCP, which allowed location of the lesion, must be used to perform endoscopic sphincterotomy, and bridging of the lost substance by a stent. Interventional radiology is used to evacuate and drain the biliary abscess via an echo-guided puncture. Bile duct intubation must be maintained for at least 60 days.

The lateral loss of substance may be significant, consisting of more than half the circumference and several centimeters in length. This is visible on ERCP or MRI cholangiography, which will show a major peribiliary effusion, which sometimes makes it difficult to ascertain whether the normal biliary axis has been maintained. In such adverse circumstances, one must seek the aid of an endoscopic gastroenterologist or surgeon to try and bridge the loss of substance with a stent, which restores the biliary axis and redirects the bile flow toward the bowel. If this fails, one must resort to open surgery. This is the worst possible time to operate, but the lesions are so serious that there is no other option. The operation will consist of a broad subcostal laparotomy followed by evacuation of the bile and pus collection, then cleansing of the subhepatic region and a search for the upper end of the injured bile duct. Of the three therapeutic aims listed above, the first two absolutely must be achieved, namely evacuation of the collection and control of the intraperitoneal bile leak. The restoration of bilioenteric continuity must be postponed. Thanks to intraoperative cholangiography, a precise map of the biliary system is obtained, which makes it possible to pinpoint the opening. It also allows one to ascertain whether the biliary junction is involved. One may then opt for one of two solutions: either control the bile leak by a complete ligation above the opening, or install external drainage that will divert the bile leak to the outside. This latter course should only be taken when the inflamed status of the bile duct is such that slippage of the entire ligation is likely. This is an emergency move to save the patient's life, but it will make it even more difficult to restore biliary continuity later on. Experience shows that in a center that specializes in conventional biliary surgery, even under such adverse circumstances, the surgeon usually succeeds through patient, painstaking, and precise dissection, in finding a normal section of the biliary tree that may be ligated pending postoperative dilation of the biliary tree above. This makes it possible, 30 to 60 days later, to perform a bilioenteric anastomosis. When performed electively, this operation can utilize all the tools available in open surgery: subglissonian dissection of the hepatic duct junction from the liver hilum, and subtotal resection of the hepatic parenchyma covering the hilum at the level of the fifth segment. The biliary junction is thus approached from above, and the entire length of the left hepatic duct can be used, so the anastomosis can be at least 10 mm in diameter. If the hilar junction is found to be sclerotic, one may also perform a double anastomosis within the hilum, on the right and left bile ducts separately. These endeavors are more likely to be successful because the operation takes place some distance from the site of acute chemical and infectious peritonitis.

Complex Traumatic Lesions

These lesions combine ligation and injury. The simplest case is a clear ligation of the CBD at the level of the pedicle, associated with a minor lateral injury of the upper segments of the bile duct (the right hepatic duct in most cases). One must not touch the ligation, but rather secure it if necessary, and insert a temporary T-tube in the injury. This rescue operation gives the patient time to get over the acute stage of peritoneal reactions and postpone the final restoration of the bilioenteric bile flow.

Unfortunately, the lesions may be more complex, with considerable damage to the bile ducts associated with major vascular injuries. We have all heard tales of near complete resection of the biliary tree. When bilistasis is achieved, even with clips applied high above the biliary junction, the situation is not desperate. On the other hand, if there are associated injuries at such a high level, there is little hope. One must try and dry up the area through bile flow diversion. One can try external ascending transhepatic transcutaneous drainage, with dead-end closure of the bile ducts entering the liver parenchyma. One can also try, as a desperate measure, to connect the destroyed hilum through a Roux-en-Y jejunal anastomosis. The intrahepatic bile ducts are catheterized with long U-shaped drains, one end of which comes out through the liver and through the skin, while the other one, according to Völker's technique, exits through the wall of the anastomosed intestinal loop, then through the abdominal wall (Fig. 91–6). Hemihepatectomies have also been described that allow anastomosis of the portion of CBD in the remaining half of the liver to a Roux-en-Y anastomosed loop. The results obtained with these acrobatic procedures are rather poor. Mortality is far from negligible (over 10%), and the risk of development of secondary stenosis is 50% at 5 years. If the lesions are located up high, in contact with the liver parenchyma, the only remaining solution is liver transplant. We do not have any personal experience with these extreme situations.

Bile Leaks in the Gallbladder Bed

Morphologic exploration may fail to show a leak at the level of the main biliary tree, although there is indeed a subhepatic bile

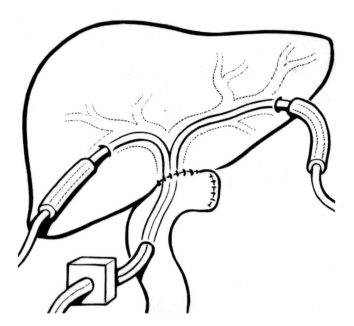

Figure 91–6. U-shaped biliary drains bridging an anastomosis between the liver hilum and a Roux-en-Y jejunal loop.

collection. Some biliary canaliculi of the fourth and fifth segment of the liver may flow directly into the gallbladder. They are probably more common than is thought, but they are easily coagulated and occluded when the gallbladder is detached from the liver. They sometimes unblock during the immediate postoperative period and create these bile collections. Repeat laparoscopy sometimes allows their visualization. If they are very thin, occluding them with electrocoagulation or laser will suffice. Some segmental canaliculi are larger, and for these one may attempt ligation reinforced with biologic glue. Only occasionally does a bile duct more than 3 mm in diameter flow directly into the gallbladder. It should be carefully isolated and occluded with a ligation, resting on Glisson's capsule if necessary. In case of failure, a Roux-en-Y anastomosis must be performed by open surgery on this important bile duct, which could be segmental (segment 5 or 6).[6–13]

Complications Due to Bleeding

In most cases, these consist of a subhepatic hematoma caused by slow oozing of blood from capillaries, which has developed silently from the hepatic bed. The clinical picture is unclear, with recurrence of subcostal pain, fatigue, and paleness and light nausea. The blood cell count shows the onset of anemia and hepatic function tests are normal. Morphologic examination is necessary; ultrasonography will reveal the collection of fluid. If there is any doubt after the onset of jaundice or a rise in temperature, one must undertake a morphological examination to explore the bile ducts and rule out a secondary biliary complication. Once the biliary tree has been shown to be patent, the most likely diagnosis is hematoma. If its volume is significant or it increases in size, echo-guided drainage must be performed.

In rare cases, acute hemorrhagic recurrences have been described after a scab falls off a venous electric burn in the portal system, especially in cases of cholecystectomy in patients with portal hypertension. Whenever signs of acute internal hemorrhage appear, the only course to take is emergency surgical exploration via laparotomy to control the bleeding.

Secondary Hollow Organ Perforations

Via the same mechanism as that of a scab falling off a burn, a clinical picture of acute peritonitis of duodenal or colonic origin may appear in the first 10 postoperative days. The picture is that of acute peritonitis due to the absence of the postoperative adhesions usually found after a laparoscopic procedure. Emergency reoperation is mandatory, using the same treatment as that described above for the early occurrence of the same complications.

LATE COMPLICATIONS AFTER POSTOPERATIVE DAY 15

Biliary Complications

The most common manifestation of biliary complications is jaundice. It can in occur as two roughly opposite clinical types, depending on the nature of the complication.

Jaundice seldom develops gradually, without regression, or without any accompanying symptoms similar to those of cancer. However, its onset 6, 12, or 18 months after cholecystectomy make one consider the possibility of gradual stenosis induced by the use of monopolar coagulation too close to the bile duct during the operation. MRI cholangiography clearly shows this type of lesion, its level, and the length of the stenosis. Such stenosis is a formal indication for an open surgical approach. Elective surgery is performed through the conventional approach as described above.

In most cases, the jaundice develops through painful, feverish recurring episodes that indicate cholangitis. The diagnosis is based on the morphologic examination of the biliary tree as described above. It will reveal the presence of a foreign body inside the bile duct lumen (a stone or other foreign body), or of partial twisting stenosis of the biliary tree over a variable length, with dilation of the biliary tree above. If the presence of a foreign body is confirmed, it must be removed through endoscopic sphincterotomy. In most cases, it is a residual stone left behind during the cholecystectomy that has remained silent for some time. Sometimes metal clips used to control the cystic duct have been found instead of a stone. We had one such case in our personal experience that was revealed 2 years after the cholecystectomy, from our early experience with cholecystectomy (1998), when Feelshie clips were used to control the cystic duct. Such complications do not seem to occur with the newer titanium clips. For cystic duct control we recommend the use of absorbable clips or ligation with absorbable suture material.

Acute episodes of cholangitis may be a sign of incomplete inflammatory stenosis. Usually, when interrogated the patient reveals that the immediately postoperative period was not totally free of symptoms, but they were overlooked at the time and eventually disappeared. This usually corresponds to a minor CBD injury that has finally healed without treatment, but at the cost of progressive sclerosis sometimes accompanied by inflammatory granulomas within the CBD, that cause repeated episodes of cholangitis. It may also be caused by a clip that partly blocks the CBD, which is only now making its presence felt. This type of complication usually occurs earlier than inflammatory stenosis due to electric burns. The main anatomic axis of the CBD is maintained. Endoscopic gastroenterologists have advocated treatment via balloon dilation of such stenoses and insertion of an internal prosthesis to maintain adequate bile flow. This can only be achieved if the prosthesis is left in place for a long time (6 to 12 months). This prosthesis may cause acute episodes of ascending cholangitis as its distal ends are in a transpapillary position, swimming in duodenal fluid. We do not advocate use of this treatment on a regular basis. It may prove useful in cases of acute cholangitis unresponsive to medical treatment, as it allows quick and efficient drainage of the CBD. In most cases, once the stenosis has been found, one must delay the operation for as long as possible by putting the patient on antibiotic therapy for each bout of cholangitis. After a few weeks, the portion of CBD upstream from the stenosis is sufficiently dilated that one can attempt a broad conventional surgical approach to definitively repair all the lesions by a Roux-en-Y bilioenteric anastomosis at a time when cholangitis is absent.

Intra-abdominal Complications

Abdominal Collections

Abscess. Abscesses may develop beyond postoperative day 15 in the usual recesses of the peritoneal cavity: the subhepatic or subphrenic space, Douglas pouch, and the mid-abdominal area. Their clinical picture does not include any specific feature related to the laparoscopic approach to cholecystectomy. It is the same as that of any suppuration occurring some distance from an intra-abdominal surgical operation. Depending on their location, they may be associated with extra-abdominal thoracic symptoms for subphrenic abscesses or urogenital symptoms for pelvic abscesses. Modern means of morphologic investigation such as sonography and CT scan allow them to be easily located. CT scan may reveal the presence of foreign bodies within the collection, such as stones expelled from the gallbladder during dissection or during its extraction. Treatment varies according to the anatomic location. Here again, one should always try to use minimally invasive treatment if possible. Some collections can be evacuated via echo-guided trans/parietal puncture. One must also use the transvaginal route to perform posterior colpotomy for pelvic collections and the transanal route for rectotomy, which also allows removal of calculous foreign bodies.

Bilioma. The symptom-free interval between the immediate postoperative course and the late collection of pus is always quite long and totally asymptomatic. This is not the case for bile collections or biliomas, which may occur during the first two postoperative weeks. As a rule, interrogating the patient reveals a few immediately postoperative symptoms that were overlooked at the time. At CT scan, the collection appears as an encysted collection of fluid. Echo-guided puncture is used to drain the bile and allows insertion of a drain to evacuate any remaining fluid. To be safe, one should also carry out a morphologic examination of the biliary tree via MRI cholangiography to make sure that there is no communication with the collection.

Postoperative Acute Bowel Obstruction.
The laparoscopic approach has a reputation for causing few postoperative adhesions, and this is true for the vast majority of laparoscopic cholecystectomies. However, late acute bowel obstructions have been described, especially when the initial operation was performed in a septic environment. One cause of the growth of adhesions is stones

that slipped out of the gallbladder during its dissection and extraction. As discussed earlier, one simple preventive measure for such an occurrence is the systematic use of an extraction bag.

Parietal Complications

At various times after the operation, infections may occur near the trocar sites. These lesions must be incised like superficial abscesses, and one should always search for bile stones within the collection. These stones can be detected either by sonography of the abdominal wall, or during incision by systematic exploration of the abscessed cavity, which also allows extraction of these foreign bodies, the only way to secure a definitive cure.

Postoperative incisional hernia may also occur along trocar routes, when the trocars used are 10 mm or more in diameter. They can also occur at the site of the incision used for the extraction of the operative specimen when the specimen was large and required extension of the aponeurotic opening, which was not properly closed afterwards. These abdominal wall ruptures represent a formal indication for surgery. An elegant and efficient solution is to use a laparoscopic approach to replace the contents of the hernia in the abdomen and closure of the aponeurotic defect via a transcutaneous approach.

Whenever an abnormal mass is found that is not a sign of suppuration or incisional hernia at the site of a former trocar port, a malignant graft should be suspected.[14] As for laparoscopic surgery for malignant tumors, laparoscopic removal of gallbladder tumors may cause cancer cell seeding of the abdominal wall. This is all the more true because gallbladder cancer is an insidious illness that is linked to lithiasis, and it may not have been diagnosed before the operation. If the gallbladder is extracted without special care, intraparietal seeding is possible. This is yet another reason for advocating the routine use of a bag for gallbladder extraction after laparoscopy. Also remember that a clear preoperative diagnosis of gallbladder cancer is a contraindication to the laparoscopic approach. If the cancer is diagnosed after pathological examination of the specimen, and if the specimen was extracted without protection, it is advisable to reoperate the patient and perform resection by open surgery of the trocar route suspected to have been contaminated.

CONCLUSION

We have just described, in chronological order, all the postoperative complications that may occur during the postoperative course of laparoscopic cholecystectomy.

TABLE 91–1. FREQUENCY OF COMPLICATIONS ACCORDING TO TIME OF DISCOVERY

	D0–D1	D2–D15	>D15
Bleeding	+++	+	0
Biliary stenosis	0	+	++
Biliary leak	+	+++	0
Bowel perforation	+	+	0
Intra-abdominal complications	0	+ Bilioma	+ Bilioma Abscess + acute bowel obstruction
Parietal complications	0	0	+

D, day

TABLE 91–2. LAPAROSCOPIC CHOLECYSTECTOMY: SOME EUROPEAN RESULTS, 1990–1993

Country	No.	Conversion (%)	Complications (%)	Mortality (%)
Belgium[1]	3244	6.5	6.4	0.2
Switzerland[1]	1091	8.1	2.8	0
France[2]	2955	4.8	3.4	0.2
Part of E.C.[3]	1236	3.6	1.6	0
France-Belgium[3]	6091	5.3	4.6	0.2
France[4]	1027	6	3	0.1

[1]Prospective studies.
[2]Retrospective studies.
[3]Compiled series.
[4]Personal series.
E.C. = European Community

Laparoscopic cholecystectomy was born in 1987 and soon became a tremendous success in the hands of its promoters because mortality and morbidity rates were from the very start similar to those obtained via open surgery. The improved postoperative comfort and shorter convalescence eventually won over most surgeons. These are the figures reported in 1990 to 1992: mortality, 0 to 0.1%; morbidity, 3 to 6%; and conversion rate, 3 to 5%.[11–15] The only problem was the percentage of CBD injuries, which was higher than with open surgery. These are the figures collected from 1990 to 1992: CBD injuries, 0.5 to 1%; and mortality related to CBD injuries, 0.08 to 0.1% (Tables 91–1, 91–2, and 91–3). There was a strong demand for laparoscopic cholecystectomy, which soon became popular worldwide. Its use spread quickly, certainly too quickly between 1990 and 1994; biliary complications became more and more frequent and peaked in 1994. Six years after this spate of complications that cast doubt on the safety of the procedure, training in laparoscopic surgery has improved, and the number of surgeons who have mastered the technique has increased. This accounts for the comparative results published in recent studies that show a gradual decrease in the complication rate, which dropped to 0.1% (Table 91–4).[16–19] As with all surgery, the results vary according to the patient's condition and the stage of the lesion. In fact, the mortality, morbidity, and conversion rates are roughly doubled when the operation is performed in an aged, underfed, or overweight patient, or when the gallbladder is surrounded with hard fibrotic tissue or is the site of acute infection.[20–22] We have reviewed the reasons other than the surgeon's

TABLE 91–3. COMMON BILE DUCT (CBD) INJURIES, 1990–1993, IN LAPAROSCOPIC CHOLECYSTECTOMY

Country	No.	CBD Injuries	%	Mortality (%)
Belgium[1]	3244	16	0.5	3 (0.09)
Switzerland[1]	1091	5	0.5	0
France[2]	2955	18	0.6	1 (0.03)
Part of E.C.[3]	1236	4	0.3	0
France-Belgium[3]	6091	12	0.2	2 (0.03)
France[4]	1027	3	0.3	0

[1]Prospective studies.
[2]Retrospective study.
[3]Compiled series.
[4]Personal series.

TABLE 91–4. BILIARY COMPLICATIONS OF LAPAROSCOPIC CHOLECYSTECTOMY

Evolution in Europe Compiled studies	
1989–1992	1993–1995
0.5% to 1%	0.2% to 0.8%
Persistence of learning curve effect	
1996–1998	
Scotland[16]	Switzerland[17]
0.8% to 0.4%	0.6% to 0.3%

lack of experience that may lead to intraoperative biliary accidents. It is obvious that biliary complications are sometimes impossible to avoid, and one must detect them as soon as possible. Here are a few rules to help in this task:

- Any symptom appearing during the postoperative course of a laparoscopic cholecystectomy should be considered as an alarm signal, and a morphologic investigation of the bile ducts must be launched immediately;
- Prevention lies in having intimate knowledge of the anatomy of Calot's triangle, in its exposure using the proper technique, and in the systematic intraoperative check of the biliary tree through cholangiography;
- Any lesion discovered must be carefully assessed and treated as follows: (1) intraperitoneal leakage demands emergency interventional treatment; (2) loss of the CBD's anatomic axis indicates mandatory open surgery; and (3) any lesion of the hilumbile duct junction indicates that the patient must be transferred to a specialized center;

Laparoscopic cholecystectomy remains the gold standard for gallstone removal.[23] If surgeons are trained properly,[24] it will truly become "a one-hour operation, followed by a one-day hospital stay, and a one-week convalescence" and lead to complete healing with no complications or sequelae. There is no such thing as surgery without risk, but if we optimize our technique and operate safely and carefully, we can keep complications to a minimum.

REFERENCES

1. Savader SJ, Lillemoe KD, Prescott CA, et al. Laparoscopic cholecystectomy related bile duct injuries: a health and financial disaster. *Ann Surg.* 1997;225:268.
2. Goodwin H. Minimal access surgery. *J Med Def Union.* 1998;14:12.
3. Moreaux J. Traitement des complications de la cholécystectomie. Ed. Tech. Encycl. Med. Chir. *Techniques Chirurgicales Généralités.* Appareil Digestif, 1993;40-960;18.
4. Salembier Y. La lithiase biliaire. Traitement chirurgical. Medsci/McGraw-Hill:1989.
5. Bismuth H. Postoperative strictures of the bile duct. In: Blumgart LH, ed. *The Biliary Tract.* Churchill Livingstone:1982;209.
6. Strasberg SM, Hertl M, Soper NJ. An analysis of the problem of biliary injury during laparoscopic cholecystetomy. *J Am Coll Surg.* 1995;180:101.
7. Mouret PH. From the first laparoscopic cholecystectomy to the frontiers of laparoscopic surgery. The future perspectives. *Dig Surg.* 1991;8:124.
8. Dubois GF, Icard P, Berthelot G, et al. Coelioscopic cholecystectomy: preliminary report of 36 cases. *Ann Surg.* 1990;191:271.
9. Perissat J, Collet D, Belliard R. Gallstones: laparoscopic treatment by intracorporeal lithotripsy followed by cholecystostomy or cholecystectomy. A personal technique. *Endoscopy.* 1989;21 Suppl:373.
10. Dubois F. Cholécystectomie et exploration de la voie biliaire principale par coelioscopie. Ed. Tech. Encycl. Med. Chir. *Techniques Chirurgicales Généralités.* Appareil Digestif, 1993:40-950;17.
11. Perissat J. Laparoscopic cholecystectomy: the European experience. *Am J Surg.* 1993;165:444.
12. Perissat J, Huibregtse K, Keane FBV, et al. Management of bile duct stones in the era of laparoscopic cholecystectomy. *Br J Surg.* 1994;81:799.
13. Couinaud C. Le foie. In: *Etudes anatomiques et chirurgicales.* Masson:1957;1.
14. Z'graggen K, Birrer S, Maurer CA, et al. Incidence of port site recurrence after laparoscopic cholecystectomy for preoperatively unsuspected gallbladder carcinoma. *Surgery* 1998:124:831.
15. Collet D. Laparoscopic cholecystectomy in 1994: Results of a prospective survey conducted by SFCERO on 4624 cases (Société Française de Chirurgie Endoscopique et Radiologie Opératoire). *Surg Endosc.* 1997;11:56.
16. MacFayden BV Jr., Vecchio R, Ricardo AE, et al. Bile duct injury after laparoscopic cholecystectomy. *Surg Endosc.* 1998;12:315.
17. Z'graggen K, Wehrli H, Metzger A, et al. Complications of laparoscopic surgery in Switzerland. A prospective 3-year study of 10,174 patients (Swiss Association of Laparoscopic and Thoracoscopic Surgery). *Surg Endosc.* 1998;12:1303.
18. Richardson MC, Bell G, Fullarton GM, et al. Incidence and nature of bile duct injuries following laparoscopic cholecystectomy: an audit of 5913 cases (West of Scotland Laparoscopic Cholecystectomy Audit Group). *Br J Surg.* 1996;83:1356.
19. Fletcher DR, Hobbs MS, Tan P, et al. Complications of cholecystectomy: risks of the laparoscopic approach and protective effects of operative cholangiography: a population-based study. *Ann Surg.* 1999;229:449.
20. Kiviluoto T, Siren J, Luukkonen P, et al. Randomized trial of laparoscopic versus open cholecystectomy for acute and gangrenous cholecystitis. *Lancet* 1998;351:321.
21. Lo CM, Liu CL, Fan ST, et al. Prospective randomized study of early versus delayed laparoscopic cholecystotomy for acute cholecystitis. *Ann Surg.* 1998;227:461.
22. Lyass S, Perry Y, Venturero M, et al. Laparoscopic cholecystectomy. What does affect the outcome? A retrospective multifactorial regression analysis. *Surg Endosc.* 2000;14:661.
23. National Institute of Health. Gallstones and Laparoscopic Cholecystectomy. NIH Consensus Statement. NIH:1992;1.
24. Calvete J, Sabater L, Camps B, et al. Bile duct injury during laparoscopic cholecystectomy: Myth or reality of the learning curve? *Surg Endosc.* 2000;14:608.

Chapter Ninety-Two • • • • • •

*C*omplications of Laparoscopic Esophageal Surgery

CRISTINA LOPEZ-PEÑALVER and MOISÉS JACOBS

The success of laparoscopic cholecystectomy[1] has driven the application of minimally invasive techniques to other disease processes. With the introduction of laparoscopic Nissen fundoplication in 1991,[2,3] laparoscopic surgery for the treatment of benign foregut diseases such as gastroesophageal reflux disease (GERD), paraesophageal hernias, and achalasia has become increasingly popular. Technological advances and the development of new equipment have facilitated this growing trend. The advantages of the minimally invasive approach have been well documented in the laparoscopic cholecystectomy literature, and include decreased pain, shorter hospitalization, and faster recovery and return to normal activity. Laparoscopy provides real benefits to the patient, provided it does not increase the surgical risk. Early criticism of this approach focused on the perceived higher incidence of complications encountered during the learning curve of each surgeon's experience. Knowledge of the anatomy and a thorough understanding of the complications associated with laparoscopic esophageal surgery should minimize the surgical risk. This chapter will outline the complications encountered with laparoscopic esophageal surgery (specifically antireflux surgery), delineate steps to prevent their occurrence, and how to manage them if they do occur.

Complications can be divided into those occurring in the perioperative and postoperative periods. Proper patient selection and preoperative evaluation are crucial and controllable factors. Every surgeon should carefully review the absolute and relative contraindications before planning any laparoscopic procedure. Factors such as morbid obesity, a hypertrophied left lobe of the liver, and previous gastric or esophageal surgery may increase conversion rates, especially during a surgeon's early experience. A thorough preoperative work-up with a history, physical examination, upper endoscopy, manometry, and 24-hour pH monitoring will improve selection of patients that respond favorably to surgery. Comorbid conditions such as coronary artery disease or severe chronic obstructive pulmonary disease (COPD) must be identified and evaluated in all prospective patients. The overall risks of general anesthesia remain the same whether the procedure is performed laparoscopically or through an open approach.

Before the operation starts, consideration must also be given to certain intraoperative details. Correct positioning of the patient is an important part of the operation. Unlike their open counterparts, most laparoscopic esophageal or upper abdominal procedures are performed in the reverse Trendelenburg or "head-up" position. Proper securing of the patient to the operating table with straps or tape prevents inadvertent movement or sliding during the procedure. Increased intra-abdominal pressure from the pneumoperitoneum and a steep reverse Trendelenburg position can impair venous return, cause pooling of blood in the legs, and increase the incidence of deep venous thrombosis.[4] To decrease this risk, sequential pneumatic compression devices are routinely employed by many surgeons.[5]

More importantly, a well-prepared team consisting of surgeon, camera operator, nursing staff, and an anesthesiologist is critical to the success of the operation. Use of laparoscopy results in a loss of depth perception and tactile sensation, and this can hamper a surgeon's ability to dissect tissue and identify important anatomic landmarks. A surgeon's experience with laparoscopic surgery and advanced laparoscopic skills such as suturing and knot tying can help prevent complications. Phillips noted that operator experience is the primary determinant of the incidence of laparoscopic complications.[6] He showed that there was an inverse relationship between the number of laparoscopic procedures performed and the incidence of complications. Proper training and credentialing of laparoscopists is essential in preventing complications, and guidelines for these criteria have been established.[7,8] Adverse outcomes associated with an individual's learning curve can be minimized with experienced supervision. In addition to surgeon experience, nurses and scrub technicians must be familiar with the equipment necessary for the procedure, including video monitors, cameras, and instrumentation. Furthermore, the anesthesiologist should be familiar with the positioning requirements of the procedure, as well as the potential complications associated with pneumoperitoneum. He or she must also be prepared to pass esophageal dilators when necessary.

INTRAOPERATIVE COMPLICATIONS

Intraoperative complications can be divided into those related to the pneumoperitoneum and those related to operative technique.

Complications of the Pneumoperitoneum

Complications related to the pneumoperitoneum can arise from CO_2 insufflation or from damage to the abdominal wall, viscera or major vessels during trocar insertion.

Laparoscopy and the insufflation of carbon dioxide into the peritoneal cavity lead to new concerns for the anesthesiologist. The physiologic effects on the pulmonary and cardiovascular systems are complex and depend on different variables such as the intra-abdominal pressure, the patient's intravascular volume status, changes in position, the anesthetic agents, and the presence of pre-existing cardiopulmonary disease. The respiratory effects with a pneumoperitoneum are caused by an elevation of the diaphragm from an increase in intra-abdominal pressure, and transperitoneal absorption of CO_2. In healthy patients, there is a mild increase in end-tidal CO_2 ($ETCO_2$) and arterial CO_2, a decrease in arterial pH and no significant change in peak airway pressure.[9] These changes are more pronounced in patients with cardiopulmonary disease and can result in significantly higher peak airway pressures. Additionally, the pneumoperitoneum decreases the functional residual capacity, which can lead to atelectasis and intrapulmonary shunting, resulting in hypoxemia. In healthy patients, the physiologic effects on the cardiovascular system are minor when the intra-abdominal pressure is maintained below 25 mm Hg.[10] However, hypovolemia, intra-abdominal pressures exceeding 20 mm Hg, and the reverse Trendelenburg position can lead to a decrease in venous return and adversely affect cardiac output. These changes may not be significant in healthy patients, but may lead to cardiovascular collapse in patients with underlying cardiac disease.

Establishment of a pneumoperitoneum is a basic prerequisite to laparoscopy. Elevation of the abdominal wall for gasless laparoscopy has been described, but is not widely used and has not been shown to decrease the complication rate. An improper insufflation technique can lead to potential complications, and therefore guidelines for safely inducing a pneumoperitoneum should be followed. Insufflation of the peritoneal cavity can be accomplished via an open or closed technique.[11,12] In the closed technique, a CO_2 pneumoperitoneum is established via blind insertion of a Veress needle through the abdominal wall into the peritoneal cavity. The abdominal wall is elevated with towel clips and the needle introduced in the midline at the level of the umbilicus and directed toward the pelvis. The aspiration and saline drop tests can then be performed to verify proper position prior to insufflation. Open laparoscopy involves entry into the abdomen via a cutdown technique, usually at the infraumbilical level, and the placement of a Hasson cannula under direct vision. This is an excellent technique to employ in patients with previous abdominal surgery because of the possibility of adhesions and the potential for injury to the bowel. Nonetheless, it can be difficult to perform in obese patients. Alternate site needle insertion (away from the scar) can also be used

in the operated abdomen. Regardless of the technique employed, abdominal wall, bowel, or vascular injuries can occur while gaining access to the abdominal cavity with a Veress needle or trocar.

Vascular injury to the abdominal wall occurs in 0.05 to 2.5% of cases and can manifest as external oozing, or blood dripping into the abdomen along the shaft of the cannula.[13] The usual source of bleeding is the epigastric artery or one of its branches. The surgeon should make every effort to identify the epigastric vessels so as to avoid injury during trocar placement. Incisions should be made lateral to the rectus abdominis muscle and trocars placed under direct vision to avoid injury to these vessels. If injury and bleeding do result, control can be obtained with electrocautery, or with a combined percutaneous/laparoscopic suture ligation technique using a Keith needle.[14] Perforating Veress needle and trocar injuries to the gastrointestinal tract and major vascular structures are equally uncommon with a combined incidence of 0.3 to 0.6% reported in both the gynecologic and surgical literature.[15–20]

Complications of the Surgical Technique

Various technical problems may be encountered that may limit the success of the laparoscopic approach to esophageal surgery. These include an enlarged left hepatic lobe, morbid obesity, large paraesophageal hernias and adhesions from previous upper abdominal surgery. In addition to this, knowledge of the anatomy and good surgical technique are essential factors in preventing complications such as bleeding and perforation.

Bleeding Complications. Every attempt should be made to minimize bleeding during a laparoscopic procedure. Blood staining can obscure tissue planes and make it difficult to identify anatomic landmarks. If bleeding occurs, it must be controlled immediately. Poor control of bleeding can rapidly obscure the operative field and lead to complications. Pooling of blood and darkening of the field as the hemoglobin-rich blood absorbs more light can make the exact bleeding site difficult to identify laparoscopically. If the precise bleeding site can be identified, definitive control can be obtained with cautery, clips, endo-loops, suture, or synthetic clotting agents such as Surgicel™. Blind clipping or suturing will invariably lead to injury of nearby structures and must be avoided. If the offending vessel is not identified, the surgeon can achieve temporary control by tamponade of the area with a 3×3 gauze. Use of the suction/irrigation device after removal of the packing can help localize the site during reassessment of the area; however, irrigation of pooled blood without first aspirating that blood will only lead to worse visualization, as the irrigant solution becomes red and will absorb light and hide the underlying anatomy. If the bleeding is severe and cannot be controlled with these maneuvers, then conversion to a laparotomy is indicated.

Intraoperative hemorrhage during laparoscopic antireflux surgery can occur from injury to the left lobe of the liver, injury to the spleen, or during dissection of the esophagus. Vascular injuries to the inferior vena cava, left hepatic vein, abdominal aorta, and inferior phrenic vessels have been reported,[21] but are fortunately rare. The left lobe of the liver is usually retracted cephalad to allow adequate visualization of the esophagus and gastroesophageal junction. Insertion and positioning of the retractor can result in a laceration or hematoma of the undersurface of the liver. Care should be taken during this maneuver and an atraumatic retractor used gently to prevent this complication. This type of bleeding is annoying, but usually minor and self-limiting. Additionally, blind

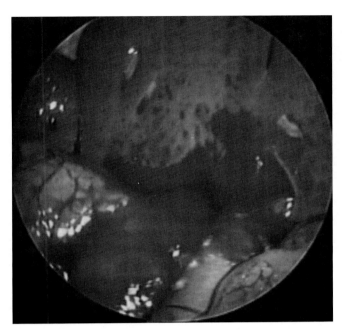

Figure 92–1. Splenic capsular tear.

insertion of laparoscopic instruments through other ports can lead to spearing of the liver if one is not cautious.

Although the spleen is not in direct contact with the hiatus, injury can occur during any laparoscopic dissection of this area. Excessive traction on surrounding tissues may cause splenic capsular tears (Fig. 92–1) or bleeding from disrupted short gastric vessels. Similarly, injury to the upper pole of the spleen may occur during dissection of the left crus or when passing instruments behind the esophagus in a right-to-left direction. Minor injury to the spleen can usually be resolved with cautery (Fig. 92–2) or the application of topical hemostatic agents (Fig. 92–3). More significant bleeding frequently requires a splenectomy, which may be performed laparoscopically or via conversion to laparotomy, depending on the skill of the surgeon. The risk of splenectomy due to

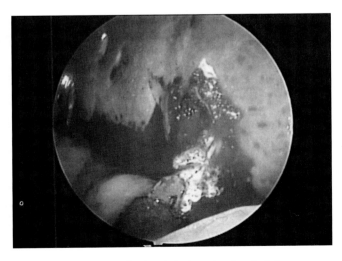

Figure 92–2. Application of electrocautery to splenic tear.

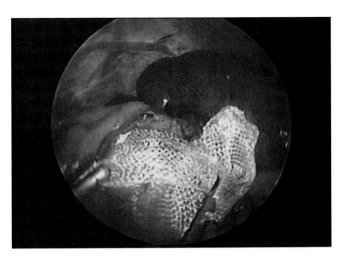

Figure 92–3. Application of topical hemostatic agent (Surgicel™).

inadvertent splenic injury during laparoscopic Nissen fundoplication is dramatically reduced by the laparoscopic method (Table 92–1).[22,23] Open fundoplication has been associated with splenectomy rates in the 1 to 4.2% range,[24–29] whereas splenectomy is seldom seen following laparoscopic fundoplication. This is likely secondary to better visualization and anatomic exposure.

Bleeding can also be encountered during dissection of the esophagus and stomach. Careful dissection allows for the identification of vessels that can be divided between clips or controlled with the harmonic scalpel or cautery. When dividing the gastrohepatic ligament to expose the distal esophagus and right crura, it is important to be aware of the possibility of an aberrant left hepatic artery. This aberrant artery is present in approximately 12% of patients, and significant hemorrhage can result from its inadvertent injury. During mobilization of the fundus, poorly secured short gastric vessels can also lead to intraoperative bleeding. Hemorrhage from injury to the short gastric vessels can be controlled with clips or the use of the harmonic scalpel.

Visceral Injury. Because of its associated high morbidity and mortality, perforation of the esophagus or stomach is the most serious complication associated with laparoscopic foregut surgery. Several mechanisms of injury have been described: injuries related to retroesophageal dissection, injuries resulting from passage of the

TABLE 92–1. SPLENECTOMY RATES IN THE SURGICAL TREATMENT OF GASTROESOPHAGEAL DISEASE

	Year	No. of Cases	Splenectomy Rate
Open Surgery			
DeMeester	1986	100	1.9%
Siewert	1989	94	4.2%
Urschel	1993	355	2%
Laparoscopic Surgery			
Cuschieri	1993	116	0%
Weerts	1993	132	0%
Hinder	1994	198	0%
Watson	1995	230	0%
Gotley	1996	200	0%
Hunter	1996	300	0%

bougie dilator or nasogastric tube, and injuries secondary to suture pullthrough.[30] Esophageal perforation can occur if there is improper dissection of the posterior esophagus. Failure to identify the esophageal border coupled with dissection in the wrong plane will undoubtedly lead to injury. Obesity, which is associated with excessive fat in the periesophageal area, and large hiatal hernias can contribute to this problem. Anterior retraction of the esophagus exposes the retroesophageal triangle, which is bounded by the posterior border of the esophagus anteriorly, the left crus superiorly and posteriorly, and the posterior gastric cardia inferiorly[13] (Fig. 92–4). Dissection outside these boundaries will usually lead to injury. For example, extension of the dissection too far anteriorly will result in esophageal perforation, too far inferiorly in gastric perforation, and too far superiorly in perforation of the pleura and pneumothorax. The majority of these injuries occur during a surgeon's early operative experience. Gastric wall injury or perforation may be a consequence of excessive traction on the anterior stomach. This risk of this injury can be lessened by gently handling the stomach with atraumatic instruments. Alternatively, injury to the fundus (Fig. 92–5) can occur secondary to electrocautery burns, primarily during division of the short gastric vessels. The surgeon must beware of cautery probes with inadequate insulation as they can cause contact injuries and subsequent perforation.

Another mechanism of intraoperative gastric or esophageal perforation involves improper passage of the bougie (Figs. 6A and 6B) or nasogastric tube. Although the incidence of injury during laparoscopic surgery is low (0.8%), it is significantly higher than the incidence of bougie perforation seen with the clinical dilatation of benign esophageal strictures (0.1%).[31,32] In contrast to open surgery, lack of direct manual palpation and guidance of the bougie tip during laparoscopic procedures may make this a more common complication. It is important that there be close communication between the anesthetist and surgeon during esophagogastric intubation. The anesthesiologist should avoid the use of excessive force and promptly inform the surgeon if any unusual resistance is

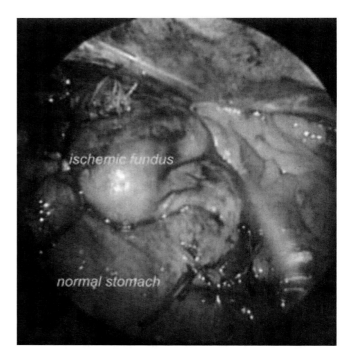

Figure 92–5. Ischemia and an electrocautery burn of the fundus.

encountered. An experienced anesthesiologist should pass the esophageal dilators slowly and under direct vision, and should exercise caution in patients with esophageal strictures. Crural closure and passage of the fundus behind the esophagus distort the gastroesophageal junction and make the passage of an esophageal dilator unsafe. Newer bougies (Fig. 92–7), such as those made by the Cook Corporation, which utilize a smaller nasogastric tube as a guide to the larger bougie, may make passage of an esophageal dilator safer. By applying caudal and anterior traction on the stomach, the surgeon minimizes distal esophageal angulation and facilitates passage of the bougie.

Disruption of full-thickness esophageal sutures accounts for another mechanism of injury. This complication usually occurs after surgery and may be associated with postoperative retching. The surgeon can prevent this by ensuring that only the muscular wall of the esophagus is penetrated during suturing. Use of a ski needle facilitates this step. Liberal use of antiemetics is also helpful in decreasing the incidence of this problem.

Perforations can be diagnosed by direct visualization of the tear or spillage of esophageal or gastric contents. If a perforation is suspected but cannot be identified, direct inspection with a gastroscope and insufflation of the esophagus and stomach under water may be helpful. Other surgeons use the technique of instilling methylene blue through the nasogastric tube to rule out a leak. Because delayed diagnosis of a perforation increases morbidity and mortality rates, some surgeons elect to perform these maneuvers routinely. If a perforation should occur and is recognized intraoperatively, laparoscopic suture repair can be carried out if the extent of the tear is clearly visualized. Surgeons experienced in advanced laparoscopic techniques can successfully manage intraabdominal esophageal perforations by laparoscopic primary closure and buttressing by the wrap. Conversion to laparotomy may be required in posterior tears if precise tissue approximation is not

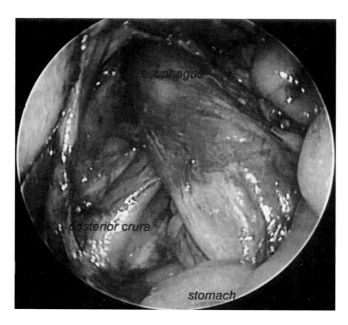

Figure 92–4. Retroesophageal anatomy.

A

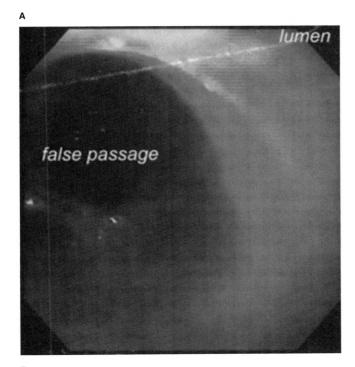

B

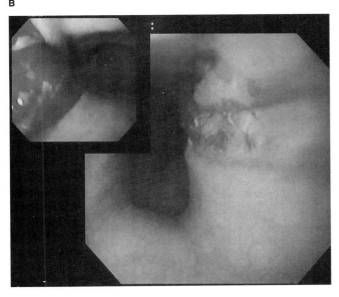

Figure 92–6. A. Creation of a false passage at the upper esophagus. **B.** Esophageal laceration.

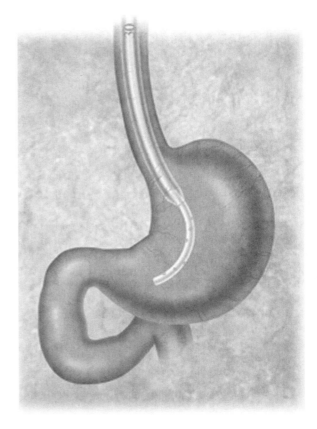

Figure 92–7. Esophageal bougie with nasogastric guidewire.

possible. If the level of skill does not permit laparoscopic repair, the surgeon should not hesitate or be faulted for converting to open repair. Thoracic esophageal perforations are best managed by thoracotomy, primary repair, mediastinal debridement, and drainage with a chest tube. Perforations that are recognized and repaired intraoperatively have a much better outcome than those with delayed diagnosis. Perforations recognized late are associated with an increased morbidity and mortality rate. Excessive postoperative pain should raise the index of suspicion and the appropriate work-up undertaken for diagnosis. Review of the literature for open antireflux

procedures reveals a 1% perforation rate with a 26% mortality rate.[33–36]

Pneumothorax. Injury to the pleura during laparoscopic esophageal surgery can lead to pneumothorax. This is usually the result of a high retroesophageal dissection. The risk of this complication may be as high as 2% in published series. Its development does not mandate the placement of a chest tube as the CO_2 gas is rapidly absorbed. Rather, it may be aspirated with a needle if it is significant enough. Pneumomediastinum has also been described, but it is rarely clinically significant.

Vagus Nerve Injury. Injury to the vagus nerves can be prevented by appropriate identification. The posterior vagus nerve (Fig. 92–8) can be identified inferiorly and to the right of the esophagus as it comes out of the hiatus. It is easy to identify because of its whitish color and positioning. Injury to this nerve can occur if an attempt is made to create a window between the esophagus and the right vagus nerve, in order to pass the gastric wrap within this location. It is an easier and safer dissection if the gastric wrap also covers the right vagus nerve.

Injury to the left or anterior vagus nerve (Fig. 92–9) can also be prevented by the appropriate identification; however, sometimes there is no true trunk, but only various branches, making this process much more difficult and inexact; alternatively, there may be more than one major trunk, which could be misidentified. Injury to the left vagus nerve can occur while anchoring the fundoplication to

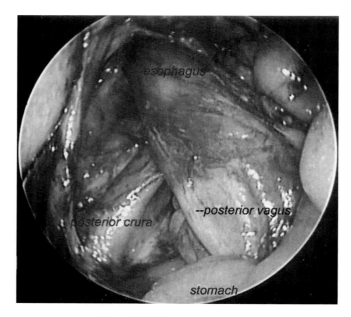

Figure 92–8. Posterior vagus nerve.

the esophagus if the sutures necrose or the needle injures the nerve directly.

POSTOPERATIVE COMPLICATIONS

Paraesophageal Hernia

Paraesophageal herniation is a rare complication following open fundoplication. The incidence of this complication has been reported to be as high as 7% in the laparoscopic fundoplication literature.[37,38] This is probably more common with the laparoscopic approach because of the tendency to extend the dissection of the esophagus further into the chest. Routine repair of the hiatus and limiting the cephalad extent of the esophageal dissection will reduce the risk of this problem.

Dysphagia

One of the most common postoperative problems after fundoplication is dysphagia. It has been reported to occur in up to 21% of patients after open surgery[39] and in an even higher percentage after laparoscopic procedures.[40] Some patients will develop dysphagia in the immediate postoperative period due to periesophageal edema and/or spasm. This usually disappears with dietary adaptations and time. Several reasons account for the persistent, troublesome dysphagia that develops in some patients postoperatively: a fundoplication that is too tight, excessive tightening of the esophageal hiatus, or a pre-existing esophageal motility disturbance. Construction of a wrap that is too tight or too long may result in a high incidence of postoperative dysphagia. Calibration of the esophagus with a bougie or dilator will ensure that the crura are not approximated too tightly and that the wrap is not too constricting. In addition to this, the length of the wrap should be kept between 1.5 and 2.0 cm to avoid this complication. Creation of a tension-free fundoplication is also a key factor in prevention. A

more generous mobilization of the fundus by division of the short gastric vessels may abolish the lateral pull of the esophagus and reduce tension on the wrap. However, the question of fundal mobilization is still controversial. In a randomized trial, Luostarinen et al[41] could not find any advantage from fundal mobilization in reducing postoperative dysphagia when compared to patients without fundal mobilization.[42] Similarly, in a prospective, randomized fashion, Watson et al[43] failed to show that routine division of the short gastric vessels improved any clinical or objective postoperative outcome. In terms of minimizing postoperative dysphagia, it seems that construction of a short, loose wrap is probably more important than whether the short gastric vessels are divided. The authors concluded that division of the short gastric vessels during laparoscopic Nissen fundoplication is indicated if a loose wrap cannot be constructed. With adequate mobilization, the wrap should reach the right side of the esophagus without traction. The decision to divide the short gastric vessels should be based on the mobility of the gastric fundus. Late stenosis of the esophageal hiatus due to diathermy dissection of the esophagus during laparoscopic mobilization and subsequent scarring has also been reported.[44] Performing a 360° fundoplication in a patient with an esophageal motor disorder will invariably lead to dysphagia. A partial wrap, or Toupet fundoplication, should be considered for patients with poor esophageal motility or for those in whom no preoperative manometry is available. Conversion of a total wrap to a partial wrap has been performed for this problem, both laparoscopically and in an open fashion, with good success.[45,46]

Wrap Migration

Another potential postoperative complication is transhiatal migration of the wrap. Postoperative retching and failure to close the hiatus are the two main reasons for wrap migration. Severe retching and vomiting in the postoperative period can cause disruption

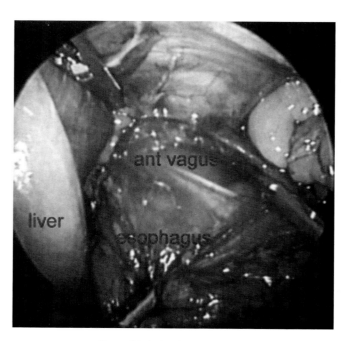

Figure 92–9. Anterior vagus nerve.

of sutures. Antiemetic prophylaxis and approximation of the crura with fixation of the wrap to the diaphragm are useful adjuncts in preventing this occurrence. However, care should be taken to avoid a hiatal closure that is too tight, or dysphagia will result.

CONCLUSION

Laparoscopic esophageal surgery is as feasible and safe as open procedures. However, as with other surgical procedures, a learning curve is required to achieve maximum benefit and minimize morbidity. Surgeons should be aware of the potential complications associated with these procedures and take the appropriate measures to prevent them. Conversion to open surgery may be necessary in certain circumstances, even for experienced laparoscopic surgeons. If the surgeon feels uncomfortable during the laparoscopy, or develops an intraoperative complication that cannot be managed laparoscopically, then conversion to open surgery is indicated. Even though the benefits of laparoscopy are well documented, the surgeon should keep in mind that the goal of the operation is to treat the disease process and not to perform a laparoscopic procedure at any cost. Proper patient selection and preoperative evaluation will increase the likelihood of a successful outcome. Safe insufflation techniques, meticulous hemostasis, and knowledge of the anatomy and surgical technique can help prevent iatrogenic injury and intraoperative mishaps. Complications will obviate the advantages of laparoscopy, so every effort should be made to prevent them.

REFERENCES

1. Reddick EA, Olsen DO. Laparoscopic cholecystectomy: A comparison with mini-lap cholecystectomy. *Surg Endosc.* 1989;3:131.
2. Dallemagne B, Weerts JM, Jehaes C, et al. Laparoscopic Nissen fundoplication: preliminary report. *Surg Laparosc Endosc.* 1991;1:138.
3. Geagea T. Laparoscopic Nissen's fundoplication: preliminary report on 10 cases. *Surg Endosc.* 1991;5:170.
4. Jorgensen JO, Lillies RB, Lalak NJ, et al. Lower limb venous hemodynamics during laparoscopy: an animal study. *Surg Laparosc Endosc.* 1994;4:32.
5. Millard JA, Hill BB, Cook PS, et al. Intermittent sequential compression in prevention of venous stasis associated with pneumoperitoneum during laparoscopic cholecystectomy. *Arch Surg.* 1993;128:914.
6. Phillips JM. Complications in laparoscopy. *Int J Gynaecol Obstet.* 1977;15:157.
7. Imbembo AL, Zucker KA. Training for laparoscopic surgery and credentialing. In: Zucker KA, Bailey RW, Reddick EJ, eds. *Surgical Laparoscopy.* Quality Medical Publishing:1991;343.
8. Society of American Gastrointestinal Endoscopic Surgeons. Granting or privileges for gastrointestinal endoscopy by surgeons. Society of American Gastrointestinal Endoscopic Surgeons, SAGES publication #0011-1/92:1992.
9. Wittgen CM, Andrus CH, Fitzgerald SD, et al. Analysis of the hemodynamic and ventilatory effects of laparoscopic cholecystectomy. *Arch Surg.* 1991;126:997.
10. Liu SY, Leighton T, Davis I, et al. Prospective analysis of cardiopulmonary responses to laparoscopic cholecystectomy. *J Laparoendosc Surg.* 1991;1:241.
11. Zucker KA, Bailey RW, Reddick EJ, eds. *Surgical Laparoscopy.* Quality Medical Publishing:1991;148.
12. Zucker KA, Bailey RW, Reddick EJ, eds. *Surgical Laparoscopy.* Quality Medical Publishing:1991;114.

13. Boswell WC, Odom JW, Rudolph R, et al. A method for controlling bleeding from abdominal wall puncture site after laparoscopic surgery. *Surg Laparosc Endosc.* 1993;3:47.
14. Haglund U, Norlen K, Rasmussen I, et al. Complications related to pneumoperitoneum. In: Bailey RW, Flowers JL, eds. *Complications of Laparoscopic Surgery.* Quality Medical Publishing:1995;33.
15. Phillips JM. Complications in laparoscopy. *Int J Gynaecol Obstet.* 1977;15:157.
16. Arian M, Appel M, Berci G, et al. Retrospective and prospective multi-institutional laparoscopic cholecystectomy study organized by the Society of American Gastrointestinal Endoscopic Surgeons. *Surg Endosc.* 1992;6:169.
17. Yuzpe AA. Pneumoperitoneum needle and trocar injuries in laparoscopy. A survey on possible contributing factors and prevention. *J Reprod Med.* 1990;35:485.
18. Loffer F, Pent D. Indications, contraindications and complications of laparoscopy. *Obstet Gynecol Surv.* 1975;30:407.
19. Scott TR, Zucker KA, Bailey RW. Laparoscopic cholecystectomy: A review or 12,397 patients. *Surg Laparosc Endosc.* 1992;2:191.
20. Byron JW, Markenson F, Miyazawa K. A randomized comparison of Veress needle and direct trocar insertion for laparoscopy. *Surg Gynecol Obstet.* 1993;177:259.
21. Baigrie RJ, Watson DI, Game PA, et al. Vascular perils during laparoscopic dissection of the oesophageal hiatus. *Br J Surg.* 1997;84:556.
22. Hinder RA, Filipi CJ, Wetscher G, et al. Laparoscopic Nissen fundoplication is an effective treatment for gastroesophageal reflux disease. *Ann Surg.* 1994;220:472.
23. Jamieson GG, Watson DI, Britten-Jones R, et al. Laparoscopic Nissen fundoplication. *Ann Surg.* 1994;220:137.
24. Hill ADK, Walsh TN, Bolger CM, et al. Randomized controlled trial comparing Nissen fundoplication and the Angelchik prosthesis. *Br J Surg.* 1994;81:72.
25. Luostarinen M, Isolauri J, Laitinen J, et al. Fate of Nissen fundoplication after 20 years. A clinical endoscopical, and functional analysis. *Gut* 1993;34:1015.
26. DeMeester TR, Bonavina L, Albertucci M. Nissen fundoplication for gastroesophageal reflux disease. Evaluation and primary repair in 100 consecutive patients. *Ann Surg.* 1986;204:9.
27. Donahue PE, Samelson S, Nyhus Lloyd M, et al. The floppy Nissen fundoplication. Effective long-term control of pathologic reflux. *Arch Surg.* 1985;120:663.
28. Siewert JR, Isolauri J, Feussner H. Reoperation following failed fundoplication. *World J Surg.* 1989;13:791.
29. Urschel JD. Complications of antireflux surgery. *Am J Surg.* 1993;166:68.
30. Schauer PR, Meyers WC, Eubanks S, et al. Mechanisms of gastric and esophageal perforations during laparoscopic Nissen fundoplication. *Ann Surg.* 1996;223:43.
31. Lowham AS, Filipi CJ, Hinder RA, et al. Mechanisms and avoidance of esophageal perforation by anesthesia personnel during laparoscopic foregut surgery. *Surg Endosc.* 1996;10:979.
32. Silvis SE, Nebel O, Rogers G, et al. Endoscopic complications—results of the 1974 American Society for Gastrointestinal Endoscopy Survey. *JAMA.* 1976;235:928.
33. Urschel JD. Complications of antireflux surgery. *Am J Surg.* 1993;166:68.
34. Shirazi SS, Schulze K, Soper RT. Long-term follow-up for treatment of complicated chronic reflux esophagitis. *Arch Surg.* 1987;122:548.
35. Polk HC. Fundoplication for reflux esophagitis: misadventures with the operation of choice. *Ann Surg.* 1976;183:645.
36. Skinner DB, Belsey RH. Surgical management of esophageal reflux and hiatus hernia: long-term results with 1030 patients. *J Thorac Cardiovasc Surg.* 1967;53:33.
37. Watson DI, Jamieson GG, Devitt PG, et al. Paraesophageal hiatus

hernia: an important complication of laparoscopic Nissen fundoplication. *Br J Surg.* 1995;82:521.

38. Johansson B, Glise H, Hallerback B. Thoracic herniation and intrathoracic gastric perforation after laparoscopic fundoplication. *Surg Endosc.* 1995;9:917.

39. DeMeester TR, Bonavina L, Albertucci M. Nissen fundoplication for gastroesophageal reflux disease. Evaluation of primary repair in 100 consecutive patients. *Ann Surg.* 1986;204:9.

40. Collard JM, Gheldere CA, De Kock M, et al. Laparoscopic antireflux surgery. What is real progress? *Ann Surg.* 1994;220:146.

41. Luostarinen M, Koskinen M, Isolauri J. Effect of fundal mobilisation in Nissen-Rossetti fundoplication on oesophageal transit and dysphagia. *Eur J Surg.* 1996;162:37.

42. Laine S, Rantala A, Gullichsen R, et al. Laparoscopic vs conventional Nissen fundoplication. *Surg Endosc.* 1997;11:441.

43. Watson DI, Pike GK, Baigrie RJ, et al. Prospective double-blind randomized trial of laparoscopic Nissen fundoplication with division and without division of short gastric vessels. *Ann Surg.* 1997;226:642.

44. Watson DI, Jamieson GG, Mitchell PC, et al. Stenosis of the esophageal hiatus following laparoscopic fundoplication. *Arch Surg.* 1995;130:1014.

45. DePaula AL, Hashiba K, Bafutto M, et al. Laparoscopic reoperations after failed and complicated antireflux operations. *Surg Endosc.* 1995; 9:681.

46. Lim JK, Moisidis E, Munro WS, et al. Re-operation for failed antireflux surgery. *Aust NZ J Surg.* 1996;66:731.

Chapter Ninety-Three ● ● ● ● ● ●

Complications of Laparoscopic Colorectal Surgery

MORRIS E. FRANKLIN, JR., JORGE E. BALLI, and MOISÉS JACOBS

INTRODUCTION

Initial laparoscopic procedures performed in the early 1900s were primarily of a diagnostic nature.[1–6] Gynecologists in the 1930s through the 1960s also utilized laparoscopy primarily as a diagnostic tool. Thoracoscopy was practiced in the 1930s for primarily diagnostic purposes, but it lost favor and essentially was not done by thoracic surgeons for many years. More intense interest in laparoscopy was kindled in the 1960s for gynecologists, who began performing tubal ligations as therapeutic procedures, and in the early 1970s began utilizing laparoscopy for other therapeutic procedures, particularly for treatment of endometriosis and ectopic pregnancy. General surgeons lagged behind and only a few diagnostic procedures were performed in the early 1980s. The first laparoscopic cholecystectomy was performed by Muhe,[7] a German surgeon, in 1985. He performed a series of laparoscopic cholecystectomies using a one-man technique utilizing bicycle frame tubing which had been modified with a home-made lens system, as well as special instrumentation. The first documented videoscopic cholecystectomy was performed by P. Mouret in France and the first publicized laparoscopic cholecystectomy was by Dubois in France in 1986.[8] McKernan, followed shortly by Reddick,[9] performed the first laparoscopic cholecystectomies in the United States in 1988 and this, initiated with the aid of video laparoscopy, led to a series of more adventuresome laparoscopic procedures. The first laparoscopically-assisted colon resection was a right colon resection by Jacobs[10] in 1990, followed very shortly by a laparoscopically-assisted left colon resection by Fowler, and a total intracorporeal resection by Franklin. The first reported laparoscopic colon resection for cancer was by Franklin in 1991 in a series published with Ed Phillips.[11] Procedures performed laparoscopically theoretically offered a variety of advantages to the patient. These proposed advantages included less pain, quicker recovery, shorter duration of ileus, quicker return to full function, and apparently, though it is still being investigated, a decreased immunologic insult to the patient. Unfortunately, performing a procedure laparoscopically does not protect the patient from a number of potential complications common to laparoscopic or any other type of surgery. These complications may be inherent to the procedure itself or in the fact that the procedure is done laparoscopically.

There are three broad categories of complications: (1) those occurring because of preoperative manipulations or lack of same; (2) those occurring intraoperatively; and (3) those occurring in the postoperative phase. Preoperative complications result primarily from either a poorly selected patient or a lack of adequate work-up in the evaluation phase. Poor patient selection may be caused by uncontrollable problems, such as multiple prior operations, the presence of a large tumor, the presence of adjacent organ involvement, obesity, or the presence of multiple adhesions. An adequate work-up should enable the surgeon to identify many of these potential problems, and an inadequate work-up to identify underlying problems is a primary cause of perioperative complications. A patient who is a poor anesthetic risk can readily be identified either by the surgeon or the anesthesiologist in the preoperative period. Among the primary concerns in this area are patients with complex cardiovascular and pulmonary problems. These patients should be readily identified and alternative therapy instituted if indicated. On the positive side, we have found that in many cases patients who are not fit for open procedures or who carry a high risk for an open procedure can tolerate a laparoscopic procedure if it is done with particular care. However, in general, any patient who is deemed unfit for general anesthesia should also be considered to be unfit for a laparoscopic procedure.

PREOPERATIVE COMPLICATIONS

Perhaps the most critical aspect of preoperative complications is in the area of preoperative planning and team preparation by the

TABLE 93–1. PREOPERATIVE COMPLICATIONS

Surgeon and team preparation to help prevent complications
  Surgeon-related
  • Knowledge and skills in laparoscopic surgery for benign and malignant disease
  • Laparoscopic knotting and tying techniques
  • Laparoscopic stapling techniques
  Team-related
  • Knowledge of steps and requirements for laparoscopic surgery
  • Knowledge of the correct set-up of patient and equipment

surgeon and his operating team. Surgeons wishing to embark upon laparoscopic colon surgery should be well prepared in a number of areas. These include having a thorough knowledge of colon disease processes, particularly metastasis, the means by which colon cancer spreads. The would-be laparoscopic surgeon should also have extensive experience in open colon surgery prior to embarking upon laparoscopic colon procedures. There should be a minimum of laparoscopic skills present, including a moderate amount of laparoscopic experience, the ability to perform laparoscopic manipulation of tissues and instrumentation, and a thorough understanding and technical skills required for laparoscopic suturing and knot tying. The surgeon should also have a working knowledge of stapling techniques, both for division of tissue as well as for creation of anastomoses. A moderate amount of planning should go into each operation, including the possible necessity for colonoscopic intervention; conversion to open surgery; orientation of the operating team, including the anesthesiologist, the circulating nurse, and the scrub nurse in the type of resection, the equipment needed, and the orientation of the patient and positioning of the monitors. Failure to perform these steps will invariably result in frustration and a very high conversion rate, which adequate preoperative planning could prevent (Table 93–1).

INTRAOPERATIVE COMPLICATIONS

The next general area of complications is that of intraoperative complications. Many experts feel that adequate preparation would certainly prevent many intraoperative complications. Consultations should be performed with the anesthesiologist regarding the type of anesthesia being contemplated, the expected duration of the procedure, and the various manipulations that will be needed during the surgery. Special attention should be paid to insertion of monitoring lines, and we recommend that a central line and an arterial line be placed in every patient, but they are absolutely mandatory in patients who have compromised cardiopulmonary systems. Long discussions should be carried out with the anesthesia personnel regarding carbon dioxide build-up intraoperatively. The patient should be properly positioned for the procedure at hand, and we recommend anal access for colonoscopy for each and every procedure. Additionally, the patient's arms should be at their sides in order to allow adequate access into and above the shoulders. The patient should be very securely fixed to the table. This can be done with a bean bag or with a series of taping maneuvers across the shoulders. We prefer taping instead of straps or table chocks, as use of the latter at the shoulders has resulted in brachial plexus injuries. Additionally, all exposed nerves or potentially exposed nerves where pressure may occur should be protected in order to

avoid (peroneal, femoral, or sciatic) nerve injury. Potential intraoperative anesthetic-related complications also include cardiovascular compromise from the pneumoperitoneum, and arrhythmia from hypothermia (particularly if the exposed extremities are not covered and if insufflated and inspired gases are not humidified). Irrigation fluid and IV fluids should also be warmed. There is a loss of body core heat from convection secondary to high CO_2 flow, and this also must be compensated for.

Particular attention should be paid to bowel preparation because inadequate or poorly planned and carried out bowel preparation will many times result in conversion of a procedure to open surgery due to unexpected and unnecessary contamination. Oral antibiotics, intraoperative antibiotics, and immediate preoperative parenteral antibiotics are also recommended.

A poorly prepared surgeon will result in a very high conversion rate and a very long procedure. The would-be laparoscopic surgeon should prepare him- or herself thoroughly by thinking through the operation and being fully aware of each step that will be performed prior to actually starting the operation. This can be accomplished by thorough reading and review of the operative techniques used by experienced laparoscopic surgeons, attending courses that teach laparoscopic surgery, and/or having a proctorship with someone who is experienced in laparoscopic colon surgery. With all other factors being equal, inexperience is probably the most common cause of conversion to open surgery and intraoperative technical errors cause most of the problems with laparoscopic colon surgery. There are a number of complications related to access to the abdominal cavity. Patients who have had prior surgery may obviously have numerous adhesions. If a Veress needle is to be used for insufflation, alternative site insufflation should be performed. If the Hasson technique is to be used, this can also be performed, but we do not recommend initially placing a trocar in an old scar site, but rather choosing an alternative site so that the old incision site (the site of previous surgery) can be visualized and adhesions taken down laparoscopically. Proper placement of trocars is imperative to successful laparoscopic surgery, and the trocars should preferably be placed outside of the rectus abdominis muscle and away from major vascular structures such as the superior and inferior epigastric arteries in the abdominal wall. After the initial trocar is placed, all others should be placed under direct vision in order to avoid abdominal wall vascular injuries as well as retroperitoneal injuries such as those of the common iliac, external iliac, and internal iliac vessels. All trocars should be fixed to the abdominal wall (preferably with sutures) to prevent slippage and dislodgment of the trocars intraoperatively. Each trocar site should be relatively snug to prevent subcutaneous emphysema. The practice of making more than one hole in the peritoneum is to be avoided, as this leads to massive subcutaneous emphysema, high CO_2 accumulation, and it also may contribute to trocar site implantation in patients with cancer.

One of the primary problems in laparoscopic colorectal surgery is that of a much wider anatomic field than is seen with laparoscopic cholecystectomy, hernia repair, or Nissen fundoplication. The colon is a four-quadrant organ and the ability to identify the anatomy in each quadrant is ever present. Lack of identification of anatomy, and in particular identification of the ureter, is a sure road to failure. Recognition of anatomy from a number of different points of view and in a wide sweeping panorama is one key to successfully performing laparoscopic colon resection for benign or malignant disease. This often takes intimate knowledge of the

TABLE 93–2. CAUSES OF INTRAOPERATIVE COMPLICATIONS

Improper anesthesia preparations
- Lack of monitoring lines

Inadequate patient positioning
- Lack of anal access
- Lack of adequate fixation to table
- Lack of measures to prevent hypothermia

Poor bowel preparation

Poor surgeon preparation

Improper insufflation site

Poor trocar placement

Lack of identification of anatomy

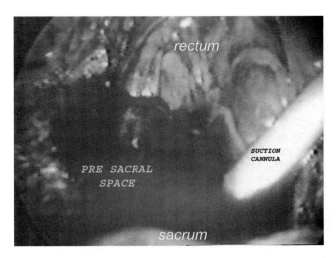

Figure 93–1. Presacral bleeding with uncontrolled pooling of blood, necessitating conversion to an open procedure.

anatomy, particularly as seen from several points of view and through various windows made in the mesentery. The ability to palpate vessels requires intricate knowledge of not only the normal anatomy, but also abnormal anatomy and vascular deviations from the norm. The key to recognition of anatomy is knowledge of certain fixed structures to which one can always refer. Among these are the ureter, the colon, the ligament of Treitz, the pancreas, and the spleen. These organs give the would-be laparoscopic surgeon a fixed structure to use as a starting point to identify a given anatomical structure in the process of performing a laparoscopic colon procedure. It is imperative that the laparoscopic colon surgeon know the course and anatomical variations of blood vessels, particularly of the major vessels, as bleeding is one of the most common causes of conversion from laparoscopic to open surgery. Getting lost anatomically, being unable to identify a given area or structure, or misidentification of a structure may result in massive bleeding, necessitating conversion to an open procedure (Table 93–2).

Laparoscopic colon surgery is perhaps the hardest laparoscopic procedure to consistently perform successfully. It is imperative that one have the very best equipment available and that this equipment be in top-notch condition. Routinely, two video sets should be available in case one set fails. It is also important to have a multitude of not only cameras, but also trocars, instrumentation, and various scopes, in order to achieve optimal angulation. It is often necessary to utilize 30°, 45°, and zero-degree scopes in the same case in order to see certain structures, particularly in obese patients or in patients who have had prior surgery with multiple adhesions. Occasionally one may also need to use a 5-mm scope in certain situations.

Bowel injuries are common for the novice surgeon who begins doing laparoscopic colon and rectal surgery. These injuries occur because of the effort put forth to achieve adequate visualization of vascular structures, and/or because of lack of ability to tilt the patient in different directions, which aids in gravitational retraction. Poor bowel preparation will result in large, edematous, fluid-filled loops of bowel, and care must be taken to do an adequate bowel prep, which results in collapse of the small bowel. The most common causes of injury to the bowel are grasping a portion of bowel with a sharp instrument or a grasper, which is similar to grabbing bowel with a hemostat and then twisting it. Occult injuries can occur from trocar injuries, cautery burns, and capatence coupling, among other means. All of these injuries can be avoided if meticulous care is taken to be absolutely certain: (1) of the location of the bowel, (2) that all instrumentation is well insu-

lated, (3) that instrumentation which promotes capatence coupling is avoided, and (4) that minor bleeding is controlled as it occurs. If this is not done, a series of events may occur. First, the exact location of the bleeding becomes harder and harder to recognize (Fig. 93–1). Second, clots that form cannot be removed and panic grips the surgical team. Next, the light begins to dim as the hemoglobin-rich blood absorbs more and more light. Vessels retract, making their identification and control even harder. The practice of blind clipping in a pool of blood is ill-advised. When bleeding occurs, it is best to stop the task at hand and control the vessel with pressure, either directly from a separate trocar and from a separate grasper, or with direct pressure from an instrument guided by the surgeon. Then a suction device can be brought in, all clots can be removed, and the exact source of bleeding can then be visualized and subsequently controlled. There are a variety of ways to control bleeding, including stapling or clipping, using endo-loops, an ultrasonic dissector, vascular clamps, bipolar cautery, an Argon beam coagulator, and on rare occasion a laser (Fig. 93–2).

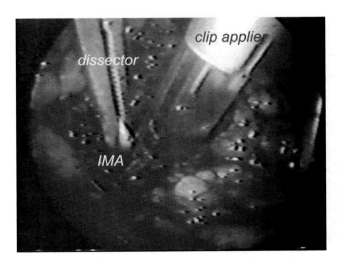

Figure 93–2. Bleeding from the inferior mesenteric artery (IMA), controlled with clips.

In addition to poor control of bleeding, another common problem for the novice surgeon is poor dissection technique. There have been a number of techniques described for dissection of various portions of the colon. Most of these revolve around identification of the individual vessels and their ligation. However, stapling techniques in which large, bulky portions of the colon are stapled into one large wad of tissue are to be entered into cautiously, because many times a structure such as a ureter, which does not need to be stapled or divided, can be included in such a wad of tissue. Frequently, unless specific types of staplers are used, bleeding will ensue between small clips. This bleeding can be stopped in most cases with careful, gentle control, such as clamping of the area or lightly touching the area with cautery. Occasionally, a suture ligature of a vessel will be needed in order to control bleeding through a staple line. We recommend identification and control of each individual vessel with either individual ligation or multiple clips. This will prevent events such as those described above, in which an unintended structure is divided because of poor dissection. A common contributing factor to poor dissection technique is the presence of adhesions. We recommend that any and all adhesions, such as those in the pelvis with a low anterior resection or a sigmoid resection, be taken down prior to initiation of dissection. Having to deal with loops of bowel stuck next to the colon makes the procedure doubly difficult, so these adhesions should be carefully taken down and all small bowel swept out of the pelvis prior to beginning a sigmoid or low anterior resection.

After dissection of the specimen, the specimen must be controlled, even if it is to be removed transabdominally. Bagging technique should be learned and utilized in order to prevent contamination of the wound, regardless of the presence of diverticulitis or a carcinomatous process. If a laparoscopically-assisted procedure is to be performed, a wound protector of some type should be used as the specimen is brought through the abdominal wall. Knowledge of stapling techniques, not only open, but laparoscopic, are imperative for a high success rate in completing laparoscopic colon procedures. While hand-sutured anastomoses can be done and are being used by several investigators, stapling remains the mainstay of laparoscopic colon resection, regardless of whether they are totally intracorporeal or laparoscopically-assisted.

Prior to division of the bowel and completion of the anastomosis, it is imperative that very small lesions be adequately localized. This can be performed either by preoperative tattooing using specific tattooing techniques, intraoperative colonoscopy, direct palpation of the lesion, or utilization of transabdominal intraluminal colonscopy. We feel that each anastomosis should be tested with the colonoscope or with air, and the anastomosis should be placed under water to detect any leaks. At the completion of the procedure, it is imperative to close all 10-mm and larger trocar sites with a fascial closure.

Bleeding can occur if the patient has not been deflated intraoperatively and all potential bleeding sites (including trocar sites) rechecked upon reinsufflation. We recommend this maneuver routinely because it results in picking up minute bleeding sites which might otherwise be missed.

POSTOPERATIVE COMPLICATIONS

Postoperative complications usually follow a pattern similar to that of intraoperative complications. However, an early and poorly rec-

TABLE 93–3. POSTOPERATIVE COMPLICATIONS

Hypothermia caused by:
- Prolonged procedures
- CO_2 leakage in trocar sites
- Lack of preventive measures

Excess administration of sedative analgesia
Early feeding
Trocar site implants and/or hernias
Anastomotic leaks and/or strictures
Bleeding

ognized complication is that of hypothermia (Table 93–3). Hypothermia is usually a result of (1) a prolonged operative time, (2) excess CO_2 leakage around trocar sites, and (3) inadequate preparation of the patient and inadequate protective measures. As previously mentioned, preventive measures include wrapping the legs, administering IV fluids and warm irrigation fluids, humidifying the inspired ventilatory gases, and covering all exposed surfaces. These steps will prevent most cases of hypothermia, but it may occur even when all these are taken, so vigilance is appropriate in the immediate postoperative period. Hypothermia will usually be evidenced by unexplained bradycardia, slow recovery from the anesthetic agents, and delayed mental response with a lower level of consciousness than would be expected. An infrequently recognized complication of hypothermia is a decrease in the ability of blood clotting mechanisms to function correctly. The body core temperature should be monitored very closely and appropriate warming devices utilized such as a Bair Hugger (Augustine Medical Inc., Eden Prairie, MN), a heating blanket, and heated IV fluids. Another problem that may occur is that of administration of an inordinate amount of analgesia for a patient undergoing laparoscopic colorectal surgery. Analgesia should be used sparingly, as the amount of pain with these procedures is usually much less than comparable procedures performed openly. The analgesia should be given sparingly, and only on demand from the patient. Similarly, a delay in ambulation can result in a multitude of problems, including thrombophlebitis, atelectasis, and delay in return of bowel activity. Thus ambulation should be initiated very early in the postoperative course, and it is usually started within the first 6

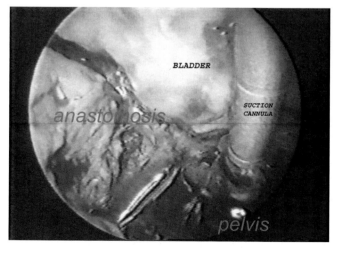

Figure 93–3. Anastomotic dehiscence in a low anterior resection.

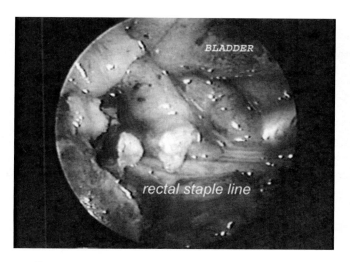

Figure 93–4. Stool leaking from the stump of the rectal staple line

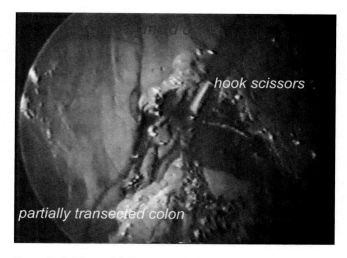

Figure 93–6. Injury to left iliac artery, which lies underneath the colon in a patient in the lithotomy, Trendelenburg, and right lateral decubitus positions.

postoperative hours. A common problem with laparoscopic surgery is that of trying to feed the patient too soon. We strongly recommend not feeding the patient before he or she is ready. Some patients are ready for feeding within 12 to 18 hours. Others need 2 to 3 days, depending on the extent of the procedure and the patient's individual response. We offer liquids when bowel sounds are present, and advance to solids after the first bowel movement.

Some later postoperative complications include trocar site implantations and hernias at trocar sites. These problems have been addressed in other publications and will not be covered in detail in this chapter. Suffice it to say, however, that adequate closure of trocar sites will almost completely prevent hernias. Other delayed complications can also occur in regard to the anastomosis, including dehiscence, if the anastomosis has not been performed correctly (Fig. 93–3). Anastomotic leaks occur for a variety of reasons, but in laparoscopic surgery the most common cause is ischemia and inadequate stapling technique.

The anastomoses should be checked intraoperatively with visualization, insufflation of air, or povidone iodine. Both stapler doughnuts should be complete. A leak at the staple line needs to be repaired, either with intracorporeal suturing, restapling, or conversion to open surgery. When in doubt, a diverting ostomy should be created. The rectal stump line should also be checked prior to anastomosis (Fig. 93–4).

SOME COMMON COMPLICATIONS

Injury to the Iliac Artery or Vein

This can occur with aggressive and wide dissection, especially at the level of the sigmoid colon, or when the anatomy is not clear to the surgeon. Prevention comes with knowledge of the laparoscopic anatomy (Figs. 93–5, 93–6, and 93–7).

Ureteral Injuries

These occur much more commonly on the left than on the right, and they can occur upon ligation and transection of the inferior

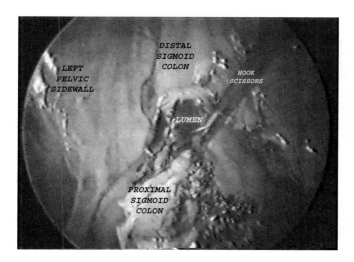

Figure 93–5. Intracorporeal transection of the sigmoid colon using hook scissors.

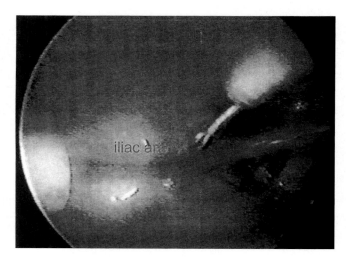

Figure 93–7. Bleeding from the iliac artery.

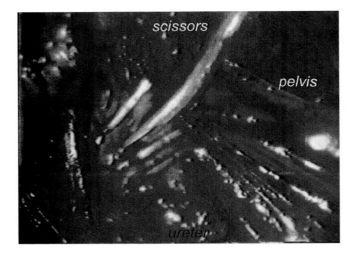

Figure 93–8. Clipped ureter.

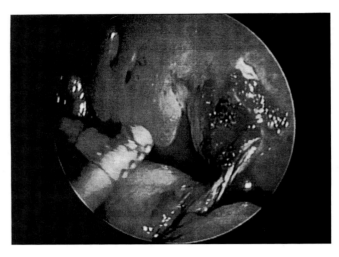

Figure 93–10. Laceration and bleeding from inferior pole of the spleen.

mesenteric artery (IMA), or with misidentification of the ureter as a blood vessel (Figs. 93–8 and 93–9). These injuries can also occur with staples, because the rectosigmoid colon is transected with an endo-stapler and the tip can catch the ureter. In addition, when closing and firing the circular stapler, the ureter can be trapped and injured.

Prevention is accomplished by identifying the ureter on all sigmoid or lower level resections. Failure to identify the left ureter may be an indication for conversion. Ureteral stents are not help-

ful in identifying the ureter as in open surgery, because of the loss of tactile sensation in laparoscopic surgery.

Splenic Injuries

As in open surgery, these can occur due to excessive pulling and traction, but they generally are much more rare in laparoscopic surgery than in open surgery because of the better visualization and more precise dissection that is possible with laparoscopy (Fig. 93–10). Again, prevention is aided by knowledge of laparoscopic anatomy.

Small Bowel Obstruction

These can occur from adhesions as in open surgery, but with laparoscopy, adhesions are usually less pronounced and more rare (Fig. 93–11). Small bowel obstruction can also occur from

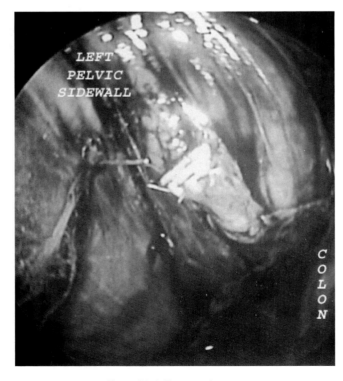

Figure 93–9. Transected ureter.

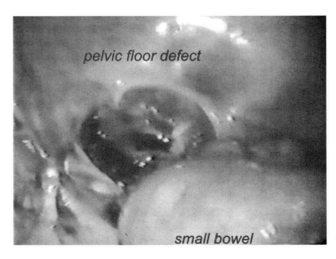

Figure 93–11. A pelvic floor defect in abdominal perineal resection, causing small bowel obstruction.

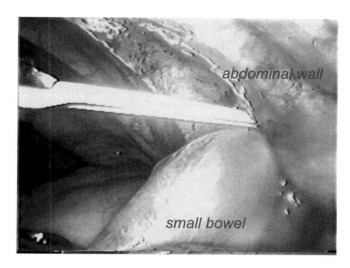

Figure 93–12. Incarcerated trocar site hernia.

incarceration at trocar sites (Fig. 93–12). All trocar sites 10 mm or larger should be closed to prevent herniation. In obese patients this may be difficult to impossible.

PREVENTION OF COMPLICATIONS

Complications can be avoided in the vast majority of laparoscopic colon and rectal surgical procedures. This begins with appropriate patient selection, avoiding the morbidly obese patient, and by allowing the surgeon to start his or her laparoscopic experience with benign disease processes that require simpler procedures (such as segmental resection for polyps), as well as doing the first operations on patients with no prior surgeries. Surgery for early-stage carcinoma may be appropriate if adequate training has been done, and if the surgeon has prior experience with benign disease. An appropriate preoperative work-up should be done, including evaluation of the cardiopulmonary system, detection of possible bleeding disorders, taking a careful history, and doing a thorough physical exam. The evaluation should also make note of prior operations, localize the lesions, and include arteriography, colonoscopy, a barium enema, and ultrasound as needed. Adequate training of the surgeon, the anesthesiologist, and the team is mandatory to minimize complications in laparoscopic colon and rectal surgery. This demands intense dedication on the part of all members of the team to prevent the many complications described here. Each operation should be carefully planned and should be discussed with the team and the anesthesiologist, and time limits should be set prior to beginning the procedure. If there is no progress made, the laparoscopic procedure should be terminated or converted to an open procedure. Appropriate equipment, including videoscopic equipment, hand-held equipment, and stapling devices and other instruments all contribute to the prevention of complications. All members of the team should be intimately familiar with the equipment and how to use it before the operation begins. The surgeon must be very adept in dissection with both hands and from all directions and all camera angles as previously discussed. High on the list of necessary equipment is an adequate operating table, one with a right and left tilt, Trendelenburg and reverse Trendelenburg positions, and preferably full body length C-arm capability.

There are other ways to prevent complications in laparoscopic colorectal surgery, including intimate knowledge of anatomy, particularly from a laparoscopic viewpoint; early control of bleeding when it occurs, bagging the specimen, using good surgical judgement, and most importantly using intraoperative colonoscopy when needed, will help prevent many problems in these operations.

CONCLUSION

Laparoscopic colorectal surgery is a safe procedure when done by an experienced surgeon. It can be less costly than an open procedure, it may be completed in a short time, and it can dramatically shorten postoperative recovery for many patients. Each operation must be meticulously planned and executed in order to derive the maximum benefit. Learning proper technique is an ongoing task, and one should begin with simpler operations and work up to the more difficult procedures. Careful preparation is essential to attaining good results in laparoscopic colorectal surgery. Many of the problems experienced are a direct result of inadequate preparation or selection of the patient, and poor preparation of the surgeon and/or the operating team.

ADDITIONAL READING

1. Kelling G. Über oesophagoskopic, gastroskopie und coelioscopie. *Munch Med Wochenschr.* 1901;49:21.
2. Kalk H. Erfahrungen mit der Laparoskopic. *Z Klin Med.* 1919;111:303.
3. Ruddock JC. Peritoneoscopy. *Surg Gynecol Obstet.* 1937;65:623.
4. Palmer R. Instrumentation et technique de la coelioscopie gynecologique. *Gynecol Obstet.* 1947;46:420.
5. Jacobaeus HC. Endopleurale Operation unter der Leitung des Thorakoskop. *Beitr Zur Krink Tuberk.* 1915;35:1.
6. Frangenheim R. History of endoscopy. In: Gordon AG, Lewis BV, eds. *Gynaecological Endoscopy.* Chapman & Hall:1988.
7. Mühe E. Die erste cholecystektomie durch das laparoskop. *Langenbecks Arch Klin Chir.* 1986;369:804.
8. Dubois F, Berthelot G, Levard H. Cholecystectomy par coelioscopy. *Nouv Presse Med.* 1989;18:980.
9. Reddick EA, Olsen DO. Laparoscopic cholecystectomy: A comparison with mini-lap cholecystectomy. *Surg Enodsc.* 1989;3:131.
10. Jacobs K, Verdeja G, Goldstein D. Minimally invasive colon resection. *Surg Laparosc Endosc.* 1991;1:144.
11. Phillips EH, Franklin ME, Carroll BJ, et al. Laparoscopic colectomy. *Ann Surg.* 1992;216:703.
12. Lumley JW, Fielding GA, Rhodes M, et al. Laparoscopic-assisted colorectal surgery. Lessons learned from 240 consecutive patients. *Dis Colon Rectum.* 1996;39:155.
13. Leroy J. Laparoscopic colorectal resection, technical aspects after 150 operations. *Osp Maggiore.* 1994;88:262.
14. Franklin ME, Rosenthal D, Abrego D, et al. Prospective comparison of open vs. laparoscopic colon surgery for carcinoma. Five-year results. *Dis Colon Rectum.* 1996;39:S35.
15. Lord SA, Larach S, Feffara A, et al. Laparoscopic resections for colorectal carcinoma. A three-year experience. *Dis Colon Rectum.* 1996;39:148.
16. Trokel MJ, Bessler K Treat MR, et al. Preservation of immune response after laparoscopy. *Surg Endosc.* 1994;8:1385.
17. Bessler K Whelan RL, Halverson A, et al. Is immune function better preserved after laparoscopic versus open colon resection? *Surg Endosc.* 1994;8:881.

18. Allendorf JDF, Bessler K Whelan RL, et al. Better preservation of immune function after laparoscopic assisted vs. open bowel resection in a murine model. *Dis Colon Rectum.* 1996;39:567.

19. Larach SW, Pantakar S, Ferrara A, et al. Complications of laparoscopic colorectal surgery. Analysis and comparison of early vs. later experience. *Dis Colon Rectum.* 1997;40:592.

20. Agachan F, Sik Joo J, Weiss E, et al. Intraoperative laparoscopic complications. Are we getting better? *Dis Colon Rectum.* 1996;39: S14.

21. Geers J, Holden C. Major vascular injury as a complication of laparoscopic surgery: A report of three cases and review of the literature. *Am Surg.* 1996;62:377.

22. Cooperman A. Complications of laparoscopic surgery. In: Arregui ME, Fitzgibbons RJJ, Katkhouda N, et al, eds. *Principles of Laparoscopic Surgery.* Springer-Verlag:1995.

23. Diemunsch P. Anesthesie Generale pour Coelioscopie. Presented at the EITS, Seminar of Laparoscopic and Thorascopic Surgery, Strasburg, France.

Chapter Ninety-Four • • • • • • •

Complications of Laparoscopic Inguinal Hernia Repair

EDWARD FELIX, JOSÉ ANTONIO VÁZQUEZ-FRIAS,
and JORGE CUETO-GARCÍA

INTRODUCTION

Each year over 700,000 hernias are repaired in the United States[1] and an increasing number are approached laparoscopically. Reports of complications and recurrences,[2–4] however, tempered the initial enthusiasm for the laparoscopic approach. As multiple hernia centers and practicing general surgeons around the world reported lower and lower recurrence and complication rates,[5–8] the number of laparoscopic repairs has again begun to increase. Improved outcomes have been the result of an accumulation of experience and knowledge of what makes the laparoscopic approach work. Understanding what factors lead to failure or complications has been the key to improving the success of the laparoscopic approach. There are situations that can be avoided altogether and others that if handled properly will result in a favorable outcome. This chapter discusses these issues, so others may benefit from the experience of surgeons who have already faced these problems.

Any discussion of laparoscopic hernioplasty must be viewed in the context of conventional repairs. The worldwide morbidity of open repairs ranges from less than 1% to more than 25% with an average recurrence rate of 10%.[9–10] The percentage of patients experiencing numbness or pain lasting more than a year after open repairs may be as great as 25%.[11] While some complications of laparoscopic repair are identical to those of open traditional or prosthetic repair, others are unique to the laparoscopic approach. In addition, there are risks that are peculiar to the both laparoscopic approaches, the transabdominal preperitoneal approach (TAPP) and the totally extraperitoneal approach (TEP).

Laparoscopic cholecystectomy taught us that surgeons thought to be experts at performing a procedure using a conventional open technique sometimes fall short of the mark when using a new laparoscopic approach.[12] Studies of laparoscopic hernioplasty[13–15] have also shown that complication rates are reduced with experience. A good measure of this experience appears to be average operative time. Stoker et al[16] and Liem et al[17] both showed that operative time correlates inversely with experience. In controlled studies that failed to show any benefit of laparoscopic hernioplasty, surgeons were usually in the early part of the learning curve, as measured by operative times that exceed 60 minutes.[18] In contrast, in a study of over 10,000 laparoscopic hernioplasties performed by surgeons with extensive experience, the average recurrence rate was less than 1%.[5] The incidence of conversion from a laparoscopic approach to an open approach, or from a TEP to a TAPP approach, also correlated with the complication[13] and recurrence rate.[15] The incidence decreased with experience. With experience, surgeons are better able to select appropriate patients for laparoscopic repair and prevent or handle peritoneal tears during TEP procedures that would have otherwise resulted in conversion. Several other studies have shown that recurrence rates as well as complication rates decrease with experience.[17,19–20] Proper training shortens the learning curve and reduces the number of complications and recurrences (Fig. 94–1).[15]

OVERVIEW OF COMPLICATIONS

In a study of patients undergoing both open and laparoscopic hernia repairs, up to 5% of patients surveyed felt that they were worse off after the hernia repair than before.[21] It is therefore important to keep complications to a minimum. The complication rate reported for laparoscopic repairs ranges from less than 3%[13] to as high 20%,[22] and is similar to that reported for open repairs.[9,23] The wide variation is due to the type and scope of complications considered and the expertise of the operating surgeons. In this chapter we will discuss only serious complications, and others that although minor, are frequent and need to be recognized.

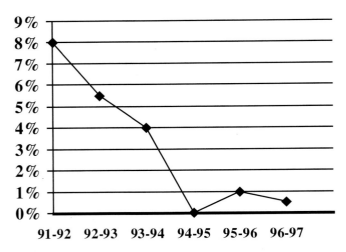

Figure 94–1. Learning curve for complications at Fresno Hernia Center, 1991–1997. The percentage of serious complications per year is shown.

COMPLICATIONS OF LAPAROSCOPIC HERNIOPLASTY

Seroma falls into the latter category. Up to 10% of patients develop a fluid collection after laparoscopic hernioplasty.[24] It presents as a recurrent mass soon after the repair and may suggest recurrence, because it sometimes transmits an impulse. Physical examination alone usually differentiates it from a recurrent hernia. If the examiner is inexperienced, an ultrasound exam will confirm the diagnosis. While 90% disappear in 6 weeks if left alone, if it persists or is symptomatic, aspiration almost always eliminates the problem.

A hydrocele may present as an enlarged testicular or scrotal mass from 2 months to several years after a hernia repair, and is always alarming to the patient. The incidence of hydrocele following laparoscopic repair is the same as after open repair, and it occurs in less than 1% of patients.[25] Only 0.4% of our laparoscopically-repaired hernias have required surgical treatment for a hydrocele. Our incidence, however, has significantly decreased since we stopped routinely using a keyhole in the mesh.[13]

The TEP repair has gained popularity because it eliminates some of the potential risks of a transabdominal approach. Injuries from trocars penetrating the peritoneal cavity, although uncommon, are extremely serious complications of the TAPP hernioplasty. Bleeding from the inferior epigastric vessels after lateral trocar placement was once common, but now is unusual because of the use of 5-mm trocars and an awareness of the location of the vessels. If bleeding does occur, it can be controlled with the use of a fascia closure device. The inferior epigastric vessels are not immune to injury during a TEP approach. The balloon dissector can take down the vessels, resulting in bleeding from small branches. The surgeon must quickly place the other trocars and rinse the space clear to find the source of bleeding and control it with bipolar cautery.

Injury to the bowel from lysis of adhesions or placement of the trocar are among the most serious complications of laparoscopic hernioplasty. The incidence of this complication is extremely low, but can be reduced even further by proper selection of patients and approach. By using a totally extraperitoneal technique, the potential for bowel injury is reduced, but not totally eliminated.[13] If the extraperitoneal space is obliterated by previous surgery, radiation, or infection, an open approach is preferred. If

bowel is incarcerated in the hernia, the transabdominal route is preferred, because it gives the surgeon the best view of the contents of the hernia and avoids inadvertent injury when reducing the incarceration. If a totally extraperitoneal approach with a balloon dissector is used, the peritoneum and possibly the bowel may be torn as the balloon expands. Also, dissection of the contents of the incarcerated hernia can be extremely difficult via the TEP approach, because of limited space and visualization. It is important to evaluate the hernia immediately before surgery to determine whether the hernia is reducible. This allows the surgeon to choose the proper approach and avoid injury to the bowel or peritoneum.

Bladder injuries can occur after both open and laparoscopic repairs. In the laparoscopic approach, it is usually due to failure to recognize that the bladder makes up part of the direct sac. Ligating the direct sac is unnecessary and can result in a delayed injury to the bladder. Injury from a balloon dissector during a TEP repair has also been described, but is rare. We have not seen this complication in over 3000 TEP repairs performed at our center.

Small bowel obstruction from inadequate closure of the peritoneum[26] was a problem in the past, because staples used to close the peritoneum following TAPP repairs left gaps in the closure. With sutured closures and more widespread use of the TEP approach, this problem is rarely seen. Schuricht et al,[27] however, stressed the importance of closing peritoneal defects even following TEP repairs, when he reported one patient with a bowel obstruction after a totally extraperitoneal approach.[27]

Trocar hernias were once common following laparoscopic hernia repair. In our early experience, the incidence of incisional or trocar hernias was greater than the incidence of recurrence after laparoscopic hernia repair.[28] After reducing the lateral trocar size to 5 mm for TAPP repairs and increasing the percentage of TEP repairs performed, trocar hernias virtually disappeared at our center. If larger ports are used, secure closure of the fascia is mandatory. There are now several commercial devices that make adequate suture closure of these wounds simple. These devices pass a suture through the fascia into the peritoneal cavity, allowing the surgeon to grasp and pull it out the opposite fascial wall. Incisions from some newer trocars do not need to be mechanically approximated because of their size and shape.

PAIN FOLLOWING HERNIA REPAIR

Pain following hernioplasty, open or laparoscopic, is still a major problem.[21] The origin of severe or chronic pain after both TEP and TAPP approaches can be due to direct injury to a nerve, entrapment of a nerve, the mesh itself, or even recurrence. The surgeon's approach to this complication should be dictated by the nature of the pain, its time course, and its severity. When severe pain in the distribution of a major nerve develops immediately after the hernia repair, re-exploration is indicated to search for and remove an offending staple or stitch. If there is delay in seeing such a patient, exploration is still indicated.[29] In contrast, patients with minor neuralgias, paresthesias, or numbness should be observed. These symptoms usually improve with time. Chronic pain that does not resolve and is disabling to the patient warrants surgical exploration. Patients referred with even longstanding severe pain that is localized or is in the distribution of a named nerve may benefit from reoperation. Exploration should be through a transabdominal laparoscopic route. If the pain is localized to the abdominal wall, it is important to mark the area of pain before beginning the laparoscopic exploration. This aids in correlating the

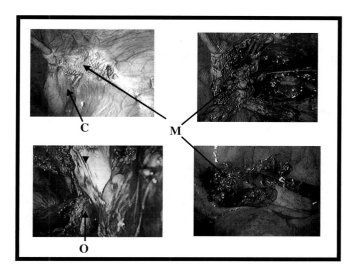

Figure 94–2 A female patient referred with 2 years of pain in the distribution of the obturator nerve following a TAPP repair. *Top left:* Peritoneal view. *Top right:* Peritoneum has been opened to expose curled mesh (M) which is irritating the obturator. *Bottom left:* The mesh has been debrided off of Cooper's ligament (C) exposing the obturator nerve (O). *Bottom right:* Debrided mesh. The patient was free of symptoms 6 months following remedial surgery.

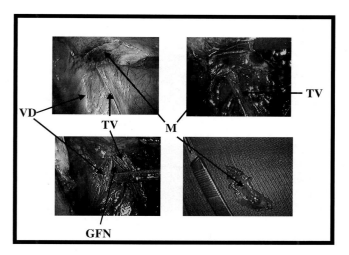

Figure 94–3. Curled mesh in a patient referred for 6 months of pain in the groin following a TEP repair. *Top left:* Peritoneal view of curled mesh (M) irritating genitofemoral nerve. *Top right:* Peritoneum has been opened to expose mesh and nerve. *Bottom left:* Dissection freeing genitofemoral nerve (GFN). *Bottom right:* Debrided mesh. The patient experienced relief of pain 1 month after remedial surgery. TV, testicular vessels; VD, vas deferens.

operative findings with the patient's symptoms. When laparoscopic exploration identifies a tack, staple, or stitch, it can be removed laparoscopically. Relief of pain may be immediate or gradual. If a neuroma has formed, neurectomy may be required in the future.

Sometimes pain is due to the mesh itself and not an anchoring device placed at the primary operation. If the polypropylene mesh curls up in the extraperitoneal space, it may form an extremely hard ridge that has the potential of irritating local nerves or surrounding tissue. The result is pain that is identical to that produced iatrogenically from a misplaced staple or tack. The offending portion of the mesh has to be removed and the nerve, if compressed by scar tissue, released. The mesh may be so hard that cautery is required to cut it free. The uninvolved mesh does not need to be removed. Using this approach, we have successfully treated several patients referred with postlaparoscopic pain, even as late as 2 years after the initial operation (Fig. 94–2). To avoid curling of the lateral mesh at the initial operation, it should be laid smoothly against the wall and held in place with a grasper as the peritoneum expands over it, if a TEP repair is performed (Fig. 94–3).

If precautions are taken at the initial laparoscopic repair, most nerve injuries are preventable. Initially, there were many serious nerve injuries, because surgeons were not aware of the location of the important nerves (Fig. 94–4).[23] Articles were written instructing surgeons to avoid dissection of the "triangle of doom."[30] Now we know

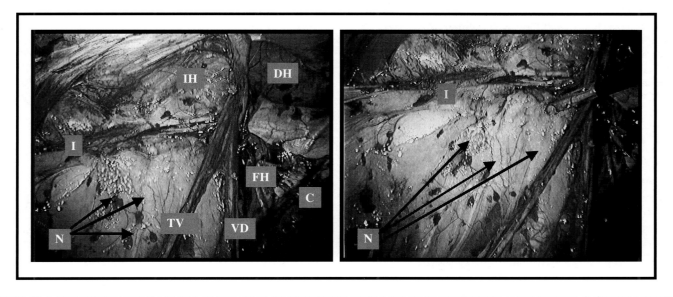

Figure 94–4. Extraperitoneal view of a 64-year-old male patient demonstrating the anatomy with special attention to the neural structures. C, Cooper's ligament; DH, direct hernia; FH, femoral hernia; IH, indirect hernia; I, iliopubic tract; N, nerves; TV, testicular vessels; VD, vas deferens.

TABLE 94–1. CRITERIA FOR CHOOSING A TAP OR TEPP HERNIAPLASTY

	Simple	Bilateral	Large Scrotal	Incarcerated	Recurrent	Diagnostic	Pelvic Incision Trans/Midline	
TAPP			X	X	X	X	X	
TEP	X	X			X			X

that the real solution is understanding the anatomy and not placing staples or other forms of fixation below the iliopubic tract lateral to Cooper's ligament. The femoral, genitofemoral, and lateral cutaneous nerve are all below the iliopubic tract and are vulnerable to injury in this area. The iliopubic tract can be identified visually, and by palpating the tacker or stapler against the abdominal wall with the opposite hand. Cautery should also be avoided in this area if possible.

The more superficial nerves, the ilioinguinal and iliohypogastric, previously were thought to be safe from injury during a laparoscopic repair. However, these nerves can be injured by overzealous placement of staples or tacks. In thin patients, anchors placed too deeply into the wall can catch and injure the anterior nerves. Localized pain in the abdominal wall or pain in the sensory distribution of one of these nerves will result. The treatment is laparoscopic removal of the offending staple or tack if it corresponds to the area marked preoperatively, as mentioned earlier in this section.

Several reports[17,31,32] have suggested that the way to avoid nerve injuries is not to anchor the mesh to the wall. This may be an overreaction to the problem, since the incidence of pain after laparoscopic repairs with fixation is now extremely low and appears to be lower than that seen after open repairs.[21] Not fixing the mesh may increase the recurrence rate[31,33] in exchange for only a small potential decrease in postoperative pain. The real answer is the proper use of fixation as outlined in this section or possibly through the use of new fixatives in the future, such as cement or glue. Meshes have recently been introduced that conform to the pelvic wall and may be less likely to roll up when not mechanically fixed. The final verdict, however, is not yet in.

SUMMARY

A randomized study from the UK suggests that only specialists should perform laparoscopic repairs.[34] It points to rare serious complications and an increased recurrence rate in the laparoscopic group as the reasons for this conclusion. In the study, however, surgeons were required to have performed only 10 cases prior to accruing patients. What this and other studies demonstrate is that laparoscopic repairs need to be performed by surgeons with a special interest in advanced laparoscopy, and experience with more than just a few hernia repairs, but not necessarily surgeons specializing only in laparoscopic hernia repair.[5,35] The key is education and supervision during the learning curve, in order to eliminate complications that stem from inexperience. There will always be complications and recurrences after any approach to hernia repair, but by following the proper steps and having proper guidance during one's early cases, one should be able to achieve the benchmarks set by experienced laparoscopic surgeons. (See an algorithm for choosing open or laparoscopic hernioplasty in Fig. 94–5.)

REFERENCES

1. Rutkow IM, Robbins AW. Demographic, classificatory, and socioeconomic aspects of hernia repair in the United States. *Surg Clin North Am.* 1993;73:413.
2. Schultz L, Graber J, Pietrafitta J, et al. Laser laparoscopic herniorrhaphy: a clinical trial and preliminary results. *J Laproendosc Surg.* 1990;1:41.
3. Bessel R, Baxter P, Ridell P, et al. A randomized controlled trial of laparoscopic repair as a day surgical procedure. *Surg Endosc.* 1996;10:495.
4. Lukaszczyk J, Preletz R, Morrow G, et al. Laparoscopic herniorrhaphy versus traditional open repair at a community hospital. *J Laparoendosc Surg.* 1996;6:203.
5. Felix E, Scott S, Crafton B, et al. Causes of recurrence after laparoscopic hernioplasty. *Surg Endosc.* 1998;12:226.
6. Liem M, Van der Graff Y, Van Steensel C, et al. Comparison of conventional anterior surgery and laparoscopic surgery for inguinal hernia repair. *N Engl J Med.* 1997;336:1541.
7. Leibl B, Schmidt J, Daubler P, et al. A single institution's experience with transperitoneal laparoscopic hernia repair. *Am J Surg.* 1998;175:446.
8. Ferzli G, Sayad P, Huie F, et al. Endoscopic extraperitoneal herniorrhaphy. A 5 year experience. *Surg Endosc.* 1998;12:1311.
9. MacFadyen B, Mathis C. Inguinal herniorrhaphy; complications and recurrences. *Semi Lap Surg.* 1994;1:128.
10. Amid P, Shulman A, Lichtenstein I. Critical scrutiny of the open "tension-free" hernioplasty. *Am J Surg.* 1993;165:369.
11. Cunningham J, Temple W, Mitchell P, et al. Cooperative study. Pain in the post-repair patient. *Ann Surg.* 1995;224:598.
12. Southern Surgeons Club. A prospective analysis of 1518 laparoscopic cholecystectomies. *N Engl J Med.* 1991;324:1073.
13. Felix E, Habertson N, Varteian S. Laparoscopic hernioplasty: Significant complications. *Surg Endosc.* 1999;13:328.
14. Frankum CE, Ramshaw BJ, White J, et al. Laparoscopic repair of bilateral and recurrent hernias. Am Surg. 1999;65:839
15. Wright D, O'Dwyer P. The learning curve for laparoscopic hernia repair. *Semi Lap Surg.* 1998;5:227.
16. Stoker D, Spiegelhalter D, Sing R, et al. Laparoscopic versus open inguinal hernia repair: randomized prospective trial. *Lancet* 1994;343:1243.

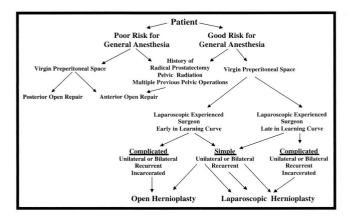

Figure 94–5. Algorithm for choosing open or laparoscopic hernioplasty.

17. Liem M, Van Steensel C, Boelhouwer R, et al. The learning curve for totally extraperitoneal laparoscopic inguinal hernia repair. *Am J Surg.* 1996;171:281.

18. Go P. Overview of randomized trials in laparoscopic inguinal hernia repair. *Semi Lap Surg.* 1998;5:238.

19. Fitzgibbons R, Camps J, Cornet D, et al. Laparoscopic inguinal herniorrhaphy. Results of a multicenter trial. *Ann Surg.* 1995;221:3.

20. Toy F, Moskowitz M, Smoot R, et al. Results of a prospective multicenter trial evaluating ePTFE peritoneal onlay laparoscopic inguinal hernioplasty. *J Laparoendosc Surg.* 1996;6:375.

21. Gillion J, Fagniez P. Chronic pain and sensory changes after hernia repair. *Hernia* 1999;3:75.

22. Tetik C, Arregui M, Dulucq J, et al. Complications and recurrences with laparoscopic repair of groin hernias. A multi-institutional retrospective analysis. *Surg Endosc.* 1994;8:1316.

23. Payne J. Complications of laparoscopic inguinal herniorrhaphy. *Semi Lap Surg.* 1997;4:166.

24. Felix E, Michas C, Gonzalez M. TAPP vs TEP laparoscopic hernioplasty. *Surg Endosc.* 1995;9:984.

25. Phillips E, Rosenthal R, Fallas M, et al. Reasons for early recurrence following laparoscopic hernioplasty. *Surg Endosc.* 1995;9:140.

26. Cueto J, V·zquez JA, SolÌs MMA, et al. Bowel obstruction in the post-operative period of laparoscopic inguinal hernia repair (TAPP). Review of the literature. *JSLS.* 1998;2:277.

27. Azurin D, Schuricht A, Stoldt H, et al. Small bowel obstruction following endoscopic extraperitoneal-preperitoneal herniorrhaphy. *J Laparoendosc Surg.* 1995;5:263.

28. Felix E, Michas C, Gonzalez M. Laparoscopic hernioplasty: TAPP vs TEP. *Surg Endosc.* 1995;9:984.

29. Seid A, Amos E. Entrapment neuropathy in laparoscopic herniorrhaphy. *Surg Endosc.* 1994;8:1050.

30. Spaw A, Ennis B, Spaw L. Laparoscopic hernia repair: The anatomic basis. *J Laparoendosc Surg.* 1991;1:269.

31. Ferzli G, Frezza E, Pecoraro A, et al. Prospective randomized study of stapled versus unstapled mesh in a laparoscopic preperitoneal inguinal hernia repair. *J Am Coll Surg.* 1999;188:461.

32. Macintyre I. Does the mesh require fixation? *Semi Lap Surg.* 1998;5:224.

33. Brooks D. Laparoscopic herniorraphy: where are we now? *Surg Endosc.* 1999;13:321.

34. The MRC Laparoscopic Groin Hernia Trial Group. Laparoscopic versus open repair of groin hernia: a randomized comparison. *Lancet* 1999;354:185.

35. Cueto GJ, Vazquez FJA, Weber SA. Complicaciones de la hernioplastÌa inguinal laparoscÛpica y como evitarlas. *Cir Gen.* 1998;20(Suppl. 1):53.

Chapter Ninety-Five • • • • • •

Complications of Laparoscopic Gynecologic Surgery

DANIEL S. SEIDMAN, CEANA H. NEZHAT, FARR NEZHAT, and CAMRAN NEZHAT

Gynecologists were among the first surgical practitioners to widely adopt the use of laparoscopy. However, until the last decade most of the procedures undertaken by gynecologists were either diagnostic laparoscopy or laparoscopic tubal sterilization. Both procedures are associated with a low risk of complications, mainly those related to the known risk of abdominal entry. Over the last decade a growing number of advanced procedures are being routinely performed by gynecologists, including laparoscopic hysterectomy, myomectomy, and bladder neck suspension. As might be expected, studies have shown that the potential for complications increases with the complexity of the procedure. For example, one recent study[1] of 6451 cases found that the complication rate rose significantly to 0.8% (39/4865) for operative laparoscopy compared with 0.19% for diagnostic laparoscopy (3/1586).

The need for greater experience and knowledge of the standard techniques contributes further to the risk of complications. Complications following operative laparoscopy appear to be low when an experienced laparoscopist performs the procedure. Since certain complications are unavoidable, surgeons must be prepared to manage them by laparotomy or laparoscopy. The incidence of conversion to laparotomy to manage complications or complete a procedure tends to be higher early in one's experience. The incidence of complications is also directly related to the severity of pelvic and abdominal pathology. In gynecologic laparoscopy, adhesions and endometriosis are common contributing factors to urinary tract and intestinal injury.

In this chapter we will describe the incidence and types of complications reported to be associated with gynecological operative laparoscopy. Complications unique to gynecologic procedures will also be reviewed.

INCIDENCE OF COMPLICATIONS

Following operative gynecologic laparoscopy the reported rate of major intraoperative and postoperative complications is less than 1%.[2-4] More specifically, the range of intestinal complications per 1000 operative gynecological procedures is 1.1 to 2.6, the rate of bladder injuries 0.2 to 1.7, the incidence of ureteral injuries is 0.1 to 1.4, while vascular injuries occur in 0.4 to 2.5 of every 1000 gynecologic laparoscopies. [2-4]

In a study encompassing 17,521 diagnostic and operative procedures performed at seven centers, an overall complication rate of 3.2/1000 was found, and the rate for diagnostic and minor procedures was 1.1/1000 and 5.2/1000 for major and advanced operations, respectively.[5] Laparotomies were performed for hemorrhage or visceral complications, and injury was most common following extensive adhesiolysis and advanced laparoscopic surgery; one fatality was reported.

Three national surveys performed in the Netherlands,[2] France,[3] and Finland,[4] included 25,764, 29,966, and 70,607 laparoscopic procedures, respectively. The total complication rate was 5.7, 4.6, and 3.6 per 1000 procedures, respectively. Laparotomy was needed in 3.3 and 3.2 per 1000 cases, respectively, in the Netherlands and France.[2,3]

The need to convert to laparotomy, notably not necessarily a complication, happens on average in 3.3 of every 1000 operative gynecologic procedures.[2-4] It is better to complete a procedure by laparotomy than to risk injury to the patient or be forced to proceed with emergency laparotomy because of a complication. However, this deviation from the surgical plan raises concerns about the adequacy of the presurgical evaluation, patient consent, and the surgeon's skill.

It should be remembered that the risk of complications for the average gynecologic surgeon might not be truly reflected by literature reports. The reports that serve as the basis for calculating the complication incidence rates are from large practices with experienced gynecologists, reports from tertiary referral clinics, and surveys of members of the American Association of Gynecologic Laparoscopists (AAGL).[5]

Mortality is extremely rare following laparoscopy.[7] However, as laparoscopic surgery increases in complexity, concern is raised regarding a possible increase in mortality rates. Fortunately, this concern is not supported by current reports, although admittedly underreporting may plague the data in light of medicolegal implications.

The AAGL 1979 membership survey, which involved primarily diagnostic laparoscopic procedures for tubal ligation, reported 2 deaths among 88,986 procedures, a death rate of 2/100,000.[5] The death rates remained essentially unchanged in subsequent AAGL surveys.[5] The 1991 AAGL membership reported 1 death from 56,536 laparoscopic procedures, a low death rate of 1.8 per 100,000 procedures.[8] The 1993 AAGL membership reported 1 death from 22,966 sterilization and none for 36,482 diagnostic procedures.[9]

In a retrospective review of the literature and the authors' experience, data revealed 15 deaths in 501,779 laparoscopic procedures, a death rate of 3/100,000.[2,9] Two recent surveys from France[3] and the Netherlands[2] revealed 3 deaths among 55,730 laparoscopic operations, a mortality rate of 5.4 per 100,000 procedures. However, in a recent Finish national study of laparoscopic complications, no deaths were reported in connection with 70,607 gynecologic laparoscopies.[4]

Twenty-nine deaths were identified by Peterson et al[10] following tubal sterilization, for a mortality rate of 3.6 per 100,000 tubal sterilizations. A stratification of the mortality cases showed that 11 resulted from anesthesia, 7 were caused by sepsis following unrecognized bowel injury, 4 were caused by hemorrhage following major vessel laceration, 3 resulted from myocardial infarction, and 4 were related to other causes. The use of endotracheal intubation for general anesthesia, safer use of unipolar coagulation or use of alternative techniques, and careful insertion of the Veress needle and trocar might have prevented some of the deaths. A more recent study found no deaths among 9475 women who had interval laparoscopic tubal sterilization.[7]

RISK FACTORS AND CONTRAINDICATIONS

Laparoscopic surgery may not be the best approach in some gynecologic cases. However, the dramatic improvement in the average surgeon's laparoscopic surgical skills and experience over the past few years, combined with the ready availability of proper instrumentation, has resulted in many once "absolute" contraindications for laparoscopy becoming obsolete. These contraindications included obesity,[11,12] severe adhesions,[13] previous abdominal surgery,[14,15] cancer,[16,17] abdominal hernia,[18] pregnancy,[19,20] hypovolemic shock,[21] and bowel perforation with generalized peritonitis.[22–24]

In patients who have generalized peritonitis, extreme caution is needed since the bowel is frequently matted and adherent to the abdominal wall. However, laparoscopic treatment of generalized peritonitis secondary to perforated sigmoid diverticulitis has been shown to be an alternative to classic surgery.[22] Furthermore, it has been shown in animal models that laparoscopic CO_2 pneumoperitoneum does not aggravate bacteremia or metabolic and hemodynamic disturbances induced by bacterial peritonitis.[23] However, applying a pneumoperitoneum during an ongoing sepsis has been found in animal models to significantly degrade hemodynamic and homeostatic variables, and therefore might enhance the risk of severe complications.[25]

The Trendelenburg position is almost always used for gynecologic laparoscopic procedures in order to allow for good exposure of the deep pelvic organs. It should be remembered that patients with class IV cardiac disease have a high risk of cardiac arrhythmias and failure as a result of Trendelenburg positioning, even for relatively short procedures.[26]

Intestinal obstruction and bowel distention are associated with an increased risk of perforation. Although laparoscopic surgery is less invasive than laparotomy and often the better of the two approaches, bowel obstruction not relieved by conservative decompression techniques may require laparotomy.

ABDOMINAL ENTRY

The most critical point of laparoscopy is abdominal cavity entry of the Veress needle and primary and secondary trocars. In a series of 2324 laparoscopies it was shown that there were more complications from Veress needle and trocar insertion than from the actual gynecologic operative procedures.[27] Another study suggested that about half of the complications occur during the installation of the laparoscopic procedure.[28]

The possibility of complications is increased in patients with multiple previous laparotomies, a body mass index greater than 30, and those who are very thin.[7,15] Bowel preparation is recommended if there is a risk of bowel injury. Veress needle and trocar insertion are modified in the presence of a large pelvic mass.

The frequency of adhesions between the abdominal wall and the underlying omentum and bowel was assessed in 360 women undergoing operative laparoscopy after a previous laparotomy.[29] Patients with prior midline incisions were found to have significantly more adhesions than those with Pfannenstiel incisions. Patients with midline incisions performed for gynecologic indications had significantly more adhesions than all types of incisions performed for obstetric indications. In addition, adhesions to the bowel were significantly more frequent after midline incisions above the umbilicus. Twenty-one women suffered direct injury to adherent omentum and bowel during the laparoscopic procedure.[29] It therefore must be realized that intra-abdominal adhesions between the abdominal scar and underlying viscera are a common consequence of laparotomy (Fig. 95–1). Great caution is required when patients undergo laparoscopy after a previous laparotomy, and the presence of adhesions between the old scar and the bowel and omentum must always be considered.

The Use of the Veress Needle

Among gynecologic surgeons the Veress needle is still commonly used to establish a pneumoperitoneum before entering the abdomen. Direct entry and the use of open (Hasson) technique for abdominal entry prior to laparoscopy are less prevalent. Intra-abdominal placement of the Veress needle is required to establish a

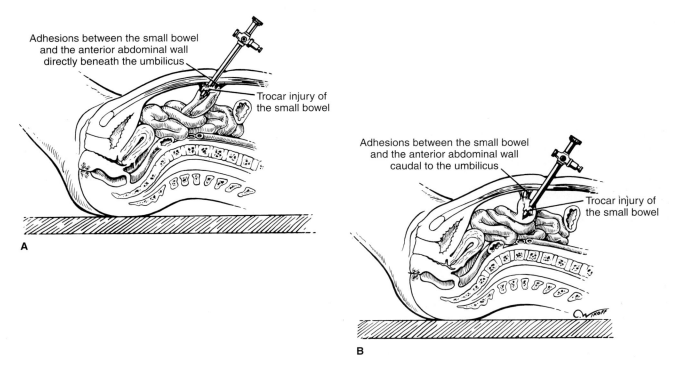

Figure 95–1. The bowel is attached to the anterior abdominal wall. **A.** The bowel is attached directly under the umbilicus. **B.** The attachment is below and distal to the umbilicus. *(Reproduced with permission from Nezhat et al.[5])*

pneumoperitoneum. Because the Veress needle is inserted blindly, the needle may enter other spaces or puncture organs. Further, instillation of CO_2 under pressure through the Veress needle can produce serious complications.

Factors that increase the risk of perforation or laceration with the Veress needle include bowel adhesions, lateral displacement of the Veress needle during insertion, too steep an insertion angle, or uncontrolled sudden entry. The patient must be horizontal so that the sacral promontory and sacral curve are identified easily. Premature Trendelenburg positioning should be avoided.

When an upper abdominal site is used in establishing a pneumoperitoneum, the Veress needle may puncture the pleural cavity, stomach, liver, or spleen. The stomach becomes distended following prolonged manual ventilation with a mask or when endotracheal intubation is difficult. Puncture of the stomach may occur even with umbilical placement of the Veress needle. A distended stomach displaces the transverse colon toward the lower abdomen, increasing the probability of intestinal puncture (Fig. 95–2). A nasogastric tube minimizes the risk of gastric distention. An overdistended bladder is also at risk for injury. Routine placement of a Foley catheter before the procedure substantially lowers the risk of inadvertent bladder injury.

Veress needle punctures generally are not apparent until CO_2 insufflation or laparoscope insertion. Abnormally high insufflation

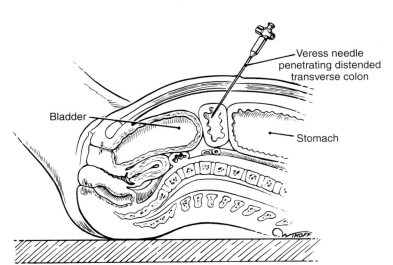

Figure 95–2. A distended stomach can displace the transverse colon toward the lower abdomen, increasing the possibility of puncture of the colon. *(Reproduced with permission from Nezhat et al.[5])*

pressures are encountered when the Veress needle is misplaced. During the initial examination of the pelvis, it is important to survey the mid and upper abdomen for signs of needle-induced trauma, such as hematomas, needle punctures, and collections of gas.

Puncture of a hollow viscus with the Veress needle generally does not require anything more than examination of the puncture site to check for a bleeding vessel or leakage from the viscus. The patient can be discharged with instructions to call the physician in case of increasing abdominal pain or fever. If puncture with the Veress needle results in laceration of a viscus, repair is indicated, and the route of repair is based on the organ involved (small or large bowel, bladder, stomach, or major blood vessels), the nature of the fluid that is leaking, and operator experience. Many injuries may require immediate laparotomy for repair and adequate irrigation of the abdomen. Some surgeons may be able to repair injuries laparoscopically.

Direct Trocar Insertion

The results of prospective randomized trials conducted by Nezhat and colleagues,[30] as well as by others,[31,32] clearly demonstrated the benefits of performing direct trocar insertion. It was found that the operating time was significantly reduced by 2.2[31] and 4.3[32] minutes. In short procedures, such as tubal ligation, this can substantially decrease the quantity of gas insufflated and the duration of exposure of the patient to the gas and to anesthesia.

Woolcott[33] reviewed the records of 6173 laparoscopies performed using the technique of direct insertion of the umbilical trocar and insufflation of carbon dioxide under vision. He found that there were 4 perforating bowel injuries (0.06%) requiring laparotomy (2 in small intestine, 2 in large intestine). Three of the four patients who had bowel injury had undergone prior abdominal surgery and had midline vertical subumbilical incisions. There were no cases of major vascular injury or gas embolus that required surgical or resuscitative measures. Woolcott[33] concluded based on his data and the published literature that the bowel or vessel perforation rates (requiring laparotomy or resuscitation) were 1 in 1000 regardless of whether the method of gaining peritoneal access was open technique, Veress needle insufflation, or direct trocar insertion. Furthermore, direct trocar insertion may reduce the risk of gas embolism by insufflating only after intraperitoneal replacement has been confirmed; moreover it allows immediate recognition and rapid treatment of major blood vessel laceration, and both of these factors have been identified as being crucial in reducing laparoscopy-associated mortality.

A large retrospective French study[34] evaluated the incidence of serious trocar accidents in 103,852 laparoscopic operations involving almost 390,000 trocars. They identified 7 perioperative deaths (mortality 0.07/1000) arising almost exclusively from vascular injuries. They subsequently concluded that the technique of open insertion of the first trocar appears to be the best means of preventing these accidents. This conclusion has been criticized by many authorities who also raised concern regarding the medicolegal implications of such recommendations. Woolcott[33] concluded that based on currently available data one cannot deduce that a particular technique of gaining peritoneal access is superior to another. The various techniques each have their individual advantages and disadvantages and similar morbidity when performed by experienced operators for appropriate indications. In view of this obser-

vation, each alternative should be considered by the individual surgeon to assess which would best suit his or her operating technique and the particular circumstances of each patient. The surgeon should give preference to the method with which he or she is most comfortable or with which he or she has the most experience.[33]

UTERINE COMPLICATIONS

Complications involving the uterus include cervical laceration or uterine perforation from sounding the uterus or use of the uterine dilator or uterine manipulator. Cervical lacerations are managed with pressure from a sponge stick or suture. Bleeding from uterine perforations is controlled with bipolar electrocoagulation. Occasionally, the uterus is repaired using laparoscopic suturing. A CO_2 laser beam can lacerate the uterine serosa and the uterus should not be used as a backstop.

BLADDER INJURIES

In gynecologic procedures bladder injury is rare and usually occurs in patients who have had laparotomies or whose bladder is not empty. Under these conditions, sharp instruments such as trocars and uterine anteverters can perforate or lacerate the bladder, electricity and lasers can cause thermal injury, and blunt instruments can lacerate the bladder. Certain laparoscopic procedures increase the risk of bladder injury. The Veress needle can perforate a distended bladder. A misplaced Rubin's cannula can perforate the vagina and bladder with upward pressure. Accessory trocar insertion can injure a full bladder, or one with anatomy distorted by previous pelvic surgery, endometriosis, or adhesions, or if insertion is less than 4 cm above the pubic symphysis. Coagulation or laser ablation of endometriosis implants or adhesiolysis in the anterior cul-de-sac can predispose the patient to bladder injury unless hydrodissection or a backstop is used with the CO_2 laser.

The bladder may be lacerated or torn during laparoscopic hysterectomy (LH) or laparoscopically-assisted abdominal hysterectomy (LAVH), if blunt dissection is used to free the bladder from the pubocervical fascia, particularly in women with prior cesarean, severe endometriosis, or lower segment myomas. Also, bladder injury can occur while entering and dissecting the space of Retzius before laparoscopic bladder neck suspension.

To prevent injuries, a Foley catheter is placed to drain the bladder. The position of the bladder should be assessed during the initial examination with the laparoscope. If the boundaries of the bladder are not clear, particularly when pelvic anatomy is distorted, the bladder should be filled with 350 mL normal saline to delineate its position. Care should be used when performing LH or LAVH and the assistant should push the uterus up during bladder dissection.

Intraoperative recognition of a bladder injury is important to prevent long-term sequelae. Signs of intraoperative bladder injury include (1) air in the urinary catheter and bag during insufflation; (2) the bladder appears to be pushed by the accessory trocar as it is advanced through the abdominal wall; (3) blood in the urine; (4) urine drainage from the accessory trocar incision; (5) postoperative urinary retention, particularly if the amount of urine obtained during catheterization is less than anticipated; (6) postoperative signs of peritonitis; and (7) leakage of indigo carmine from the injured site. Because trocar injury often involves entry and exit punctures, locating both is important.

Small holes generally heal without sequelae. However, trocar injuries to the bladder dome require closure followed by urinary drainage for 5 to 7 days. Drainage promotes healing, encourages spontaneous closure, and minimizes further complications.

Lacerations may require a laparotomy, although some laparoscopists can repair the laceration laparoscopically.[35] Laparoscopic closure of intentional or unintentional bladder lacerations during operative laparoscopy was described in 19 women.[35] The defect was repaired laparoscopically in one layer using interrupted absorbable polyglycolic suture (17 patients) or polydioxanone suture (2 patients) and followed by 7 to 14 days of transurethral drainage. Complications were limited to one vesicovaginal fistula that required reoperation. After 6 to 48 months of follow-up all patients were well with a good outcome.[35]

URETER INJURY

The development of the ureter is embryologically associated with the development of the female genital tract. This close association persists postnatally, predisposing women to ureteral injury. Knowledge of the ureter's path through the pelvis and its vulnerable points are key to preventing injuries. The intrapelvic segment of the ureter is near the broad ligament, ovaries, and uterosacral ligaments, and injuries occur often in these areas. The ureter seems to be most at risk during laparoscopic surgery when the cardinal ligament is dissected and divided below the uterine vessels.[36] The surgeon should note the ureter's course through the peritoneum. Endometriosis and severe pelvic adhesions can thicken the peritoneum, obscuring the location of the ureter, especially near the uterosacral ligaments.[37]

Until recently, more reported cases of ureteral injury during laparoscopic procedures involved electrocoagulation because it is the most reliable technique to arrest bleeding. As the use of stapling devices increases, additional injury to the ureters is being reported. Laparoscopic placement of transmural sutures at the bladder neck has also been reported to lead to entrapment of the intramural portion of ureter.[38]

Ureteral injury can occur during sharp dissection of an ovary adherent to the pelvic sidewall, in uterosacral transection, with ligation/transection/coagulation of the uterine arteries, when removing endometriotic implants or fibrosis from the ureter, and while trying to control bleeding vessels.

The routine use of preoperative intravenous pyelogram (IVP) is not recommended and no prospective study substantiates that it prevents ureteral injury. However, for selected patients, it may help diagnose ureteral obstruction and allow appropriate surgical planning.

Lighted ureteral catheters are now available and are designed to provide a visual roadmap of the ureter during laparoscopy.[39] The prophylactic use of ureteral catheters, including the use of lighted catheters during laparoscopic surgery, was found to be safe and the insertion technically simple.[40] The ureteral catheters were found to enhance identification of ureters and facilitate ureteral dissection.[40] However, the use of prophylactic ureteral catheters was not found to reduce the rate of ureteral injury.[41] Furthermore, it has been suggested that the routine use of ureteral catheters in LH may result in unnecessary complications.[42] Thus we agree with Wood et al[42] that as long as surgical techniques meticulously avoid

ureteral injury, routine ureteral catheterization during LH is not warranted. Nevertheless, we do find ureteral catheters useful in some cases of severe endometriosis and adhesions.[37]

Intraoperative ureter damage is suspected when urine leakage or blood-tinged urine is noted and indigo carmine dye is spilled intraperitoneally following intravenous administration. When surgical procedures involve the ureter, postoperative ureteral integrity can be ascertained by cystoscopy, ureteral catheterization, or intravenous retrograde pyelogram. A new technique using transvaginal color Doppler ultrasound has recently been introduced for postoperative detection of ureteral jets into the bladder when ureteral integrity is in question.[43] Stenting of the ureter or repair by laparotomy is generally indicated, but laparoscopic repair of partial- and full-thickness injuries is an option for some laparoscopists.

A laparoscopist highly experienced with laparoscopic suturing can repair ureteral injuries laparoscopically with good results.[35] Nezhat and coworkers[5] managed a case of long-term ureteral obstruction caused by endometriosis and incidental partial resection of the ureter laparoscopically. The ureter's course was distorted by a 2-cm fibrotic nodule on the ureter, approximately 4 cm above the bladder, corresponding to the level of obstruction (Fig. 95–3A). Hydrodissection aided in entering the retroperitoneal space at the pelvic brim. The ureter was dissected with the CO_2 laser (Fig. 95–3B). Under cystoscopic guidance, a 7F ureteral catheter was passed through the ureterovesical junction (Fig. 95–3C). The catheter was advanced through the proximal portion of the ureter to the left renal pelvis (Fig. 95–3D). The edges of the ureter were reapproximated using four interrupted 4-0 polydioxanone sutures (Fig. 95–3E). The postoperative course was uncomplicated and a postoperative IVP confirmed ureteral patency.

BOWEL INJURY

During gynecologic procedures small bowel injuries most commonly occur if the bowel is immobilized by adhesions. The bowel can be injured during Veress needle or trocar insertion, bowel manipulation, or enterolysis (Fig. 95–1). Electrosurgery and stray laser beams can result in unrecognized thermal injuries to the bowel. Injury to the gastrointestinal tract is a serious complication. Whether discovered intraoperatively or several days following surgery, small bowel injuries result in unplanned laparotomy, serious morbidity, and even death.

A recent survey of the surgical and gynecologic literature revealed 266 laparoscopic bowel perforation injuries in 205,969 laparoscopic cases. The combined incidence of bowel complications in the literature was 1.3/1000 cases.[44] It should be noted that most of these injuries (69%) were not recognized at surgery.[44] Of the injuries, 58% were of small bowel and 32% were of colon.[44] Only 50% were caused by electrocautery. Of these patients, 80% required laparotomy to repair the bowel injuries.

Laparoscopic surgery involving the sigmoid colon is commonly performed by gynecologists for treatment of severe pelvic endometriosis and adhesions.[45,46] Prompt and accurate diagnosis of proctosigmoid injury is crucial since any bowel injury should be treated at the time of recognition to avoid associated severe and potentially fatal morbidity.[47] Chapron et al[48] concluded that prevention of bowel injury relies on the surgeon's experience, strict observance of the safety rules, a high degree of familiarity with the

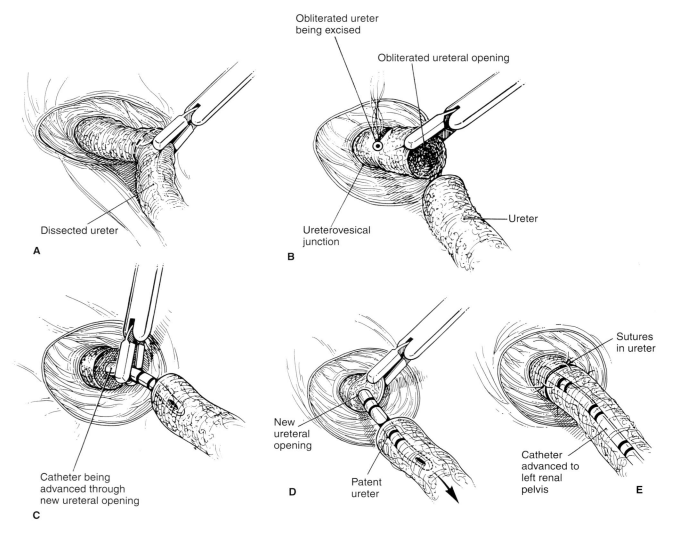

Figure 95–3. A uterolysis is done. **A.** The involved endometriosis is dissected and pulled medially. **B.** The obliterated portion of the ureter is excised. **C.** Under cystoscopic guidance, a 7F ureteral catheter is passed through the uterovesical junction. **D.** The catheter is advanced through the proximal part of the ureter to the renal pelvis. **E.** The edges of the ureter are approximated and sutured. *(Reproduced with permission from Nezhat et al.[5])*

physical characteristics of the instruments used, systematic use of bowel preparation for patients presenting a risk of bowel complications, close supervision of the route taken by the trocars, meticulous inspection on completion of surgery of all areas where bowel adhesiolysis has been done, and in case of any doubt, tests for leakage involving the rectosigmoid.

Complications from small bowel injury are related to the extent of damage and the time that elapses before the injury is discovered. Sharp trocar injuries to the bowel may be limited to the serosa or may be deep, involving the entire wall. Small punctures or superficial lacerations seal readily and require no further treatment, assuming that careful inspection of the affected bowel reveals no leakage of bowel contents or bleeding. Small (less than 5 mm) superficial lacerations need to be inspected to ensure that only the serosa is involved. In such a case the patient may be treated conservatively and discharged the day of surgery with instructions to report any untoward reaction.

Patients with obvious peritoneal soiling require intervention and perhaps laparotomy. The bowel should be inspected on both sides to detect through-and-through injuries, especially if produced by a trocar. If only one site of entry is found and repaired, peritonitis may develop postoperatively. If the laparoscope has been inserted through the bowel laceration and laparotomy is performed, the defect is identified and closed using a purse-string suture as the laparoscope is withdrawn to minimize peritoneal contamination.

When the cul-de-sac is dissected, identification of the vagina and rectum is facilitated by placing a probe or an assistant's finger in both the vagina and rectum. Dissection should begin lateral to the uterosacral ligaments, where the anatomy is less distorted, and proceed toward the obliterated cul-de-sac. Similarly, when posterior culdotomy is performed for tissue removal or during laparoscopic hysterectomy, correct identification of vagina and rectum is important.

When a difficult pelvic operation is contemplated, such as cul-de-sac nodularity in a patient with endometriosis or a history suggesting significant pelvic adhesions, preoperative bowel preparation is indicated.

Intraoperative sigmoidoscopy may assist in early detection and prompt intraoperative management of proctosigmoid injury, thereby preventing a potentially catastrophic outcome. Sigmoidoscopy is a relatively simple procedure during laparoscopy and aids in the diagnosis of bowel perforation and in assessment of bowel wall invasion, and can detect any potential stricture caused by endometriosis. It is a safe procedure, even when performed immediately after extensive laparoscopic surgical treatment of rectosigmoid endometriosis and adhesions. Sigmoidoscopy may be used with discretion as a diagnostic and risk management tool during laparoscopic surgery of the rectosigmoid colon, allowing the surgeon to proceed with immediate corrective action.

The knowledge that the bowel can be repaired successfully by laparoscopic techniques in the properly prepared patient should increase the confidence of the surgeon operating in the deep pelvis.

VAGINAL CUFF DEHISCENCE

Vaginal vault rupture with intestinal herniation, although rare, is a recognized postoperative complication of both vaginal and abdominal hysterectomies, and may occur spontaneously or postcoitally. The incidence after LH is unknown. We reported on 3 women, ages 40 to 43 years, who presented to the emergency room with bleeding and pain 2 to 5 months after total LH.[50] The small bowel was visible through the introitus or protruding into the vagina. One occurred following vaginal intercourse, and the other two were apparently spontaneous. Inspection of the bowel revealed no evidence of trauma. Two vaginal cuff repairs were completed transvaginally and one laparoscopically, all with interrupted sutures of 0 polydioxanone or polyglactin. In a follow-up period of 12 to 17 months, the patients were doing well. Based on our preliminary report[50] it was suggested that total LH might be associated with an increased risk of vaginal vault evisceration.

BLEEDING

Following gynecologic surgery, bleeding and hemorrhage are the cause of most emergency laparotomies.[51] Bleeding occurs during sharp dissection of adhesions, transection of vessels during laser excision or dissection (the laser effectively coagulates very small vessels), uterosacral ablation, or with rough handling of tissues.[45] Lacerations of the oviduct, mesosalpinx, and infundibulopelvic ligament can bleed profusely.

Distorted anatomy is an important compounding factor in many cases of major retroperitoneal vascular injuries.[52] Equipment and drugs, including unipolar or bipolar electrocoagulators, vasopressin, clips, sutures, and loop ligatures, should be on hand to help control bleeding. The choice of method depends on the surgeon's preference. Most bleeding can be controlled with bipolar forceps. Infertility surgeons should use fine bipolar forceps to minimize thermal damage and adhesion formation. Pressure enables evacuation of blood and minimizes blood loss until the necessary equipment is placed in the abdomen.

The increased intra-abdominal pressure from CO_2 insufflation, the decreased venous pressure caused by Trendelenburg positioning, and retroperitoneal hematoma can tamponade bleeding from small or large vessels. When pressure gradients return to normal, bleeding into the retroperitoneal space may begin, eventually leading to hematoma and hypovolemic shock.[52] All exposed vessels should be evaluated at the end of the procedure with the patient supine and intra-abdominal pressure reduced. The adequacy and safety of laparoscopic control of major vessel bleeding should be investigated further and consultation with a vascular surgeon should be considered in all cases.[52]

Hemoperitoneum in an unstable patient has long been considered a contraindication because the bleeding source may be difficult to find and treat laparoscopically. However, laparoscopy offers many theoretical advantages for the immediate diagnosis and management of a patient presenting with hemodynamic instability and suspected active intra-abdominal bleeding due to conditions such as ectopic pregnancy.[21] These features include superior visualization of the entire abdomen, decreased intra-abdominal bleeding due to compression by creation of a pneumoperitoneum, and ability to effectively control the source of bleeding with minimal tissue damage. Thus it seems appropriate to diagnose and treat suspected intra-abdominal bleeding caused by ectopic pregnancies or a bleeding hemorrhagic corpus luteum.

INTRAOPERATIVE SPILLAGE

Spillage of ovarian cyst contents during surgery, potentially leading to complications such as chemical peritonitis and spread of malignancy, remains an ongoing concern. A recent review of the literature summarized the safety of laparoscopic management of ovarian dermoid cysts.[54] A review of 14 studies revealed spillage in 310 (66%) of the 470 reported cases of dermoid cyst excision. Despite this high rate of spillage only a single case of chemical peritonitis following laparoscopic removal of dermoid cysts was reported, an incidence of 0.2%. It was concluded that laparoscopic management of dermoid cysts is a safe and beneficial method in selected patients when performed by an experienced laparoscopic surgeon.

More recently, a series was reported of 390 patients who had surgery for removal of a teratoma of the ovary.[55] Two malignant teratomas were observed in this group. Enucleation of the dermoid cyst in toto using a salvage bag for removal was only possible in few cases without contamination of the abdominal cavity by spillage of cyst contents. However, here again, there were no serious complications in any patients including those with laparoscopic cystectomies and intraperitoneal spill.

A current prospective randomized trial compared the results of removing mature teratoma using culdotomy with laparoscopy or without laparoscopy.[56] Laparoscopically-assisted cystectomy was found to be associated with a significantly lower rate of tumor spillage and less blood loss during the operation.[56] It therefore seems that laparoscopic treatment of benign teratomas is a safe procedure.

The safety of managing adnexal cysts laparoscopically when suspicion of malignancy exists remains unresolved.[56] There are limited reports on the potential risk of cancer dissemination. From experimental data, the laparoscopic treatment of gynecologic cancer has potential risk for dissemination under certain conditions.[56]

After a careful preoperative evaluation, the laparoscopic diagnosis of malignancy is reliable.[57] It therefore seems at that by using strict guidelines, laparoscopic diagnosis can be proposed for both non-suspicious and complex tumors, thus avoiding many unnecessary laparotomies for benign tumors suspicious at ultrasound.[56,57]

REFERENCES

1. Wang PH, Lee WL, Yuan CC, et al. Major complications of operative and diagnostic laparoscopy for gynecologic disease. *J Am Assoc Gynecol Laparosc.* 2001;8:68.
2. Jansen FW, Kapiteyn K, Trimbos-Kemper T, et al. Complications of laparoscopy: a prospective multicentre observational study. *Br J Obstet Gynaecol.* 1997;104:595.
3. Chapron C, Querleu D, Bruhat MA, et al. Surgical complications of diagnostic and operative gynaecological laparoscopy: a series of 29,966 cases. *Hum Reprod.* 1998;13:867.
4. Härkki-Sirén P, Kurki T. A nationwide analysis of laparoscopic complications. *Obstet Gynecol.* 1997;89:108.
5. Nezhat CR, Siegler AM, Nezhat FR, et al (eds.). *Operative Gynecologic Laparoscopy: Principles and Techniques*, 2nd ed. McGraw-Hill:2000.
6. Hulka JF, Levy BS, Luciano AA, et al. 1997 American Association of Gynecologic Laparoscopists (AAGL) membership survey: practice profiles. *J Am Assoc Gynecol Laparosc.* 1998;5:93.
7. Jamieson DJ, Hillis SD, Duerr A, et al. Complications of interval laparoscopic tubal sterilization: findings from the United States Collaborative Review of Sterilization. *Obstet Gynecol.* 2000;96:997.
8. Hulka JF, Peterson HB, Phillips JM, et al. Operative laparoscopy. American Association of Gynecologic Laparoscopists 1991 membership survey. *J Reprod Med.* 1993;38:569.
9. Hulka JF, Phillips JM, Peterson HB, et al. Laparoscopic sterilization: American Association of Gynecologic Laparoscopists' 1993 membership survey. *J Am Assoc Gynecol Laparosc.* 1995;2:137.
10. Peterson HB, DeStefano F, Rubin GL, et al. Deaths attributable to tubal sterilization in the United States, 1977 to 1981. *Am J Obstet Gynecol.* 1983;146:131.
11. Fried M, Peskova M, Kasalicky M. The role of laparoscopy in the treatment of morbid obesity. *Obes Surg.* 1998;8:520.
12. Eltabbakh GH, Shamonki MI, Moody JM, et al. Hysterectomy for obese women with endometrial cancer: laparoscopy or laparotomy? *Gynecol Oncol.* 2000;78:329.
13. Clough KB, Ladonne JM, Nos C, et al. Second look for ovarian cancer: laparoscopy or laparotomy? A prospective comparative study. *Gynecol Oncol.* 1999;72:411.
14. Brill AI, Nezhat F, Nezhat CH, et al. The incidence of adhesions after prior laparotomy: a laparoscopic appraisal. *Obstet Gynecol.* 1995; 85:269.
15. Lecuru F, Leonard F, Philippe Jais J, et al. Laparoscopy in patients with prior surgery: results of the blind approach. *JSLS.* 2001;5:13.
16. Malur S, Possover M, Michels W, et al. Laparoscopic-assisted vaginal versus abdominal surgery in patients with endometrial cancer—a prospective randomized trial. *Gynecol Oncol.* 2001;80:239.
17. Eltabbakh GH, Shamonki MI, Moody JM, et al. Laparoscopy as the primary modality for the treatment of women with endometrial carcinoma. *Cancer* 2001;91:378.
18. Moreno-Egea A, Liron R, Girela E, et al. Laparoscopic repair of ventral and incisional hernias using a new composite mesh (Parietex): initial experience. *Surg Laparosc Endosc Percutan Tech.* 2001;11:103.
19. Soriano D, Yefet Y, Seidman DS, et al. Laparoscopy versus laparotomy in the management of adnexal masses during pregnancy. *Fertil Steril.* 1999;71:955.
20. Nezhat FR, Tazuke S, Nezhat CH, et al. Laparoscopy during pregnancy: a literature review. *J Soc Laparoendosc Surg.* 1997;1:17.
21. Soriano D, Yefet Y, Oelsner G, et al. Operative laparoscopy for management of ectopic pregnancy in patients with hypovolemic shock. *J Am Assoc Gynecol Laparosc.* 1997;4:363.
22. Rizk N, Barrat C, Faranda C, et al. Laparoscopic treatment of generalized peritonitis with diverticular perforation of the sigmoid colon. Report of 10 cases. *Chirurgie* 1998;123:358.
23. Collet e Silva FD, Ramos RC, Zantut LF, et al. Laparoscopic pneumoperitoneum in acute peritonitis does not increase bacteremia or aggravate metabolic or hemodynamic disturbances. *Surg Laparosc Endosc Percutan Tech.* 2000;10:305.
24. Navez B, Tassetti V, Scohy JJ, et al. Laparoscopic management of acute peritonitis. *Br J Surg.* 1998;85:32.
25. Nagelschmidt M, Holthausen U, Goost H, et al. Evaluation of the effects of a pneumoperitoneum with carbon dioxide or helium in a porcine model of endotoxemia. *Langenbecks Arch Surg.* 2000;385:199.
26. Stone J, Dyke L, Fritz P, et al. Hemodynamic and hormonal changes during pneumoperitoneum and Trendelenburg positioning for operative gynecologic laparoscopy surgery. *Prim Care Update Ob Gyns.* 1998;5:155.
27. Bateman BG, Kolp LA, Hoeger K. Complications of laparoscopy—operative and diagnostic. *Fertil Steril.* 1996;66:30.
28. MacCordick C, Lecuru F, Rizk E, et al. Morbidity in laparoscopic gynecological surgery: results of a prospective single-center study. *Surg Endosc.* 1999;13:57.
29. Brill AI, Nezhat F, Nezhat CH, et al. The incidence of adhesions after prior laparotomy: a laparoscopic appraisal. *Obstet Gynecol.* 1995; 85:269.
30. Nezhat FR, Silfen SL, Evans D, et al. Comparison of direct insertion of disposable and standard reusable laparoscopic trocars and previous pneumoperitoneum with Veress needle. *Obstet Gynecol.* 1991;78:148.
31. Borgatta L, Gruss L, Barad D, et al. Direct trocar insertion versus Veress needle use for laparoscopic sterilization. *J Reprod Med.* 1990; 35:891.
32. Byron JW, Markenson G, Miyazawa K. A randomized comparison of Veress needle and direct trocar insertion for laparoscopy. *Surg Gynecol Obstet.* 1993;177:259.
33. Woolcott R. The safety of laparoscopy performed by direct trocar insertion and carbon dioxide insufflation under vision. *Aust N Z J Obstet Gynaecol.* 1997;37:216.
34. Champault G, Cazacu F, Taffinder N. Serious trocar accidents in laparoscopic surgery: a French survey of 103,852 operations. *Surg Laparosc Endosc.* 1996;6:367.
35. Nezhat CH, Seidman DS, Nezhat F, et al. Laparoscopic management of intentional and unintentional cystotomy. *J Urol.* 1996;156: 1400.
36. Tamussino KF, Lang PF, Breinl E. Ureteral complications with operative gynecologic laparoscopy. *Am J Obstet Gynecol.* 1998;178:967.
37. Nezhat C, Nezhat F, Nezhat CH, et al. Urinary tract endometriosis treated by laparoscopy. *Fertil Steril.* 1996;66:920.
38. Ferland RD, Rosenblatt P. Ureteral compromise after laparoscopic burch colpopexy. *J Am Assoc Gynecol Laparosc.* 1999;6:217.
39. Teichman JM, Lackner JE, Harrison JM. Comparison of lighted ureteral catheter luminance for laparoscopy. *Tech Urol.* 1997;3:213.
40. Quinlan DJ, Townsend DE, Johnson GH. Are ureteral catheters in gynecologic surgery beneficial or hazardous? *J Am Assoc Gynecol Laparosc.* 1995;3:61.
41. Kuno K, Menzin A, Kauder HH, et al. Prophylactic ureteral catheterization in gynecologic surgery. *Urology* 1998;52:1004.
42. Wood EC, Maher P, Pelosi MA. Routine use of ureteric catheters at laparoscopic hysterectomy may cause unnecessary complications. *J Am Assoc Gynecol Laparosc.* 1996;3:393.
43. Timor-Tritsch IE, Haratz-Rubinstein N, Monteagudo A, et al. Transvaginal color Doppler sonography of the ureteral jets: a method to detect ureteral patency. *Obstet Gynecol.* 1997;89:113.
44. Bishoff JT, Allaf ME, Kirkels W, et al. Laparoscopic bowel injury: incidence and clinical presentation. *J Urol.* 1999;161:887.

45. Nezhat C, Nezhat F, Ambroze W, et al. Laparoscopic repair of small bowel and colon. A report of 26 cases. *Surg Endosc.* 1993;7:88.

46. Jerby BL, Kessler H, Falcone T, et al. Laparoscopic management of colorectal endometriosis. *Surg Endosc.* 1999;13:1125.

47. Schrenk P, Woisetschlager R, Rieger R, et al. Mechanism, management, and prevention of laparoscopic bowel injuries. *Gastrointest Endosc.* 1996;43:572.

48. Chapron C, Pierre F, Harchaoui Y, et al. Gastrointestinal injuries during gynaecological laparoscopy. *Hum Reprod.* 1999;14:333.

49. Saidi MH, Sadler RK, Vancaillie TG, et al. Diagnosis and management of serious urinary complications after major operative laparoscopy. *Obstet Gynecol.* 1996;87:272.

50. Nezhat CH, Nezhat F, Seidman DS, et al. Vaginal vault evisceration after total laparoscopic hysterectomy. *Obstet Gynecol.* 1996;87:868.

51. Chapron CM, Pierre F, Lacroix S, et al. Major vascular injuries during gynecologic laparoscopy. *J Am Coll Surg.* 1997;185:461.

52. Nezhat C, Childers J, Nezhat F, et al. Major retroperitoneal vascular injury during laparoscopic surgery. *Hum Reprod.* 1997;12:480.

53. Seidman DS, Nasserbakht F, Nezhat F, et al. Delayed recognition of iliac artery injury during laparoscopic surgery. *Surg Endosc.* 1996;10:1099.

54. Nezhat CR, Kalyoncu S, Nezhat CH, et al. Laparoscopic management of ovarian dermoid cysts: ten years' experience. *JSLS.* 1999;3:179.

55. Mecke H, Savvas V. Laparoscopic surgery of dermoid cysts—intraoperative spillage and complications. *Eur J Obstet Gynecol Reprod Biol.* 2001;96:80.

56. Wang PH, Lee WL, Juang CM, et al. Excision of mature teratoma using culdotomy, with and without laparoscopy: a prospective randomised trial. *BJOG.* 2001;108:91.

57. Canis M, Rabischong B, Botchorishvili R, et al. Risk of spread of ovarian cancer after laparoscopic surgery. *Curr Opin Obstet Gynecol.* 2001;13:9.

58. Mettler L, Jacobs V, Brandenburg K, et al. Laparoscopic management of 641 adnexal tumors in Kiel, Germany. *J Am Assoc Gynecol Laparosc.* 2001;8:74.

Chapter Ninety-Six ● ● ● ● ● ●

*C*omplications of Intervertebral Disk Surgery

RONALD J. ARONOFF

As spinal surgery becomes part of the minimally invasive discipline, there are going to be growing pains. Just as other specialties have experienced, not only do the old complications remain, but new problems are lurking around the corner. Some of the complications seem to be universal and are shared with all minimally invasive procedures, while others are particular to the organ system involved. The intent of this chapter is to explore both the universal and unique complications of minimally invasive surgery of the lumbar spine.

The complications can be divided into those involving anesthetic, access, and exposure, and can be vascular, neurologic, and postoperative in nature. Each of these will be addressed in the sections that follow.

ACCESS

The introduction of laparoscopy into the field of surgery poses certain risks. These seem to be lessened by using an open technique or by direct observation through use of an optical trocar. Entrance into the peritoneal cavity using the Hasson technique has greatly reduced the fear of accidental bowel or vessel perforation, and optical trocars have facilitated entrance into the extraperitoneal space.

EXPOSURE

In order for the surgeon to have a clear field in which to work, the small and large bowel must be moved out of the pelvis. This can be accomplished by using a steep Trendelenburg position and gentle mobilization with atraumatic forceps. It is essential that all adhesions between the bowel and pelvic sidewalls be lysed. Preoperative bowel preparation with clear liquids and an oral cathartic agent such as magnesium citrate are usually adequate. Often the sigmoid colon falls into the field. This is best managed by sewing the cut edge of the colonic mesentery to the left lower quadrant. It is best to sew the edge because this lessens the risk of vessel or bowel injury. In some individuals it is necessary to use multiple

sutures if the sigmoid is particularly fatty or large. This technique has been used to keep a large cecum out of the field of view. On rare occasions the small bowel may be massively dilated, and this can be reduced by spraying 1% lidocaine on the bowel. This will reduce the size sufficiently to proceed with the operation.[1]

Adhesions from prior procedures are problematic. Most adhesions can be lysed and the pelvis cleared. The only significant considerations are those of accidental bowel perforation and the time required to clear the pelvis. These factors have to be taken into consideration preoperatively and discussed with the patient, since perforation of the bowel would lead to early termination of the procedure.

VASCULAR INJURY

Injury to an artery or vein can occur at several points during the procedure. Injury during access should be rare unless a closed technique of peritoneal entry is used. During dissection of the interspace, the surgeon needs to be aware of anomalous structures as well as normal ones. The surgeon should always work from identified structures toward those that are unknown.

Most complications have been from venous injuries. These seem to stem from either avulsion or entrapment of the vein with the trocar. If the iliac vein is carefully identified on its medial surface, accessory or medial branches can be identified before they are injured. In many individuals there are branches off the posterior surface of the vena cava, which must be occluded or troublesome bleeding can occur. These branches should be sought in the initial dissection to prevent bleeding. The origin of the median sacral vein should be handled carefully so as not to tear it off the left common iliac vein. A simple way to prevent entrapment injuries is to dissect enough of the vein so that it may be elevated as well as retracted. These injuries are common to both types of access, but obviously are more difficult to manage in a laparoscopic procedure. A completely avoidable source of bleeding is loss of ligature. Though it is not often reported, clips becoming dislodged from vascular branches is a common occurrence. Since these vessels are handled during the course of the procedure, it is prudent to back-up clips with a ligature (endo-loop) on high pressure vessels. In my experience, I have had no intraoperative or postoperative bleeding when this technique was employed. It is obvious that repair of a significant iliac vein laceration may lead to other complications.

Arterial injuries are fortunately rare. Since the artery is lateral to the vein at L5–S1, injury should be extremely rare if the anatomy is carefully identified. Only in an obese patient should the surgeon stray from the proper spot. Retraction of the artery is only rarely needed. At the L4–L5, it is often necessary to retract either the aorta or the left iliac artery. This is an area of concern, since a diseased artery is less pliable and more fragile than a normal one. There have been a few reports of iliac thrombosis after laparoscopic approach for interbody fusion (LAIF).[6,7] One can easily surmise that an atherosclerotic plaque could easily be fractured and lead to immediate or delayed thrombosis. The plain films, CT scan, and MRI can be inspected for calcification of the iliac vessels and aorta. If these are found, the surgeon will have to look for other methods of exposure of the disc space. Often there is no preoperative history of vascular disease, but it should be sought nonetheless. Obviously, peripheral pulses should be documented pre- and postoperatively.

NEUROLOGIC

Neurologic injuries can be divided into those to the autonomic and sensory systems. Both have been well described in the literature. Interestingly, many of the lessons learned in the minimally invasive experience are also applicable to open surgery. It seems that most, but not all, injuries can be avoided by using careful technique and having a thorough knowledge of anatomy.[8–10]

Autonomic

The autonomic nervous system has two components: the parasympathetic and the sympathetic. When performing lumbar spine procedures both can be injured. The sympathetic nerve fibers consistently run along the lateral aspect of the vertebral bodies, and it is quite simple to see the ganglia as the disc space is dissected. The parasympathetic fibers are much more difficult to see and protect. The parasympathetic nerves run along the anterolateral surface of the aorta and divide into left and right branches at the level of the lower lumbar vertebrae. These two branches eventually form the superior and inferior hypogastric plexus. The hypogastric plexus occurs in three different forms: a true plexus (84%), a single nerve (8%), and two parallel nerve trunks (8%). The shape of the plexus is also varied, and may be triangular (46%), narrow (25%), broad (25%), arch-shaped (1.5%), or spider web-like (1%). The key to the location of the superior plexus is a triangle with the apex at the aortic bifurcation, and the sides consisting of the pelvic side walls to the level of the sacroiliac joint or iliac bifurcation. The plexus is just below the peritoneum in the connective tissue. It tends to cross toward the left side of the pelvis after the sacral promontory. Some people have a long mesosigmoid, and in them the plexus can be close to the inferior mesenteric or superior hemorrhoidal artery.[2]

With this configuration, it is easy to see how injury to parasympathetic fibers could occur. The obvious outcome is development of retrograde ejaculation. This complication has been reported with varying degrees of frequency, depending on the

approach used by the surgeon. The high incidence reported in some reports from practitioners using a transperitoneal approach does not seem to be borne out by the current series. There have also been reports of this complication with the use of an extraperitoneal approach.

The best strategy for avoidance of retrograde ejaculation is twofold. First, and most important, is to avoid use of monopolar cautery, especially from the level of the peritoneum down. It has been our policy not to use monopolar cautery except on the skin and subcutaneous tissues. We have had no cases of retrograde ejaculation since we stopped using monopolar cautery inside the body cavity. The second technique is to start the peritoneal dissection just to the right of the right ureter and bluntly sweep all of the areolar tissues to the left, dividing only the medial sacral artery. This technique has been described in the vascular literature with good preservation of ejaculation.[3–5]

Injury to the sympathetics should be rare at the L5–S1 level since they do not need to be retracted for cage placement. At higher levels, it is often necessary to retract the sympathetic on the left for cage placement. This seems to be more affected by patient anatomy than by approach. Obviously, traction on the nerve has consequences different from transection or ligation. The other area of injury is during division of the ascending iliolumbar vein, which crosses over the sympathetic. Care must be taken not to include the sympathetic in a clip or ligature at this level.

Autonomic nervous system injury seems to occur if the surgery proceeds into the pelvis below the sacral promontory. This obviously puts the inferior plexus in jeopardy. In several reports there was an association between excessive bleeding and the incidence of not only retrograde ejaculation, but also permanent sympathectomy.[4]

Sensory

The sensory nervous system can be injured during the mobilization of the colon or during trocar placement. Trocar placement might cause an injury to a cutaneous nerve, but this should be extremely rare. The genitofemoral and ilioinguinal nerves lie on the anterior surface of the psoas muscle and could be injured during mobilization. There should not be much difference here between an open and a laparoscopic procedure. Once again, this dissection is blunt and not sharp, so transection should be rare.

POSTOPERATIVE

Most postoperative complications are not unique to the use of laparoscopic technique, and many can be avoided by using careful technique. The incidence of ileus has been equal in open and laparoscopic patients. Our policy has been not to feed if there are no bowel sounds and to keep the patient on clear liquids until bowel function has returned.

Postoperative bleeding can be avoided by careful intraoperative technique. It is important to cautiously secure all significant vessels. We also view the operative field after the patient has been placed flat and all CO_2 has been released to allow all venous structures to distend, in the hope of revealing any structure that needs ligation. Finally, it is important to view all trocar sites to check for bleeding. If an epigastric vessel has been injured, it should be readily apparent early in the procedure.

It is important to close the peritoneum with a running stitch. My preference is to use absorbable suture material. The use of clips or staples may leave gaps or injure posterior structures. There has been at least one instance of small bowel obstruction in which the small bowel became adherent to the raw surfaces of the fusion site.

Trocar-site hernias can easily be avoided by closing the peritoneum and the anterior rectus fascia at any trocar site larger than 10 mm. This may take a few extra minutes, but will circumvent the unpleasant complication of postoperative small bowel obstruction.

REFERENCES

1. John RM, McGuire EJ. Urogenital complications of anterior approaches to the lumbar spine. *Clin Orthoped Related Res.* 1981;154: 114.

2. Duncan HJM, Jonck LM. The presacral plexus in anterior fusion of the lumbar spine. *S Afr J Surg.* 1965;3:93.

3. Weinstein MH, Machleder HI. Sexual function after aorto-iliac surgery. *Ann Surg.* 1974;6:787.

4. Flynn JC, Price CT. Sexual complications of anterior fusion of the lumbar spine. *Spine* 1984;5:489.

5. Flanigan DP, Schuler JJ, Keifert T, et al. Elimination of iatrogenic impotence and improvement of sexual function after aortoiliac revascularization. *Arch Surg.* 1982;117:544.

6. Regan JJ, Aronoff R, et al. Laparoscopic approach to interbody fusion using BAK cages: Experience in the first 58 cases. *Spine* 1999;24:2171.

7. Heini PF, Krahenbuhl L, Schwarzenbach O, et al. Laparoscopic assisted spine surgery. *Dig Surg.* 1998;15:185.

8. Zelko JR, Misko J, Swanstrom L, et al. Laparoscopic lumbar discectomy. *Am J Surg.* 1995;169:496.

9. Kathkouda N, Campos GM, Mavor RJ, et al. Is laparoscopic approach to lumbar spine fusion worthwhile? *Am J Surg.* 1999;178:458.

10. Mahvi DM, Zdeblick TA. A prospective study of laparoscopic spinal fusion. Technique and operative complications. *Ann Surg.* 1996;224:85.

Occupational Injuries and Ambulatory Surgery

Chapter Ninety-Seven ● ● ● ● ● ●

*O*ccupational Injuries of the Laparoscopic Surgeon

DAVID LASKY-MARCOVICH, PABLO TARAZONA-VELUTINI, PABLO CASTAÑEDA, and LUIS G. CASTAÑEDA

As in any other craft, in medicine, and more specifically in surgery, there is always the risk of suffering a work-related injury. This fact has been recognized since ancient times, and has been pointed out on many occasions. In the University College Hospital in London, professor Robert Liston, (1794–1847) while amputating the gangrenous leg of a patient, cut the fingers of his assistant, and with the same knife injured one spectator: the patient, the assistant, and the spectator died, which represents a mortality of 300%.[1] Semmelweis and Pfannenstiel died due to hand infections acquired practicing surgery.[2] Marie Curie, whose original name was Manya Sklodowska, died of leukemia due to chronic and excessive exposure to radiation.[3] Brenkel et al reported a metacarpal fracture in a surgeon sustained while trying to reduce a hip hemiprosthesis during a surgical procedure.[4]

Surgeons are exposed to injuries from traditional instruments (needles, knives, etc.) or from high-technology instruments (electrocautery, laser, etc.) and to infectious diseases like hepatitis in all its forms and AIDS.[5–14] All surgical specialties have reported impairments caused by the constant use of certain muscles or due to tension in ligaments and tendons during long periods of work; these are generally classified as tenosynovitis.[15] For example, the anesthesiologist, while keeping the thumb in forced abduction for a long period while handling the mask, may sustain an avulsion fracture of the ulnar collateral ligament of the thumb in the metacarpophalangeal joint (gamekeeper's thumb). The treatment may require surgery (Fig. 97–1).[16–17]

General surgeons, while using the nondominant hand to retract the bowel during long, open procedures of the biliary tract, may cause constant pressure and trauma of the carpal tunnel and reduction of its diameter due to fibrosis and inflammation of the anterior carpal ligament, resulting in compression injury of the median nerve which produces paresthesia in the index, middle, and ring fingers, and also pain and weakness of the hand. At first, the treatment is conservative, but some cases will require surgery.[18]

Plastic surgeons, while performing an external capsulotomy of the breast for spherical contracture after implants, make great effort with their pectoralis major muscles, which may cause pain and tendinitis; this is known as "breast augmentor's arm." They may also develop "tennis elbow syndrome" (lateral epicondylitis).[19]

In the 1960s, gynecologists introduced laparoscopy into their diagnostic and therapeutic practice. Realizing that the procedures brought positive and efficient results, they kept practicing and perfecting their techniques. Since then, there have been reports of specific injuries such as bursitis and tendinitis among those who practice this technique.[20–21] Since publication of the report of Dubois et al,[22] laparoscopic surgery has been used all over the world for removal of the gallbladder, and its use has become common practice. As the confidence in the procedure grew, surgeons demanded better instrument quality, and the procedures became more complicated, resulting in advanced laparoscopic surgery. When surgeons used bimanual techniques, they had to make postural changes of their body, arms, and hands in order to adapt to these new procedures.

Today, in spite of the benefits of staplers and other mechanical suturing devices that facilitate these techniques, the surgeon must further hone his or her skills in order to obtain similar or even better results with laparoscopic surgery than with traditional methods.

In laparoscopic surgery the mechanisms for occupational injuries are similar to those described in traditional surgery, but are more frequent because of the use of endoscopic instruments and the different positions that the surgeon and assistants have to maintain.

When some surgeons noticed discomfort in the hand, wrist, elbow, shoulder, and spine (in particular, paresthesias of the digital nerves, pain in the carpal tunnel area, and pain in the elbow or lateral epicondylitis), they didn't pay much attention at the beginning;[23] however, research reports were soon published

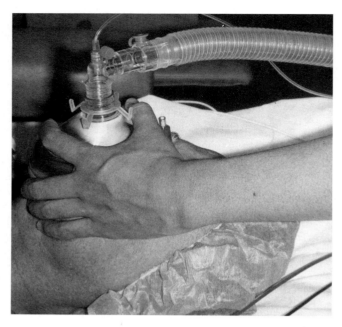

Figure 97–1. Forced abduction of the metacarpophalangeal joint of the thumb. Potential lesion: "Gamekeeper's thumb" (rupture of medial collateral metacarpophalangeal ligament).

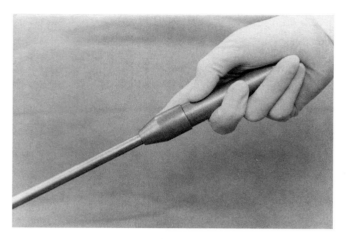

Figure 97–3. Pressure on the carpal tunnel caused by gripping an instrument. Potential lesion: Carpal tunnel syndrome.

detailing the injuries caused by adoption of unnatural and stressful postures, and awareness of this problem has increased. Sustained tension of the flexor muscles can generate medial epicondylitis or "golfer's elbow" by overuse of the palmaris longus, flexor superficialis of the fingers, flexor carpi ulnaris, and pronator teres (Fig. 97–2). Carpal tunnel syndrome can be caused by direct trauma (at the time of introducing a trocar), or by dynamic tension that persists when forcefully gripping instruments for long periods of time, which puts direct pressure on the flexor retinaculum at the wrist and the median nerve (Fig. 97–3). Sustained tension of the extensor pollicis brevis and abductor pollicis longus

causes increased muscle volume, which in turn produces inflammation of the tendon sheath at the base of the thumb (stenosing tenosynovitis or de Quervain's syndrome).

In tennis elbow, the constant tension of the extensor muscles of the wrist, especially over the second radial, the common extensor digiti, the extensor minimi digiti, and the extensor carpi ulnaris, causes inflammation and degeneration of the insertion site of the tendons at the lateral epicondyle (Fig. 97–4).

Any position that maintains tension on a tendon or a group of tendons tends to produce inflammation of these elements and of the synovial lining that covers them. In some surgeons, tension on the biceps when performing constant and forced supination of the forearm leads to the development of tendinitis, especially in the long head of this muscle (Fig. 97–5).

Repeated and forced abduction of the arm above 90° or 100° may produce bursitis between the acromion and the humerus on the subacromial bursa. The supraspinatus muscle may also be injured, causing pain if the movement is repeated. In chronic cases, calcification of the tendons, bursae, or capsule may develop. Such

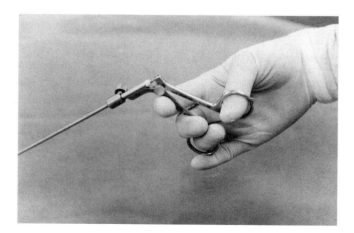

Figure 97–2. Forced flexion of the wrist, causing tension of the flexor muscles. Potential lesion: "Golfer's elbow" (tenosynovitis at the medial epicondyle).

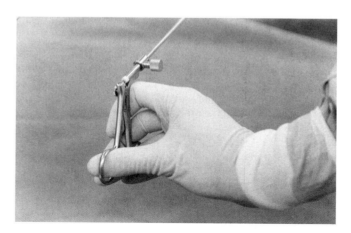

Figure 97–4. Tension of the extensor muscles of the wrist. Potential lesion: Tennis elbow (tenosynovitis of the lateral epicondyle).

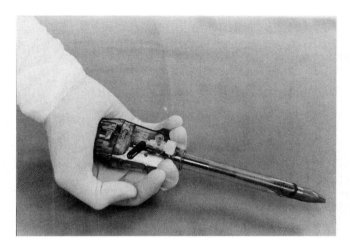

Figure 97–5. Tension of the first carpometacarpal joint (abductor pollicis longus and extensor pollicis brevis). Potential lesion: Stenosing tenosynovitis or de Quervain syndrome.

lesions may extend to the rotator cuff and are usually incapacitating, requiring surgical treatment[24] (arthroscopic debridement of partial-thickness tears, acromioplasty, or division of coracoacromial ligaments), or extracorporeal shock wave lithotripsy (Figs. 97–6 and 97–7).[25–26]

The tension required to maintain the surgeon's head in certain positions during surgery can give rise to contraction of the paravertebral muscles of the cervical spine (trapezius and levator scapulae) that tends to cause pain in the neck and head. If any degenerative or traumatic problem is present in the spine, it may worsen due to the muscle strain required by performing a surgical procedure (Fig. 97–8). The prolonged position of fixed flexion of the upper back and neck produces pain due to strain on the trapezius and rhomboideus. This can be avoided by frequent and gentle stretching and extension exercises.

Some ways of avoiding these injuries include the use of instruments with a rack (auto-locking instruments) or in-line in-

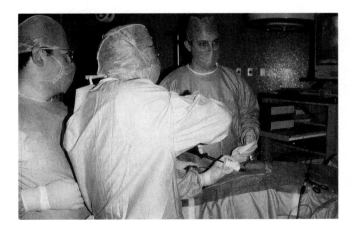

Figure 97–6. Forced tension over the anterior portion of the deltoid muscle. Potential lesion: Anterior deltoid myalgia.

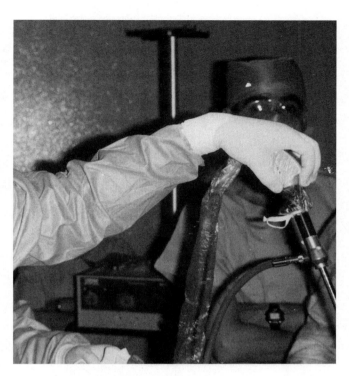

Figure 97–7. Arm in abduction causing tension over the medial portion of the deltoid muscle. Potential lesion: Subacromial bursitis, myalgia of the medial portion of the deltoid, lesions of the rotator cuff, and impingement syndrome.

struments[27] to avoid prolonged effort when handling them. Other possibilities include the use of instruments with increased distal angulation and rotation of the jaws, as well as different types of articulated instruments like the kinematic system or the endo-hand.[28]

Another helpful measure may be to adjust the height of the operating table so the work can be done in a more natural and comfortable way. It is important to seek professional assistance if the symptoms described above appear, otherwise a permanent disability may result. Simple measures used in physiotherapy, such as exercises, heat pads, ultrasound, and massage can improve the symptoms and prevent further damage. Allowing some precious time for the surgeon ("physician heal thyself") will enable him or her to perform better for his patients. There are several surgical manufacturers (Karl-Storz, Endoscopy-America, and Microsurge Inc., among others) that have made efforts to improve instruments to help avoid these injuries. These new designs include such innovations as instruments with handles with dual interchangeable positions.[29–30]

Important reviews have been made of the risks and potential mechanisms which may cause injury to the laparoscopic surgeon, as well as recommendations about ways to avoid them. On the other hand, it has been shown that when performing laparoscopic procedures the surgeon is protected from suffering cuts or exposure to smoke and bodily fluids, thus limiting the possibility of acquiring infectious diseases such as hepatitis or AIDS.

A

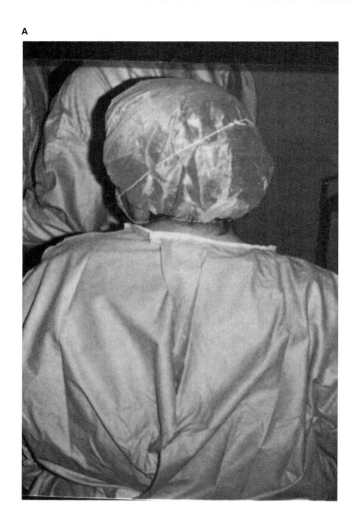

B

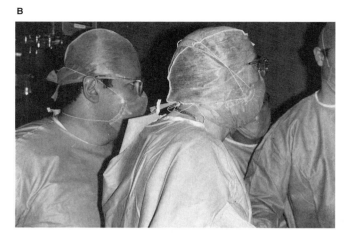

C

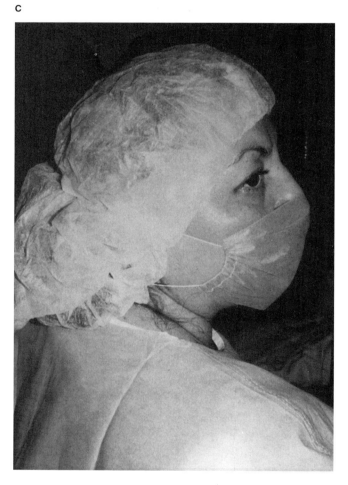

Figure 97–8. Three different positions of the head that put stress on muscles of the neck (**A, B,** and **C**). Potential lesion: Painful syndromes of muscular groups of the neck and upper back.

REFERENCES

1. Fleming P. Robert Liston: the first professor of clinical surgery at UCH. *University College Magazine* 1926;1:76.
2. Williams B. Some surgeons and their hand injuries. *Practitioner* 1974; 23:717.
3. Compton's Interactive Encyclopedia. Compton's NewMedia, Inc.: 1993–1994.
4. Brenkel U, Pearse M, Gregg P. A cracking complication of hemiarthroplasty of the hip. *Br Med J.* 1986;293:1649.
5. Mohr RM, McDonell BC. Safety considerations and safety protocol for laser surgery. *Surg Clin North Am.* 1984;64:851.
6. Gerberding JL, Littell C. Role of exposure of surgical personnel to patient's blood: surgery at San Francisco General Hospital. *N Engl J Med.* 1990;322:1788.
7. Marcus R. CDC Cooperative needlestick surveillance group: surveillance of health care workers exposed to blood of patients infected with the human immunodeficiency virus. *N Engl J Med.* 1988;319:1118.
8. Lipsett PA, Allo M. AIDS and surgeon. *Surg Clin North Am.* 1988;68:73.
9. Bartlet JG. HIV infection and surgeons. *Curr Prob Surg.* 1992;29:197.
10. Frieland GH, Klein RS. Transmission of the human immunodeficiency virus. *N Engl J Med.* 1987;317:1125.
11. Weber SA, Serrano BF. El SIDA y el cirujano. *Rev Cirujano Gen.* 1991;13:155.
12. Manzano-Trovamala JR, Guerrero MG. SIDA y cirugía (Parte I). *Rev Cirujano Gen.* 1994;16:97.
13. Manzano-Trovamala JR, Guerrero MG. SIDA y cirugía (Parte II). *Rev Cirujano Gen.* 1994;16:187.
14. Fry DE, Elford GL, Fecteau DL, et al. Prevention of blood exposure. Body and facial protection. *Surg Clin North Am.* 1995;75:1141.
15. Campbell-Semple J. Tenosynovitis, repetitive strain injury, cumulative trauma disorder and overuse syndrome, etc. *J Bone Joint Surg (Am).* 1991;73:536.
16. Campbell CS. Gamekeeper's thumb. *J Bone Joint Surg (Br).* 1955;37:148.
17. Parkish M, Nahigian S, Froimson A. Gamekeeper's thumb. *Plast Reconstr Surg.* 1976;58:24.
18. Belsole RJ, Greeleyt JM. Surgeon's acute carpal tunnel syndrome: an occupational hazard? *J Fla Med Assoc.* 1988;75:369.
19. Weistreich M. Breast augmentor's arm. *JAMA.* 1978;239:401.
20. Almazan DM. Laparoscopía diagnóstica y operatoria en ginecología. *Ginecol y Obstet de México.* 1976;39:337.
21. Almazan DM. Personal communication, 1978.
22. Dubois F, Berthelot G, Levard H. Cholécystectomie par coelioscopie. *Nouv Presse Med.* 1989;18:980.
23. Regier H. Game, set and (almost) match: laparoscopist deals with the incapacity of "tennis elbow." *Laparoscopy News* 1994:11.
24. Budoff JE, Nirshi RP, Guidi EJ. Debridement of partial thickness tears of the rotator cuff without acromioplasty. *J Bone Joint Surg.* 1998;80:733.
25. Haupt G. Use of extracorporeal short wave lithotripsy in the treatment of pseudoarthroses, tendinopathy and other ortho-paedic diseases. *Am J Urol.* 1997;158:4.
26. Berjano P. Personal communication, 1998.
27. Berguer R, Gerber S, Kilpatrick G, Beckley D. An ergonomic comparison of in line vs. pistol grip handle configuration in laparoscopic grasper. *Surg Endosc.* 1998;12:805.
28. Melzer A, Kipfmüller K, Halfar B. Deflectable endoscopic instrument system DENIS. *Surg Endosc.* 1997;11:1045.
29. Berguer R, Remler M, Beckley D. Laparoscopic instruments cause increased forearm fatigue: a subjective comparison of open and laparoscopic techniques. *Minimally Invasive Ther Allied Technol.* 1997;6:36.
30. Berguer R. Surgical technology and the ergonomics of laparoscopic instruments. *Surg Endosc.* 1998;12:458.

Chapter Ninety-Eight . . . .

Ambulatory Endoscopic Surgery

**JOSÉ ANTONIO VÁZQUEZ-FRÍAS, ANGELES FUENTES DEL TORO,
ALEXANDER RASCHKE-FEBRES, and JORGE CUETO-GARCÍA**

INTRODUCTION

Ambulatory surgery, day-case surgery, and outpatient surgery are all synonyms. By definition, the terms mean that the patient is discharged the same day of surgery.[1] In this chapter, extended care (23-hour stay) will also be used as an equivalent term.

The likely first report of ambulatory surgery was done by Nicholl of the Royal Glasgow Hospital for Children in 1909. After several other efforts, the first modern successful ambulatory surgery center was established by Reed in Phoenix, Arizona in 1970.[2,3] Today, the number of hospitals and freestanding units providing ambulatory surgery, the number of patients undergoing such surgery, and the percentage of surgical patients choosing the ambulatory route are all constantly increasing.[4,5] Perhaps the most important reason for this growth are the increasing costs of inpatient hospital care,[2,3] but there is no doubt that more efficiently operated facilities, new surgical techniques, and improved anesthetic agents and practices have also made it possible.[4]

Ambulatory surgery has demonstrated its usefulness, cost-effectiveness, and safety throughout the world and already extends its benefits to patients that undergo different types of mini-invasive surgery.

OBJECTIVES

The main goal of ambulatory laparoscopic surgery is to offer safe, quality medical services at a low cost with a high level of patient satisfaction. The main factor that allows an ambulatory surgery program to achieve this and be successful with mini-invasive surgical procedures is smooth interaction of medical staff, nursing services, administration personnel, and the governing body. A surgical group experienced in mini-invasive surgery and a well equipped ambulatory surgical unit are needed, as well as modern and appropriate means of communication and transportation between the facility and a hospital for emergency cases.

By reaching these goals, several advantages are gained, including:[6,7]

- More efficient operating rooms and hospital services;
- Readily available hospital beds for hospitalization when needed;
- Optimized medical and paramedical personnel;
- A rapid return of the patient to everyday activities;
- The patient receives more individual attention and anxiety is lessened;
- A decreased risk of acquiring nosocomial infections;
- The patient enjoys the many benefits of mini-invasive surgery.

PREOPERATIVE EVALUATION

A patient that submits to an outpatient mini-invasive surgical procedure must generally meet the same criteria that other surgical patients do. Obviously, a complete medical history and a meticulous physical examination should be done preoperatively. Laboratory tests, ECG, and radiographic studies should also be obtained as needed. Anesthetic consultation some days before the surgical procedure is also recommended. Selected individuals should constitute an ASA class I or II anesthetic surgical risk, although some papers report successful procedures in higher-risk patients.[8] The following issues must be addressed:[3,7]

- Cardiopulmonary evaluation in patients 40 years of age and older and when otherwise indicated;
- Correction of metabolic disorders;
- The patient should not be suffering from any intercurrent infection;
- The patient must be given explicit written instructions, including preoperative indications, the pros and cons of the endoscopic procedure, and the possibility of conversion to open laparotomy, and the patient's signature must be obtained on a copy to make sure he or she understands the risks and benefits;
- Support of the patient's family should be obtained;

- The patient and his or her relatives should be reachable by phone at the home.

SELECTION OF THE SURGICAL PROCEDURE

In order to carry out an ambulatory laparoscopic procedure, it must be elective, preferably be less than 2 hours in duration, should not require blood transfusion, and it must be terminated at a convenient hour.

It is the surgeon's responsibility to make an individual judgement for every ambulatory surgical patient by taking into account: (1) the patient's age and physical and mental condition; (2) the anesthetic risk; (3) the attitude toward having the operation on an outpatient basis; (4) the social and family situation; and (5) whether the magnitude of the operation falls within the current standards for ambulatory surgery in that community.[9]

LAPAROSCOPIC PROCEDURES THAT CAN BE CARRIED OUT IN THE AMBULATORY SURGICAL UNIT

General Surgery

- Cholecystectomies (uncomplicated cases only);[8,10–15]
- Diagnostic procedures such as biopsies,[16] fever of unknown origin,[17] or persistent chronic pain;[18]
- Inguinal hernioplasty;[19,20]
- Insertion and salvage of peritoneal dialysis catheters;[21]
- Evaluation of the patient with lower abdominal pain: Differential diagnosis between appendicitis and adnexal inflammatory processes.[22–24] Today, even perforated appendicitis can be managed as an outpatient procedure;[25]
- Tumor staging using a carefully controlled protocol (selected cases only);[26]
- Gastrostomy and jejunostomy (selected cases only);[27]
- Evaluation of the patient with blunt abdominal trauma (carefully selected patients only);
- Antireflux procedures: Although these have been done in ambulatory units,[28–30] the opinion of the authors is that this policy should not be generally adopted, because any situation that stresses the diaphragm after an antireflux operation could result in failure. Nausea and vomiting may be one of these stressors;[31,32]
- Adrenalectomies have been performed as outpatient procedures for certain selected patients.[33]

Gynecologic Surgery[34,35]

- Infertility;
- Sterilization;
- Endometriosis;
- Diagnostic and therapeutic procedures: Ovarian cysts, lysis of adhesions, tubal occlusion, etc.;
- Differential diagnosis in pelvic peritonitis (selected cases only).

Some of these procedures have been performed in an office setting under local anesthesia.[36]

Urologic Surgery

- Varicocelectomy;[37]
- Orchiopexy and orchiectomy;[38]

- Renal biopsy;[39]
- Pelvic lymphadenectomy;[40]

Thoracic Surgery

- Lung and pleural biopsies (selected cases only);[41]
- Ligation of patent ductus arteriosus (selected cases only);[42]
- Thoracic sympathectomy (selected cases only).[43]

Other Procedures

Several other minimally invasive procedures from other surgical specialties such as otolaryngology, reconstructive surgery, and orthopedic surgery are sometimes performed in the ambulatory surgical unit.

POSTOPERATIVE CARE

Once the procedure is completed, the patient should be closely monitored in the recovery room. Postoperative pain, nausea and/or vomiting appear to be key factors in determining inpatient or outpatient status. Endoscopic and laparoscopic surgical procedures are known to produce less pain than open operations; thus the use of opioids can be limited, diminishing postoperative nausea and vomiting (PONV). Multimodal analgesia (local analgesics plus nonsteroidal anti-inflammatory drugs [NSAIDs]) should be first-line therapy, with opioids used only for more extensive operations.[44] Should PONV occur, it must be effectively managed. In a recent randomized study, antiemetic prophylaxis (ondansetron 4 mg and cyclizine 50 mg) for outpatient gynecologic laparoscopic surgery proved to be effective.[45]

The patient may be discharged by the surgeon and/or the anesthesiologist if the following criteria are met:[3,7]

- No signs of respiratory abnormalities are present;
- Vital signs are stable and near preoperative levels;
- The patient is alert, oriented to person, place, and time, with no dizziness;
- Vision is adequate;
- Surgical wounds are without bleeding, inflammation, or excessive drainage;
- There is no severe pain;
- There is no nausea or vomiting;
- The patient should be able to void and tolerate a liquid diet;
- The patient should be able to get out of bed and sit by him- or herself and to walk with the help of a single person.

At the time of discharge, postoperative instructions must be reviewed with the patient and a family member to make sure they are clearly understood. Also, the patient should be contacted by phone at least twice a day until the next office visit. The surgeon's pager number should also be given to the patient in case an emergency should arise.

CONCLUSION

The many well-known advantages of laparoscopic surgery—diminished postoperative pain, absent or decreased ileus and respiratory complications, better preserved immune function, reduced surgical trauma, the potential for almost immediate ambulation, and improved cosmetic results, among others—must be exploited to benefit the many patients that can be operated on successfully with outpatient surgery. Significant cost savings can also be realized. Provided the patient was correctly evaluated, the proper procedure was chosen, and it was performed by an experienced surgical team working in a well-equipped and staffed ambulatory surgical unit, the patient should enjoy these benefits of minimally invasive surgery. New developments in surgical technology will expand the possibilities of minimally invasive ambulatory surgery to benefit the many patients that today are not ideal candidates for such procedures.

REFERENCES

1. Cuschieri A. Day-case (ambulatory) laparoscopic surgery. Let us sing from the same hymn sheet. Editorial. *Surg Endosc.* 1997;11:1143.
2. Cueto GJ. *Manual de Cirugía Ambulatoria.* Secretaría de Salud y Asistencia. 1993.
3. Detmer DE. Ambulatory surgery. *N Engl J Med.* 1981;305:1406.
4. Davis JE. Ambulatory surgery. . . . How far can we go? *Med Clin North Am.* 1993;77:365.
5. Hill CJ. Ambulatory surgery: 10 frequently asked questions. *Bull Am Coll Surg.* 1998;83:10.
6. Davis JE. The major ambulatory surgical center and how it is developed. *Surg Clin North Am.* 1987;67:671.
7. Cueto J, Rodríguez M, Weber A. Cirugía laparoscópica ambulatoria. In: Cueto J, Weber A, eds. *Cirugía Laparoscópica*, 2nd ed. McGraw-Hill Interamericana:1997;617.
8. Voitk AJ. Is outpatient cholecystectomy safe for the higher-risk elective patient? *Surg Endosc.* 1997;11:1147.
9. Davis JE, Sugioka K. Selecting the patient for major ambulatory surgery. *Surg Clin North Am.* 1987;67:721.
10. Fiorillo MA, Davidson PG, Fiorillo M, et al. 149 ambulatory laparoscopic cholecystectomies. *Surg Endosc.* 1996;10:52.
11. Tan LR. Early discharge standard at California HMO following laparoscopic cholecystectomy. *Gen Surg Laparosc News.* 1996;Feb.:17.
12. Zegarra II RF, Saba AK, Peschiera JL. Outpatient laparoscopic cholecystectomy: safe and cost effective? *Surg Laparosc Endosc.* 1997;7:487.
13. Smith II M, Wheeler W, Ulmer MB. Comparison of outpatient laparoscopic cholecystectomy in a private nonteaching hospital versus a private teaching community hospital. *JSLS.* 1997;1:51.
14. Voyles CR, Berch BR. Selection criteria for laparoscopic cholecystectomy in an ambulatory care setting. *Surg Endosc.* 1997;11:1145.
15. Richardson WS, Fuhrman GS, Burch E, et al. Outpatient laparoscopic cholecystectomy. Outcomes of 847 planned procedures. *Surg Endosc.* 2001;15:193.
16. Unal G, van Buuren HR, de Man RA. Laparoscopy as a day-case procedure in patients with liver disease. *Endoscopy* 1998;30:3.
17. Langer, HE. Laparoscopy in fever of unknown origin. *Dtsch Med Wochenschr.* 1988;113:616.
18. Salky BA, Edye MB. The role of laparoscopy in the diagnosis and treatment of abdominal pain syndromes. *Surg Endosc.* 1998;12:911.
19. Evans DS, Ghanesh P, Khan IM. Day-case laparoscopic hernia repair. *Br J Surg.* 1996;83:1361.
20. O'Riordain DS, Kelly P, Horgan PG, et al. Laparoscopic extraperitoneal inguinal hernia repair in the day-care setting. *Surg Endosc.* 1999;13:914.
21. Leung LC, Yiu MK, Man CW, et al. Laparoscopic management of Tenchkoff catheters in continuous ambulatory peritoneal dialysis. A one-port technique. *Surg Endosc.* 1998;12:891.
22. Join A, Mercado PD, Grafton KP, et al. Outpatient laparoscopic appendectomy. *Surg Endosc.* 1995;9:424.
23. Schreiber JH. Results of outpatient laparoscopic appendectomy in women. *Endoscopy* 1994;26:292.
24. Steege JF. Repeated clinic laparoscopy for the treatment of pelvic adhesions: A pilot study. *Obstet Gynecol.* 1994;83:276.
25. Alvarez C, Voitk AJ. The road to ambulatory laparoscopic management of perforated appendicitis. *Am J Surg.* 2000;179:63.
26. Sand J, Marnela K, Airo I, et al. Staging of abdominal cancer by local anesthesia outpatient laparoscopy. *Hepatogastroenterology* 1996; 43:1685.
27. Edelman DS, Unger SW. Laparoscopic gastrostomy and jejunostomy: review of 22 cases. *Surg Laparosc Endosc.* 1994;4:297.
28. Milford MA, Paluch TA. Ambulatory laparoscopic fundoplication. *Surg Endosc.* 1997;11:1150.
29. Trondsen E, Mjaland O, Raeder J, et al. Day-case laparoscopic fundoplication for gastro-oesophageal reflux disease. *Br J Surg.* 2000; 87:1708.
30. Narain PK, Moss JM, DeMaria EJ. Feasibility of 23-hour hospitalization after laparoscopic fundoplication. *J Laparoendosc Adv Surg Tech.* 2000;10:5.
31. Soper NJ, Dunnegan D. Anatomic fundoplication failure after laparoscopic antireflux surgery. *Ann Surg.* 1999;229:676.
32. Hunter GJ, Smith D, Branum GD, et al. Laparoscopic fundoplication. *Ann Surg.* 1999;230:595.
33. Gill IS, Hobart MG, Schweizer D, et al. Outpatient adrenalectomy. *J Urol.* 2000;163:717.
34. Risquez F, Pennehoaut G, McCorvey R, et al. Diagnostic and operative microlaparoscopy: a preliminary multicentre report. *Hum Reprod.* 1997;12:1645.
35. Frenzel D, Burkart WC, Cirkel U. Ambulatory versus inpatient laparoscopy: decision aids for choice of management. *Zentralbl Gynakol.* 1998;120:165.
36. Palter SF. Office microlaparoscopy under local anesthesia. *Obstet Gynecol Clin North Am.* 1999;26:109.
37. Dahisfroud C, Thune A, Hedelin H, et al. Laparoscopic ligature of the spermatic veins: A comparison between outpatient and hospitalized treatment. *Scand J Urol Nephrol.* 1994;28:159.
38. Thomas MD, Mercer LC, Soltzstein EC. Laparoscopic orchiectomy for unilateral intra-abdominal testis. *J Urol.* 1992;148:1251.
39. Gimenez LF, Micali S, Chen RN, et al. Laparoscopic renal biopsy. *Kidney Int.* 1998;54:525.
40. Buizza C, Mandressi A. Urologic laparoscopy in day hospital. *Arch Ital Urol Androl.* 1998;70:137.
41. Garcha I, Conn J. Outpatient thoracoscopy: a case report and discussion. *Am Surg.* 1995;61:229.
42. Hines MH, Bensky AS, Hammon JW, et al. Video-assisted thoracoscopic ligation of patent ductus arteriosus: safe and outpatient. *Ann Thorac Surg.* 1998;66:353.
43. Reardon PR, Preciado A, Scarborough T, et al. Outpatient endoscopic thoracic sympathectomy using 2-mm instruments. *Surg Endosc.* 1999; 13:1139.
44. Smith I. Anesthesia for laparoscopy with emphasis on outpatient laparoscopy. *Anesthesiol Clin North Am.* 2001;19:21.
45. Ahmed AB, Hobbs GJ, Curran JP. Randomized, placebo-controlled trial of combination antiemetic prophylaxis for day-case gynaecological laparoscopic surgery. *Br J Anaesth.* 2000;85:675.

*I*ndex

Page numbers followed by *t* and *f* indicate tables and figures, respectively.